Seidel's Guide to

PHYSICAL
EXAMINATION

EIGHTH EDITION

CONTENTS

1 The History and Interviewing Process, *1*

2 Cultural Competency, *21*

3 Examination Techniques and Equipment, *30*

4 Vital Signs and Pain Assessment, *50*

5 Mental Status, *64*

6 Growth and Measurement, *79*

7 Nutrition, *95*

8 Skin, Hair, and Nails, *114*

9 Lymphatic System, *166*

10 Head and Neck, *184*

11 Eyes, *204*

12 Ears, Nose, and Throat, *231*

13 Chest and Lungs, *260*

14 Heart, *294*

15 Blood Vessels, *332*

16 Breasts and Axillae, *350*

17 Abdomen, *370*

18 Female Genitalia, *416*

19 Male Genitalia, *466*

20 Anus, Rectum, and Prostate, *485*

21 Musculoskeletal System, *501*

22 Neurologic System, *544*

23 Sports Participation Evaluation, *581*

24 Putting It All Together, *594*

25 Taking the Next Steps: Critical Thinking, *610*

26 Recording Information, *616*

27 Emergency or Life-Threatening Situations, *632*

Photo and Illustration Credits, *645*

References and Readings, *647*

Glossary, *666*

Appendix A Height/Weight Growth Charts, *675*

Appendix B Pediatric Blood Pressure Tables, *679*

Appendix C Conversion Tables and Anthropometric Measurements, *684*

Index, *686*

Seidel's Guide to

PHYSICAL EXAMINATION

EIGHTH EDITION

Jane W. Ball, DrPH, RN, CPNP
Trauma Systems Consultant
American College of Surgeons
Gaithersburg, Maryland

Joyce E. Dains, DrPH, JD, RN, FNP-BC, FAANP
Associate Professor
Department of Nursing
The University of Texas
The University of Texas MD Anderson Cancer Center
Houston, Texas

John A. Flynn, MD, MBA, MEd
Clinical Director and Professor of Medicine
Division of General Internal Medicine
The Johns Hopkins University
School of Medicine
Baltimore, Maryland

Barry S. Solomon, MD, MPH
Associate Professor of Pediatrics
Medical Director, Harriet Lane Clinic
Division of General Pediatrics and Adolescent Medicine
The Johns Hopkins University
School of Medicine
Baltimore, Maryland

Rosalyn W. Stewart, MD, MS, MBA
Associate Professor of Pediatrics and Medicine
Departments of Pediatrics and Internal Medicine
The Johns Hopkins University
School of Medicine
Baltimore, Maryland

3251 Riverport Lane
St. Louis, Missouri 63043

SEIDEL'S GUIDE TO PHYSICAL EXAMINATION ISBN: 978-0-323-11240-6

Notices

Knowledge and best practice in this field are constantly changing. As new research and experience broaden our understanding, changes in research methods, professional practices, or medical treatment may become necessary.

Practitioners and researchers must always rely on their own experience and knowledge in evaluating and using any information, methods, compounds, or experiments described herein. In using such information or methods, they should be mindful of their own safety and the safety of others, including parties for whom they have a professional responsibility.

With respect to any drug or pharmaceutical products identified, readers are advised to check the most current information provided (i) on procedures featured or (ii) by the manufacturer of each product to be administered to verify the recommended dose or formula, the method and duration of administration, and contraindications. It is the responsibility of practitioners, relying on their own experience and knowledge of their patients, to make diagnoses, to determine dosages and the best treatment for each individual patient, and to take all appropriate safety precautions.

To the fullest extent of the law, neither the Publisher nor the authors, contributors, or editors, assume any liability for any injury and/or damage to persons or property as a matter of products liability, negligence or otherwise, or from any use or operation of any methods, products, instructions, or ideas contained in the material herein.

Library of Congress Cataloging-in-Publication Data

Ball, Jane (Jane W.), author.
  Seidel's guide to physical examination / Jane W. Ball, Joyce E. Dains, John A. Flynn, Barry S. Solomon, Rosalyn W. Stewart.—Eighth edition.
    p. ; cm.
  Guide to physical examination
  Preceded by Mosby's guide to physical examination / Henry M. Seidel ... [et al.]. 7th ed. c2011.
  Includes bibliographical references and index.
  ISBN 978-0-323-11240-6 (pbk. : alk. paper)
  I. Dains, Joyce E., author.   II. Flynn, John A. (Physician), author.   III. Solomon, Barry S., author.
IV. Stewart, Rosalyn W., author.   V. Title.   VI. Title: Guide to physical examination.
  [DNLM: 1. Physical Examination–methods.   2. Medical History Taking–methods. WB 205]
  RC76
  616.07'54–dc23
                    2013043592

Executive Content Strategist: Kristin Geen
Content Manager: Jamie Randall
Associate Content Development Specialist: Melissa Rawe
Marketing Manager: Traci Cahill
Publishing Services Manager: Deborah L. Vogel
Project Manager: Bridget Healy
Designer: Jessica Williams

Printed in Canada

Last digit is the print number: 9 8 7 6 5 4 3 2

We dedicate the eighth edition of this text to our colleague, Henry M. Seidel, MD who passed away in 2010. For seven editions the text has been known as Mosby's Guide to Physical Examination. *In Henry's honor and memory we have renamed it* Seidel's Guide to Physical Examination.

Henry spent all of his professional life (except for time served in the U.S. Army), from college through his appointment as Professor Emeritus of Pediatrics, at The Johns Hopkins University. He received numerous awards and a named scholarship at The Johns Hopkins University, testimony of his service at the bedside, in the lecture and seminar rooms, and as Associate Dean for Student Affairs in the School of Medicine.

As an original author we are indebted to him as he contributed greatly to the initial text design as well as to its ongoing development. He understood the importance of communication, sensitivity, and connection with patients, and he was able to share these concepts during the initial book development. He often reminded us that human interaction, sensitivity during history taking, and excellent physical examination skills enable health professionals to understand a patient and develop a healing relationship.

This text was one of the earliest collaborations of a physician and nurse author team, in this case to develop a text targeted to students of medicine, nursing, and other allied health professions. Henry's vision for this text meshed with those of the nurse authors, as well as that of William Benedict, MD, the fourth original author. Through Henry's leadership and collaboration, the authors were able to shape this text and share these important values with students. Henry also wisely planned to have the text's vision remain on course by identifying Barry, John and Rosalyn, the current physician authors, to continue that vision. We hope we have fulfilled his vision with this edition.

About The Authors

Jane W. Ball, DrPH, RN, CPNP

Jane W. Ball graduated from The Johns Hopkins Hospital School of Nursing and subsequently received her master's and doctoral degrees in public health from The Johns Hopkins University Bloomberg School of Public Health. She began her nursing career as a pediatric nurse and pediatric nurse practitioner in The Johns Hopkins Hospital. Since completing her public health degrees, she has held several positions that enable her to focus on improving the health care of children, such as serving as the chief of Child Health for the Commonwealth of Pennsylvania Department of Health and as Assistant Professor at the University of Texas at Arlington School of Nursing. For the next 20 years Jane focused her efforts on improving the system of emergency medical care for children while employed by Children's National Medical Center in Washington, DC. She served as the executive director of the National Resource Center at Children's

National Medical Center providing support to two federal programs: Emergency Medical Services for Children and the Trauma-Emergency Medical Services Systems Program. Dr. Ball serves as a consultant to the American College of Surgeons' Committee on Trauma to help states improve their trauma care systems, an investigator for an Emergency Medical Services for Children Program grant awarded to Wake Forest University School of Medicine, and a consultant to the Uniformed Services University of the Health Sciences for the development of a pediatric emergency education program. She is also the author of several pediatric nursing textbooks. Dr. Ball was recognized as a distinguished alumnus of The Johns Hopkins University in 2010.

Joyce E. Dains, DrPH, JD, RN, FNP-BC, FAANP

As a board-certified family nurse practitioner with doctorates in both public health and law, Joyce E. Dains has had a rich and productive career in education and clinical practice. She graduated as Valedictorian from the New England Baptist Hospital School of Nursing in Boston and subsequently earned a baccalaureate degree in nursing from Boston College, graduating magna cum laude; a master's degree in nursing from Case Western Reserve University; and a doctorate in public health from the University of Texas–Houston. She also completed a post-graduate nurse practitioner program at the Texas Woman's University. She earned her law degree at the University of Houston and practiced law for a brief period. Dr. Dains has been in clinical practice, teaching, and leadership positions at major universities and medical institutions including Ohio State University, the University of Texas-Houston, and Baylor College of

Medicine. She has been instrumental in the education of nursing students, medical students, and other health care professionals. As a family nurse practitioner, she has maintained a clinical practice in a variety of primary care settings. She is currently at the University of Texas MD Anderson Cancer Center where she is Program Director for Advanced Practice Nursing and a Family Nurse Practitioner in the Cancer Prevention Center. Dr. Dains is a Fellow of the American Association of Nurse Practitioners and is the recipient of other distinguished honors, including election to the National Academies of Practice. Dr. Dains is also the author of Elsevier's *Advanced Health Assessment and Clinical Diagnosis in Primary Care.*

John A. Flynn, MD, MBA, MEd

John A. Flynn completed his undergraduate work at Boston College, graduating magna cum laude with a bachelor's degree in mathematics. He attended medical school at the University of Missouri–Columbia where he was recognized in 2004 with the "Outstanding Young Alumni" award. Dr. Flynn completed his internship and residency at The Johns Hopkins University School of Medicine, followed by a fellowship in rheumatology, and was selected to serve as an assistant chief of service for the Longcope Firm of the Osler Medical Service. Dr. Flynn also completed a master's degree in business administration at The Johns Hopkins University. Dr. Flynn is currently the Director of Clinical Practice Improvement within the Clinical Practice Association, Chief Administrative Officer within the Office of Johns Hopkins Physicians, and Associate Dean of Johns Hopkins University School of Medicine. He holds the D. William Schlott, MD, Professorship in Medicine. Dr. Flynn also serves as the medical director of the spondyloarthritis program at The Johns Hopkins University and is the co-director of the Osler Center for Clinical Excellence. He is a founding member of the Vivien T. Thomas College within

The Johns Hopkins University School of Medicine Colleges Advisory Program. Dr. Flynn is a Fellow with The American College of Rheumatology and a Diplomat of The American Board of Rheumatology, as well as a Fellow to The American College of Physicians. Dr. Flynn holds memberships in The American College of Physicians, the American College of Rheumatology, the Society of General Internal Medicine, the Association of Chiefs of General Internal Medicine, the Spondyloarthritis Research and Treatment Network, and the Group for Research and Assessment of Psoriasis and Psoriatic Arthritis. He has served as an editor of *Cutaneous Medicine: Cutaneous Manifestations of Systemic Disease* and the *First and Second Editions of the Oxford American Handbook of Clinical Medicine*. Dr. Flynn's clinical interest is arthritis and his research interests include ambulatory education, the delivery of ambulatory care in an academic setting, and the care of patients with spondyloarthritis.

Barry S. Solomon, MD, MPH

Barry Solomon graduated from the University of Pennsylvania School of Medicine and completed his residency at the Children's Hospital of Pittsburgh. He subsequently completed a fellowship in general academic pediatrics at The Johns Hopkins University School of Medicine, during which time he received a master of public health degree from The Johns Hopkins University Bloomberg School of Public Health. His interests include the integration of children's mental health services in pediatric primary care, injury prevention, community pediatrics training, and medical education. He has given many research presentations and educational workshops at regional and national meetings and has authored numerous publications in peer-reviewed journals. Barry is currently an associate professor of pediatrics in the Division of General Pediatrics and Adolescent Medicine in the School of Medicine, a core faculty member in the Women's and Children's Health Policy Center, and an adjunct faculty member in the Center for Injury Research and Policy in the Bloomberg School of Public Health. He is the medical director

of the Harriet Lane Clinic, a large pediatric primary care practice that serves as the main outpatient training site for pediatrics residents at The Johns Hopkins University. As medical director, Barry has focused his efforts on enhancing the ability of the Harriet Lane Clinic to serve as a true medical home for urban children and families by providing an array of on-site health and social services, including an interdisciplinary mental health program. As a general pediatrician, he provides primary care in the Harriet Lane Clinic and serves as an inpatient attending in The Johns Hopkins Children's Center. Barry is an admired teacher and mentor to residents and medical students. He is an associate program director for the Johns Hopkins pediatric residency program and a faculty co-leader in the Colleges Advisory Program. In these roles, he serves as a longitudinal faculty advisor to medical students and residents.

Rosalyn W. Stewart, MD, MS, MBA

Rosalyn Stewart began her career at the University of Texas Medical Branch where she earned her medical degree and subsequently completed her combined internal medicine–pediatrics residency and a master of science degree in preventive medicine. She is currently an associate professor in internal medicine and pediatrics at The Johns Hopkins University and is also a member of the faculty in the Bloomberg School of Public Health and The Johns Hopkins School of Nursing. She completed a master of business administration degree with an emphasis on health care. She practices both general internal medicine and general pediatrics. Her academic focus is on medical education, primary care, and health disparities. She holds many positions centered on these interests and has been recognized for her ability to carry forth the Osler philosophy, discipline, and practice of medicine. She is associate director of the Longitudinal Ambulatory

Clerkship, a clinical clerkship devoted to primary care and systems of health practice. As the associate director of both Johns Hopkins University Internal Medicine–Pediatrics Urban Health Residency Program and the Osler Internal Medicine Urban Primary Track, she focuses her efforts on assembling a cadre of excellent teachers, training the very best students of medicine in the ongoing continuity of patient care developing new curriculum for the education of the best clinicians. Her goal is to create physician leaders who will serve as primary care systems–level change agents and will provide effective, longitudinal, comprehensive, coordinated, person-focused care for the underinsured inner-city patient.

Reviewers

Craig S. Boisvert, D.O.
Professor and Chair of Clinical Sciences
West Virginia School of Osteopathic Medicine
Lewisberg, West Virginia

Jason Ferguson, BPA, AAS NREMT-Paramedic
EMS Program Head
Central Virginia Community College
Lynchburg, Virginia

Rebecca A. Fountain, RN, PhD
Assistant Professor
College of Nursing and Health Sciences
University of Texas at Tyler
Tyler, Texas

Alicia C. Henning, RN, BSN, SANE
Member of ACFEI: American College of Forensic Examiners
Member of IAFN: International Association of Forensic Nurses
Breckenridge Memorial Hospital
Hardinsburg, Kentucky

Carla Lynch, BSN, MS
Clinical Assistant Professor of Nursing
School of Nursing
The University of Tulsa
Tulsa, Oklahoma

Kristin Ramirez, MSN, RN, ACNS-BC
Assistant Clinical Professor of Nursing
Department of Nursing
Angelo State University
San Angelo, Texas

Anita K. Reed, MSN, RN
Department Chair Adult and Community Health Practice
Remington, Indiana

Susan K. Rice, PhD, RN, CPNP, CNS
Professor
College of Nursing
University of Toledo
Toledo, Ohio

Susan D. Rymer, MSN, RN
Assistant Professor
School of Nursing
Bellin College
Green Bay, Wisconsin

Pamella Stockel, PhD, RN, CNE
Associate Professor of Nursing
Loretto Heights School of Nursing
Regis University
Denver, Colorado

Karen Vanbeek, MSN, CCNS
Assistant Professor of Nursing
School of Nursing
Bellin College
Green Bay, Wisconsin

Lynn Wimett, APRN-C, EdD, BSN, MS
Professor of Nursing
Loretto Heights School of Nursing
Regis University
Denver, Colorado

Preface

Seidel's Guide to Physical Examination is written primarily for students beginning their careers as a healthcare professional. The core message of our book is that patients are primary and must be served well. Learning how to take histories and perform physical examinations is necessary but not sufficient for the full understanding of patients. The relationship with your patients and the development of trust most often begins with conversation. You need reliable information if you are to serve your patients well. You are, after all, learning the stories of unique individuals, and they involve far more than the sum of body parts and systems. The art and skills involved in history taking and the physical examination are common to all of us, regardless of our particular health profession.

Organization

The achievement of a constructive relationship with a patient begins with your mastery of sound history taking and physical examination. Chapter 1 offers vital "getting to know you" guidelines to help you learn about the patient as the patient learns about you. Chapter 2 stresses that "knowing" is incomplete without the mutual understanding of cultural backgrounds and differences. Chapter 3 gives an overview of examination processes and the equipment you will need.

Chapters 4, 5, 6, and 7 introduce important elements of assessment: vital signs and pain, mental status, growth and development, and nutrition. Chapters 8 through 22 discuss specific body systems and body parts, with each chapter divided into four major sections:

+ Anatomy and Physiology
+ Review of Related History
+ Examination and Findings
+ Abnormalities

Each of these sections begins with consideration of the adult patient and ends, when appropriate, with variations for infants, children, and adolescents; pregnant women; older adults; and individuals with disabilities.

To help you get organized, each chapter starts with a preview of the step-by-step examination process. The Anatomy and Physiology sections begin with the physiologic basis for the interpretation of findings, and they describe the key anatomic landmarks to guide physical examination. The Review of Related History sections detail a specific method of inquiry when a system or organ-related problem is discovered during the interview or examination. The Examination and Findings sections list needed equipment and then describe in detail the procedures for the examination and the expected findings. These sections encourage you to develop an approach and sequence that is comfortable for you and, particularly, for the patient. In some chapters advanced examination procedures are described for use in specific circumstances or when specific conditions exist. Sample write-up of findings conclude these sections. You will note that the terms "normal" and "abnormal" are avoided whenever possible to describe findings because, in our view, these terms suggest a value judgment that may or may not prove valid with experience and additional information. The Abnormalities sections provide an overview of diseases and associated problems relevant to the particular system or body part. The Abnormalities sections include three-column tables clearly listing pathophysiology, subjective data, and objective data for selected conditions and often include full-color photos and illustrations.

Chapter 23 details the issues relevant to the sports participation evaluation. Chapter 27 provides guidelines for the change in standard examination approaches in emergency and life-threatening situations. This information is only a beginning and is intended to be useful in your clinical decision making. You will need to add other resources to your base of knowledge.

The remaining chapters put it all together. Chapter 24 points the way to integrating what you have learned, making it useful in decision making and problem solving. Chapter 25 provides guidelines in thinking critically about clinical challenges. All you have learned and thought about regarding the patient, along with your decisions must be carefully recorded. Chapter 26 describes how to do this, with particular emphasis on the Problem Oriented Medical Record (POMR) and the use of SOAP (**S**ubjective findings, **O**bjective findings, **A**ssessment, and **P**lan) to document your patients' problems completely.

The thoroughly updated appendixes and companion website content provide clinical tools and resources to document observations or problems and complete the physical examination, preserving a continuous record.

Special Features

The basic structure of the book—with its consistent chapter organization and the inclusion of special considerations sections for infants, children, adolescents, pregnant women, and older adults—facilitates learning.

+ Physical Variations boxes highlight variations from expected findings.
+ Differential Diagnosis content—a hallmark of this text—is highlighted throughout.
+ Evidence-Based Practice in Physical Examination boxes are reminders that our clinical work—as much as possible—should be supported by sound, proven information.
+ Risk Factors boxes highlight modifiable and nonmodifiable risk factors for a variety of conditions.
+ Sample Documentation and Examination Summary boxes at the end of each Examination and Findings section model good documentation practice and provide a convenient summary of examination steps.
+ Functional Assessment boxes help readers consider specific physical problems and their effect on patient function.
+ Staying Well boxes provide a focus on patient wellness and health promotion for a holistic approach.

New to This Edition

The entire book has been thoroughly updated for this edition. This includes the replacement of illustrations of abnormal findings with updated photos and the use of new full-color photos and drawings to replace one- and two-color illustrations in the seventh edition. There are a total of approximately 1200 illustrations in addition to the numerous tables and boxes that have traditionally given readers easy access to information. Among the many changes:

+ Evidence-Based Practice in Physical Examination boxes have been thoroughly updated. These boxes focus on the ongoing need to incorporate recent research into clinical practice and decision making.
+ Clinical Pearls and Physical Variations boxes have been updated and revised.
+ Mnemonics have been integrated into text where appropriate to assist with history and physical examination assessments.
+ The Abnormalities section now includes a summary of the pathophysiology and subjective and objective data associated with the condition or disorder.
+ The Techniques and Equipment chapter includes updated recommendations for Standard Precautions.
+ A new chapter on vital signs assessment is integrated with pain assessment, considered the fifth vital sign.
+ Cancer screening controversies and summary evidence are included in the abdomen, breast, and prostate chapters
+ The emergency or life-threatening situations chapter has been updated.
+ The sports participation chapter includes recommendations for assessing and managing patients with sports-related concussions.

Our Ancillary Package

Seidel's Physical Examination Handbook is a concise, pocket-sized companion for clinical experiences. It summarizes, reinforces, and serves as a quick reference to the core content of the textbook.

Student Laboratory Manual for Seidel's Guide to Physical Examination is a practical printed workbook that helps readers integrate the content of the textbook and ensure content mastery through a variety of engaging exercises.

ⓔ *Instructor Resources* on the companion Evolve website (http:/evolve.elsevier.com/Seidel) include an extensive electronic image collection and two PowerPoint lecture slide collections that included integrated animations, case studies, and a series of audience response questions. In addition, *TEACH* provides learning objectives, key terms, nursing curriculum standards, content highlights, student and instructor resource lists, teaching strategies, and case studies. Also now available on the Evolve website are two thoroughly revised and expanded Test Banks, in ExamView® format, which faculty can use to create customized exams for medical, allied health, or nursing programs. Together these resources provide the complete building blocks needed for course preparation.

ⓔ *Student Resources* on the companion Evolve website include a wide variety of interactive activities, case studies, audio clips of heart, lung, and abdominal sounds, video clips of selected examination procedures, animations depicting content and processes, 270 NCLEX style review questions, and downloadable student checklists and key points. Audio, video, and animations icons have been added throughout the text chapters to highlight physical exam–related media segments provided on the comprehensive Evolve website.

Also available is the thoroughly revised and expanded online course library titled *Physical Examination and Health Assessment Online*, which is an exhaustive multimedia library of online resources, including animations, video clips, interactive exercises, quizzes, and much more. Comprehensive self-paced learning modules offer flexibility to faculty or students, with tutorial learning modules and in-depth capstone case studies for each body system chapter in the text. Also included in this online course are advanced practice case studies that put the student in the exam room and test information gathering and differential diagnosis skills. Animations, heart and lung sounds, images, interactive activities, and video clips are embedded in the learning modules and cases to provide a dynamic, multimodal learning environment for today's learners. Available for individual student purchase or as a required course supplement, *Physical Examination and Health Assessment Online* unlocks a rich online learning experience.

An additional electronic offering is the inclusion of this book in *Pageburst®*, a next-generation electronic book platform that allows for highlighting and annotating text content, adding notes, and sharing with other *Pageburst®* users, as well as linking and cross-referencing with other online Elsevier textbooks. This text will also be available in other electronic book formats.

The existing physical examination video series comprises 14 examination videos, each of which features an examination of a

PREFACE

specific body system with animations and illustration overlays to demonstrate examination techniques in greater depth, and a fifteenth "Putting It All Together" video that shows a head-to-toe examination of an adult along with appropriate life span variations. The series has been expanded to include three special topics: *Effective Communication and Interviewing Skills*, *Physical Examination of the Hospitalized Patient*, and *Putting It All Together: Physical Examination of the Child*. All 18 videos in this video series are offered in three formats: DVD, streaming (online), and networkable (for institutional purchase).

Our Core Values

In the eighth edition of *Seidel's Guide to Physical Examination*, we have made every attempt to consider patients in all of their variety and to preserve the fundamental messages explicit in earlier editions. These include the following:

* Respect the patient.
* Achieve the complementary forces of competence and compassion.
* The art and skill essential to history taking and physical examination are the foundation of care; technologic resources complement these processes.
* The history and physical examination are inseparable; they are one.
* The computer and technology cannot replace you. You, your care and skills are what builds a trusting, fruitful relationship with the patient.
* That relationship can be indescribably rewarding.

We hope that you will find this a useful text and that it will continue to serve as a resource as your career evolves.

Acknowledgments

The eighth edition of our textbook is possible only because of the professionalism and skills of so many others who really know how to fashion a book and its ancillaries so that it is maximally useful to you. First, there are those instructors and students who have so thoughtfully and constructively offered comment over the years. Improvements in content and style stem in large part from their suggestions.

We have, of course, provided the content, but it has to be accessible to the reader. A textbook needs a style that ensures readability, and our partners at Elsevier have made that happen. Sally Schrefer, our friend and also managing director, nursing and health professions, has been with us and guided us from the first day of planning for the first edition. She continued to exercise the wisdom she demonstrated early on without trampling our sometimes tender sensibilities. We wish her well in retirement, but we are sad that she will not be there to guide the ninth edition.

Each word, figure, and page needs the artful attention of skilled professionals. The whole is a demanding project requiring effective editing and design. This was ensured by Debbie Vogel, publishing services manager, and Bridget Healy, project manager. Bridget did a spectacular job of keeping everything moving with

her qualitative eye for detail throughout. Jessica William's design is visually appealing and showcases the content.

We also want to recognize the indispensable efforts of the entire marketing team led by Pat Crowe and Kim Eaves, as well as the sales representatives, who make certain that our message is honestly portrayed and that comments and suggestions from the field are candidly reported. Indeed, there are so very many men and women who are essential to the creation and potential success of our eighth edition, and we are indebted to each of them.

The remarkable teaching tools we call the ancillaries need special attention. These are the laboratory manual, handbook, instructor's resource manual, test banks, health assessment online, and video series, all demanding an expertise—if they are to be useful—that goes beyond that of the authors. Dr. Denise Vanacore-Chase offers hers for the laboratory manual, the nursing test bank, nursing PowerPoint slides, and TEACH; Frank Bregar offers his for the medical test bank and medical PowerPoint slide collection. The careful attention to all ⊜volve asset development is overseen by David Rushing. The development of *Health Assessment Online* is led by Chris Lay; Nancy Priff, Glenn Harman, and Paul Trumbore's efforts are essential to the success of the video series. And then there is Kristin Geen, our executive content specialist, and Michele Hayden and Jamie Randall, our content managers, who were always quietly there, a firm hand in a velvet glove. A phone call from Shelly or Jamie always ends with the feeling that their suggestions had really originated with us. They made our book better and we thought we were doing it.

Kristin, Shelly and Jamie worked hand in glove with splendid allies. Melissa Rawe, our content development specialist, maintained professional skill and calm and taught us that it is possible to do this and keep life at home and office in proper balance. And Hannah Corrier ensured that, when we used the work of others, it was appropriately acknowledged and recognized.

In addition, we offer many thanks to the following individuals for their contributions of time, talent, expertise, and resources: Craig S. Boisvert; Jason Ferguson; Alicia Greenwell; Carla Lynch; Kristin Ramirez; Anita K. Reed; Susan K. Rice; Susan D. Rymer; Pamella Stockel; Lynn Wimett; and Karen Vanbeek.

Thanks, too, to the following contributors to previous editions: John S. Andrews, Barbara Cousins, Candis Morrison, Kevin Murphy, Donald P. O'Connor, Adam Seidel, Samuel Seidel, Sharon Lechter Smalling, Leah Payne Smith, Allen Walker, Diane Wind Wardell, George J. Wassilchenko, and Patrick Watson.

And finally—our families! They are patient with our necessary absences, support what we do, and are unstinting in their love. They have our love and our quite special thanks.

Jane W. Ball, DrPH, RN, CPNP
Joyce E. Dains, DrPH, JD, RN, FNP-BC, FAANP
John A. Flynn, MD, MBA, MEd
Barry S. Solomon, MD, MPH
Rosalyn W. Stewart, MD, MS, MBA

Contents

About The Authors, *vii*

Reviewers, *ix*

Preface, *x*

1 The History and Interviewing Process, *1*
  Developing a Relationship with the Patient, *1*
    Effective Communication, 2
  The Patient History, *6*
    Setting for the Interview, 6
    Structure of the History, 6
  Building the History, *6*
    Sensitive Issues, 7
    Outline of the History, 10
    Adaptations for Age, Gender, and Possible
      Disabilities, 14
  The Next Step, *20*

2 Cultural Competency, *21*
  A Definition of Culture, *21*
  Distinguishing Physical Characteristics, *21*
  Cultural Competence, *22*
  Cultural Humility, *23*
  The Impact of Culture, *23*
  The Blurring of Cultural Distinctions, *23*
  The Primacy of the Individual in Health Care, *24*
  Professional Cultures within the Health
    Professions, *24*
  The Impact of Culture on Illness, *24*
  The Components of a Cultural Response, *25*
    Modes of Communication, 26
    Health Beliefs and Practices, 27
    Family Relationships, 27
    Diet and Nutritional Practices, 28
  Summing Up, *28*

3 Examination Techniques and Equipment, *30*
  Precautions to Prevent Infection, *30*
  Latex Allergy, *30*
  Examination Technique, *32*
    Patient Positions and Draping, 32
    Inspection, 32
    Palpation, 33

    Percussion, 34
    Auscultation, 35
  Modifications for Patients with Disabilities, *35*
    Patients with Mobility Impairments, 35
    Patients with Sensory Impairment, 36
    Special Concerns for Patients with Spinal Cord Injury
      or Lesion, 37
  Equipment, *37*
    Weight Scales and Height Measurement Devices, 37
    Thermometer, 39
    Stethoscope, 39
    Sphygmomanometer, 40
    Pulse Oximeter, 40
    Doppler, 41
    Portable Ultrasound, 41
    Fetal Monitoring Equipment, 41
    Ophthalmoscope, 42
    PanOptic Ophthalmoscope, 43
    StrabismoScope, 43
    Photoscreening, 43
    Visual Acuity Charts, 43
    Near Vision Charts, 44
    Amsler Grid, 44
    Otoscope, 45
    Tympanometer, 45
    Nasal Speculum, 45
    Tuning Fork, 45
    Percussion (Reflex) Hammer, 46
    Neurologic Hammer, 46
    Tape Measure, 46
    Transilluminator, 47
    Vaginal Speculum, 47
    Goniometer, 48
    Wood's Lamp, 48
    Dermatoscope, 48
    Calipers for Skinfold Thickness, 49
    Monofilament, 49
    Scoliometer, 49

4 Vital Signs and Pain Assessment, *50*
  Anatomy and Physiology, *50*
    Temperature, 50

CONTENTS

Pulse Rate, 50
Respiratory Rate, 50
Blood Pressure, 50
Pain, 50
Review of Related History, 52
Present Problem, 52
Personal and Social History, 52
Examination and Findings, 52
Temperature, 52
Pulse Rate, 53
Respiratory Rate, 53
Blood Pressure, 53
Pain Assessment, 56
Self-Report Pain Rating Scales, 56
Assessing Pain Behaviors, 56
Abnormalities, 62

5 Mental Status, 64
Anatomy and Physiology, 64
Review of Related History, 65
History of Present Illness, 65
Past Medical History, 66
Family History, 66
Personal and Social History, 66
Examination and Findings, 66
Physical Appearance and Behavior, 66
Grooming, 66
Emotional Status, 67
Nonverbal Communication (Body Language), 67
State of Consciousness, 67
Cognitive Abilities, 67
Analogies, 67
Abstract Reasoning, 69
Arithmetic Calculation, 69
Writing Ability, 69
Execution of Motor Skills, 69
Memory, 70
Attention Span, 70
Judgment, 70
Speech and Language Skills, 70
Voice Quality, 70
Articulation, 70
Comprehension, 70
Coherence, 70
Emotional Stability, 71
Mood and Feelings, 71
Thought Process and Content, 71
Perceptual Distortions and Hallucinations, 71
Abnormalities, 75

6 Growth and Measurement, 79
Anatomy and Physiology, 79
Differences in Growth by Organ System, 80
Review of Related History, 82
History of Present Illness, 82
Past Medical History, 82
Family History, 82
Personal and Social History, 82
Examination and Findings, 83
Equipment, 83
Weight and Standing Height, 83

Body Mass Index, 83
Recumbent Length, 83
Weight, 84
Head Circumference, 84
Chest Circumference, 85
Gestational Age, 85
Stature and Weight, 86
Upper-to-Lower Segment Ratio, 87
Arm Span, 87
Sexual Maturation, 87
Abnormalities, 91

7 Nutrition, 95
Anatomy and Physiology, 95
Macronutrients, 95
Carbohydrate, 95
Protein, 96
Fat, 96
Micronutrients, 96
Water, 96
Energy Requirements, 97
Resting Energy Expenditure, 97
Physical Activity, 97
Thermogenesis, 97
Review of Related History, 97
History of Present Illness, 97
Past Medical History, 97
Family History, 98
Personal and Social History, 98
Infants and Children, 98
Adolescents, 99
Pregnant Women, 99
Older Adults, 99
Examination and Findings, 99
Equipment, 99
Anthropometrics, 100
Waist Circumference and Waist-Height Ratio, 100
Waist-to-Hip Circumference Ratio, 100
Determination of Diet Adequacy, 101
Twenty–Four-Hour Recall Diet, 101
Food Diary, 101
Measures of Nutrient Analysis, 101
ChooseMyPlate.gov, 101
Vegetarian Diets, 102
Ethnic Food Guide Pyramids, 102
Measures of Nutrient Adequacy, 102
Special Procedures, 107
Triceps Skinfold Thickness, 107
Mid-Upper Arm Circumference, 108
Midarm Muscle Circumference/Midarm Muscle Area, 108
Biochemical Measurement, 108
Abnormalities, 110

8 Skin, Hair, and Nails, 114
Anatomy and Physiology, 114
Epidermis, 115
Dermis, 115
Hypodermis, 115
Appendages, 115

Review of Related History, *117*
    History of Present Illness, *117*
    Past Medical History, *118*
    Family History, *118*
    Personal and Social History, *118*
Examination and Findings, *119*
    Equipment, *119*
    Skin, *119*
      Inspection, 119
      Palpation, 124
      Skin Lesions, 125
    Hair, *133*
    Nails, *134*
      Inspection, 134
      Palpation, 135
Abnormalities, *144*

9   Lymphatic System, *166*
Anatomy and Physiology, *166*
    Lymph Nodes, *167*
    Lymphocytes, *169*
    Thymus, *170*
    Spleen, *170*
    Tonsils and Adenoids, *170*
    Peyer Patches, *170*
Review of Related History, *171*
    History of Present Illness, *171*
    Past Medical History, *171*
    Family History, *172*
    Personal and Social History, *172*
Examination and Findings, *172*
    Equipment, *172*
    Inspection and Palpation, *172*
    Head and Neck, *174*
    Axillae, *175*
    Epitrochlear Lymph Nodes, *175*
    **Inguinal and Popliteal Lymph
      Nodes,** *176*
    Spleen, *176*
Abnormalities, *178*

10 Head and Neck, *184*
Anatomy and Physiology, *184*
Review of Related History, *186*
    History of Present Illness, *187*
    Past Medical History, *188*
    Family History, *188*
    Personal and Social History, *188*
Examination and Findings, *188*
    Equipment, *188*
    Head and Face, *189*
      Inspection, 189
      Palpation, 192
      Percussion, 192
      Auscultation, 192
    Neck, *192*
      Inspection, 192
      Palpation, 193
      Lymph Nodes, 193
      Thyroid Gland, 193
      Inspection, 195
      Palpation, 196
      Transillumination, 196
Abnormalities, *198*

11 Eyes, *204*
Anatomy and Physiology, *204*
    External Eye, *205*
      Eyelid, 205
      Conjunctiva, 205
      Lacrimal Gland, 205
      Eye Muscles, 205
    Internal Eye, *205*
      Sclera, 206
      Cornea, 206
      Uvea, 206
      Lens, 206
      Retina, 206
Review of Related History, *207*
    History of Present Illness, *207*
    Past Medical History, *208*
    Family History, *208*
    Personal and Social History, *208*
Examination and Findings, *208*
    Equipment, *208*
    Visual Acuity Testing, *208*
    External Examination, *209*
      Surrounding Structures, 210
      Eyelids, 210
      Palpation, 211
      Conjunctiva, 211
      Cornea, 212
      Iris and Pupil, 212
      Lens, 214
      Sclera, 214
      Lacrimal Apparatus, 214
    Extraocular Muscles, *214*
    Ophthalmoscopic Examination, *216*
      Unexpected Findings, 218
Abnormalities, *223*

12 Ears, Nose, and Throat, *231*
Anatomy and Physiology, *232*
    Ears and Hearing, *232*
    Nose, Nasopharynx, and Sinuses, *233*
    Mouth and Oropharynx, *234*
Review of Related History, *236*
    History of Present Illness, *236*
    Past Medical History, *237*
    Family History, *237*
    Personal and Social History, *238*
Examination and Findings, *238*
    Equipment, *238*
    Ears and Hearing, *238*
      External Ear, 238
      Otoscopic Examination, 239
      Hearing Evaluation, 241

Nose, Nasopharynx, and Sinuses, *242*
  External Nose, *242*
  Nasal Cavity, *242*
  Sinuses, *243*
Mouth and Oropharynx, *244*
  Lips, *244*
  Buccal Mucosa, Teeth, and Gums, *244*
  Oral Cavity, *246*
  Oropharynx, *248*
Abnormalities, *254*

13 Chest and Lungs, *260*
Anatomy and Physiology, *260*
  Anatomic Landmarks, *262*
Review of Related History, *264*
  History of Present Illness, *264*
    Coughs, *264*
  Sputum, *265*
  Past Medical History, *265*
  Family History, *266*
  Personal and Social History, *266*
  Equipment, *267*
Examination and Findings, *267*
  Inspection, *267*
    Observing Respiration, *267*
    Looking for Clues at the Periphery, *271*
  Palpation, *271*
    Tactile Fremitus, *272*
    Examining the Trachea, *273*
  Percussion, *273*
    Diaphragmatic Excursion, *274*
  Auscultation, *276*
    Breath Sounds, *276*
    Vocal Resonance, *279*
Abnormalities, *283*

14 Heart, *294*
Anatomy and Physiology, *294*
  Structure, *295*
  Cardiac Cycle, *297*
  Electrical Activity, *298*
Review of Related History, *301*
  History of Present Illness, *301*
  Past Medical History, *302*
  Family History, *303*
  Personal and Social History, *303*
Examination and Findings, *304*
  Equipment, *304*
  Inspection, *304*
  Palpation, *305*
  Percussion, *306*
  Auscultation, *306*
    Basic Heart Sounds, *307*
    Extra Heart Sounds, *310*
    Heart Murmurs, *311*
    Rhythm Disturbance, *318*
Abnormalities, *320*

15 Blood Vessels, *332*
Anatomy and Physiology, *332*
  Blood Circulation, *332*

  Arterial Pulse and Pressure, *336*
  Jugular Venous Pulse and Pressure, *336*
Review of Related History, *337*
  History of Present Illness, *337*
  Past Medical History, *337*
  Family History, *338*
  Personal and Social History, *338*
Examination and Findings, *338*
  Equipment, *338*
  Peripheral Arteries, *338*
    Palpation, *338*
    Auscultation, *340*
    Assessment for Peripheral Arterial Disease, *340*
  Peripheral Veins, *342*
    Jugular Venous Pressure, *342*
    Hepatojugular Reflux, *343*
    Evaluation of Hand Veins, *343*
    Assessment for Venous Obstruction and
      Insufficiency, *343*
Abnormalities, *346*

16 Breasts and Axillae, *350*
Anatomy and Physiology, *350*
Review of Related History, *353*
  History of Present Illness, *353*
  Past Medical History, *353*
  Family History, *355*
  Personal and Social History, *355*
Examination and Findings, *355*
  Equipment, *355*
  Inspection, *355*
    Breasts, *355*
    Nipples and Areolae, *356*
    Reinspection in Varied Positions, *357*
  Palpation, *358*
    Patient in Seated Position, *360*
    Patient in Supine Position, *360*
Abnormalities, *365*

17 Abdomen, *370*
Anatomy and Physiology, *370*
  Alimentary Tract, *370*
  Liver, *372*
  Gallbladder, *373*
  Pancreas, *373*
  Spleen, *373*
  Kidneys, Ureters, and Bladder, *373*
  Musculature and Connective Tissues, *373*
  Vasculature, *373*
Review of Related History, *375*
  History of Present Illness, *375*
  Past Medical History, *377*
  Family History, *377*
  Personal and Social History, *377*
Examination and Findings, *377*
  Equipment, *377*
  Preparation, *377*
  Inspection, *378*
    Surface Characteristics, *378*
    Contour, *379*
    Movement, *381*

CONTENTS

Auscultation, *381*
    Bowel Sounds, *381*
    Additional Sounds and Bruits, *381*
Percussion, *381*
    Liver Span, *381*
    Spleen, *383*
    Gastric Bubble, *383*
    Kidneys, *383*
Palpation, *383*
    Light Palpation, *383*
    Moderate Palpation, *383*
    Deep Palpation, *384*
    Masses, *384*
    Umbilical Ring, *385*
    Palpation of Specific Organs and
        Structures, *385*
    Ascites Assessment, *388*
    Pain Assessment, *388*
    Abdominal Signs, *391*
    Rebound Tenderness, *391*
    Iliopsoas Muscle Test, *393*
    Obturator Muscle Test, *393*
    Ballottement, *393*
Abnormalities, *399*

18 Female Genitalia, *416*
Anatomy and Physiology, *416*
    External Genitalia, *416*
    Internal Genitalia, *418*
    Bony Pelvis, *419*
Review of Related History, *423*
    History of Present Illness, *423*
    Past Medical History, *424*
    Family History, *425*
    Personal and Social History, *425*
Examination and Findings, *427*
    Equipment, *427*
    Preparation, *427*
    Positioning, *428*
    Draping and Gloving, *428*
    External Examination, *428*
        Inspection and Palpation, *428*
        Labia Majora, *428*
        Labia Minora, *429*
        Clitoris, *429*
        Urethral Orifice, *429*
        Vaginal Introitus, *429*
        Skene and Bartholin Glands, *429*
        Muscle Tone, *430*
        Perineum, *430*
        Anus, *430*
    Internal Examination, *430*
        Preparation, *430*
        Insertion of Speculum, *430*
        Cervix, *431*
        Withdrawal of Speculum, *435*
    Bimanual Examination, *435*
        Cervix, *436*
        Uterus, *437*
        Adnexa and Ovaries, *437*

Rectovaginal Examination, *438*
    Preparation, *438*
    Anal Sphincter, *438*
    Rectal Walls and Rectovaginal
        Septum, *439*
    Uterus, *439*
    Adnexa, *439*
    Stool, *439*
    Completion, *439*
Abnormalities, *450*

19 Male Genitalia, *466*
Anatomy and Physiology, *466*
Review of Related History, *468*
    History of Present Illness, *468*
    Past Medical History, *469*
    Family History, *469*
    Personal and Social History, *469*
Examination and Findings, *471*
    Equipment, *471*
    Inspection and Palpation, *471*
        Genital Hair Distribution, *471*
        Penis, *471*
        Urethral Meatus, *472*
        Penile Shaft, *472*
        Scrotum, *472*
        Hernia, *472*
        Testes, *473*
        Cremasteric Reflex, *474*
        Prostate, *474*
Abnormalities, *476*

20 Anus, Rectum, and Prostate, *485*
Anatomy and Physiology, *485*
Review of Related History, *487*
    History of Present Illness, *487*
    Past Medical History, *488*
    Family History, *488*
    Personal and Social History, *488*
Examination and Findings, *489*
    Equipment, *489*
    Preparation, *489*
    Positioning, *489*
    Sacrococcygeal and Perianal Areas, *489*
    Anus, *489*
    Sphincter, *489*
    Anal Ring, *489*
    Lateral and Posterior Rectal Walls, *490*
    Bidigital Palpation, *490*
    Anterior Rectal Wall, *490*
    Prostate, *491*
    Uterus and Cervix, *491*
    Stool, *491*
Abnormalities, *494*

21 Musculoskeletal System, *501*
Anatomy and Physiology, *501*
    Upper Extremities, *505*
    Head and Spine, *505*
    Lower Extremities, *507*

Review of Related History, *508*
   History of Present Illness, *508*
   Past Medical History, *509*
   Family History, *509*
   Personal and Social History, *509*
Examination and Findings, *510*
   Equipment, *510*
   Inspection, *510*
   Palpation, *510*
   **Range of Motion and Muscle
      Tone,** *511*
   Muscle Strength, *511*
   Specific Joints and Muscles, *512*
      Hands and Wrists, 512
      Elbows, 513
      Shoulders, 514
      Temporomandibular Joint, 516
      Cervical Spine, 516
      Thoracic and Lumbar Spine, 518
      Hips, 519
      Legs and Knees, 520
      Feet and Ankles, 522
   Advanced Skills, *524*
      Hand and Wrist Assessment, 524
      Shoulder Assessment, 524
      Lower Spine Assessment, 526
      Hip Assessment, 526
      Knee Assessment, 527
      Limb Measurement, 529
Abnormalities, *535*

22 Neurologic System, *544*
Anatomy and Physiology, *544*
   Brain, *545*
      Cerebrum, 545
      Cerebellum, 546
      Brainstem, 546
      Cranial Nerves, 547
   Spinal Cord and Spinal Tracts, *547*
   Spinal Nerves, *547*
Review of Related History, *550*
   History of Present Illness, *550*
   Past Medical History, *551*
   Family History, *551*
   Personal and Social History, *551*
Examination and Findings, *552*
   Equipment, *552*
   Cranial Nerves, *553*
      Olfactory (I), 553
      Optic (II), 554
      *Oculomotor, Trochlear, and Abducens (III, IV,
        and VI), 554*
      Trigeminal (V), 554
      Facial (VII), 555
      Acoustic (VIII), 556
      Glossopharyngeal (IX), 556
      Vagus (X), 556
      Spinal Accessory (XI), 556
      Hypoglossal (XII), 556

   Proprioception and Cerebellar Function, *556*
      Coordination and Fine Motor Skills, 556
      Balance, 559
   Sensory Function, *559*
      Primary Sensory Functions, 561
      Cortical Sensory Functions, 561
   Reflexes, *562*
      Superficial Reflexes, 562
      Deep Tendon Reflexes, 564
   Advanced Skills, *565*
      Protective Sensation, 565
      Meningeal Signs, 565
      Jolt Accentuation of Headache, 566
      Posturing, 566
Abnormalities, *573*

23 Sports Participation Evaluation, *581*

24 Putting It All Together, *594*
At the Start, *594*
Accuracy, *595*
The Potential for Error, *596*
Uncertainty, *596*
Examination Sequence, *596*
General Inspection, *597*
Preparation, *597*
Measurements, *597*
   Patient Seated, Wearing Gown, 597
   Patient Seated, Back Exposed, 599
   Patient Seated, Chest Exposed, 599
   Patient Reclining 45 Degrees, 599
   Patient Supine, Chest Exposed, 600
   Patient Supine, Abdomen Exposed, 600
   Patient Supine, Legs Exposed, 600
   Patient Sitting, Lap Draped, 600
   Patient Standing, 601
   Female Patient, Lithotomy Position, 601
   *Male Patient, Bending Forward (Lateral Decubitus or
      Knee-Chest Positions Are Also Possible), 601*
   Newborns, 602
   Older Infants, 602
Examination Sequence with Infants, *603*
   General Inspection, 603
   General Inspection, 606
   Child Playing, 606
   Child on Parent's Lap, 606
   *Child Relatively Supine, Still on Lap, Diaper
      Loosened, 607*
   Child Standing, 607
   Child Returns to Parent's Lap, 607
The Closing Discussion, *608*

25 Taking the Next Steps: Critical Thinking, *610*
The Clinical Examination, *610*
Critical Thinking, *610*
   Assessment, Judgment, and Evidence, 610
   Problem Identification, 610
   Valid Hypotheses, 611
   Possible Barriers to Critical Thinking, 611
   Validity of the Clinical Examination, 613

Bayes Theorem, *613*

Evidence-Based Practice, *614*

Evaluation and Management Plan and Setting Priorities, *614*

26 Recording Information, *616*

General Guidelines, *616*

EMR Replicating Functions, *617*

Organization of the Note, *617*

Organizing the Patient's Health Record with SOAP Notes, *618*

Subjective Data, *618*

Objective Data, *618*

Illustrations, *619*

Problem-Oriented Medical Record, *619*

Comprehensive Health History and Physical Examination, *619*

Problem List, *619*

Assessment, *620*

Plan, *620*

SOAP Notes, *620*

APSO Notes, *621*

Notes from Subsequent Evaluations, *621*

Problem-Oriented Medical Record Format, *621*

The History, *621*

Review of Systems, *622*

Physical Examination Findings, *624*

Assessment (for Each Problem on Problem List), *625*

Plan (for Each Problem on Problem List), *625*

Sample Records, *628*

Inpatient Admission Note, *628*

Summary, *631*

27 Emergency or Life-Threatening Situations, *632*

Emergency Assessment of the Injured Patient, *632*

The Primary Survey, *632*

Secondary Assessment of the Injured Patient, *635*

Injury Mechanisms, *636*

Blunt Trauma, *637*

Penetrating Trauma, *637*

Burns, *637*

Assessment of an Acute Medical Emergency, *637*

Advanced Cardiac Life Support Survey, *637*

Legal Considerations, *641*

Records, *641*

Consent for Treatment, *641*

Trauma Due to Violence, *641*

Medical Orders for Life-Sustaining Treatment, *642*

Summary, *642*

Abnormalities, *642*

Photo and Illustration Credits, *645*

References and Readings, *647*

Glossary, *666*

Appendix A Height/Weight Growth Charts, *675*

Appendix B Pediatric Blood Pressure Tables, *679*

Appendix C Conversion Tables and Anthropometric Measurements, *684*

Conversion Tables, *684*

Anthropometric Measurements, *685*

Index, *686*

CHAPTER 1

The History and Interviewing Process

This chapter discusses the development of your relationships with patients and the building of the histories of your patients. We write of it as "building" a history rather than "taking" one because you and your patient are involved in a joint effort, a partnership, which should have among other outcomes a history that truly reflects the patient's perspectives and unique status (Haidet and Paterniti, 2003; Haidet 2010). The chapter discusses the context of the relationship in emotional, physical, and ethical terms, and offers suggestions in verbal and nonverbal behavior that you may adapt to your individual comfort and style. Finally, we offer widely accepted, time-tested approaches to the structure of a history with adaptations suggested for age, gender, and disability. The history is vital to the appropriate interpretation of the physical examination.

evolve *http://evolve.elsevier.com/Seidel*
- NCLEX Review Questions
- Student Checklist

Developing a Relationship with the Patient

Our purpose is to offer instruction in learning about the well and the sick as they seek care. History and physical examination are at the heart of this effort. It is not easy to get the sense of another person or to fully appreciate someone else's orientation in the world. You and the patient may seem to have a similar experience but may in all likelihood interpret it differently (see Clinical Pearl, "Unique," Originally Derived from Latin "Unus," Meaning "One"). If you are to prevent misinterpretations and misperceptions, you must make every effort to sense the world of the individual patient as that patient senses it. (See Chapter 2 for additional discussion.)

Clinical Pearl

"Unique," Originally Derived from Latin "Unus," Meaning "One"
We use it in that sense of *being the only one.* Each of us is unique, incomparably different from anyone in the past, present, or future. No relationship, then, has an exact counterpart. Each moment is unique, different from the time before with the same patient.

From Merriam-Webster Online, 2012.

The first meeting with the patient sets the tone for a successful partnership as you inform the patient that you really want to know all that is needed and that you will be open, flexible, and eager to deal with questions and explanations. You can also explain the boundaries of your practice and the degree of your availability in any situation. Trust evolves from honesty and candor.

A primary objective is to discover the details about a patient's concern, explore expectations for the encounter, and display genuine interest, curiosity, and partnership. Identifying underlying worries, believing them, and trying to deal with them optimizes your ability to be of help. You need to understand what is expected of you. Your judgment and flexibility will confirm that each interaction is unique. If you are successful, the intimate nature of the interview and physical examination will be reinforced. You will savor frequent sweet moments with patients when you recognize that your efforts are going well and that trust and promise are there. We want to help you ensure those moments.

Clinical Pearl

The Patient Relationship
You will, in the course of your career, have numerous relationships with patients. Never forget that each time they are having an experience with you that is important to them. Think of actors in a long-running play. Every performance is new for the actors and the persons paying to be in the audience.

Much has been written about technology replacing the physical examination and history in some part, but the care of patients goes far beyond the merely technical. Health care providers are enabled by society to offer advice and the potential of healing to fellow human beings. Appropriate care satisfies a need that can be fully met only by a human touch, intimate conversation, and the "laying on of hands." This actual realization of your relationships with patients, particularly when illness compounds vulnerability, cannot be replaced (see Clinical Pearl, "The Patient Relationship").

Because cost containment is also essential, the well-performed history and physical examination can, in an advantaged society, justify the appropriate and cost-effective use of technological resources. In a disadvantaged society, it can help compensate for their absence. This underscores the need for judgment and the use of resources in a balance appropriate for the individual patient and for the utilitarian needs of society.

At a first meeting, you are in a position of strength and your patients are vulnerable. You do not necessarily have similar perspectives but you need to grasp theirs if you are to establish a meaningful partnership. This partnership has been conceptualized as patient-centered care, identified by the Institute of Medicine (IOM) as an important element of high-quality care. The report defined patient-centered care as "respecting and responding to patients' wants, needs and preferences, so that they can make choices in their care that best fit their individual circumstances" (IOM, 2001). Box 1-1 identifies questions that represent a patient-centered approach in building a history. Your own beliefs, attitudes, and values cannot be discarded, but you do have to discipline them. You have to be aware of your cultural beliefs, faith, and conscience so that they do not inappropriately intrude as you discuss with patients a variety of issues. That means *knowing yourself* (Curlin et al, 2007; Gold, 2010; see also Chapter 2).

You react differently to different people. Why? How? Do you want to be liked too much? Does thinking about how you are doing get in the way of your effort? Why does a patient make you angry? Is there some frustration in your life? Which of your prejudices may influence your response to a patient? Talk about such questions with others you trust rather than make this a lonely, introspective effort. You will better control possible barriers to a successful outcome.

Effective Communication

Establishing a positive patient relationship depends on *communication* built on *courtesy, comfort, connection,* and *confirmation* (Box 1-2).

Be courteous; ensure comfort, both physical and emotional; be sure that you have connected with the patient with trust and candor; and confirm that all that has happened during the interaction is clearly understood and your patient is able to articulate the agreed upon plan. That is communication.

Seeking Connection. Examine your habits and modify them when necessary so that you are not a barrier to effective communication. Stiff formality may inhibit the patient; a too-casual attitude may fail to instill confidence. Do not be careless with words—what you think is innocuous may seem vitally important to a patient searching for meaning in everything you say. Consider intellectual and emotional constraints related to how you ask questions and offer information, how fast you talk, and how often you punctuate speech with "uh huh" and "you know." The interaction requires the active encouragement of patient participation with questions and responses addressed to social and emotional issues as much as the physical nature of health problems.

At the start, greet the patient and those with the patient. Begin by asking open-ended questions ("How have you been feeling since we last met?" "What questions would you like to

---

Box 1-1 Patient-Centered Questions

The following questions represent a patient-centered approach in building a history:

- How would you like to be addressed?
- How are you feeling today?
- What would you like for us to do today?
- What do you think is causing your symptoms?
- What is your understanding of your diagnosis? Its importance? Its need for management?
- How do you feel about your illness? Frightened? Threatened? Angry? As a wage earner? As a family member? (Be sure, though, to allow a response without putting words in the patient's mouth.)
- Do you believe treatment will help?
- How are you coping with your illness? Crying? Drinking more? Tranquilizers? Talking more? Less? Changing lifestyles?
- Do you want to know all the details about your diagnosis and its effect on your future?
- How important to you is "doing everything possible"?
- How important to you is "quality of life"?
- Have you prepared advance directives?
- Do you have people you can talk with about your illness? Where do you get your strength?
- Is there anyone else we should contact about your illness or hospitalization? Family members? Friends? Employer? Religious advisor? Attorney?
- Do you want or expect emotional support from the health care team?
- Are you troubled by financial questions about your medical care? Insurance coverage? Tests or treatment you may not be able to afford? Timing of payments required from you?
- If you have had previous hospitalizations, does it bother you to be seen by teams of physicians, nurses, and students on rounds?
- How private a person are you?
- Are you concerned about the confidentiality of your medical records?
- Would you prefer to talk to an older/younger, male/female health care provider?
- Are there medical matters you do not wish to have disclosed to others?

We suggest that use of the questions should be determined by the particular situation. For example, talking about a living will might alarm a patient seeking a routine checkup but may relieve a patient hospitalized with a life-threatening disease. Cognitive impairment, anxiety, depression, fear, or related feelings as well as racial, gender, ethnic, or other differences should modify your approach.

---

discuss?" "What do you want to make sure we cover in today's visit?"). Later, as information accumulates, you will need to be more specific. However, early on, it is entirely appropriate to check the patient's agenda and concerns and let the information flow. It is important to not interrupt the patient at the start of the interview and to ask if there is "anything else" to be sure the patient's primary concerns are identified early in the visit. Thus, you and the patient can collaboratively set the current visit's agenda.

Having clear and agreed upon goals for each of our patient interactions often leads to successful communication. You must

Box 1-2 Communication

Courtesy, Comfort, Connection, Confirmation

Courtesy
- Knock before entering a room.
- Address, first, the patient formally (e.g., Miss, Ms., Mrs., Mr.) It is all right to shake hands.
- Meet and acknowledge others in the room and establish their roles and degree of participation.
- Learn their names.
- Ensure confidentiality.
- Be in the room, sitting, with no effort to reach too soon for the doorknob.
- Make notes sparingly; note key words as reminders but do not let note-taking distract from your observing and listening.
- Respect the need for modesty.
- Allow the patient time to be dressed and comfortably settled after the examination. Follow-up discussion with the patient still "on the table" is often discomfiting.

Comfort
- Ensure physical comfort for all; yours, too.
- Try to have a minimum of furniture separating you and the patient.
- Maintain privacy, using available curtains and shades.
- Ensure a comfortable room temperature or provide a blanket—a cold room will make a patient want to cover up.
- Ensure good lighting.
- Ensure necessary quiet. Turn off the television set.
- Try not to overtire the patient. It is not always necessary to do it all at one visit.

Connection
- Look at the patient; maintain good eye contact if cultural practices allow.
- Watch your language. Avoid professional jargon. Do not patronize with what you say.

- Do not dominate the discussion. Listen alertly. Let the patient order priorities if several issues are raised.
- Do not accept a previous diagnosis as a chief complaint. Do not too readily allow a predetermined path.
- Find out if the patient has turned from others to come to you.
- Take the history and conduct the physical examination before you look at previous studies or tests. Consider first what the patient has to say.
- Avoid leading or direct questions at first. Open-ended questions are better for starters. Let specifics evolve from these.
- Avoid being judgmental.
- Respect silence. Pauses can be productive.
- Be flexible. Rigidity limits the potential of an interview.
- Assess the patient's potential as a partner.
- Seek clues to problems from the patient's verbal behaviors and body language (e.g., talking too fast or too little).
- Look for the hidden concerns underlying chief concerns.
- Never trivialize any finding or clue.
- Problems can have multiple causes. Do not leap to one cause too quickly.
- Define any concern completely: Where? How severe? How long? In what context? What soothes or aggravates the problem?

Confirmation
- Ask the patient to summarize the discussion. There should be clear understanding and uncertainty should be eased.
- Allow the possibility of more discussion with another open-ended question: "Anything else you want to bring up?"
- If there is a question that you cannot immediately answer, say so. And be sure to follow up later if at all possible.
- If you seem to have made a mistake, make every effort to repair it. The candor is important for development of a trusting partnership. Most patients respect it.

---

be a skilled listener and observer with a polished sense of timing and a kind of repose that is at once alert and reassuring. Your nonverbal behavior complements your listening. Your face need not be a mask. You can be expressive and nod in agreement, but it is better to avoid the extremes of reaction (e.g., startle, surprise, or grimacing). Eye contact should be assured and comfortable, and your body language should show that you are really in the room, open to and engaged with the patient, comfortably seated, not standing and not reaching for the doorknob (see Clinical Pearl, "Professional Dress and Grooming").

Remember too that patients also communicate nonverbally, and understanding this is advantageous to both you and the patient (Henry et al, 2012).

Clinical Pearl

Professional Dress and Grooming
Appropriate dress and grooming go a long way toward establishing a first good impression with the patient. Although clean fingernails, modest clothing, and neat hair are imperative, you need not be stuffy to be neat. You can easily avoid extremes so that appearance does not become an obstacle in the patient's response to care.

Confidentiality, which is important in all aspects of care, is another essential element. The patient should provide the information. It is important to identify everyone in the room to be sure the patient is comfortable with and wants others to participate in the visit. You may want to ask the parent, spouse, or other person to step out of the room so you can have a confidential discussion with the patient. If language is a barrier, a professional interpreter—rather than a family member—should be utilized (Fig. 1-1).

Gentle guidance and polite re-direction are sometimes necessary to keep the visit focused and moving forward (e.g., "But now let's also talk about …" or "I'm sorry to interrupt, but let me make sure I understand …"). Be prepared with questions you think are important to address based on the patient's history and main concerns. If the patient touches on something that does not seem to be immediately relevant to your purposes (e.g., introducing a possible problem not previously mentioned), be flexible enough to clarify at least the nature of the concern. Some apparent irrelevancies may contain clues to the care-seeking behaviors or concerns that may be hidden beneath the primary concern. The patient's body language, as well as words, will suggest the intensity of an underlying feeling. Although too many

FIGURE 1-1 Interviewing a patient with the help of an interpreter. Someone other than a family member should act as interpreter to bridge the language difference between the health care provider and the patient.

digressions can lead to misspent time, paying attention may save a lot of time later, and information learned may be important to the future plan of care.

Enhancing Patient Responses.   Carefully phrased questions can lead to more accurate responses. Ask one question at a time, avoiding a barrage that discourages the patient from being more complete or that limits answers to a simple yes or no:

+ The *open-ended question* gives the patient discretion about the extent of an answer: "And then what happened?" "What are your feelings about this?" "Tell me more about ..." "What else do you need to talk about?"
+ The *direct question* seeks specific information: "How long ago did that happen?" "Where does it hurt?" "Please put a finger where it hurts." "How many pills did you take each time?" and "How many times a day did you take them?"
+ The *leading question* is the most risky because it may limit the information provided to what the patient thinks you want to know: "It seems to me that this bothered you a lot. Is that true?" "That wasn't very difficult to do, was it?" "That's a horrible-tasting medicine, isn't it?" Also, ask how often something happened, allowing the patient to define "often," rather than asking, "It didn't happen too often, did it?"

Sometimes the patient does not quite understand what you are asking and says so. Recognize the need when it is appropriate to:

+ *Facilitate:* Encourage your patient to say more, either with your words or with a silence that the patient may break when given the opportunity for reflection.
+ *Reflect:* Repeat what you have heard to encourage more detail.
+ *Clarify:* Ask "What do you mean?"
+ *Empathize:* Show your understanding and acceptance. Do not hesitate to say "I understand," or "I'm sorry" if the moment calls for it.
+ *Confront:* Do not hesitate to discuss a patient's disturbing behavior.
+ *Interpret:* Repeat what you have heard to confirm the patient's meaning.

What you ask is complemented by how you ask it. Take the following actions, if necessary, to clarify the patient's point of view:

+ Ask what the patient *thinks* and *feels* about an issue.
+ Make sure you know what the chief *concern* is.
+ Ask about the patient's life situation, so that nothing seemingly extraneous to the chief concern and present illness has gone unnoticed.
+ Suggest at appropriate times that you have the "feeling" that the patient could say more or that things may not be as well as they are reported.
+ Suggest at appropriate times that it is all right to be angry, sad, or nervous, and it is all right to talk about it.
+ Make sure that the patient's expectations in the visit are met and that there are no further questions.

Make sure your questions are clearly understood. Define words when necessary and choose them carefully. Avoid technical terms if possible. Adapt when necessary to the patient's education level language. Ask the patient to stop you if he or she does not understand what you are talking about. Similarly, do the same if you do not grasp the patient's meaning. For example, a patient may report that he had "low blood" (anemia), "high blood" (hypertension), "bad blood" (syphilis), and "thin blood" (he was taking anticoagulants)! It can take a bit of exploring to sort it all out. Do not assume every question needs a complex and technical answer. Learn when enough is enough. Remember, too, that a patient who is a professional colleague may not be familiar with the jargon of your particular discipline.

Moments of Tension: Potential Barriers to Communication

Curiosity About You.   Patients will sometimes ask about you. Although you are not the point, you may be comfortable revealing some relevant aspects of your experience ("I have trouble remembering to take medicines, too.") A direct answer will usually do. Often, simply informing your patients that you have experienced similar life events (e.g., illness, pregnancy, and childbirth) can help alleviate fears and—with further exploration—can help in the identification of the patient's concerns. The message that you are a "real" person can lead to a trust-enhancing or even therapeutic exchange. At the same time, it would be wise to exercise caution and remain professional in what and how much you disclose (Lussier and Richard, 2007).

Anxiety.   Anxiety has multiple sources, such as an impending procedure or anticipated diagnosis. Some disorders will be more likely to cause an intense response, such as those associated with crushing chest pain or difficulty in breathing; with other disorders, just seeing a health care professional can cause anxiety. You can help by avoiding an overload of information, pacing the conversation, and presenting a calm demeanor.

Silence.   Sometimes intimidated by silence, many health care providers feel the urge to break it. Be patient. Do not force the conversation. You may have to move the moment along with an open-ended question ("What seems to worry you?") or a mild nudge ("And after that?"). Remember, though, that silence allows the patient a moment of reflection or time to summon courage.

Some issues can be so painful and sensitive that silence becomes necessary and should be allowed. Most people will talk when they are ready. The patient's demeanor, use of hands, possible teary eyes, and facial expressions will help you interpret the moment. Silence may also be cultural: for example, some cultural groups take their time, ponder their responses to questions, and answer when they feel ready. Do not push too hard. Be comfortable with silence but give it reasonable bounds.

Depression. Being sick or thinking that you are sick can be enough to provoke situational depression. Indeed, serious or chronic, unrelenting illness or taking certain prescription drugs (e.g., steroids) is often accompanied by depression. A sense of sluggishness in the daily experience, disturbances in sleeping, eating, and social contact, and feelings of loss of self-worth can be clues. Pay attention. First ask, "When did you start feeling this way?" Then ask, "How do you feel about it?" "Have you stopped enjoying the things you like to do?" "Do you have trouble sleeping?" "Have you had thoughts about hurting yourself?" "Are you depressed?" A patient in this circumstance cannot be hurried and certainly cannot be relieved by superficial assurance. You need not worry about introducing the idea of suicide (see Clinical Pearl, "Adolescent Suicide"). It has most often been considered, if only briefly (see Chapter 5, Risk Factors box, "Suicide").

> **Clinical Pearl**
>
> **Adolescent Suicide**
> Suicide is a major cause of mortality in the preteen and teen years, more often in boys. If the thought of it occurs to you, you can be pretty sure that it has to the patient, too. You can mention it and thus give permission to talk about it. You will not be suggesting anything new. You may actually help prevent it.

Crying and Compassionate Moments. People will cry. Let the emotion proceed at the patient's pace. Resume your questioning only when the patient is ready. If you suspect a patient is holding back, give permission. Offer a tissue or simply say, "It seems like you're feeling bad. It's OK to cry." Name the emotion. Be direct about such a tender circumstance, but gently, not too aggressively or insistently. Do not hesitate to say that you feel for the patient, that you are sorry for something that happened, and that you know it was painful. At times, the touch of a hand or even a hug is in order. Sometimes, a concern—a difficult family relationship, for example—must be confronted. You may have to check an assumption and hope that you have guessed right in bringing the patient's feelings to the surface. If uncertain, ask without presupposing what the response might be.

Physical and Emotional Intimacy. It is not easy to be intimate with the emotions and the bodies of others. Cultural norms and behaviors are at once protective of and barriers to trusting relationships. The patient is in a dependent status as well. You can acknowledge this while explaining clearly and without apology what you must do for the patient's benefit. Of course, respect modesty, using covers appropriately without hampering a complete examination. Be careful about the ways in which you use words or frame questions. You cannot be sure of the degree to which a given patient has been "desensitized" to the issues of intimacy. However, respect for modesty carried too far, such as skipping examination of the genitals, can be a trap delaying or barring access to much needed information. You can keep the necessary from becoming too big an issue by being calm and asking questions with professional poise.

Seduction. Some patients can be excessively flattering and manipulative and even seductive. Their illness and insecurity beg for extra-special attention. Do not be taken in by this. There are limits to warmth and cordiality. Certainly not all touch is sexually motivated; a heartfelt hug is sometimes just right. Nevertheless, beware of that trap. Avert it courteously and firmly, delivering the immediate message that the relationship is and will remain professional. It takes skill to do this while maintaining the patient's dignity but there is no room for sexual misconduct in the relationship, and there can be no tolerance for exploitation of the patient in this regard.

Anger. Sometimes the angriest patients (or persons with them) are the ones who may need you the most. Of course, it can be intimidating. Confront it. It is all right to say, "It seems like you're angry. Please tell me why. I want to hear." Speak softly and try not to argue the point. You may not know if or why you made someone angry. Most often, you have done nothing wrong. Still, the stress of time, heavy workload, and the tension of caring for the acutely—even terminally—ill can generate your own impatience and potential for anger. Avoid being defensive, but acknowledge the problem. Only when appropriate, apologize and ask how to make things better. Explore the feelings. Often, you can continue on a better footing after anger is vented. On occasion, nothing will seem to help. It is then all right to defer to another time or even to suggest a different professional (Thomas, 2003).

Afterward, do not hesitate to talk about the episode with a trusted colleague. It helps. Discussing the incident later may lend insight into behaviors and help prevent the occurrence again. Better ways of responding can be explored.

Avoiding the Full Story. Patients may not always tell the whole story or even the truth, either purposely or unconsciously. Dementia, illness, alcoholism, sexual uncertainties, domestic violence, and child abuse are among the reasons. Do not push too hard when you think this is happening. Allow the interview to go on and then come back to a topic with gentle questioning. You might say, "I think that you may be more concerned than you are saying" or "I think you're worried about what we might find out." Unless there is concern about the safety of the patient or another individual learning all that is necessary may not come in one sitting. You may have to pursue the topic at a later visit or perhaps with other members of the family or friends or your professional associates.

Financial Considerations. The cost of care and the resulting drain on resources (and the potential impact on employment) are often sources of stress for the patient. Talk about them with candor and accurate knowledge. Otherwise, an appropriate care plan acceptable to the patient cannot be devised or implemented. Pressing circumstances and obligations may still present barriers to appropriate care.

FIGURE 1-2 Interviewing a young adult. Note the absence of an intervening desk or table.

The Patient History

A first objective in building the history is to identify those matters the patient defines as problems, the subtle as well as the obvious. You need to establish a sense of the patient's reliability as an interpreter of events. Consider the potential for intentional or unintentional suppression or underreporting of certain experiences that may give context to a problem that is at odds with your expectation. Constantly evaluate the patient's words and behavior. The history is built on the patient's perspective, not yours. *Make modifications as required for the patient's age, pregnancy, and physical and emotional disabilities.*

Setting for the Interview

Regardless of the setting, make everyone as comfortable as possible. Position yourself so that there are no bulky desks, tables, or electronic equipment between you and the patient. (Fig. 1-2). If possible, have a clock placed where you can see it without obviously looking at your watch (preferably behind the patient's chair). Sit comfortably and at ease, maintaining eye contact and a conversational tone of voice. Your manner can assure the patient that you care and that relieving worry or pain is one of your prime concerns. You can do this only by concentrating on the matter at hand, giving it for that moment primacy in your life, and putting aside both personal and professional distractions.

Structure of the History

You build the history to establish a relationship with the patient, so that you jointly discover the issues and problems that need attention and priority. A widely accepted approach is provided that can and should be modified to fit the individual circumstance:

+ First, the identifiers: name, date, time, age, gender, race, occupation, and referral source
+ Chief concern (CC)
+ History of present illness or problem (HPI)
+ Past medical history (PMH)

+ Family history (FH)
+ Personal and social history (SH)
+ Review of systems (ROS)

The *chief concern* is a brief statement about why the patient is seeking care. Direct quotes are helpful. It is important, however, to go beyond the given reason and to probe for underlying concerns that cause the patient to seek care rather than just getting up and going to work. If the patient has a sore throat, why is help sought? Is it the pain and fever, or is it the concern caused by past experience with a relative who developed rheumatic heart disease? Many interviewers include the *duration of the problem* as part of the chief concern.

Understanding the *present illness* or *problem* requires a step-by-step evaluation of the circumstances that surround the primary reason for the patient's visit. The full history goes beyond this to an exploration of the patient's *overall health before the chief concern*, including past medical and surgical experiences. The spiritual, psychosocial, and cultural contexts of the patient's life are essential to an understanding of these events. The patient's *family* also requires attention—their health, past medical history, illnesses, deaths, and the genetic, social, and environmental influences. One question should underlie all of your inquiry: *Why is this happening to this particular patient at this particular time?* In other words, if many people are exposed to a potential problem and only some of them become ill after the exposure, what are the unique factors in this individual that led to that outcome? Careful inquiry about the *personal and social experience of the patient* should include work habits and the variety of relationships in the family, school, and workplace. Finally, the ROS includes a detailed inquiry of possible concerns in each of the body's systems, looking for complementary or seemingly unrelated symptoms that may not have surfaced during the rest of the history. Flexibility, the appreciation of subtlety, and the opportunity for the patient to ask questions and to explore feelings are explicit needs in the process.

Building the History

Introduce yourself to the patient and accompanying persons if you have not already met, clearly stating your name and your role. If you are a student, say so. Be certain that you know the patient's full name and that you pronounce it correctly. Ask if you are not certain.

Address the patient properly (e.g., as Mr., Miss, Mrs., Ms., or the manner of address preferred by the patient) and repeat the patient's name at appropriate times. Avoid the familiarity of using a first name when you do not expect familiarity in return. Do not use a surrogate term for a person's name; for example, when the patient is a child, do not address the parent as "Mother" or "Father." It is respectful and courteous to take the time to learn each name.

It is respectful, too, to look at the patient and not at the electronic device that is usually close at hand. Use it if you must, but position it so that it does not distract from the patient. More and more the electronic device in the examination room is being introduced into the patient-physician dynamic for educational purposes (e.g., demonstrating the findings on an imaging study, showing the trend of a laboratory result over time, or reviewing a website together). Unless you already know the patient and know that there is urgency, proceed at a reasonable pace, asking for the reason for the visit with the intent of learning what their specific expectations of the visit are. *Listen, but do not be too directive* at this point. You will often be surprised at how much of the story and details you will hear without pushing. *Let the patient spill it all out* and, after the first flow of words, probe for the reason for seeking health care. If 100 people wake up with a bad headache, and 97 go to work while 3 seek care, what underlying dimension prompted those decisions?

You have by then begun *to give structure to the present illness or problem*, giving it a chronologic and sequential framework. Unless there is urgency, go slowly, hear the full story, and refrain from striking out too quickly on what seems the obvious course of questioning. The patient will take cues from you on the leisure you will allow. You must walk a fine line between permitting this leisure and meeting the many time constraints you are sure to have. Fix your attention on the patient, avoid interrupting as much as possible, and do not ask the next question before you have heard the complete answer to the prior one.

The patient's responses may at times be unclear. Seek certainty:
+ "Of what you've told me, what concerns you the most?"
+ "What do you want to make sure we pay attention to today?"
+ "Do you have any ideas about what we ought to do?"
+ Or, a leading question sometimes, "I think _____ worries you the most. Am I right? Shall we talk about that first?"

As the interview proceeds, thoroughly explore each positive response with the following questions:
+ *Where?* Where are symptoms located, as precisely as possible? If they seem to move, what is the range of their movement? Where is the patient when the complaint occurs—at work or play, active or resting?
+ *When?* Everything happens in a chronologic sequence. When did it begin? Does it come and go? If so, how often and for how long? What time of day? What day of the week?
+ *What?* What does it mean to the patient? What is its impact? What does it feel like? What is its quality and intensity? Has it been bad enough to interrupt the flow of the patient's life, or has it been dealt with rather casually? What else happened during this time that might be related? What makes it feel better? Worse?
+ *How?* The background of the symptom becomes important in answering the "how" question. How did it come about? Are other things going on at the same time, such as work, play, mealtime, or sleep? Is there illness in the family? Have there been similar episodes in the past? If so, how was it treated or did it resolve without treatment? Is there concern about similar symptoms in friends or relatives? Are there companion complaints? How is the patient coping? Are there social supports? Nothing ever happens in isolation.
+ *Why?* Of course, the answer to "why" is the solution to the problem. All other questions lead to this one.

Once you have understood the patient's chief concern and present problem and have a sense of underlying issues, you may

go on to other segments of the history: the *family and past medical histories, emotional, spiritual, and cultural concerns,* and *social and workplace accompaniments to the present concerns.* Remember that nothing in the patient's experience is isolated. Aspects of the present illness or problem require careful integration with the medical and family history. The life of the patient is not constructed according to your outline, with many factors giving shape to the present illness and with any one chief concern possibly involving more than one illness.

A visit should conclude with a review:
+ Ask the patient to try to satisfy gaps in your understanding.
+ Ask for questions.
+ Interpret and summarize what you have heard.
+ Ask the patient to summarize for you to ensure complete understanding.
+ Repeat instructions and ask to hear them back.
+ Explain the next steps: needed examinations and/or studies, appointment times, keeping in touch.

Sensitive Issues

Sensitive issues, which may be difficult to discuss (e.g., sex, drug or alcohol use, or concerns about death), are important to address. The following guidelines, keys to any successful interview, are essential in an approach to sensitive issues.
+ Provide privacy.
+ Do not waffle. Be direct and firm. Avoid asking leading questions.
+ Do not apologize for asking a question.
+ Do not preach. Avoid confrontation. You are not there to pass judgment.
+ Use language that is understandable to the patient, yet not patronizing (see Clinical Pearl, "Watch the Use of Jargon").
+ Do not push too hard.
+ Afterward, document carefully, using the patient's words (and those of others with the patient) whenever possible. It is all right to take notes, but try to do this sparingly, especially when discussing sensitive issues.

Clinical Pearl

Watch the Use of Jargon
Unfortunately, many of us may too often lapse into the use of jargon, the language of our particular professions that is not accessible to the patient. Patient-demeaning words are worse. Stress, frustration, fatigue, and anger are common underlying causes for these lapses. Know yourself. Understand why you might fall into the habit, and do your best to avoid it.

You must always be ready to explain again why you examine sensitive areas. A successful approach will have incorporated four steps:
1. An introduction, the moment when you bring up the issue, alluding to the need to understand its context in the patient's life.
2. Open-ended questions that first explore the patient's feelings about the issue—whether, for example, it is alcohol, drugs,

THE HISTORY AND INTERVIEWING

sex, cigarettes, education, or problems at home—and then the direct exploration of what is actually happening.

3. A period in which you thoughtfully attend to what the patient is saying and then repeat the patient's words or offer other forms of feedback. This permits the patient to agree that your interpretation is appropriate, thus confirming what you have heard.

4. And finally, an opportunity for the patient to ask any questions that might be relevant.

Alcohol. The CAGE questionnaire is one model for discussing the use of alcohol (Box 1-3). CAGE is an acronym for **C**utting down, **A**nnoyance by criticism, **G**uilty feeling, **E**ye-openers. Its use does not ensure absolute sensitivity in the detection of a problem. It can be complemented or supplemented by the TACE model (Box 1-4), particularly in the identification of alcoholism in a pregnant woman (because of the potential for damage to the infant), or by CRAFFT, for identification of an alcohol problem in adolescents (Box 1-5). There is similarity in all of these questionnaires. You can adapt them to your style and to the particular patient. You can also adapt them to concerns about drugs or substances other than alcohol (see Clinical Pearl, "Screening").

Box 1-3   CAGE Questionnaire

The CAGE questionnaire was developed in 1984 by Dr. John Ewing, and it includes four interview questions designed to help diagnose alcoholism.

The CAGE acronym helps practitioners quickly recall the main concepts of the four questions (Cutting down, Annoyance by criticism, Guilty feeling, Eye-openers).

Probing questions may be asked as follow-up questions to the CAGE questionnaire.

Many online resources list the complete questionnaire (e.g., http://addictionsandrecovery.org/addiction-self-test.htm). The exact wording of the CAGE Questionnaire can be found in: Ewing JA: Screening for Alcoholism using CAGE: cut down, annoyed, guilty, eye opener, JAMA 280(2): 1904-1905, 1984.

Clinical Pearl

Screening
There is a difference between a screening and an assessment interview. The goal of screening is to find out if a problem exists. This is particularly true of CAGE, CRAFFT, and TACE screening tools. They are effective, but they are only the start, and assessment goes on from there. Discovering a problem early may lead to a better treatment outcome.

Box 1-4   TACE Questionnaire

The following questions are included in the TACE model:
T How many drinks does it *T*ake to make you feel high? How many when you first started drinking? When was that? What do you prefer: beer, wine, or liquor? (More than two drinks suggests a tolerance to alcohol that is a red flag.)
A Have people *A*nnoyed you by criticizing your drinking?
C Have you felt you ought to *C*ut down on your drinking?
E Have you ever had an *E*ye-opener drink first thing in the morning to steady your nerves or get rid of a hangover?
   An answer to T alone (more than two drinks) or a positive response to two of A, C, or E may signal a problem with a high degree of probability. Positive answers to all four signal a problem with great certainty.

From Sokol et al, 1989.

Box 1-5   CRAFFT Questionnaire

The CRAFFT questionnaire was developed in 2002 as a screening tool for alcohol and substance abuse in adolescents.

The CRAFFT acronym helps practitioners remember the main concepts of the six questions: Car, Relax, Alone, Forget, Friends, Trouble.

The exact wording of the CRAFFT questions can be found here: Knight JR et al., Validity of the CRAFFT Substance Abuse Screening Test Among Adolescent Clinic Patients. Arch Pediatr Adolesc Med 156:607-614, 2002 (available online at http://archpedi.jamanetwork.com/article.aspx?articleid=203511).

Intimate Partner Violence. We too often underestimate the incidence of intimate partner violence (IPV) in the experience of our patients of any age or gender. IPV includes a range of abusive behaviors perpetrated by someone who is or was involved in an intimate relationship with the victim. It affects primarily women, children, and dependent older adults as victims and, in lesser frequency, men. Intimate partners are usually the perpetrators. Same-sex partners probably have the same prevalence, although underreporting may be more of a problem in this population. Alcohol is a common facilitator. Children exposed to IPV are at increased risk for social and emotional problems. There is significant overlap between IPV and child abuse so when IPV is detected, child abuse should be considered.

Reluctance to screen for fear of offending patients and families is a misplaced concern. This is occasionally compounded by an inappropriate response to an abused woman, such as making too little of her experience or even laying the blame on her. She is, then, twice a victim. The "she" is used advisably. Although IPV affects both men and women as victims and perpetrators, more women experience IPV and most studies about screening and interventions for intimate violence enroll women. (Nelson et al, 2012). Only a relatively few will discuss IPV willingly with a health care provider and, in that event, the patient is almost always the initiator of the discussion. If a health care provider makes the initial inquiry, it is usually asked in an emergency department of a person who may have difficulty getting out of an abusive relationship, a minority woman, or one who is obviously vulnerable. All female patients should be routinely screened (U.S. Preventive Services Task Force, 2012). A validated brief Partner Violence Screen (PVS) uses three questions to detect partner violence (Feldhaus, 1997):

+ Have you been hit, kicked, punched, or otherwise hurt by someone within the past year?
+ Do you feel safe in your current relationship?
+ Is there a partner from a previous relationship who is making you feel unsafe now?

These cover two dimensions of partner violence, and a positive response to any one of them constitutes a positive screen. The first question addresses physical violence. The latter two questions evaluate the woman's perception of safety and estimate her short-term risk of further violence and need for counseling.

Additionally, you may see something suggestive on physical examination and ask the following: "The bruises I see. How did you get them?"

Positive answers require accurate documentation, using words, drawings, and, if possible, photographs and the preservation of any tangible evidence. Positive answers require that the patient's safety be ensured. Ask the following:

+ Are you afraid to go home?
+ Are there guns or knives at home?
+ Is alcohol (or other drugs) part of the problem?
+ Has it gotten worse lately?
+ Are children involved?

A "yes" answer mandates an intervention that requires utilization of other health care professionals such as social workers and mental health providers who may be able to provide more in-depth assessment and linkage to resources. Get the patient's viewpoint. Let her speak; assure her that she is not alone and that you will do your best to help her.

A "no" answer may still leave you uncomfortable. Get permission from the patient to document your concern and your suspicion of injury. Be unafraid to ask direct questions about your suspicion ("Where did that bruise come from?"). Ask her to come back to see you again.

The same approach works for men but it is not necessarily used routinely. His statements or a suspicious injury may trigger your action. Infants and children have the protection of the legal mandate for you to report your suspicions. Questioning a child about abuse suffered or witnessed at home can be problematic because you want to avoid suggestion. In general, open-ended questions are comfortably asked of the young or of a parent in their presence (Zink et al, 2006):

+ Why did you come to see me today? (Do not mention the concern directly.)
+ Tell me everything that happened to you, please. (No leading questions.)

With infants, a bruise or burn with an odd shape or unexpected location usually suggests a problem. It is difficult for an infant who is not yet crawling or toddling to break a femur, for example.

Evidence-Based Practice in Physical Examination

Screening for Abuse and Intimate Partner Violence

Data from a systematic review indicates that screening practices by health care professionals are inconsistent for several reasons, including the existence of a variety of screening instruments, a lack of consensus on which instrument to use, lack of specificity of risk factors, lack of training, lack of effectiveness studies about what to do if violence is identified, discomfort with screening, and time constraints. Several instruments have been developed for intimate partner violence screening, and their diagnostic accuracy has been evaluated in studies of different populations using various reference standards. Six instruments with 1 to 8 items demonstrated sensitivity and specificity >80% in clinical populations of asymptomatic women; results varied between studies and across instruments. The Feldhaus PVS 3-item screening instrument had a higher sensitivity and specificity when compared to two longer instruments. The HITS 4-item screening instrument for abuse (Box 1-6) demonstrated 86% sensitivity and 99% specificity (English version) and 100% percent sensitivity and 86% specificity (Spanish version).

Studies to develop and evaluate tools are generally lacking to assess screening older and vulnerable adults for abuse. Existing instruments to detect child abuse are not designed for direct administration to the child, missing opportunities to screen older children in the context of usual health care.

Data from Nelson et al, 2004; 2012.

Box 1-6 Brief Screening Tool for Domestic Violence: HITS

Verbal abuse is as intense a problem as physical violence. **HITS** stands for *H*urt, *I*nsult, *T*hreaten, or *S*cream. The wording of the question is, "In the last year, how often did your partner:
*H*urt you physically?"
*I*nsult or talk down to you?"
*T*hreaten you with physical harm?"
*S*cream or curse at you?"

From Sherin et al, 1998.

Adolescents may endure violence, particularly sexual, at home or away. The clue may be changes in behavior, such as dress and makeup, school effort, sleeping, and eating. Alcohol or drug use can become an issue. Former friends may be avoided. Most important, take your time and ask the following questions:

+ Have you ever had sex?
+ When did you start?
+ Did you want to, or were you forced or talked into it?
+ Do the people you are with ever scare you?
+ Did anyone ever touch you in your private places?

Always be available for more conversation. The questions are just a start. Note, too, that the young may also witness as well as endure violence at home, with a profound effect on their lives and behavior. These problems should be dealt with as if the patient were the direct victim.

The risk of abuse of older adults, often underreported, is greater if the older adult has had a history of mental illness, is physically or cognitively impaired, or is living in a dependent situation with inadequate financial resources. The abusers may have similar risks, perhaps alcohol or drug related. Both groups may well have a past history of domestic violence. In any event, confront the issue with an approach modeled on that for women in difficulty.

Spirituality. The basic condition that life imposes is death. It stirs in us a spiritual or "sacred" feeling—always with us, often sublimated, sometimes not. Illness, however mild, may stir that feeling and may carry with it a sense of dread. Faith may be an intimate contributor to one's perspective. An understanding of "spirituality" is, then, integral to the care we offer but it is complicated by the fact that there is no universally agreed upon definition and each of us brings our own to the care provided.

Many patients want attention paid to spirituality, and faith can be a key factor in the success of a management plan. Others may prefer that you not broach the subject. This requires the same degree of sensitivity and caution as talking about drugs, cigarettes, sex, and alcohol. The questions suggested by Puchalski and Romer (2000) with the acronym FICA and adapted by us suggest an approach:

+ Faith, Belief, Meaning
  + What is your spiritual or religious heritage? Is the Bible, the Quran, or similar writings important to you?
  + Do these beliefs help you cope with stress?
+ Importance and Influence
  + How have these beliefs influenced how you handle stress? To what extent?
+ Community
  + Do you belong to a formal spiritual or religious community? Does this community support you? In what way? Is there anyone there with whom you would like to talk?
+ Address/Action in Care
  + How do your religious beliefs affect your health care decisions (e.g., choice of birth control)? How would you like me to support you in this regard when your health is involved?

Answers to these questions may guide you to involve the clergy or other spiritual care providers or to become more deeply involved. There is some evidence that prayer can aid in healing. You may, if you are asked and if you are inclined, pray with a patient, although it is best that you not lead the prayer. You may even suggest it if the patient is sorely troubled and you understand the need. There are, however, boundaries. Except for very few of us, we are not theologians, and it is inappropriate to go beyond the limits of our professional expertise.

Auster (2004) suggests sensitivity on our part when patients ask about our personal beliefs and express their wish to talk of this only with someone of their own faith. You might say, "I want to help you as best I can, so please tell me why you ask about my faith" or, more directly, "I understand your feeling. Would it help if I found another person for you?" Let your sense of the situation guide you (Fosarelli, 2003; Puchalski and Romer, 2000).

Sexuality. Questions about the patient's sexual history may first be indirect, addressing feelings rather than facts. "Are you satisfied with your sexual life, or do you have worries or

concerns? Many people do." Although this is a leading question, it does not suggest what the patient's feelings should be. Rather, if there are concerns about sex, it may be comforting to know that one is not alone. The age of the patient should not deter discussion. Do not assume more or less for a given age, particularly older adults.

Patients should be told that discussion is routine and confidential. You might say: "I am going to ask you some questions about your sexual health and sexuality that I ask all my patients. The answers to these questions are important for me to know to help keep you healthy. Like the rest of this visit, this information is confidential." (Makadon, 2011).

The sexual orientation of a patient must be known if appropriate continuity of care is to be offered. About 10% of the persons you serve are likely to be other than heterosexual (i.e., gay men, lesbian women, bisexual men and women, or transgendered persons) (Makadon, 2011). Working with these persons demands knowing yourself regarding any potential feelings about heterosexism and homophobia that you may have. The apprehension these patients may feel in revealing their preferences should be respected. Reassuring, nonjudgmental words help: "I'm glad you trust me. Thank you for telling me." It is also supportive if the health care setting offers some recognition of the patients involved (e.g., by making relevant informational pamphlets available in waiting areas).

Trust can be better achieved if questions are "gender neutral":
+ Tell me about your living situation.
+ Are you sexually active?
+ In what way?
  Rather than:
+ Are you married?
+ Do you have a boyfriend/girlfriend?

If you use a nonjudgmental approach a variety of questions applicable to any patient and any sexual circumstance becomes possible. The patient's vernacular may be necessary. Once the barrier is broken, you can be more direct, asking, for example, about frequency of sexual intercourse, problems in achieving orgasm, variety and numbers of "partners" (a non–gender-linked term), masturbation, and particular likes and dislikes. Identifying risk factors for unintentional pregnancy and sexually transmitted infections (STIs) are an important part of the sexual history.

Outline of the History

The outline offered is a guide derived over time from multiple sources, formal and informal. It is not rigid and you can decide what meets the needs of your patient and your style. Take advantage, too, of old family photographs, digital cameras, video, baby books, and more recent visualizing techniques to complement, not replace, what you learn in the history.

Chief Concern or the Reason for Seeking Care. This answers the question, "Why are you here?" (see Clinical Pearl, "Chief Concern"). Follow-up questions ask about duration (e.g., "How long has this been going on?" or "When did these symptoms begin?"). The patient's age, gender, marital status, previous hospital admissions, and occupation should be noted for the record. Other concerns may surface. A seemingly secondary issue

Clinical Pearl

Chief Complaint or Chief Concern?
Many of us do not view patients as "complainers" and prefer to express the "chief complaint" differently, adopting "chief concern," "presenting problem," or "reason for seeking care" as a more appropriate term. Feel free to use the words that suit you best or are most appropriate in your health care setting.

Box 1-8 Factors That Affect the Patient's Expression of Illness

Disease is real. Illness is the unique way in which a disease is expressed by the afflicted individual. An infinite number of variables come into play and may even cause illness without disease:
- Recent termination of a significant relationship because of death, divorce, or other stressors such as moving to a new city
- Physical or emotional illness or disability in family members or other significant individuals
- Inharmonious spousal or family relationships
- School problems and stresses
- Poor self-image
- Drug and alcohol misuse
- Poor understanding of the facts of a physical problem
- Influence from social media
- Peer pressure (among adults as well as adolescents and children)
- Secondary gains from the complaints of symptoms (e.g., indulgent family response to complaints, providing extra comforts or gifts, solicitous attention from others, distraction from other intimidating problems)

At any age, such circumstances can contribute to the intensity and persistence of symptoms or, quite the opposite, the denial of an insistent, objective complaint. The patient may then be led to seek help or, at other times, to avoid it.

may have greater significance than the original concern because the driving force for the chief concern may be found in it. What really made the patient seek care? Was it a possibly unexpressed fear or concern? Each hint of a care-seeking reason should be thoroughly explored (Box 1-7).

Box 1-7 The Basis of Understanding

The following are vital questions that probe the *unique* experience of each patient:
- Why is this happening in the life of this particular person at this time?
- How is this patient different from all other patients?
- Can I assume that what is generally true for others is necessarily true for this patient?
- How does this bear on my ultimate interpretation of possible problems and solutions?

History of Present Illness or Problem. You will often find that it is easiest to question the patient on the details of the current problem immediately after hearing the chief concern. Sometimes, it may be of value to take the patient's past and family history before returning to the present. The specific order is not critical. You want the patient's version without the use of leading questions. Box 1-8 suggests many of the variables that can influence the patient's version.

A complete HPI will include the following:
+ *Chronologic ordering of events*
+ *State of health just before the onset of the present problem*
+ *Complete description of the first symptoms.* The question "When did you last feel well?" may help define the time of onset and provide a date on which it might have been necessary to stop work or school, miss a planned event, or be confined to bed.
+ *Symptom analysis:* Questions in the following categories assist the patient in specifying characteristics of the presenting symptom(s): location, duration, intensity, description/character, aggravating factors, alleviating factors.
+ *Description of a typical attack, including its persistence.* If the present problem involves intermittent attacks separated by an illness-free interval, ask the patient to describe a typical attack (e.g., onset, duration, variation in intensity and associated symptoms, such as pain, chills, fever, jaundice, hematuria, or seizures) and any variations. Then ask the patient to define inciting, exacerbating, or relieving factors such as specific activities, positions, diet, or medications.
+ *Possible exposure to infection, toxic agents or other environmental hazards*

+ *Impact of the illness on the patient's usual lifestyle* (e.g., sexual experience, leisure activity, ability to perform tasks or cope with stress), an assessment of the ability to function in the expected way with an indication of the limitations imposed by illness
+ *Immediate reason that prompted the patient to seek care,* particularly if the problem has been long-standing
+ *Appropriate relevant system review*
+ *Medications:* current and recent, including dosage of prescription and home remedies and nonprescription medications
+ *Use of complementary or alternative therapies and medications*
+ A review, at the end of the interview, of the *chronology of events,* seeking the patient's confirmations and corrections. (If there appears to be more than one problem, the process should be repeated for each problem.)

Past Medical History. The past medical history is the baseline for assessing the present concern.
+ *General health and strength*
+ *Childhood illnesses:* measles, mumps, whooping cough, chickenpox, scarlet fever, acute rheumatic fever, diphtheria, poliomyelitis, asthma
+ *Major adult illnesses or chronic diseases:* tuberculosis, hepatitis, diabetes, hypertension, myocardial infarction, heart disease, stroke, respiratory disease, tropical or parasitic diseases, other infections; any nonsurgical hospital admissions
+ *Immunizations:* polio; diphtheria, pertussis, and tetanus toxoid; influenza; hepatitis A; hepatitis B; rotavirus, measles, mumps, rubella; varicella; herpes zoster vaccine; pneumococcus; meningococcus; human papillomavirus; bacille Calmette-Guérin (BCG); last tuberculosis or other skin tests; unusual

reactions of any sort to immunizations or antisera (travel-related immunizations [e.g., typhoid, cholera, yellow fever] should be considered in the special circumstance of the destinations)

- *Surgery:* dates, hospital, diagnosis, complications
- *Serious injuries and resulting disability;* obtain complete details if present problem has potential medicolegal relation to an injury
- *Limitation of ability to function as a result of past events*
- *Medications:* past, current, and recent medications, including dosage of prescription and home remedies and nonprescription medications (when not mentioned in present problem)
- *Allergies and the nature of reactions,* especially to medications, but also to environmental allergens and foods
- *Transfusions:* reactions and the nature of reactions, date, and number of units transfused
- *Recent screening tests* (e.g., cholesterol, Pap smear, colonoscopy, mammogram)
- *Emotional status:* mood disorders, psychiatric attention

Evidence-Based Practice in Physical Examination

History Taking

There is evidence that the risk for type 2 diabetes or cardiovascular disease is detectable in childhood and that the diseases share risk factors, including obesity and dyslipidemia. Other studies suggest that these risks can be reduced in childhood. The pathway to detecting risk is the family history. Adults with one or more second-degree relatives with diabetes or cardiovascular disease are at high risk. So, too, are the young with similar histories. The family history provides insight into the genomic influence on health and disease and offers the clue that can lead to prevention strategies.

From Yang et al, 2010.

Family History

- Blood relatives in the immediate or extended family with illnesses with features similar to the patient's are an immediate concern. If a disease "runs in the family," such as sickle cell disease, ask about everyone from grandparents to cousins. A pedigree diagram helps illustrate the family members with the disorder (see Chapter 26). A thorough and well-done family history is the essence of genomic medicine (Pyeritz, 2012). Determine the health and, if applicable, the cause of death of first-degree relatives (parents, children, and siblings), including age at death; after that, second-degree relatives (grandparents, grandchildren, aunts, nieces, uncles, and nephews); and then third-degree relatives (first cousins). There should be at least three generations for the pedigree.
- Include in your list of concerns: heart disease, high blood pressure, cancer (including the type), tuberculosis, stroke, sickle cell disease, cystic fibrosis, epilepsy, diabetes, gout, kidney disease, thyroid disease, asthma or other allergic condition, forms of arthritis, blood diseases, STIs, familial hearing, and visual or other sensory problems.
- In particular, determine if cancers have been multiple, bilateral, and occurring more than once in the family and at a young age (younger than age 50).

- Note the age and outcome of any illness.
- Note the ethnic and racial background of the family.
- Note the age and health of the patient's spouse/partner or the child's parents.

Personal and Social History

- *Personal status:* birthplace, where raised, home environment when young (e.g., parental divorce or separation, socioeconomic class, cultural and ethnic background), education, position in family, marital status, general life satisfaction, hobbies and interests, sources of stress or strain (see Clinical Pearl, "Who Are You?")

Clinical Pearl

Who Are You?

We cannot assume how patients define themselves ethnically or culturally without asking them. "Hispanic," "non-Hispanic," "black," "white," "Latino," and "Asian," among many other designations, are subject to a variety of interpretations. The individual patient is the final judge. Just ask, "How do you see yourself?" "How do you define yourself?" "What do you tell others you are?" What do I need to know to provide care for you as I respect your values and beliefs?" And remember not to stereotype just because a patient is a member of a culture. Each person is his or her own unique culture.

- *Habits:* nutrition and diet; regularity and patterns of eating and sleeping; quantity of coffee, tea, tobacco, alcohol; use of street drugs (e.g., frequency, type, and amount); ability to perform activities of daily living (see Functional Assessment for All Patients, p. 19). The extent of cigarette use can be reported in "pack-years," that is, the number of packs a day multiplied by the number of years (e.g., 1.5 packs per day × 10 years = 15 pack-years; see Evidence-Based Practice in Physical Examination, "Smoking Cessation").
- *Self-care:* breast and/or testicular self-examination; use of home, herbal, natural, complementary or alternative therapies/exercise (quantity and type)
- *Sexual history:* concerns with sexual feelings and performance, frequency of intercourse, ability to achieve orgasm, number and variety of partners, specific sexual practices, modes of birth control, protection against STIs and past STIs. "Partner" is a gender-free term, appropriate in the early stages of discussion (see Clinical Pearl, "The Five Ps of a Sexual History")

Clinical Pearl

The Five Ps of a Sexual History.
The five Ps stand for:
- Partners
- Practices
- Protection from STIs
- Past history of STIs
- Prevention of pregnancy

These are the areas that you should openly discuss with your patients. You probably will need to ask additional questions that are appropriate to each patient's special situation or circumstances.

From Centers for Disease Control (2012), *Guide to Taking a Sexual History.* http://http://www.cdc.gov/std/treatment/SexualHistory.pdf.

- *Home conditions:* housing, economic condition, types of furnishings (e.g., carpeting and drapes), pets and their health
- *Occupation:* description of usual work (and present work if different); list of job changes; work conditions and hours; physical or mental strain; duration of employment; present and past exposure to heat and cold or industrial toxins (especially lead, arsenic, chromium, asbestos, beryllium, poisonous gases, benzene, and polyvinyl chloride or other carcinogens and teratogens); any protective devices required (e.g., goggles or masks)
- *Environment:* travel and other exposure to contagious diseases, residence in tropics, water and milk supply, other sources of infection if applicable
- *Military record:* dates and geographic area of assignments
- *Religious and cultural preferences:* any religious proscriptions concerning food, medical care; spiritual needs
- *Access to care:* transportation and other resources available to patient, type of health insurance coverage (if any), worries in this regard, primary care provider, customary pattern of seeking care, candid discussion of issues

Evidence-Based Practice in Physical Examination
Smoking Cessation

There is abundant evidence that patients in a trusting relationship with nurses, physicians, or other health professionals will respond positively to even brief, simple advice about smoking cessation. Pooled data from 17 trials of brief advice versus no advice (or usual care) detected a significant increase in the rate of quitting (relative risk, 1.66). Among 11 trials where the intervention was more intensive the estimated effect was higher (relative risk, 1.84) but there was no statistical difference between the intensive and minimal subgroups. A systematic review evaluating randomized trials of smoking cessation interventions delivered by nurses also provides reasonable evidence that intervention is effective. The bottom line is that it pays to offer even minimal advice if given respectfully and earnestly. Of course, not everyone will respond, but any gain is important. The challenge is to incorporate smoking cessation interventions as part of standard practice.

Data from Rice & Stead, 2008; Stead et al, 2008.

Review of Systems (ROS). Identify the presence or absence of health-related issues in each body system. You may not ask all of the questions relevant to each system each time you take a given patient's history. Nevertheless, many should be, particularly at the first interview. More comprehensive questions for particular circumstances in each system are detailed in subsequent chapters. Negative responses to ROS questions are as important as positive responses.

- *General constitutional symptoms:* pain, fever, chills, malaise, fatigue, night sweats, sleep patterns, weight (i.e., average, preferred, present, change)
- *Skin, hair, and nails:* rash or eruption, itching, pigmentation or texture change; excessive sweating, abnormal nail or hair growth
- *Head and neck*
  - *General:* frequent or unusual headaches, their location; dizziness, syncope, severe head injuries; concussions, periods of loss of consciousness (momentary or prolonged)
  - *Eyes:* visual acuity, blurring, diplopia, photophobia, pain, recent change in appearance or vision; glaucoma; use of eye drops or other eye medications; history of trauma
  - *Ears:* hearing loss, pain, discharge, tinnitus, vertigo, infections
  - *Nose:* sense of smell, frequency of colds, obstruction, epistaxis, postnasal discharge, sinus pain
  - *Throat and mouth:* hoarseness or change in voice, frequent sore throats, bleeding or swelling of gums, recent tooth abscesses or extractions, soreness of tongue or buccal mucosa, ulcers, disturbance of taste, dental care
- *Lymph nodes:* enlargement, tenderness, suppuration
- *Chest and lungs:* pain related to respiration; dyspnea, cyanosis, wheezing, cough, sputum (character and quantity), hemoptysis, night sweats, exposure to tuberculosis; date and result of last chest x-ray examination
- *Breasts:* development, pain, tenderness, discharge, lumps, galactorrhea, mammograms (screening or diagnostic), breast self-awareness/breast self-examination
- *Heart and blood vessels:* chest pain or distress, precipitating causes, timing and duration, relieving factors, palpitations, dyspnea, orthopnea (number of pillows needed), edema, hypertension, previous myocardial infarction, estimate of exercise tolerance, past electrocardiogram or other cardiac tests
- *Peripheral vasculature:* pain in legs with walking or activity (claudication)—frequency, severity, tendency to bruise or bleed, thromboses, thrombophlebitis
- *Hematologic:* anemia, bruising, any known abnormality of blood cells
- *Gastrointestinal:* appetite, digestion, intolerance for any class of foods, dysphagia, heartburn, nausea, vomiting, hematemesis; regularity of bowels, constipation, diarrhea, change in stool color or contents (e.g., clay-colored, tarry, fresh blood, mucus, undigested food); flatulence, hemorrhoids; jaundice, history of ulcer, gallstones, polyps, tumor; previous diagnostic imaging (where, when, findings)
- *Diet:* appetite, likes and dislikes, restrictions (e.g., because of religion, allergy, or other disease), vitamins and other supplements, use of caffeine-containing beverages (e.g., coffee, tea, and cola); an hour-by-hour detailing of food and liquid intake (sometimes a written diary covering several days of intake may be necessary)
- *Endocrine:* thyroid enlargement or tenderness, heat or cold intolerance, unexplained weight change, diabetes, polydipsia, polyuria, distribution and changes in facial or body hair, increased hat and glove size, skin striae
- *Genitourinary:* dysuria, flank or suprapubic pain, urgency, frequency, nocturia, hematuria, polyuria, dark or discolored urine, hesitancy, dribbling, loss in force of stream, passage of stone; edema of face; stress incontinence; hernias; STIs (type, laboratory confirmations, and treatment)
- *Musculoskeletal:* joint stiffness, pain, restriction of motion, swelling, redness, heat, bony deformity

+ *Neurologic:* syncope, seizures, weakness or paralysis, abnormalities of sensation or coordination, tremors, loss of memory
+ *Psychiatric:* depression, mood changes, difficulty concentrating, anxiety, agitation, tension, suicidal thoughts, irritability, sleep disturbances

Females

+ *Menses:* age at menarche, regularity, duration and amount of flow, dysmenorrhea, last menstrual period (LMP), intermenstrual discharge or bleeding, itching, date of last Pap smear, age at menopause, libido, frequency of intercourse, pain during intercourse, sexual difficulties, infertility
+ *Pregnancies:* number, living children, multiple births, miscarriages, abortions, duration of pregnancy, each type of delivery, any complications during any pregnancy or postpartum period or with neonate; use of oral or other contraceptives

Males

+ Puberty onset, difficulty with erections, emissions, testicular pain, libido, infertility

Concluding Questions. Give the patient further opportunity. "Is there anything else that you want me to know?" If there are several issues, ask "What problem concerns you most?" When situations are vague, complicated, or contradictory, it may be helpful to ask "What do you think is the matter with you?" or "What worries you the most about how you are feeling?"

Adaptations for Age, Gender, and Possible Disabilities

There are pervasive concerns common to all patients, particular concerns common to some, and unique concerns that distinguish any one individual.

✤ Infants and Children

Children love it when you get down on the floor to play with them. They have anxieties and fears that must be eased (Fig. 1-3). Use language that they understand. When they are old enough, allow them to actively participate in the interview. Children at age 7 years can be dependable reporters on aspects of their health (Olson et al, 2007). The older the child, the more productive it becomes to ask questions directly and to give information directly.

FIGURE 1-3 Interviewing a child with his parent. Note that the interviewer is sitting close to the patient and that the child is secure on his father's lap.

The older child and the adolescent may seem passive, and sometimes appear hostile to some degree. This may suggest a wish to be alone with you, which may help to get a more accurate history. Be proactive and arrange for this routinely (see Clinical Pearl, "Twins or More").

Clinical Pearl

Twins or More

Your patients may be twins, triplets, or more! Each is an individual entitled to separate consideration and a separate record. Ensure that each has separate time with you and confidentiality.

Family dynamics become evident during history taking and may even lead to clues that a parent is in need. For example, an excessively tearful mother who does not seem to be having much pleasure in her child and who seems self-absorbed, unresponsive, and uncommunicative—or even hostile—may be depressed. Your responsibility goes beyond that for the child. Acknowledge your concern and suggest pathways to help (Olson et al, 2006). Respect, too, parental concerns about their children, whatever the source, and do what is needed to ease the worry.

There are aspects of the history concerning the young that may complement the approach suggested for adults or vary from it. They are as follows:

Chief Concern. A parent or other responsible adult (Box 1-9) most often makes a threesome. The relationship of that person should be recorded. However, the child should be included as much as is possible and as is age appropriate. The latent fears underlying any chief concerns of both parents and children should be explored.

Box 1-9 **Consent by Proxy**

Infants, children, and many adolescents are minors. They may come to you accompanied by someone other than their custodial parent or guardian, often a grandparent or other member of their extended family. Sometimes, your informant might be an au pair or nanny or, in the event of divorce and remarriage, a noncustodial parent or stepparent. Does that person have the right to consent to your care for the child? You need to know. Learn about the policy and procedure for consent in your health care setting.

History of Present Illness. The degree and character of the reaction to the problem on the part of parent and child should be noted.

Past Medical History

+ *Note general health and strength:* Age of the child and/or the nature of the problem determine the approach to questioning. Mother's health during pregnancy:
  + General health as related by the mother if possible, extent of prenatal care, gravidity, parity
  + Specific diseases or conditions: infectious disease (approximate gestational month), weight gain, edema,

hypertension, proteinuria, bleeding (approximate gestational month), preeclampsia
+ Medications, hormones, vitamins, special or unusual diet, general nutritional status
+ Quality of fetal movements and time of onset
+ Emotional and behavioral status (e.g., attitudes toward pregnancy and children)
+ Radiation exposure
+ Use of illicit drugs
+ *Birth*
  + Duration of pregnancy
  + Place of delivery
  + Labor: spontaneous or induced, duration, analgesia or anesthesia, complications
  + Delivery: presentation, forceps, vacuum extraction, spontaneous, or cesarean section; complications
  + Condition of infant, time of onset of cry, Apgar scores if available
  + Birth weight of infant

Staying Well
Putting Prevention into Practice

Take time to consider prevention. Consider how you can include prevention-related advice when talking with your patient or a surrogate. For example, infants should sleep alone on their backs in a crib to decrease the risk of sudden infant death syndrome. And, too often, child safety seats are used incorrectly. Their correct use should be reviewed.

+ *Neonatal period*
  + Congenital anomalies; baby's condition in hospital, oxygen requirements, color, feeding characteristics, vigor, cry; duration of baby's stay in hospital and whether infant was discharged with mother; bilirubin phototherapy; prescriptions (e.g., antibiotics)
  + First month of life: jaundice, color, vigor of crying, bleeding, convulsions, or other evidence of illness
  + Degree of early bonding: opportunities at birth and during the first days of life for the parents to hold, talk to, and caress the infant (i.e., opportunities for both parents to relate to and develop a bond with the baby)
  + The mother's feelings: loss of laughter; unreasonable anxiety or sense of panic; excessive crying and sadness; sleeplessness; feelings of guilt; suicidal ideation, clues singly but most often in combination may be related to postpartum depression
+ *Feeding*
  + Formula or breast, reason for changes, if any; type of formula used and how it is prepared, amounts offered and consumed; frequency of feeding and weight gain
  + Present diet and appetite; age of introduction of solids; age when child achieved three feedings per day; present feeding patterns, with elaboration of any feeding problems; age weaned from bottle or breast; type of milk and daily intake; food preference; ability to feed self; cultural variations

+ *Development:* Obtain the age when the child achieved common developmental milestones:
  + Holds head erect while in sitting position
  + Rolls over from front to back and back to front
  + Sits alone and unsupported
  + Stands with support and alone
  + Walks with support and alone
  + Uses words
  + Talks in sentences
  + Dresses self

Expand the list when indicated. Parents may have baby books, which can stimulate recall, or photographs may be helpful. Additional developmental information to inquire about includes:
+ Age when toilet-trained: approaches to and attitudes regarding toilet training
+ School: grade, performance, problems
+ Dentition: age of first teeth, loss of deciduous teeth, eruption of first permanent teeth; last dental visit
+ Growth: height and weight in a sequence of ages; changes in rates of growth or weight gain
+ Pubertal development: present status. In females, development of breasts, nipples, sexual hair, menstruation (onset, cycle, regularity, pain, description of menses), acne; in males, development of sexual hair, voice changes, acne, nocturnal emissions
+ Illnesses: immunizations, communicable diseases, injuries, hospitalizations

Family History
+ *Maternal gestational history* listing all pregnancies, together with the health status of living children. For *deceased children,* include date, age, cause of death, and dates and duration of pregnancies in the case of miscarriages.
+ *Mother's health* during pregnancies and the *ages of parents* at the birth of this child.
+ *Are the parents consanguineous?* Again, a pedigree diagram helps (see Chapter 26).

Personal and Social History
+ *Behavioral status:* child care or school adjustment; masturbation, nail biting, thumb sucking, breath holding, temper tantrums, pica, tics, rituals; bed wetting, constipation or fecal soiling of pants; playing with fire; reactions to prior illnesses, injuries, or hospitalization
+ An account of a *day in the life of the patient* (from parent, child, or both) is often helpful in providing insights. Box 1-10 emphasizes the particular needs of children who are adopted or are in foster care.
+ *Family circumstances:* father's and mother's occupations, the principal caretakers of child, whether parents are divorced or separated, educational attainment of parents; spiritual orientation; cultural heritage; food preparation and by whom; adequacy of clothing; dependence on relief or social agency
+ *Setting of the home:* number of rooms in house and number of persons in household; sleep habits, sleeping arrangements available for the child, possible environmental hazards

Box 1-10   Adoption and Foster Care

Patients who are adopted or in foster care may not have a sufficient history available. Learn as much as you can. Our outline for history taking is a starter and should be filled out by an exploration of the circumstances that led to adoption or foster care. Do this with care. Some adoptive parents may not yet have shared the knowledge with their children. The trials of the adoptive parents as they sought a child, the process of adoption, the country of origin of the adoptee, and the particular concerns of all involved must be explored.

The needs of foster children vary considerably from those who are adopted. The history may be offered by a social worker, and the issues you encounter will differ in variety and intensity. Foster parents have varying experience, and foster children have often lived in more than one home. Invariably, difficult social circumstances underlie the separation from their parents. The probable lack of stability and security and incomplete knowledge of past illnesses or other conditions make it more difficult to understand the full range of the child's complex and urgent needs.

Box 1-11   Violence or Traumatic Events in Childhood

Witnessing or experiencing violence or injury is a fact of life for many children and is a barrier to appropriate growth and development. Talk about the event in a straightforward, simple, and direct fashion:

- Can you tell me what happened?
- What did you see? What did you hear?
- What scared you the most?
- What were you doing when it happened?
- Do you ever dream about it?
- Do you think about it during the day?
- Do you worry it will happen again?
- Whom do you talk to when you feel worried or scared?
- Why do you think it happened?
- For the older child and adolescent:
- How do you think it changed your life?

These questions are not value-laden and are not too constraining. The child is free to talk if you can be comfortable with the silences that may often ensue. Parents can also respond to the same questions to fill out the story, and you can then learn how they dealt with the circumstance and what they observed in their child's behavior.

Modified from Augustyn et al, 1995.
Reprinted with permission from *Contemporary Pediatrics*, vol 12, 1995. *Contemporary Pediatrics* is a copyrighted publication of Advanstar Communications Inc. All rights reserved.

Review of Systems. In addition to the usual concerns, inquire about any past medical or psychologic testing of the child (Box 1-11). Ask about the following:

- *Skin:* eczema, seborrhea, "cradle cap"
- *Ears:* otitis media (frequency, laterality)
- *Nose:* snoring, mouth breathing, allergic reaction
- *Teeth:* dental care
- *Genitourinary:* bedwetting

✤ Adolescents

Adolescence, the time during the second decade of life from puberty to maturity, is different from childhood and adulthood both physically and psychosocially. It is a time made vulnerable by a tendency to experiment with risky behaviors. Adolescents may be reluctant to talk and have a clear need for confidentiality. All adolescent patients should be given the opportunity to discuss their concerns with you privately. It is wise to let the parent or other caregiver know you will be asking them to step out of the room to provide this important opportunity for the adolescent. The visit can be an opportunity to provide a safe space for teens to talk with their caregivers about sensitive issues with your support. Every effort should be made to maintain confidentiality. The limits on what can be guaranteed should be clearly discussed. Information that suggests that the adolescent's safety or the safety of another is at risk may be reasons to "break" confidentiality.

If a parent is present, first acknowledge the patient. It is helpful in the beginning to talk about what is happening in the patient's day-to-day experiences. Do not force conversation, because adolescents do not readily respond to confrontation. On the other hand, you will often sense a need to talk and an inability to get the words out. Silences can be long, sometimes sheepish, occasionally angry, and not always constructive.

The peer group and the desire to be like peers take on a dominant role during *middle adolescence.* Experimentation with risky behaviors begins, and frequent arguments with parents are common. Immature decision making can lead to destructive, life-changing experiences and lifelong bad habits. During *late adolescence with approaching* adulthood, a more thoughtful consideration of consequences ordinarily occurs, along with a more secure sense of self and an ability to establish intimate relationships and to start planning a career.

Essentially, the eternal questions, "Who am I?" and "Where am I going?" are at the heart of the teenage experience. The adoption of risky behaviors depends on a number of factors:

- Peer pressure
- Loosening attachment to parents
- Poor school performance
- Nonparticipation in school extracurricular activities
- Poor self-esteem
- Need to act older
- Susceptibility to advertising or social media

These issues may make it difficult to transcend the barrier imposed by age in caring for the adolescent (see Clinical Pearl, "Identification of Concerns by Adolescents"). Make generous use of open-ended questions, and do not force an adolescent to talk.

Clinical Pearl

Identification of Concerns by Adolescents:
Pre-visit screeners or questionnaires allow the adolescent to identify his or her concerns prior to the start of the visit. Sometimes allowing an opportunity to write a concern or allowing a choice of concerns presented in written, silent fashion may help (Box 1-12). Then you can phrase the appropriate questions and make the transition to a verbal discussion reasonably comfortable. Take an open-ended approach, always indicating a sense of alliance and partnership.

Box 1-12 Adolescents' Concerns

The following subjects list may be of concern to adolescents. These are highly charged issues mandating the effort for discussion but requiring sensitivity, knowledge of adolescent language, and an unforced approach.

- Bed wetting
- Menstrual pain
- Concern with height or weight: too short, too tall, underweight, overweight
- Concern with breast size: too big, too small
- Concern with penis size: too small
- Worry about pregnancy
- Worry about sexual preference
- Sex? Ready or not?
- HIV, AIDS
- Gambling
- Smoking
- Substance use and abuse
- Parents' attitudes and demands
- Friends and their pressures
- Bullying
- School: not doing well, excessive work
- What am I going to do in life?
- Thoughts about dying

Box 1-13 Screening Tools for Adolescent Issues

HEEADSSS

- *H*ome environment
- *E*ducation, employment
- *E*ating
- *A*ctivities (peer-related), affect, ambitions, anger
- *D*rugs
- *S*exuality
- *S*uicide/depression
- *S*afety from injury and violence

PACES

- *P*arents, peers
- *A*ccidents, alcohol/drugs
- *C*igarettes
- *E*motional issues
- *S*chool, sexuality

NOTE: HEEADSSS and PACES are screening tools and are not substitutes for earnest conversation in a trusting relationship.
From Goldenring and Rosen, 2004; DiFrancesco, 1992. Reprinted with permission from *Contemporary Pediatrics*, vol 12, 2004, pp. 64-90. *Contemporary Pediatrics* is a copyrighted publication of Advanstar Communications Inc. All rights reserved.

Flexibility, respect, and confidentiality are key; otherwise, little productive discussion will result. On occasion, the patient may ask to talk with someone of the same gender, and this should be facilitated if possible. Box 1-13 provides useful screening tools for adolescent issues. You can use them as a guide for an exploratory interview. Some questions that you can ask to structure the interview include:

- "How are things going at home?" "Tell me about your living situation." Do not assume the traditional family structure. Do not ask directly about who else lives in the house. The open-ended question at the start can lead to greater specifics later on.
- "How is school going?" "Are you working?" "What is it about school that appeals to you?" "What is it about school that doesn't appeal to you?" You may expect to hear somewhat more about jobs outside of school and ideas about the future when the patient approaches the age of 20 years.
- "Tell me about your friends." "Where do you go with them?" "What do you do with them?" "What groups do you belong to?" "How would a friend describe you?"
- "What types of computer and electronic games do you play?"
- "What are you good at doing?"

Open-ended conversations about home, school, jobs, and friends can suggest the areas that may trouble the adolescent (e.g., sex, drugs, and suicidal ideation). Talk does not always flow easily as the adolescent moves from dependency to independency, from parents to peer group, and ultimately to self, but you can help (Friedman, 2006).

❀ Pregnant Women

Care during the prenatal period depends on the commitment of the woman to her health and that of her fetus, in partnership with the care provider. Her approach to pregnancy is influenced by many factors, including previous experiences with childbearing and childrearing; her relationship with her mother and other significant individuals in her life; her desire for children; and her present life circumstances. The interaction of the mother with her fetus increases the complexity of care. The initial interview includes past history, assessment of health practices, identification of potential risk factors, and assessment of the patient's knowledge, expectations, and perceptions as they affect pregnancy.

If you use an electronic device or preprinted history form to gather the history, bridge the distance by talking comfortably and at some length with the patient, particularly her expectations and concerns. There will, of course, be much "laying on of hands" as the pregnancy matures.

Basic Information

- Patient's age, ethnicity
- Marital status, partner, or relationship
- Last menstrual period (LMP)
- Previous usual/normal menstrual period (PUMP or PNMP)
- Expected date of confinement/delivery (EDC)
- Occupation
- Father of the baby and his occupation

History of Present Illness or Problem. Obtain a description of the current pregnancy, and identify previous medical care. Identify specific problems (e.g., bleeding or spotting, nausea, vomiting, fatigue, or edema). Include information about illness, injuries, surgeries, or accidents or other injuries since conception.

Obstetric History. Information on each previous pregnancy (gravidity and parity) includes the date of delivery; length of pregnancy; weight and gender of infant(s); type of delivery (e.g., spontaneous vaginal; cesarean section and type of scar [an evaluation of the competency of the scar is needed for women attempting vaginal birth after cesarean section]); or spontaneous, therapeutic, or elective abortion and the type of procedure; length of labor; and complications in pregnancy or labor, postpartum, or with the infant.

Menstrual History. In addition to previous information, include age at menarche, characteristics of the cycle, unusual bleeding, and associated symptoms. If known, include dates of ovulation and conception, and the use of contraceptives before or during conception.

Gynecologic History. Record the date of the most recent Pap smear and human papilloma virus (HPV) test along with any history of abnormalities, treatments, or gynecologic surgery. A sexual history includes age of first intercourse and whether it was consensual, number of sex partners, safe-sex methods, partner orientation, and, if a minor, age of partner. Information regarding the types of contraceptives used and reason for discontinuing them, along with plans for use postpartum, is obtained. Any history of infertility should be explored. If any STIs are reported, discuss the type, dates, treatments, and complications. Give full attention to any history of sexual assault.

Past Medical History. The same information identified previously for adults is obtained, with the addition of risk factors for HIV, hepatitis, tuberculosis, and exposure to environmental and occupational hazards.

Family History. Obtain a family history of genetic conditions, multiple births, gestational diabetes, preeclampsia/eclampsia or pregnancy-induced hypertension (PIH), and/or congenital anomalies.

Personal and Social History. Obtain information about feelings toward the pregnancy, whether it was planned, consideration of adoption or abortion, gender preference, social and spiritual resources, experiences with mothering (of being both mothered and a mother), experience with and plans for labor and breast-feeding, and history of past or present abuse in relationships (intimate partner violence).

Review of Systems. Perform a complete review of all systems because the effects of pregnancy are seen in all systems. Give special attention to the reproductive system (including breasts) and cardiovascular systems (documentation of prepregnancy blood pressure if possible). Assess the endocrine system for signs of diabetes and thyroid dysfunction. Assess the urinary tract for infection, and review kidney function. Assess respiratory function because it may be compromised later in pregnancy or with tocolytic therapy for preterm labor. Evaluate dental care needs because treatment of periodontitis can prevent preterm birth and/or low birth weight (George et al, 2011).

Risk Assessment. Identify conditions from the history and physical examination or circumstances that threaten the well-being of the mother and/or fetus. These include maternal diabetes, preterm labor, preeclampsia/eclampsia, maternal malnutrition and vitamin deficiency, and use of potentially teratogenetic agents such as lithium and valproic acid.

Postpartum. Postpartum depression occurs in about one of every five women after delivery. The clues are similar to those of depression in other circumstances—feeling down, depressed, or hopeless, sleep disturbance, loss of energy, eating disturbance, trouble concentrating, restlessness, sad mood, anxiety, fatigue, feelings of worthlessness, inappropriate guilt, and suicidal ideation. A cluster of these symptoms should strongly suggest the need for assessment for postpartum depression (Gjerdingen et al, 2009; O'Hara et al, 2012).

❀ Older Adults

A change in knowledge, experience, cognitive abilities, and personality may occur with aging (Box 1-14). It is important to anticipate the effect these changes may have on the interview. However, physiologic age and chronologic age may not match. It is equally important to recognize that not all adults experience the same changes, they do not occur at the same rate, and some abilities may not decline with age.

Some older adults have sensory losses, such as hearing, that make communication more difficult. Position yourself so that the patient can see your face. Speak clearly and slowly, taking care to always face the patient while you are talking. Shouting magnifies the problem by distorting consonants and vowels. In some instances, a written interview may be less frustrating. If this is necessary, include only pertinent questions because this approach can be tedious and exhausting. Impaired vision and light-dark

---

Box 1-14   Competency to Make Medical Decisions

Patients or their surrogates have the right to decide the extent of care they will accept under your guidance. Many may have lost the ability to make relevant *competent* decisions. To give informed consent, patients must be well informed about what is proposed, and they must be able to voluntarily give consent. Competency to make medical decisions is used interchangeably with the word capacity. In a report from the President's Commission for the Study of Ethical Problems in Medicine, clinical decision-making capacity includes three specific elements: the patient has a set of values and goals, the patient is able to understand and communicate information, and the patient is able to reason and deliberate about the choice being made by the patient. Competency may fluctuate from hour to hour or day to day, depending on the age and the physical/emotional circumstance. It is often necessary to seek consultative help in deciding a patient's status. The law in your state may require this, and it may ultimately be left to a judge to decide on legal competence. It is important to recognize that *the patient who disagrees with you is not necessarily incompetent, and the patient who agrees with you is not necessarily competent.*

From Appelbaum, 2007; Magauran, 2009; President's Commission for the Study of Ethical Problems in Medicine and Biomedical and Behavioral Research, 1982.

adaptation are a problem with written interview forms. Ensure large print and ample lighting with a source that does not glare or reflect in the eyes.

Some older adults may be confused or experience memory loss, particularly for recent events. Take whatever extra time is needed. Ask short (but not leading) questions, and keep your language uncomplicated and free of double negatives. Consult other family members to clarify discrepancies or to fill in the gaps. On the other hand, the older patient has a lifetime of experience that may be a rich source of wisdom and perspective. Listen for it.

The history is more complex and increasingly subtle with the chronic, progressive, and debilitating problems that occur with aging. Symptoms may be less dramatic, vague or nonspecific. Confusion may be the only indication of a major problem. Pain may be unreliably reported because, with age, its perception varies from the expected. The excruciating pain usually associated with pancreatitis, for example, may be perceived as a dull ache, and myocardial infarction can occur without any perception of pain. Some patients may not report symptoms because they attribute them to old age or because they believe that nothing can be done. They may have lived with a chronic condition for so long that it has been part of their expectation of daily living.

Multiple problems needing multiple drugs increase risk for iatrogenic disorders. A medication history with attention to interactions of drugs, diseases, and aging is needed for prescribed and over the counter medications and herbal preparations. It is particularly helpful to have patients (of all ages) bring in their medication bottles. Encourage patients with complex medication needs or several providers to use a single pharmacy so that the computer database available to the pharmacist can flag drug–drug interactions.

Routinely include functional assessment as part of the older adult's history (see Functional Assessment for All Patients box and individual chapters with functional assessment specific to systems). Questions concerning the ability to take care of one's daily needs are part of the ROS. The personal and social history should include other dimensions of functional capacity such as social, spiritual, and economic resources; recreational activity; sleep patterns; environmental control; and use of the health care system. Maintaining function is a compelling concern of older adults.

For all ages, a cognitive impairment that deprives the patient of the ability to join in the decision-making process emphasizes the need for a designated health care agent (medical power of attorney for health care) and/or advance directives (a document outlining the patient's wishes regarding extraordinary means of life support). Be aware of the specific rules governing these issues in your state. Encourage the patient and family to pursue these documents if steps have not yet been taken.

The Frail. Frailty has its onset with the loss of physical reserve and the increased risk for loss of physical function

---

FUNCTIONAL ASSESSMENT

Functional Assessment for All Patients

Quite simply, functional assessment is an attempt to understand a patient's ability to achieve the basic activities of daily living. This assessment should be made for all older adults and for any person limited by disease or disability, acute or chronic. A well-taken history and a meticulous physical examination can bring out subtle influences, such as tobacco and alcohol use, sedentary habits, poor food selection, overuse of medications (prescribed and nonprescribed), and less than obvious emotional distress. Even some physical limitations may not be readily apparent (e.g., limitations of cognitive ability or of the senses). Keep in mind that patients tend to overstate their abilities and, quite often, to obscure reality.

When performing a functional assessment consider a variety of disabilities: physical, cognitive, psychologic, social, and sexual. An individual's social and spiritual support system must be as clearly understood as the physical disabilities. There are a variety of physical disabilities, including:

- Mobility
  Difficulty walking standard distances: ½ mile, 2 to 3 blocks, ⅓ block, across a room
  Difficulty climbing stairs, up and down
  Problems with balance
- Upper extremity function
  Difficulty grasping small objects, opening jars
  Difficulty reaching out or up overhead, such as taking something off a shelf

- Housework
  Heavy (vacuuming, scrubbing floors)
  Light (dusting)
  Meal preparation
  Shopping
  Medication use
  Money management
- Instrumental activities of daily living
  Bathing
  Dressing
  Toileting
  Moving from bed to chair, chair to standing
  Eating
  Walking in home
  Any limitations, even mild, in any of these areas will affect a patient's independence and autonomy and, to the extent of the limitation, increase reliance on other people and on assistive devices. These limitations indicate the loss of physical reserve and the potential loss of physical function and independence that indicate the onset of frailty. The patient's social support system and material resources are then integral to the development of reasonable management plans.

FIGURE 1-4 Interviewing a patient with a physical disability. Note the uncluttered surroundings; be sure the patient in a wheelchair has room to maneuver.

and independence. Its prevalence increases with age, particularly past 80 years. Frailty is characterized by weakness, weight loss, low activity, and diminished ability to respond to stress and is associated with adverse health outcomes. It is considered an at-risk state caused by the age-associated accumulation of deficits. With multisystem dysregulation, decreased physiologic reserves, and increased vulnerability to stressors, frailty shares features of normal aging (Fedarko, 2011; Rockwood and Minitski, 2011). Nonetheless, age and frailty are not necessarily synonymous.

Patients with Disabilities

You must adapt to the needs of all patients *of any age* with disabling physical or emotional states (e.g., deafness, blindness, depression, psychosis, developmental delays, or neurologic impairments). They may or may not be effective historians, but respect them regardless. Their perspectives and attitudes matter. Involve each fully to the limit of emotional and mental capacity or physical ability (Fig. 1-4). Still, when necessary, use the family other health professionals involved in care, and the patient's record as resources for a more complete story. Some of the most common communication barriers can be overcome by keeping the following in mind:

- Family members are often available to make the patient more comfortable and to provide you with information.
- Persons with impaired hearing often read, write, sign, and/or read lips, but you must speak slowly and enunciate each word clearly and in full view. A translator who signs may be available.

Persons with visual impairment usually can hear, but talking louder to make a point does not help. Remember, however, that you must always vocalize what you are trying to communicate; gestures may not be seen.

Aging, debilitating illness, and the onset of frailty increase dependency on others, worry about tomorrow, and grieving for what has been lost. Recognize these vast concerns and the sense of loss in both the patient and the immediate caregiver. You can acknowledge this and offer to talk about it.

The Next Step

Once the history (Box 1-15) has been built, move on to the physical examination, the laying on of hands, which is discussed in subsequent chapters. These chapters are necessarily segmented and are not meant to reflect the natural flow that you will develop with experience. Do not be intimidated because your patients expect you to be perfect. Just be disciplined, alert, and recognize that your value judgments are not necessarily imbued with wisdom.

CHAPTER 2

Cultural Competency

Achieving cultural competence is a learning process that requires self-awareness, reflective practice, and knowledge of core cultural issues. It involves recognizing one's own culture, values, and biases, and using effective patient-centered communication skills. A culturally competent health care provider adapts to the unique needs of patients of backgrounds and cultures that differ from his or her own. This adaptability, coupled with a genuine curiosity about a patient's beliefs and values, lay the foundation for a trusting patient-provider relationship.

---

evolve *http://evolve.elsevier.com/Seidel*
• NCLEX Review Questions

A Definition of Culture

Culture, in its broadest sense, reflects the whole of human behavior, including ideas and attitudes; ways of relating to one another; manners of speaking; and the material products of physical effort, ingenuity, and imagination. Language is a part of culture. So, too, are the abstract systems of belief, etiquette, law, morals, entertainment, and education. Within the cultural whole, different populations may exist in groups and subgroups. Each group is identified by a particular body of shared traits (e.g., a particular art, ethos, or belief; or a particular behavioral pattern) and is rather dynamic in its evolving accommodations with internal and external influences. Any individual may belong to more than one group or subgroup, such as ethnic origin, religion, gender, sexual orientation, occupation, and profession.

Distinguishing Physical Characteristics

The use of physical characteristics (e.g., gender or skin color) to distinguish a cultural group or subgroup can be a trap. There is a sharp difference between distinguishing cultural characteristics and distinguishing physical characteristics. Do not confuse the physical with the cultural or allow the physical to symbolize the cultural. To assume homogeneity in the beliefs, attitudes, and behaviors of all individuals in a particular group leads to misunderstandings about the individual. The *stereotype*, a fixed image of any group that denies the potential of originality or individuality within the group, should be rejected. People can and do respond differently to the same stimuli. Stereotyping occurs through two cognitive phases. In the first phase, a stereotype becomes activated when an individual is categorized into a social group. When this occurs, the beliefs and feelings (prejudices) come to mind about what members of that particular group are like. Over time, this first phase occurs without effort or awareness. In the second phase, people use these activated beliefs and feelings when they interact with the individual, even when they explicitly deny these stereotypes. Multiple studies have shown that health care providers activate these implicit stereotypes, or non-conscious bias, when communicating with and providing care to minority patients (Stone and Moskowitz, 2011). With this in mind, you can begin the learning process of achieving cultural competence by acknowledging your implicit, or nonconscious, biases toward patients based on physical characteristics.

At the same time, this does not minimize the value of understanding the cultural characteristics of groups, nor does this deny the interdependence of the physical with the cultural. Genotype, for example, precedes the development of the intellect, sensitivity, and imagination that leads to unique cultural achievements, such as the creation of classical or jazz music. Similarly, a person's phenotype, like skin color, precedes most of the experience of life and the subsequent interweaving of that phenotype with cultural experience. Although commonly used in clinical practice, the use of phenotypic traits to classify an individual's race is problematic. The term *race* has been used to categorize individuals based on their continent or subcontinent of origin (e.g., Asian, Southeast Asian). However, there is ongoing debate about the usefulness of race, considering the degree of phenotypic and genetic variation of individuals from the same geographic region (Relethford, 2009). In addition, the origins of race date back to the 17th century, long before scientists identified genetic similarities. Over time, beliefs about particular racial groups were shaped by economic and political factors and many believe race has become a social construct (Harawa and Ford, 2009).

There is a growing body of research examining genetic markers associated with racial and ethnic groups and potential interactions with environmental determinants in predicting disease susceptibility and response to medical treatment (Risch,

2006). An explosion of genome-wide association studies (GWAS) are attempting to link genomic loci, or single-nucleotide polymorphisms (SNPs) with common diseases like rheumatoid arthritis, type 1 and type 2 diabetes mellitus, and Crohn disease (Visscher et al, 2012). Clinical care in the 21st century will focus on disease prevention by the integration of genetic individuality within the context of environmental and cultural influence (Valle, 2004). Health care providers will need to become fluent in the language of genomics and learn how to discuss risks and benefits of gene testing with their patients (Feero and Green, 2011). During this time, it will be perhaps even more important to acknowledge implicit biases and seek to understand the patient's unique cultural and personal health beliefs and expectations.

Cultural Competence

Culturally competent care requires that health care providers be sensitive to patients' heritage, sexual orientation, socioeconomic situation, ethnicity, and cultural background (Cuellar et al, 2008). Many models have been proposed to teach cultural competence. Most include the domains of acquiring knowledge (e.g., understanding the meaning of culture), shaping attitudes (e.g., respecting differences of individuals from other cultures) and developing skills (e.g., eliciting patients cultural beliefs about health and illness) (Saha et al, 2008). Some of these domains overlap with core aspects of the patient-centered care model (Fig. 2-1). Seeleman et al have proposed a framework for teaching cultural competence that emphasizes an awareness of the social context in which specific ethnic groups live. For ethnic minority individuals,

assessing the social context includes inquiring about stressors and support networks, sense of life control, and literacy. In doing so, health care providers will need to be flexible and creative in working with patients (Seeleman et al, 2009). Campinha-Bacote's Process of Cultural Competence Model is another approach and includes five cultural constructs: awareness, knowledge, skill, encounters, and desire (Campinha-Bacote, 2011). Box 2-1 defines these five constructs.

Box 2-1 Dimensions of Cultural Competence

CULTURAL ENCOUNTERS—The continuous process of interacting with patients from culturally diverse backgrounds in order to validate, refine or modify existing values, beliefs, and practices about a cultural group and to develop cultural desire, cultural awareness, cultural skill, and cultural knowledge.

CULTURAL DESIRE—The motivation of the health care professional to "want to" engage in the process of becoming culturally competent, not the "have to."

CULTURAL AWARENESS—The deliberate self-examination and in-depth exploration of one's biases, stereotypes, prejudices, assumptions and "isms" that one holds about individuals and groups who are different from them.

CULTURAL KNOWLEDGE—The process of seeking and obtaining a sound educational base about culturally and ethnically diverse groups.

CULTURAL SKILL—The ability to collect culturally relevant data regarding the patient's presenting problem, as well as accurately performing a culturally-based physical assessment in a culturally sensitive manner.

From Campinha-Bacote, 2011.

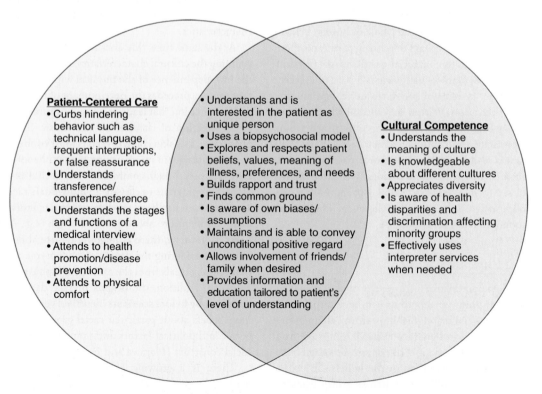

FIGURE 2-1 Overlapping concepts of patient-centered care and cultural competence. *(From Saha S, Beach MC, Cooper LA, 2008.)*

Cultural Humility

Cultural humility involves the ability to recognize one's limitations in knowledge and cultural perspective and be open to new perspectives. Rather than assuming all patients of a particular culture fit a certain stereotype, the health care provider should view each patient as an individual. In doing so, cultural humility helps equalize the imbalance in the patient-provider relationship. (Borkan et al, 2008). A provider may know many specific details about a patient's particular culture yet not show cultural humility. Cultural humility involves self-reflection and self-critique with the goal of having a more balanced, mutually beneficial relationship. Being open to understanding a patient's belief systems and developing a partnership is much more important than knowing everything about a patient's specific culture (Juarez et al, 2006).

The Impact of Culture

The information in Box 2-2 suggests that racial and ethnic differences, as well as social and economic conditions, may affect the provision of specific health care services to certain groups and subgroups in the United States. Poverty and inadequate education disproportionately affect various cultural groups (e.g., ethnic minorities and women); socioeconomic disparities negatively affect the health and medical care of individuals belonging to these groups. Although death rates have declined overall in the United States over the past 50 years, the poorly educated and those in poverty still die at higher rates from the same conditions than those who are better educated and economically advantaged. Morbidity, too, is greater among the poor. Data from the 2011 CDC Health Disparities and Inequalities Report reveals a variety of health care disparities, including a significantly higher rate of uninsured Hispanic and non-Hispanic blacks compared to Asian/Pacific Islanders and whites and a 2.4 times higher infant mortality rate among infants born to non-Hispanic black women compared to non-Hispanic white women. Compared to white women, a much higher percentage of black women die from coronary heart disease before age 75 (37.9% versus 19.4%). This same difference was observed between black and white men (61.5% versus 41.5%) (CDC, 2011). These rather stark facts are sufficient to underscore the need for cultural awareness in health and medical care professionals. Cultural and practice differences exist among health care professionals as well. Allopathic providers often demonstrate skepticism regarding the use of complementary and alternative medicine (CAM) without considering the possibility of potential benefit to patients (see Box 2-2).

The Blurring of Cultural Distinctions

Some cultural differences may be malleable in a way that physical characteristics may not be. For example, one group of people can be distinguished from another by language (see Clinical Pearl, "Language Is Not All"). However, globalization, the growing diversity of the U.S. population, and evidence of health care disparities mandate more and more that we learn one another's languages. Although modern technology and economics may

---

Box 2-2 | The Influence of Age, Race, Ethnicity, Socioeconomic Status, and Culture

Age, gender, race, ethnic group and, with these variables, cultural attitudes, regional differences, and socioeconomic status influence the way patients seek medical care and the way clinicians provide care. Consider, for example, the ethnic and racial differences in the treatment of depression in the United States. The prevalence of depression is similar across groups; however, compared with white Americans, black and Latino patients are less likely to receive treatment. Although some of the disparity is related to differing attitudes and perceptions of counseling and medication, other cultural and personal factors are likely to be major determinants. Black and Latino children in the United States also experience health disparities, including lower overall health status and lower receipt of routine medical care and dental care compared to white children. Flores and colleagues (2010), in a systematic literature review, demonstrated that compared to white children, black children have lower rates of preventive and population health care (e.g., breastfeeding and immunization coverage), higher adolescent health risk behaviors (e.g., sexually transmitted diseases), higher rates of asthma emergency visits, and lower mental health service use. There is a clear need to better understand why these differences exist more globally, but removing cultural blindness at the individual patient level is an important first step.

Furthermore, the possible beneficial and harmful effects of many culturally important herbal medicines, which are used but not always acknowledged, must be understood and, in trusting relationships, reported to us if we are to guide their appropriate use. Crossing the cultural divide helps, but skepticism is a barrier. For example, many allopathic medical providers question the notion that complementary and alternative medicine might be a helpful adjuvant therapy for the prevention and treatment of acute otitis media. However, in several randomized controlled studies, xylitol, probiotics, herbal ear drops, and homeopathic treatments have been shown, compared with placebo, to have a greater effect in reducing pain duration and decreasing the use of antibiotics. Although skepticism can be put aside, evidence-driven guidance is still essential. Cultural competence is entirely consistent with that.

Data from Bukutu et al, 2008; Miranda and Cooper, 2004; Flores, 2010.

---

eventually lead to universality in language, we can begin by acknowledging and overcoming our individual biases and cultural stereotypes. Because it is impossible to learn the native languages of all of our patients, when language barriers arise, we must become aware of our resources and know how to effectively use interpreters (Seeleman et al, 2009). Use of medical interpreters has a positive impact on health care quality, but we haven't yet begun using these services regularly (Flores, 2005; Kuo, 2007).

Clinical Pearl

Language Is Not All
A patient who knows the English language, however well, cannot be assumed to know the culture. Consider the diversity of the populations in Britain, India, American Samoa, and South Africa who are English speaking. The absence of a language barrier does not preclude a cultural barrier. You will likely still need to achieve a "cultural translation."

The Primacy of the Individual in Health Care

The individual patient may be visualized as being at the center of an indefinite number of concentric circles. The outermost circles represent constraining universal experiences (e.g., death). The circles closest to the center represent the various cultural groups or subgroups to which anyone must, of necessity, belong. The constancy of change forces adaptation and acculturation. The circles are constantly interweaving and overlapping. For example, a common experience in the United States has been the economic gain at the root of the assimilation of many ethnic groups. Although this results in greater homogeneity among the population, an individual's traditions and ethnic behaviors will likely be unique. Predicting the individual's character merely on the basis of the common cultural behavior, or stereotype, is not appropriate; rather, understanding and taking the common cultural behavior into account are appropriate (Box 2-3).

Nevertheless, ethical issues often arise when the care of an individual comes into conflict with the utilitarian needs of the larger community, particularly with the recognition of limited resources and, in the United States, rising health care costs. Cultural attitudes of our patients, at times vague and poorly understood, may constrain our professional behavior and may confuse the context in which we serve the individual. Box 2-4 offers a guide to help understand the patient's beliefs and practices that can lead to individualized, culturally competent care.

Box 2-3　Questions That Explore the Patient's Culture

These questions may be addressed directly to the patient or modified for third persons, such as parents and other caregivers who are responsible for and/or involved with the patient. These questions, appropriate in any culture, allow you to gain insights about an individual. They help you to avoid the stereotype and lead to a true individualization of care.

- What do you call your problem?
- What do you think caused it?
- Why do you think it started when it did?
- What does your sickness do to you?
- How does it work?
- How bad is your sickness?
- How long do you think it will last?
- What should be done to get rid of it?
- Why did you come to me for treatment?
- What benefit will you get from the treatment?
- What are the most important problems your sickness has caused for you?
- What worries you and frightens you the most about your sickness?
- Who else or what else might help you get better?
- Has anyone else helped you with this problem?

Modified from Kleinman et al, 1978; and Taylor and Willies-Jacobo, 2003, who remind us that we can substitute "your child" for "your" to adapt these questions for the young.

Professional Cultures within the Health Professions

There is a harmony—a unity—in the care of patients that is not constricted by the cultural and administrative boundaries of the individual health professions. To the extent that we stake out territories of care by allowing individual professional cultures and needs to take precedence over patient needs, we may impede the achievement of harmony. The blurring of professional cultural borders may work to the advantage of the patient as long as the blurring is motivated by the best interests of the patient. Each of us must understand our professional role and must be adaptable as cultural shifts suggest greater homogeneity in a number of those roles. In addition, Box 2-5 indicates that there are health beliefs and practices that are different from the long-institutionalized Western perspective that dominates health education in the United States. Health care providers in different parts of the world make different decisions. Your ability to understand and to respect differences, and to allow for the blurring of borders, will be a measure of your ability to form reinforcing relationships with other professionals and to care for a wide range of individuals.

The Impact of Culture on Illness

Disease is shaped by illness, and illness—the full expression of the impact of disease on the patient—is shaped by the totality of the patient's experience. Cancer is a disease. The patient dealing with, reacting to, and trying to live with cancer is having an illness—is "ill" or "sick." The definition of "ill" or "sick" is based on the individual's belief system and is determined in large part by his or her enculturation. This is so for a brief, essentially mild episode or for a chronic, debilitating, life-altering condition. If we do not consider the substance of illness—the biologic, emotional, and cultural aspects—we will too often fail to offer complete care. To make the point, imagine that while taking a shower you have conducted a self-examination and, still young, still looking ahead to your career, you have discovered an unexpected mass in a breast or a testicle. How will you respond? How might other individuals respond?

Staying Well

Consider the "Norm" with Care

We often use a variety of screening questionnaires to identify concerns and help our patients stay well. These screening tools are based on norms that, as Rhodes says, "Tell us how to place individuals in relation to one another according to some agreed on and standardized measure." Norms, however, may not be consistent across cultures. Screening tools may contain cultural biases and result in misleading information. Problems in one may be the expected in another. Whenever possible, we should use instruments that have been adapted for and tested with individuals from our patients' specific cultural groups. When this is not possible, we must be cautious and use these tools, recognizing that they may well not be universally applicable.

From Rhodes, 2003; Center for Substance Abuse Treatment, 2009.

Box 2-4 **Cultural Assessment Guide: The Many Aspects of Understanding**

Health Beliefs and Practices
- How does the patient define health and illness? How are feelings concerning pain, illness in general, or death expressed?
- Are there particular methods used to help maintain health, such as hygiene and self-care practices?
- Are there particular methods being used for treatment of illness?
- What is the attitude toward preventive health measures such as immunizations?
- Are there health topics that the patient may be particularly sensitive to or considered taboo?
- Are there restrictions imposed by modesty that must be respected; for example, are there constraints related to exposure of parts of the body, discussion of sexual health, and attitudes toward various procedures such as termination of pregnancy or vasectomy?
- What are the attitudes toward mental illness, pain, handicapping conditions, chronic disease, death, and dying? Are there constraints in the way these issues are discussed with the patient or with reference to relatives and friends?
- Is there a person in the family responsible for various health-related decisions such as where to go, whom to see, and what advice to follow?
- Does the patient prefer a health professional of the same gender, age, ethnic and racial background?

Faith-Based Influences and Special Rituals
- Is there a religion or faith to which the patient adheres?
- Is there a significant person to whom the patient looks for guidance and support?
- Are there any faith-based special practices or beliefs that may affect health care when the patient is ill or dying?
- What events, rituals, and ceremonies are considered important within the life cycle of birth, puberty, marriage, and death? What is the culturally appropriate way to respond to these life events? To what extent is an overt expression of emotion and spirituality inherent in that response?

Language and Communication
- What language is spoken in the home?
- How well does the patient understand English, both spoken and written?
- Are there special signs of demonstrating respect or disrespect?
- Is touch involved in communication?
- Are there culturally appropriate ways to enter and leave situations (e.g., greetings and farewells) and convenient times to make a home visit?

- Is an interpreter needed? (If so, this person ideally should be a trained professional and not a family member.)

Parenting Styles and Role of Family
- Who makes the decisions in the family?
- What is the composition of the family? How many generations are considered to be a single family, and which relatives compose the family unit?
- When the marriage custom is practiced, what is the attitude about separation and divorce?
- What is the role of and attitude toward children in the family?
- When do children need to be disciplined or punished, and how is this done (if physical means are used, in what way)?
- Do family members demonstrate physical affection toward their children and each other?
- What major events are important to the family, and how are they celebrated?
- Are there special beliefs and practices surrounding conception, pregnancy, childbirth, lactation, and childrearing? Is co-sleeping practiced? (If so, further inquiry is necessary regarding safe sleep practices for infants 12 months and younger.)

Sources of Support beyond the Family
- Are there ethnic or cultural organizations that may have an influence on the patient's approach to health care?
- Are there individuals in the patient's social network that can influence perception of health and illness?
- Is there a particular cultural group with which the patient identifies? Can this be clarified by where the patient was born and has lived?
- What is the patient's need for relationships with others?
- Is the patient socially gregarious or introverted, and is the preference indicated by behaviors displayed before the illness?

Dietary Practices
- What does the family like to eat? Does everyone in the family have similar tastes in food?
- Who is responsible for food preparation?
- Are any foods forbidden by the culture, or are some foods a cultural requirement in observance of a rite or ceremony?
- How is food prepared and consumed?
- Are there specific beliefs or preferences concerning food, such as those believed to cause or to cure an illness?
- Are there periods of required fasting? What are they?

Modified from Stulc, 1991.

The Components of a Cultural Response

When cultural differences exist, be certain that you grasp exactly what the patient means and know exactly what the patient thinks you mean in words and actions. Asking the patient if you are not sure is far better than making a damaging mistake. Avoid assumptions about cultural beliefs and behaviors made without validation from the patient.

Beliefs and behaviors that will have an impact on patient assessment include the following:
- Modes of communication: the use of speech, body language, and space
- Health beliefs and practices that may vary from your own
- Diet and nutritional practices
- The nature of relationships within a family

A variety of ethnic attitudes toward autonomy may exist. The patient-centered model, still firmly respected in the United States, could be at odds with a more family-centered model that is more likely dominant elsewhere. In Japan, for example, the family is generally considered the legitimate decision-making authority for competent and incompetent patients. Persons of some cultures (e.g., Middle Eastern and Navajo Native American) believe that a patient should not be told of a diagnosis of a metastatic cancer or a terminal prognosis for any reason, but this attitude is not likely to be shared by Americans with European or African traditions. Traditionally, the members of the Navajo culture believe that thought and language have the power to shape reality. Talking about a possible outcome is thought to ensure the outcome. It is important, then, to avoid thinking or speaking in a negative way. The situation can be dealt with by talking in terms of a third person or an abstract possibility. You might even refer to an experience you have had in your own family. Obviously, the conflicts that may arise from differing views of autonomy, religion, and information sharing require an effort that is dominated by a clear understanding of the patient's goals. However, it is important to remember that a patient may not typify the attitudes of the group of origin.

Box 2-5 Comparison of Value Orientations among Cultural Groups

Value Orientation

Time Orientation
Present oriented: Accepts each day as it comes; future unpredictable
Past oriented: Maintains traditions that were meaningful in the past; worships ancestors
Future oriented: Anticipates bigger and better future; places high value on change

Activity Orientation
"Doing" orientation: Emphasizes accomplishments that are measurable by external standards
"Being" orientation: Spontaneous expression of self
"Being-in-becoming": Emphasizes self-development of all aspects of self as an integrated whole

Human Nature Orientation
Human being basically imperfect but with perfectible nature; constant self-control and discipline necessary
Human being as neutral, neither good nor evil

People-to-Nature Orientation
Human being subject to environment with very little control over own destiny
Human being in harmony with nature
Human being master over nature

Relational Orientation
Individualistic: Encourages individualism; interpersonal relationships occur more with outsiders and less with family
Lineal: Group goals dominant over individual goals; ordered positional succession (father to son)
Collateral: Group goals dominant over individual goals: more emphasis on relationship with others on one's own level

Modified from Kluckhohn, 1976.

Modes of Communication

Communication and culture are interrelated, particularly in the way feelings are expressed verbally and nonverbally. The same word may have different meanings for different people. For example, in the United States, a "practicing physician" is an experienced, trained person. "Practicing," however, suggests inexperience and the status of a student to an Alaskan Native or to some Western Europeans. Similarly, touch, facial expressions, eye movement, and body posture all have varying significance.

In the United States, for example, people tend to talk more loudly and to worry less about being overheard than others do. The English, on the other hand, tend to worry more about being overheard and speak in modulated voices. In the United States, people are direct in conversation and are eager to be thought logical, preferring to avoid the subjective and to come to the point quickly. The Japanese tend to do the opposite, using indirection, talking around points, and emphasizing attitudes and feelings. Silence, although sometimes uncomfortable for many of us, affords patients who are Native American time to think; the response should not be forced and the quiet time should be allowed.

Many groups use firm eye contact. The Spanish meet one another's eyes and look for the impact of what is being said. The French, too, have a firm gaze and often stare openly at others. This, however, might be thought rude or immodest in some Asian or Middle Eastern cultures. Americans are more apt to let the eyes wander and to grunt, nod the head, or say, "I see," or "uh huh," to indicate understanding. Americans also tend to avoid touch and are less apt to pat you on the arm in a reassuring way than are, for example, Italians.

These are but a few examples of cultural variation in communication. They do, however, suggest a variety of behaviors within groups. As with any example we might use, they are not to be thought of as rigidly characteristic of the indicated groups. Still, the questions suggested in Box 2-4 can at times provide insight to particular situations and can help avoid misunderstanding and miscommunication.

The cultural and physical characteristics of both patient and health care provider may significantly influence communication (Fig. 2-2). Social class, age, and gender are variables that characterize everyone; they can intrude on successful communication

FIGURE 2-2 Being sensitive to cultural differences that may exist between you and the patient can help avoid miscommunication.

if there is no effort for mutual knowledge and understanding (see Clinical Pearl, "The Impact of Gender"). The young student or health care provider and the older adult patient may have to work harder to develop a meaningful relationship. Recognizing the possible problem and talking about it, evoking feelings sooner rather than later, makes it easier. It is permissible to ask if the patient is uncomfortable with you or your background and to talk about it. Also, when any aspect of the patient's person disturbs you, you must try to understand why.

Clinical Pearl

The Impact of Gender
In a qualitative study examining videotapes of primary care visits, compared to male physicians, women physicians were more "patient-centered" in their communication skills. The greatest amount of patient-centeredness was observed when female physicians interacted with female patients. On the flip side, compared to a female physician, obese men seen by a male physician were more likely to receive diet and exercise counseling.

From Bertakis and Azari, 2012; Pickett-Blakely et al, 2011.

Health Beliefs and Practices

The patient may have a view of health and illness and an approach to cure that are shaped by a particular cultural and/or faith belief or paradigm. If that view is "scientific," in the sense that a cause can be determined for every problem in a very precise way, the patient is more apt to be comfortable with Western approaches to health and medical care.

However, the scientific view is reductionist and looks to a very narrow, specific cause and effect. A more naturalistic or "holistic" approach broadens the context. It views our lives as part of a much greater whole (the entire cosmos) that must be in harmony. If the balance is disturbed, illness can result. The goal, then, is to retrieve balance and harmony. Aspects of this concept are evident among the beliefs of many Hispanics, Native Americans, Asians, and Middle Eastern groups, and they are increasingly evident in people of all ethnic groups in the United States today (Box 2-6). Other groups believe in the supernatural or forces of good and evil that determine individual fate. In such a context, illness may be thought of as a punishment for wrongdoing.

Clearly, there can be a confusing ambivalence in many of us, patient and health care provider alike, because our genuine faith-based or naturalistic beliefs may conflict with the options available for the treatment of illness. Consider, for example, a child with a broken bone, the result of an accident that occurred while the child was under the supervision of a babysitter. The first need is to tend the fracture. That done, there is a need to talk with the mother about the guilt she may feel because she was away working. She might think this accident must be God's punishment. It is important to be aware of, to respect, and to discuss without belittlement a belief that may vary from yours in a manner that may still allow you to offer your point of view. This can apply to the guilt of a parent and to the use of herbs, rituals, and religious artifacts. After all, the pharmacopoeia of Western medicine is replete with plants and herbs that we now call drugs

---

Box 2-6   The Balance of Life: The "Hot" and the "Cold"

A naturalistic or holistic approach often assumes that there are external factors—some good, some bad—that must be kept in balance if we are to remain well. The balance of "hot" and "cold" is a part of the belief system in many cultural groups (e.g., Middle Eastern, Asian, Southeast Asian, and Hispanic). To restore a disturbed balance, that is, to treat, requires the use of opposites (e.g., a "hot" remedy for a "cold" problem and vice versa). Different cultures may define "hot" and "cold" differently. It is not a matter of temperature, and the words used might vary: for example, the Chinese have named the forces yin (cold) and yang (hot). The bottom line: We cannot ignore the naturalistic view if many of our patients are to have appropriate care.

Hot and Cold Conditions and Their Corresponding Treatments

Cold Conditions	Hot Treatments	Hot Conditions	Cold Treatments
Conditions	*Foods*	*Conditions*	*Foods*
Cancer	Beef	Constipation	Barley water
Cold	Cereals	Diarrhea	Chicken
Earaches	Chili	Fever	Dairy products
Headaches	peppers	Infection	Fresh vegetables
Joint pain	Chocolate	Kidney	Fruits
Malaria	Eggs	problems	Honey
Menses	Goat's milk	Rash	Goat meat
Pneumonia	Liquor	Sore throat	Raisins
Stomach	Onions		
cramps	Peas		
Teething			
Tuberculosis			
	Medicines and Herbs		*Medicines and Herbs*
	Anise		Bicarbonate of
	Aspirin		soda
	Castor oil		Milk of Magnesia
	Cinnamon		Orange flower
	Cod liver oil		water
	Garlic		Sage
	Ginger root		
	Iron		
	Tobacco		
	Penicillin		
	Vitamins		

Modified from Purnell and Paulanka, 2008.

(see Clinical Pearl, "Complementary and Alternative Treatments for the Common Cold"). Our difficulty in understanding the belief of another does not invalidate its substance, nor does a patient's adherence to a particular belief preclude concurrent reliance on allopathic or osteopathic health practitioners.

Family Relationships

Family structure and the social organizations to which a patient belongs (e.g., faith-based organizations, clubs, and schools) are among the many imprinting and constraining cultural forces. The expectations of children and how they grow and develop are key in this regard and often culturally distinct. Determining these

---

Clinical Pearl

Complementary and Alternative Treatments for the Common Cold
Home-based remedies for common colds are widely used. In children, the following therapies may be effective: buckwheat honey, vapor rub, geranium, and zinc sulfate. In adults, *Echinacea purpurea*, geranium extract, and zinc gluconate may be effective. When asking about medications, always remember to ask about use of complementary and alternative therapies. Using a nonjudgmental approach, you may wish to start with the question, "What else have you tried?"

From Fashner et al, 2012.

---

family and social structures needs emphasis in the United States today, with its shift toward dual-income families, single-parent families, and a significant number of teenage pregnancies. The prevalence of divorce (nearly one for every two marriages) and the increasing involvement of fathers in child care in two-parent families suggest cultural shifts that need to be recognized.

One type of already known behavior may predict another type of behavior. For example, low-income urban mothers who take advantage of appropriate prenatal care generally take advantage of appropriate infant care, regardless of educational level (Van Berckelaer et al, 2011). Adolescents who are unsupervised after school are more likely to smoke, use alcohol and marijuana, perform poorly in school, be depressed, and take risks than are those who are well supervised (DeVore and Ginsburg, 2005). Being aware of this sequence of related behaviors is especially important because it may be unrelated to the integrity of the family structure, gender, or background. Parenting style and child-rearing practices like setting boundaries and expectations may also be culturally driven. Many adolescents and young adults find comfort in their families' cultural traditions and practices and benefit from their connectedness. In a large study of U.S. college students from immigrant families, compared to their peers, students who retained their heritage practices reported fewer health risk behaviors like substance use, unsafe sex, and

impaired driving (Schwartz et al, 2011). These examples remind us that one individual may belong to many subgroups and that the behaviors and attitudes of a subgroup—for example, the college student who remains connected to his cultural heritage—can override the impact of the cultural values of the larger group (e.g., college student peers engaged in risk-taking behaviors).

Diet and Nutritional Practices

Beliefs and practices related to food, as well as the social significance of food, play an obvious vital role in everyday life. Some of these beliefs of cultural and/or faith-based significance may have an impact on the care you provide to patients. An Orthodox Jewish patient will not take some medicines, particularly during a holiday period like Passover, because the preparation of a drug does not meet the religious rules for food during that time. The woman who is Muslim must respect Halal (prescribed diet), even throughout pregnancy. A Chinese person with hypertension and a salt-restricted diet may need to consider a limited use of monosodium glutamate (MSG) and soy sauce. Attitudes toward vitamins vary greatly, with or without scientific proof, in many of the subgroups in the United States. It is still possible to work out a mutually agreed upon management plan if the issues are recognized and freely discussed. This is possible, too, with attitudes toward home, herbal, and natural—complementary or alternative—therapies. Many will have benefit; others may be dangerous. For example, dietary supplements containing ephedra alkaloids may increase the risk of stroke (Keisler and Hosey, 2005), whereas other herbal preparations interact with prescribed medications.

Summing Up

As health care providers, we face a compelling need to meet each patient on his or her own terms and to resist forming a sense of the patient based on prior knowledge of the culture or cultures from which that patient comes. That knowledge should not be formative in arriving at conclusions; rather, we

---

Box 2-7 | **Communication**

This list of questions, derived over the years from our experience and multiple resources, illustrates the variation in human responses. Try not to be intimidated by the mass of "need to know" cultural issues, but begin reflecting on them as you work with patients to raise your cultural awareness.
- How important are nonverbal clues?
- Are moments of silence valued?
- Is touching to be avoided?
- Are handshakes, or even embracing, avoided or desired at meeting and parting?
- What is the attitude toward eye contact?
- Is there a greater than expected need for "personal space?"
- What is the verbal or nonverbal response if your suggestions are not understood?
- Is there candor in admitting lack of understanding?
- What are the attitudes concerning respect for self and for authority figures?

- What are the attitudes toward persons in other groups, such as minorities, majorities?
- What are the language preferences?
- What is the need for "chit-chat" before getting down to the primary concern?
- Is there a relaxed or rigid sense of time?
- What is the degree of trust of health care professionals?
- How easily are personal matters discussed?
- Is there, even with you, a wish to avoid discussing income and other family affairs?

Health Customs/Health Practices
- What is the degree of dependence on the health care system, for illness alone or also for preventive and health maintenance needs?
- What is generally expected of a health professional and what defines a "good one?"

Box 2-7 **Communication—cont'd**	
<ul><li>What defines health?</li><li>Are there particularly common folk practices?</li><li>Is there a greater (or lesser) inclination to invoke self-care and use home remedies?</li><li>Is there a particular suspicion or fear of hospitals?</li><li>What is the tendency to use alternative care approaches and/or herbal remedies exclusively or as a complement?</li><li>What are the tendencies to invoke the magical or metaphysical?</li><li>Who is ultimately responsible for outcomes, you or the patient?</li><li>Who is ultimately responsible for maintaining health, you or the patient?</li><li>Is there a particular fear of painful or intrusive testing?</li><li>Is there a tendency toward stoicism?</li><li>What is the dependence on prayer?</li><li>Is illness thought of as punishment and a means of penance?</li><li>Is there "shame" attached to illness?</li><li>What is the belief about the origins of illness?</li><li>Is illness thought to be preventable and, if so, how?</li><li>What is the attitude toward autopsy?</li><li>Does a belief in reincarnation mandate that the body be left intact?</li><li>Are there particular cultural cooking habits that can influence diagnosis or management?</li><li>Is the degree of modesty in both men and women more than you would generally expect?</li><li>Do women, considering modesty, need a much more cautious and protected approach than usual—for example, during the examination?</li></ul>	**Family, Friends, and the Workplace**<ul><li>How tightly organized (and multigenerational) is the family hierarchy?</li><li>How tight is the family?</li><li>Is social life extended beyond the family and, if so, to what degree?</li><li>Does the family tend to be matriarchal or patriarchal?</li><li>What are the relative roles of women and men?</li><li>Are there particular tasks assigned to individual genders—for example, who does the laundry, family finances, grocery shopping?</li><li>To what extent are older adults and other authority figures given deference, and how?</li><li>Who makes decisions for the family?</li><li>To what extent is power shared?</li><li>Who makes decisions for the children and adolescents?</li><li>How strongly are children valued?</li><li>Is there a greater value placed on one of the genders?</li><li>How much are self-reliance and personal discipline valued?</li><li>What is the work ethic?</li><li>What is the sense of obligation to the community?</li><li>How is education sought, from school, reading and/or experience?</li><li>What is the emphasis on tradition and ritual practice?</li></ul>

must draw on it to help make the questions we ask more constructively probing to avoid viewing the patient as a stereotype (Box 2-7).

You need to understand yourself well. Your involvement with any patient gives that interaction a unique quality and your contribution to that interaction, to some extent, makes it different from what it might have been with anyone else. Remember that your attitudes and prejudices, which are largely culturally derived, may interfere with your understanding of the patient, and increase the probability of non-conscious bias and stereotypic judgment. When you're able to adapt to the unique needs of your patients and display genuine curiosity about their beliefs and values, you will be making strides toward cultural competence.

It is not unusual to find tables of information about health care–related cultural attitudes for a variety of religious and ethnic groups in reference materials. Although this provides quick access to information about various population groups, our experience suggests that the rigid superficiality in this information often does not adequately describe the beliefs and attitudes of a particular individual. Our purpose in this chapter is to review many of the questions and frameworks that might be relevant as you prepare to meet your patients. Patient by patient, your insights will develop as you avoid stereotypes, consider the individual, and become increasingly culturally competent. View cultural competence as a lifelong journey and not a destination or endpoint in and of itself.

CHAPTER 3

Examination Techniques and Equipment

This chapter provides an overview of the techniques of inspection, palpation, percussion, and auscultation that are used throughout the physical examination. In addition, general use of the equipment for performing physical examination is discussed (Box 3-1). Specific details regarding utilization of techniques and equipment as they relate to specific parts of the examination can be found in the relevant chapters. This chapter also addresses special issues related to the physical examination process.

evolve *http://evolve.elsevier.com/Seidel*
• NCLEX Review Questions   • Student Checklist

Precautions to Prevent Infection

Because persons of all ages and backgrounds may be sources of infection, it is important to take proper precautions when examining patients. Standard Precautions are to be used for the care of all patients in any setting in which health care is delivered. These precautions are designed to reduce the risk of infection based on the principle that all blood, body fluids, secretions, excretions except sweat, nonintact skin, and mucous membranes may contain transmissible infectious agents. Standard Precautions include the following:

+ Hand hygiene
+ Personal protective equipment (PPE): use of gloves, gown, mask, eye protection, or face shield, depending on the anticipated exposure
+ Respiratory hygiene/cough etiquette
+ Safe injection practices
+ Use of sterile procedures for invasive procedures (e.g., lumbar puncture, pleuracentesis, thoracentesis, central line placement)
+ Equipment or items in the patient environment likely to have been contaminated with infectious body fluids must be handled in a manner to prevent transmission of infectious agents.

Guidelines for Standard Precautions are summarized in Table 3-1. Use precautions to protect yourself and patients.

A second tier of precautions, Transmission-Based Precautions, is designed for the care of specified patients who are known or suspected to be infected by epidemiologically important pathogens that are spread by airborne or droplet transmission or by contact with dry skin or contaminated surfaces. Further information regarding the recommendations for Transmission-Based Precautions can be obtained from the Centers for Disease Control and Prevention (Seigel et al, 2007).

Latex Allergy

The incidence of serious allergic reaction to latex has increased dramatically in recent years. Latex allergy occurs when the body's immune system reacts to proteins found in natural rubber latex. Latex products also contain added chemicals, such as antioxidants, that can cause irritant or delayed hypersensitivity reactions. Box 3-2 describes the different types of latex reactions.

Health care providers are at risk for developing latex allergy because of exposure to latex in the form of gloves and other equipment and supplies. Sensitization to the latex proteins occurs by direct skin or mucous membrane contact or through airborne exposure. Box 3-3 contains a summary of recommendations to protect you from latex exposure in the workplace. Also be aware that some patients who have had multiple procedures or surgeries performed are at higher risk for the development of latex allergy. Snapping off powder-filled latex gloves disperses latex molecules into the air and increases the chance for inhalation, putting those with latex allergy at risk for severe reactions.

Staying Well

The Vulnerability of the Health Professional

Health care providers do not have better immune systems than other people, although we sometimes behave as if we think we do. Nor are we invincible against the everyday work-related injuries. We stand a much better chance of staying well if we are scrupulous in protecting ourselves:

• Follow Standard Precautions.
• Use personal protective equipment (PPE) when appropriate.
• Minimize latex exposure.
• Use good body mechanics or lift devices in transferring or assisting patients into various positions. NO EXCEPTIONS!

Box 3-1 What Equipment Do You Need to Purchase?

Students are confronted by a large number and variety of pieces of equipment for physical examination. A commonly asked question is "What do I really need to buy?" The answer depends somewhat on where you will be practicing. If you are in a clinic setting, for example, wall-mounted ophthalmoscopes and otoscopes are provided. This is not necessarily true in a hospital setting.

The following list is intended only as a guideline to the equipment that you will use most often and should personally own. The price of stethoscopes, otoscopes, ophthalmoscopes, and blood pressure equipment can vary markedly. Different models, many with optional features, can affect the price. Because these pieces of equipment represent a significant monetary investment, evaluate the quality of the instrument, consider the manufacturer's warranty and support, and decide on the features that you will need.

- Stethoscope
- Ophthalmoscope or PanOptic ophthalmoscope
- Otoscope
- Blood pressure cuff and manometer
- Centimeter ruler
- Tape measure
- Reflex hammer
- Tuning forks: 500 to 1000 Hz for auditory screening; 100 to 400 Hz for vibratory sensation
- Penlight
- Near vision screening chart

Table 3-1 Recommendations for Application of Standard Precautions for the Care of All Patients in All Health Care Settings

Component	Recommendations
Hand hygiene	After touching blood, body fluids, secretions, excretions, contaminated items; immediately after removing gloves; between patient contacts
Personal protective equipment (PPE)	
Gloves	For touching blood, body fluids, secretions, excretions, contaminated items; for touching mucous membranes and nonintact skin
Gown	During procedures and patient-care activities when contact of clothing/exposed skin with blood/body fluids, secretions, and excretions is anticipated
Mask, eye protection (goggles), face shield*	During procedures and patient-care activities likely to generate splashes or sprays of blood, body fluids, secretions, especially suctioning, endotracheal intubation
Soiled patient-care equipment	Handle in a manner that prevents transfer of microorganisms to others and to the environment; wear gloves if visibly contaminated; perform hand hygiene.
Environmental control	Develop procedures for routine care, cleaning, and disinfection of environmental surfaces, especially frequently touched surfaces in patient-care areas.
Textiles and laundry	Handle in a manner that prevents transfer of microorganisms to others and to the environment.
Needles and other sharps	Do not recap, bend, break, or hand-manipulate used needles; if recapping is required, use a one-handed scoop technique only; use safety features when available; place used sharps in puncture-resistant container.
Patient resuscitation	Use mouthpiece, resuscitation bag, other ventilation devices to prevent contact with mouth and oral secretions.
Patient placement	Prioritize for single-patient room if patient is at increased risk of transmission, is likely to contaminate the environment, does not maintain appropriate hygiene, or is at increased risk of acquiring infection or developing adverse outcome following infection.
Respiratory hygiene/cough etiquette (source containment of infectious respiratory secretions in symptomatic patients, beginning at initial point of encounter, e.g., triage and reception areas in emergency departments and physician offices)	Instruct symptomatic persons to cover mouth/nose when sneezing/coughing; use tissues and dispose in no-touch receptacle; observe hand hygiene after soiling of hands with respiratory secretions; wear surgical mask if tolerated or maintain spatial separation, >3 feet if possible.

From Seigel et al, 2007.

*During aerosol-generating procedures on patients with suspected or proven infections transmitted by respiratory aerosols, wear a fit-tested N95 or higher respirator in addition to gloves, gown, and face/eye protection.

Box 3-2 Types of Latex Reactions

Irritant contact dermatitis—Chemical irritation that does not involve the immune system. Symptoms are usually dry, itching, irritated areas on the skin, typically the hands.

Type IV dermatitis (delayed hypersensitivity)—Allergic contact dermatitis that involves the immune system and is caused by the chemicals used in latex products. The skin reaction usually begins 24 to 48 hours after contact and resembles that caused by poison ivy. The reaction may progress to oozing skin blisters.

Type I systemic reactions—True allergic reaction caused by protein antibodies (IgE antibodies) that form as a result of interaction between a foreign protein and the body's immune system. The antigen-antibody reaction causes release of histamine, leukotrienes, prostaglandins, and kinins. These chemicals cause the symptoms of allergic reactions. Type I reactions include the following symptoms: local urticaria (skin wheals), generalized urticaria with angioedema (tissue swelling), asthma, eye/nose itching, gastrointestinal symptoms, anaphylaxis (cardiovascular collapse), chronic asthma, and permanent lung damage.

Box 3-3 Summary of Recommendations for Workers to Prevent Latex Allergy

- Use nonlatex gloves for activities not likely to involve infectious materials. Hypoallergenic gloves are not necessarily latex free, but they may reduce reactions to chemical additives in the latex.
- For barrier protection when handling infectious materials, use powder-free latex gloves with reduced protein content.
- When wearing latex gloves, do not use oil-based hand creams or lotions unless they have been shown to reduce latex-related problems.
- After removing gloves, wash hands with mild soap and dry thoroughly.
- Use good housekeeping practices to remove latex-containing dust from the workplace.
- Take advantage of all latex allergy education and training provided.
- If you develop symptoms of latex allergy, avoid direct contact with latex gloves and products until you can see a health care provider experienced in treating latex allergy.

From DHHS (NIOSH) Publication Number 98-113, 1998. www.cdc.gov/niosh/docs/98-113.

Examination Technique

Patient Positions and Draping

Most of the physical examination is conducted with the patient in seated and supine positions. Other positions are used for specific aspects of the examination. Special positioning requirements are discussed in the relevant chapters.

Seated. When seated, position the drape to cover the patient's lap and legs. You can move it to uncover parts of the body as they are examined.

Supine. In the supine position, the patient lies on his or her back, with arms at the sides and legs extended. The drape should cover the patient from chest to knees or toes. Again, you can move or reposition the drape to give appropriate exposure.

Prone. The patient lies on his or her stomach. This position may be used for special maneuvers as part of the musculoskeletal examination. Drape the patient to cover the torso.

Dorsal Recumbent. This position may be used for examination of the genital or rectal areas. The patient lies supine with knees bent and feet flat on the table. Place the drape in a diamond position from chest to toes. Wrap each leg with the corresponding lateral corner of the "diamond." Turn back the distal corner of the drape to perform the examination.

Lateral Recumbent. This is a side-lying position, with legs extended or flexed. The left lateral recumbent position (patient's left side is down) may be used in listening to heart sounds or palpating the spleen.

Lithotomy. The lithotomy position is generally used for the pelvic examination. Variations of positioning are discussed in Chapter 18. Begin with the patient in the dorsal recumbent position, with feet at the corners of the table. Help the patient to stabilize her feet in the stirrups and slide her buttocks down to the edge of the table. Drape in the diamond position as with the dorsal recumbent position.

Sims. The Sims position can be used for examination of the rectum or obtaining rectal temperature. The patient starts in a lateral recumbent position. The torso is rolled toward a prone position; the top leg is flexed sharply at the hips and knee and the bottom leg is flexed slightly. Drape the patient from shoulders to toes.

Inspection

Inspection is the process of observation. Your eyes and nose are sensitive tools for gathering data throughout the examination (Box 3-4). Take time to practice and develop this skill. Challenge yourself to see how much information you can collect through inspection alone. As the patient enters the room, observe the gait and stance and the ease or difficulty with which undressing and getting onto the examining table are accomplished. These observations alone will reveal a great deal about the patient's neurologic and musculoskeletal integrity. Is eye contact made? Is the demeanor appropriate for the situation? Is the clothing appropriate for the weather? The answers to these questions provide clues to the patient's emotional and mental status. Color and moisture of the skin or an unusual odor can alert you to the possibility of underlying disease. These preliminary observations require only a few seconds, yet they provide basic information that can influence the rest of the examination.

Inspection—unlike palpation, percussion, and auscultation—can continue throughout the history-taking process and during the physical examination. With this kind of continuity, observations about the patient can constantly be modified until a complete picture is created. Be aware of both the patient's verbal statements and body language right up to the end of the

Box 3-4 The Sense of Smell: The Nose as an Aid to Physical Examination

The first observation when entering an examining room may be an odor, obvious and pervasive. A foreign body that has been present in a child's nose may cause this. Distinctive odors provide clues leading to the diagnosis of certain conditions, some of which need early detection if life-threatening sequelae are to be avoided. However, do not rush to premature diagnosis. Appreciate these odors for what they are—clues that must be followed up with additional investigation. Examples of odor clues follow:

Condition	Source of Odor	Type of Odor
Inborn errors of metabolism	Phenylketonuria	Mousy
	Tyrosinemia	Fishy
Infectious diseases	Tuberculosis	Stale beer
	Diphtheria	Sweetish
Ingestions of poison or intoxication	Cyanide	Bitter almond
	Chloroform and salicylates	Fruity
Physiologic nondisease states	Sweaty feet	Cheesy
Foreign bodies (e.g., in the nose or vagina)	Organic material (e.g., bead in a child's nose)	Foul-smelling discharge

The odors may range from objectionable to bland to rather pleasant. The examiner often is the one to determine the characterization of the odor.

From Kippenberger et al, 2012.

Table 3-2 Areas of the Hand to Use in Palpation

To Determine	Use
Position, texture, size, consistency, fluid, crepitus, form of a mass, or structure	Palmar surface of the fingers and finger pads
Vibration	Ulnar surfaces of hand and fingers
Temperature	Dorsal surface of hand

Knowing what to look for is, of course, essential to the process of focused attention. Be willing to validate inspection findings with your patient. The ability to narrow or widen your perceptual field selectively will come with time and experience, but the process must begin right now and will develop only through practice.

Palpation

Palpation involves the use of the hands and fingers to gather information through the sense of touch. Certain parts of your hands and fingers are better than others for specific types of palpation (Table 3-2). The palmar surface of the fingers and finger pads is more sensitive than the fingertips. Use this surface whenever discriminatory touch is needed for determining position, texture, size, consistency, masses, fluid, and crepitus. The ulnar surface of the hand and fingers is the most sensitive area for distinguishing vibration. The dorsal surface of the hands is best for estimating temperature. Of course, this estimate provides only a crude measure—use it to compare temperature differences among parts of the body.

Specific techniques of palpation are discussed in more detail as they occur in each part of the examination (see Clinical Pearl, "Right-Sided Examination?"). Palpation may be either light or deep and is controlled by the amount of pressure applied with the fingers or hand. Short fingernails are essential to avoid discomfort or injury to the patient

encounter. The stance, stride, firmness of handshake, and eye contact can tell you a great deal about the patient's perception of the encounter (see Clinical Pearl, "The Handshake").

Clinical Pearl

The Handshake
Although a nice gesture (coupled with appropriate hand washing), we need to be careful not to harm our patients by squeezing too tightly, especially those patients with conditions that may involve their hands—rheumatoid arthritis or osteoarthritis, for example.

Some general guidelines will be helpful as you proceed through the examination and inspect each area of the body. Adequate lighting is essential. The primary lighting can be either daylight or artificial light, as long as the light is direct enough to reveal color, texture, and mobility without distortion from shadowing. Secondary, tangential lighting from a lamp that casts shadows is also important for observing contour and variations in the body surface. Inspection should be unhurried. Give yourself time to carefully observe what you are inspecting. Pay attention to detail and note your findings. An important rule to remember is that you have to expose what you want to inspect. All too often, necessary exposure is compromised for modesty at the cost of important information. Part of your job is to look and observe critically.

Clinical Pearl

Right-Sided Examination?
It is the convention, at least in the United States, to teach students to examine patients from the right side and to palpate and percuss with the right hand. We have continued with this convention, if only to simplify description of a procedure or technique. We feel no obligation to adhere strictly to the right-sided approach. Our suggestion is that students learn to use both hands for examination and that they be allowed to stand on either side of the patient, depending on both the patient's and examiner's convenience and comfort. The important issue is to develop an approach that is useful and practical and yields the desired results.

Touch is in many ways therapeutic, and palpation is the actuality of the "laying on of hands." Our advice that your approach be gentle and your hands warm is not only practical but also symbolic of your respect for the patient and for the privilege the patient gives you.

EXAMINATION TECHNIQUE

Table 3-3 | **Percussion Tones**

Tone	Intensity	Pitch	Duration	Quality	Example Where Heard
Tympanic	Loud	High	Moderate	Drumlike	Gastric bubble
Hyperresonant	Very loud	Low	Long	Boomlike	Emphysematous lungs
Resonant	Loud	Low	Long	Hollow	Healthy lung tissue
Dull	Soft to moderate	Moderate to high	Moderate	Thudlike	Over liver
Flat	Soft	High	Short	Very dull	Over muscle

Percussion

Percussion involves striking one object against another to produce vibration and subsequent sound waves. In the physical examination, your finger functions as a hammer, and the impact of the finger against underlying tissue produces the vibration. Sound waves are heard as percussion tones (called *resonance*) that arise from vibrations 4 to 6 cm deep in the body tissue. The density of the medium through which the sound waves travel determines the degree of percussion tone. The more dense the medium, the quieter the percussion tone. The percussion tone over air is loud, over fluid less loud, and over solid areas soft. The degree of percussion tone is classified and ordered as listed in Table 3-3 and as follows:

+ Tympany
+ Hyperresonance
+ Resonance
+ Dullness
+ Flatness

Tympany is the loudest, and flatness is the quietest. Quantification of the percussion tone is difficult, especially for the beginner. For points of reference, as noted in Table 3-3, the gastric bubble is considered to be tympanic; air-filled lungs (as in emphysema) to be hyperresonant; healthy lungs to be resonant; the liver to be dull; and muscle to be flat. Degree of percussion is more easily distinguished by listening to the sound change as you move from one area to another. Because it is easier to hear the change from resonance to dullness (rather than from dullness to resonance), proceed with percussion from areas of resonance to areas of dullness. A partially full milk carton is a good tool for practicing percussion skills. Begin with percussion over the air-filled space of the carton, appreciating its resonant quality. Work your way downward and listen for the change in sound as you encounter the milk. This principle applies in percussion of body tissues and cavities.

The techniques of percussion are the same regardless of the structure you are percussing. Immediate (direct) percussion involves striking the finger or hand directly against the body. Most health care providers use indirect or mediate percussion. In this technique the finger of one hand acts as the hammer (plexor) and a finger of the other hand acts as the striking surface. To perform indirect percussion, place your nondominant hand on the surface of the body with the fingers slightly spread. Place the distal phalanx of the middle finger firmly on the body surface with the other fingers slightly elevated off the surface. Snap the wrist of your other hand downward, and with the tip of the

FIGURE 3-1 Percussion technique: tapping the interphalangeal joint. Only the middle finger of the examiner's nondominant hand should be in contact with the patient's skin surface.

middle finger, sharply tap the interphalangeal joint of the finger that is on the body surface (Fig. 3-1). You may tap just distal to the interphalangeal joint if you choose, but decide on one and be consistent because the sound varies from one to the other. Percussion must be performed against bare skin. If you are not able to hear the percussion tone, try pressing harder against the patient's skin with your finger that lies on the body surface. Failing to press firmly enough is a common error. On the other hand, pressing too hard on an infant or very young chest can obscure the sound.

Several points are essential in developing the technique of percussion. The downward snap of the striking finger originates from the wrist and not the forearm or shoulder. Tap sharply and rapidly; once the finger has struck, snap the wrist back, quickly lifting the finger to prevent dampening the sound. Use the tip and not the pad of the plexor finger (hence short fingernails are again a necessity). Percuss one location several times to facilitate interpretation of the tone. Like other techniques, percussion requires practice to obtain the skill needed to produce the desired result. Box 3-5 describes common percussion errors. In learning to distinguish between the tones, it may be helpful to close your eyes to block out other sensory stimuli, concentrating exclusively on the tone you are hearing.

You can also use your fist for percussion. Fist percussion is most commonly used to elicit tenderness arising from the liver, gallbladder, or kidneys. In this technique, use the ulnar aspect of the fist to deliver a firm blow to the area. Too gentle a blow will

Box 3-5 | **Common Percussion Errors**

Percussion requires practice. In learning percussion, beginning health care providers often make the following errors:
- Failing to exert firm pressure with the finger placed on the skin surface
- Failing to separate the hammer finger from other fingers
- Snapping downward from the elbow or shoulder rather than from the wrist
- Tapping by moving just the hammer finger rather than the whole hand
- Striking with the finger pad rather than the fingertip of the hammer finger
- Failing to trim the fingernail of the hammer finger

not produce enough force to stimulate the tenderness, but too much force can cause unnecessary discomfort, even in a well patient. The force of a direct blow can be mediated by use of a second hand placed over the area. Practice on yourself or a colleague until you achieve the desired middle ground.

Auscultation

Auscultation involves listening for sounds produced by the body. Some sounds, such as speech, are audible to the unassisted ear. Most others require a stethoscope to augment the sound. Specific types of stethoscopes, their use, and desired characteristics are discussed later in the section on stethoscopes.

Although what you are listening for will depend on the specific part of the examination, there are some general principles that apply to all auscultatory procedures. The environment should be quiet and free from distracting noises. Place the stethoscope on the naked skin, because clothing obscures the sound. Listen not only for the presence of sound but also its characteristics: intensity, pitch, duration, and quality. The sounds are often subtle or transitory, and you must listen intently to hear the nuances. Closing your eyes may prevent distraction by visual stimuli and narrow your perceptual field to help you focus on the sound. Try to target and isolate each sound, concentrating on one sound at a time. Take enough time to identify all the characteristics of each sound. Auscultation should be carried out last, except with the abdominal examination, after other techniques have provided information that will assist in interpreting what you hear (see Clinical Pearl, "Unexpected Findings").

Clinical Pearl

Unexpected Findings
Respect your judgment and your instinct when you identify a physical examination finding you had not expected to find. Pay attention when this occurs, even if it does not seem to make sense or you cannot explain it easily. The flip side—not finding a previously documented "abnormal" finding—may simply be a learning opportunity, or it may reflect a change in the patient's condition. It is OK to say "I couldn't hear that" or "I'm not sure I felt that." If in doubt have someone else check it with you.

One of the most difficult achievements in auscultation is learning to isolate sounds. You cannot hear everything all at once. Whether it is a breath sound, or a heartbeat, or the sequence of respirations and heartbeats, each segment of the cycle must be isolated and listened to specifically. After the individual sounds are identified, they are put together. Do not anticipate the next sound; concentrate on the one at hand. Auscultation of the lungs is discussed in Chapter 13, of the heart in Chapter 14, and of the abdomen in Chapter 17.

Modifications for Patients with Disabilities

Each disability affects each person differently; therefore, it is important for health care providers to educate themselves about relevant aspects of a patient's disability. Sensitivity in asking only pertinent questions about the disability will increase the patient's comfort and cooperation.

Keep some considerations in mind about the environment and the encounter. Speak directly to the patient. Often people will address a disabled person's spouse, friend, an attendant, or an interpreter instead of speaking directly to the person. Remove or rearrange the furnishings in the examination room to provide space, such as that needed for a wheelchair. Take the paper covering off the examination table if it is a bother during transfers and positioning. Equipment such as a high-low examination table or a particularly wide examination table or a slide board can be obtained to facilitate safer, easier transfers and positioning. Obstetric or foot stirrups can be padded or equipped with a strap to increase the patient's comfort and safety during a pelvic examination. For the pelvic examination, a woman can wear an easily removable skirt or pair of pants. A button-up or zippered shirt will facilitate the breast examination. It is appropriate to suggest to your patient or the caregiver that such clothing be worn for future visits.

Patients with Mobility Impairments

The patient is the expert in transferring from the wheelchair or in using assistants to climb onto the examination table. Transfers are relatively simple if the patient, assistant, and health care provider all understand the method that will best suit the patient's disability, the room space, and the examination table (Box 3-6). You need to know your own physical limits for lifting or moving a patient—always seek assistance if uncertain. This will avoid falls and injuries to both you and the patient.

Pivot Transfer. Stand in front of the patient, take the patient's knees between your own knees, grasp the patient around the back and under the arms, raise the patient to a vertical position, and then pivot from wheelchair to the table. The examination table must be low enough for the patient to sit on; therefore, a hydraulic high-low table may be needed when using this transfer method.

Cradle Transfer. While bending or squatting beside the patient put one arm under both of the patient's knees and the other arm around the back and under the armpits. Stand and carry the patient to the table.

Box 3-6   Transfer Guidelines

Guidelines for the Assistant

The patient/parent/caregiver should direct the transfer and positioning process.

Assistants should not overestimate their ability to lift.

Keep in mind that not all nonambulatory patients need assistance.

Assistants should keep their backs straight, bend their knees, and lift with their legs.

It may be helpful to perform a test lift or to practice the transfer by lifting the patient just over the wheelchair before attempting a complete transfer.

Assistants who feel that they may drop a patient during a transfer should not panic. It is important, whenever possible, to explain what is happening to reassure the patient throughout the situation. Assistants will usually have time to lower the patient safely to the floor until they can get additional help.

Guidelines for the Patient

Explain clearly the preferred transfer method and direct the health care provider and assistants during the process.

Assistants can help by preparing equipment. Because many people are not familiar with wheelchairs or supportive devices, the patient may need to explain to the health care providers and assistants how they can handle belongings. Patients who use wheelchairs should explain how to apply the brakes, detach the footrests and armrests, or turn off the motor of an electric wheelchair. Have the patient who wears adaptive devices (e.g., leg braces or supportive undergarments) explain how to remove them, if necessary, and where to put them if the patient cannot do so.

Patients who use urinary equipment should direct assistants in the moving or straightening of catheter tubing. The patient may wish to unstrap the leg bag and place it on the table beside or across the abdomen for proper drainage while supine. Assistants should be reminded not to pull on the tubing or allow kinks to develop.

Have the patient inform the health care provider and assistants when he or she is comfortable and balanced after the transfer is completed.

All parties should be aware of jewelry, clothing, tubing, or equipment that might catch or otherwise interfere with the transfer.

Two-Person Transfer. In all two-person transfers, the assistants must be careful to work together to lift the patient over the arms of the wheelchair from a sitting position onto the examination table. A stronger, taller person should always lift the upper half of the patient's body.

+ *Method 1* requires the patient to fold the arms across the chest. The assistant standing behind the patient kneels down, putting his or her elbows under the patient's armpits, and grasps the patient's opposite wrists. The second assistant lifts and supports the patient under the knees.
+ *Method 2* can be used if the patient cannot fold the arms. The assistant standing behind the patient puts his or her own hands together around the patient, if possible, so there is less likelihood of losing hold of the patient. The second assistant lifts and supports the patient under the knees.

+ *Cradle Transfer*—a variation of the one-person cradle transfer. Two assistants grasp each other's arms behind the patient's back and under the knees and then stand and carry the patient to the table.

Equipment. Some persons with mobility impairments use a slide board, which forms a bridge to slide across from the wheelchair to the examination table. For this method to work, the table and chair must be approximately the same height. Most examination tables, however, are quite a bit higher than wheelchairs. Some examining rooms have high-low examination tables that can be adjusted to a height that will facilitate the safest and easiest transfer. A wider table, even if it is not adjustable in height, can also make transfers and positioning easier.

Patients with Sensory Impairment

At the beginning of the visit by a patient with a hearing or speech impairment, discuss the communication system that will be used (e.g., a sign language interpreter, word board, or talk box). Specialized educational materials (e.g., Braille or audio-taped information, or three-dimensional anatomic models) can be acquired to make information accessible to sensory-impaired patients.

Impaired Vision. Remember to identify yourself upon entering the examination room and inform the patient when you are leaving the room. A red-tipped white cane and guide animal are mobility aids used by many persons with visual impairments. If a patient is accompanied by a guide animal, do not pet or distract the animal, which is trained to respond only to its owner. A patient may prefer to keep the guide animal or white cane nearby in the examination room. Do not move either of these without the patient's permission. Before the examination, ask whether the patient would like to examine any equipment or instruments that will be used during the examination. If three-dimensional models are available, they can be used to acquaint the patient with the examination process (e.g., with the genital examination). During the examination, the patient may feel more at ease if you maintain continuous tactile or verbal contact (e.g., by keeping a hand on the arm or by narrating what is taking place during the examination).

Some patients with visual impairments will want to be oriented to their surroundings, whereas others may not. Each should be encouraged to specify the kind of orientation and assistance needed. Verbally describe and assist the patient in locating where to put the clothes, where the various furnishings are positioned, how to approach the examination table, and how to get positioned on the table.

Impaired Hearing or Speech. The patient should choose which form of communication to use during the examination (e.g., a sign language interpreter, lipreading, or writing). Although a patient may use an interpreter throughout most of the visit, she or he may decide not to use the interpreter during parts of the actual examination. If an interpreter is used, you and the patient should decide where the interpreter should stand or sit. When working with an interpreter, speak at a regular speed and directly to the patient instead of to the interpreter. If a patient wishes to lip-read, be careful not to move your face out of sight of the patient without first explaining what you are doing. Look directly at the patient and enunciate words clearly. Some patients may wish to view a pelvic examination with a mirror while it is happening.

Special Concerns for Patients with Spinal Cord Injury or Lesion

Bowel and bladder concerns and other conditions such as hyperreflexia, hypersensitivity, and spasticity should be given special attention during the examination process.

Bowel and Bladder Concerns. Some patients do not have voluntary bladder or bowel movements. A bladder or bowel routine could affect the pelvic or rectal examination. The physical stimulation of a speculum, bimanual, or rectal examination can mimic the stimulation for the bowel routine and cause a bowel movement during the examination. An indwelling catheter need not be removed during the examination unless it is not working; if it is removed, another catheter should be available for insertion. If a woman is catheterized, it is not necessary to remove the catheter during the pelvic examination because it will not interfere in any way.

If a patient uses intermittent catheterization to manually open the bladder sphincter at regular intervals during the day, tactile stimulation in the pelvic area during the examination could cause the bladder sphincter to open and produce incontinence.

Autonomic Hyperreflexia. Autonomic hyperreflexia, also called dysreflexia, is a potentially life-threatening condition associated with spinal cord injury. Symptoms include severe high blood pressure, sweating, blotchy skin, nausea, or goose bumps due to stimulation of the bowel, bladder, or skin below the spinal lesion. Some causes of hyperreflexia that may occur during the physical examination include reactions to a cold, hard examination table or cold stirrups; insertion and manipulation of a speculum; pressure during the bimanual or rectal examination; or tactile contact with hypersensitive areas. If the patient experiences hyperreflexic high blood pressure, identify and remove the source of the stimulation. Once the hyperreflexia ceases, you and the patient should mutually decide whether to continue the examination. If the examination is continued and hyperreflexia recurs, stop the examination and reschedule for another time. If the blood pressure does not decrease with removal of stimulus, or if the hyperreflexic symptoms persist and lead to a throbbing headache or nasal obstruction, treat the situation as a medical emergency. Do not leave a patient experiencing any degree of hyperreflexia unaccompanied.

Hypersensitivity. To help prevent possible discomfort or spasms, ask the patient about hypersensitive areas of the body before the examination. Some patients may experience variable responses (e.g., spasms or pain) to ordinary tactile stimulation. Often, you can avoid sensitive areas or use an extra amount of lubricant jelly to decrease friction or pressure.

Spasticity. Spasms may range from slight tremors to quick, violent contractions. Spasms may occur during a transfer, while assuming an awkward or uncomfortable position, or from stimulation of the skin with an instrument. If spasm occurs during the examination, gently support the area (usually a leg, an arm, or the abdominal region) to avoid any injury to the patient. Allow the spasms to resolve before continuing the examination. A feeling of physical security can decrease spasm intensity or frequency. A patient who experiences spasms should never be left alone on the examination table. Have an assistant stand near the examination table and maintain physical contact with the patient to provide a feeling of safety.

Equipment

Weight Scales and Height Measurement Devices

Height and weight of adults are measured on a standing platform scale with a height attachment. The scale uses a system of adding and subtracting weight in increments as small as ¼ lb or 0.1 kg to counterbalance the weight placed on the scale platform. Manually calibrate the scale each time it is used to ensure its accuracy.

For manual scales, calibrate the scale to zero before the patient mounts the platform by moving both the large and small weights to zero. Level and steady the balance beam by adjusting the calibrating knob. Pull up the height attachment, before the patient steps on the scale, and then position the headpiece at the patient's crown (Fig. 3-2). Place a paper towel on the platform before the patient steps on it to avoid the potential transmission of organisms from bare feet.

FIGURE 3-2 Platform scale with height attachment.

With electronic scales, weight is calculated electronically and provided as a digital readout. These scales are automatically calibrated each time they are used. Always note what the patient is wearing—adults and older children should wear lightweight clothing for more accurate measurement

The infant platform scale is used for measuring weights of infants and small children (Fig. 3-3). It works the same as the adult scale but can measure in ounces or grams. The scale has a platform with curved sides in which the child may sit or lie. Place paper under the child, and never leave the child unattended on the scale. Weigh the infant either nude or with only a diaper for accuracy of weight.

FIGURE 3-4 Devices used to measure length of an infant. **A,** Infant length board. **B,** Measure mat. *(A, Courtesy Perspective Enterprises, Inc., Portage, MI. B, Courtesy Seca North America, Medical Scales and Measuring Systems, Seca Corp.)*

Once a child is able to stand erect without support, use a stadiometer, a stature-measuring device, to measure height. The device consists of a movable headpiece attached to a rigid measurement bar and platform. Standing height is measured barefoot. With the child standing with the shoulders, buttocks, and heels against the wall, lower the head piece to the crown of the child's head (Fig. 3-5).

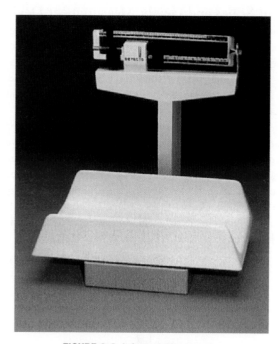

FIGURE 3-3 Infant platform scale.

Infant lengths can be measured by using an infant measuring device that comes with a rigid headboard and movable footboard (Fig. 3-4, *A*). An alternative to the rigid measuring device is a commercially available measure mat, consisting of a soft rubber graduated mat attached to a plastic headboard and footboard (Fig. 3-4, *B*). Place the measuring board on the table so that the headboard and footboard are perpendicular to the table. Position the infant supine on the measuring board with the head against the headboard and knees held straight. Move the footboard until it touches the bottom of the infant's feet. The baby's length can be read in either inches or centimeters. Be sure to clean the mat between uses.

An infant can also be measured by placing the baby on a pad, putting one pin into the pad at the top of the head and another at the heel of the extended leg. Then measure the length from pin to pin. The same technique can be used with a marking pen if the infant is lying on a disposable paper sheet.

FIGURE 3-5 Device used to measure height of a child. *(Courtesy Perspective Enterprises, Portage, MI.)*

FIGURE 3-6 Devices for electronic temperature measurement. **A,** Rectal, oral, or axillary thermometer. **B** and **C,** Tympanic membrane thermometers.

Thermometer

Electronic temperature measurement has decreased the time required for accurate temperature readings. One piece of equipment that contains an electronic sensing probe can be used for measurement of rectal, oral, and axillary temperatures (Fig. 3-6, *A*). The probe, covered by a disposable sheath, is placed under the tongue with the mouth tightly closed, in the rectum, or in the axillary space with the arm held close to the torso. A temperature reading (in either Fahrenheit or Celsius) is revealed on a liquid crystal display (LCD) screen within 15 to 60 seconds, depending on the model used.

The measurements obtained from tympanic thermometers vary somewhat from those obtained by oral or rectal routes (Fig. 3-6, *B* and *C*). In some situations, as with very young infants, traditional routes of measurement may be more accurate; in other situations, such as with children in an outpatient setting, the tympanic route is preferred. A systematic review of the evidence suggests that tympanic thermometry provides the best means of measuring temperature in children ages 2 months to 16 years both in and out of the hospital (Dew, 2006).

For tympanic membrane temperature measurement, a specially designed probe similar in shape to an otoscope is required. Gently place the covered probe tip at the external opening of the ear canal. Do not try to force the probe into the canal or to occlude it. Infrared technology provides a temperature reading on the LCD screen in approximately 2 seconds. Ear temperature reflects the body's temperature because the tympanic membrane shares its blood supply with the hypothalamus in the brain.

Infrared axillary thermometers for neonates are available. A recessed reflective cup on the probe protects the measurement from the effects of external heat sources, making these thermometers suitable for use in incubators and under radiant warmers or phototherapy lights.

Stethoscope

Auscultation of most sounds requires a stethoscope. Three basic types are available: acoustic, magnetic, and electronic.

The acoustic stethoscope is a closed cylinder that transmits sound waves from their source and along its column to the ear

FIGURE 3-7 Acoustic stethoscope.

(Fig. 3-7). Its rigid diaphragm has a natural frequency of around 300 Hz. It screens out low-pitched sounds and best transmits high-pitched sounds such as the second heart sound. The bell end piece has a natural frequency that varies with the amount of pressure exerted. It transmits low-pitched sounds when very light pressure is used. With firm pressure, the skin converts it to a diaphragm end piece. The chest piece contains a closure valve so that only one end piece, either the diaphragm or bell, is operational at any one time (thus preventing inadvertent dissipation of sound waves).

The stereophonic stethoscope, a type of acoustic stethoscope, is used to differentiate between the right and left auscultatory sounds using a two-channel design (Fig. 3-8). With a single tube, diaphragm, and bell, it looks and functions like an acoustic stethoscope. However, the right and left ear tubes are independently connected to right and left semicircular microphones in the chest piece.

The magnetic stethoscope has a single end piece that is a diaphragm. It contains an iron disk on the interior surface; behind this is a permanent magnet. A strong spring keeps the diaphragm bowed outward when it is not compressed against a

FIGURE 3-8 Stereophonic stethoscope. Note divided bell and diaphragm.

FIGURE 3-9 Position the stethoscope between the index and middle fingers against the patient's bare skin.

body surface. Compression of the diaphragm activates the air column as magnetic attraction is established between the iron disk and the magnet. Rotation of a dial adjusts for high-, low-, and full-frequency sounds.

The electronic stethoscope picks up vibrations transmitted to the surface of the body and converts them into electrical impulses. The impulses are amplified and transmitted to a speaker, where they are reconverted to sound. Newer versions of the electronic stethoscope can also provide additional features such as extended listening ranges, digital readout, sound recording and storage, playback, and electronic device linkage.

The most commonly used is the acoustic stethoscope, which comes in several models. The ability to auscultate accurately depends in part on the quality of the instrument, so it is important that the stethoscope have the following characteristics:
+ The diaphragm and bell are heavy enough to lie firmly on the body surface.
+ The diaphragm cover is rigid.
+ The bell is large enough in diameter to span an intercostal space in an adult and deep enough so that it will not fill with tissue.
+ The bell and diaphragm are pediatric-sized for use in children
+ A rubber or plastic ring is around the bell edges to ensure secure contact with the body surface.
+ The tubing is thick, stiff, and heavy; this conducts better than thin, elastic, or very flexible tubing.
+ The length of the tubing is between 30.5 and 40 cm (12 and 18 inches) to minimize distortion.
+ The earpieces fit snugly and comfortably. Some instruments have several sizes of earpieces and some have hard and soft earpieces. The determining factors are how they fit and feel to the examiner. The earpieces should be large enough to occlude the auditory canal, thus blocking outside sound. If

they are too small, they will slip into the ear canal and be painful.
+ Angled binaurals point the earpieces toward the nose so that sound is projected toward the tympanic membrane.

To stabilize the stethoscope when it is in place, hold the end piece between the fingers, pressing the diaphragm firmly against the skin (Fig. 3-9). The diaphragm piece should never be used without the diaphragm. Because the bell functions by picking up vibrations, it must be positioned so that the vibrations are not dampened. Place the bell evenly and lightly on the skin, making sure there is skin contact around the entire edge. To prevent extraneous noise, do not touch the tubing with your hands or allow the tubing to rub against any surfaces.

Sphygmomanometer

Blood pressure is measured indirectly with a stethoscope and either an aneroid or mercury sphygmomanometer. Electronic sphygmomanometers, which do not require the use of a stethoscope, are also available. Each sphygmomanometer is composed of a cuff with an inflatable bladder, a pressure manometer, and a rubber hand bulb with a pressure control valve to inflate and deflate the bladder. The electronic sphygmomanometer senses vibrations and converts them into electric impulses. The impulses are transmitted to a device that translates them into a digital readout. The instrument is relatively sensitive and is also capable of simultaneously measuring the pulse rate. It does not, however, indicate the quality, rhythm, and other characteristics of a pulse and should not be used in place of your touch in assessing pulse.

Pulse Oximeter

Pulse oximetry measures the percentage of hemoglobin saturated with oxygen (oxyhemoglobin). Oxygen saturation is a measure of how much oxygen the blood is carrying as a percentage of the maximum it could carry. A sensor attached to a digit or earlobe has two light-emitting diodes, one that sends out invisible infrared light and one that sends out red light. Oxygenated hemoglobin absorbs more infrared light and allows more red light to pass through. Deoxygenated hemoglobin absorbs more red light and allows more infrared light to pass through. The ratio of the

FIGURE 3-10 Pulse oximeter monitor and sensor. *(Image used by permission from Nellcor Puritan Bennett LLC, Boulder, CO, part of Covidien.)*

FIGURE 3-11 Doppler.

absorption is used to calculate the oxy/deoxyhemoglobin ratio. The difference between the two gives a measure of the fraction of the oxyhemoglobin in the blood. The readout displays the result as a percentage.

Pulse oximetry requires a reasonably translucent site with good blood flow. Typical adult/pediatric sites are the finger, toe, pinna (top) or lobe of the ear. Infant sites are the foot or palm of the hand and the big toe or thumb (Fig. 3-10). The oximeter detects the slight change in color of the arterial blood caused by the beat of the heart when blood is pushed into the finger (or earlobe or toe). Because the change in color is so minute, it is imperative to ensure a strong pulse during testing. When the pulse is weak, the results may be inaccurate.

Doppler

Some sounds are so difficult to auscultate that a regular stethoscope will not suffice. Dopplers are useful at these times (Fig. 3-11). Dopplers are ultrasonic stethoscopes that detect blood flow rather than amplify sounds, and they vary in frequency from 2 to 10 MHz. The use of a Doppler requires that you first place transmission gel over the skin area where you will be listening. Then place the tip of the instrument directly over the area being examined. Tilt the tip at an angle along the axis of blood flow to obtain the best signal. Arterial flow is heard as a pulsatile pumping sound, and venous flow resembles the sound of rushing wind. When using a Doppler, do not press so hard as to impede blood flow.

The Doppler can be used to detect systolic blood pressures in patients with weak or difficult-to-hear sounds (e.g., patients in shock, infants, or obese persons). It is used to auscultate fetal heart activity, locate vessels, take weak pulses, and assess vessel patency. Other uses include localization of acute and chronic arterial occlusions in the extremities, assessment of deep vein thrombosis and valvular incompetency, and assessment of testicular torsion and varicocele.

Portable Ultrasound

Compact portable units (CPUs) are used for bedside ultrasonography. The ultrasound unit uses a transducer to emit sounds and detect returning echoes that are produced when the sound wave strikes an object. The returning echoes identify the distance, size and shape of the object. A CPU analyzes the echoes and transforms them into a 2- or 3-dimensional image of the organs or tissues being examined. Ultrasound waves pass easily through fluids and soft tissues, making the procedure especially useful for assessing fluid-filled organs such as the urinary bladder for fullness, distention, and incomplete emptying, and soft organs such as the gallbladder and liver. Because ultrasound produces dynamic moving images, it can show the structure and movement of the body's internal organs, as well as blood flowing through blood vessels. Abnormalities that can be detected by ultrasound include cysts, tumors, and infections. Blockages in major blood vessels can also be detected. Ultrasound provides a visual aid to improving targeted clinical procedures such as aspiration and drainage of pleural effusions, abscesses, and biopsies. Use of the ultrasound device for diagnostic purposes requires training and skilled operation.

Fetal Monitoring Equipment

The fetal heart rate is determined by the use of specially designed instruments called the fetoscope and Leff scope; by use of the clinical stethoscope, addressed previously; or with an electronic instrument that uses the Doppler effect. The fetoscope has a band that fits against the head of the listener and makes handling of the instrument unnecessary (Fig. 3-12). The metal band also aids in bone conduction of sound, so that the heart tones are heard more easily. The Leff scope has a weighted end that, when placed on the abdomen, does not need stabilization by the health care provider. These instruments can detect the fetal heart rate at 17 to 19 weeks of gestation.

The Doppler method employs a continuous ultrasound that picks up differing frequencies from the beating fetal heart. It is a more sensitive method and can detect the fetal heart at 10 to 12 weeks of gestation, and even earlier in some individuals. These instruments are often supplied with amplifiers so that both the

FIGURE 3-12 Fetoscope.

Table 3-4	Apertures of the Ophthalmoscope
Aperture	**Examination Use**
Small aperture	Small pupils
Red-free filter	Produces a green beam for examination of the optic disc for pallor and minute vessel changes; also permits recognition of retinal hemorrhages, with blood appearing black
Slit	Examination of the anterior eye and determination of the elevation of lesions on the retina
Grid	Estimation of the size of fundal lesions

FIGURE 3-13 Ophthalmoscope.

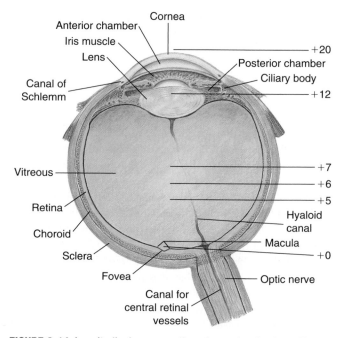

FIGURE 3-14 Longitudinal cross section of eye showing lens diopters to focus eye structures.

health care provider and parents can hear the fetal heartbeat at the same time.

Ophthalmoscope

The ophthalmoscope has a system of lenses and mirrors that enables visualization of the interior structures of the eye (Fig. 3-13). The instrument has a light source that projects through various apertures while you focus on the inner eye. The large aperture, the one used most often, produces a large round beam. The various apertures (described in Table 3-4) are selected by rotating the aperture selection dial.

The lenses in varying powers of magnification are used to bring the structure under examination into focus by converging or diverging light. An illuminating lens indicator displays the lens number positioned in the viewing aperture. The number, ranging from about ±20 to ±140, corresponds to the magnification power (diopter) of the lens. The positive numbers (plus lenses) are shown in black, and the negative numbers (minus lenses) are shown in red. A way to remember this is that when you are using a minus lens, you are in the red. Clockwise rotation of the lens selector brings the plus sphere lenses into place. Counterclockwise rotation brings the minus sphere lenses into place. Figure 3-14 shows the expected lens diopters to focus on eye structures. The system of plus and minus lenses can compensate for myopia or hyperopia in both the examiner and the patient. There is no compensation for astigmatism.

Seat the ophthalmoscope head in the handle by fitting the adapter of the handle into the head receptacle and pushing downward while turning the head in a clockwise direction. The two pieces lock into place.

FIGURE 3-15 PanOptic ophthalmoscope. *(Courtesy Welch Allyn, Skaneateles Falls, NY.)*

ABS housing

3.5v halogen lamp

Semi-silvered (one-way) mirror— allows direct observation of occluded eye

FIGURE 3-16 StrabismoScope. *(Courtesy Welch Allyn, Skaneateles Falls, NY.)*

Turn on the ophthalmoscope by depressing the on/off switch and turning the rheostat control clockwise to the desired intensity of light. Turn the instrument off when you have finished using it to preserve the life of the bulb.

The ophthalmoscopic examination is discussed in more detail in Chapter 11.

PanOptic Ophthalmoscope

The "panoramic" ophthalmoscope head uses an optical design that allows a larger field of view (25 degrees versus the standard 5 degrees), and increases magnification. As a result, the view of the fundus is five times larger than the view achieved with the standard ophthalmoscope in an undilated eye. The PanOptic head connects to a standard handle (Fig. 3-15).

StrabismoScope

The StrabismoScope is used for detecting strabismus (eye misalignment) and can be used as part of eye testing in children (Fig. 3-16). Instruct the child to focus on an accommodative target, such as the wall poster that comes with the instrument. Turn on the StrabismoScope and place it over the patient's eye. Because of a one-way mirror, you are able to see in but the patient is not able to see out. As a result, subtle eye movements associated with strabismus are more easily detected. With the StrabismoScope in place, watch for movement in both the covered and the uncovered eye. Repeat with the other eye. The instrument comes with test instructions and a guide to interpretation of test results.

Photoscreening

Photoscreening is used to detect amblyopia ("lazy eye") and strabismus in children through the use of an appropriately equipped camera or video system to obtain images of pupillary reflexes and red reflexes. Various optical systems can be used for photoscreening. The child need only visually fixate on the appropriate target long enough for the photoscreening to occur. Data are then analyzed by the evaluator, reviewing center, or computer.

Visual Acuity Charts

Snellen Alphabet. The Snellen alphabet chart is used for a screening examination of far vision (Fig. 3-17, *A*) for literate, verbal, and English-speaking adults and school-age children. The chart contains letters of graduated sizes with standardized numbers at the end of each line of letters. These numbers indicate the degree of visual acuity when read from a distance of 20 feet. Some charts are standardized for use at 10 feet.

Test visual acuity for each eye using the standardized numbers on the chart. Visual acuity is recorded as a fraction, with the numerator of 20 (the distance in feet between the patient and the chart) and the denominator as the distance from which a person with normal vision could read the lettering. The larger the denominator, the poorer is the vision. The standard used for normal vision is 20/20. Measurement other than 20/20 indicates either a refractive error or an optic disorder. Record the smallest complete line that the patient can read accurately without missing any letters. If the patient is able to read some but not all letters of the next smaller line, indicate this by adding the number of letters read correctly on that next line (e.g., 20/25 + 2). This would indicate that the patient read all of the letters in the 20/25 line correctly and also two of the letters of the 20/20 line correctly.

For young children or adults not able to use the Snellen chart, several options are available. The highest difficulty of test that the child is capable of performing should be used. In general, the Tumbling E or the HOTV test should be used for children 3 to 5 years of age and Snellen letters or numbers for children 6 years and older. For children, cover the nontested eye by an occluder held by the examiner or by an adhesive occluder patch applied to eye. Ensure that it is not possible to peek with the nontested eye. Children usually stand 10 feet (3 m) away from the visual chart to minimize distraction (one standardized for that distance). Young children require training before testing.

EQUIPMENT

FIGURE 3-17 Charts for testing distant vision. A, Snellen chart. B, Tumbling E chart.

Tumbling E. A nonalphabet version of the Snellen chart, the Tumbling E chart has the capital letter "E" facing in different directions (Fig. 3-17, *B*). The person being tested must determine which direction the "E" is pointing—up, down, left, or right—by holding out three or four fingers to mimic the letter.

HOTV. This test consists of a wall chart composed only of H's, O's, T's, and V's. The child is given a testing board containing a large H, O, T, and V. Point to a letter on the wall chart, and ask the child to point to (match) the correct letter on the testing board.

LH Symbols (LEA Symbols). The LEA Symbols chart consists of four optotypes (circle, square, apple, house) that blur equally. The child has to find a matching block or point to the shape that matches the target presented. The visual acuity is determined by the smallest symbols that the child is able to identify accurately at 10 feet. For example, if the child is able to identify the 10/15 symbols at 10 feet, then the child's visual acuity is 10/15 or 20/30. If it is not possible to perform testing at 10 feet, move closer to the child until he or she correctly identifies the largest symbol. Proceed down in size to the smallest symbols that the child is consistently able to correctly identify. Record the acuity as the smallest symbol identified (bottom number) at the testing distance (top number). For example, correctly identifying the 10/15 symbols at 5 feet is recorded as 5/15 or 20/60.

Broken Wheel Cards. The Broken Wheel test consists of six pairs of cards with the following acuities: 20/100, 20/80, 20/60, 20/40, 20/30, and 20/20. In each pair, one card has solid wheels while the other has Landolt C or "broken" wheels. The child identifies the card that has the broken wheels on the pictured car. Record the acuity of the card with the smallest car for which the child can distinguish the broken wheels.

Near Vision Charts

To assess near vision, a specially designed chart such as the Rosenbaum or Jaeger chart can be used, or simply use newsprint. The Rosenbaum chart contains a series of numbers, E's, X's, and O's in graduated sizes. Test and record vision for each eye separately. Acuity is recorded as either distance equivalents such as 20/20 or Jaeger equivalents such as J-2. Both these measures are indicated on the chart. If newsprint is used, the patient should be able to read it without difficulty.

Amsler Grid

A screening test for use with individuals at risk of macular degeneration is provided with the Amsler grid. The grid monitors about 10 degrees of central vision and is used when retinal drusen bodies are seen during an ophthalmologic examination or when there is a strong family history of macular degeneration. The grid consists of straight lines that resemble graph paper. At the center of the grid is a black dot that acts as a fixation point. The patient views the grid with one eye at a time and

FIGURE 3-18 Otoscope with various sizes of specula and a pneumatic attachment.

FIGURE 3-19 Tympanometer.

notes the occurrence of line distortion or actual scotoma (see Chapter 11).

Otoscope

The otoscope provides illumination for examining the external auditory canal and the tympanic membrane (Fig. 3-18). The traditional otoscope head is seated in the handle in the same manner as the ophthalmoscope and is turned on the same way. Newer models can provide a macro view and operate slightly differently. An attached speculum narrows and directs the beam of light. Select the largest size speculum that will fit comfortably into the patient's ear canal. Chapter 12 discusses the specific techniques of examination.

You can also use the otoscope for the nasal examination if a nasal speculum is not available. Use the shortest, widest otoscope speculum and insert it gently into the patient's naris.

The pneumatic attachment for the otoscope is used to evaluate the fluctuating capacity of the tympanic membrane. A short piece of rubber tubing is attached to the head of the otoscope. A handbulb attached to the other end of the tubing, when squeezed, produces puffs of air that cause the tympanic membrane to move.

Tympanometer

Various instruments are used to perform screening tympanometry. Tympanometry is a simple, reliable, and objective means of assessing the functions of the ossicular chain, eustachian tube, and tympanic membrane, as well as the interrelation of these parts.

Position the probe at the opening of the ear canal (Fig. 3-19). When a tight seal is obtained, a known quantity of sound energy is introduced into the ear. The amount of the sound energy transmitted is the amount of sound energy introduced minus the amount of sound energy that returns to the probe microphone. The amount of energy transmitted is directly related to the compliance of the system. Compliance (measured in milliliters or cubic centimeters of equivalent volume) indicates the amount of

mobility in the middle ear. A low compliance measurement indicates that more energy has returned to the probe, with less energy admitted to the middle ear. A high compliance reading indicates a flaccid or highly mobile system.

At this point, the probe introduces a pressure of 200 daPa (decaPascals; a measurement of air pressure) to the middle ear canal. This positive pressure forces the tympanic membrane inward, and the approximate ear canal volume is recorded. This volume gives a baseline from which the compliance curve is drawn. The pressure is then varied in the negative direction, constantly monitoring the compliance of the system. The pressure continues toward the negative direction until a pressure peak has been detected or until a pressure of 2400 daPa is present in the ear canal, whichever comes first. The point of peak compliance occurs once the pressure is equalized on both sides of the tympanic membrane.

A tympanogram is a graphic representation of the change in compliance of the middle ear system as air pressure is varied. The tympanogram results are displayed on the probe monitor or can be printed out for a hard copy.

Nasal Speculum

Use the nasal speculum with a penlight to visualize the lower and middle turbinates of the nose (Fig. 3-20). Be sure that the patient is in a comfortable position. You may need to support the patient's head, or you can have the patient lie down. You will need to tilt the patient's head at various angles for a complete nasal examination. Stabilize the speculum with your index finger to avoid contact of the blades with the nasal septum, which can cause discomfort. Squeezing the handles of the instrument opens the blades.

Tuning Fork

Tuning forks are used in screening tests for auditory function and for vibratory sensation as part of the neurologic examination (Fig. 3-21). As tuning forks are activated, vibrations are created that produce a particular frequency of sound wave, expressed as

FIGURE 3-20 Nasal specula.

FIGURE 3-21 Tuning forks for testing vibratory sensation *(top)* and auditory screening *(bottom)*.

FIGURE 3-22 Squeezing and stroking the tuning fork to activate it. Hold the fork only by the handle so as not to dampen the sound.

cycles per second (cps) or Hertz (Hz). Thus, a fork of 512 Hz vibrates at 512 cycles per second.

For auditory evaluation, use a fork with a frequency of 500 to 1000 Hz, as it estimates hearing loss in the range of normal speech, approximately 300 to 3000 Hz. Forks of lower frequency can cause you to overestimate bone conduction and can be felt as vibration as well as heard. Activate the fork by gently squeezing and stroking the prongs or by tapping them against the knuckles of your hand so that they ring softly (Fig. 3-22). Because touching the tines will dampen the sound, you must hold the fork by the handle. Hearing is tested at near-threshold level; this is the lowest intensity of sound at which an auditory stimulus can be heard. Striking the prongs too vigorously results in a loud tone that is above the threshold level and requires time to quiet to a tone appropriate for auditory testing. The specific tuning fork tests for hearing are described in Chapter 12.

For vibratory sensation, use a fork of lower frequency. The greatest sensitivity to vibration occurs when the fork is vibrating between 100 and 400 Hz. Activate the tuning fork by tapping it against the heel of your hand, then apply the base of the fork to a bony prominence. The patient feels the vibration as a buzzing or tingling sensation. The specific areas of testing are described in Chapter 22.

Percussion (Reflex) Hammer

The percussion hammer is used to test deep tendon reflexes. Hold the hammer loosely between the thumb and index finger so that the hammer moves in a swift arc and in a controlled direction. As you tap the tendon, use a rapid downward snap of the wrist, tap quickly and firmly, and then snap your wrist back so that the hammer does not linger on the tendon (Fig. 3-23). The tap should be brisk and direct. Practice this action to achieve smooth, rapid, and controlled motion. You can use either the pointed or flat end of the hammer. The flat end is more comfortable when striking the patient directly; the pointed end is useful in small areas, such as on your finger placed over the patient's biceps tendon. Chapter 22 contains a detailed discussion of evaluation of deep tendon reflexes.

Your finger can also act as a reflex hammer; this can be particularly useful when you are examining very young patients. Certainly it is less threatening to a child than a hammer. Many pediatric specialists let the child hold the hammer while they use their fingers.

Neurologic Hammer

A variant of the percussion hammer is the neurologic hammer, which is also used for testing deep tendon reflexes. The hammer has two additional features that make it a multipurpose neurologic instrument. The base of the handle unscrews, revealing a soft brush. A tiny knob on the head also unscrews, to which is attached a sharp needle. These additional implements were designed to determine sensory perception as part of the neurologic examination. The brush can still be used for that purpose; however, because of the possibility of cross infection, the needle should not be used at all. Instead, use a disposable needle, a pin, or the sharp end of a broken tongue blade. Some models come with a rotating wheel to test sharp sensation. The procedure for testing sensory perception is described in detail in Chapter 22.

Tape Measure

Use a tape measure 7 to 12 mm wide for determining circumference, length, and diameter. It may be helpful to have one that measures in both inches and metric units. Tape measures are available in a variety of materials, including paper (disposable), plastic or vinyl, and cloth. The tape measure should be nonstretchable for accuracy and pliable for circumference measurement. Because it is placed against the skin, beware of edges that are sharp and can cut.

When measuring, make sure that the tape is not caught or wrinkled beneath the patient. Pull the tape closely but not tightly enough to cause depression of the skin when measuring circumference.

FIGURE 3-23 A, Reflex hammer. **B,** Use a rapid downward snap of the wrist.

When monitoring serial measures, such as head circumferences or abdominal girth, it is important to place the tape measure in the same position each time. If serial measures are made over a period of days, an easy way to ensure accurate placement is to use a pen to mark the borders of the tape at several intervals on the skin. Subsequently, the tape can be placed within the markings (see Clinical Pearl, "The Transience of Memory"). Accurate placement of the tape for specific measurements is described in Chapter 5 and related chapters.

> **Clinical Pearl**
>
> The Transience of Memory
> I saw a patient today who had a swollen elbow. Was it less swollen than when I first saw him 2 days ago? Hard to tell. It would have been much better if I had measured the circumference of the elbow and also of the other one. Use a tape measure! It should always be with you. (A small ruler, too!) Do not rely on memory for judging such observations.

Transilluminator

A transilluminator consists of a strong light source with a narrow beam. The beam is directed to a particular body cavity and is used to differentiate between various media present in that cavity. Air, fluid, and tissue differentially transmit light; this allows you to detect the presence of fluid in sinuses or the presence of blood or masses in the scrotum (see Clinical Pearl, "Transillumination").

Specific transilluminating instruments are available, or a flashlight with a rubber adapter can be used. It is fine, when situations demand, to use a plain flashlight or penlight. Do not use a light source with a halogen bulb because this can burn the patient's skin. Perform transillumination in a darkened room. Place the beam of light directly against the area to be observed, shielding the beam with your hand if necessary. Watch for the red glow of light through the body cavity. Note the presence or absence of illumination and any irregularities.

Vaginal Speculum

A vaginal speculum is composed of two blades and a handle. There are three basic types of vaginal specula, which are used to

> **Clinical Pearl**
>
> Transillumination
> Compared to imaging technology, transillumination may seem archaic and imprecise. Imaging is used when necessary, but transillumination maintains its value as a clinical tool and is far less expensive.

view the vaginal canal and cervix. The Graves speculum is available in a variety of sizes with blades ranging from 3½ to 5 inches in length and ¾ to 1¼ inches in width. The blades are curved, with a space between the closed blades. The bottom blade is about ¼ inch longer than the top blade to conform to the longer posterior vaginal wall and to aid in visualization. The Pederson speculum has blades that are as long as those of the Graves speculum but are both narrower and flatter. It is used for women with small vaginal openings. Pediatric or virginal specula are smaller in all dimensions, with short, narrow, flat blades (Fig. 3-24).

Specula are available in either disposable plastic or reusable metal. The metal speculum has two positioning devices. The top blade is hinged and has a positioning thumb piece lever attached. When you press down on the thumb piece, the distal end of the blade rises, thus opening the speculum. To lock the blade in an open position, tighten the thumbscrew on the thumb piece. Moving the top blade up or down controls the degree of opening of the proximal end of the blades; it is locked in place by another thumbscrew, which is on the handle.

The plastic speculum operates in a different way. The bottom blade is fixed to a posterior handle, and an anterior lever handle controls the top blade. As you press on the lever, the distal end of the top blade elevates. At the same time, the base of the speculum also widens. Lock the speculum into position with a catch on the lever handle that snaps into place in a positioning groove.

You will need to become familiar with and practice with both types of specula to feel comfortable with them. Do not wait until you are in the process of doing your first examination, or you are likely to be embarrassed and cause discomfort to the woman because of your initial clumsiness in handling the instrument. The procedure for performing the speculum examination is described in detail in Chapter 18.

FIGURE 3-24 **Vaginal specula.** *(From Wilson and Giddens, 2009.)*

FIGURE 3-25 Goniometer.

FIGURE 3-26 **Wood's lamp.** The purple color on the skin indicates no fungal infection is present. *(From Thompson and Wilson, 1996.)*

Goniometer

The goniometer is used to determine the degree of joint flexion and extension. The instrument consists of two straight arms that intersect and that can be angled and rotated around a protractor marked with degrees (Fig. 3-25). Place the center of the protractor over the joint and align the straight arms with the long axes of the extremities. The degree of angle flexion or extension is indicated on the protractor. The specific joint examinations are discussed in Chapter 21.

Wood's Lamp

The Wood's lamp contains a light source with a wavelength of 360 nm (Fig. 3-26). This is the black light that causes certain substances to fluoresce. It is used primarily to determine the presence of fungi on skin lesions. Darken the room, turn on the Wood's lamp, and shine it on the area or lesion you are evaluating. A yellow-green fluorescence indicates the presence of fungi.

Darkening the room can sometimes be intimidating, particularly to children. Children and their parents react positively when they know what to expect. You can accomplish this by shining the lamp on something fluorescent (e.g., a nondigital watch) to give them the sense of what you are looking for.

Dermatoscope

A dermatoscope is a skin surface microscope that uses epiluminescence microscopy (ELM) with or without the application of oil on a skin lesion to illuminate and magnify a lesion to allow for a more detailed inspection of the surface of pigmented skin

lesions (Fig. 3-27, *A*). Digital epiluminescence microscopy (DELM) uses technology to not only examine the skin's surface but also to view, image, record, and document subsurface layers and structures of the skin (Fig. 3-27, *B*). Dermoscopy requires special training and expertise and is used to confirm a diagnosis or determine which skin lesions require biopsy or removal.

FIGURE 3-27 **Dermatoscopes. A,** Epiluminescence microscope. **B,** Digital epiluminescence microscope. *(A, Courtesy Welch Allyn, Skaneateles Falls, NY. B, Courtesy of 3Gen LLC, Dana Point, CA.)*

FIGURE 3-28 Triceps skinfold caliper. Grasp the handle and depress the lever with thumb.

FIGURE 3-29 **A,** Monofilament. **B,** Press the monofilament against the skin hard enough to allow it to bend.

Calipers for Skinfold Thickness

Skinfold thickness calipers are designed to measure the thickness of subcutaneous tissue at certain points of the body (Fig. 3-28). Specifically calibrated and tested calipers, such as the Lange and Harpenden models, are used. The skinfold is pinched up so the sides of the skin are parallel. Place the caliper edges at the base of the fold, being careful not to capture bone or muscle. Tighten the calipers so that they are grasping the skinfold but not compressing it. The specific technique for triceps skinfold thickness measurement is described in Chapter 5.

Monofilament

The monofilament is a device designed to test for loss of protective sensation, particularly on the plantar surface of the foot (Fig. 3-29, *A*) such as with diabetic or other peripheral neuropathy and nerve damage. It bends at 10 g of linear pressure. Patients who cannot feel the application of the monofilament at the point that it bends have lost their protective sense and are at increased risk for injury.

Test intact skin on the plantar surface of the foot at various areas, including the great toe, heel, and ball of the foot (Fig. 3-29, *B*). Lock the monofilament in its handle at a 90-degree angle. With the patient's eyes closed, apply the monofilament perpendicular to the surface of the skin. Press hard enough to allow the monofilament to bend, holding pressure for approximately 1.5 seconds. Test at various locations in random order. Ask the patient to indicate whether the monofilament is felt. Vary the interval between applications. Note the response at each location in the patient record. Dispose of or clean the monofilament with alcohol. For a further discussion of skin testing with the monofilament, see Chapter 22.

FIGURE 3-30 The scoliometer. *(Courtesy Ortholutions, 2013.)*

Scoliometer

A scoliometer measures the degree of rotation of the spine to screen for scoliosis. Ask the patient to bend forward slowly, stopping when the shoulders are level with the hips. View from the back. Note any rib elevation and/or symmetry in the low back area. Before measuring with the scoliometer, adjust the height of the patient's bending position to the level at which the deformity of the spine is most pronounced. This position will vary depending upon the location of the curvature. Lay the scoliometer across the deformity at right angles to the body, with the "0" mark over the top of the spinous process (Fig. 3-30). Let the scoliometer rest gently on the skin. Do not push down. Read the number of degrees of rotation. The screening examination is considered positive if the reading on the scoliometer is 7 degrees or more at any level of the spine. Lesser degrees of rotation may or may not indicate a mild degree of scoliosis.

CHAPTER 4

Vital Signs and Pain Assessment

The vital signs include assessment of temperature, pulse, respiration, and blood pressure. They are considered the baseline indicators of a patient's health status.

Pain assessment is now considered the fifth vital sign. Pain is a subjective unpleasant symptom of many conditions and injuries. The pain experience, its characteristics, and intensity are unique for each person. The Joint Commission (2013) requires that all patients in all health care facilities have a documented pain assessment. Repeat assessment of pain is performed to evaluate the treatment response and to identify the presence of new or recurring pain.

evolve *http://evolve.elsevier.com/Seidel*
• NCLEX Review Questions • Student Checklist

Physical Examination Preview

The following is a preview of the steps involved in conducting an assessment of vital signs and pain. ⊖ These procedures are explained in detail in this chapter and are available on Evolve in printable formats.
Temperature (p. 52)
Pulse rate (p. 53)
Respiratory rate (p. 53)
Blood pressure (p. 53-56)
Self-report pain rating scales (pp. 56-57)
Assessing pain behaviors (pp. 56-57)
Pain scales for children (pp. 59-60)

ANATOMY AND PHYSIOLOGY

Temperature

Body temperature is regulated by the hypothalamus. When microorganisms invade the body endogenous pyrogens are released and travel to the hypothalamus. The fever (also called pyrexia) response is then triggered by the production and release of prostaglandins. The body generates heat by shivering, a rapid contraction and relaxation of the skeletal muscles, and by vasoconstriction, which reduces heat loss through the skin. Body cooling occurs by vasodilation, which increases heat loss through the skin and evaporation of perspiration.

Pulse Rate

The arterial pulse results when the ventricular heart contraction pushes a pressure wave of blood throughout the arterial system.

Respiratory Rate

The primary muscles of respiration are the diaphragm and the intercostal muscles. The diaphragm is the dominant muscle. It contracts and moves downward during inspiration to increase the intrathoracic space. The external intercostal muscles increase the AP chest diameter during inspiration, and the internal intercostals decrease the lateral diameter during expiration. Air is drawn into the lungs during inspiration and expelled during expiration due to elastic recoil and force of muscular contraction.

Blood Pressure

The arterial blood pressure is the force of the blood against the wall of an artery as the ventricles of the heart contract and relax. Systolic pressure, the force exerted when the ventricles contract, is largely the result of cardiac output, blood volume, and compliance of the arteries. Diastolic pressure is the force exerted by peripheral vascular resistance when the heart is in the filling or relaxed state. Blood pressure is highest during systole and falls to the lowest point during diastole. The pulse pressure is the difference between the systolic and diastolic pressures.

Pain

Pain is an uncomfortable sensation and emotional experience associated with actual or potential tissue damage. *Acute pain* is of short duration and has a sudden onset in association with injury, surgery, or an acute illness episode. Inflammation helps sustain the pain response. Persistent (*chronic*) pain lasts several months or longer, and is often sustained by a pathophysiologic process (e.g., joint disease, chronic inflammation, headache, or cancer). Neuropathic pain is long-term pain associated with damage or dysfunction of the central or peripheral nervous system (e.g., amputation, complex regional pain syndrome).

ANATOMY AND PHYSIOLOGY

FIGURE 4-1 Transmission of pain impulses from pain receptors to the central nervous system. Nociceptors transmit pain impulses from the periphery along A-delta (Aδ) and C fibers to the dorsal horn of the spinal cord.

Nociceptors are free nerve endings that are activated to transmit pain impulses from the site of injury. Biochemical mediators such as bradykinin, prostaglandins, serotonin, histamine, and substance P help transmit the pain impulses from the nerve endings along nerve pathways. Pain impulses travel from the site of injury to the dorsal horn of the spinal cord through the ascending spinal tracts to the thalamus and cerebral cortex. Two specialized nerve fibers transmit pain impulses (nociception). Sharp, well-localized pain is quickly transmitted by the large, myelinated A-delta fibers. Dull, burning, diffuse, and chronic pain is slowly transmitted by the small, unmyelinated C-polymodal fibers (Fig. 4-1).

A two-way control of pain transmission occurs in the spinal nerve pathways. After the pain impulses reach the spinal cord's dorsal horn, the pain signal may be modified when other stimuli are present from either the brain or the periphery. Substances, such as *endorphins* (exogenous opioids), serotonin, and norepinephrine can change or inhibit the pain perceived. Pain impulse transmission may be reduced when nonpain impulses (e.g., ice, massage) compete to transmit sensations along the same spinal pathways to the brain.

Response to pain is individualized because it is a physiologic, behavioral, and emotional phenomenon. Individuals have different thresholds at which pain is perceived and different pain tolerance levels. Emotions, cultural background, sleep deprivation, previous pain experience, and age are some factors that have an impact on a person's perception and interpretation of pain.

✤ Infants

Infants are more susceptible to hypothermia because of their large body surface area for weight ratio, thinner skin, and limited ability to cope with cold stress. Infants have a higher pulse rate and respiratory rate than adults, and the rates decrease as the child ages. Infants have a lower blood pressure than adults, and blood pressure increases as the child ages.

The peripheral and central nervous systems are adequately developed for neonates to feel pain. The ability to process pain develops early in fetal life. The immaturity of the neurologic system results in some differences in pain transmission and processing. Most pain impulses are transmitted along the nonmyelinated slower C fibers because myelination of the A-delta fibers continues to develop after birth. The transmission distance to the brain is short. Infants are less able to modify pain impulses because the descending pathways from the brain to the dorsal horn of the spinal cord are not fully developed at birth (Kennedy et al, 2008).

✤ Pregnant Women

Blood pressure commonly decreases beginning at about 8 weeks' gestation, gradually falling until a low point is reached at midpregnancy. The diastolic blood pressure gradually rises to prepregnant levels by term (Gabbe, 2012).

During pregnancy, some women may experience pain due to several physiologic processes:
+ Back pain may be related to lax ligaments, weight gain, hyperlordosis, and anterior tilt of the pelvis.

+ Cramping or pressure may be signs of premature labor or Braxton Hicks contractions (sporadic uterine contractions that start at around 6 weeks of pregnancy).
+ Pressure from the gravid uterus may cause epigastric pain.
+ Round ligament pain may be due to the stretching of the ligaments by the enlarging uterus.
+ Pressure on the bladder may occur from the weight of the enlarging uterus.

During labor, pain may be related to dilation of the cervix, stretching of the lower uterine segment, and pressure on adjacent structures. During delivery additional pain is caused by pressure of the fetal head against of the pelvic floor, vagina, and perineum.

⚘ Older Adults

No evidence exists that older adults have a diminished perception of pain. Many have chronic health conditions associated with pain, such as arthritis, or osteoporosis—which can lead to fractures, and diabetic neuropathy. They may not report pain for several reasons (Bruckenthal, 2007):

+ It is believed to be a normal part of aging.
+ They do not want to be a nuisance.
+ Reporting pain will lead to expensive testing or hospitalization.
+ They are hesitant to take pain medications.

REVIEW OF RELATED HISTORY

For each of the conditions discussed in this section, topics to include in the history of the present illness are listed. Responses to questions about these topics help to assess the patient's condition and provide clues for focusing the physical examination.

Present Problem

+ Fever
  + *Onset:* date of onset, duration, cyclic nature, variability; related to injury or exposure to illness
  + *Associated symptoms:* sweating, chills, irritability, nausea, vomiting, fatigue
  + *Medications:* acetaminophen or nonsteroidal antiinflammatory drugs (NSAIDs)
+ Pain
  + *Onset:* date of onset, sudden or gradual, time of day, duration, precipitating factors, variation, rhythm (constant or intermittent)
  + *Quality:* throbbing, shooting, stabbing, sharp, cramping, gnawing, hot or burning, aching, heavy, tender, splitting, tiring or exhausting, sickening, fear producing, punishing or cruel
  + *Intensity:* ranges from slight to severe using a pain scale from 1 to 10 or from little to worst pain ever felt
  + *Location:* Identify all sites. Can the patient point a finger to it? Does it travel or radiate?
  + *Associated symptoms:* nausea, fatigue, behavior change, irritability, disturbed sleep, distress caused by pain
  + *What the patient thinks is causing the pain*

+ *Effect of pain on daily activities:* activity limitation, sleep disruption, need for increased rest, appetite change
+ *Effect of pain on psyche:* change in mood or social interactions, poor concentration, can think only about pain; irritability
+ *Pain control measures:* distraction, relaxation, ice, heat, massage, electrical stimulation, acupuncture
+ *Medications:* opioids, anxiolytics, NSAIDs, nonprescription medications

Personal and Social History

+ Previous experiences with pain and its effect; typical coping strategies for pain control
+ Family's concerns and cultural beliefs about pain: expect or tolerate pain in certain situations
+ Attitude toward the use of opioids, anxiolytics, and other pain medications for pain control; fear of addiction
+ Current or past use of illicit substances

⚘ Children

+ Word(s) the child uses for pain, such as "owie," "ouch," "ache," or "hurt"
+ What do you tell your mother or father when you hurt? What do you want him or her to do for the hurt?
+ What kinds of things caused hurt in the past? What made the hurt feel better?
+ Pain behaviors (facial expressions, grimacing, protective posture) the parent identifies in the infant or child

⚘ Pregnant Women

+ Discomforts associated with increasing fetal size, description of discomfort, location, and when it occurs
+ Investigate all known medical conditions and physical limitations to identify sources for persistent or acute pain.

⚘ Older Adults

+ Investigate all known medical conditions and physical limitations to identify potential sources for persistent or acute pain.
+ Word used by the older adult for pain, such as "achy," "sore," or "discomfort." Use this word consistently during the pain assessment.
+ When the older adult is cognitively impaired, have a family member describe cues to the patient's expression of pain.

EXAMINATION AND FINDINGS

Temperature

The assessment of body temperature may often provide an important clue to the severity of a patient's illness. Temperature measurement is most commonly performed by oral, rectal, axillary, tympanic, and forehead routes. The temperature is read in either Fahrenheit or Celsius. The expected temperature range is 97.2° to 99.9° F (36.2° to 37.7° C) with an average of 98.6° F or 37.0° C (McCance, 2011). The body temperature normally varies over a 24-hour period and in response to activity.

FIGURE 4-2 Location of the sites to palpate the pulse.

Pulse Rate

The pulse rate is best palpated over an artery close to the surface of the body that lies over bones, such as the carotid, brachial, radial, femoral, popliteal, dorsalis pedis, and posterior tibial arteries (Fig. 4-2). The radial pulse is most often used to assess the heart rate. With the pads of your second and third fingers, palpate the radial pulse on the flexor surface of the wrist laterally. If you have difficulty finding a pulse, vary your pressure, feeling carefully throughout the area (see Fig. 15-8, C, on page 339). Count the pulsations for 60 seconds (or count for 30 seconds and multiply by 2).

The average resting pulse rate in adults is 70 beats per minute, and ranges between 60 and 100 beats per minute. Well-conditioned athletes or individuals taking beta-blockers may have a resting pulse rate of 50 to 60 beats per minute. In adults, tachycardia is a pulse rate that exceeds 100 beats per minute, and bradycardia is a pulse rate less than 60 beats per minute.

Determine the steadiness of the heart rhythm; it should be regular. If an irregular rhythm is detected, count for a full 60 seconds. See Chapter 14 for more information about heart rhythm assessment. While counting the heart rate, also note the contour (waveform) and amplitude (force) of each pulsation. See Chapter 15 for a more detailed discussion of arterial pulse evaluation.

Respiratory Rate

Assess the respiratory rate (number of breaths per minute) by inspecting the rise and fall of the chest. Count the number of breaths (inspiration and expiration) that occur in 1 minute, or count the number of breaths for 30 seconds and multiply by 2. Avoid telling the patient that you are counting the respiratory rate so the patient will not vary the rate or pattern of breathing. A good way to do this is to count the respirations just after counting the pulse, while you are still palpating the radial artery.

The expected adult resting respiratory rate is 12 to 20 breaths per minute. The ratio of the respiratory rate to the heart rate is approximately 1:4. Respiratory rates can vary between waking and sleep states. The normal rate of respirations (breaths per minute) depends on a number of factors, including the age of the individual and the amount of activity. Tachypnea is a faster-than-normal respiratory rate. Bradypnea is a slower-than-normal respiratory rate. See Chapter 13, page 260 to further evaluate respiratory patterns.

Blood Pressure

The blood pressure is most often measured in the arm when the patient is seated. Blood pressures taken in supine position tend to be lower than those taken in sitting position. Standards for blood pressure readings are based upon the seated position using the right arm.

Free the arm of clothing and apply a cuff of appropriate size around the upper arm (Box 4-1). Center the deflated bladder over the brachial artery, just medial to the biceps tendon, with the lower edge 2 to 3 cm above the antecubital crease. Make sure the cuff is snug and secure because a loose cuff will give an inaccurate diastolic reading. Flex the patient's arm to be at the level of the heart and support it comfortably on a table, pillow, or your hand.

Check the palpable systolic blood pressure first to avoid being misled by an auscultatory gap when using the stethoscope. Place the fingers of one hand over the brachial or radial artery and palpate the pulse. Rapidly inflate the cuff with the hand bulb 20 to 30 mm Hg above the point at which you no longer feel the peripheral pulse. Deflate the cuff slowly at a rate of 2 to 3 mm Hg per second until you again feel at least two beats of the pulse. This point is the palpable systolic blood pressure. Immediately deflate the cuff completely (Fig. 4-4, *A*).

Pause for 30 seconds, and then place the *bell of the stethoscope* over the brachial artery. Inflate the cuff until it is 20 to 30 mm Hg

EXAMINATION AND FINDINGS

Box 4-1	Selecting the Correct Cuff Size

Cuffs are available in several sizes to match the size of the patient's limb (Fig. 4-3). The correct cuff size ensures that equal pressure will be exerted around the artery, resulting in an accurate measurement. If the cuff is too wide the blood pressure will be underestimated. If the cuff is too narrow an artificially high blood pressure reading will result. The size of the cuff is measured by the width and length of bladder, not the material covering the bladder.

- For adults, choose a width that is one-third to one-half the circumference of the limb.

- The length of the bladder should be twice the width or about 80% of the limb circumference. The bladder should not completely encircle the limb.
- If the patient has an obese arm, attempt to find a cuff size appropriate for the arm size. If a sufficiently large cuff is not available, wrap a standard-size cuff around the forearm and auscultate over the radial artery.
- If the adult patient is very thin, a pediatric cuff may be necessary. Record the size of the cuff used and the site of auscultation.

FIGURE 4-3 Select the correct size blood pressure cuff. **A,** Large adult, adult, and child cuffs. **B,** Infant cuff *(top)* and neonatal cuff for use with electronic vital signs monitor *(bottom).* (**A,** From Thompson and Wilson, 1996.)

FIGURE 4-4 Blood pressure measurement. **A,** Checking the systolic blood pressure by palpation. **B,** Using bell of stethoscope to auscultate the blood pressure.

above the palpable systolic blood pressure (Fig. 4-4, *B*). The bell of the stethoscope is more effective than the diaphragm in transmitting the low-pitched sound produced by the turbulence of blood flow in the artery (Korotkoff sounds). Deflate the cuff slowly 2 to 3 mm Hg per second, listening for the following sounds (Fig. 4-5):

- Two consecutive beats indicate the systolic pressure reading, and the beginning of the Korotkoff sounds, phase 1.
- Sometimes the Korotkoff sounds will be heard, will disappear, and will reappear 10 to 15 mm Hg below the systolic

pressure reading (Korotkoff sounds, phase 2). The period of silence is the auscultatory gap. Be aware of the possibility of this gap to avoid underestimation of the systolic pressure or overestimation of the diastolic pressure. The auscultatory gap widens with systolic hypertension in older persons due to the loss of arterial pliability. It also widens with a drop in diastolic pressure when chronic severe aortic regurgitation is present. The auscultatory gap narrows in the case of pulsus paradoxus due to cardiac tamponade or other constrictive cardiac events.

FIGURE 4-5 Phases of Korotkoff sounds, including an example of auscultatory gap.

Table 4-1	Categories for Blood Pressure Levels for Adults

Category	Systolic (mm Hg)		Diastolic (mm Hg)
Normal	Less than 120	*And*	Less than 80
Prehypertension	120-139	*Or*	80-89
High blood pressure			
Stage 1	140-159	*Or*	90-99
Stage 2	160 or higher	*Or*	100 or higher

From National Institutes of Health, 2004.

+ Note the point at which the initial crisp sounds (Korotkoff sounds, phase 3) become muffled (Korotkoff sounds, phase 4). The muffled sound is the first diastolic sound, and it is considered to be the closest approximation of direct diastolic arterial pressure. It signals disappearance of the Korotkoff sounds.

+ Note the point at which the sounds disappear (Korotkoff sounds, phase 5). This is the second diastolic sound. Now deflate the cuff completely.

The two blood pressure readings recorded are the first systolic and the second diastolic sounds (e.g., 110/68). The systolic pressure is expected to be below 120 mm Hg and less than 80 mm Hg for the (second) diastolic sound. The difference between the systolic and diastolic pressures is the pulse pressure. The pulse pressure should range from 30 to 40 mm Hg, even to as much as 50 mm Hg. Some studies suggest that the pulse pressure may be a more important predictor of heart disease than either the systolic or diastolic pressure alone.

The Seventh Report of the Joint National Committee on Prevention, Detection, Evaluation, and Treatment of High Blood Pressure (JNC 7) (National Institutes of Health, 2004) has classified blood pressure for adults (Table 4-1). Because the systolic pressure is labile and responsive to a wide range of physical, emotional, and pharmacologic (e.g., caffeine) stimuli, high blood pressure or hypertension is usually diagnosed on the basis of several measurements taken over time.

Repeat the process in the other arm. Readings between the arms may vary by as much as 5 to 10 mm Hg. Record both sets of measurements. The higher reading should be used as

Box 4-2 Pointers for Taking the Blood Pressure

- Keep the mercury sphygmomanometer vertical and make all readings at eye level, no more than 3 feet away.
- Position the dial of the aneroid sphygmomanometer so it faces you directly, no more than 3 feet away. An aneroid manometer needs periodic calibration.
- Slow or repeated inflations of the cuff can cause venous congestion and result in inaccurate readings. Wait at least 15 seconds between readings, with the cuff fully deflated.
- Electronic sphygmomanometers with a Doppler or oscillometric device work by sensing vibrations, converting them to electrical impulses, and transmitting the information to a digital readout. These devices are more sensitive than a stethoscope to the first Korotkoff sound. The electronic device systolic reading is thus somewhat higher than the auscultatory systolic reading. The two techniques are not interchangeable. If the electronic reading and clinical impression are not consistent, take a manual blood pressure to validate the electronic reading.
- When documenting a patient's blood pressure measurements over time, use the same position and the same arm.
- The accuracy of the blood pressure reading may be undermined by some conditions, even when using impeccable technique:
  - *Cardiac dysrhythmias.* If heart rate irregularity is sustained take the average of several blood pressure readings and document the problem.
  - *Aortic regurgitation.* If the sounds of aortic regurgitation do not disappear, the diastolic pressure reading will be obscured.
  - *Venous congestion.* If sluggish venous flow occurs due to a pathologic event or repeated slow inflations of the cuff, the systolic pressure will be heard lower than it actually is and the diastolic pressure will be higher.
  - *Valve replacement.* If the sounds are heard all the way down to a zero gauge reading, listen carefully for the first muffling of the sound (Korotkoff phase 4) to determine the diastolic pressure. More modern valves do not cause this discrepancy.

the patient's blood pressure. Measure the blood pressure in both arms at least once annually and during a hospitalization (Box 4-2).

Most cases of hypertension in adults have no discoverable cause and are referred to as essential hypertension. An elevated blood pressure may be the only significant clinical finding and persons with hypertension are often asymptomatic. Individuals who complain of frequent nose bleeds (epistaxis) or recurrent morning headaches that disappear as the day progresses should have their blood pressure carefully monitored.

If the diastolic pressure reading in the arm is above 90 mm Hg, or if you suspect coarctation of the aorta, measure the blood pressure in the legs. Place the patient in prone position (if the patient is in supine position, flex the leg as little as possible). Center the thigh cuff bladder over the popliteal artery and wrap the cuff securely on the distal third of the femur. Auscultate the blood pressure over the popliteal artery. A Doppler measurement may be helpful in this regard. Leg blood pressures are expected to be higher than arm pressures. The leg blood pressure will be lower than the arm blood pressure in cases of coarctation of the aorta or aortic stenosis.

If the patient is taking antihypertensive medications, has a depleted blood volume, or complains of fainting or postural light-headedness, measure the blood pressure in the arm within 3 minutes after the patient stands. Compare this reading to the sitting blood pressure. As a patient changes position from sitting to standing, a slight drop or no drop in systolic pressure and a slight rise in diastolic pressure occurs. If orthostatic (postural) hypotension is present, expect to see a significant drop in systolic pressure (greater than 20 mm Hg) and a 10 mm Hg drop in diastolic pressure (National Institutes of Health, 2004). An increase in heart rate often occurs as well. Mild blood loss (e.g., blood donation), drugs, autonomic nervous system disease, or prolonged time in a recumbent position can contribute to orthostatic hypotension. Patients with active gastrointestinal bleeding will often have dramatic changes in blood pressure with postural change.

Pain Assessment

When the chief concern is pain, the location and related symptoms may assist in the diagnosis of a patient's condition. If the pain is related to a diagnosed condition (e.g., trauma, surgery, sickle cell disease, cancer, or arthritis), assessment of its character and intensity is necessary for pain management (see Clinical Pearl, "The Fifth Vital Sign"). Remember that more than one cause of pain may exist.

Clinical Pearl

The Fifth Vital Sign
Pain is often referred to as the fifth vital sign because of its association with tissue damage, the pathophysiologic effect of pain on body systems, and the patient's emotional response, which may worsen the pain perceived.

Self-Report Pain Rating Scales

Because of the subjective nature of pain, assessment is often based on history and patient responses to various tools that evaluate pain intensity and quality. The patient's report of pain is the most reliable indicator of pain and should be believed, even when observed behaviors do not seem to correspond. Encourage patients to report the presence, intensity, and character of discomfort.

Several pain rating scales have been developed for patients to rate and report their pain intensity and quality; only a sample is presented here (Figs. 4-6, 4-7, 4-8, and 4-9). The patient's rating of pain may not compare with another person's pain rating for an equivalent injury or condition. The patient's own rating should be used as the standard for future comparison after pain treatment. It is often helpful for a facility or group of health care providers to select a few self-report pain scales to use routinely. If all providers use the same set of pain scales, more consistent interpretation of patient pain ratings is likely occur.

Introduce the patient to a pain scale by explaining its purpose and clearly describing the meaning of the numbers or figures on the scale (see Clinical Pearl, "Selection of Pain Scale"). Ask about the patient's usual terms for different kinds of pain (e.g., "aching," "burning," "stabbing," "sharp," or "dull"). Allow the patient to practice using the pain scale to rate a prior painful episode (e.g., headache or specific injury) before evaluating the current pain level. Remember that the patient may have multiple sites of pain and the pain rating may vary by site. The pain rating may also vary with procedures and activities such as moving, coughing, and deep breathing. Body drawings may help patients to identify painful sites. Document the pain rating for each site of pain.

Clinical Pearl

Selection of Pain Scale
When more than one pain scale is available and used in a facility, ask the patient to select a pain scale. Use the same pain scale to evaluate and document the patient's pain for the entire painful episode so pain rating comparisons are interpreted accurately.

Assessing Pain Behaviors

Throughout your examination of the patient, be alert to behaviors indicating acute pain, such as the following:

+ Guarding, protective behavior, hands over the painful area, distorted posture, reluctance to be moved
+ Facial mask of pain: lackluster eyes, "beaten look," wrinkled forehead, tightly closed or opened eyes, fixed or scattered movement, grimace or other distorted expression, a sad or frightened look
+ Vocalizations: grunting, groaning, crying, talkative patient becomes quiet
+ Body movements such as head rocking, pacing, or rubbing; an inability to keep the hands still
+ Changes in vital signs: blood pressure, pulse, respiratory rate and depth, with acute onset of pain. Fewer changes in vital signs are found in patients with persistent pain or after they adapt to acute pain.
+ Pallor and diaphoresis
+ Pupil dilation
+ Dry mouth
+ Decreased attention span, greater confusion, irritability

Cognitively impaired adults who are unable to use a self-rating pain scale should have pain evaluated as described for older adults with cognitive impairment (see p. 62).

| None | Slight | Mild | Moderate | Severe | Worst Pain |

FIGURE 4-6 Descriptive pain intensity scale.

0   1   2   3   4   5   6   7   8   9   10

No Pain   Moderate   Worst Pain
                       Pain

FIGURE 4-7 Numeric pain intensity scale.

No Pain   Worst Pain

FIGURE 4-8 **Visual analogue scale.** Use a 10-cm line with word anchors ("No pain" and "Worst pain") on each end. Ask the patient to mark the level of pain felt on the line. A centimeter ruler is then used to identify a numeric pain rating for future comparison.

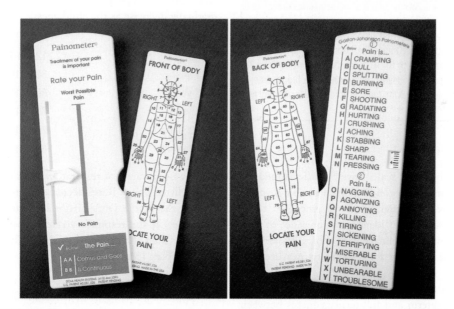

FIGURE 4-9 **The Painometer.** A multidimensional measure of pain, allowing a measure of intensity and quality and an opportunity for localization. It is the first handheld instrument that meets the standards of The Joint Commission. (Courtesy Dr. Fannie Gaston-Johansson, School of Nursing, Johns Hopkins University, Baltimore.)

A number of classic pain patterns may provide valuable clues to underlying conditions, such as the following:

+ Bone and soft tissue pain may be tender, deep, and aching.
+ Heavy, throbbing, and aching pain may be associated with a tumor pressing on a cavity.
+ Burning, shocklike pain may indicate nerve tissue damage.
+ A clenched fist over the chest with diaphoresis and grimacing is the classic picture of myocardial infarction. Even a mild pain can require immediate attention in this regard.
+ Cramping spasms may define visceral or colic pain.

� Newborns and Infants

The pulses of the newborn are easily palpable. Rates close to 200 beats per minute may occur in neonates. The decrease in pulse rate is relatively rapid, and the rate may be closer to 120 at a few hours of age. The newborn's pulse rate is more variable than that of older infants with activities such as feeding, sleeping, and waking. The variation is greatest around the time of birth and is even more marked in premature infants. A sustained tachycardia in a neonate may be the first indication of infection or it may be a clue to an underlying cardiac rhythm disturbance, such as paroxysmal atrial tachycardia. See Chapter 14 for more information.

Count the respiratory rate for 1 minute. The expected rate for neonates varies from 40 to 60 breaths per minute, but a rate of up to 80 may be noted. Babies delivered by cesarean section may have a more rapid respiratory rate than babies delivered vaginally.

The blood pressure of infants is often determined using an electronic sphygmomanometer with a Doppler or other oscillometric technique. The expected newborn blood pressure ranges from 60 to 96 mm Hg systolic and 30 to 62 mm Hg diastolic. A sustained increase in blood pressure is almost always significant (see Clinical Pearl, "Blood Pressure in Infants"). Hypertension in the newborn may be the result of many conditions, such as thrombosis after the use of an umbilical catheter, coarctation of the aorta, renal disorders (e.g., renal artery stenosis, cystic disease, or hydronephrosis), congenital adrenal hyperplasia, or central nervous system disease.

Clinical Pearl

Blood Pressure in Infants
A very ill baby can maintain a "normal blood pressure" and quickly develop hemodynamic instability. Check the capillary refill, which is usually less than 2 seconds (see p. 345). It can be as long as 6 to 7 seconds (indicating very poor perfusion), even when the blood pressure seems normal. The lesson: Both measurements are needed to fully evaluate the infant.

Pain Assessment

Valid and reliable pain behavior scales have been developed for the assessment of pain in neonates and infants. Physiologic measures and behaviors are combined for development of these scales. A pain behavior score helps identify the presence of pain and can be used to evaluate pain management efforts (Pasero and McCaffery, 2011). These scales are not designed to measure pain intensity.

- The Premature Infant Pain Profile (PIPP) is used to assess procedural pain in preterm and full-term neonates between 28 and 40 weeks' gestation. It measures physiologic signs (heart rate and oxygen saturation), pain behaviors (brow bulge, eye squeeze, and nasolabial furrow), gestational age, and behavioral state (Stephens, 2010).
- The Neonatal Infant Pain Scale is used to assess procedure pain in preterm and full-term infants up to 6 weeks of age. The infant's facial expression, cry, breathing pattern, arm and leg movements, and state of arousal are observed and scored (Twycross et al, 2009).
- The CRIES scale (Crying, Requires oxygen to keep saturation above 95, Increased vital signs, Expression, and Sleeplessness) is used to evaluate procedure and surgical pain in newborns and infants. The infant's behaviors (crying, expression, and sleeplessness) as well as physiologic signs (oxygen saturation, heart rate, and blood pressure) are scored (Twycross et al, 2009).

Staying Well

Think Sugar Water!

One way to keep well is to be freed of the prospect of pain. This is as true for newborns as it is for persons of all ages. Infants let us know that venipunctures hurt by crying. When given 2 mL of 24% sucrose solution by mouth, neonates up to 1 month of age have reduced pain during procedures. Infants up to 12 months of age have pain relief for immunizations (Harrison et al, 2010). When in contact with the oral mucosa, the sucrose solution is believed to activate the endogenous opioid system (Taddio et al, 2008).

Various pain-free local anesthetic options (e.g., vapocoolant sprays, lidocaine cream, or anesthetic patches) also exist to reduce procedure pain perceived by children and adults.

Children

The heart rates of children are more variable than those of adults, and react with wider swings related to exercise, fever, or stress. A child may have an increased heart rate of 10 to 14 beats per minute for each Celsius degree of temperature elevation (Thompson, 2009). The expected heart rate ranges gradually decrease as the child ages:

Age	Heart Rate (Beats Per Minute)
Newborn	120 to 170
1 year	80 to 160
3 years	80 to 120
6 years	75 to 115
10 years	70 to 110
17 years	60 to 100

The usual range of respiratory rates for children of different ages is listed below. Rates decrease with age with a greater variation in the first 2 years of life and without significant gender difference. If the respiratory rate is sustained at a level higher or lower than the expected range, further evaluation is needed (see Chapter 13).

Age	Respirations per Minute
Newborn	30 to 80
1 year	20 to 40
3 years	20 to 30
6 years	16 to 22
10 years	16 to 20
17 years	12 to 20

Select the correct cuff size to obtain an accurate blood pressure reading (Box 4-3). Children become more cooperative for the blood pressure measurement at 2 to 3 years of age. Allow the child to explore the sphygmomanometer. Explain that the cuff is a balloon that will squeeze the arm and then slowly stop squeezing. Take time to allow the child to play with the equipment and squeeze the bulb to gain better cooperation. Use Korotkoff phase 5 (disappearance of sound) as the diastolic reading unless the sounds are heard down to zero or very low. In that case use the Korotkoff phase 4 sound (muffling) as the

Box 4-3	Selecting a Blood Pressure Cuff for the Child

Choosing the correct blood pressure cuff for a child is more than selecting a cuff for the age of the child. Children, even those of the same age, are very different in build. Blood pressure cuffs for children also differ in dimensions by manufacturer. Use the following guidelines to select an appropriately sized cuff to obtain the most accurate blood pressure reading:

- The cuff width should cover approximately 70% of the distance between the acromion and the olecranon (tip of the elbow).
- The bladder length should be 80% to 100% of the upper arm circumference, and the bladder width should be at least 40% of the arm circumference at the midpoint of the acromion–olecranon distance.

From Brady et al, 2008.

diastolic reading (National High Blood Pressure Education Program Working Group on High Blood Pressure in Children and Adolescents, 2004).

Blood pressure standards for children are provided by gender, age, and height percentiles. Compare the reading to standards for normal blood pressure (less than 90th percentile), prehypertension (90th to 95th percentile), and hypertension (more than 95th percentile). After measuring the child's height, determine the child's height percentile using the standard length or height growth curve (see Appendix A). Then select the correct table for the child's gender, age, and percentile for height to determine if the child's systolic and diastolic blood pressure reading is below, at, or above the 90th or 95th percentile values (see Appendix B). The child's systolic and diastolic blood pressure values should be below the 90th percentile for age and height percentile (see Clinical Pearl, "Obesity in Children and Adolescents").

Do not make the diagnosis of hypertension based on one reading. Take at least three readings over several visits. If the systolic pressure is elevated and the diastolic is not, anxiety may be the cause. Take time to reassure the child and reduce anxiety. If the blood pressure is in the 90th to 95th percentile range, repeat the blood pressure later during the same visit and average the systolic and diastolic readings. If the pressure is more than

the 95th percentile, have the child return soon for additional blood pressure measurements. The majority of children with a diagnosis of hypertension have an identifiable cause, most often renal disease (Viera and Neutze, 2010).

Clinical Pearl

Obesity in Children and Adolescents
Because of the increase in numbers of children and adolescents who are obese, primary or essential hypertension is becoming more common. Studies have revealed that a third of obese children with a body mass index greater than 90th percentile have hypertension (Kavey et al, 2010).

Pain Assessment

Some children as young as 3 years of age have adequate communication skills to self-report their pain perception. Assess the child's ability to use a self-report pain scale by determining if the child understands concepts of higher/lower and more/less. Give the child a chance to practice using the chosen pain scale by describing a prior painful episode (e.g., finger stick, earache, or skinned knee).

Valid and reliable self-rating pain scales for young children include the Wong/Baker Faces Rating Scale (Fig. 4-10) and the Oucher Scale (Fig. 4-11). Give the child clear instructions about the amount of pain each face means, beginning with the face with no pain/hurt and ending with the last face that is the most pain/hurt ever felt. Ask the child to select the face that is the best match for the amount of pain felt. Do not compare the child's facial expression to that on the pain scale to evaluate the child's pain. Older children and adolescents may use these pain scales or those listed for adults.

For nonverbal children the FLACC Behavioral Pain Assessment Scale can be used (Fig. 4-12 on page 61). FLACC is an acronym for the five assessment categories: *f*ace, *l*egs, *a*ctivity, *c*ry, and *c*onsolability. This scale is used most commonly to assess acute pain associated with surgery in children between 2 months and 7 years of age.

The FLACC in combination with a numeric pain scale can also be used to develop a customized pain behavioral scale for children with intellectual disability. Parents can be asked to recall

FIGURE 4-10 The Wong/Baker FACES Rating Scale. Explain to the patient that each face is for a person who feels happy because he has no pain (hurt) or sad because he has some or a lot of pain. Face 0 is very happy because the person does not hurt at all. Face 1 hurts just a little bit. Face 2 hurts a little more. Face 3 hurts a little more. Face 4 hurts a whole lot. Face 5 hurts as much as you can imagine, although you do not have to be crying to feel this bad. Ask the patient to choose the face that best describes how he or she is feeling. Recommended for persons 3 years of age and older. (From Hockenberry MJ, Wilson D: *Wong's essentials of pediatric nursing*, ed 9, St. Louis, 2013, Mosby. Used with permission. Copyright Mosby.)

EXAMINATION AND FINDINGS

OUCHER!   OUCHER!   OUCHER!

FIGURE 4-11 A, Version of the Oucher for white children. (**A,** Developed and copyrighted in 1983 by Judith E. Beyer, PhD, RN [University of Missouri-Kansas City School of Nursing].) **B,** Version of the Oucher for black children. (**B,** Developed and copyrighted in 1990 by Mary J. Denyes, PhD, RN [Wayne State University], and Antonia M. Villarruel, PhD, RN [University of Michigan]. Cornelia P. Porter, PhD, RN, and Charlotta Marshall, RN, MSN, contributed to the development of this scale.) **C,** Version of the Oucher for Hispanic children. (**C,** Developed and copyrighted in 1990 by Antonia M. Villarruel, PhD, RN [University of Michigan], and Mary J. Denyes, PhD, RN [Wayne State University].)

one of the child's prior painful episodes and think about unique pain clues in association with the FLACC categories. The parent can then rate the behavior for each of the categories on a scale of 1 to 10 (Voepel-Lewis et al, 2005).

✿ Pregnant Women

Vital Signs

The heart rate gradually increases throughout pregnancy until it is 10% to 30% higher at term.

To identify the onset of hypertension during pregnancy, measure the blood pressure consistently in the right arm in the sitting position. Document both Korotkoff phase 4 (muffling) and Korotkoff phase 5 (disappearance of sounds) at each visit (Gabbe, 2012). A gradual increase in blood pressure is common from the second to the third trimester. Gestational hypertension (blood pressure reading of greater than or equal to 140 mm Hg

systolic **or** 90 mm Hg diastolic) develops in 6% to 29% of nulliparous women and in up to 4% of multiparous women, often late in pregnancy. The rate is higher in women with multiple gestations (Gabbe, 2012). Hypertension (blood pressure reading greater than or equal to 160 mm Hg systolic **or** 110 mm Hg diastolic) is one sign of preeclampsia; see Chapter 15 for more information.

Pain Assessment

The majority of women have significant pain during labor, often described as sharp, cramping, aching, throbbing, stabbing, shooting, heavy, and exhaustive. Childbirth training is not associated with very different perceptions of pain. Socioeconomic status and prior menstrual difficulties may be a better predictor of pain severity (Gabbe, 2012).

✿ Older Adults

Vital Signs

The heart rate may be slower because of increased vagal tone, or more rapid, with a wide range that may vary from the low 40s to more than 100 beats per minute.

Because of stiffness of the blood vessels and increased vascular resistance during the process of aging, the systolic blood pressure often increases. Hypertension in older adults is defined as a blood pressure greater than 140/90. Recent studies suggest that individuals who are normotensive at 55 years of age will have a 90% lifetime risk of developing hypertension (Aronow, 2009).

Pain Assessment

Use self-report pain scales with older adults, but make sure the patient can hear and understand the instructions for use of the scale. Repeat the instructions if necessary. If the patient has vision problems, use a scale with large print and give verbal descriptors for the self-report pain scale. To help the older adult focus and indicate where pain is located, touch or point to the body part when asking about the patient's current pain (Ferris, 2008).

Many patients with mild or moderate cognitive impairment can use a simple pain rating scale (e.g., the numeric rating scale, faces scale, verbal descriptor scale, and pain thermometer) to report pain reliably. Many can describe their pain when asked (Ware et al, 2006). When a self-report pain rating scale cannot be used, observe for pain behaviors when a condition that can cause pain is present. The Checklist of Nonverbal Pain Indicators (Fig. 4-13 on page 62) provides guidelines to observe and score pain behaviors, but no pain intensity rating is calculated. An analgesia trial may help confirm that the observed behaviors are caused by pain (Herr et al, 2006).

EXAMINATION AND FINDINGS

CATEGORIES	SCORING		
	0	**1**	**2**
Face	No particular expression or smile	Occasional grimace or frown; withdrawn, disinterested	Frequent to constant frown, clenched jaw, quivering chin
Legs	Normal position or relaxed	Uneasy, restless, tense	Kicking or legs drawn up
Activity	Lying quietly, normal position, moves easily	Squirming, shifting back and forth, tense	Arched, rigid, or jerking
Cry	No cry (awake or asleep)	Moans or whimpers, occasional complaint	Crying steadily, screams or sobs; frequent complaints
Consolability	Content, relaxed	Reassured by occasional touching, hugging, or being talked to; distractable	Difficult to console or comfort

Guidelines for Scoring the FLACC
Face
Score 0 if the patient has a relaxed face, makes eye contact, shows interest in surroundings.
Score 1 if the patient has a worried facial expression, with eyebrows lowered, eyes partially closed, cheeks raised, mouth pursed.
Score 2 if the patient has deep furrows in the forehead, closed eyes, an open mouth, deep lines around nose and lips.

Legs
Score 0 if the muscle tone and motion in the limbs are normal.
Score 1 if patient has increased tone, rigidity, or tension; if there is intermittent flexion or extension of the limbs.
Score 2 if patient has hypertonicity, the legs are pulled tight, there is exaggerated flexion or extension of the limbs, tremors.

Activity
Score 0 if the patient moves easily and freely, normal activity or restrictions.
Score 1 if the patient shifts positions, appears hesitant to move, demonstrates guarding, a tense torso, pressure on a body part.
Score 2 if the patient is in a fixed position, rocking; demonstrates side-to-side head movement or rubbing of a body part.

Cry
Score 0 if the patient has no cry or moan, awake or asleep.
Score 1 if the patient has occasional moans, cries, whimpers, sighs.
Score 2 if the patient has frequent or continuous moans, cries, grunts.

Consolability
Score 0 if the patient is calm and does not require consoling.
Score 1 if the patient responds to comfort by touching or talking in 30 seconds to 1 minute.
Score 2 if the patient requires constant comforting or is inconsolable.

Interpreting the Behavioral Score
Each category is scored on the 0–2 scale, which results in a total score of 0–10.

0 = Relaxed and comfortable   **4–6** = Moderate pain
1–3 = Mild discomfort   **7–10** = Severe discomfort or pain or both

FIGURE 4-12 FLACC Behavioral Pain Assessment Scale for nonverbal children. (From Merkel et al, 1997.)

Signs	With Movement	At Rest
Vocal Complaints—nonverbal expression of pain demonstrated by moans, groans, grunts, cries, gasps, sighs		
Facial Grimaces and Winces—furrowed brow, narrowed eyes, tightened lips, dropped jaw, clenched teeth, distorted expression		
Bracing—clutching or holding onto siderails, bed, tray table, or affected area during movement		
Restlessness—constant or intermittent shifting of position, rocking, intermittent or constant hand motions, inability to keep still		
Rubbing—massaging affected area		
Vocal Complaints—verbal expression of pain using words such as "ouch" or "that hurts;" cursing during movement, or exclamations of protest, such as "stop" or "that's enough."		
TOTAL SCORE		

Instructions: Score a 0 if the behavior was not observed; score a 1 if the behavior was observed even briefly during activity or rest. The total score ranges from 0 to 5.

FIGURE 4-13 The Checklist of Non-Verbal Pain Indicators with movement and at rest. (From Feldt, 2000.)

ABNORMALITIES

HYPERTENSION

Hypertension is one of the most common diseases in the world; it is often responsible for stroke, renal failure, and congestive heart failure.

Pathophysiology
- Defined as a blood pressure consistently at 140/90 mm Hg or higher.
- For essential hypertension, its pathologic origin is poorly understood.
- For secondary hypertension, potential causes include renal disease, renal artery stenosis, aldosteronism, thyroid disorders, coarctation of the aorta, or pheochromocytoma.

Subjective Data
- Essential hypertension is asymptomatic.
- In malignant (severe) hypertension, headache, blurred vision, dyspnea, or encephalopathy may be present.

Objective Data
- Multiple confirmed blood pressure readings at or above 140/90 or in children greater than 95th percentile for age, gender, and height percentile.
- End-organ damage (e.g., papilledema and evidence of heart failure) may be present with long-standing hypertension.

NEUROPATHIC PAIN

A form of chronic pain caused by a primary lesion or dysfunction of the central nervous system that persists beyond expected after healing

Pathophysiology
- Potential causes include postherpetic neuralgia, diabetic peripheral neuropathy, trigeminal neuralgia, or radiculopathy.
- Damaged peripheral nerves fire repeatedly. Dorsal horn neurons are hyperexcited and transmit enhanced pain to the brain. This causes sustained pain.

Subjective Data
- Burning, intense tightness, shooting, stabbing, shocklike sensations
- Pain sensations may worsen at night.
- Exaggerated pain response to pain stimuli (hyperalgesia)
- Pain response to stimuli that are not typically painful (allodynia)
- Sleep disturbance
- Interference with activities of daily living, work, or social activities

Objective Data
- Confirmed self-report of pain for all painful body regions
- Distribution of pain sensations (e.g., glove or stocking, leg)
- Pain response to nonpainful stimulus (e.g., stroking skin)
- Light touch, pin prick, vibration sense, and proprioception may be diminished in affected area; numbness, weakness, and loss of deep tendon reflexes in affected area (Gilron et al, 2006)

COMPLEX REGIONAL PAIN SYNDROME

A syndrome in which regional pain extends beyond a specific peripheral nerve injury in an extremity with motor, sensory, and autonomic changes

Pathophysiology

- No relationship between the original trauma severity and the severity and cause of the symptoms
- Cause is unknown, but the sympathetic nervous system helps maintain symptoms.

Subjective Data

- Burning, shooting, or pain with aching character
- Exaggerated sensitivity to cold or sweating changes
- Pain increases or persists after light pressure.
- Allodynia
- Numbness may be present.

Objective Data

- Edema
- Changes in skin blood flow: abnormal skin color; red and hot, cyanotic, temperature difference of up to 1° C between the affected and unaffected extremity
- Increased sweating may be seen

ABNORMALITIES

Mental Status

The mental status portion of the neurologic examination is one of the most complex examinations. Mental status is the total expression of a person's emotional responses, mood, cognitive functioning (ability to think, reason, and make judgments), and personality. A major focus of the examination is identification of the individual's strengths and capabilities for interaction with the environment. This chapter will focus on mental status evaluation of the individual's overall cognitive state. See Chapter 22 for the assessment of neurologic lesions that cause alterations in mental status.

evolve *http://evolve.elsevier.com/Seidel*
• NCLEX Review Questions   • Videos   • Student Checklist

Physical Examination Preview

Here is a preview of the steps involved in conducting a mental status examination. ⓔ These procedures are explained in detail in this chapter and are available on Evolve in printable formats.
1. Observe physical appearance and behavior (pp. 66-67).
2. Investigate cognitive abilities (pp. 67-70):
    • State of consciousness
    • Response to analogies
    • Abstract reasoning
    • Arithmetic calculation
    • Memory
    • Attention span
3. Observe speech and language for the following (pp. 70-71):
    • Voice quality
    • Articulation
    • Coherence
    • Comprehension
4. Evaluate emotional stability for the following (pp. 71-72):
    • Signs of depression or anxiety
    • Disturbance in thought content
    • Hallucinations

ANATOMY AND PHYSIOLOGY

The cerebrum of the brain is primarily responsible for a person's mental status. Many areas in the cerebrum contribute to the total functioning of a person's mental processes. Two cerebral hemispheres, each divided into lobes, comprise the cerebrum. The gray outer layer—the cerebral cortex—houses the higher mental functions and is responsible for perception and behavior (Fig. 5-1).

The frontal lobe, containing the motor cortex, is associated with speech formation (in the Broca area). This lobe is responsible for decision making, problem solving, the ability to concentrate, and short-term memory. Associated areas—related to emotions, affect, drive, and awareness of self and the autonomic responses related to emotional states—also originate in the frontal lobe.

The parietal lobe is primarily responsible for receiving and processing sensory data.

The temporal lobe is responsible for perception and interpretation of sounds as well as localizing their source. It contains the Wernicke speech area, which allows a person to understand spoken and written language. The temporal lobe is also involved in the integration of behavior, emotion, and personality, as well as long-term memory.

The limbic system mediates certain patterns of behavior that determine survival (e.g., mating, aggression, fear, and affection). Reactions to emotions such as anger, love, hostility, and envy originate here, but the expression of emotion and behavior is mediated by connections between the limbic system and the frontal lobe.

The reticular activating system (RAS) in the brainstem regulates awareness and arousal. Disruption of the ascending RAS can lead to altered mental status (e.g., confusion and delirium).

⚜ Infants and Children

All brain neurons are present at birth in a full-term infant, but brain development continues with myelinization of nerve cells over several years. Brain insults, such as infection, trauma, or metabolic imbalance, can damage brain cells, which may result in serious permanent dysfunction in mental status.

⚜ Adolescents

Intellectual maturation continues, with greater capacity for information and vocabulary development. Abstract thinking (i.e., the ability to develop theories, use logical reasoning, make future plans, use generalizations, and consider risks and possibilities)

FIGURE 5-1 **Functional subdivisions of the cerebral cortex.** *(Modified from Thibodeau and Patton, 2003.)*

develops during this period. Judgment begins to develop with education, intelligence, and experience.

❧ Older Adults

Cognitive function should be intact in the healthy older adult, but declines in cognitive abilities occur in some older adults after 60 or 70 years of age. Speed of information processing and psychomotor speed begin declining at a modest rate after 30 years of age. However, verbal skills and general knowledge continue to increase into the 60s and often remain stable into the 80s. Cognitive declines in executive functioning (the ability to plan and develop strategies, organize, concentrate and remember details, and manage activities) often preceded memory loss and other cognitive impairments in a recent study of highly functioning older women (Carlson et al, 2009). The cognitive decline leading to dementia may occur over 20 to 30 years, and it may begin as early as 45 years of age in some persons (Singh-Manoux et al, 2012).

REVIEW OF RELATED HISTORY

For each of the symptoms or conditions discussed in this section, targeted topics to include in the history of the present illness are listed. Responses to questions about these topics provide clues for focusing the physical examination and the development of an appropriate diagnostic evaluation. Questions regarding medication use (prescription and over the counter preparations) as well as complementary and alternative therapies are relevant for each area.

History of Present Illness

- **Disorientation and confusion**
  - Abrupt or insidious onset: intermittent, fluctuating, or persistent; association with time of day or overwhelming emotional crisis
  - Associated health problems: new hearing or vision impairment; neurologic disorder, vascular occlusion, or brain

injury; systemic infection; withdrawal from alcohol; metabolic or electrolyte disorder
  - Associated symptoms: delusions, hallucinations (imaginary perceptions), mood swings, anxiety, sadness, lethargy or agitation, insomnia, change in appetite, drug toxicity
  - Medications: anticholinergics, benzodiazepines, opioid analgesics, tricyclic antidepressants, levodopa or amantadine, diuretics, digoxin, antiarrhythmics, sedatives, hypnotics, or alternative and complementary therapies such as gingko biloba and St. John's wort
- **Depression**
  - Troubling thoughts or feelings, constant worry; change in outlook on life or change in feelings; feelings of hopelessness; inability to control feelings
  - Low energy level, awakens feeling fatigued, agitation, feels best in the morning or at night
  - Recent changes in living situation, death or relocation of friends or family members, changes in physical health
  - Thoughts or plans for hurting self and/or others, thoughts about dying, hopelessness, no plans for the future
  - Medications: antidepressants; medications that may cause or worsen depression (e.g., antihypertensive agents, corticosteroids, beta-blockers, calcium channel blockers, barbiturates, phenytoin, anabolic steroids)
- **Anxiety**
  - Sudden, unexplained episodes of intense fear, anxiety or panic for no apparent reason; afraid will be unable to get help or will be unable to escape in certain situations; unable to control worrying; spends more time than necessary repeatedly doing or checking things
  - Feels uncomfortable in or avoids situations or events that involve being with people
  - Prior experience with a frightening or traumatic event
  - Associated symptoms: panic attacks, obsessive thoughts, or compulsive behaviors
  - Medications: antidepressants, steroids, benzodiazepines

Past Medical History

+ Neurologic disorder, brain surgery, brain injury, residual effects, chronic disease, or debilitating condition
+ Psychiatric disorder or hospitalization

Family History

+ Psychiatric disorders, mental illness, alcoholism
+ Alzheimer disease
+ Learning disorders, intellectual disability, autism

Personal and Social History

+ Emotional status: feelings about self; anxious, restless, or irritable; discouraged or frustrated; problems with money, job, legal system, spouse, partner, or children; ability to cope with current stressors in life
+ Life goals, attitudes, relationship with family members
+ Intellectual level: educational history, access to information, mental stimulation
+ Communication pattern, able to understand questions, coherent and appropriate speech, change in memory or cognitive thought processes
+ Changes in sleeping or eating patterns; change in appetite or diet, weight loss or gain; decreased sexual activity
+ Use of alcohol or illicit drugs, especially mood-altering drugs

✤ Children

+ Speech and language: first words, words understood, progression to phrases and sentences
+ Behavior: temper tantrums, ease in separating from family or adjusting to new situations
+ Performance of self-care activities: dressing, toileting, feeding
+ Personality and behavior patterns: changes related to any specific event, illness, or trauma
+ Learning or school difficulties: associated with interest, hyperactivity, or ability to concentrate

✤ Adolescents

+ Risk-taking behaviors
+ School performance and peer interactions
+ Family interactions, reluctance to talk about attitudes, behaviors and experience

✤ Older Adults

+ Changes in cognitive functioning, thought processes, memory; association with medications prescribed (e.g., opiates, benzodiazepines, antidepressants, corticosteroids, muscle relaxants)
+ Depression: somatic complaints, hopelessness, helplessness, lack of interest in personal care

EXAMINATION AND FINDINGS

Mental status is assessed continuously throughout the entire interaction with a patient by evaluating the patient's alertness,

---

Box 5-1 Procedures of the Mental Status Screening Examination

The shorter screening examination is commonly used for health visits when no known neurologic problem is apparent. Information is generally obtained during the history in the following areas (pp. 66-71):

Appearance and Behavior
- Grooming
- Emotional status
- Body language

Emotional Stability
- Mood and feelings
- Thought processes

Cognitive Abilities
- State of consciousness
- Memory
- Attention span
- Judgment

Speech and Language
- Voice quality
- Articulation
- Comprehension
- Coherence
- Aphasia

FIGURE 5-2 During the initial greeting, observe the patient for behavior, emotional status, grooming, and body language. Note the patient's body posture and ability to make eye contact.

orientation, cognitive abilities, and mood (Box 5-1). Observe the patient's physical appearance, behavior, and responses to questions asked during the history (Fig. 5-2). Note any variations in response to questions of differing complexity. Speech should be clearly articulated. Questions should be answered appropriately, with ideas expressed logically, relating current and past events.

Physical Appearance and Behavior

Grooming

Assess the patient's hygiene, grooming, and appropriateness of dress for age and season. Poor hygiene, lack of concern with appearance, or inappropriate dress for season or occasion in a

EXAMINATION AND FINDINGS

previously well-groomed individual may indicate depression, a psychiatric disorder, or dementia.

Emotional Status

Note the patient's behavior, which is usually cooperative and friendly. The patient's manner should demonstrate concern appropriate for the topics discussed. Consider cultural variations when assessing emotional responses. Note patient behavior that conveys carelessness, apathy, loss of sympathetic reactions, unusual docility, hostility, rage reactions, or excessive irritability.

Nonverbal Communication (Body Language)

Note the patient's posture, eye contact, and facial expression. Some cultural groups will not maintain eye contact with you. Slumped posture and a lack of facial expression may indicate depression or a neurologic condition such as Parkinson disease. Excessively energetic movements or constantly watchful eyes suggest tension, mania, anxiety, a metabolic disorder, or the effects of illicit or prescription drug use (e.g., methamphetamine, amphetamine salts, cocaine, and steroids).

State of Consciousness

The patient should be oriented to person, place, and time and make appropriate responses to questions, as well as physical and environmental stimuli. Person disorientation results from cerebral trauma, seizures, or amnesia. Place disorientation occurs with psychiatric disorders, delirium, and cognitive impairment. Time disorientation is associated with anxiety, delirium, depression, and cognitive impairment. See Table 5-1 for potential causes of unresponsiveness. The Glasgow Coma Scale is used to quantify the level of consciousness after an acute brain injury or medical condition (see Chapter 27).

Cognitive Abilities

Evaluate cognitive functions as the patient responds to questions during the history-taking process. Specific questions and tasks

Table 5-1	Common Causes of Unresponsiveness
Type of Disorder	**Cause**
Focal lesions of the brain	Hemorrhage, hematoma, infarction, tumor, abscess, trauma
Diffuse brain disease	Drug intoxications Disturbances of glucose, sodium, or calcium metabolism, renal failure, myxedema, pulmonary insufficiency Hypothermia, hyperthermia Hypoxic or anoxic event, such as strangulation, drowning, cardiac arrest, pulmonary embolism Encephalitis, meningitis Seizures
Psychogenic unresponsiveness	Dementia

can provide a detailed assessment of cognition, the execution of complex mental processes (e.g., learning, perceiving, decision making, and memory). Several screening tests are available to assess cognition, but the Mini-Mental State Examination (MMSE) is the most studied to date (see Evidence-Based Practice in Physical Examination, "Mini-Mental State Examination").

The Mini-Cog is a brief screening tool for measuring cognitive function that takes up to 5 minutes to administer (Fig. 5-5). Ask the patient to listen carefully to and remember three unrelated words (e.g., "red," "plate," and "milk") and then immediately repeat the words. Do not help if a word is not repeated. Next the patient is asked to draw the face of a clock and draw the hands to read a specific time. The patient has 3 minutes to draw the clock. Once the clock face drawing is completed, ask the patient to repeat the 3 words (1 point for each recalled word). The patient scores 2 points when all numbers of the clock face are near the rim, in correct sequence, and hands point to the specific time requested. A total of 0 to 5 points is possible, and a score of 2 or less may be associated with dementia. The Mini-Cog has a sensitivity of 76% to 99% and a specificity of 89% to 96% for detecting probable dementia (McGee, 2012). It has been used successfully in non–English-speaking and culturally diverse populations, as well as those with varying educational levels (Doerflinger, 2007).

Signs of possible cognitive impairment include the following: significant memory loss, confusion (impaired cognitive function with disorientation, attention and memory deficits, and difficulty answering questions or following commands), impaired communication, inappropriate affect, personal care difficulties, hazardous behavior, agitation, and suspiciousness (see Clinical Pearl, "The Importance of Validation").

Clinical Pearl

The Importance of Validation

If you have concerns about any of the patient's responses or behaviors, it is important to interview a family member or other independent observer and ask if the patient has had any problems with the following activities: remembering important appointments or events, paying bills, shopping independently for food or clothing, taking medication, getting lost while walking or driving, making decisions about daily life, or asking the same thing again and again (Maslow and Mezey, 2008).

Analogies

Ask the patient to describe simple analogies first and then more complex analogies:

+ What is similar about these objects: Peaches and lemons? Ocean and lake? Trumpet and flute?
+ Complete this comparison: An engine is to an airplane as an oar is to a _____.
+ What is different about these two objects: A magazine and a telephone book? A bush and a tree?

Correct responses should be given when the patient has average intelligence. An inability to describe similarities or differences may indicate a lesion of the left or dominant cerebral hemisphere.

EXAMINATION AND FINDINGS

Evidence-Based Practice in Physical Examination

Mini-Mental State Examination

The Mini-Mental State Examination (MMSE) is a standardized tool to assess cognitive function changes over time (Fig. 5-3). The 11 items—measuring orientation, registration, attention and calculation, recall, and language—take approximately 5 to 10 minutes to administer (Folstein et al, 1985). The maximum score is 30. A score of 20 or less may be associated with dementia (sensitivity of 71% to 92%, specificity of 52% to 96%) and a score of 26 or higher is not associated with dementia.

Higher education is associated with higher MMSE scores, even when dementia is present (McGee, 2012; Snyderman and Rovner, 2009). The MMSE has been translated into 15 languages and adapted for many cultures, and in some cases external validity, sensitivity, and specificity have been evaluated (Steis and Schrauf, 2009). Figure 5-4 shows testing of the copying skill under the language portion of the MMSE. See www.minimental.com for access to the full tool.

Mini-Mental State Examination Sample Items

Orientation to Time
"What is the date?"

Registration
"Listen carefully, I am going to say three words. You say them back after I stop.
Ready? Here they are . . . HOUSE (pause), CAR (pause), LAKE (pause).
Now repeat those words back to me."
[Repeat up to five times, but score only the first trial.]

Naming
"What is this?" [Point to a pencil or pen.]

Reading
"Please read this and do what it says." [Show examinee the words on the stimulus form.]
CLOSE YOUR EYES

FIGURE 5-3 **Sample items from the Mini-Mental State Examination (MMSE).** *(Reproduced by special permission of the publisher, Psychological Assessment Resources, Inc., 16204 North Florida Avenue, Lutz, Florida 33549, from the Mini-Mental State Examination by Marshal Folstein and Susan Folstein, Copyright 1975, 1998, 2001 by Mini Mental LLC, Inc. Published 2001 by Psychological Assessment Resources, Inc. Further reproduction is prohibited without permission of PAR, Inc. The MMSE can be purchased from PAR, Inc. online at www.parinc.com or by calling [813]968-3003.)*

FIGURE 5-4 **Copying intersecting pentagons and drawing a clock face are tasks on the Mini-Mental State Examination.**

EXAMINATION AND FINDINGS

The Mini-Cog Assessment Instrument for Dementia

The Mini-Cog assessment instrument combines an uncued 3-item recall test with a clock-drawing test (CDT). The Mini-Cog can be administered in about 3 minutes, requires no special equipment, and is relatively uninfluenced by level of education or language variations.

Administration

The test is administered as follows:

1. Instruct the patient to listen carefully to and remember 3 unrelated words and then to repeat the words.

2. Instruct the patient to draw the face of a clock, either on a blank sheet of paper or on a sheet with the clock circle already drawn on the page. After the patient puts the numbers on the clock face, ask him or her to draw the hands of the clock to read a specific time, such as 11:20. These instructions can be repeated, but no additional instructions should be given. Give the patient as much time as needed to complete the task. The CDT serves as the recall distractor.

3. Ask the patient to repeat the 3 previously presented words.

Scoring

Give 1 point for each recalled word after the CDT distractor. Score 1–3.

A score of O indicates positive screen for dementia.

A score of 1 or 2 with an abnormal CDT indicates positive screen for dementia.

A score of 1 or 2 with a normal CDT indicates negative screen for dementia.

A score of 3 indicates negative screen for dementia.

The CDT is considered normal if all numbers are present in the correct sequence and position, and the hands readably display the requested time.

Source: Borson S, Scanlan J, Brush M, Vitaliano P, Dokmak A. The mini-cog: a cognitive "vital signs" measure for dementia screening in multi-lingual elderly. *Int J Geriatr Psychiatry* 2000; 15(11):1021–1027.

FIGURE 5-5 **The Mini-Cog is a brief screening tool for measuring cognitive function.**

Abstract Reasoning

Ask the patient to tell you the meaning of a fable, proverb, or metaphor, such as the following:
+ A stitch in time saves nine.
+ A bird in the hand is worth two in the bush.
+ A rolling stone gathers no moss.

When the patient has average intelligence, an adequate interpretation should be given. Inability to explain a phrase may indicate poor cognition, dementia, brain damage, or schizophrenia.

Arithmetic Calculation

Ask the patient to do simple arithmetic, without paper and pencil, such as the following:
+ Subtract 7 from 50, subtract 7 from that answer, and so on, until the answer is 8.
+ Add 8 to 50, add 8 to that total, and so on, until the answer is 98.

The calculations should be completed with few errors and within 1 minute when the patient has average intelligence.

Impairment of arithmetic skills may be associated with depression and diffuse brain disease.

Writing Ability

Ask the patient to write his or her name and address or a dictated phrase. Omission or addition of letters, syllables, words, or mirror writing may indicate aphasia (impairment in language function). Alternatively, if poor literacy is a concern, ask the patient to draw simple geometric figures (e.g., a triangle, circle, or square) and then more complex figures such as a clock face, a house, or a flower. Uncoordinated writing or drawing may indicate dementia, parietal lobe damage, a cerebellar lesion, or peripheral neuropathy.

Execution of Motor Skills

Ask the patient to unbutton a shirt button or to comb his or her hair. Apraxia (the inability to translate an intention into action that is unrelated to paralysis or lack of comprehension) may indicate a cerebral disorder.

Video: Assessing Memory

Memory

Immediate recall or new learning: Ask the patient to listen and then repeat a sentence or a series of numbers. Five to eight numbers forward or four to six numbers backward can usually be repeated.

Recent memory: Give the patient a short time to view four or five test objects, telling him or her that you will ask about them in a few minutes. Ten minutes later, ask the patient to list the objects. All objects should be remembered. See Clinical Pearl, "Testing Memory in the Visually Impaired."

Remote memory: Ask the patient about verifiable past events such as mother's maiden name, high school attended, or a subject of common knowledge.

Memory loss may result from disease, infection, or temporal lobe trauma. Impaired memory occurs with various neurologic or psychiatric disorders, such as anxiety and depression. Loss of immediate and recent memory with retention of remote memory suggests dementia.

Clinical Pearl

Testing Memory in the Visually Impaired
When a patient is visually impaired, test recent memory with unrelated words rather than observed objects. Pick four unrelated words that sound distinctly different, such as "green," "daffodil," "hero," and "sofa" or "bird," "carpet," "treasure," and "orange." Tell the patient to remember these words. After 5 minutes, ask the patient to list the four words.

Attention Span

Ask the patient to follow a short set of commands. Alternatively, ask the patient to say either the days of the week or to spell the word "world" forward or backward. The ability to perform arithmetic calculations is another test of attention span. Appropriate response to directions is expected. Easy distraction, confusion, negativism, and impairment of recent and remote memory may all indicate a decreased attention span. This may be related to fatigue, depression, delirium, or toxic or metabolic causes that result in confusion.

Judgment

Determine the patient's judgment and reasoning skills by exploring the following topics:

+ How is the patient meeting social and family obligations?
+ What are the patient's plans for the future? Do they seem appropriate?
+ Ask the patient to provide solutions to hypothetical situations, such as: "What would you do if you found a stamped envelope?" "What would you do if you were stopped by a police officer after you drove through a red light?"

If the patient is meeting social and family obligations and adequately dealing with financial obligations, judgment is considered intact. The patient should be able to evaluate the situations presented and recognize the consequences of action. Impaired judgment may indicate intellectual disability, emotional disturbance, frontal lobe injury, dementia, or psychosis.

Speech and Language Skills

Detailed evaluation of the patient's communication skills, both receptive and expressive, should be performed if the patient has difficulty communicating during the history. The patient's voice should have inflections, be clear and strong, and be able to increase in volume. Determine if the patient's rate of speech is excessively fast or slow, normal, or has hesitations. Speech should be fluent with clear expression of thoughts.

Voice Quality

Determine if there is any difficulty or discomfort in phonation, or if laryngeal speech sounds are present. Dysphonia, a disorder of voice volume, quality (e.g., harsh, nasal, or breathy), or pitch (e.g., monotony of pitch or loudness), suggests a problem with laryngeal innervation or disease of the larynx.

Articulation

Evaluate spontaneous speech for pronunciation and ease of expression. Abnormal articulation includes imprecise pronunciation of consonants, slurring, difficulty articulating a single speech sound, hesitations, repetitions, and stuttering. Dysarthria, a motor speech disorder, is associated with many conditions of the nervous system such as stroke, inebriation, cerebral palsy, and Parkinson disease.

Comprehension

Ask the patient to follow simple one- and two-step directions during the examination, such as during the attention span assessment. The patient should be able to follow simple instructions.

Coherence

The patient's intentions or perceptions should be clearly conveyed to you. Communication characteristics that may be associated with a psychiatric disorder include:

+ Circumlocution—Pantomime or word substitution to avoid revealing that a word was forgotten
+ Perseveration—Repetition of a word, phrase, or gesture
+ Flight of ideas or use of loose associations—Disordered words or sentences
+ Word salad—Meaningless, disconnected word choices
+ Neologisms—Made up words; have meaning only to the patient
+ Clang association—Word choice based on sound so that words rhyme in a nonsensical way (e.g., The far car mar to the star)
+ Echolalia—Repetition of another person's words
+ Utterances of unusual sounds

Aphasia, a speech disorder that can be receptive (understanding language) or expressive (speaking language) may be indicated by hesitations and other speech rhythm disturbances, omission of syllables or words, word transposition, circumlocutions, and neologisms. Aphasia can result from facial muscle or tongue weakness or from neurologic damage to brain regions controlling speech and language. Characteristics of different types of aphasia are listed in the Differential Diagnosis table on page 71.

DIFFERENTIAL DIAGNOSIS
Distinguishing Characteristics of Aphasias

Characteristics	Broca Aphasia (Expressive)	Wernicke Aphasia (Receptive)	Global Aphasia (Expressive and Receptive)
Word comprehension	Fair to good	Can hear words but cannot relate them to previous experiences	Absent or reduced to person's own name, few select words
Spontaneous speech	Impaired speech flow; laborious effort to speak; know what they want to say but cannot articulate properly; telegraphic speech (mostly nouns and verbs)	Fluent speech but uses words inappropriately, such as neologisms or word substitutions; may be totally incomprehensible	Absent or reduced to only a few words or sounds
Reading comprehension	Intact	Impaired	Severely impaired
Writing	Impaired	Impaired	Severely impaired

Emotional Stability

Emotional stability is evaluated when the patient does not seem to be coping well or does not have resources to meet his or her personal needs.

Mood and Feelings

During the history and physical examination, observe the mood and emotional expression evident from the patient's verbal and nonverbal behaviors. Note any mood swings or behaviors indicating anxiety, depression, anger, hostility, or hypervigilance.

Ask the patient how he or she feels right now, whether feelings are a problem in daily life, and whether there are times or experiences that are particularly difficult for the patient. The following questions, recommended for depression screening by the U.S. Preventive Health Task Force, have a sensitivity of 96% and specificity of 57% (Snyderman and Rovner, 2009):

+ Over the past 2 weeks, have you felt down, depressed, or hopeless?
+ Over the past 2 weeks, have you felt little interest or pleasure in doing things?

A positive response to both questions is an indication to ask more questions about depression symptoms such as fatigue, restlessness, and poor concentration.

Be concerned if the patient does not express appropriate feelings that correspond to the situation. For example, does the patient laugh when talking about a seriously ill family member? Unresponsiveness, hopelessness, agitation, aggression, anger, euphoria, irritability, or wide mood swings indicate disturbances in mood, affect, and feelings. Identify the potential for suicide.

Thought Process and Content

Observe the patient's thought patterns, especially the appropriateness of sequence, logic, coherence, and relevance to the topics discussed. The patient's thought process should be easy to follow with logical and goal-directed ideas expressed. Illogical, disorganized, or unrealistic thought processes, flight of ideas (rapid disconnected thoughts), blocking (i.e., an inappropriate pause in the middle of a thought, phrase, or sentence), or an impaired stream

Risk Factors
Suicide

- Social isolation, older men or women, divorced or widowed, living alone
- Mental health disorder, depression, hopelessness
- Serious chronic or terminal health condition (e.g., HIV infection, cancer, renal failure)
- Family history of suicide or suicide attempt; knowing someone who recently attempted or committed suicide
- Significant personal losses or challenges (e.g., bereavement, financial or legal problems, unemployment, adolescent feeling disrespected, recent break up with partner)
- Has thought about a plan for suicide; previous suicide attempt
- Alcohol and substance use disorders
- Access to firearms or other means of self-harm

of thinking (e.g., repetition of a word, phrase, or behavior) indicates an emotional disturbance or a psychiatric disorder.

Evaluate disturbance in thought content by asking about obsessive thoughts related to fears, guilt, or making decisions. Does the patient ever feel like he or she is being watched or followed, is controlled or manipulated, or loses touch with reality? Does the patient compulsively repeat actions or check and recheck to make sure something is done? Obsessive thoughts, compulsive behaviors, phobias, or anxieties that interfere with daily life may indicate mental dysfunction or a psychiatric disorder.

Does the patient have delusions (false personal beliefs not shared by others in the same culture), such as delusions of grandeur or of being controlled by an outside force? Does the patient feel unrealistic persecution, jealousy, or paranoia? Delusions are often associated with psychiatric disorders, delirium, and alcohol or drug intoxication. See Clinical Pearl, "Distorted Thinking."

Perceptual Distortions and Hallucinations

Determine whether the patient perceives any sensations that are not caused by external stimuli (e.g., hears voices, sees vivid images

Clinical Pearl

Distorted Thinking
A patient who demonstrates an unrealistic sense of persecution, jealousy, grandiose ideas, or ideas of reference (e.g., neutral things in the environment have a special meaning to the person) may be experiencing distorted thinking.

or shadowy figures, smells offensive odors, tastes offensive flavors, feels worms crawling on the skin). Find out when these experiences occur. Auditory and visual hallucinations are associated with psychiatric disorders, severe depression, acute intoxication, delirium, and dementia. Tactile hallucinations are most commonly associated with alcohol withdrawal.

✤ Infants and Children

Evaluate an infant's general behavior and level of consciousness by observing the level of activity and responsiveness to environmental stimuli. Note whether the baby is lethargic, drowsy, stuporous, alert, active, or irritable (Fig. 5-6, *A*). By 2 months of age, the infant should appear alert, quiet, and content, and should recognize the face of a primary caregiver (Fig. 5-6, *B*). The examiner who devotes time to developing a relationship with a 2- to 3-month old infant should be able to coax a smile. When it is difficult or impossible to elicit a social smile in an infant who appears ill, be concerned about a neurologic condition or infection, such as meningitis. Be concerned if the mother or primary caregiver is depressed because the infant's social and emotional development is influenced by interaction with that person.

Crying and other vocal sounds are evaluated when language has not yet developed. The infant's cry should be loud and angry. A shrill or whiny, high-pitched cry or catlike screeching cry suggests a central nervous system deficit. Cooing and babbling are expected after 3 and 4 months of age, respectively.

Evaluate the types of words and speech patterns used by the child. Language development should be appropriate for age and speech should be more clearly understandable as the child ages. Table 5-2 describes expressive language milestones for toddlers. Articulation milestones in children between 2.5 and 6 years of age may be evaluated with the Denver Articulation Screening Exam (DASE) (see www.denverii.com/DASE.html).

Questionnaires completed by parents (e.g., Ages and Stages Questionnaire [see www.agesandstages.com] and Parent's Evaluation of Developmental Status (PEDStest.com) [see www.pedstest.com]) are effective screening tools for developmental assessment. These questionnaires have good sensitivity and specificity for detecting developmental concerns. The Denver II tool is useful for determining whether the child is developing fine and gross motor skills, language, and personal-social skills as expected. Ask children 5 years and older to draw a picture of a person, doing the best job possible. Scores for the detail in 14 body part attributes are available to assess cognitive development (Perniciano, 2012) (Fig. 5-7).

Observe the child's behaviors during the patient history to identify mood, activity level, communication pattern, preferences, responsiveness to the parent, and ability to separate. Does

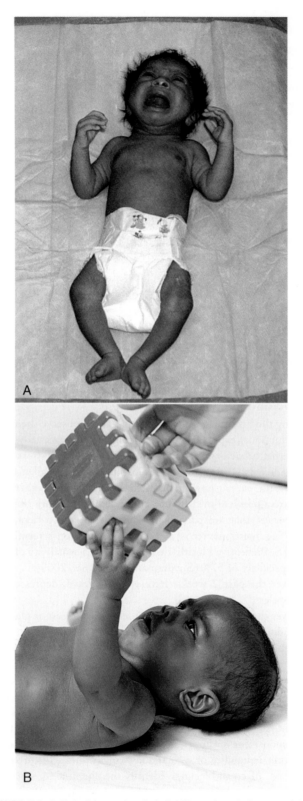

FIGURE 5-6 **A,** Note this newborn's irritability and posturing associated with cocaine withdrawal. **B,** Note this infant's level of alertness and interest in various objects and people.

Table 5-2	Expressive Language Milestones for Toddlers and Preschoolers
Age (mo)	Expressive Language Milestones
4 to 6	Babbles speech-like sounds, including p, b, and m
10 to 12	Has 1 or 2 words, such as "mama," "dada," "bye-bye"
12 to 24	Increases words each month, 2-word combinations (e.g., "Where baby?" and "Want cookie")
24 to 36	Uses two- to three-word sentences to ask for things or talk about things, large vocabulary, speech understood by family members
36 to 48	Sentences may have four or more words, speech understood by most people
48 to 60	Says most sounds correctly except a few like l, s, r, v, z, ch, sh, th. Tells stories and uses same grammar as rest of family

Data from American Speech and Language Association (2011). *How does your child hear and talk?* Retrieved from www.asha.org/public/speech/development/chart.htm.

FIGURE 5-8 Test a child's memory recall by using familiar objects.

FIGURE 5-7 Ask the child to draw a picture of a man or woman. The presence and form of body parts provide a clue about the child's development when following the scoring criteria of the Goodenough-Harris Drawing Test.

the child have self-comforting measures? Does the child play and have fun?

Attempt memory testing at about 4 years of age if the child pays attention and is not too anxious. Expected memory skills vary with the age of the child. When testing immediate recall, a 4-year-old can repeat three digits or words, a 5-year-old can repeat four digits or words, and a 6-year-old can repeat five digits or words. Test recent memory in a child starting at 5 to 6 years by showing the child familiar objects and waiting no longer than 5 minutes to ask the child to recall the objects (Fig. 5-8). Remote memory is tested by asking the child what he or she had for dinner the previous night or what his or her address is, or asking the child to recite a nursery rhyme.

Concerns about behaviors and mood disorders may be assessed in children 4 to 18 years of age with tools like the Pediatric Symptom Checklist (www2.massgeneral.org/allpsych/psc/psc_home.htm). Positive responses should prompt questions about school, family, friends, moods, and activities.

⚙ Pregnant Women

The prevalence of depression during pregnancy and postpartum is estimated to be 10% to 16%, whereas postpartum "blues" may be found in up to 70% of women. Postpartum psychosis occurs in 0.2% of women (Muzik et al, 2009). Risk factors for postpartum depression include a history of depression, prior postpartum depression, and poor social support. Because the depression may interfere with the mother's health, ability to work, attachment to the newborn, and the infant's subsequent development, all new mothers should be screened for depressive symptoms.

One approach to such screening is to phrase open-ended questions in a positive and validating manner at least once during each trimester and postpartum. Examples are "Many pregnant women get sad or depressed. Have you felt this way?" or "Lots of new moms are overwhelmed by having a new baby around. How are you doing?" Use of the two depression screening questions on p. 71 is also an appropriate screening method. A positive response to questions should lead to additional questions to determine if depression is present.

⚙ Older Adults

Mental function as a whole may be evaluated in about 5 minutes with the Isaac Set Test. Ask the patient to name 10 items in each of four groups: Fruits, Animals, Colors, and Towns/cities (FACT) without prompting or rushing (Chopard et al, 2007; Isaacs and Akhtar, 1972). The patient's ability to respond demonstrates executive functioning, alertness, attention span, and recent memory. The patient has to categorize, count, name, and remember the items listed. Give each item 1 point for a possible total score of 40. Expect a score greater than 25. Dementia is associated with a score less than 15. Scores between 15 and 25 may be associated with mental changes and cultural, educational, or social factors.

Recent memory for important events and conversations is usually not impaired. The older adult may complain about memory loss but this is not predictive of cognitive decline.

EXAMINATION AND FINDINGS

Staying Well

Promoting Memory and Cognitive Functioning

Encourage patients to engage in a variety of cognitive exercises such as using the computer, various games, reading books, and craft activities such as knitting or sewing because such activities are associated with a significantly reduced risk of developing mild cognitive impairment (Geda et al, 2011). Lifestyles that include physical activities and extensive social interactions in addition to cognitive stimulation are believed to offer the best opportunity to preserve cognitive function (La Rue, 2010).

Individuals who report that memory loss interfered with daily activities were at higher risk for cognitive decline (Sargent-Cox et al, 2011). When close family members are more concerned about memory loss than the patient, be concerned about cognitive impairment and dementia (Rabins, 2004).

Determine whether any changes in cerebral function could be the result of cardiovascular, hepatic, renal, or metabolic disease. Medications can also impair central nervous system function, causing slowed reaction time, disorientation, confusion, loss of memory, tremors, and anxiety. Problems may develop because of the dosage, number, or interaction of prescribed and over the counter medications. Review the patient's ability to perform activities of daily living associated with mental status functioning.

Older adults are expected to maintain the same level of interpersonal skills and have no personality changes. Depression, one of the most common conditions in older adults, may contribute to cognitive impairment. Depression can be identified with the Geriatric Depression Scale (Fig. 5-9). Paranoid thought may be a striking alteration in personality. Attempt to determine whether the thought process is accurate or a paranoid ideation, keeping in mind the incidence of elder abuse. Facial expressions that are masklike or overly dramatic, or a stance that is stooped and fearful, may indicate a progressive disease in the older adult.

FUNCTIONAL ASSESSMENT

Activities of Daily Living Related to Mental Status

The ability to perform instrumental activities of daily living (ADLs), or the ability to live independently, is an important assessment. When assessing the patient's mental status, attempt to determine the patient's ability to perform the following:

- Shop, cook, and prepare nutritious meals
- Use problem-solving skills
- Manage medications (purchase, understand, and follow directions)
- Manage personal finances and business affairs
- Speak, write, and understand spoken and written language
- Remember appointments, family occasions, holidays, household tasks

Sample Documentation

History and Physical Examination

Subjective

66 year-old female accompanied by spouse who expresses concern about his wife's memory loss. One week ago she got lost in a shopping mall she frequently visited. Previously was a good cook, but over the last few months either does not have necessary ingredients or has difficulty following recipes. Needs help to ensure that she takes correct daily medications. Able to dress and undress self independently, but now needs help to select clothes appropriate for the occasion. Spouse has assumed more household work and some meal preparation. Patient recognizes all family members and social contacts and is able to talk with them.

Objective

Pleasant woman with clear speech who responds to simple questions correctly. Turns to spouse frequently for answers to some history questions. Follows one-step directions, but needs reminder with two-step directions. Immediate and recent memory impaired, but remote memory is intact. Arithmetic calculation impaired. Mini-Cog score = 2, and Set Test score = 14. For additional sample documentation, see Chapter 26, pp. 628-631.

Ask the patient to choose the best answer for how he or she felt over the preceding week.

1. Are you basically satisfied with your life?	Yes/No
2. Have you dropped many of your activities and interests?	Yes/No
3. Do you feel that your life is empty?	Yes/No
4. Do you often get bored?	Yes/No
5. Are you in good spirits most of the time?	Yes/No
6. Are you afraid that something bad is going to happen to you?	Yes/No
7. Do you feel happy most of the time?	Yes/No
8. Do you feel helpless?	Yes/No
9. Do you prefer to stay at home rather than going out and doing new things?	Yes/No
10. Do you feel you have more problems with memory than most people?	Yes/No
11. Do you think it is wonderful to be alive now?	Yes/No
12. Do you feel pretty worthless the way you are now?	Yes/No
13. Do you feel full of energy?	Yes/No
14. Do you feel that your situation is hopeless?	Yes/No
15. Do you think most people are better off than you are?	Yes/No

Correct responses are the following:
Yes for questions 2, 3, 4, 6, 8, 9, 10, 12, 14, and 15.
No for questions 1, 5, 7, 11, and 13.
Give 1 point for each correct answer. A score greater than 5 suggests depression.

FIGURE 5-9 Geriatric Depression Scale (short form). *(From www.stanford.edu/~yesavage.)*

ABNORMALITIES

MENTAL STATUS

DISORDERS OF ALTERED MENTAL STATUS

Concussion

An alteration in mental status resulting from a blow to the head, face, or neck

Pathophysiology

- A blow causes acceleration-deceleration and rotational forces that may stretch, compress, or shear nerve fibers as the brain moves within the skull, and disrupts the brain chemicals responsible for brain functioning; often caused by sports injuries (see Chapter 23).

Subjective Data

- Headache
- Dazed or dizzy
- Nausea and vomiting
- Blurred vision
- Ringing in ears
- Amnesia
- Restless or irritable
- May or may not have lost consciousness

Objective Data

- Dazed expression
- Slow motor and verbal responses, slurred speech
- Emotional lability
- Hypersensitivity to stimuli
- Deficits in coordination, cognition, memory, and attention
- Coma (sign of a more severe injury)
- Symptoms may disappear within 15 minutes or persist for several weeks

Delirium

Impaired cognition, consciousness, mood and behavioral dysfunction of acute onset

Pathophysiology

- Risk factors in older adults include serious illness or injury, impaired vision or hearing, or age-related changes in how medications are metabolized (Smith and Serafi, 2009)

Subjective Data

- Suspicious, fearful
- Mood swings
- See Differential Diagnosis table on p. 76

Objective Data

- Altered consciousness
- Incoherence, illogical flow of ideas
- Illusions, hallucinations, delusions
- Poor memory

ABNORMALITIES

DIFFERENTIAL DIAGNOSIS

Distinguishing Characteristics of Delirium, Dementia, and Depression

Characteristic	Delirium	Dementia	Depression
Onset	Sudden	Insidious, relentless	Sudden or insidious
Duration	Hours, days	Persistent	For longer than 2 wk
Time of day	Fluctuates during the day	Stable, no change	Throughout most of the day
Consciousness	Altered	Not impaired except in severe cases	Not impaired
Cognition	Impairment of memory, attentiveness, numerous errors in assessment tasks	Minimal cognitive impairment initially, progresses to impaired abstract thinking, judgment, memory, thought patterns, calculations, agnosia	Impaired concentration, reduced attention span, indecisiveness, slower thought processes, impaired short-term and long-term memory
Activity	Increased or decreased activity, may fluctuate	Unchanged from usual behavior	Insomnia or excessive sleeping, fatigue, restlessness, anxiety, increased or decreased appetite
Speech/language	Rambling and irrelevant conversation, illogical flow of ideas, incoherent	Disordered, rambling, incoherent; struggles to find words	Slower speech
Mood and affect	Rapid mood swings; fearful, suspicious	Depressed, apathetic, uninterested	Sad, hopeless, feels worthless, loss of interest or pleasure
Delusions/hallucinations	Misperceptions, illusions, hallucinations, and delusions	Misperceptions usually absent, delusions, no hallucinations	Usually no delusions or hallucinations
Reversibility	Potential	No, progressive	Can be treated, may recur
Pathophysiology	Associated with infections, medications, electrolyte and metabolic disorders, major organ failure, brain injury, and acute alcohol withdrawal (Smith and Serafi, 2009)	Usually related to structural diseases of the brain	Associated with grief, a stressful life event, reaction to medical or neurologic diseases, or a change in lifestyle

DISORDERS OF MOOD

Depression

A mood disorder in which feelings of sadness, loss, anger, or frustration interfere with everyday life for an extended period (weeks or longer)

Pathophysiology
- Associated with a neurochemical imbalance, a decreased level of monoamines, or increased plasma cortisol
- Associated with stressful life event, grief, or change in lifestyle

Subjective Data
- Feels sad, hopeless, worthless
- No interest or pleasure in what was previously of interest or pleasurable
- Insomnia or excessive sleeping
- Increased or decreased appetite

Objective Data
- Poor concentration
- Slowed thought processes and speech
- Agitation or restlessness
- See Differential Diagnosis table above

Mania

A persistently elevated, expansive, euphoric or irritable and agitated mood lasting longer than a week; one phase of the bipolar psychiatric disorder

Pathophysiology
- Associated with abnormal levels of neurotransmitters, norepinephrine, serotonin, dopamine, glutamate, and gamma-aminobutyric acid (GABA) (Wieseke et al, 2011)

Subjective Data
- Hyperactivity
- Overconfidence, exaggerated view of own abilities
- Impaired occupational, social, and interpersonal functioning
- Excessive involvement in pleasurable activities with high potential for serious or painful consequences
- Decreased need for sleep
- Racing thoughts
- Lack of impulse control

Objective Data
- Grandiose or persecutory delusions, euphoria
- Increased talkativeness or pressure to keep talking, may involve excessive rhyming or puns; flight of ideas
- Impaired attention, easily distracted
- Impaired judgment

Anxiety Disorder

A group of disorders with such marked anxiety or fear that it causes significant interference with personal, social, and occupational functioning

Pathophysiology	Subjective Data	Objective Data

• Abnormalities in the norepinephrine and serotonin systems
• Specific disorders include:
  • Panic attacks
  • Generalized anxiety disorder
  • Specific phobias
  • Obsessive-compulsive disorder (OCD)
  • Posttraumatic stress disorder (PTSD)
	• *Panic attacks:* palpitations, sweating, shaking, dizziness, faintness, chest pain, nausea, abdominal distress, chronic social avoidance
	• *Generalized anxiety disorder:* chronic worry, restless, irritable, tense, fatigue, poor concentration, sleep disturbance
	• *OCD:* preoccupation with contamination, religious, or sexual themes; belief that failure to perform a specific act will lead to a bad outcome
	• *PTSD:* recurrent intrusive flashbacks, dreams, thoughts; avoidance behavior; sleeping difficulty; hypervigilance; poor concentration
		• *Panic attacks:* tachycardia, diaphoresis, tremors
		
		• *Generalized anxiety disorder:* impaired attention, motor tension, tremors
		
		• *OCD:* Ritualized acts performed compulsively (washing, cleaning, hoarding, organizing, counting)
		
		• *PTSD:* anger or rage reactions, impulsive behavior, hyperarousal, condition persists for more than 4 weeks

Schizophrenia

A severe, persistent, psychotic syndrome with impaired reality that relapses throughout life

Pathophysiology	Subjective Data	Objective Data
• A genetic susceptibility interacts with environmental considerations such as intrauterine infection, maternal nutritional deficiencies, brain injury, substance use (e.g., cannabis). Neurochemical and brain cell changes may account for symptom onset (Freudenreich et al, 2008).	• Hears voices • Unpleasant tastes or odors • Sees images • Paranoid thoughts • Unable to experience emotions, blunted affect, apathy, detached from environment • Poor personal hygiene	• Incoherent speech, loose associations, illogical answers to questions • Hallucinations (tactile, auditory, visual, somatic, gustatory, or olfactory) • Delusions • Repetitive or aimless behavior • Inappropriate affect in response to a situation

✿ Infants and Children

Intellectual Disability

A developmental, cognitive, or intellectual deficit that begins before 18 years of age, with accompanying deficits in adaptive behavior, academic performance, and adaptive functioning; previously called mental retardation

Pathophysiology	Subjective Data	Objective Data
• May be associated with structural brain defects, genetic disorders, fetal alcohol syndrome, or serious brain insult (infection or injury) during childhood • Genetic link (e.g., parents have intellectual disability) • Cause may not be identified	• Delayed motor development • Delayed speech and language skills	• Delayed developmental milestones • Impaired cognitive function and short-term memory • Poor academic performance • Lack of motivation

Attention-Deficit/Hyperactivity Disorder (ADHD)

A neurobehavioral problem of impaired attention and hyperactive behavior affecting 5% to 10% of school-age children

Pathophysiology	Subjective Data	Objective Data
• Disorder with genetic component potentially affecting dopamine transport and reception; also may be associated with severe traumatic brain injury or functional brain abnormalities (Kelly and Natale, 2011)	• Short attention span, easily distracted, fails to complete school assignments or follow instructions • Fidgets and squirms, often moving, running, climbing • Disruptive behavior, talks excessively, temper outbursts, labile moods, poor impulse control	• Onset before 7 years of age • Increased motor activity • Difficulty organizing tasks • Difficulty sustaining attention • Poor school performance • Low self-esteem • Has problems in more than one setting

ABNORMALITIES

Autism

A pervasive neurodevelopmental disorder of unknown etiology; refers to a wide spectrum of disorders typically identified prior to 3 years of age and in more boys than girls

Pathophysiology

- A strong genetic influence that inactivates areas of the genome that affect early brain development; potential intrauterine toxic insults leading to abnormal brain growth in the frontal, temporal, cerebellar and limbic areas (Raviola et al, 2011)
- Active research continues to clarify the pathophysiology

Subjective Data

- Does not make eye contact or point to objects for the purpose of sharing experiences with others
- Resists being held or touched
- Odd and repetitive behaviors
- Ritualized play, preoccupation with parts of objects
- Motor development appropriate for age

Objective Data

- Impaired social interactions
- Impaired language, either delayed or undeveloped
- Odd intonation to speech, pronoun reversal, nonsensical rhyming
- Impaired symbolic and imaginative play
- Lacks awareness of others
- Cognitive impairment in many cases
- Macrocephaly apparent by 1 year of age (Chawarska et al, 2011)

� Older Adults

Dementia

A chronic, slowly progressive disorder of failing memory, cognitive impairment, behavioral abnormalities, and personality changes that often begins after age 60 years

Pathophysiology

- Usually related to structural diseases of the brain

DEMENTIA OF ALZHEIMER TYPE

- Up to 70% of cases; presence of senile plaques and neurofibrillary tangles may be associated with abnormal amyloid processing or deposition (Castellani et al, 2010)

VASCULAR DEMENTIA

- Up to 20% of cases; acute or recurrent embolic strokes, cerebral hemorrhage due to hypertension (Wright et al, 2008)

OTHER DEMENTIAS

- Associated with diffuse Lewy bodies in the brain, Parkinson disease, and frontal lobe degeneration (Wright et al, 2008)

Subjective Data

- Impaired memory, forgets appointments
- Gets lost in familiar areas, wanders
- Unable to manage shopping, food preparation, medication, finances, and driving
- Behavioral changes, such as socially inappropriate dress or conduct, impaired grooming, impulsiveness, disinhibition
- Aphasia, agnosia, apraxia
- Apathy, withdrawal
- Anxiety, irritability
- Changes in mood (depression, uncharacteristic anger, anxiety, agitation)
- See Differential Diagnosis table on p. 76

Objective Data

- Memory impairment
- Disturbance in executive functioning
- Impairment in social and occupational functioning
- Impaired use of language
- Impaired functioning in activities of daily living
- Eventual profound disintegration of personality and complete disorientation
- Failure to identify odors may be early indication of Alzheimer disease onset (Wilson et al, 2007)
- Stepwise deterioration of cognitive function with plateaus and occasional episodes of improvement characteristic of vascular dementia

CHAPTER 6

Growth and Measurement

Weight and body composition offer information about an individual's health status and may provide a clue to the presence of disease when they are out of balance. This chapter focuses on the evaluation of an individual's body size and the examination for growth, gestational age, and pubertal development. Nutritional assessment is discussed in Chapter 7. Neurologic and motor development of children is discussed in Chapters 21 and 22.

evolve *http://evolve.elsevier.com/Seidel*
• NCLEX Review Questions   • Videos

Physical Examination Preview

Here is a preview of the steps involved in conducting an examination of growth and measurement.

1. From the history, assess the patient's size (pp. 82-83), including the following:
   • Recent growth, weight gain, or weight loss
   • Chronic illnesses affecting weight gain or loss
2. Obtain the following body size measurements (p. 83):
   • Standing height
   • Weight
   • Calculate the body mass index

ANATOMY AND PHYSIOLOGY

Growth, the increase in size of an individual or of a single organ, is dependent on a sequence of endocrine, genetic, environmental, and nutritional influences.

Many hormones must interact and be in balance for normal growth and development to proceed (Fig. 6-1). Two hypothalamic hormones control growth hormone synthesis and secretion in the anterior pituitary gland. Growth hormone–releasing hormone (GHRH) stimulates the pituitary to release growth hormone. Somatostatin inhibits the secretion of both GHRH and thyroid-stimulating hormone. Growth hormone is secreted in pulses, with 70% of secretion occurring during deep sleep (Sam and Frohman, 2008). Growth hormone promotes growth and increase in organ size, and it regulates carbohydrate, protein, and lipid metabolism.

Thyroid hormone stimulates growth hormone secretion and the production of insulin-like growth factor 1 (IGF-1) and interleukins 6 and 8 (IL-6 and IL-8), which have an important role in bone formation and resorption. Thyroid hormones also affect the growth and maturation of other body tissues.

IGF-1 is a growth hormone–dependent peptide primarily produced by the liver. Insulin regulates its synthesis (Clemmons, 2007). IGF-1 exerts a negative feedback effect on growth hormone secretion and mediates the effect of growth hormone on the peripheral tissues (Goldenberg and Barkan, 2007). IGF-1 stimulates the target cells that control connective tissue growth and ossification. Ghrelin, a peptide synthesized in the peripheral tissues and gastric mucosa, helps control growth hormone release and influences food intake and obesity development (Melmed and Kleinbert, 2008).

Leptin has a key role in regulating body fat mass, and its concentration is thought to be a trigger for puberty by informing the central nervous system that adequate nutritional status and body fat mass are present to support pubertal changes and growth (Low, 2011). During puberty the gonads begin to secrete testosterone and estrogen. Rising levels of these hormones trigger the release of gonadotropins (luteinizing hormone [LH] and follicle-stimulating hormone [FSH]) that stimulate the gonads to release more sex hormones. The genitalia begin growing to adult proportions. Testosterone enhances muscular development and sexual maturation, and it promotes bone maturation and epiphyseal closure. Estrogen stimulates the development of female secondary sexual characteristics, regulating the timing of the growth spurt and the acceleration of skeletal maturation and epiphyseal fusion. Androgens, secreted by the adrenal glands, promote masculinization of the secondary sex characteristics and skeletal maturation.

Growth at puberty is dependent on the interaction of growth hormone, IGF-1, and the sex steroids (androgens). The sex steroids stimulate an increased secretion of the growth hormone, which in turn mediates the dramatic increase in IGF-1. This leads to the adolescent growth spurt.

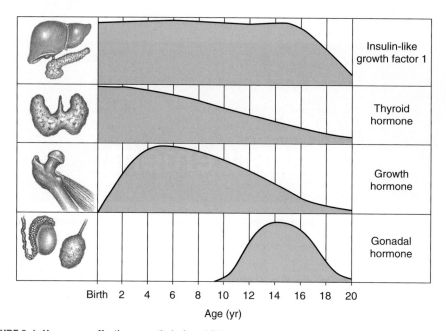

FIGURE 6-1 Hormones affecting growth during childhood and the ages at which they are most influential. *(Redrawn from Hughes, 1984.)*

Differences in Growth by Organ System

Each organ or organ system has its particular period of rapid growth, marked by rapid cell differentiation. Each individual has a unique growth timetable and final growth outcome, but the sequential growth patterns are consistent. An external environmental or abnormal pathophysiologic process may intervene and influence the expected growth pattern (Fig. 6-2).

The growth of the musculoskeletal system and most organs such as the liver and kidneys follows the growth curves described for stature. Skeletal growth is considered complete when the epiphyses of long bones have completely fused during late puberty. More than 90% of skeletal mass is present by 18 years of age (Reiter and Rosenfield, 2008).

Weight is closely related to growth in stature and organ development. Growth and development are influenced by nutritional adequacy, which contributes to the number and size of adipose cells. The number of adipose cells increases throughout childhood. Gender-related differences in fat deposition appear in infancy and continue through adolescence.

Lymphatic tissues (i.e., lymph nodes, spleen, tonsils, adenoids, and blood lymphocytes) are small in relation to total body size, but are well developed at birth. These tissues grow rapidly to reach adult size by 6 years of age. By age 10 to 12 years, the lymphatic tissues are at their peak, about double adult size. During adolescence, they decrease to adult size.

The internal and external reproductive organs grow slowly prior to puberty. The reproductive organs double in size during adolescence, achieving maturation and function.

The brain, along with the skull, eyes, and ears, completes physical development more quickly than any other body part. The most rapid and critical period of brain growth occurs between conception and 3 years of age. By 34 weeks' gestation, 65% of the weight of a newborn's brain is present. Gray matter

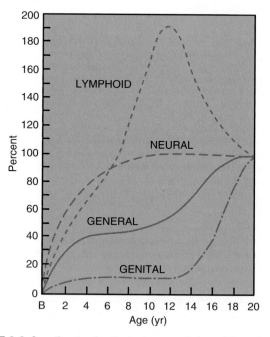

FIGURE 6-2 Growth rates for the body as a whole and three types of tissues. Lymphoid type: thymus, lymph nodes, and intestinal lymph masses. Neural type: brain, dura, spinal cord, optic apparatus, and head dimensions. General type: body as a whole; external dimensions; and respiratory, digestive, renal, circulatory, and musculoskeletal systems. Genital type: includes the reproductive organ system. *(From Wong, 1999; modified from Harris et al, 1930.)*

and myelinated white matter increase dramatically between the 34th and 40th weeks of gestation. At the time of full-term birth, the brain's structure is complete and an estimated 1 billion neurons are present. Glial cells, dendrites, and myelin continue to develop after birth, and by 3 years of age, most brain growth

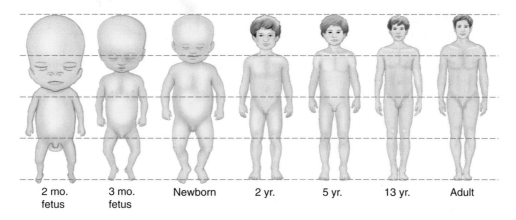

FIGURE 6-3 Changes in body proportions from 8 weeks of gestation through adulthood.

is completed (Feigelman, 2011). The head circumference increases in infants and toddlers as brain growth occurs. During adolescence, the size of the head further increases because of the development of air sinuses and thickening of the scalp and skull.

Infants and Children

As infants and children grow the change in body proportion is related to the pattern of skeletal growth (Fig. 6-3).

Growth of the head predominates during the fetal period. Fetal weight gain follows growth in length, but weight reaches its peak during the third trimester with the increase in organ size. An infant's birth weight is influenced by the mother's prepregnancy weight, weight gain during pregnancy, function of the placenta, gestational age, and maternal complications such as gestational diabetes.

During infancy, the growth of the trunk predominates. Weight gain is initially rapid, but the speed with which weight is gained decreases over the first year of life. The fat content of the body increases slowly during early fetal development and then increases during infancy.

The legs are the fastest growing body part during childhood, and weight is gained at a steady rate. Fat tissue increases slowly until 7 years of age, at which time a prepubertal fat spurt occurs before the true growth spurt.

The trunk and the legs lengthen during adolescence and lean body mass averages 80% in males and females (Cromer, 2011). During adolescence about 50% of the individual's ideal weight is gained, and the skeletal mass and organ systems double in size.

During adolescence, males develop broader shoulders and greater musculature; females develop a wider pelvic outlet. Males have a slight increase in body fat during early adolescence and then have an average gain in lean body mass to 90%. Females accumulate subcutaneous fat and have a slight decrease in lean body mass to an average of 75% (Cromer, 2011).

Pregnant Women

Progressive weight gain is expected during pregnancy, but the amount varies among women. The growing fetus accounts for 6

to 8 pounds of the total weight gained. The remainder results from an increase in maternal tissues (Gregory et al, 2012):

+ Fluid volume—2 to 3 pounds
+ Blood volume—3 to 4 pounds
+ Breast enlargement—1 to 2 pounds
+ Uterine enlargement—2 pounds
+ Amniotic fluid—2 pounds
+ Maternal fat and protein stores—4 to 6 pounds

The rate of desirable weight gain follows a curve through the trimesters of pregnancy, slowly during the first trimester and more rapidly during the second and third trimesters. Maternal tissue growth accounts for most of the weight gained in the first and second trimesters. Fetal growth accounts for most weight gained during the third trimester.

Maternal nutrition before and during pregnancy and during lactation may have subtle effects on the developing brain of the infant and on the outcome of the pregnancy. Women who have inadequate weight gain are at greater risk for delivering a low-birth-weight infant (Gregory et al, 2012). Epigenetic research is revealing the potential consequences of inadequate maternal nutrition on the adult health of the fetus (Gluckman et al, 2008) (Box 6-1).

Box 6-1   **Epigenetic Research and Nutrition**

Epigenetic research is revealing an association between an individual's genome and environmental exposures during fetal life and adult health. Under-nutrition during the second and third trimesters of pregnancy is believed to influence the fetus during the critical growth stages. Under-nutrition (poor maternal nutrition or poor intrauterine environment) stresses the fetus, leading to adaptive and permanent changes in the infant's endocrine and metabolic processes. Restricted fetal growth and a low birth weight for gestational age are associated with increased adult cardiovascular risk factors such as hypertension, insulin resistance, and abnormal lipid metabolism. These risk factors are further influenced by nutrition and growth after birth. Increased nutrition can lead to compensatory growth in these higher risk infants during the first 2 years of life, resulting in a child who has an increased body mass index and body fat by 5 years of age (Cota & Allen, 2010).

Postpartum weight loss often occurs over the first 6 months after birth, with most weight loss occurring by 3 months after delivery (Katz, 2012). Women who gained more than the recommended weight during pregnancy are less likely to return to their prepregnancy weight. They may be susceptible to future obesity and its health consequences.

❀ Older Adults

Physical stature declines in older adults beginning at approximately 50 years of age. The intervertebral disks thin and kyphosis develops with osteoporotic vertebral compression.

Individuals older than 60 years often have a decrease in weight for height and body mass index (BMI) and a loss of 5% body weight over several years. An increase in body fat also occurs as skeletal muscle declines and anabolic steroid secretion is reduced (Chapman, 2007). Older adults also frequently have decreased exercise, which also contributes to skeletal muscle loss. An increase in overweight and obese older adults has been documented over the past 15 to 20 years. An age-associated reduction in size and weight of various organs has been identified, especially of the liver, lungs, and kidneys (McCance et al, 2010).

REVIEW OF RELATED HISTORY

For each of the symptoms or conditions discussed in this section, topics to include in the history of the present illness are listed. Responses to questions about these topics provide clues for focusing the physical examination and developing an appropriate diagnostic evaluation. Questions regarding medication use (prescription and over the counter preparations) as well as complementary and alternative therapies are relevant for each area.

History of Present Illness

+ Weight loss and weight gain (see Chapter 7 for nutrition-related targeted topics)
  + Undesired weight loss: over what time period; anorexia; vomiting or diarrhea, difficulty swallowing, excessive thirst, frequent urination; change in lifestyle, activity, and stress levels
  + Medications: chemotherapy, diuretics, insulin, fluoxetine (Prozac), nonprescription diet pills, laxatives, steroids, oral contraceptives
+ Changes in body proportions
  + Coarsening of facial features, enlargement of hands and feet, moon facies
  + Change in fat distribution: trunk-girdle versus generalized
  + Medication: steroids

Past Medical History

+ Chronic illness: gastrointestinal, renal, pulmonary, cardiac, cancer, human immunodeficiency virus (HIV) or other infections, allergies
+ Previous weight loss or gain efforts: weight at 21 years, maximum body weight

Family History

+ Obesity
+ Constitutionally short or tall stature, precocious or delayed puberty
+ Genetic or metabolic disorder: cystic fibrosis, dwarfism

Personal and Social History

+ Usual weight and height
+ Physical activity or exercise pattern
+ Use of alcohol
+ Use of illicit drugs

❀ Infants

+ Estimated gestational age, birth weight, length, head circumference
+ Following an established percentile growth curve
  + Unexplained changes in length, weight, or head circumference
  + Poor growth/failure to thrive: falling one or more standard deviations off growth curve pattern; below fifth percentile for weight and height; infant small for gestational age; quality of mother-infant bond and interaction; psychosocial stressors and food insecurity
  + Rapid weight gain: overfeeding
+ Development: achieving milestones at appropriate ages
+ Congenital anomaly or chronic illness: heart defect, hydrocephalus, microcephaly, malabsorption syndrome or chronic diarrhea, formula intolerance, urinary tract infection, others

❀ Children and Adolescents

+ Initiation of sexual maturation of girls: early (before 7 years) or delayed (beyond 13 years); signs of breast development and pubic hair, age at menarche
+ Initiation of sexual maturation of boys: early (before 9 years) or delayed (beyond 14 years); signs of genital development and pubic hair
+ Short stature: not growing as fast as peers, change in shoe and clothing size in past year, extremities short or long for size of trunk, height of parents, size of head disproportionate to body
+ Tall stature: height of parents, growing faster than peers, signs of early sexual maturation
+ Chronic disease, such as inflammatory bowel disease, cystic fibrosis, malignancy
+ Medications: steroids, growth hormones, anabolic steroids

❀ Pregnant Women

+ Prepregnancy weight, dietary intake (see Chapter 7 for more information)
+ Age at menarche
+ Date of last menstrual period, weight gain pattern, following established weight gain curve for gestational course
+ Eating disorders
+ History of pica (cravings for and eating non-nutritive substances such as laundry starch, ice, clay, raw icing)
+ Nausea and vomiting

✤ Older Adults

+ Chronic debilitating illness: problems with meal preparation; difficulty feeding self, chewing, or swallowing; poorly fitting dentures; ability to follow prescribed diet; difficulty with digestion
+ See Chapter 7 for nutrition topics to discuss.

EXAMINATION AND FINDINGS

Equipment

+ Standing platform scale with height attachment
+ Measuring tape
+ Infant scale
+ Recumbent measuring device (for infants)
+ Stature measuring device (for children)

Weight and Standing Height

To measure the weight, ask the patient to remove excess clothing and shoes. Have the patient stand in the middle of the scale platform and note the digital reading. If using a balance scale move the largest weight to the last 50-pound or 10-kg increment under the patient's weight. Adjust the smaller weight to balance the scale. Read the weight to the nearest 0.1 kg or ¼ pound. Weight variations occur during the day and from day to day with changes in body fluid and intestinal contents. When monitoring a patient's weight daily or weekly, weigh the patient at the same time each day using the same scale.

To measure height, have the patient stand erect with his or her back to the stature-measuring device. Pull up the height attachment and position the headpiece on the top of the head. Make the reading at the nearest centimeter or ½ inch.

Body Mass Index

The BMI is the most common method used to assess nutritional status and total body fat. It correlates to body fat measures using underwater body measuring and dual energy x-ray absorptiometry. See Box 6-2 for the formulas to calculate the BMI. For adult men and women, the following are classifications of weight for height by BMI values (in kg/m²):

+ Undernutrition—under 18.5
+ Appropriate weight for height—18.5 to 24.9
+ Overweight—25 to 29.9
+ Obese—30 to 39.9
+ Extreme obesity—40 and higher

Box 6-2 **Calculating the Body Mass Index**

The formula to calculate the BMI using pounds (be sure to convert ounces to a decimal) and inches:

$$[\text{Weight [in pounds]} \div \text{Height [in inches]}^2] \times 703$$

The formula to calculate the BMI using kilograms and centimeters:

$$\text{Weight [in kg]} \div \text{Height [in meters]}^2$$

Track the change of a patient's BMI over time to identify nutritional problems and obesity (see Physical Variations, "Obesity"). The prevalence of obesity among adults 20 years of age and older in 2009-2010 was 35.7%. The prevalence of obesity varies by age group: 32.2% in adults 20 to 39 years old, 36.6% in adults 40 to 59 years old, and 39.7% in adults 60 years and older (Ogden et al, 2012) (see Chapter 7). Severe weight loss and wasting are usually associated with a debilitating disease or self-starvation.

Physical Variations

Obesity

The prevalence of obesity, defined as a body mass index of 30 or higher, was 32.2% in adult men and 35.5% in adult women ages 20 years and older in 2007-2008. The rate of obesity varies by race and ethnicity. The rate of obesity is highest among non-Hispanic blacks (44.1%), followed by Hispanics (37.9%) and non-Hispanic whites (32.8%) (Flegel et al, 2010).

Staying Well

Controlling Weight

Exercise is a key factor in maintaining body weight or in reducing body weight. Aerobic exercise such as 30 minutes of walking at least 3 times a week is recommended. Look for ways to increase activity, such as using the stairs rather than an elevator or parking farther from the doors to businesses and workplaces. Limit the time children sit and view videos, television, computer screens or play with electronic devices. Encourage children to walk, ride a bicycle, and participate in sports or recreational activities.

See Chapter 7 for triceps skinfold thickness information.

✤ Infants

The care of children is exciting because of the continuous change that accompanies growth and development. Give careful attention to measuring weight and height and the sequence of developmental achievements as you get to know a child over time.

The newborn with the best chance to be a healthy infant is born at term, is an appropriate size for gestational age, and has no history of prenatal or perinatal difficulty. Most babies born at term to the same parents weigh within 6 ounces of their siblings at birth. Pay close attention to an unexpected birth weight difference. If the baby has a lower birth weight than older siblings, suspect an undisclosed congenital abnormality or intrauterine growth restriction. Newborns with a greater birth weight than older siblings, at 10 pounds or greater, are at risk for hypoglycemia. A more rapid weight gain than expected during early infancy (e.g., the infant's weight percentile level keeps increasing rather than following a specific growth curve) is associated with increased cardiovascular disease risk as an adult (Singhal, 2006).

Recumbent Length

Measure the length of infants between birth and 24 months of age in supine position on a measuring device (Fig. 6-4). Have the

EXAMINATION AND FINDINGS

FIGURE 6-4 Measurement of infant length. *(Courtesy Seca Corporation, Hanover, MD.)*

parent hold the infant's head against the headboard. Hold the infant's legs straight at the knees and place the footboard against the bottom of the infant's feet. Read the length measurement to the nearest 0.5 cm or ¼ inch. Plot the infant's length on the World Health Organization growth curve for age and gender, and identify the infant's percentile placement (see Appendix A, Figs. *A-1* and *A-2*). Use the same growth curve to plot future length measurements and to monitor the infant's growth over time. Beginning at 2 years of age, use the Centers for Disease Control and Prevention (CDC) growth curve for gender (see Appendix A, Figs. A-3 and A-4 and Clinical Pearl, "Using the Correct Growth Chart").

At birth, healthy term newborns have length variations between 45 and 55 cm (18 and 22 inches). Length increases by 50% in the first year of life (see Clinical Pearl, "Reliability of Length Measurements").

Clinical Pearl

Using the Correct Growth Chart
Despite the toddler's ability to stand, continue measuring length until 24 months of age and continue plotting the length on the World Health Organization growth curve. Measurements of length are 0.7 to 0.8 cm greater than height or stature (Grummer-Strawn et al, 2010). Using the child's height rather than length on the World Health Organization growth curve will give an incorrect impression of poor growth. At 24 months of age, begin measuring the child's height and plotting the child's measurements on the Centers for Disease Control growth curves for children ages 2 to 18 years.

Clinical Pearl

Reliability of Length Measurements
Obtaining a reliable length measurement in newborns is difficult because of the natural flexion of the infant and the molding of the head. In infants, reliability of the length measurement is difficult if the infant resists and moves. Use a consistent technique to increase reliability between examiners, and verify the length with a second measurement.

Weight

Use an infant scale, measuring weight in grams for infants and small children. Infants and children are weighed on a scale that measures only in grams and kilograms to reduce medication errors because pediatric dosages are calculated per kilogram of body weight (The Joint Commission, 2008). Use distraction to help keep the infant quiet and still until the digital reading appears or until the scale is balanced. Read the weight to the nearest 10 g when the infant is most still. Plot the infant's weight on the World Health Organization growth curve for age and gender, comparing the infant's weight to the population standard. Identify the infant's percentile placement (see Appendix A, Figs. A-1 and A-2). As with length, monitor the child's weight by plotting future measurements on the same growth curve. Beginning at 2 years of age, convert to the CDC growth curve for the child's gender (see Appendix A, Figs. A-3 and A-4). Use conversion tables to give parents the infant's weight in pounds and ounces (see Appendix C).

Most term newborns vary in weight between 2500 and 4000 g (5 lb and 8 oz to 8 lb and 13 oz). After losing up to 10% of their birth weight, newborns regain that weight within 2 weeks, and then gain weight at a rate of approximately 30 g (1 oz) per day. This rate of weight gain decreases starting at about 3 months of age (Fiegelman, 2011). In general, infants double their birth weight by 4 to 5 months of age and triple their birth weight by 12 months of age.

After obtaining the length and weight, plot the infant's weight for length on the World Health Organization growth curve. This provides information about whether the infant's weight is proportional to length (see Clinical Pearl, "Uses of Growth Charts").

Clinical Pearl

Uses of Growth Charts
Growth charts are designed to plot and track anthropometric data to screen for unusual size and growth patterns and to make an overall clinical assessment. For example, growth charts for children between birth and 24 months of age make it possible to identify excessive weight gain for length. A separate growth curve for very-low-birth weight infants compares the growth of these infants with growth of other low-birth-weight infants, although the World Health Organization growth charts may also be used to evaluate the growth of these infants. See Appendix A.

Head Circumference

Measure the infant's head circumference at every health visit until 2 to 3 years of age. Wrap a paper measuring tape snugly around the child's head at the occipital protuberance and the supraorbital prominence to find the point of largest circumference (Fig. 6-5). Make the reading to the nearest 0.5 cm or ¼ inch. Confirm the accuracy of the head circumference measurement at least once. Plot the measurement on the appropriate growth curve, and identify the child's percentile in comparison with the population standard. Compare measurements over time to

FIGURE 6-5 Place the measuring tape around the largest circumference of the infant's head, across the occiput and the forehead.

FIGURE 6-6 Measurement of infant chest circumference with the measuring tape at the level of the nipple line.

monitor the head circumference growth pattern (see Appendix A, Figs. A-1 and A-2).

Expected head circumferences for term newborns range between 32.5 and 37.5 cm (12.5 to 14.5 inches) with a mean of 33 to 35 cm (13 to 14 inches). At 2 years of age, the child's head circumference is two-thirds its adult size. If the head circumference increases rapidly and plots in higher percentile curves, increased intracranial pressure may be present. If the head circumference does not grow as expected and plots in lower percentile curves, microcephaly may be present.

Chest Circumference

Although the chest circumference is not used routinely, it is a useful measurement for comparison with the head circumference when a problem is suspected with either the head size or chest size. Wrap the measuring tape around the infant's chest at the nipple line, firmly but not tight enough to cause an indentation of the skin (Fig. 6-6). Read the chest circumference measurement midway between inspiration and expiration to the nearest 0.5 cm or ¼ inch.

The newborn's head circumference may equal or exceed the chest circumference by 2 cm (¾ inch) until 5 months of age. Between the ages of 5 months and 2 years, the infant's chest circumference and head circumference are close to the same size. If an infant's head circumference is smaller than the chest circumference, consider evaluating the infant for microcephaly. After 2 years of age, the chest circumference exceeds the head circumference because the chest grows faster than the head.

Gestational Age

Gestational age is an indicator of a newborn's maturity. One method of determining gestational age is to calculate the number of completed weeks between the first day of the mother's last menstrual period and the date of birth. An estimate of gestational age is used to evaluate an infant's developmental progress. It is also used to identify preterm newborns of appropriate size and term newborns who are small for gestational age.

The Ballard Gestational Age Assessment Tool evaluates six physical and six neuromuscular newborn characteristics within 36 hours of birth to establish or confirm the newborn's gestational age. The assessment is accurate within 2 weeks of the assigned gestational age. Scores are more accurate for extremely preterm newborns when the assessment occurs within 12 hours of birth.

The gestational ages of 37 through 41 weeks are considered term and are associated with the best health outcomes. Infants born before 37 weeks of gestation are preterm, and infants born after 41 completed weeks of gestation are postterm.

Size for Gestational Age. A newborn's fetal growth pattern and size for gestational age can be determined once gestational age is assigned. An intrauterine growth curve is used to plot the newborn's birth weight, length, and head circumference. The infant is then classified as small, appropriate, or large for gestational age by percentile curve placement for weeks of gestation (Fig. 6-7). The classification system is as follows:

+ Appropriate for gestational age: 10th to 90th weight percentile
+ Small for gestational age: less than 10th weight percentile
+ Large for gestational age: greater than 90th weight percentile

FIGURE 6-7 A, Small for gestational age infant and appropriate for gestational age infant. **B,** Large for gestational age infant. *(From Zitelli, 2007.)*

Infants who are small or large for gestational age have an increased risk for morbidity and mortality. Small for gestational age infants who are full term have an increased risk for respiratory distress, hypoglycemia, and other health problems (see Physical Variations, "Low Birth Weight"). Large for gestational age infants are at higher risk for birth injuries such as shoulder dystocia, as well as health conditions such as respiratory distress syndrome, intraventricular hemorrhage, and bronchopulmonary dysplasia (Reinold et al, 2011).

Physical Variations

Low Birth Weight

In 2009, 8.2% of infants were born at low birth weight (less than 2500 g, or 5 lb 8 oz). The low-birth-weight rate varies by race and ethnicity. The highest percentage of low birth weight occurred in non-Hispanic black infants (11.9%), followed by Asian/Pacific Islander infants (7.4%), American Indian/Alaskan Native infants (7.4%), non-Hispanic white infants (7.2%), and Hispanic infants (7.0%) (Reinold et al, 2011).

FIGURE 6-8 Measuring the stature of a child.

�急 Children

Stature and Weight

Standing height (stature) is obtained beginning at 24 months when the child is walking well. Remove the child's shoes and heavy clothing. To get the most accurate measurement, use a stature-measuring device (stadiometer) mounted on the wall rather than the height-measurement device on a scale. Have the child stand erect with heels, buttocks, and shoulders against the wall or freestanding stadiometer, looking straight ahead (Fig. 6-8). The outer canthus of the eye should be on the same horizontal plane as the external auditory canal while you position the headpiece at the top of the head. The stature reading is made to the nearest 0.5 cm or ¼ inch (see Clinical Pearl, "Special Growth Charts").

Clinical Pearl

Special Growth Charts

Special growth charts exist for children with specific conditions such as Down syndrome and Turner syndrome, but use them in association with the World Health Organization and Centers for Disease Control and Prevention standardized charts. These special growth charts may be obtained online at www.magicfoundation.org/www/docs/7.

To calculate height velocity, determine the change in height over a time interval (e.g., 1 year). Shorter time intervals may reflect seasonal variations in growth. Make height measurements as close to 12 months apart as possible, no fewer than 10 months and no more than 14 months. (See the website for gender-specific height velocity growth curves during adolescence.)

Weigh young children older than 2 years of age on a standing scale in light garments. Read the weight to the nearest 0.1 kg.

Plot the child's height and weight on the CDC growth curves for gender and age, comparing the child's growth with the other children the same age. (See Appendix A, Figs. A-3 and A-4, for physical growth curves for height and weight of children 2 through 20 years of age.)

The BMI is now standardized for use in children and adolescents, and it is calculated the same way as for adults (see Physical Variations, "Body Mass Index in Children and Youth"). In children and adolescents the amount of body fat changes with age, and the body fat values differ between males and females. As a result, the BMI is interpreted using age and gender-specific percentiles. Once the BMI is calculated, plot the value on the appropriate growth chart for gender found in Appendix A. Established cutoff points used to identify underweight and overweight children and adolescents are based on the following percentiles:

+ Underweight—BMI for age under the 5th percentile
+ At risk of overweight—BMI for age greater than the 85th percentile
+ Overweight—BMI for age greater than the 95th percentile

Evaluate the child's growth pattern over time by placing all weight and height measurements on the growth curve. The child is expected to consistently follow a percentile curve on the growth curve. Children adopted from other countries may not fit the U.S. population standard, but they should have a consistent growth pattern (percentile), even if it is near or below the fifth percentile. Infants and children who suddenly fall below or rise above their established percentile growth curve should be examined more closely to determine the cause.

Upper-to-Lower Segment Ratio

The upper-to-lower segment ratio is calculated when a child's body may have inappropriate proportions between the head and trunk to the lower extremities. Measure the lower body segment (distance from the symphysis pubis to the floor when a child stands). Calculate the upper body segment by subtracting the lower body segment from the total height. Then divide the upper body segment by the lower body segment to calculate the ratio. Expected ratios by age are as follows (Keane, 2011):

*   At birth—1.7
*   At 3 years—1.3
*   After 7 years—1.0

A higher upper-to-lower body segment ratio than expected may be associated with dwarfism or bone disorders.

Arm Span

The arm-span measurement is not routinely obtained, but may be useful when evaluating a child with tall stature. Have the child hold his or her arms fully extended from the sides of the body. Measure the distance from the middle fingertip of one hand to that of the other hand. The arm span should equal the child's height or stature. Arm span that exceeds height is associated with Marfan syndrome.

Sexual Maturation

Assessment of children and adolescents involves evaluation of secondary sexual characteristic development. In girls, breast and pubic hair development is evaluated; in boys, genital and pubic hair development is evaluated. The duration and tempo of each stage vary between individuals (see Physical Variations, "Sexual Maturation").

Have the girl sit while assessing the stage of breast development. Breast tissue may be seen and possibly palpated below a slightly enlarging areola (1 cm in diameter of palpable glandular tissue) is stage 2 (Hermann-Giddens et al, 2011). Most girls start puberty between 9 and 12 years of age with breast enlargement. A girl's breasts often develop at different rates and appear asymmetric. Stage 2 pubic hair is lightly pigmented, sparse, and straight along the labia majora. See Figures 6-9 and 6-10 for expected stages of female sexual maturation.

Ask the boy to stand to assess pubertal development. Most boys start puberty between 10 and 13 years of age with testicular enlargement. Pubic hair development, enlargement of the penis, and the growth spurt follow. See Figure 6-11 and 6-12 for expected stages of male sexual maturation.

After the secondary sexual characteristics are examined and staged, a sexual maturity rating (SMR) may be assigned to determine the child's overall pubertal development. The height growth spurt and timing of other physiologic events occurring during puberty (e.g., menarche or nocturnal emissions) are associated with the stage of secondary sexual characteristic development. An SMR is calculated by averaging the girl's stages of pubic hair and breast development or the boy's stages of pubic hair and genital development.

The onset of puberty in females is the age at which breast stage 2 or public hair stage 2 is reached, whichever occurs first. Most girls have breast development before pubic hair appears. Completion of puberty is when breast stage 4 or public hair stage 5 has been reached. Menarche generally occurs in SMR 4 or breast stage 3 to 4. Even though the mean age at which stage 2 breast development occurs has become younger over time, the average age at menarche has remained fairly constant, between 12 and 13 years (Walvoord, 2010). The peak height velocity usually occurs before menarche. These events may be plotted on the standardized height velocity growth chart for adolescents. Higher BMI scores and higher rates of change in BMI from 3 to 6 years of age are associated with early puberty in childhood (Lee et al, 2007). Breast development may begin as early as 6 years in black girls and 7 years in white girls. Breast development before these ages is abnormal and needs further evaluation (Biro et al, 2010).

The stage of genital and pubic hair development in males is related to age and the height spurt. External genital changes usually precede pubic hair development. Ejaculation generally occurs at SMR 3, with semen appearing between SMR 3 and 4. The peak height velocity occurs at a mean age of 13.5 years, usually in SMR 4 or genital development stage 4 to 5. These events may be plotted on the standardized height velocity growth chart for adolescents. Development of genitals or pubic hair in prepubertal boys younger than 9 years should be further investigated for cause.

Delayed onset of puberty and secondary sexual characteristic development (at an age later than the average) may be a normal variant in both boys and girls. It is usually accompanied by a

EXAMINATION AND FINDINGS

M₁—Tanner 1 (preadolescent). Only the nipple is raised above the level of the breast, as in the child.

M₂—Tanner 2. Budding stage; bud-shaped elevation of the areola; areola increased in diameter and surrounding area slightly elevated.

M₃—Tanner 3. Breast and areola enlarged. No contour separation.

M₄—Tanner 4. Increasing fat deposits. The areola forms a secondary elevation above that of the breast. This secondary mound occurs in approximately half of all girls and in some cases persists in adulthood.

M₅—Tanner 5 (adult stage). The areola is (usually) part of general breast contour and is strongly pigmented. Nipple projects.

FIGURE 6-9 Five stages of breast development in females. *(Growth diagrams 1965 Netherlands: second national survey on 0-24-year-olds, by J. C. Van Wieringen, F. Wafelbakker, H. P. Verbrugge, J. H. DeHaas. Groningen: Noordhoff Uitgevers BV, The Netherlands.)*

lag of stature growth. A parent or sibling often may have had a similar adolescent growth pattern. Once pubertal changes begin, the sequence of development is the same as for other adolescents, but it may occur over a different time span. Ultimate height may still be the same. Further evaluation is needed if no evidence of pubertal development is seen in a boy by 14 years of age or a girl by 13 years of age (Kaplowitz, 2010).

Early development of sexual hair without signs of sexual maturation may be an indication of premature pubarche. In these children, pubescence usually occurs at the expected time, as with healthy children.

✤ Pregnant Women

Calculate the weight gain during pregnancy from the woman's prepregnant weight. To provide guidance in weight gain during pregnancy, first determine the prepregnancy BMI (see Box 6-2). Then monitor the woman's weight throughout pregnancy using the BMI weight gain curve guidelines on the prenatal weight gain chart (see page 90 for Fig. 6-13).

Guidelines for recommended weight gain during pregnancy are based on the woman's prepregnancy BMI to improve reproductive outcomes. Women with a prepregnancy BMI of 19.8 to

P₁—Tanner 1 (preadolescent). No growth of pubic hair.

P₂—Tanner 2. Initial, scarcely pigmented straight hair, especially along medial border of the labia.

P₃—Tanner 3. Sparse, dark, visibly pigmented, curly pubic hair on labia.

P₄—Tanner 4. Hair coarse and curly, abundant but less than adult.

P₅—Tanner 5. Lateral spreading; type and triangle spread of adult hair to medial surface of thighs.

P₆—Tanner 6. Further extension laterally, upward, or dispersed (occurs in only 10% of women).

FIGURE 6-10 **Six stages of pubic hair development in females.** *(Growth diagrams 1965 Netherlands: second national survey on 0-24-year-olds, by J. C. Van Wieringen, F. Wafelbakker, H. P. Verbrugge, J. H. DeHaas. Groningen: Noordhoff Uitgevers BV, The Netherlands.)*

26.0 should gain 11.5 to 16 kg (25 to 35 pounds) over the entire pregnancy. Underweight women should gain up to 12.2 to 18.2 kg (28 to 40 pounds). Overweight women (BMI 26.1 to 29) should gain 7 to 11.5 kg (15 to 25 pounds). Those who are obese (BMI greater than 29) should gain no more than 5 to 9.1 kg (11 to 20 pounds) (Institute of Medicine and National Research Council, 2009). Adjust the recommended weight gain for women with twin or triplet pregnancy.

Obese women are at increased risk of maternal complications such as gestational hypertension, preeclampsia, gestational diabetes, cesarean delivery, and failure to initiate breast-feeding (Reinold et al, 2011). Pregnant adolescents younger than 16 years, or less than 2 years after menarche, may still be in their growth spurt. They may require higher weight gains during pregnancy to achieve an optimal infant birth weight (Fernandez et al, 2008).

Note any variation from the expected weight gain. First trimester gain is variable, from 1.4 to 2.7 kg (3 to 6 lbs). In the second and third trimesters, weekly weight gain should be approximately 0.23 to 0.45 kg (0.5 to 1 lb) per week. Women who gain too little weight during pregnancy are at risk for having a low-birth-weight infant. Women who gain too much weight are at risk for having a high-birth-weight infant, which may lead to a difficult delivery (Reinold et al, 2011).

⚛ Older Adults

Measurement procedures for the older adult are the same as those used for other adults. Calculate the BMI. Identify any problems with underweight that could be associated with a health condition or food insecurity. Of older adults in the U.S. in 2009 and 2010, 36.6% of men and 42.3% of women were obese (Ogden et al, 2012).

G₁—Tanner 1. Testes, scrotum, and penis are the same size and shape as in the young child.

G₂—Tanner 2. Enlargement of scrotum and testes. The skin of the scrotum becomes redder, thinner, and wrinkled. Penis no larger or scarcely so.

G₃—Tanner 3. Enlargement of the penis, especially in length; further enlargement of testes; descent of scrotum.

G₄—Tanner 4. Continued enlargement of the penis and sculpturing of the glans; increased pigmentation of scrotum. This stage is sometimes best described as "not quite adult."

G₅—Tanner 5 (adult stage). Scrotum ample, penis reaching nearly to bottom of scrotum.

FIGURE 6-11 Five stages of penis and testes/scrotum development in males. *(Growth diagrams 1965 Netherlands: second national survey on 0-24-year-olds, by J. C. Van Wieringen, F. Wafelbakker, H. P. Verbrugge, J. H. DeHaas. Groningen: Noordhoff Uitgevers BV, The Netherlands.)*

Prepregnancy BMI <19.8   Prepregnancy BMI 19.8-26.0   Prepregnancy BMI >26.0

FIGURE 6-13 Prenatal weight gain curve by weeks of gestation. *(From Food and Nutrition Board, 2003.)*

Sample Documentation

History and Physical Examination

Subjective

A 4-month-old female infant in for routine health visit. Breast-fed, no other foods introduced. Feeds eagerly every 2 to 3 hours. Good appetite. No illnesses.

Objective

Weight 6.2 kg (13.5 lbs) is above 25th percentile; length 62 cm (24.5 inches) is at 50th percentile; head circumference 41 cm (16 inches) is above 25th percentile; weight for length ratio is above 50th percentile; following the same growth curves since the health visit 2 months ago.

For additional sample documentation, see Chapter 26, pp. 628-631.

P₁—Tanner 1 (preadolescent). No growth of pubic hair; that is, hair in pubic area no different from that on the rest of the abdomen.

P₂—Tanner 2. Slightly pigmented, longer, straight hair, often still downy; usually at base of penis, sometimes on scrotum. Stage is difficult to photograph.

P₃—Tanner 3. Dark, definitely pigmented, curly pubic hair around base of penis. Stage 3 can be photographed.

P₄—Tanner 4. Pubic hair definitely adult in type but not in extent (no further than inguinal fold).

P₅—Tanner 5 (adult distribution). Hair spread to medial surface of thighs, but not upward.

P₆—Hair spread along linea alba (occurs in 80% of men).

FIGURE 6-12 **Six stages of pubic hair development in males.** *(Growth diagrams 1965 Netherlands: second national survey on 0-24-year-olds, by J. C. Van Wieringen, F. Wafelbakker, H. P. Verbrugge, J. H. DeHaas. Groningen: Noordhoff Uitgevers BV, The Netherlands.)*

ABNORMALITIES

GROWTH AND MEASUREMENT

Acromegaly

A rare disease of excessive growth and distorted proportions caused by hypersecretion of growth hormone and insulin-like growth factor after closure of the epiphyses

Pathophysiology	Subjective Data	Objective Data
• A benign pituitary adenoma or other rare tumor is the most common cause; familial syndromes (e.g., multiple endocrine neoplasia type 1 and McCune-Albright syndrome) • Growth hormone excess leads to slow skeletal growth and soft tissue enlargement. • Most common in middle-aged adults	• Slow progressive changes in facial feature exaggeration • Increased shoe size, ring size • No change in height • Oily and sweaty skin • Excessive snoring, sleep apnea • Decreased exercise tolerance • Pain in joints and hands • See Figure 6-14.	• Face and skull—frontal skull bossing, cranial ridges, mandibular overgrowth, maxillary widening, teeth separation, malocclusion, overbite • Skin thickening on the face (tongue, lips and nose), hands and feet leading to enlargement • Joint enlargement, swelling, pain; vertebral enlargement, kyphoscoliosis • Cardiac ventricular enlargement bilaterally with decreased exercise tolerance

ABNORMALITIES

FIGURE 6-14 **Acromegaly.** Note the large head, forward projection of jaw, protrusion of frontal bone, and the large hands. *(From images.rheumatology.org).*

Cushing Syndrome

A disorder associated with a prolonged and excessively high exposure to glucocorticoids

Pathophysiology

- Caused most commonly by the use of medically prescribed corticosteroids
- Other causes include adrenal gland oversecretion leading to excessive production of cortisol or a pituitary tumor leading to excessive secretion of adrenocorticotropic hormone (ACTH).
- Conditions caused by the excess cortisol such as diabetes, hypertension, depression, and menstrual irregularities

Subjective Data

- Weight gain, changes in appetite
- Depression, irritability, decreased libido
- Decreased concentration, impaired short-term memory
- Bruises easily
- Menstrual abnormalities
- Weight gain but slow height velocity in children
- See Figure 10-8, *A* and *B*

Objective Data

- Obesity, "buffalo hump" fat pad, supraclavicular and pendulous abdominal fat distribution
- Facial plethora or moon facies
- Thin skin, reddish purple striae, poor skin healing
- Proximal muscle weakness
- Hirsutism or female balding
- Peripheral edema
- In children—short stature, abnormal genital virilization, delayed puberty, or pseudo-precocious puberty

Turner Syndrome

A genetic disorder in which there is partial or complete absence of a second X chromosome

Pathophysiology

- Signs result from a reduced complement of genes that are typically expressed from both X chromosomes in females.
- Turner syndrome incidence is 1 per 2500 to 3000 live births.

Subjective Data

- Poor height growth
- Lack of breast development and amenorrhea
- Have normal intelligence
- See Figure 6-15.

Objective Data

- Short stature
- Webbed neck
- Broad chest with widely spaced nipples
- Wide carrying angle of elbow (cubitus valgus)
- Low posterior hairline, misshapen or rotated ears, narrow palate with crowded teeth
- Coarctation of aorta, bicuspid aortic valve
- Sensorineural hearing loss
- Infertility
- Karyotype or chromosome analysis is performed.

FIGURE 6-15 **Turner syndrome.** *(From Patton and Thibodeau, 2010.)*

Hydrocephalus

An excess volume of cerebrospinal fluid (CSF) in the brain leading to an enlarged head circumference or increased intracranial pressure

Pathophysiology

- May be caused by an infection or obstruction in the subarachnoid space that interferes with the reabsorption of CSF, or from an infection or injury that obstructs the flow of CSF to the subarachnoid space where it can be reabsorbed
- Often occurs in association with meningomyelocele

Subjective Data

- Enlarged head
- Difficulty holding head up or inability to lift head off bed
- Irritable, lack of energy, poor feeding
- After sutures close: severe headache, diplopia or other vision problems, vomiting not associated with an illness
- See Figure 6-16.

Objective Data

- Rapidly increasing head circumference
- Tense, full, or bulging fontanel; split sutures
- Bossing (protrusion) of frontal area, face disproportionate to the skull size
- Prominent, distended scalp veins, translucent scalp skin
- Increased tone or hyperreflexia, brisk deep tendon reflexes, positive Babinski sign
- Once skull sutures are closed, increased intracranial pressure, papilledema
- Paralysis of upward gaze (6th cranial nerve palsy)

FIGURE 6-16 **Infantile hydrocephalus.** Paralysis of the upward gaze is seen in an infant with hydrocephalus resulting from aqueductal stenosis. It appears more apparent on the right. This phenomenon is often termed the *sunsetting sign. (From Zitelli and Davis, 1997. Courtesy Dr. Albert Biglan, Children's Hospital of Pittsburgh.)*

Failure To Thrive

Growth in an infant or child below the 3rd to 5th percentiles on a growth chart, or a slower than expected rate of growth in a short period of time (e.g., from the 50th percentile to below the 10th percentile on the growth chart)

Pathophysiology

- Psychosocial causes include poverty and inadequate food, errors in food preparation, or a poor parent–child interaction (e.g., maternal depression, child abuse or neglect, or family dysfunction)
- Organic causes include an underlying medical condition such as major infection or organ system disease.
- May result from a combination of organic disease and psychosocial stressors

Subjective Data

- Insufficient food for infant or child, poor dietary intake
- Breast-feeding failure, tires or sweats when feeding, refuses food
- Smaller than infants or children of same age
- See Figure 6-17.

Objective Data

- Does not meet expected weight and length (height) norms for age
- Reduced muscle mass, loss of subcutaneous fat, wasted buttocks, thin extremities, prominent ribs, alopecia
- Signs of neglect (diaper rash, unwashed skin, skin infections, unwashed clothing)
- Developmental delay

FIGURE 6-17 **Psychosocial failure to thrive as the result of neglect.** This 4-month-old infant was brought to the emergency department because of congestion. She was found to be below weight expectations and suffering from severe developmental delay. Note the marked loss of subcutaneous tissue manifested by the wrinkled skinfolds over the buttocks, shoulders, and upper arms. *(From Zitelli and Davis, 1997.)*

ABNORMALITIES

Growth Hormone Deficiency

Failure of the anterior pituitary to secrete adequate growth hormone to support growth in stature

Pathophysiology

- May be congenital or develop from a pituitary tumor, radiation therapy for a tumor, or brain trauma

Subjective Data

- Normal birth weight and growth during the first year
- Smaller than child of same age
- See Figure 6-18.

Objective Data

- Short stature; growth begins leveling off at 9 to 12 months
- Body proportions of younger age child, cherubic or elfin appearance, child appears younger than chronologic age
- Excess subcutaneous fat
- High-pitched voice

FIGURE 6-18 The normal 3-year-old boy is in the 50th percentile for height. The short 3-year-old girl exhibits the characteristic "Kewpie doll" appearance, suggesting a diagnosis of growth hormone deficiency. *(From Zitelli and Davis, 1997.)*

Precocious Puberty

The onset of secondary sexual characteristics before 7 years of age in white girls, 6 years in black girls, and 9 years of age in males with progressive sexual maturation (Lobo, 2012; Kaplowitz, 2008)

Pathophysiology

- A brain tumor or lesion (e.g., hypothalamic hamartoma) may activate the hypothalamic-pituitary-gonadal axis with gonadotropins triggering the growth of the gonads, secretion of the sex hormones, and progressive sexual maturation. It may also be related to McCune-Albright syndrome.

Subjective Data

- Development of breast tissue or pubic hair at earlier age than expected in girls
- Enlargement of testes, then the penis, and appearance of pubic hair at an earlier age than expected in boys
- See Figure 6-19.

Objective Data

- In young girls—breast development, pubic hair, maturation of external genitalia, axillary hair development, and onset of menses
- In boys—progressive signs of sexual maturation with testicular and penis enlargement, pubic hair, acne, erections, and nocturnal emissions
- Accelerated height growth at an early age
- Sex hormone concentrations are appropriate for stage of puberty.

FIGURE 6-19 Precocious puberty with pubic hair development in a young girl. *(From Zitelli and Davis, 2007.)*

CHAPTER 7

Nutrition

Nutrition may be defined as the science of food as it relates to promoting optimal health and preventing chronic disease. Nutritional intake and status offer insight into an individual's total health status. A nutrition assessment is an analysis of an individual's approximate nutrient intake and relates it to the history, physical examination findings, body size measurements (see Chapter 6) and biochemical measures. This chapter reviews the use of nutrients for growth, development, and maintenance of health. It also provides guidelines for assessing an individual's intake.

evolve *http://evolve.elsevier.com/Seidel*
• NCLEX Review Questions

Physical Examination Preview

Here is a preview of the steps involved in conducting a nutrition assessment.

Nutrition Assessment
1. From the history and physical examination, assess the patient's nutritional status, including the following:
   • Recent growth, weight loss, or weight gain (p. 97)
   • Chronic illnesses affecting nutritional status or intake (pp. 97-98)
   • Medication and supplement use (p. 100)
   • Nutrition screen
   • Assessment of nutrient intake (pp. 100-107)
   • Clinical signs or symptoms of nutrient or energy deficiency (p. 107)
   • Laboratory values (p. 109)
2. Obtain the following anthropometric measurements and compare them to standardized tables:
   • Standing height (p. 100, see Chapter 6)
   • Weight (p. 100, see Chapter 6)
   • Calculated BMI (p. 100, see Chapter 6)
   • Waist circumference (p. 100)
   • Calculate waist-height ratio and waist-hip circumference ratio (pp. 100-101)
   • Triceps skinfold (TSF) thickness and mid–upper arm circumference measurements; calculate midarm muscle circumference (MAMC) and cross-sectional midarm muscle area (MAMA) (pp. 107-108)

ANATOMY AND PHYSIOLOGY

Food nourishes the body by supplying necessary nutrients and calories to function in one or all of three ways:
* To provide energy for necessary activities
* To build and maintain body tissues
* To regulate body processes

The nutrients necessary to the body are classified as macronutrients, micronutrients, and water. Energy requirements are based on the balance of energy expenditure associated with body size, composition, and the level of physical activity. An appropriate balance contributes to long-term health and allows for the maintenance of optimal physical activity.

Macronutrients

Carbohydrate, protein, and fat are the main sources of calories in the diet and are referred to as macronutrients. These three macronutrients provide the calories needed to produce energy in the human body.

Carbohydrate

Carbohydrate, a nutrient found mostly in plants and in milk, is considered the body's main source of energy. Carbohydrates provide 4 calories per gram and are classified as simple (sugars) or complex (starches and fibers). Sugars can be natural (e.g., lactose in milk) or added to foods and beverages (e.g., high fructose corn syrup in some beverages). Fiber can also be natural (e.g., whole grains). Most carbohydrates are consumed in starches (e.g., refined grains and potatoes). About 365 g are stored as glycogen in the liver and muscle tissues, which provides energy for only about 13 hours of moderate activity. Moderate amounts of carbohydrate must be ingested at frequent intervals to meet the energy demands of the body. Carbohydrate also serves major functions in vital organs:
* The liver—sparing the use of protein for energy and participating in specific detoxifying metabolic pathways
* The heart—as glycogen stored in cardiac muscle
* The central nervous system—as the only energy source to the brain

Although most individuals consume an adequate level of carbohydrates, typical diets include an excess of sugar and not

ANATOMY AND PHYSIOLOGY

Box 7-1	Nine Essential Amino Acids

Histidine	Phenylalanine
Isoleucine	Threonine
Leucine	Tryptophan
Lysine	Valine
Methionine	

enough fiber. When more carbohydrate is consumed than is needed for energy, the excess is stored in fatty tissues throughout the body. The recommended carbohydrate content of the diet for children and adults is 45% to 65% of total calories, with no less than 130 g being consumed per day for adults. Refer to the Food and Nutrition Information Center of the U.S. Department of Agriculture (USDA) at fnic.nal.usda.gov for the Dietary Reference Intakes (DRIs) for carbohydrate needs from birth to adult, as established by the Food and Nutrition Board, Institute of Medicine.

Protein

Protein provides 4 calories per gram and is present in all animal and plant products. It is a part of more than half the organic matter in the body, including hair, skin, nails, muscle, glandular organs, connective tissue, blood plasma, and hemoglobin. During digestion, protein is broken down into amino acids, the building blocks of the protein molecule, and absorbed into the bloodstream, where they are carried to the tissues. Each tissue uses a specific group of amino acids to build its individual protein. In all, 20 different amino acids combine in different ways to form proteins. Nine amino acids are considered essential because they cannot be manufactured by the body and are essential for normal growth and development (see Box 7-1). The major functions of protein include the following:

+ Building and maintaining tissues
+ Regulating internal water and acid-base balances
+ Acting as a precursor for enzymes, antibodies, and several hormones

Excess protein is either used to supply energy or is stored as body fat if total calorie intake exceeds the body's needs. The recommended protein content of the diet for adults is 10% to 35% of total calories, with a Recommended Daily Allowance (RDA) goal of 46 g in adult women and 56 g in adult men. Refer to fnic.nal.usda.gov for the DRIs for protein needs, from birth to adult, as established by the Food and Nutrition Board, Institute of Medicine.

Fat

Fat provides 9 calories per gram (more than any other calorie source) and is present in fatty fish, animal, and some plant products (particularly the seeds of plants). Fats are classified as saturated, trans, monounsaturated, and polyunsaturated. Fat is necessary as the main source of linoleic acid (omega-6 fatty acid) and alpha-linolenic acid (omega-3 fatty acid), fatty acids essential

for normal growth and development. Other major functions of fat include the following:

+ Synthesis and regulation of certain hormones
+ Absorption of fat-soluble vitamins (A, D, E, and K)
+ Maintenance of tissue structure
+ Nerve impulse transmission
+ Memory storage
+ Energy metabolism

When excess fat is consumed it is stored in fatty tissues throughout the body. Some of these fatty tissues, especially those under the skin and around the abdominal organs, serve a purpose (e.g., as a fuel reserve to be used when calorie intake does not meet demand, to support and protect organs from injury, and to prevent undue loss of heat from the body surface). The recommended fat content of the adult diet is 20% to 35% of total calories. Refer to fnic.nal.usda.gov for the DRIs for fat from birth to adult as established by the Food and Nutrition Board, Institute of Medicine.

Micronutrients

Vitamins, minerals (elements), and electrolytes are known as *micronutrients* because they are required and stored in very small quantities by the body. Even though they are not used as a source of energy, they are essential for growth, development, and hundreds of metabolic processes that occur daily. Vitamins and minerals must be taken in either through food or by supplement. With the exception of vitamin D (synthesized from cholesterol), niacin (synthesized from tryptophan), vitamin K, and biotin (produced by certain intestinal microorganisms), micronutrients cannot be metabolized by the body. Refer to fnic.nal.usda.gov for the DRIs as established by the Food and Nutrition Board, Institute of Medicine, for selected vitamins and minerals, including updated 2010 recommendations for calcium and vitamin D.

Water

Water, although listed last in this section, is the most vital nutrient. An individual can exist without food for several weeks, but without water only a few days. The body of an adult is about 55% to 65% water. The major functions of water include the following:

+ Providing turgor to body tissues
+ Altering dissolved substances to make them available for metabolic processes
+ Transporting dissolved nutrients and wastes throughout the body
+ Maintaining a stable body temperature

Water is continuously lost from the body in the urine, in water vapor of expired air, and by perspiration. Approximately 2 to $2\frac{1}{2}$ liters of water are lost daily. This loss of water is replaced by fluids taken in, water contained in solid foods eaten, and water produced in the body as a result of oxidative processes. The body has a harder time maintaining a fluid balance during some acute and chronic illnesses. Because individual water needs vary by physical activity level and exposure to heat stress, a universally recommended dietary allowance for water intake does not exist.

REVIEW OF RELATED HISTORY

Table 7-1	Equations for Predicting Resting Energy Expenditure (REE) from Body Weight*		
Gender and Age (yr)		**Equation to Derive REE in kcal/Day**	
Males	**Females**	**Males**	**Females**
0 to 3	0 to 3	$(60.9 \times wt^\dagger) - 54$	$(61.0 \times wt) - 51$
3 to 10	3 to 10	$(22.7 \times wt) + 495$	$(22.4 \times wt) + 499$
10 to 18	10 to 18	$(17.5 \times wt) + 651$	$(12.2 \times wt) + 746$
18 to 30	18 to 30	$(15.3 \times wt) + 679$	$(14.7 \times wt) + 496$
30 to 60	30 to 60	$(11.6 \times wt) + 879$	$(8.7 \times wt) + 829$
>60	>60	$(13.5 \times wt) + 487$	$(10.5 \times wt) + 596$

Modified from Subcommittee on the Tenth Edition of the RDAs, 1989.
*From World Health Organization, 1985. These equations were derived from BMR data.
†Weight of person in kilograms.

Energy Requirements

Sustaining an appropriate body weight requires an individual to balance calories consumed from foods and beverages with calories, or energy, expended. A day's total energy expenditure includes the energy used at rest, energy used in physical activity, and energy used as a result of thermogenesis, the metabolic response to food intake. Affecting these components are age, gender, body size and composition, genetics, physiologic state (e.g., rapid growth, pregnancy, or lactation), presence of disease, and body temperature.

Resting Energy Expenditure

Resting energy expenditure (REE) contributes the largest proportion of total energy expenditure by the body. REE represents energy expended at rest under conditions of stable temperature. Although basal metabolic rate (BMR) is defined as the REE measured soon after awakening in the morning (12 hours after the last meal), these two values are often interchangeable (their variability is less than 10%). Table 7-1 presents equations developed by the World Health Organization (WHO, 1985). These equations are meant to serve as a guide; they are not completely accurate for all individuals but can be helpful in determining approximate energy needs. The table accounts for age, weight, and gender but not height. Height does not appear to affect the accuracy of the calculation.

Physical Activity

Physical activity constitutes the second largest proportion of total energy expenditure. The energy expended by a given activity varies greatly among individuals and is most affected by body weight and muscle mass. A heavier person will expend more energy for a given task than a lighter individual. This often makes calculating exact energy expenditure difficult and time consuming. Physical activity recommendations vary by age. See Table 7-2 for guidelines for physical activity by age group from the U.S. Department of Health and Human Services (HHS).

Thermogenesis

After eating, the metabolic rate increases, depending on the size and composition of the meal. This accounts for about 7% of the total energy expended during a day. The increased rate peaks after about 1 hour and disappears after 4 hours. It has little long-term effect on energy requirements, being lost in the day-to-day variations in energy metabolism.

REVIEW OF RELATED HISTORY

For each of the symptoms or conditions discussed in this section, topics necessary for inclusion in the history of the present illness are listed. Responses to these questions provide clues for focusing the physical examination and developing an appropriate diagnostic evaluation. Questions regarding medication use (prescription and over the counter preparations) as well as complementary and alternative therapies are relevant for each.

History of Present Illness

+ Weight loss
  + Total weight lost, compared with usual weight; time period (sudden, gradual); intentional or unintentional
  + Desired weight loss: eating pattern, diet plan used, food preparation, food group avoidance, average daily calorie intake, appetite, exercise pattern, support group participation, weight goal
  + Undesired weight loss: anorexia; vomiting or diarrhea, difficulty swallowing, other illness symptoms, time period; frequent urination, excessive thirst; change in lifestyle, activity, mood and stress level
  + Preoccupation with body weight or body shape: never feeling thin enough, fasting, unusually strict caloric intake; unusual food restrictions or cravings; laxative abuse, induced vomiting; amenorrhea; excessive exercise; alcohol intake
  + Medications: chemotherapy, diuretics, insulin, fluoxetine; prescription and nonprescription appetite suppressants; laxatives; oral hypoglycemics; herbal supplements
+ Weight gain
  + Total weight gained: time period, sudden or gradual, desired or undesired, possibility of pregnancy
  + Change in lifestyle: change in social aspects of eating; more meals eaten out of the home; meals eaten quickly and "on the go"; change in meal preparation patterns; change in exercise patterns, mood, stress level, or alcohol intake
  + Medications: steroids, oral contraceptives, antidepressants, insulin
+ Increased metabolic requirements
  + Infancy, prematurity
  + Fever, infection, burns, trauma, pregnancy, hyperthyroidism, cancer
  + External losses (e.g., fistulas, wounds, abscesses, chronic blood loss, chronic dialysis)

Past Medical History

+ Chronic illness: liver disease, diabetes, congestive heart failure, hypothyroidism, hyperthyroidism, pancreatic insufficiency, chronic infection (e.g., human immunodeficiency virus [HIV]

Table 7-2	Guidelines For Physical Activity by Age
Age Group	
6 to 17 years	≥60 minutes of physical activity daily Aerobic: Most of the time should be spent in moderate*- or vigorous†-intensity aerobic physical activity, and should include vigorous-intensity physical activity 3 days per week. Muscle-strengthening:‡ At least 3 days per week as part of the time spent in daily physical activity Bone-strengthening:§ At least 3 days per week as part of the time spent in daily physical activity Encourage children and adolescents to participate in a variety of age-appropriate and enjoyable physical activities.
18 to 64 years	Avoid inactivity; adults who participate in any amount of physical activity gain some health benefits. For substantial health benefits, adults should participate in at least 150 minutes a week of moderate-intensity, or 75 minutes a week of vigorous-intensity aerobic physical activity, or an equivalent combination of moderate- and vigorous-intensity activity. Aerobic activity should be performed in episodes of at least 10 minutes, and preferably, it should be spread throughout the week. For additional and more extensive health benefits, adults should participate in aerobic physical activity for 300 minutes a week of moderate-intensity, or 150 minutes a week of vigorous-intensity aerobic physical activity, or an equivalent combination of moderate- and vigorous-intensity activity. Additional health benefits are gained by engaging in physical activity beyond this amount. Adults should include muscle-strengthening activities that involve all major muscle groups on 2 or more days a week.
65 years and older	Follow adult guidelines, but if this is not possible older adults should be as physically active as their abilities and conditions will allow. Older adults should do exercises that maintain or improve balance if at risk of falling. Older adults should determine their level of effort for physical activity relative to their fitness level. Older adults with chronic conditions should understand whether and how their conditions affect their ability to do regular physical activity safely.

*Moderate-intensity physical activity: Aerobic activity that increases heart rate and breathing; on a scale relative to an individual's capacity, usually a 5 or 6 on a 0 to 10 scale; examples include brisk walking, dancing, swimming and bicycling.

†Vigorous-intensity physical activity: Aerobic activity that greatly increases heart rate and breathing; on a scale relative to an individual's capacity, usually a 7 or 8 on a 0 to 10 scale; examples include jogging, singles tennis, swimming continuous laps, or bicycling uphill.

‡Muscle-strengthening activity: Physical activity, including exercise, that increases skeletal muscle strength, power, endurance and mass; includes strength training, resistance training, and muscular strength and endurance exercises.

§Bone-strengthening activity: Physical activity that produces an impact or tension force on bones, which promotes bone growth and strength; examples include running, jumping rope, and lifting weights.

Modified from *Dietary Guidelines for Americans*, 2010.

and tuberculosis), celiac disease, inflammatory bowel disease, surgical resection of the gastrointestinal tract
+ Previous weight loss or gain efforts: weight at 21 years, maximum body weight, minimum weight as an adult
+ Previously diagnosed eating disorder, hypoglycemia

Family History

+ Obesity, dyslipidemia (see Box 7-2)
+ Constitutionally short or tall stature
+ Genetic or metabolic disorder: diabetes (see list of chronic illnesses under Past Medical History)
+ Eating disorder: anorexia, bulimia
+ Alcoholism

Personal and Social History

+ Nutrition: appetite; usual calorie intake; vegetarianism; medical nutrition therapy guidelines followed; religious/cultural food practices; proportion of fat, protein, carbohydrate in the diet; intake of major vitamins and minerals (e.g., vitamins A, C, D, iron, calcium, folate)
+ Use of vitamin, mineral, and herbal supplements

+ Usual weight and height; current weight and height; ability to maintain weight, goal weight
+ Use of alcohol
+ Use of illicit drugs
+ Food insecurity (i.e., limited or uncertain availability of nutritionally adequate and safe foods); limited/fixed income; eligibility for the Supplemental Nutrition Assistance Program (SNAP; formerly the Food Stamp Program); financial and psychosocial stressors
+ Functional assessment (i.e., ability to shop and prepare foods); access to healthy foods in neighborhood; access to food storage/preparation equipment (refrigerator, stove, oven)
+ Typical mealtime situations, companions, living environment
+ Use of oral supplements, tube feedings, parenteral nutrition
+ Dentition: dentures, missing teeth, gum disease

Infants and Children

+ Nutrition: breastfeeding frequency and duration; type and amount of infant formula; method of formula preparation; time it takes to drink one feeding; intake of protein, calories, vitamins, and minerals adequate for growth; vegetarianism;

| Box 7-2 | Statistics on Obesity and Diet-Related Chronic Diseases in the United States |

Over one-third of adults in the Unites States are obese and an additional 30% to 40% are overweight. Poor diet and physical inactivity (regardless of weight status) are associated with serious chronic diseases including type 2 diabetes, hypertension, cardiovascular disease, osteoporosis, and some types of cancer.

- About 26 million adults (8.3% of the U.S. population) have diabetes. Most of these individuals have type 2 diabetes. An additional 79 million adults have prediabetes.
- About 81 million adults (37% of the U.S. population) have cardiovascular disease and 16% have high cholesterol. Just over one-third of adults have hypertension and an additional 36% have prehypertension.
- Half of women and 25% of men over 50 years of age will have a fracture related to osteoporosis.
- Cancers linked to poor diet include breast (postmenopausal), endometrial, colon, kidney, mouth, pharynx, larynx, and esophageal.

The Division of Nutrition, Physical Activity, and Obesity at the Centers for Disease Control and Prevention has a wealth of information and useful resources patients and healthcare professionals (www.cdc.gov/nccdphp/dnpao/index.html).

From the Centers for Disease Control and Prevention, 2011 and the 2010 *Dietary Guidelines for Americans.*

| Risk Factors |

Eating Disorders

- Weight preoccupation
- Poor self-esteem, perfectionist personality
- Self-image perceptual disturbances
- Chronic medical illness (insulin-dependent diabetes)
- Family history of eating disorders, obesity, alcoholism, or affective disorders
- Cultural pressure for thinness or outstanding performance
- Athlete driven to excel in sports (gymnasts, ice skaters, boxers, and wrestlers)
- Food cravings, restrictions
- Compulsive/binge eating
- Difficulties with communication and conflict resolution; separation from families
- Use of appetite suppressants and/or laxatives

| Clinical Pearl |

Eating Disorders

A major risk factor for developing an eating disorder (e.g., anorexia or bulimia) is having a first-degree relative with an eating disorder.

---

cow's milk protein and other food allergies; vitamin and mineral supplements; number of fast food meals eaten per week; eligibility for Women, Infants, and Children (WIC) program or school breakfast and lunch programs
- Hours of screen time per day (i.e., television, computer use, video and electronic games); access to safe areas for physical activity
- Chronic illness: cystic fibrosis, phenylketonuria (PKU), celiac disease, inborn errors of carbohydrate metabolism, amino acid and fatty acid oxidation disorders, tyrosinemia, homocystinuria, Prader-Willi syndrome
- Congenital anomalies, prematurity, prolonged neonatal hospitalization, cleft palate, malformed palate, tongue thrust, feeding and swallowing disorders, prolonged enteral tube feeding (gastrostomy and gastrojejunostomy), neurologic disorders, gastroesophageal reflux, congenital heart disease

Adolescents

- Nutrition: intake of protein, calories, vitamins, and minerals adequate for growth; vegetarianism; number of fast food meals eaten per week; food allergies; vitamin and mineral supplements; herbal supplements; appetite suppressants; laxative use; alcohol use
- Preoccupation with weight; overly concerned with developing muscle mass, losing body fat; excessive exercise; weighs self daily, boasts about weight loss, weight goals; omits perceived fattening foods and food groups from diet (see Clinical Pearl, "Eating Disorders")

Pregnant Women

- Prepregnancy weight and body mass index (BMI), age, eating patterns/disorders
- Weight gain during pregnancy; nutrient intake during pregnancy (particularly protein, calories, iron, folate, calcium); supplementation with vitamins, iron, folic acid; eligibility for WIC program
- Potential risks: pica, alcohol, inadequate weight gain
- Lactation: nutrient intake during lactation (particularly protein, calories, calcium, vitamins A and C); fluid intake (water, juice, milk, caffeine)
- Chronic illness: diabetes, renal disease, others

Older Adults

- Nutrition: weight gain or loss, adequate income for food purchases, interest and capability in preparing meals, participant in older adult feeding programs, social interaction at mealtime, number of daily meals and snacks, transportation to grocery stores and access to healthy foods
- Energy level, regular exercise/activities
- Chronic illness: diabetes, renal disease, cancer, heart disease, swallowing dysfunction after stroke
- Food/nutrient/medication interactions (Box 7-3)

EXAMINATION AND FINDINGS

Equipment

- Tape measure with millimeter markings
- Calculator
- Standing platform scale with height attachment

Box 7-3 Food–Nutrient–Medication Interactions

Medications can affect nutritional intake and status just as some foods, and the nutrients contained in them, can affect absorption, metabolism, and excretion of medications. For example, a consistently high intake of grapefruit juice while taking simvastatin increases the bioavailability of the medication, often resulting in an increased risk of myopathy. It is important to assess the medications that a patient is taking to determine appropriateness and whether there are any possible interactions. The term *medications* includes those prescribed as well as those purchased over the counter. Often patients do not remember to list vitamin, mineral, herbal, and protein supplements during the history unless specifically asked about them.

Risk Factors

Possible Medication Effects on Nutritional Intake and Status

- Altered food intake resulting from altered taste/smell, gastric irritation, bezoars (food-ball found in the stomach and/or intestines), appetite increase/decrease, nausea/vomiting
- Modified nutrient absorption resulting from altered gastrointestinal pH, increased/decreased bile acid activity, altered gastrointestinal motility, inhibited enzymes, damaged mucosal cell walls, insoluble nutrient-drug complexes
- Modified nutrient metabolism resulting from vitamin antagonism (e.g., warfarin is a vitamin K antagonist)
- Modified nutrient excretion resulting from urinary loss, fecal loss

Anthropometrics

Procedures for accurately measuring height and weight, and the tables of the norms for the pediatric age and gender groups are addressed in Chapter 6. These measures are useful in assessing a patient's nutritional status and possible disease risk. Refer to Box 6-2 in Chapter 6 for calculating BMI using pounds and inches and Appendix B, Table B-3, for a BMI quick reference guide. Refer to Box 7-4 to assess desirable weight and percent weight change.

Waist Circumference and Waist-Height Ratio

Waist circumference and waist-height ratio are indicators of visceral fat or abdominal obesity. Waist circumference should be measured at the high point of the iliac crest when the individual is standing and at minimal respiration. Persons of normal weight who have increased waist circumferences often fall into a higher disease risk classification. A large waist circumference (>35 inches in women, >40 inches in men) is associated with increased risk for type 2 diabetes, dyslipidemia, hypertension, and cardiovascular disease (Klein et al, 2007). Monitoring changes in a person's waist circumference over time, with or without changes in BMI, may aid in predicting relative disease risk in terms of cardiovascular risk factors and obesity-related diseases.

Waist-height ratio is calculated as a ratio of the waist circumference (cm) and height (cm). Like waist circumference, waist-height ratio has been shown to be a strong predictor for diabetes and cardiovascular disease in adults (Ashwell et al, 2012). A waist-height ratio >0.5 is associated with increased risk.

Box 7-4 Assessing Height and Weight

Current Weight _____   Current Height _____

Usual Weight _____

Desirable Body Weight _____

(Women: 100 pounds for first 5 feet; plus 5 pounds for each inch thereafter)

(Men: 106 pounds for first 5 feet; plus 6 pounds for each inch thereafter)

This is a quick method for determining desirable weight.

(See Chapter 6, Box 6-2, for body mass index measurements.)

Add 10% for a large frame; subtract 10% for a small frame. Refer to Chapter 6 for methods used to determine body frame size.

% Desirable Weight _____   Current weight × 100 ÷ Desirable body weight

% Usual Weight _____   Current weight × 100 ÷ Usual weight

% Weight Change _____   (Usual weight − Current weight) × 100 ÷ Usual weight

A significant weight loss equals or exceeds:
1% to 2% in 1 week
5% in 1 month
7.5% in 3 months
10% in 6 months

For pediatric patients (birth to age 18), refer to the growth charts in Appendix A.

See Centers for Disease Control and Prevention (CDC) Waist Circumference tables at www.cdc.gov/nchs/data/series/sr_11/sr11_252.pdf.

Waist-to-Hip Circumference Ratio

The waist-to-hip circumference ratio is another measure of fat distribution by body type, but it is not as helpful as the BMI in assessing total body fat. An excess proportion of trunk and abdominal fat (i.e., an ovoid or apple-shaped body) has a higher risk association with diabetes, dyslipidemia, metabolic syndrome, stroke, and ischemic heart disease than does a greater proportion of gluteal fat (i.e., a pear-shaped body). Measure the waist at a midpoint between the costal margin and the iliac crest (inches or millimeters may be used). Then measure the hip at the widest part of the gluteal region (Fig. 7-1). Divide the waist circumference by the hip circumference to obtain the waist-to-hip ratio.

FIGURE 7-1 Measurement of waist circumference **(A)** and hip circumference **(B)** to calculate the waist-to-hip circumference ratio: waist circumference (cm)/hip circumference (cm) = waist-to-hip ratio.

FIGURE 7-2 Choose My Plate. *(From US Department of Agriculture: ChooseMyPlate, 2011, http://www.choosemyplate.gov.)*

24-hour recall method provides a very limited view of an individual's actual intake over time and may be misleading. Individuals may be unable to accurately remember everything they ate the day before, causing further inaccuracies in interpreting the information. There are now a variety of web-based and electronic device 24-hour recall tools. Patients report minimal burden and high rates of satisfaction with these types of tools compared to a typical diet history assessment (Arab et al, 2010).

Food Diary

The food diary can be an accurate but time-consuming method for the patient and health professional. It provides a retrospective view of an individual's eating habits and dietary intake, recorded as it happened. It can also collect relevant data that may aid in identifying problem areas. The USDA ChooseMyPlate.gov website has a useful web-based tool for tracking daily food and beverage intake by food groups (grains, vegetables, fruits, dairy, and protein foods) at www.choosemyplate.gov/SuperTracker/foodtracker.aspx.

Measures of Nutrient Analysis

Complete a nutrient analysis by using a method of diet history or recall. Nutrition screening forms and web-based tools can be found on the USDA Food and Nutrition Information Center website (fnic.nal.usda.gov). The questions can be modified for infants, children, older adults, or particular circumstances. Other web-based nutrient analysis programs and electronic device applications offer the quickest and most efficient method of analyzing an individual's nutrient intake. Analysis may be performed for 1 or more days to obtain averages for all or selected nutrients.

ChooseMyPlate.gov

ChooseMyPlate.gov provides practical information, tips, and web-based tools to help individuals build healthier diets (Fig. 7-2). ChooseMyPlate.gov is based on the most up to date

Ratios greater than 1.0 in men and greater than 0.85 in women indicate central fat distribution and risk for obesity-related disorders.

Determination of Diet Adequacy

The history of an individual's food and beverage intake allows estimation of the adequacy of the diet. Histories may be obtained through 24-hour diet recalls or with a 3- or 4-day food diary that includes 1 weekend day. Various methods for measuring nutrient intake are available.

Twenty–Four-Hour Recall Diet

The 24-hour recall is a frequently used method for obtaining a food intake history. Ask the patient to complete a 24-hour food recall, listing all foods, beverages, and snacks eaten during the last 24 hours. Ask specific questions about the method of food preparation, portion sizes, amount of sugar-sweetened beverages, and use of salt or other additives. The Automated Multiple Pass Method (AMPM), developed by the USDA, is a standardized method for collecting 24-hour dietary recalls in studies of the U.S. population, such as the National Health and Nutrition Examination Survey. In this method, for each food, individuals are asked a variety of questions about the type of food, additions to the food (e.g., cream in coffee), amount consumed, and the location and time when the food was eaten. Other questions include the use of salt in foods, water and beverage consumption, and whether the amount consumed was much more than usual, usual, or less than usual (www.ars.usda.gov). Some believe the

EXAMINATION AND FINDINGS

recommendations from the 2010 Dietary Guidelines for Americans. The Guidelines, published every 5 years by HHS and the USDA, provide evidence-based information and advice for choosing a healthy eating pattern that focuses on nutrient-dense foods and beverages and helps individuals achieve and maintain a healthy weight. The full guidelines are available at www.cnpp.usda.gov/Publications/DietaryGuidelines/2010/PolicyDoc/PolicyDoc.pdf. Individuals can use the ChooseMyPlate.gov website to create a Daily Food Plan based on age, gender, weight, height, and physical activity level. Individuals can track and analyze their diet and physical activity habits and check the nutritional value of specific foods.

ChooseMyPlate.gov emphasizes the following key messages:

- Balancing Calories
  - Enjoy your food, but eat less.
  - Avoid oversized portions.
- Foods to Increase
  - Make half your plate fruits and vegetables.
  - Make at least half your grains whole grains.
  - Switch to fat-free or low-fat (1%) milk.
- Foods to Reduce
  - Compare sodium in foods like soup, bread, and frozen meals—and choose the foods with lower numbers.
  - Drink water instead of sugary drinks.

Vegetarian Diets

Vegetarian diets can meet all the recommendations for nutrients. The key is to consume a variety of foods and the right amount of foods to meet an individual's caloric needs. Five nutrients may be deficient in a vegetarian diet if it is not carefully planned: protein, calcium (lacto-ovo and vegan), iron, vitamin B_{12} (vegan), and vitamin D. The Office of Dietary Supplements at the National Institutes of Health has a variety of useful educational materials for patients and health care providers about the effectiveness, safety, and quality of dietary supplements (ods.od.nih.gov).

Ethnic Food Guide Pyramids

Food Guide Pyramids for ethnic populations are available (e.g., Mediterranean, Indian, Mexican, and Asian). To see examples of ethnic and cultural food guide pyramids, go to the USDA Food and Nutrition Information Center (fnic.nal.usda.gov/dietary-guidance/myplatefood-pyramid-resources/ethniccultural-food-pyramids). In addition, Oldways Preservation Trust (www.oldwayspt.org) is a useful resource.

Measures of Nutrient Adequacy

Nutrition can be assessed through many body systems. Summaries of the functions/metabolism/utilization, deficiency/toxicity symptoms, and food sources of fat- and water-soluble vitamins and minerals are provided in Tables 7-3, 7-4, and 7-5. The clinical findings often associated with nutrient deficiencies are indicated in Table 7-6. The following section discusses methods of measuring nutrient intake and adequacy along with specific anthropometric and biochemical measures of nutritional status.

An individual's diet can be measured for nutritional adequacy based on energy needs and/or a variety of macronutrients or micronutrients (see Clinical Pearl, "'Rule of Thumb' Estimates for Calculating Daily Energy Needs").

Clinical Pearl

"Rule of Thumb" Estimates for Calculating Daily Energy Needs

Healthy Adults	kcal/kg Body Weight
To promote weight loss	25
To promote weight maintenance	30
To promote weight gain	35
To promote weight maintenance and/or weight gain in hypermetabolic and malnourished patients	35 to 50

Use adjusted weight for patients who are greater than 125% of their DBW.

Adjustment for obese patients (for energy if 125% of DBW):

Adjusted weight − [(ABW − DBW) × 25%] + DBW

Pediatric Patients: 1000 kcal + 100 kcal/yr of age up to age 12

ABW, Actual body weight; *DBW,* desirable body weight.

- *Energy:* A variety of methods can be used for calculating an individual's energy needs. The "rule of thumb" calculations also offer a quick estimate for energy needs for those needing to gain, maintain, or lose weight. Adjustments to the calculations may be made to meet the needs of certain individuals (e.g., those who appear to have a higher metabolic rate and continue to lose weight even when the higher calculation is used). It is important to note that overweight individuals underreport their energy intake by 30% to 55% and lean individuals by only 0% to 20%.
- *Carbohydrates:* Children and adults should have 45% to 65% of their daily calorie intake from carbohydrates. The Adequate Intake (AI) for fiber is 25 g per day for an adult female and 38 g per day for an adult male. In children and adolescents 1 to 18 years of age, recommended fiber intake ranges from 14 to 31 g. Refer to fnic.nal.usda.gov for the suggested DRIs for total fiber for all individuals, including infants, children, and adolescents.
- *Fat:* Recommendations for daily fat intake decreases with age. For children 1 to 3 years of age, 30% to 40% of daily calories should come from fat. Children and adolescents 4 to 18 years of age should have 25% to 35% of daily calories and adults should have 20% to 35% of daily calories from fat. For all ages, less than 10% of calories should be from saturated fat. Refer to fnic.nal.usda.gov for the DRIs for fat for all individuals, including infants, children, and adolescents.
- *Protein:* For children 1-3 years of age, protein intake should be 5% to 20% of daily calories. Children and adolescents 4 to

Text continued on p. 107

Table 7-3 Fat-Soluble Vitamin Summary

Vitamins	Function	Deficiency Symptoms	Toxicity Symptoms	Food Sources
Vitamin A Retinol Retinal Retinoic acid	Preserves integrity of epithelial cells Formation of rhodopsin for vision in dim light Necessary for wound healing, growth, and normal immune function	Night blindness Dry eyes Poor bone growth Impaired resistance to infection Severe drying and scaling of the skin	Fatigue, night sweats Vertigo, headaches Dry and fissured skin and lips Retarded growth, bone pain Abdominal pain, vomiting, jaundice	Breast milk, infant formula Liver, butter, fortified margarine, egg yolk Dark green and deep yellow vegetables and fruits
Vitamin D Precursors: Ergosterol in plants 7-dehydrocholesterol; in skin	Mobilization and mineralization of bone Promotes the absorption of calcium and phosphorus in the intestine	Rickets Costochondral beading Epiphyseal enlargement Enlarged skull Cranial bossing Bowed legs Osteomalacia Renal osteodystrophy	Retarded growth, vomiting Hypercalcemia Nephrocalcinosis	Infant formula Egg yolk Liver, fatty fish, sunlight
Vitamin E Tocopherols	Functions as an antioxidant in the intestines and elsewhere Protects cell membranes and red blood cells May have a role in preventing the development of cardiovascular disease	Red cell hemolysis in malnourished infants Hyporeflexia Retinal degeneration	May interfere with vitamin K activity leading to prolonged clotting and bleeding time Suppresses the normal response to iron in patients with anemia	Breast milk, infant formula Vegetable oils, egg yolk Liver, butter, fortified margarine Green leafy vegetables Whole-grain breads, cereals, and other fortified or enriched grain products
Vitamin K	Forms prothrombin for normal blood clotting Synthesized by bacteria in the intestines	Prolonged bleeding and prothrombin time Hemorrhagic manifestations (especially in newborns)	Possible hemolytic anemia; hyperbilirubinemia (jaundice)	Infant formula, vegetable oils Green leafy vegetables Pork, liver

Modified from Robinson et al, 1993; and from *Infant Nutrition and Feeding*, U.S. Department of Agriculture Food and Nutrition Service, 2008.

Table 7-4 Water-Soluble Vitamin Summary

Vitamins	Function	Deficiency Symptoms	Toxicity Symptoms	Food Sources
Ascorbic acid Vitamin C	Forms collagen (which strengthens tissues and improves wound healing and resistance to infection) Keeps teeth firm in gums Hormone synthesis Improves iron absorption and transport	Poor wound healing Poor bone, tooth development Scurvy Bruising and hemorrhage Bleeding gums Loose teeth	Nausea, abdominal cramping, diarrhea Possible formation of kidney stones	Breast milk, infant formula Citrus fruits Papaya, cantaloupe, strawberries Tomatoes, broccoli, potatoes Raw green vegetables
Thiamin Vitamin B$_1$	Coenzyme for breakdown of glucose for energy Normal digestion Normal appetite Healthy nervous system Positive mental outlook	Beriberi Fatigue Poor appetite Constipation Depression Neuropathy Polyneuritis Edema Heart failure	Toxicity extremely rare	Breast milk, infant formula Pork, liver, other meats, poultry Dry beans and peas, peanut butter Whole-grain or enriched breads, cereals Milk, eggs

Continued

EXAMINATION AND FINDINGS

Table 7-4	Water-Soluble Vitamin Summary—cont'd			
Vitamins	Function	Deficiency Symptoms	Toxicity Symptoms	Food Sources
Riboflavin Vitamin B$_2$	Coenzymes for protein and glucose metabolism Fatty acid synthesis Healthy skin Normal vision in bright light	Cheilosis, glossitis Photophobia Burning, itching, sensitive eyes Poor growth Scaling skin	Toxicity extremely rare	Breast milk, infant formula and dairy products Meat, poultry, fish Egg yolk, legumes Dark-green leafy vegetables Whole-grain or enriched breads, cereals
Niacin Nicotinic acid Niacinamide	Coenzymes for energy metabolism Normal digestion Healthy nervous system Healthy skin	*Pellagra* Dermatitis Angular stomatitis Diarrhea Depression Disorientation Delirium	Transient symptoms due to the vasodilating effects of niacin (does not occur with niacinamide) include flushing, tingling, dizziness, nausea Liver function abnormalities, hyperuricemia	Breast milk, infant formula Meat, poultry, fish Egg yolk Dark-green leafy vegetables Whole-grain or enriched breads, cereals
Vitamin B$_6$ Pyridoxine Pyridoxal Pyridoxamine	Coenzymes for protein synthesis and breakdown Conversion of tryptophan to niacin Normal growth Formation of heme	Cheilosis Gastrointestinal symptoms Weak gait Irritability Neuropathy Convulsions Microcytic anemia	Sensory neuropathy with progressive ataxia Photosensitivity	Breast milk, infant formula Meat Whole-grain or enriched breads, cereals Dark-green leafy vegetables Potatoes
Vitamin B$_{12}$	Synthesis of DNA, RNA Maturation of red blood cells Involved with central nervous system metabolism Requires intrinsic factor from stomach for absorption	Pernicious anemia: lack of intrinsic factor, or after gastrectomy Macrocytic anemia: neurologic degeneration, pallor	Toxicity extremely rare	Breast milk, infant formula Animal foods only: milk, egg yolk, cheese, meat, poultry, fish
Folate Folacin Folic acid	Synthesis of DNA, RNA Maturation of red blood cells	Poor growth Macrocytic anemia in pregnancy, sprue (concurrent vitamin B$_{12}$ deficiency should be suspected)	Masking of vitamin B$_{12}$ deficiency symptoms in those with pernicious anemia not taking cyanocobalamin	Breast milk, infant formula Dark-green leafy vegetables Lean beef, liver, fish, poultry, eggs Whole-grain or enriched breads, cereals Oranges, cantaloupe
Biotin	Essential component of enzymes Coenzyme carrier of carbon dioxide Role in metabolism of fatty acids and amino acids	Seborrheic dermatitis, loss of hair Glossitis, nausea Insomnia	Diarrhea Water retention	Breast milk, infant formula Liver, meats Egg yolk Bananas, strawberries, grapefruit, watermelon Most vegetables Legumes, nuts
Pantothenic acid	Component of coenzyme A Synthesis and breakdown of many vital body compounds Essential in metabolism of carbohydrate, fat, and protein	Deficiency rare Neuritis of arms, legs; burning sensation of feet; impaired coordination Fatigue, sleep disturbances Muscle cramps	Diarrhea Water retention	Breast milk, infant formula Meat, poultry, fish, liver Egg yolk Legumes, whole-grain breads and cereals Vegetables

Modified from Robinson et al, 1993; and from *Infant Nutrition and Feeding*, U.S. Department of Agriculture Food and Nutrition Service, 2008.

Table 7-5 | **Mineral Summary**

Element	Function	Utilization and Deficiency Symptoms	Toxicity Symptoms	Food Sources
Calcium	Builds and maintains bones and teeth Nerve transmission and muscle contraction Blood clotting Activates enzymes	10% to 40% absorbed Aided by vitamin D and lactose; hindered by oxalic acid Regulates parathyroid hormone blood levels *Deficiency:* fragile bones, osteoporosis	Hypercalcemia Excessive calcification of bone and soft tissues Vomiting, lethargy	Breast milk, infant formula Dairy products (yogurt, cheese) Fortified or enriched grain products Collards, kale, mustard greens, and turnip greens Cabbage, broccoli Clams, oysters, sardines, salmon
Phosphorus	Builds and maintains bones and teeth Component of nucleic acids, phospholipids Transport of fats Coenzyme function in energy metabolism; protein synthesis	Vitamin D favors absorption and use by bones *Deficiency:* rare	Toxicity rare Hypocalcemia (with parathyroid gland dysfunction)	Breast milk, infant formula Dairy products, cheese Egg yolk Meat, poultry, fish Whole-grain cereals, nuts, legumes
Magnesium	Nerve transmission and muscle contraction Enzymes for energy metabolism	Muscle tremors, convulsions, irritability, tetany, hyperreflexia Acid favors absorption *Deficiency:* rare; occurs in alcoholism, renal failure	Toxicity rare Hyporeflexia, prolonged AV conduction, and heart block, hypocalcemia	Breast milk, infant formula Milk Tofu Meat, green leafy vegetables, legumes, whole-grain cereals
Sodium	Helps regulate osmotic pressure of body fluids Influences cell permeability Acid-base balance Nervous stimulation and muscle contraction	Almost completely absorbed Body levels regulated by adrenal; excess excreted in urine and by skin Nausea, vomiting, dizziness *Deficiency:* rare; occurs with excessive perspiration	Hypernatremia Edema, hypertension	Sodium chloride (table salt) Baking powder, baking soda Milk, meat, poultry, fish, eggs Ample amounts in most foods except fruits
Potassium	Helps regulate osmotic pressure of body fluids Protein and glycogen synthesis Transmits nerve impulses and muscle contraction (especially cardiac muscle)	Almost completely absorbed Body levels regulated by adrenal glands; excess excreted in urine *Deficiency:* occurs with starvation, diuretic therapy Muscle weakness, decreased intestinal tone and distension Cardiac arrhythmias	Hyperkalemia Nausea, fatigue, muscle weakness Cardiac arrhythmias	Breast milk, infant formula Ample amounts in meat, cereals, fruits (especially bananas and dried fruits), fruit juices (especially orange juice), vegetables Soy products
Iron	Essential for hemoglobin formation and oxygen transport Muscle myoglobin Oxidizing enzymes for release of energy	5% to 20% absorption Ascorbic acid (vitamin C) aids absorption Daily losses in urine and feces Menstrual loss *Deficiency:* hypochromic microcytic anemia, cheilosis, pallor, lethargy, anorexia	Hemochromatosis Hemosiderosis	Breast milk, infant formula Meat, liver, fish, poultry Whole-grain, fortified, and enriched breads and cereals Green vegetables, dried fruits

Continued

EXAMINATION AND FINDINGS

Table 7-5   Mineral Summary—cont'd

Element	Function	Utilization and Deficiency Symptoms	Toxicity Symptoms	Food Sources
Iodine	Needed for the production of thyroid hormones Cellular oxidation and growth	Chiefly in thyroid gland *Deficiency:* endemic goiter, symptoms of hypothyroidism (constipation, depressed mood)	Hypothyroidism due to feedback inhibition of thyroid hormone synthesis	Breast milk, infant formula Iodized salt Shellfish, saltwater fish
Fluoride	Protects teeth from tooth decay	Storage in bones and teeth *Deficiency:* increased risk of dental caries	Teeth mottling and dark brown staining	Fluoridated water or fluoride supplement
Copper	Utilization of iron for hemoglobin formation Involved in collagen synthesis	In form of ceruloplasmin in blood *Deficiency:* rare; anemia, pallor, retarded growth, edema, anorexia	Wilson disease: copper deposits in cornea, liver cirrhosis, impaired neurologic functioning	Liver, shellfish, meats, nuts, legumes, whole-grain cereals, and other grain products
Selenium	Essential for cell growth and development Associated with fat metabolism and vitamin E Antioxidant	*Deficiency:* rare Myalgia, muscle tenderness Cardiac myopathy Increased fragility of red blood cells Degeneration of pancreas	Nausea, vomiting, fatigue Diarrhea Loss of hair and nails Peripheral neuropathy	Whole-grain breads, cereals, and other fortified or enriched grain products Onions and other vegetables (dependent on soil content) Meats, seafood
Zinc	Cofactor for enzymes involved with metabolism of protein, carbohydrate, fat, and alcohol Protein synthesis and integrity of cell membranes Tissue growth and repair, wound healing Taste	*Deficiency:* decreased wound healing, hypogonadism, anemia, growth retardation, hair loss, diarrhea, altered taste	Gastrointestinal disturbance, vomiting, sweating, dizziness Decreased levels of HDL, white blood cells, and copper	Breast milk, infant formula Meat, liver Egg yolk Oysters and other seafood Whole-grain breads, cereals, and other fortified or enriched grain products Plant and animal proteins

Modified from Robinson et al, 1993; and from *Infant Nutrition and Feeding*, U.S. Department of Agriculture Food and Nutrition Service, 2008.

Table 7-6   Clinical Signs and Symptoms of Various Nutrient Deficiencies

Examination	Sign/Symptom	Deficiency
Hair	Alopecia Easy pluckability Lackluster "Corkscrew" hair Decreased pigmentation	Zinc, essential fatty acids Protein, essential fatty acids Protein, zinc Vitamin C, vitamin A Protein, copper
Eyes	Xerosis of conjunctiva Keratomalacia Bitot spots Corneal vascularization	Vitamin A Vitamin A Vitamin A Riboflavin
Gastrointestinal tract	Nausea, vomiting Diarrhea Stomatitis Cheilosis Glossitis	Pyridoxine Zinc, niacin Pyridoxine, riboflavin, iron Pyridoxine, iron Pyridoxine, zinc, niacin, folate, vitamin B_{12} Riboflavin Vitamin C Protein

Table 7-6   Clinical Signs and Symptoms of Various Nutrient Deficiencies—cont'd

Examination	Sign/Symptom	Deficiency
Skin	Dry and scaling	Vitamin A, essential fatty acids, zinc
	Petechiae/ecchymoses	Vitamin C, vitamin K
	Follicular hyperkeratosis	Vitamin A, essential fatty acids
	Nasolabial seborrhea	Niacin, pyridoxine, riboflavin
	Atopic dermatitis	Niacin, zinc
Extremities	Subcutaneous fat loss	Calories
	Muscle wastage	Calories, protein
	Edema	Protein
	Osteomalacia, bone pain, rickets	Vitamin D
	Arthralgia	Vitamin C
Neurologic	Disorientation	Niacin, thiamin
	Confabulation	Thiamin
	Neuropathy	Thiamin, pyridoxine, chromium
	Paresthesia	Thiamin, pyridoxine, vitamin B_{12}
Cardiovascular	Congestive heart failure, cardiomegaly, tachycardia	Thiamin
	Cardiomyopathy	Selenium

18 years of age should consume 10% to 30% of daily calories and adults 19 years of age and older should consume 10% to 35% of their calories from protein. Refer to fnic.nal.usda.gov for the DRIs for protein needs for all individuals, including infants, children, and adolescents.

+ *Vitamins, minerals, and electrolytes:* An individual who eats a variety of foods from the food groups will meet his or her needs for most vitamins and minerals. Several that may be of concern if food intake is restricted include vitamins A, C, and E; calcium; iron; and folate. Refer to fnic.nal.usda.gov for the suggested DRIs for all individuals, including infants, children, and adolescents.

Special Procedures

Triceps Skinfold Thickness

The measurement of skinfold or fatfold thickness provides another parameter to evaluate the nutritional status of the patient. The jaws of skinfold thickness calipers must be correctly placed to get an accurate reading.

To determine the site of the triceps skinfold (TSF) thickness measurement, have the patient flex the right arm at a right angle. Position yourself behind the patient and, using a measuring tape, make a horizontal mark halfway between the tips of the olecranon and acromial processes on the posterior aspect of the arm. Then draw a line along the vertical plane of the arm to cross the midpoint. Allowing the patient's arm to hang relaxed, use your thumb and forefinger to grasp and lift the TSF about ½ inch (1.27 cm) proximal to the marked cross. Make sure you feel the main bulk of the triceps muscle, identifying the muscle's subcutaneous interface between your fingers deep to the skinfold. (If you do not feel the muscle bulk, you may be too medial or lateral to the muscle mass and need to reposition your fingers.) Place the caliper jaws on each side of the raised skinfold at the marked cross, but not so tightly as to cause an indentation (Fig. 7-3).

FIGURE 7-3 Placement of calipers for triceps skinfold thickness measurement.

With the gauge at eye level, make two readings to the nearest millimeter at the same site and derive an average.

Because approximately 50% of the body fat is present in the subcutaneous tissue layers, a correlation exists between the TSF thickness and the body's fat content. Therefore, the TSF measurement may be used in the diagnosis of obesity. Compare the patient's measurement with the percentiles of TSF thickness by age and gender, which can be found on the CDC National Center for Health Statistics website (www.cdc.gov/nchs). Measuring skinfold thickness in the very obese is difficult because calipers are not large enough for some skinfolds. The thickness of adipose tissue in obese patients also makes it more difficult to raise the

EXAMINATION AND FINDINGS

FIGURE 7-4 Measurement of mid–upper arm circumference.

skinfold with parallel sides for the measurement. In addition, measurement is not routinely recommended for children, and has been reported to have limited value in assessing overweight children because measures are poorly predictive of abdominal and total fat (Watts et al, 2006).

Mid-Upper Arm Circumference

The mid-upper arm circumference (MAC), not routinely obtained, provides a rough estimate of muscle mass and available fat and protein stores. A depressed value, however, is usually found only in the most severe forms of protein-calorie malnutrition. The measurement is of more value in the calculation of arm muscle circumference and arm muscle mass, both of which are sensitive to changes in muscle and/or protein stores. Select the patient's bare right arm for measurement. (NOTE: Use the same side of the body for all anthropometric measures.) Place the millimeter measuring tape around the patient's upper arm, midway between the tips of the olecranon and acromial processes (Fig. 7-4), the same location where the TSF thickness measurement is made. Hold the measuring tape snugly, but not tight enough to cause an indentation, and measure to the nearest 5 mm (0.5 cm). Anthropometric reference data, including percentiles for MAC for infants, children, men, and women can be found on the CDC National Center for Health Statistics website (www.cdc.gov/nchs).

Midarm Muscle Circumference/ Midarm Muscle Area

Midarm muscle circumference (MAMC) and midarm muscle area (MAMA) are estimated from measures of MAC and TSF. The MAMC is well accepted as a sensitive index of body protein reserves. Both measures are commonly decreased in the presence of protein malnutrition. MAMA is useful in children because the muscle area changes more with age than does arm muscle circumference. This measure of arm muscle is only an estimate because the thickness of the humerus is not taken into account and upper arms are not perfectly round as the formula assumes. Reference tables for these two measures can be found on the Internet and in many nutrition assessment textbooks.

Calculations:

$$\text{MAMC}: \text{MAC (in mm)} - [3.14 \times \text{TSF (in mm)}]$$

$$\text{MAMA}: \{\text{MAC (in mm)} - [3.14 \times \text{TSF (in mm)}]\}^2 \div 12.56$$

Biochemical Measurement

The following list is intended as a guideline. Not all indicators may be necessary or appropriate to assess nutritional adequacy for a given patient. Likewise, other laboratory measures not listed here may be useful or necessary in a particular situation. Compare laboratory data to the norms for the relevant age and gender group (Table 7-7). A laboratory may have established different reference ranges based on testing equipment and procedure.

- Hemoglobin (g/dL)
- Hematocrit (%)
- Transferrin saturation (%)
- Serum albumin (g/dL)
- Serum cholesterol (CHOL) (mg/dL)
- Serum triglycerides (TRI) (mg/dL)
- High-density lipoproteins (HDL) (mg/dL)
- Low-density lipoproteins (LDL) (mg/dL)
- CHOL/HDL ratio
- Serum glucose (mg/dL)
- Hemoglobin A1c (%)
- Serum folate (ng/mL)

Sample Documentation

History and Physical Examination

Subjective

A 45-year-old man with steady weight gain over the past 5 years seeks nutrition and physical activity counseling. Eats three full meals per day with snacking in between eats breakfast and dinner at home, wife prepares meals. Often eats lunch (fast foods) on the run. Sugar beverage intake: 1 or 2 cans of non-diet soda per day. No regular exercise. Has never kept a meal log. No change in lifestyle, moderate stress.

Objective

Height: 173 cm (68 inches); weight: 90.9 kg (200 pounds); 123% of desirable body weight; BMI 30.5 kg/m²; triceps skinfold thickness 20 mm (90th percentile), midarm circumference 327.8 mm; midarm muscle circumference 265 mm (25th percentile); waist circumference 42 inches; hip circumference 41 inches; waist-hip ratio 1.02; 2200 calories daily, estimated for appropriate weight loss

For additional sample documentation, see Chapter 26, pp. 628-631.

Table 7-7	**Biochemical Indicators of Good Nutrition Status**			
Nutrient or Measurement	**Test**	**Age Group**	**Male**	**Female**
Iron	Hemoglobin (g/dL)			
		Adults	≥14.0	≥12.0
		Newborns	≥13.7	≥13.7
		Infants and young children (6 mo to 6 yr)	≥12.0	≥12.0
		Children (7 to 12 yr)	≥11.0	≥11.0
		Adolescents (13 to 16 yr)	≥13.5	≥11.5
		Pregnancy		
		(2nd trimester)		≥11.0
		(3rd trimester)		≥10.5
	Hematocrit (%)	Adults	≥40.0	≥37.0
		Newborns	≥45.0	≥45.0
		Infants and young children (6 mo to 6 yr)	≥33.0	≥33.0
		Children (7 to 12 yr)	≥34.0	≥34.0
		Adolescents (13 to 16 yr)	≥40.0	≥36.0
	Transferrin saturation (%)	Adults	≥20.0	≥20.0
		Infants (<2 yr)	≥15.0	≥15.0
		Children (2 to 12 yr)	≥20.0	≥15.0
		Adolescents (12+ yr)	≥20.0	≥15.0
Protein	Serum albumin (g/dL)	Adults	3.4 to 5.4	3.4 to 5.4
		Children and adolescents	3.0 to 5.0	3.0 to 5.0
Normal lipid metabolism	Serum cholesterol (mg/dL)	Adults	<200	<200
		Children and adolescents	<170	<170
	Serum triglyceride (mg/dL)		<150	<150
		Children (0 to 10 years)	<75	<75
		Children and adolescents (10 to 19 years)	<90	<90
	High-density lipoprotein (mg/dL)		>40	>40
		Children and adolescents	>45	>45
	Low-density lipoprotein (mg/dL)	Adults	<130	<130
		Children and adolescents	<110	<110
	Cholesterol/high-density lipoprotein ratio		<4.5	<4.5
Normal carbohydrate metabolism	Serum glucose (mg/dL)		75 to 110	75 to 110
	Hemoglobin A1c (%)		≤6	≤6
Folate (ng/mL)	Serum folate		3.6 to 20	3.6 to 20

ABNORMALITIES

ABNORMALITIES

NUTRITION

Obesity

Excessive proportion of total body fat

Pathophysiology

- Genetic, behavioral, and environmental factors contribute to the development of obesity.
- Excess body fat develops as a result of energy imbalance of caloric intake and energy expenditure (physical activity).
- Disproportionately affects some racial groups (e.g., blacks) and those of low socioeconomic status
- Body fat, especially visceral fat, increases the risk for numerous health problems including type 2 diabetes, cardiovascular disease, dyslipidemia, and cancer.
- Medications (e.g., steroids) and certain disease processes (e.g., Cushing disease and polycystic ovarian syndrome) may cause weight gain and contribute to obesity.

Subjective Data

- Weight gain; increase in daily caloric intake and high-fat foods
- Decrease in physical activity
- Medications
- Recent life change or stressors
- Obesity-related symptoms or conditions include snoring and sleep apnea, shortness of breath, headaches, musculoskeletal symptoms, depression, irregular menses, polyuria, and polydipsia.

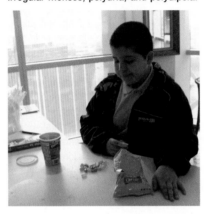

Objective Data

- Excess fat tissue generally located in breasts, buttocks, and thighs
- May have acanthosis nigricans (see Fig. 8-57) and pale striae
- Physical exam findings of obesity-related conditions can be found in Table 7-8.
- Characteristic features of genetic disorders should be assessed (e.g., Prader-Willi syndrome).
- Adult classification of BMI: overweight 25 to 29.9; obesity 30 to 39.9; extreme obesity >40
- Children and adolescents 2 to 18 years old: obesity is a BMI ≥95th percentile for age and gender or BMI >30; overweight is a BMI ≥85th percentile but less than 95th percentile for age and gender or BMI 25 to 29.9 (Fig. 7-5)
- See Table 7-10 for cholesterol and LDL cutoffs in children and adolescents.

FIGURE 7-5 Childhood obesity has become a major public health problem in the United States. (From Hockenberry and Wilson, 2009.)

Table 7-8	Physical Examination Findings in Obesity Assessment and Possible Causes	
System	**Findings**	**Possible Explanations**
Anthropometric features	High BMI percentile	Overweight or obesity
	Short stature	Underlying endocrine or genetic condition
Vital signs	Elevated blood pressure	Hypertension if systolic blood pressure ≥140 or diastolic blood pressure ≥90 on ≥3 occasions; for children and adolescents systolic or diastolic blood pressure ≥95th percentile for age, gender, and height percentile on ≥3 occasions
Skin	Acanthosis nigricans	Common in obese children, especially when skin is dark; increased risk of insulin resistance
	Excessive acne, hirsutism	Polycystic ovary syndrome
	Irritation, inflammation	Consequence of severe obesity
	Violaceous striae	Cushing syndrome
Eyes	Papilledema, cranial nerve VI paralysis	Pseudotumor cerebri
Throat	Tonsillar hypertrophy	Obstructive sleep apnea
Neck	Goiter	Hypothyroidism
Chest	Wheezing	Asthma (may explain or contribute to exercise intolerance)
Abdomen	Tenderness	Gastroesophageal reflux disorder, gallbladder disease, NAFLD
	Hepatomegaly	NAFLD
Reproductive system	Tanner stage	Premature puberty in <7-yr-old white girls, <6-yr-old black girls, and <9-yr-old boys
	Apparent micropenis	May be normal penis that is buried in fat
	Undescended testes	Prader-Willi syndrome
Extremities	Abnormal gait, limited hip range of motion	Slipped capital femoral epiphysis
	Bowing of tibia	Blount disease
	Small hands and feet, polydactyly	Some genetic syndromes

From Barlow et al, 2007.
NAFLD, Nonalcoholic fatty liver disease, a condition that is usually without signs.

Table 7-9	Comparison of Laboratory Test Results for Anemias				
Test	Normal Value	Iron Deficiency Anemia	Folic Acid Deficiency Anemia	Vitamin B$_{12}$ Deficiency Anemia
Hemoglobin, g/dL	Men: 14 to 16 Women: 12 to 14	Decreased	Decreased	Decreased
Hematocrit, %	Men: 40 to 54 Women: 37 to 47	Decreased	Decreased	Decreased
MCV, fL	82 to 92	Decreased	Increased	Increased
MCH, pg/cell	27 to 31	Decreased	Increased	Increased
MCHC, %	32 to 36	Decreased	Normal	Normal
Serum iron, mcg/dL	60 to 180	Decreased	Increased	Increased
TIBC, mcg/dL	250 to 450	Increased	Normal	Normal
Transferrin saturation, %	20 to 55	Decreased	Normal	Normal

MCH, Mean corpuscular hemoglobin; *MCHC,* mean corpuscular hemoglobin concentration; *MCV,* mean corpuscular volume; *TIBC,* total iron binding capacity.

Table 7-10	Cutoffs for Total and LDL Cholesterol Levels in Children and Adolescents				
Category	Total Cholesterol	LDL Cholesterol	Non-HDL Cholesterol	Triglycerides 0 to 9 Years	Triglycerides 10 to 19 Years
Acceptable (mg/dL)	<170	<110	<120	<75	<90
Borderline-High (mg/dL)	170 to 199	110 to 129	120 to 144	75 to 99	90 to 129
High (mg/dL)	≥200	≥130	≥145	≥100	≥130

Modified from Expert Panel on Integrated Guidelines for Cardiovascular Health and Risk Reduction in Children and Adolescents, 2011.

Anorexia Nervosa

Eating disorder classified by the *Diagnostic and Statistical Manual of Mental Disorders (DSM-IV)* as a psychiatric disease, characterized by low body weight and body image distortion

Pathophysiology
- Cause unknown, but genetic, environmental, and sociocultural factors likely to contribute to development of anorexia
- Adolescent and young adult women, usually from middle and upper class families, most commonly affected; also occurs in adolescent boys and men
- Two types: restricting (food intake is voluntarily limited) and purging (patients engage in purging after eating)

Subjective Data
- May report preoccupation with weight, excessive exercise and unusual eating habits including voluntary starvation, purging, vomiting, and weight control measures such as diet pills, use of laxatives, and diuretics
- May report being overweight as a child and unhappiness with current weight as well as poor body image
- Symptoms may include fatigue, dizziness, low energy, amenorrhea, weight loss or gain, constipation, bloating, abdominal discomfort, heartburn, intolerance to cold, palpitations, depression or irritability, decreased libido, and interrupted sleep

Objective Data
- Physical examination findings may include dry skin, lanugo hair, brittle nails, bradycardia, hypothermia, orthostatic hypotension, and loss of muscle mass and subcutaneous fat.
- May have hypoglycemia, elevated liver enzymes, and thyroid hormone abnormalities
- *DSM-IV* criteria for diagnosis includes refusal to maintain body weight at or above a minimally normal weight for age and height (failure to maintain weight at 85% of ideal body weight); intense fear of gaining weight; disturbance in self-perception of body weight; and amenorrhea in females
- BMI ≤17.5 also characteristic

Bulimia Nervosa

Eating disorder classified by the *DSM-IV* as psychiatric disease

Pathophysiology

- Cause unknown, but genetic, environmental, and sociocultural factors likely to contribute to the development of bulimia
- Adolescent and young adult women most commonly affected
- Two types are purging and nonpurging type episodes followed by fasting or excessive exercising.

Subjective Data

- Binge-eating episodes on average 2 times a week, usually high-calorie or high-carbohydrate foods in purging type; followed by purging behaviors (e.g., vomiting, laxatives, diuretics)
- Bloating, fullness, lethargy, abdominal pain, heartburn, and sore throat

Objective Data

- Body weight can be normal, underweight or overweight.
- Knuckle calluses, dental enamel erosion, salivary gland enlargement
- Metabolic alkalosis from vomiting, hypokalemia from laxative or diuretic use, and elevated salivary amylase
- *DSM-IV* criteria for diagnosis includes recurrent binge-eating episodes over a discrete period of time and lack of control over eating; recurrent compensatory behaviors to prevent weight gain (e.g., self-induced vomiting); and behaviors occur on average twice per week for 3 months.

Anemia

Lower than normal number of circulating red blood cells

Pathophysiology

- Iron deficiency is most common cause
- Other causes: nutrient deficiency states including vitamin B_{12} and folate (see Table 7-9 to determine type of anemia based on laboratory values)

Subjective Data

- Based on degree of anemia, symptoms may include skin pallor, weakness, fatigue, lack of energy, headaches, dizziness, sensitivity to cold, paresthesia, and loss of appetite
- Severe anemia: palpitations and shortness of breath
- Behavioral and cognitive manifestations include pica (consumption of nonfood items) and decreased intellectual functioning

Objective Data

- Frequently no physical findings
- May see skin and conjunctival pallor, cheilosis, angular stomatitis, glossitis, and concave fingernails with longitudinal ridging (koilonychia)
- Severe anemia: vital sign changes, including tachycardia and hypotension
- Diagnosis made when hemoglobin and hematocrit concentrations are lower than normal, based on age and gender

---

Staying Well

Therapeutic Lifestyle Changes

The Third Report of the Expert Panel on Detection, Evaluation, and Treatment of High Blood Cholesterol in Adults (Adult Treatment Panel III) from the National Cholesterol Education Program recommends a multifaceted lifestyle approach to reduce risk for coronary heart disease (CHD). This approach is designated *therapeutic lifestyle changes* (TLCs). Its essential features are the following:

- Reduced intake of saturated fats (<7% of total calories) and cholesterol (<200 mg per day) (see nutrient composition of the TLC Diet, below)
- Therapeutic options for enhancing LDL lowering such as plant stanols/sterols (2 g/day) and increased viscous (soluble) fiber (10 to 25 g/day)
- Weight reduction
- Increased physical activity

Nutrient Composition of the TLC Diet

Nutrient	Recommended Intake
Saturated fat*	Less than 7% of total calories
Polyunsaturated fat	Up to 10% of total calories
Monounsaturated fat	Up to 20% of total calories
Total fat	25% to 35% of total calories
Carbohydrate†	50% to 60% of total calories
Fiber	20 to 30 g/day
Protein	Approximately 15% of total calories
Cholesterol	Less than 200 mg/day
Total calories (energy)‡	Balance energy intake and expenditure to maintain desirable body weight/prevent weight gain

Trans-fatty acids are another LDL-raising fat that should be kept at a low intake.
†Carbohydrate should be derived predominantly from foods rich in complex carbohydrates, including grains, especially whole grains, fruits, and vegetables.
‡Daily energy expenditure should include at least moderate physical activity (contributing approximately 200 kcal per day).
From U.S. Department of Health and Human Services. *Your guide to lowering your cholesterol with TLC.* December 2005 found at www.nhlbi.nih.gov/health/public/heart/chol/chol_tlc.pdf.

ABNORMALITIES

Staying Well

Dietary Guidelines for Americans 2010

Dietary Guidelines for Americans is published jointly every 5 years by the Department of Health and Human Services (HHS) and the U.S. Department of Agriculture (USDA). The guidelines provide updated evidence-based recommendations to help individuals attain and maintain a healthy weight and reduce risk for major chronic diseases through diet and physical activity. The Guidelines take into account customs and cultural traditions of a diverse U.S. population, as well as the nearly 15% of Americans experiencing food insecurity. In prior years, the recommendations have targeted healthy Americans older than 2 years. Recognizing the significant impact of poor diet and physical inactivity on the obesity epidemic in the United States, the 2010 Guidelines are also intended for individuals at increased risk of chronic disease. The two main concepts include the importance of "maintaining calorie balance over time to achieve and sustain a healthy weight" and a "focus on consuming nutrient-dense foods and beverages." The Guidelines are used to develop educational materials for the public as well as for policymakers responsible for developing and implementing nutrition-related programs. The full document is available at www.cnpp.usda.gov/DGAs2010-PolicyDocument.htm.

CHAPTER 8

Skin, Hair, and Nails

$\mathcal{S}$kin provides an elastic, rugged, self-regenerating, protective covering for the body. In addition, the skin and its appendages are our primary physical presentation to the world. Examination of the skin, hair, and nails is performed as part of a comprehensive examination, and as part of a focused examination when the patient presents with a particular concern. The skin, hair, and nails can provide external clues to systemic disease that may not otherwise be apparent.

evolve *http://evolve.elsevier.com/Seidel*
- Physical Exam Key Points
- NCLEX Review Questions
- Interactive Activities
- Animations
- Videos
- Student Checklist

Physical Examination Preview

Here is a preview of the steps involved in conducting a physical examination of the skin, hair, and nails. ⓔ These procedures are explained in detail in this chapter and are available on Evolve in printable formats.

Skin, Hair, and Nails

Skin
1. Perform overall inspection of entire skin surface (p. 119). During evaluation of each organ system, evaluate the overlying skin for the following characteristics:
   - Color
   - Uniformity
   - Thickness
   - Symmetry
   - Hygiene
   - Lesions
   - Odors
2. Palpate skin surfaces for the following (p. 124):
   - Moisture
   - Temperature
   - Texture
   - Turgor (fullness or tension produced by the fluid content of the cells and tissue)
   - Mobility

Hair
1. Inspect hair for the following (p. 133):
   - Color
   - Distribution
   - Quantity
2. Palpate hair for texture (p. 133)

ANATOMY AND PHYSIOLOGY

The skin is a stratified structure composed of several functionally related layers. Figure 8-1 shows the main structural components and their approximate spatial relationships. The anatomy of the skin varies somewhat from one part of the body to another.

Skin structure and physiologic processes perform the following integral functions:
- Protect against microbial and foreign substance invasion and minor physical trauma
- Restrict body fluid loss by providing a mechanical barrier

Nails
1. Inspect for the following (p. 134):
   - Pigmentation of nails and beds
   - Length
   - Symmetry
   - Ridging, beading, pitting, peeling
2. Inspect and palpate proximal and lateral nail folds for the following (p. 135):
   - Redness
   - Swelling
   - Pain
   - Exudate
   - Warts, cysts, tumors
3. Palpate nail plate for the following (p. 135):
   - Texture
   - Firmness
   - Thickness
   - Uniformity
   - Adherence to nail bed
4. Measure nail base angle (p. 135)

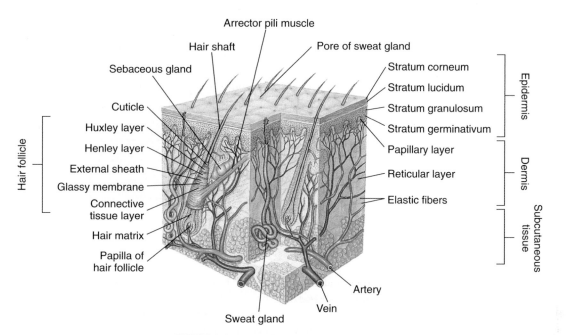

FIGURE 8-1 Anatomic structures of the skin.

- Regulate body temperature through radiation, conduction, convection, and evaporation
- Provide sensory perception via free nerve endings and specialized receptors
- Produce vitamin D from precursors in the skin
- Contribute to blood pressure regulation through constriction of skin blood vessels
- Repair surface wounds by exaggerating the normal process of cell replacement
- Excrete sweat, urea, and lactic acid
- Express emotions

Epidermis

The epidermis, the outermost portion of the skin, consists of two major layers: the stratum corneum, which protects the body against harmful environmental substances and restricts water loss, and the cellular stratum, in which the keratin cells are synthesized. The basement membrane lies beneath the cellular stratum and connects the epidermis to the dermis. The epidermis is avascular and depends on the underlying dermis for its nutrition.

The stratum corneum consists of closely packed, dead squamous cells that contain the waterproofing protein keratin; these form the protective barrier of the skin. These keratin cells are formed in the deepest sublayer of the cellular stratum, the stratum germinativum. The keratinocytes mature as they make their way to the surface through the stratum spinosum and stratum granulosum to replace the cells in the stratum corneum. The stratum germinativum also contains melanocytes, the cells that synthesize melanin, which gives the skin its color. An additional sublayer of the cellular stratum, the stratum lucidum, is present only in the thicker skin of the palms and soles and lies just below the stratum corneum.

Dermis

The dermis is the richly vascular connective tissue layer of the skin that supports and separates the epidermis from the cutaneous adipose tissue. Upward projecting papillae penetrate the epidermis and provide nourishment for the living epidermal cells. Elastin, collagen, and reticulum fibers provide resilience, strength, and stability. Sensory nerve fibers located in the dermis form a complex network to provide sensations of pain, touch, and temperature. The dermis also contains autonomic motor nerves that innervate blood vessels, glands, and the arrectores pilorum muscles.

Hypodermis

The dermis is connected to underlying organs by the hypodermis, a subcutaneous layer that consists of loose connective tissue filled with fatty cells. This adipose layer generates heat and provides insulation, shock absorption, and a reserve of calories.

Appendages

The epidermis invaginates into the dermis at various points and forms the following appendages: eccrine sweat glands, apocrine sweat glands, sebaceous glands, hair, and nails.

The eccrine sweat glands open directly onto the surface of the skin and regulate body temperature through water secretion. The glands are distributed throughout the body except at the lip margins, eardrums, nail beds, inner surface of the prepuce, and glans penis.

The apocrine glands are specialized structures found only in the axillae, nipples, areolae, anogenital area, eyelids, and external ears. These glands are larger and located more deeply than the eccrine glands. In response to emotional stimuli, the glands

FIGURE 8-2 Anatomic structures of the nail. *(Modified from Thompson et al, 1997.)*

secrete a white fluid containing protein, carbohydrate, and other substances. Secretions from these glands are odorless; body odor is produced by bacterial decomposition of apocrine sweat.

The sebaceous glands secrete sebum, a lipid-rich substance that keeps the skin and hair from drying out. Secretory activity, which is stimulated by sex hormones (primarily testosterone), varies according to hormonal levels throughout the life span.

Hair consists of a root, a shaft, and a follicle (i.e., the root and its covering). The papilla, a loop of capillaries at the base of the follicle, supplies nourishment for growth. Melanocytes in the shaft provide its color. Adults have both vellus and terminal hair. Vellus hair is short, fine, soft, and nonpigmented. Terminal hair is coarser, longer, thicker, and usually pigmented. Each hair goes through cyclic changes: anagen (growth), catagen (atrophy), and telogen (rest), after which the hair is shed. Males and females have about the same number of hair follicles that are stimulated to differential growth by hormones.

The nails are epidermal cells converted to hard plates of keratin. The highly vascular nail bed lies beneath the plate, giving the nail its pink color. The white crescent-shaped area extending beyond the proximal nail fold marks the end of the nail matrix, the site of nail growth. The stratum corneum layer of skin covering the nail root is the cuticle, or eponychium, which pushes up and over the lower part of the nail body. The paronychium is the soft tissue surrounding the nail border. Figure 8-2 shows the structures of the nail.

Infants and Children

The skin of infants and children appears smoother than that of adults, partly because of the relative absence of coarse terminal hair and partly because the skin has not been subjected to years of exposure to the elements. Desquamation of the stratum corneum may be present at birth or very shortly after. The degree of desquamation varies from mild flakiness to shedding of large sheets of cornified epidermis. Postterm infants often have cracked, peeling skin. Vernix caseosa, a mixture of sebum and cornified epidermis, covers the infant's body at birth. The subcutaneous fat layer is poorly developed in newborns, predisposing them to hypothermia. The newborn's body, particularly the shoulders and back, can be covered with fine, silky hair called lanugo. More commonly seen in preterm infants, this hair is shed within 10 to 14 days. Some newborns are bald, whereas others have a large amount of head hair. Either way, most of the hair is shed by about 2 to 3 months of age, to be replaced by more permanent hair with a new texture and often a different color.

The eccrine sweat glands begin to function after the first month of life. Apocrine function has not yet begun, giving the skin a less oily texture and resulting in characteristic inoffensive perspiration.

Adolescents

During adolescence, the apocrine glands enlarge and become active, causing increased axillary sweating and sometimes body odor. Sebaceous glands increase sebum production in response to increased hormone levels, primarily androgen, giving the skin an oily appearance and predisposing the individual to acne.

Coarse terminal hair appears in the axillae and pubic areas of both female and male adolescents and on the face of males. Hair production is one response to changing androgen levels. Refer to Chapter 6 for a more thorough discussion of maturational changes during adolescence.

Pregnant Women

Increased blood flow to the skin, especially to the hands and feet, results from peripheral vasodilation and increased numbers of capillaries. Acceleration of sweat and sebaceous gland activity occurs. Both processes assist in dissipating the excess heat caused by increased metabolism during pregnancy. Vascular spiders and hemangiomas that are present may increase in size.

The skin thickens, and fat is deposited in the subdermal layers. Because of increased fragility of connective tissues, separation may occur with stretching. Most pregnant women have some degree of increased pigmentation that is seen on the face, nipples, areolae, axillae, vulva, perianal skin, and umbilicus. During pregnancy, some nevi may grow and new nevi may appear.

Older Adults

Sebaceous and sweat gland activity decreases in older adults, and as a result the skin becomes drier with less perspiration produced. The epidermis begins to thin and flatten, taking on the look of parchment as the vascularity of the dermis decreases.

Epidermal permeability is increased, reducing the efficiency of the barrier function of the stratum corneum.

The dermis becomes less elastic, loses collagen and elastic fibers, and shrinks, causing the epidermis to fold and assume a wrinkled appearance. A lifetime of exposure to the sun also predisposes the skin to wrinkling. Whites have an earlier onset and greater skin wrinkling and sagging signs than others (Rawlings, 2006).

Subcutaneous tissue also decreases, particularly in the extremities, giving joints and bony prominences a sharp, angular appearance. The hollows in the thoracic, axillary, and supraclavicular regions deepen.

Gray hair results from a decrease in the number of functioning melanocytes. Axillary and pubic hair production declines because of reduced hormonal functioning. The density and rate of scalp hair growth (anagen phase) decline with age. The size of hair follicles also changes, and terminal scalp hair progressively transitions into vellus hair, causing age-associated baldness in both men and women. The opposite transition, from vellus to terminal, occurs in the hair of the nares and on the tragus of men's ears. Women produce increased coarse facial hair because of higher androgen-estrogen ratios. Both genders experience overall loss of hair from the trunk and extremities. Peripheral extremity hair loss may also occur when peripheral vascular disease is present.

Nail growth slows because of decreased peripheral circulation. The nails, particularly the toenails, become thicker, brittle, hard, and yellowish. They develop longitudinal ridges and are prone to splitting into layers.

REVIEW OF RELATED HISTORY

For each of the symptoms or conditions discussed in this section, targeted topics to include in the history of the present illness are listed. Responses to questions about these topics provide clues for focusing the physical examination and developing an appropriate diagnostic evaluation. Questions regarding medication use (prescription and over the counter preparations) as well as complementary and alternative therapies are relevant for each.

History of Present Illness

- Skin
  - Changes in skin: dryness, pruritus, sores, rashes, lumps, color, texture, odor, amount of perspiration; changes in wart or mole; lesion that does not heal or is chronically irritated (see Risk Factors boxes)
  - Temporal sequence: date of initial onset; time sequence of occurrence and development; sudden or gradual onset; date of recurrence, if any
  - Symptoms: itching, pain, exudate, bleeding, color changes, seasonal or climate variations
  - Location: skinfolds, extensor or flexor surfaces, localized or generalized
  - Associated symptoms: presence of systemic disease or fever, relationship to stress or leisure activities

- Recent exposure to environmental or occupational toxins or chemicals, new skin or personal care products, new household cleaning products
- Recent exposure to persons with similar skin condition
- Apparent cause of problem, patient's perception of cause
- Travel history: where, when, length of stay, exposure to diseases, contact with travelers
- What the patient has been doing for the problem, response to treatment, what makes the condition worse or better
- How the patient is adjusting to the problem
- Medications: antibiotics, any new medications, topical preparations to treat—steroids, antifungals

---

Risk Factors

Melanoma

- Previous personal history of melanoma
- Family history of melanoma (first-degree relative)
- Moles
  - Dysplastic or atypical nevi
  - Numerous nondysplastic nevi
  - Large congenital nevus (>15 cm)
- Exposure to sunlight or ultraviolet radiation (UVA and UVB)
  - Severe blistering sunburns as child or teenager
  - Indoor tanning device usage
  - Geographic exposure (people who live in areas that get large amounts of UV radiation from the sun)
- Immune suppression
- Fair skin, light eyes
- Sun sensitivity, relative inability to tan

From Abeloff et al, 2008; American Cancer Society, 2012; Habif, 2010; National Cancer Institute, 2012.

You can use the National Cancer Institute's Melanoma Risk Assessment Tool to estimate a person's absolute risk of developing invasive melanoma at: www.cancer.gov/melanomarisktool.

Risk Factors

Basal and Squamous Cell Cancer

- Age (older than 50 years)
- Exposure to sunlight or ultraviolet radiation (UVA and UVB)
  - Indoor tanning device usage
  - Blistering sunburns as a child
  - Chronic and cumulative exposure – squamous cell carcinoma
  - Intermittent exposure – basal cell carcinoma
- Fair, freckled, ruddy complexion
- Light-colored hair or eyes
- Tendency to sunburn easily
- Geographic location: near equator or at high altitudes
- Exposure to arsenic, creosote, coal tar, and/or petroleum products
- Overexposure to radium, radioisotopes, or x-rays
- Repeated trauma or irritation to skin
- Precancerous dermatoses

From Abeloff et al, 2008; American Cancer Society, 2012; Habif, 2010.

+ Hair
  + Changes in hair: loss or growth, distribution, texture, color
  + Occurrence: sudden or gradual onset, symmetric or asymmetric pattern, recurrence
  + Associated symptoms: pain, itching, lesions, presence of systemic disease or high fever, recent stress, hair-pulling
  + Exposure to drugs, environmental or occupational toxins or chemicals, commercial hair care chemicals
  + Nutrition: dietary changes, dieting
  + What the patient has been doing for the problem, response to treatment, what makes the problem worse or better
  + How the patient is adjusting to the problem
  + Medications: drugs or preparations for hair loss (minoxidil, finesteride, dihydrotestosterone [DHT] inhibitors)
+ Nails
  + Changes in nails: splitting, breaking, discoloration, ridging, thickening, markings, separation from nail bed
  + Recent history: systemic illness, high fever, trauma, stress
  + Associated symptoms: pain, swelling, exudate
  + Temporal sequence: sudden or gradual onset, relationship to injury of nail or finger
  + Recent exposure to drugs, environmental or occupational toxins or chemicals; frequent immersion in water
  + What the patient has been doing for the problem, response to treatment, what makes the problem worse or better
  + Medications: chemotherapy (taxanes, anthracyclines), psoralens, retinoids, tetracyclines, antimalarials

Past Medical History

+ Skin
  + Previous skin problems: sensitivities, allergic skin reactions, allergic skin disorders (e.g., infantile eczema), lesions, treatment
  + Tolerance to sunlight (Box 8-1)
  + Diminished or heightened sensitivity to touch
  + Cardiac, respiratory, liver, endocrine, or other systemic diseases
+ Hair
  + Previous hair problems: loss, thinning, unusual growth or distribution, brittleness, breakage, treatment

Box 8-1   Skin Type

People burn or tan depending on their skin type, the time of year, and how long they are exposed to UV rays. The six types of skin, based on how likely it is to tan or burn, are:
• I: Always burns, never tans, sensitive to UV exposure
• II: Burns easily, tans minimally
• III: Burns moderately, tans gradually to light brown
• IV: Burns minimally, always tans well to moderately brown
• V: Rarely burns, tans profusely to dark
• VI: Never burns, deeply pigmented, least sensitive
   Although everyone's skin can be damaged by UV exposure, people with skin types I and II are at the highest risk.

From Centers for Disease Control (2013): *Skin cancer risk factors.* Retrieved from: http://www.cdc.gov/cancer/skin/basic_info/risk_factors.htm

+ Systemic problems: thyroid disorder, rheumatologic disease, any severe illness, malnutrition, associated skin disorder
+ Nails
  + Previous nail problems: injury; bacterial, fungal, or viral infection
  + Systemic problems: associated skin disorder; congenital anomalies; respiratory, cardiac, endocrine, hematologic, or other systemic disease

Family History

+ Current or past dermatologic diseases or disorders in family members; melanoma; psoriasis; allergic skin disorders; infestations; bacterial, fungal, or viral infections
+ Allergic hereditary diseases such as asthma or hay fever
+ Familial hair loss or pigmentation patterns

Personal and Social History

+ Skin care habits: cleansing routine; soaps, oils, lotions, or local applications used; cosmetics; home remedies or preparations used; sun exposure patterns and history; sunburn history; use of sunscreen agents; recent changes in skin care habits (see Clinical Pearl, "Sunscreen")
+ Skin self-examination (Box 8-2)

Box 8-2   Patient Instructions for Skin Self-Examination

• Always use a good light, positioned to minimize distracting glare. Look for a new growth or any skin change.
• Be aware of the locations and appearance of moles and birthmarks.
• Examine your back and other hard-to-see areas of the body using full-length and handheld mirrors. Ask a friend or relative to help inspect those areas that are difficult to see, such as the scalp and back.
• Begin with your face and scalp using one or more mirrors. Proceed downward, focusing on neck, chest, and torso. Women, check under breasts. With back to the mirror, use hand mirror to inspect back of neck, shoulders, upper arms, back, buttocks, legs. Concentrate especially on areas where dysplastic nevi (those with unexpected changes) are most common—the shoulders and back; and areas where ordinary moles are rarely found—the scalp, breast, and buttocks. Check hands, including nails. In a full-length mirror, examine elbows, arms, underarms. Sitting down, check legs and feet, including soles, heels, nails, and between the toes. Use a hand mirror to examine genitals. See rather than feel any early signs of a mole change. Compare photographs of your moles (if you have them) with the appearance of those same moles on self-examination. Monitor change in size by measuring. It can be done simply with a small ruler or even by comparing the moles to the size of your thumb or fingernail.
• Consult your health care provider promptly if any pigmented skin spots look like melanoma, if new moles have appeared, or if any existing moles have changed. See also the ABCDE changes in moles (Melanoma, in Abnormalities).

- Hair care habits: cleansing routine, shampoos and rinses used, coloring preparations used, permanents, recent changes in hair care habits
- Nail care habits: any difficulty in clipping or trimming nails, instruments used; biting nails; use of artificial nail overlays
- Exposure to environmental or occupational hazards: dyes, chemicals, plants, toxic substances, frequent immersion of hands in water, frequent sun exposure
- Recent psychologic or physiologic stress
- Use of alcohol, tobacco
- Sexual history: sexually transmitted infections (syphilis, gonorrhea, human immunodeficiency virus [HIV])
- Use of recreational drugs

Clinical Pearl

Sunscreen

Surprise! Do you ask if your patients use sunscreen? Keep this in mind when they respond: Those who use sunscreen with a protection factor of 30 or higher are still at risk for significant sunburn. Why? Those who are users do not use enough, they think they are protected, and they stay out in the noonday sun too long. It is necessary to apply sunscreen generously and frequently. Apply it 15 to 20 minutes before exposure. Reapply after swimming, and reapply after 2 to 3 hours of exposure.

❀ Infants

- Feeding history: breast or formula, type of formula, what foods introduced and when (see Clinical Pearl, "Carotenemia")
- Diaper history: type of diapers used, skin cleansing routines, and methods of cleaning
- Types of clothing and washing practices: soaps and detergents used, new blanket or clothing
- Bathing practices: types of soap, oils, or lotions used
- Dress habits: amount and type of clothing in relation to environmental temperature
- Temperature and humidity of the home environment: air conditioning, heating system (drying or humidified)
- Rubbing head against mattress, rug, furniture, wall

Clinical Pearl

Carotenemia

Carotenemia, common in infants who have started eating baby foods, is yellow pigmentation of the skin and increased beta-carotene levels in the blood. Carotenemia does not cause orange discoloration of the sclerae, and thus is usually easy to distinguish from jaundice. In most cases, the condition follows increased consumption of carotene-rich foods, such as carrots, squash, and sweet potatoes.

❀ Children and Adolescents

- Eating habits and types of food
- Food allergies

- Exposure to infectious diseases at day care, school: impetigo; viruses that produce skin rashes; measles, mumps, rubella in unvaccinated children
- Allergic disorders: eczema, urticaria, pruritus, hay fever, asthma, other chronic respiratory disorders
- Pets or animal exposure
- Outdoor exposures such as play areas, hiking, camping, picnics, gardening
- Skin injury history: frequency of falls, cuts, abrasions; repeated history of unexplained injuries
- Chronic hair-pulling or manipulation
- Nail biting

❀ Pregnant Women

- Weeks of gestation or postpartum
- Hygiene practices
- Exposure to irritants
- Presence of skin problems before pregnancy (e.g., acne may worsen)
- Effects of pregnancy on preexisting conditions (e.g., psoriasis may remit; condylomata acuminata commonly become larger and more numerous)

❀ Older Adults

- Increased or decreased sensation to touch or to the environment
- Generalized chronic itching; exposure to skin irritants, detergents, lotions with high alcohol content, woolen clothing, humidity of environment
- Susceptibility to skin infections
- Healing response: delayed or interrupted
- Frequent falls resulting in multiple cuts or bruises
- Risk for pressure ulcers secondary to immobilization or nonambulatory status
- History of diabetes mellitus or peripheral vascular disease
- Hair loss history: gradual versus sudden onset, loss pattern (symmetric or asymmetric)

EXAMINATION AND FINDINGS

Equipment

- Centimeter ruler (flexible, clear)
- Flashlight with transilluminator
- Handheld magnifying lens or dermatoscope
- Wood's lamp (to view fluorescing, hypopigmented or hyperpigmented lesions)

Skin

Use inspection and palpation to examine the skin. The most important tools are your own eyes and powers of observation. Sometimes, when gross inspection leaves you uncertain, a handheld magnifying glass or dermatoscope may help.

Inspection

Adequate lighting is essential. Daylight provides the best illumination for determining color variations, particularly jaundice. If daylight is unavailable or insufficient, supplement it with overhead fluorescent lighting. Inadequate lighting can result in inadequate assessment. Tangential lighting is helpful in assessing contour.

Although the skin is commonly observed as each part of the body is examined, it is important to make a brief but careful overall visual sweep of the entire body. This "bird's-eye view" gives a good idea of the distribution and extent of any lesions. It also allows you to observe skin symmetry, to detect differences between body areas, and to compare sun-exposed to non–sun-exposed areas. You can also be alert for special conditions that require attention as the examination progresses (Box 8-3).

Adequate exposure of the skin is necessary. It is essential to remove clothing and to fully remove drapes or coverings as each section of the body is examined. Make sure that the room temperature is comfortable. Look carefully at areas not usually exposed, such as the axillae, buttocks, perineum, backs of thighs, and inner upper thighs. Remove shoes and socks to look at the feet. Pay careful attention to intertriginous surfaces (areas where two skin surfaces may touch, e.g., axillae and groin), especially in infants, older adults and bedridden patients. As you complete the examination for each area, re-drape or cover the patient. Begin by inspecting the skin and mucous membranes (especially oral) for color and uniform appearance, thickness, symmetry, hygiene, and the presence of any lesions.

Skin thickness varies over the body, with the thinnest skin on the eyelids and the thickest at areas of pressure or rubbing, most notably the soles, palms, and elbows. Note calluses on the hands or feet. Look for corns on pressure points. Corns are flat or slightly elevated, circumscribed, painful lesions with a smooth, hard surface. "Soft" corns are caused by the pressure of a bony prominence against softer tissue; these appear as whitish thickenings, commonly between the fourth and fifth toes. "Hard" corns are sharply delineated and have a conical appearance; they occur most often over bony prominences where pressure is exerted, such as from shoes pressing on the interphalangeal joints of the toes (Fig. 8-3). A superficial area of hyperkeratosis is called a callus. Calluses usually occur on the weight-bearing areas of the feet and on the palmar surface of the hands. Calluses are less well demarcated than corns and are usually not tender (Fig. 8-4).

The range of expected skin color varies from dark brown to light tan with pink or yellow overtones. Although color should

FIGURE 8-3 Corn. *(From White, 1994.)*

Box 8-3   Cutaneous Manifestations of Traditional Health Practices

The use of certain traditional health practices by various cultural groups can produce cutaneous manifestations that could be wrongly confused with disease or physical abuse. Two such practices are "coining" and "cupping" as used by some Asian subcultures. In coining, a coin dipped in mentholated oil is vigorously rubbed across the skin in a prescribed manner, causing a mild dermabrasion. This practice is believed to release excess force from the body and hence restore balance. In cupping, a series of small, heated glasses are placed on the skin, forming a suction that leaves a red or purpuric circular mark, drawing out the bad force. The skin markings may alarm the health care provider who is unaware of such practices. The lesson: In the history, ask about home remedies or practices.

FIGURE 8-4 Calluses are common on both the sole (heels and metatarsal heads) and the dorsum of the foot (especially in women). *(From Lawrence and Cox, 1993.)*

assume an overall uniformity, there may be sun-darkened areas and darker skin around knees and elbows. Knuckles may be darker in dark-skinned patients. Callused areas may appear yellow. Vascular flush areas (e.g., cheeks, neck, upper chest, and genital area) may appear pink or red, especially with anxiety or excitement. Be aware that skin color may be masked by cosmetics and tanning agents. Look for localized areas of discoloration (see Physical Variations, "Pigmentary Demarcation Lines").

Nevi (moles) occur in forms that vary in size and degree of pigmentation (see Physical Variations, "Nevi"). Nevi are present on most persons regardless of skin color, and may occur anywhere on the body. They may be flat, slightly raised,

Physical Variations

Pigmentary Demarcation Lines

Individuals with dark skin may show pigmentary demarcation lines. These lines, a normal variation, mark the border between deeply pigmented skin and lighter pigmented skin. They are most commonly seen on the arms, legs, chest, and back and have been reported most often in black and Japanese populations. Accentuation of preexisting lines or appearance of new lines may occur during pregnancy.

From Amichai and Grunwald, 2007; James et al, 1984; James et al, 1987; Nakama et al, 2009; Peck et al, 2011.

dome-shaped, smooth, rough, or hairy. Their color ranges from pink, tan, gray, and shades of brown to black. Table 8-1 describes the features and occurrence of various types of pigmented nevi.

Physical Variations

Nevi

Nevi occur more often in lighter-skinned than in darker-skinned individuals. Blacks have the fewest nevi, whites have the most, and Asians and Native Americans have intermediate numbers. There is a strong association between sun exposure and the number of nevi. They increase in number throughout infancy and childhood, with peak incidence in the fourth to fifth decades. Nevi diminish in number with advancing age.

Data from Gallagher et al, 1991; Habif, 2010; Rampen 1988; Rampen and de Wit, 1989.

Although most nevi are harmless, some may be dysplastic, precancerous, or cancerous. Table 8-2 describes differences in the features of normal and dysplastic moles. Dysplastic nevi tend to occur on the upper back in men and on the legs in women (see Box 8-4, "Dysplastic Mole or Melanoma?").

Several variations in skin color occur in almost all healthy adults and children, including nonpigmented striae (i.e., silver or pink "stretch marks" that occur during pregnancy or weight gain),

EXAMINATION AND FINDINGS

Video: Skin, Hair, and Nails: Assessing a Mole

Table 8-1	Features and Occurrence of Various Types of Pigmented Nevi		
Type	**Features**	**Occurrence**	**Comments**
Halo nevus	Sharp, oval, or circular; depigmented halo around mole; may undergo many morphologic changes; usually disappears and halo repigments (may take years)	Usually on back in young adult	Usually benign; biopsy indicated because same process can occur around melanoma
Intradermal nevus	Dome-shaped; raised; flesh to black color; may be pedunculated or hair bearing	Cells limited to dermis	No indication for removal other than cosmetic
Junction nevus	Flat or slightly elevated; dark brown	Nevus cells lining dermoepidermal junction	Should be removed if exposed to repeated trauma
Compound nevus	Slightly elevated brownish papule: indistinct border	Nevus cells in dermis and lining dermoepidermal junction	Should be removed if exposed to repeated trauma
Hairy nevus	May be present at birth; may cover large area; hair growth may occur after several years		Should be removed if changes occur

From Wilson and Giddens, 2005.

Table 8-2	Features of Normal and Dysplastic Moles	
Feature	**Normal Mole**	**Dysplastic Mole**
Color	Uniformly tan or brown; all moles on one person tend to look alike	Mixture of tan, brown, black, and red/pink; moles on one person often do not look alike
Shape	Round or oval with a clearly defined border that separates the mole from surrounding skin	Irregular borders may include notches; may fade into surrounding skin and include a flat portion level with skin
Surface	Begins as flat, smooth spot on skin; becomes raised; forms a smooth bump	May be smooth, slightly scaly, or have a rough, irregular, "pebbly" appearance
Size	Usually less than 6 mm (size of a pencil eraser)	Often larger than 6 mm and sometimes larger than 10 mm
Number	Typical adult has 10 to 40 moles scattered over the body	Many persons do not have increased number; however, persons severely affected may have more than 100 moles
Location	Usually above the waist on sun-exposed surfaces of the body; scalp, breast, and buttocks rarely have normal moles	May occur anywhere on the body, but most commonly on back; may also appear below the waist and on scalp, breast, and buttocks

Box 8-4 Dysplastic Mole or Melanoma?

Dysplastic nevi (atypical moles) occur predominantly on the trunk. They tend to be large, usually greater than 5 mm, with a flat component. The border is typically ill-defined. The shape can be round, oval, or irregular. The color is usually brown but can be mottled with dark brown, pink, and tan. Some individuals have only 1 to 5 moles; others have more than 100.

In melanoma, the border is more irregular. Lesions tend to be larger, often greater than 6 mm. Color variation within the lesion is characteristic, ranging from tan-brown, dark brown, or black to pink, red, gray, blue, or white.

Any lesion suggestive of a melanoma must be biopsied. Individuals with dysplastic moles are at increased risk for melanoma.

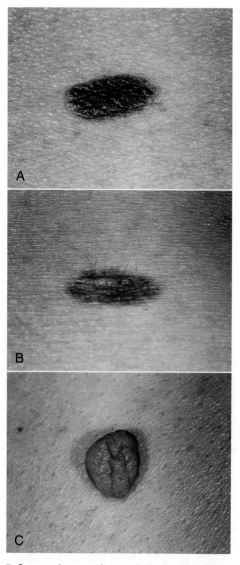

FIGURE 8-5 **Commonly occurring nevi. A,** Junction nevus. Color and shape of this black lesion are uniform. **B,** Compound nevus. Center is elevated and surrounding area is flat, retaining features of a junction nevus. **C,** Dermal nevus. Papillomatous with soft, flabby, wrinkled surface. *(From Habif, 2004.)*

FIGURE 8-6 **Vitiligo.** *(From Lemmi and Lemmi, 2009.)*

freckles in sun-exposed areas, some birthmarks, and some nevi (Fig. 8-5). Adult women will commonly have chloasma (also called melasma; see Fig. 8-34), areas of hyperpigmentation on the face and neck that are associated with pregnancy or the use of hormones. This condition is more noticeable in darker-skinned women. The absence of melanin produces patches of unpigmented skin or hair, such as with vitiligo (Fig. 8-6).

Color hues in dark-skinned persons are best seen in the sclera, conjunctiva, buccal mucosa, tongue, lips, nail beds, and palms. Be

Table 8-3 Cutaneous Color Changes

Color	Cause	Distribution	Select Conditions
Brown	Darkening of melanin pigment	Generalized Localized	Pituitary, adrenal, liver disease Nevi, neurofibromatosis
White	Absence of melanin	Generalized Localized	Albinism Vitiligo
Red (erythema)	Increased cutaneous blood flow Increased cutaneous blood flow Increased intravascular red blood cells	Localized Generalized Generalized	Inflammation Fever, viral exanthem, urticaria Polycythemia
Yellow	Increased bile pigmentation (jaundice) Increased carotene pigmentation	Generalized Generalized (except sclera)	Liver disease Hypothyroidism, increased intake of vegetables containing carotene
Blue	Increased unsaturated hemoglobin secondary to hypoxia	Lips, mouth, nail beds	Cardiovascular and pulmonary diseases

aware, however, that heavily callused palms in dark-skinned persons have an opaque yellow cast. Particular variations in skin color may be the result of physiologic pigment distribution. The palms and soles are lighter in color than the rest of the body. Hyperpigmented macules on the soles of the feet are common. Freckling of the buccal cavity, gums, and tongue is common. The sclera may appear yellowish brown (often described as "muddy") or may contain brownish pigment that looks like petechiae. A bluish hue of the lips and gums can be a normal finding in persons with dark skin. Some dark-skinned persons have very blue lips, giving a false impression of cyanosis.

Systemic disorders can produce generalized or localized color changes; these are described in Table 8-3. Localized redness often results from an inflammatory process. Pale, shiny skin of the lower extremities may reflect peripheral changes that occur with systemic diseases such as diabetes mellitus and cardiovascular disease. Injury, steroids, vasculitis, and several systemic disorders can cause localized hemorrhage into cutaneous tissues, producing red-purple discolorations. The discolorations produced by injury are called ecchymoses; when produced by other causes they are called petechiae if smaller than 0.5 cm in diameter (Fig. 8-7) or purpura if larger than 0.5 cm in diameter (Fig. 8-8). Vascular skin lesions are characterized in Figure 8-9 (see Clinical Pearl, "Telangiectasias: Capillary Spider/Spider Angioma"). Box 8-5 describes some characteristic odors that you may note as you examine the skin.

FIGURE 8-7 **Petechiae.** *(From Weston et al, 2007.)*

Clinical Pearl

Telangiectasias: Capillary Spider/Spider Angioma

Telangiectasias are permanently dilated, small blood vessels consisting of venules, capillaries, or arterioles. How do you tell the difference between a capillary spider and a spider angioma? Capillary spiders are little masses of venules. When you blanch them, they will refill in an erratic, not-at-all-organized way. Spider angiomas are arterial. Blanch the center and they will refill in a very organized way, from the center out and evenly in all directions (see Figure 8-9).

FIGURE 8-8 **Senile purpura.** *(From Lemmi and Lemmi, 2000.)*

Purpura—red-purple nonblanchable discoloration greater than 0.5 cm in diameter
Cause: Intravascular defects, infection

Petechiae—red-purple nonblanchable discoloration less than 0.5 cm diameter
Cause: Intravascular defects, infection

Ecchymoses—red-purple nonblanchable discoloration of variable size
Cause: Vascular wall destruction, trauma, vasculitis

Spider angioma—red central body with radiating spider-like legs that blanch with pressure to the central body
Cause: Liver disease, vitamin B deficiency, idiopathic

Venous star—bluish spider, linear or irregularly shaped; does not blanch with pressure
Cause: Increased pressure in superficial veins

Telangiectasia—fine, irregular red line
Cause: Dilation of capillaries

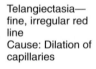

Capillary hemangioma (nevus flammeus)—red irregular macular patches
Cause: Dilation of dermal capillaries

FIGURE 8-9 Characteristics and causes of vascular skin lesions.

Palpation

As you inspect, palpate the skin for moisture, temperature, texture, turgor, and mobility. Palpation may yield additional data for describing lesions, particularly in relation to elevation or depression.

Minimal perspiration or oiliness should be present. Increased perspiration may be associated with activity, warm environment, obesity, anxiety, or excitement; it may be especially noticeable on the palms, scalp, forehead, and in the axillae (usually the dampest areas). The intertriginous areas should evidence minimal dampness. Pay particular attention to areas that get little or no exposure to circulating air such as in the folds of large breasts or obese abdomens or in the inguinal area (Fig. 8-10).

The skin should range from cool to warm to the touch. Use the dorsal surface of your hands or fingers because these areas are most sensitive to temperature perception. At best, this assessment is a rough estimate of skin temperature; what you are really looking for is bilateral symmetry. Environmental conditions, including the temperature of the examining room, may affect surface temperature.

Box 8-5 | Smell the Skin

Even the skin may have odors suggesting a variety of problems: infectious, metabolic, or neurologic. Sweatiness intensifies the smell.

Cause of Odor	Type of Odor
Clostridium gas gangrene	Rotten apples
Proteus infection	Mousy
Pseudomonas infection (especially burns)	Grapelike
Tuberculous lymphadenitis (scrofula)	Stale beer
Anaerobic infection; scurvy	Putrid
Intestinal obstruction, peritonitis	Feculent
Phenylketonuria	Mousy, musty

FIGURE 8-11 Testing skin turgor.

FIGURE 8-10 Examining an intertriginous area. *(From Paller and Mancini, 2011.)*

The texture should feel smooth, soft, and even. Roughness on exposed areas or areas of pressure (particularly the elbows, soles, and palms) may be caused by heavy or woolen clothing, cold weather, or soap. Extensive or widespread roughness may be the result of a keratinization disorder or healing lesions. Hyperkeratoses, especially of the palms and soles, may be the sign of a systemic disorder such as exposure to arsenic or other toxins.

To assess turgor and mobility, gently pinch a small section of skin on the forearm or sternal area between the thumb and forefinger and then release the skin (Fig. 8-11). Turgor is the fullness or tension produced by the fluid content of the cells and tissue. The skin should feel resilient, move easily when pinched, and return to place immediately when released. Turgor should not be tested on the back of a patient's hand because of the looseness and thinness of the skin in that area. Turgor will be altered if the patient is substantially dehydrated or if edema is present. For example, turgor is decreased in a dehydrated patient as evidenced by the pinched skin's failing to spring back to place after release. Some connective tissue diseases, notably the forms of scleroderma, affect skin mobility.

Skin Lesions

As you assess the skin, pay particular attention to any lesions that may be present. *Skin lesion* is a general term that collectively describes any pathologic skin change or occurrence. Lesions may be primary (i.e., those that occur as initial spontaneous manifestations of a pathologic process) or secondary (i.e., those that result from later evolution of or external trauma to a primary lesion).

Tables 8-4 and 8-5 show the characteristics of primary and secondary lesions. The nomenclature is often used inaccurately; if you are uncertain about a lesion, use the descriptors rather than the name. Be aware that several types of lesions may occur concurrently and that secondary changes may obscure primary characteristics.

Describe lesions according to characteristics (Table 8-6), exudates, configuration, and location and distribution:

Characteristics

* Size (measure all dimensions)
* Shape
* Color
* Texture
* Elevation or depression
* Attachment at base: pedunculated (having a stalk) or sessile (without a stalk)
* Exudates
  * Color
  * Odor
  * Amount
  * Consistency
* Configuration
  * Annular (rings)
  * Grouped
  * Linear
  * Arciform (bow-shaped)
  * Diffuse
* Location and distribution
  * Generalized or localized
  * Region of the body (Box 8-6 on page 132)
  * Patterns (Figs. 8-12, 8-13, and 8-14 on page 133)
  * Discrete or confluent

A small, clear, flexible ruler is necessary for measuring the size of lesions. Examiners often rely on household measures such as

Text continued on p. 133

EXAMINATION AND FINDINGS

Table 8-4   Primary Skin Lesions

Description	Examples		
Macule A flat, circumscribed area that is a change in the color of the skin; less than 1 cm in diameter	Freckles, flat moles (nevi), petechiae, measles		Measles. (From Hockenberry and Wilson, 2007.)
Papule An elevated, firm, circumscribed area; less than 1 cm in diameter	Wart (verruca), elevated moles, lichen planus		Lichen planus. (From Weston et al, 1996.)
Patch A flat, nonpalpable, irregularly-shaped macule greater than 1 cm in diameter	Vitiligo, port-wine stains, Mongolian spots, café au lait patch		Vitiligo. (From Weston and Lane, 1991.)
Plaque Elevated, firm, and rough lesion with flat top surface greater than 1 cm in diameter	Psoriasis, seborrheic, and actinic keratoses		Plaque. (From James et al, 2000.)

Table 8-4 **Primary Skin Lesions—cont'd**

Description	Examples	
Wheal Elevated, irregular-shaped area of cutaneous edema; solid, transient, variable diameter	Insect bites, urticaria, allergic reaction	 Wheal. (From Farrar et al, 1992.)

Description	Examples	
Nodule Elevated, firm, circumscribed lesion; deeper in dermis than a papule; 1 to 2 cm in diameter	Erythema nodosum, lipoma	 Hypertrophic nodule. (From Goldman and Fitzpatrick, 1994.)
Tumor Elevated and solid lesion; may or may not be clearly demarcated; deeper in dermis; greater than 2 cm in diameter	Neoplasms, benign tumor, lipoma	 Lipoma. (From Lemmi and Lemmi, 2000.)
Vesicle Elevated, circumscribed, superficial, not into dermis; filled with serous fluid; less than 1 cm in diameter	Varicella (chickenpox), herpes zoster (shingles)	 Vesicles caused by varicella. (From Farrar et al, 1992.)

Continued

Table 8-4 Primary Skin Lesions—cont'd

Description	Examples
Bulla Vesicle greater than 1 cm in diameter	Blister, pemphigus vulgaris

Blister.
(From White, 1994.)

| **Pustule**
Elevated, superficial lesion; similar to a vesicle but filled with purulent fluid | Impetigo, acne |

Acne.
(From Weston et al, 1996.)

| **Cyst**
Elevated, circumscribed, encapsulated lesion; in dermis or subcutaneous layer; filled with liquid or semisolid material | Sebaceous cyst, cystic acne |

Sebaceous cyst.
(From Weston et al, 1996.)

| **Telangiectasia**
Fine, irregular, red lines produced by capillary dilation | Telangiectasia in rosacea |

Telangiectasia.
(From Lemmi and Lemmi, 2000.)

TABLE 8-5	Secondary Skin Lesions		

Description	Examples		
Scale Heaped-up, keratinized cells; flaky skin; irregular; thick or thin; dry or oily; variation in size	Flaking of skin with seborrheic dermatitis or following a drug reaction; dry skin		 Fine scaling. (From Baran et al, 1991.)
Lichenification Rough, thickened epidermis secondary to persistent rubbing, itching, or skin irritation; often involves flexor surface of extremity	Chronic dermatitis		 Lichenification. (From Lemmi and Lemmi, 2000.)
Keloid Irregularly shaped, elevated, progressively enlarging scar; grows beyond the boundaries of the wound; caused by excessive collagen formation during healing	Keloid formation following surgery		 Keloid. (From Weston et al, 1996.)
Scar Thin to thick fibrous tissue that replaces normal skin following injury or laceration to the dermis	Healed wound or surgical incision		 Hypertrophic scar. (From Goldman and Fitzpatrick, 1994.)

Continued

Table 8-5 Secondary Skin Lesions—cont'd

Description	Examples
Excoriation Loss of the epidermis; linear hollowed-out, crusted area	Abrasion or scratch, scabies

Excoriation from a tree branch.
(From Lemmi and Lemmi, 2000.)

| **Fissure**
Linear crack or break from the epidermis to the dermis; may be moist or dry | Athlete's foot, cracks at the corner of the mouth |

Scaling and fissures of tinea pedis.
(From Lemmi and Lemmi, 2000.)

| **Erosion**
Loss of part of the epidermis; depressed, moist, glistening; follows rupture of a vesicle or bulla | Varicella, variola after rupture |

Erosion.
(From Cohen, 1993.)

| **Ulcer**
Loss of epidermis and dermis; concave; varies in size | Decubiti, stasis ulcers |

Stasis ulcer.
(From Swartz 2009.)

Table 8-5	Secondary Skin Lesions—cont'd	
Description	**Examples**	
Crust Dried serum, blood, or purulent exudates; slightly elevated; size varies; brown, red, black, tan, or straw-colored	Scab on abrasion, eczema	Scab.
Atrophy Thinning of skin surface and loss of skin markings; skin translucent and paper-like	Striae; aged skin	Striae. (Courtesy Antoinette Hood, MD, Department of Dermatology, University of Indiana, Department of Medicine, Indianapolis.)

Table 8-6	Morphologic Characteristics of Skin Lesions	
Characteristic	**Description**	**Examples**
Distribution		
Localized	Lesion appears in one small area	Impetigo, herpes simplex (e.g., labialis), tinea corporis (ringworm)
Regional	Lesions involve a specific region of the body	Acne vulgaris (pilosebaceous gland distribution), herpes zoster (nerve dermatomal distribution), psoriasis (flexural surfaces and skin folds)
Generalized	Lesions appear widely distributed or in numerous areas simultaneously	Urticaria, disseminated drug eruptions
Shape/Arrangement		
Round/discoid	Coin-shaped (no central clearing)	Nummular eczema
Oval	Ovoid shape	Pityriasis rosea
Annular	Round, active margins with central clearing	Tinea corporis, sarcoidosis
Zosteriform (dermatomal)	Following a nerve or segment of the body	Herpes zoster
Polycyclic	Interlocking or coalesced circles (formed by enlargement of annular lesions)	Psoriases, urticaria
Linear	In a line	Contact dermatitis
Iris/target lesion	Pink macules with purple central papules	Erythema multiforme
Stellate	Star-shaped	Meningococcal septicemia
Serpiginous	Snakelike or wavy line track	Cutanea larva migrans
Reticulate	Netlike or lacy	Polyarteritis nodosa, lichen planus lesions of erythema infectiosum
Morbilliform	Measles-like: maculopapular lesions that become confluent on the face and body	Measles, roseola, drug eruptions

Continued

Table 8-6 Morphologic Characteristics of Skin Lesions—cont'd

Characteristic	Description	Examples
Border/Margin		
Discrete	Well demarcated or defined, able to draw a line around it with confidence	Psoriasis
Indistinct	Poorly defined, have borders that merge into normal skin or outlying ill-defined papules	Nummular eczema
Active	Margin of lesion shows greater activity than center	Tinea eruptions
Irregular	Nonsmooth or notched margin	Malignant melanoma
Border raised above	Center of lesion depressed compared to the edge	Basal cell carcinoma center
Advancing	Expanding at margins	Cellulitis
Associated Changes Within Lesions		
Central clearing	An erythematous border surrounds lighter skin	Tinea eruptions
Desquamation	Peeling or sloughing of skin	Rash of toxic shock syndrome
Keratotic	Hypertrophic stratum corneum	Calluses, warts
Punctation	Central umbilication or dimpling	Basal cell carcinoma
Telangiectasias	Dilated blood vessels within lesion blanch completely, may be markers of systemic disease	Basal cell carcinoma, actinic keratosis
Pigmentation		
Flesh	Same tone as the surrounding skin	Neurofibroma, some nevi
Pink	Light red undertones	Eczema, pityriasis rosea
Erythematous	Dark pink to red	Tinea eruptions, psoriasis
Salmon	Orange-pink	Psoriasis
Tan-brown	Light to dark brown	Most nevi, pityriasis versicolor
Black	Black or blue-black	Malignant melanoma
Pearly	Shiny white, almost iridescent	Basal cell carcinoma
Purple	Dark red-blue-violet	Purpura, Kaposi sarcoma
Violaceous	Light violet	Erysipelas
Yellow	Waxy	Lipoma
White	Absent of color	Lichen planus

Box 8-6 Regional Distribution of Skin Lesions

Sun-Exposed Areas
- Sunburn
- Lupus erythematosus
- Viral exanthem
- Porphyria

Cloth-Covered Areas
- Irritant contact dermatitis
- Miliaria

Flexural Aspects of Extremities
- Atopic dermatitis
- Intertrigo
- Candidiasis
- Tinea cruris

Extensor Aspects of Extremities
- Psoriasis

Stocking and Glove (Acrodermatitis)
- Viral exanthem/atopic dermatitis
- Tinea pedis with "id" reaction*
- Poststreptococcal infection

Truncal
- Pityriasis rosea (Christmas tree pattern)
- Atopic dermatitis
- Drug reaction

Face, Shoulder, Back
- Acne vulgaris
- Drug-induced acne
- Cushing syndrome

*"id" reaction: a generalized acute cutaneous reaction, probably immunologic in origin, to a variety of stimuli, including fungal infection.

FIGURE 8-12 Clustering of lesions. *(Reproduced by permission of the Wellcome Foundation, Ltd.)*

FIGURE 8-13 Linear formation of lesions (herpes zoster). *(From Lemmi and Lemmi, 2000.)*

FIGURE 8-14 Annular formation of lesions (granuloma annulare). An annular plaque or plaques may occur on the dorsa of the feet or hands as a manifestation of granuloma annulare. *(From White, 1994.)*

fruit, vegetables, and coins to estimate the size of lesions, nodules, or eruptions, but the resulting descriptions can be as inaccurate as they are interesting. Subjective estimates should not be used as measures of size; instead, use the ruler and report sizes in centimeters (inches may also be used, but centimeters is the preferred unit of measure). Try to measure size in all dimensions (i.e., height, width, and depth) when possible.

Use a light for closer inspection of a particular lesion to detect its nuances of color, elevation, and borders. A ×5 to ×10 power handheld magnifying lens is useful in evaluating the subtle details

of a lesion. Transillumination may be used to determine the presence of fluid in cysts and masses. Darken the room and place the tip of the transilluminator against the side of the cyst or mass. Fluid-filled lesions will transilluminate with a red glow, whereas solid lesions will not.

The Wood's lamp can be used to evaluate epidermal hypopigmented or hyperpigmented lesions and to distinguish fluorescing lesions. Darken the room and shine the light on the area to be examined. Look for the characteristic well-demarcated hypopigmentation of vitiligo, hyperpigmentation of café au lait spots, and the yellow-green fluorescence that indicates the presence of some types of fungal infection.

Hair

Palpate the hair for texture while at the same time inspecting it for color, distribution, and quantity. The scalp hair may be coarse or fine, curly or straight, and should be shiny, smooth, and resilient. Palpate the scalp hair for dryness and brittleness that could indicate a systemic disorder. Color will vary from very light blond to black to gray and may show alterations with rinses, dyes, or permanents.

The quantity and distribution of hair vary according to individual genetic makeup. Hair is commonly present on the scalp, lower face, neck, nares, ears, chest, axillae, back and shoulders, arms, legs, toes, pubic area, and around the nipples. Note hair loss, which can be either generalized or localized. Inspect the feet and toes for hair loss that may indicate poor circulation or nutritional deficit. Look for any inflammation or scarring that accompanies hair loss, particularly when it is localized. Diffuse hair loss usually occurs without inflammation and scarring. The presence of scarring is helpful in diagnosis. Note whether the hair shafts are broken off or are completely absent.

Genetically predisposed men often display a gradual symmetric hair loss on the scalp during adulthood as a response to androgens. Asymmetric hair loss may indicate a pathologic condition. Women in their 20s and 30s may also develop adrenal androgenic female-pattern alopecia (hair loss), with a gradual loss of hair from the central scalp.

Fine vellus hair covers the body, whereas coarse terminal hair occurs on the scalp, pubic, and axillary areas, on the arms and legs (to some extent), and in the beard of men. The male pubic hair configuration is an upright triangle with the hair extending midline to the umbilicus (Chapter 6, Fig. 6-12). The female pubic configuration is an inverted triangle; the hair may extend midline to the umbilicus (Chapter 6, Fig. 6-10). Look for hirsutism in women—growth of terminal hair in a male distribution pattern on the face, body, and pubic area. Hirsutism, by itself or associated with other signs of virilization, may be a sign of an endocrine disorder.

Nails

Inspection

Inspect the nails for color, length, configuration, symmetry, and cleanliness. The condition of the fingernails can provide important insight to the patient's sense of self. Are they bitten down to the quick? Are they clean? Are they kept smooth and neat, or do they look unkempt? The condition of the hair and nails gives a clue about the patient's level of self-care and some sense of emotional order and social integration.

Nail edges should be smooth and rounded. Jagged, broken, or bitten edges or cuticles are indicators of poor care habits and may predispose the patient to localized infection. Peeling nails (from the plate splitting into layers) are usually found in individuals whose hands are subject to repeated water immersion.

Examine the proximal and lateral nail folds for redness, swelling, pus, warts, cysts, and tumors. Pain usually accompanies ingrown nails and infections.

Color. The shape and opacity of nails vary considerably among individuals. Nail bed color should be variations of pink. There are physical clues in the nails that may indicate pathophysiologic problems. Pigment deposits or bands may be present in the nail beds of persons with dark skin (Fig. 8-15) (see Physical Variations, "Pigment in the Nail Beds"). Yellow discoloration occurs with several nail diseases, including psoriasis and fungal infections, and may also occur with chronic respiratory disease. Proximal subungual fungal infection is associated with HIV infection. Diffuse darkening of the nails may arise from antimalarial drug therapy, candidal infection, hyperbilirubinemia, and chronic trauma, such as occurs from tight-fitting shoes. Green-black discoloration, which is associated with *Pseudomonas* infection, may be confused with similar discoloration caused by injury to the nail bed (subungual hematoma). Pain accompanies a subungual hematoma, whereas *Pseudomonas* infection is painless. Nail beds that are blue may be a transient response to a cold examining room. A single blue or black nail may indicate melanoma or bruising/bleeding from trauma. Generalized blue nails may be

FIGURE 8-15 Pigmented bands in nails are expected in persons with dark skin. *(From Johr et al, 2004.)*

FIGURE 8-16 White spots on nail from injury (leukonychia punctata). *(From Scher and Daniel, 2005.)*

caused by conditions that produce cyanosis such as asthma, cardiac disorders, or severe anemia. Other causes of blue nails include silver poisoning, medication side effects, and Wilson disease, an inherited disorder of copper metabolism. Splinter hemorrhages, longitudinal red or brown streaks, may occur in endocarditis, vasculitis, with severe psoriasis of the nail matrix or as the result of minor injury to the proximal nail fold (habit-tic deformity). White spots in the nail plate (leukonychia punctate), a common finding, result from cuticle manipulation or other forms of mild trauma that injure the nail matrix (Fig. 8-16). These spots need to be differentiated from longitudinal white streaks or transverse white bands that are indicative of a systemic disorder. Separation of the nail plate from the bed produces a white, yellow, or green tinge on the nonadherent portion of the nail.

Physical Variations

Pigment in the Nail Beds

Pigmented deposits or bands may be present in the nail beds of persons with dark skin. The sudden appearance of such a band in whites may indicate melanoma.

FIGURE 8-17 **Aging nails.** Longitudinal ridging of the nail is a common expected variation. *(From White, 1994.)*

FIGURE 8-18 **Median nail dystrophy.** *(From James et al, 2011.)*

Nail Plate. The nail plate should appear smooth and flat or slightly convex. Complete absence of the nail (anonychia) may occur as a congenital condition. Look for nail ridging, grooves, depressions, and pitting. Longitudinal ridging and beading are common expected variants (Fig. 8-17). Longitudinal ridges and grooves may also occur with lichen planus of the nail. Transverse grooves result from repeated injury to the nail, usually the thumb, as with chronic manipulation to the proximal nail fold (Fig. 8-18). The most common cause is picking at the thumb with the index finger (habit-tic deformity). Chronic inflammation, such as occurs with chronic paronychia or chronic eczema, produces transverse rippling of the nail plate. Transverse depressions that appear at the base of the lunula occur after stress that temporarily interrupts nail formation.

Involvement of a single nail usually points to an injury to the nail matrix. Assure the patient that the nail will grow out and assume normal appearance in about 6 months. Depressions that occur in all the nails are usually a response to systemic disease, including syphilis, disorders producing high fevers, peripheral vascular disease, and uncontrolled diabetes mellitus. Pitting is seen most commonly with psoriasis. Broadening and flattening

of the nail plate may be seen in secondary syphilis. Figure 8-19 illustrates unexpected nail findings.

Inward folding of the lateral edges of the nail causes the nail bed to draw up; this often becomes painful. Curvature is most common in the toenails and is thought to be caused by shoe compression.

Nail Base Angle. The nail base angle should measure 160 degrees. One way to observe this is to place a ruler or a sheet of paper across the nail and dorsal surface of the finger and examine the angle formed by the proximal nail fold and nail plate. In clubbing, the angle increases and approaches or exceeds 180 degrees. Another method of assessment is the Schamroth technique (Fig. 8-20). Have the patient place together the nail (dorsal) surfaces of the thumbs from the right and left hands. When the nails are clubbed, the diamond-shaped window at the base of the nails disappears, and the angle between the distal tips increases. Clubbing is associated with a variety of respiratory and cardiovascular diseases, cirrhosis, colitis, and thyroid disease (Fig. 8-21).

Palpation

The nail plates should feel hard and smooth with a uniform thickness. Thickening of the nail may occur from tight-fitting shoes, chronic trauma, and some fungal infections. Thinning of the nail plate may also accompany some nail diseases. Pain in the area of a nail groove may be secondary to ischemia.

FIGURE 8-20 **Schamroth technique. A,** Patient with healthy nails, illustrating window. **B,** Patient with nail clubbing, illustrating loss of the window and prominent distal angle. *(From Spicknall et al, 2005.)*

EXAMINATION AND FINDINGS

Clubbing—early   almost 180°

Darkening of nail

Clubbing—middle   180°

Terry nails

Clubbing—severe   >180°

Splinter hemorrhages

Transverse grooving (Beau lines)

Nail pitting

Curvature of nail

Onycholysis

Spoon nail (koilonychia)

Anonychia (absence of nail)

Broadening of nail

Paronychia

FIGURE 8-19 Nails: unexpected findings and appearance.

FIGURE 8-21 **Finger clubbing.** Nail is enlarged and curved. *(From Lawrence and Cox, 1993.)*

FIGURE 8-22 **Testing nail bed adherence.**

Gently squeeze the nail between your thumb and the pad of your finger to test for adherence of the nail to the nail bed. Separation of the nail plate from the bed is common with psoriasis, trauma, candidal or *Pseudomonas* infections, and some medications. The nail base should feel firm (Fig. 8-22). A boggy nail base accompanies clubbing.

�֍ Infants and Children

In the first few hours of life, the infant's skin may look very red. The gentle pink coloring that predominates in infancy usually surfaces in the first day after birth. Skin color is partly determined by the amount of subcutaneous fat: the less subcutaneous fat, the redder and more transparent the skin. Dark-skinned newborns do not always manifest the intensity of melanosis that will be readily evident in 2 to 3 months. The exceptions in this regard are the nail beds and skin of the scrotum. The expected color changes in newborns are described in Box 8-7.

Physiologic jaundice may be present to a mild degree in many newborn infants. It usually starts after the first day of life and disappears by the eighth to tenth day but may persist for as long as 3 to 4 weeks. Intense and persistent jaundice suggests liver disease, a hemolytic process, or severe, overwhelming infection. Risk factors for hyperbilirubinemia in the newborn are listed in the Risk Factors box.

In examining the newborn for hyperbilirubinemia, look at the whole body. Be sure to examine the oral mucosa and sclera of the eyes, where jaundice can be detected more easily. Examine the baby in natural daylight if possible. Both artificial light

---

Box 8-7	Expected Color Changes in the Newborn

- **Acrocyanosis:** Cyanosis of hands and feet
- **Cutis marmorata:** Transient mottling when infant is exposed to decreased temperature
- **Erythema toxicum:** Pink papular rash with vesicles superimposed on thorax, back, buttocks, and abdomen; may appear in 24 to 48 hours and resolves after several days
- **Mongolian spots:** Irregular areas of deep blue pigmentation, usually in the sacral and gluteal regions; seen predominantly in newborns of African, Native American/American Indian, Asian, or Latin descent
- **Salmon patches ("stork bites"):** Flat, deep pink localized areas usually seen on the mid-forehead, eyelids, upper lip, and back of neck

---

Risk Factors

Major Risk Factors for Severe Hyperbilirubinemia in Infants of 35 or More Weeks' Gestation

- Total serum bilirubin (TSB) or transcutaneous bilirubin (TcB) greater than 75th percentile
- Jaundice observed in the first 24 h
- Blood group incompatibility with positive direct antiglobulin test, other known hemolytic disease (e.g., G6PD [glucose-6-phosphate dehydrogenase] deficiency), elevated $ETCO_c$ (End-Tidal Carbon Monoxide concentration)
- Gestational age 35-36 wk
- Previous sibling received phototherapy
- Cephalohematoma or significant bruising (e.g., from vacuum assisted delivery)
- Exclusive breast-feeding, particularly if nursing is not going well and weight loss is excessive
- East Asian race

From the American Association of Pediatrics, 2004.

---

and environmental colors (e.g., orange drapes) can produce a false color.

Check the skin of the newborn carefully for small defects, especially over the entire length of the spine; the midline of the head, from the nape of the neck to the bridge of the nose; and the neck extending to the ear. This may offer a clue to brachial sinus tracts or brachial cleft cysts. The skin should feel soft and smooth. Also look for skin findings that may signal underlying systemic conditions (Box 8-8).

Inspect the skin for distortions in contour suggestive of hygromas, fluid-containing masses, subcutaneous angiomas, lymphangiomas, hemangiomas, nodules, and tumors. Transillumination may help if there is a question about the density of the mass or the amount of fluid. With more density and less fluid, there is less tendency to glow on transillumination.

Examine the hands and feet of newborns for skin creases. Flexion results in creases that are readily discernible on the fingers, palms, and soles (Fig. 8-23). One indicator of maturity is the number of creases; the older the baby, the more creases there are. Examine the crease patterns of the fingers and palms because abnormalities are associated with specific patterns. The most commonly recognized pattern is a single transverse crease

Box 8-8 Skin Lesions: External Clues to Internal Problems

Many systemic conditions or disorders may present congenital external clues that are apparent on physical examination. The following are a few examples of cutaneous markers that may signal underlying disease. A thorough evaluation is necessary, although some clues may be isolated findings and may require no intervention, follow-up, or treatment.

- **Faun tail nevus:** Tuft of hair overlying the spinal column at birth, usually in the lumbosacral area; may be associated with spina bifida occulta
- **Epidermal verrucous nevi:** Warty lesions in a linear or whorled pattern that may be pigmented or skin colored; present at birth or in early childhood; associated most commonly with skeletal, central nervous system, and ocular abnormalities
- **Café au lait macules:** Flat, evenly pigmented spots varying in color from light brown to dark brown or black in dark skin; larger than 5 mm in diameter; present at birth or shortly thereafter; may be associated with neurofibromatosis or miscellaneous other conditions including pulmonary stenosis, temporal lobe dysrhythmia, and tuberous sclerosis
- **Freckling in the axillary or inguinal area:** Multiple flat pigmented macules associated with neurofibromatosis; may occur in conjunction with café au lait macules
- **Ash leaf macule:** White macules present at birth associated with tuberous sclerosis. Occur most commonly on the trunk, but may also appear on the face and limbs
- **Facial port-wine stain:** When it involves the ophthalmic division of trigeminal nerve, may be associated with ocular defects, most notably glaucoma; or may be accompanied by angiomatous malformation of the meninges (Sturge-Kalischer-Weber syndrome), resulting in atrophy and calcification of the adjacent cerebral cortex
- **Port-wine stain of limb and/or trunk:** When accompanied by varicosities and hypertrophy of underlying soft tissues and bones, may be associated with orthopedic problems (Klippel-Trenaunay-Weber syndrome)
- **Congenital lymphedema with or without transient hemangiomas:** May be associated with gonadal dysgenesis caused by absence of an X chromosome, producing an XO karyotype (Turner syndrome)
- **Supernumerary nipples:** Congenital accessory nipples with or without glandular tissue, located along the mammary ridge (see Chapter 16); may be associated with renal abnormalities, especially in the presence of other minor anomalies, particularly in whites
- **"Hair collar" sign:** A ring of long, dark, coarse hair surrounding a midline scalp nodule in infants is usually an isolated cutaneous anomaly that may indicate neural tube closure defects of the scalp.

FIGURE 8-23 Expected creases of newborn's hands (A) and feet (B).

FIGURE 8-24 Unexpected palmar crease. Single transverse crease in child with Down syndrome. Compare to Figure 8-23, *A. (From Zitelli and Davis, 1997.)*

in the palm that is commonly seen in children with Down syndrome (trisomy 21) (Fig. 8-24).

All newborn infants are covered to some degree by vernix caseosa, a whitish, moist, cheeselike substance. Transient puffiness of the hands, feet, eyelids, legs, pubis, or sacrum occurs in some newborns. It has no discernible cause, and it should not create concern if it disappears within 2 to 3 days.

Newborn infants are particularly susceptible to hypothermia, partly because of their poorly developed subcutaneous fat. In addition, infants have a relatively large body surface area, providing greater area for heat loss. Combined with an inability to shiver, these factors cause term newborns to lose heat.

Cutis marmorata, a mottled appearance of the body and extremities, is part of the newborn's response to changes in

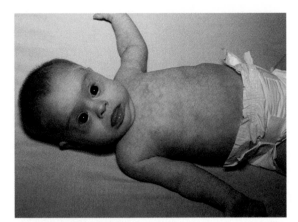

FIGURE 8-25 **Mottling (cutis marmorata).** *(From Hockenberry and Wilson, 2007.)*

FIGURE 8-27 Hyperpigmented patches (Mongolian spots) are common in babies with dark skin. *(From Lemmi and Lemmi, 2000.)*

FIGURE 8-26 **Acrocyanosis of hands in newborn.**

FIGURE 8-28 **Hemangiomas in infant.** *(From Zitelli and Davis, 2007.)*

FIGURE 8-29 **Café au lait patches.** *(From Lemmi and Lemmi, 2009.)*

ambient temperature, whether cooling or heating. It is more common in premature infants and children with Down syndrome or hypothyroidism (Fig. 8-25). Cyanosis of the hands and feet (acrocyanosis) may be present at birth and may persist for several days or longer if the newborn is kept in cool ambient temperatures. It often recurs when the baby is chilled. If cyanosis persists, suspect an underlying cardiac or pulmonary defect (Fig. 8-26).

Bluish black to slate gray spots are sometimes seen on the back, buttocks, shoulders, and legs of well babies. These hyperpigmented patches (Mongolian spots) occur most often in babies with dark skin and usually disappear in the preschool years. Mongolian spots are easily mistaken for bruises by the inexperienced examiner (Fig. 8-27).

Several vascular lesions are common in infancy. Superficial and subcutaneous hemangiomas are true neoplasms, which develop in the first 1 to 2 months of life, grow for 2 to 6 months, and regress over the next 5 to 10 years (Fig. 8-28). A salmon patch ("stork bite") represents a common capillary vascular formation, found most frequently on the mid-forehead, eyelids, upper lip, and back of neck

Coffee-colored patches (café au lait macules) may be either harmless or indicative of underlying disease. Be suspicious of neurofibromatosis (NF-1) if there are six or more café au lait macules more than 5 mm in greatest diameter in prepubertal individuals or more than 15 mm in greatest diameter after puberty (National Institute of Neurological Disorders and Stroke, 2012) (Fig. 8-29).

FIGURE 8-30 Milia in infant. *(From Lemmi and Lemmi, 2009.)*

FIGURE 8-31 Testing skin turgor in an infant.

Table 8-7	Estimating Dehydration
Return to Normal After the Pinch	**Degree of Dehydration**
<2 seconds	<5% loss of body weight
2 to 3 seconds	5% to 8% loss of body weight
3 to 4 seconds	9% to 10% loss of body weight
>4 seconds	>10% loss of body weight

Milia are small whitish, discrete papules on the face; they are commonly found during the first 2 to 3 months of life. The sebaceous glands function in an immature fashion at this age and are easily plugged by sebum (Fig. 8-30).

Sebaceous hyperplasia produces numerous tiny yellow macules and papules in the newborn, probably the result of androgen stimulation from the mother. It commonly occurs on the forehead, cheeks, nose, and chin of the full-term infant. Sebaceous hyperplasia disappears quickly within 1 to 2 months of life.

The skin and subcutaneous tissues of an infant and young child, more readily than in the older child and adolescent, can give an important indication of the state of hydration and nutrition (Table 8-7). The tissue turgor is best evaluated by gently pinching a fold of the abdominal skin between the index finger and thumb. As with the adult, resiliency allows it to return to its undisturbed state when released. A child who is seriously dehydrated (i.e., more than 10% of body weight) or very poorly nourished will have skin that retains "tenting" after it is pinched. How quickly the tent disappears provides a clue to the degree of dehydration or malnutrition (Fig. 8-31).

Because the normal range of skin moisture is broad, look at other factors that may suggest a problem. Excessive sweating or dryness alone rarely has pathologic significance in infants or children.

Children with atopic dermatitis or chronic skin changes involving the face will commonly rub their eyes, sufficiently sometimes to cause an extra crease or pleat of skin below the eye. This is known as the Dennie-Morgan fold; it is probably secondary to chronic rubbing and inflammation. Also see Clinical Pearl, "Bald Spots in Infants and Children."

Clinical Pearl

Bald Spots in Children and Infants

Bald spots in children? Typically, it is ringworm of the scalp (tinea capitis), alopecia areata, or trichotillomania (compulsive hair-pulling). Infants who sleep on their backs can develop areas of alopecia from pressure on occiput.

Adolescents

The examination of the adolescent's skin is the same as that for the adult. The adolescent's skin may have increased oiliness and perspiration, and hair oiliness may also be increased. Increased sebum production predisposes the adolescent to develop acne.

As a reflection of maturing apocrine gland function, increased axillary perspiration occurs, and the characteristic adult body odor develops during adolescence. Hair on the extremities darkens and becomes coarser. Pubic and axillary hair in both males and females develops and assumes adult characteristics. Males develop facial and chest hair that varies in quantity and coarseness. Chapter 6 provides a more thorough discussion of the maturational changes that occur during adolescence.

Pregnant Women

Striae gravidarum (stretch marks) may appear over the abdomen, thighs, and breasts during the second trimester of pregnancy. They fade after delivery but never disappear (Fig. 8-32). There is an increase in telangiectasias (vascular spiders), which may be found on the face, neck, chest, and arms; these appear during the second to fifth months of pregnancy and usually resolve after delivery. Hemangiomas that were present before pregnancy may increase in size, or new ones may develop. Cutaneous tags (molluscum fibrosum gravidarum) are either pedunculated or sessile skin tags that are most often found on the neck and upper chest. They result from epithelial hyperplasia and are not inflammatory. Most resolve spontaneously.

An increase in pigmentation is common and is found to some extent in all pregnant women. The areas usually affected include the areolae and nipples, vulvar and perianal regions, axillae, and the linea alba. Pigmentation of the linea alba is called the linea nigra. It extends from the symphysis pubis to the top of the fundus in the midline (Fig. 8-33). Preexisting pigmented moles

FIGURE 8-32 **Striae.** *(Courtesy Antoinette Hood, MD, Department of Dermatology, Indiana University School of Medicine, Indianapolis.)*

FIGURE 8-33 **Linea nigra on abdomen of pregnant woman.**

FIGURE 8-34 **Facial hyperpigmentation: chloasma (melasma).** *(From White and Cox, 2006.)*

(nevi) and freckles may darken, with some nevi increasing in size. New nevi may form. The chloasma, or "mask of pregnancy," occurs frequently in pregnant women and is found on the forehead, cheeks, bridge of the nose, and chin. It is blotchy in appearance and is usually symmetric (Fig. 8-34).

Palmar erythema is a common finding in pregnancy. A diffuse redness covers the entire palmar surface or the thenar and hypothenar eminences. The cause is unknown, and it usually disappears after delivery.

Itching over the abdomen and breasts resulting from skin stretching is common and not a cause for concern; however,

FIGURE 8-35 **Hands of older adult.** Note prominent veins and thin appearance of skin.

itching accompanied by a rash may signal a pregnancy-specific dermatosis, which requires further investigation. Itching during pregnancy can also be caused by impaired flow of bile from the liver, which may also produce jaundice. The itching is generalized but may be more severe on the palms and soles. Be alert to these serious manifestations of underlying pathology. Hair growth is altered in pregnancy by the circulating hormones. The growing phase of the hair is lengthened and hair loss is decreased. Two to 4 months after delivery, increased hair shedding occurs. Regrowth will occur in 6 to 12 months. Acne vulgaris may be aggravated during the first trimester of pregnancy but often improves in the third trimester.

⚘ Older Adults

The skin of the older adult may appear more transparent and paler in light-skinned individuals. Pigment deposits, increased freckling, and hypopigmented patches may develop, causing the skin to take on a less uniform appearance.

Flaking or scaling, associated with the drier skin that comes with aging, occurs most commonly over the extremities. The skin also thins (especially over bony prominences, the dorsal surface of hands and feet, forearms, and lower legs) and takes on a parchment-like appearance and texture (Fig. 8-35).

The skin often appears to hang loosely on the bony frame as a result of a general loss of elasticity, loss of underlying adipose tissue, and years of gravitational pull (Fig. 8-36). You may observe tenting of the skin when testing for turgor (Fig. 8-37) (see Clinical Pearl, "Hydration Status in Older Adults").

Clinical Pearl

Hydration Status in Older Adults

Since loss of skin turgor is a common finding in older adults, it is not a good indicator of hydration status. To determine hydration status use other assessments such as amount of saliva, urine output, and urine specific gravity.

Table 8-8	Staging of Pressure Ulcers (Decubitus Ulcers)
Stage	**Characteristics**
Suspected deep tissue injury	Localized area of discolored intact skin (purple or maroon) or blood-filled blister due to damage of underlying soft tissue from pressure and/or shear. The area may be preceded by tissue that is painful, firm, mushy, boggy, warmer, or cooler as compared to adjacent tissue.
I	Red intact skin that does not blanch, usually localized over a bony prominence. Darkly pigmented skin may not have visible blanching; its color may differ from the surrounding area.
II	Partial-thickness loss of dermis presenting as a shallow open ulcer with a red-pink wound bed, without slough. May also present as an intact or open/ruptured serum-filled blister.
III	Full-thickness tissue loss. Subcutaneous fat may be visible but bone, tendon or muscle are not exposed. Slough may be present but does not obscure the depth of tissue loss. May include undermining and tunneling.
IV	Full-thickness tissue loss with exposed bone, tendon or muscle. Slough or eschar may be present on some parts of the wound bed. Often include undermining and tunneling.
Unstageable	Full-thickness tissue loss in which the base of the ulcer is covered by slough (yellow, tan, gray, green or brown) and/or eschar (tan, brown or black) in the wound bed.

From National Pressure Ulcer Advisory Panel, 2007.

FIGURE 8-36 Skin hanging loosely, especially around bony prominences.

FIGURE 8-38 Cherry angioma in older adult. *(From Habif, 2004.)*

FIGURE 8-37 **Skin turgor in older adult.** Note tenting.

The immobility of some older adults, especially when combined with decreased peripheral vascular circulation, increases their risk for pressure ulcers (decubitus ulcers). During examination, pay particular attention to bony prominences and areas subject to persistent pressure or shearing forces. Heels and the sacrum are common sites in patients who are confined to bed. Do not neglect to examine less obvious areas such as the elbows, scapulae, and back of the head. Assess the diameter and depth of the ulcer and stage it accordingly. The staging criteria are described in Table 8-8.

Increased wrinkling is evident, especially in areas exposed to sun and in expressive areas of the face. Sagging or drooping is most obvious under the chin, beneath the eyes, and in the earlobes, breasts, and scrotum. Purpura, particularly dorsal surfaces of hands and lower arm that get tapped or bumped, is commonly seen in older adults on aspirin therapy.

Several types of lesions may occur on the skin of healthy older adults. The following lesions are considered expected findings:

+ Cherry angiomas are tiny, bright ruby-red, round papules that may become brown with time. They occur in virtually everyone older than 30 years and increase numerically with age (Fig. 8-38).
+ Seborrheic keratoses are pigmented, raised, warty lesions, usually appearing on the face or trunk. These must be distinguished from actinic keratoses, which have malignant potential. Because the lesions may look similar, seek the assistance of an experienced practitioner for differential diagnosis (Fig. 8-39).
+ Sebaceous hyperplasia occurs as yellowish, flattened papules with central depressions (Fig. 8-40).

FIGURE 8-39 Seborrheic keratoses in older adult. *(From Lawrence and Cox, 1993.)*

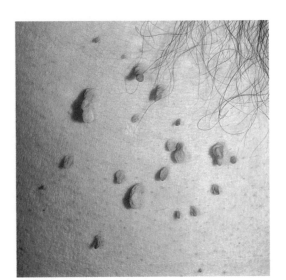

FIGURE 8-41 Multiple cutaneous tags in axilla. *(From Salvo, 2009.)*

FIGURE 8-40 Sebaceous hyperplasia. *(From Carey, 2010.)*

The hair turns gray or white as melanocytes cease functioning. Head, body, pubic, and axillary hair thins and becomes sparse and drier. Men may show an increase in coarse aural, nasal, and eyebrow hair; women tend to develop coarse facial hair. Symmetric balding, usually frontal or occipital, often occurs in men.

The nails thicken, become more brittle, and may be deformed, misshapen, striated, distorted, or peeling. They can take on a yellowish color and may lose their transparency. These changes occur most often in the toenails.

Audio: Steps involved in conducting a physical examination of skin, hair, and nails

EXAMINATION AND FINDINGS

Sample Documentation
History and Physical Examination

Subjective
A 23-year-old woman reports body rash that she first noticed 4 days ago. Thinks it may be from drinking new citrus juice. Describes rash as red, itchy, transient bumps on face, neck, arms, legs, and torso. No known food allergies. Denies exposure to new contact irritants. No new medications; is currently taking antihistamine for allergic rhinitis. Denies respiratory difficulty, difficulty swallowing, and edema. Denies fever, cough, and malaise.

Objective
Skin: Dark pink papules on face, torso, and extremities; large urticarial wheal on right cheek. No excoriation or secondary infection. Turgor resilient. Skin uniformly warm and dry. No edema.
Hair: Curly, black, thick with female distribution pattern. Texture coarse.
Nails: Opaque, short, well-groomed, uniform and without deformities. Nail bed pink. Nail base angle 160 degrees. No redness, exudates, or swelling in the surrounding folds, and no tenderness to palpation.
  For additional sample documentation, see Chapter 26, pp. 628-631.

- Cutaneous tags (acrochordon) are small, soft tags of skin, usually appearing on the neck and upper chest. They are attached to the body by a narrow stalk (pedunculated) and may or may not be pigmented (Fig. 8-41).
- Cutaneous horns are small, hard projections of the epidermis, usually occurring on the forehead and face (Fig. 8-42).
- Solar lentigines are irregular, round, gray-brown macules with a rough surface that occur in sun-exposed areas. These are often referred to as "age spots" or incorrectly as "liver spots" (Fig. 8-43). They are epidermal proliferations and are early signs of photoaging of the skin.

FIGURE 8-42 Cutaneous horn. *(From White, 1994.)*

FIGURE 8-43 Lentigo, a brown macule that appears in sun-exposed areas. *(From Ignatavicius and Workman, 2006.)*

ABNORMALITIES

SKIN, HAIR, NAILS

SKIN: INFLAMMATORY AND INFECTIOUS CONDITIONS

Eczematous Dermatitis

Most common inflammatory skin disorder; several forms, including irritant contact dermatitis, allergic contact dermatitis, and atopic dermatitis

Pathophysiology

- Common factor of the various forms are intercellular edema and epidermal breakdown
- Eczematous dermatitis has three stages: acute, subacute, and chronic.
- Excoriation from scratching predisposes to infection and causes crust formation (Fig. 8-44).

Subjective Data

- Itching may or may not be present.
- Those with atopic dermatitis often report allergy history (allergic rhinitis, asthma).

Objective Data

- Acute phase characterized by erythematous, pruritic, weeping vesicles
- Subacute eczema characterized by erythema and scaling
- Chronic stage characterized by thick, lichenified, pruritic plaques
- Atopic dermatitis: during childhood, lesions involve flexures, the nape, and the dorsal aspects of the limbs; in adolescence and adulthood, lichenified plaques affect the flexures, head, and neck.

FIGURE 8-44 Contact dermatitis. *(From Morison and Moffatt, 1994.)*

Folliculitis

Inflammation and infection of the hair follicle and surrounding dermis

Pathophysiology

- Presence of inflammatory cells within the wall and ostia of the hair follicle creates a follicular-based pustule.
- Inflammation can be either superficial or deep; deep folliculitis can result from chronic lesions of superficial folliculitis or from lesions that are manipulated.
- Persistent or recurrent lesions may result in scarring and permanent hair loss.

Subjective Data

- Acute onset of papules and pustules associated with pruritus or mild discomfort; may have pain with deep folliculitis
- Risk factors: frequent shaving, immunosuppression, hot tubs without adequate chlorine, preexisting dermatoses, long-term antibiotic use, occlusive clothing and/or occlusive dressings, exposure to hot humid temperatures, diabetes mellitus, obesity, and use of EGFR (epithelial growth factor receptor) inhibitor medications

Objective Data

- Primary lesion: small pustule 1 to 2 cm in diameter that is located over a pilosebaceous orifice and may be perforated by a hair
- Pustule may be surrounded by inflammation or nodular lesions; after the pustule ruptures, a crust forms (Fig. 8-45).
- May have suppurative drainage with deep folliculitis
- Any hair-bearing site can be affected; the sites most often involved are the face, scalp, thighs, axilla, and inguinal area.

FIGURE 8-45 Beard folliculitis. *(From Lemmi and Lemmi, 2000.)*

Furuncle (Boil)

A deep-seated infection of the pilosebaceous unit

Pathophysiology

- *Staphylococcus aureus* most common organism
- Initially, a small perifollicular abscess that spreads to the surrounding dermis and subcutaneous tissue
- May occur singly or in multiples; when infection involves several adjacent follicles, a coalescent purulent mass or carbuncle forms.

Subjective Data

- Acute onset of tender red nodule that becomes pustular

FIGURE 8-46 Furuncle. *(From Lemmi and Lemmi, 2009.)*

Objective Data

- Skin red, hot, and tender
- Center of the lesion fills with pus and forms a core that may rupture spontaneously or require surgical incision (Fig. 8-46)
- Sites commonly involved are the face and neck, arms, axillae, breasts, thighs, and buttocks.

Cellulitis

Diffuse, acute, infection of the skin and subcutaneous tissue

Pathophysiology

- Majority of cases caused by *Streptococcus pyogenes* or *Staphylococcus aureus*

Subjective Data

- Break in the skin, such as a fissure, cut, laceration, insect bite, or puncture wound
- Pain and swelling at the site
- May have fever

Objective Data

- Skin red, hot, tender, and indurated; borders are not well demarcated (Fig. 8-47).
- Lymphangitic streaks and regional lymphadenopathy may be present.

FIGURE 8-47 Cellulitis of the leg. *(From Wilson and Giddens, 2013.)*

Tinea (Dermatophytosis)

Group of noncandidal fungal infections that involve the stratum corneum, nails, or hair

Pathophysiology

- Infection by dermatophytes, typically acquired by direct contact with infected humans or animals; invade the skin and survive on dead keratin
- Lesions usually classified according to anatomic location and can occur on nonhairy parts of the body (tinea corporis), on the groin and inner thigh (tinea cruris), on the scalp (tinea capitis), on the feet (tinea pedis), and on the nails (tinea unguium)

Subjective Data

- May report pruritus

Objective Data

- Lesions vary in appearance and may be papular, pustular, vesicular, erythematous, or scaling (Fig. 8-48).
- Secondary bacterial infection may be present.
- Microscopic examination of skin scraping with KOH solution shows presence of hyphae.
- Infected nails are yellow and thick and may separate from the nail bed.

FIGURE 8-48 A, Tinea corporis. **B,** Tinea cruris. **C,** Tinea capitis. **D,** Tinea pedis. (**A** and **B** from Callen et al, 2000; **C** and **D** from White, 2004.)

Pityriasis Rosea

Self-limiting inflammation of unknown cause

Pathophysiology

- Possible infectious etiology (Drago et al, 2009)
- Not contagious

Subjective Data

- Sudden onset with occurrence of a primary (herald) oval or round plaque
- Herald lesion often missed
- Eruption occurs 1 to 3 weeks later and lasts for several weeks.
- Pruritus may be present with the generalized eruption.

Objective Data

- Lesions usually pale, erythematous, and macular with fine scaling, but may be papular or vesicular (Fig. 8-49)
- Lesions develop on the extremities and trunk; palms and soles are not involved, and facial involvement is rare.
- Trunk lesions characteristically distributed in parallel alignment following the direction of the ribs in a Christmas tree–like pattern

FIGURE 8-49 Pityriasis rosea. *(From Salvo, 2009.)*

Psoriasis

Chronic and recurrent disease of keratin synthesis

Pathophysiology

- Multifactorial origin with genetic component and immune regulation
- Characterized by increased epidermal cell turnover, increased numbers of epidermal stem cells, and abnormal differentiation of keratin expression leading to thickened skin with copious scale

Subjective Data

- May have pruritus
- Concerns about appearance

Objective Data

- Characterized by well-circumscribed, dry, silvery, scaling papules and plaques (Fig. 8-50)
- Lesions commonly occur on the back, buttocks, extensor surfaces of the extremities, and the scalp.
- Can be associated with psoriatic arthritis in up to 30% of patients.

FIGURE 8-50 Psoriasis. Note characteristic silver scaling. *(From Lemmi and Lemmi, 2009.)*

ABNORMALITIES

Rosacea

Chronic inflammatory skin disorder

Pathophysiology

- Cause unknown; occurs most often in persons with a fair complexion
- Lasts for years, with episodes of activity followed by quiescent periods of variable length

Subjective Data

- Itching always absent
- Many patients report a stinging pain associated with flushing episodes.
- Common triggers: exposure to the sun, cold weather, sudden emotion, including laughter or embarrassment, hot beverages, spicy foods, and alcohol consumption

Objective Data

- Eruptions appear on the forehead, cheeks, nose, and occasionally about the eyes.
- Characterized by telangiectasia, erythema, papules, and pustules that occur particularly in the central area of the face (Fig. 8-51)
- Although rosacea resembles acne, comedones are never present.
- Tissue hypertrophy of the nose (rhinophyma) may occur, characterized by sebaceous hyperplasia, redness, prominent vascularity, and swelling of the skin of the nose (Fig. 8-52).

FIGURE 8-51 Rosacea. *(From White, 1994.)*

FIGURE 8-52 Rhinophyma. *(Courtesy Michael O. Murphy, MD; from White, 1994.)*

Herpes Zoster (Shingles)

Varicella-zoster viral (VZV) infection

Pathophysiology

- VZV morphologically and antigenically identical to the virus causing varicella (chickenpox)
- Dormant viral particles (since the original episode of varicella) in the posterior spinal ganglia or cranial sensory ganglia become activated

Subjective Data

- Pain, itching, or burning of the dermatome area usually precedes eruption by 4 to 5 days.

Objective Data

- Single dermatome that consists of red, swollen plaques or vesicles that become filled with purulent fluid (Fig. 8-53)

FIGURE 8-53 Herpes zoster (shingles) confined to one dermatome. *(From Lemmi and Lemmi, 2000.)*

Herpes Simplex

Infection by herpes simplex virus (HSV)

Pathophysiology

- Two different virus types cause the infection: type 1, usually associated with oral infection, and type 2, with genital infection.
- Crossover infections are becoming common.

Subjective Data

- Tenderness, pain, paresthesia, or mild burning at the infected site before onset of the lesions

Objective Data

- Grouped vesicles appear on an erythematous base and then erode, forming a crust (Fig. 8-54).
- Lesions last 2 to 6 weeks.

FIGURE 8-54 Herpes simplex. **A,** Oral. **B,** Female genital. **C,** Male genital. *(A, from Salvo, 2009; B, from Swartz, 2010; C, from Morse et al, 1996.)*

Lyme Disease

A tick-borne disease that can lead to multisystemic infection

Pathophysiology

- Spirochetal infection caused by *Borrelia burgdorferi*
- Most common tick-borne disease in the United States
- The spirochete is deposited by the tick into the skin rather than directly into the bloodstream.
- Three phases of the disease are recognized: early localized, early disseminated, and late disease.
- The objective clinical manifestations are thought to be due to an inflammatory response to live spirochetes or to their antigens.

Subjective Data

- Exposure to ticks
- Constitutional symptoms of fatigue, anorexia, and headache may develop.

Objective Data

- Early localized infection typically manifested by a single erythema migrans skin lesion, a flat to slightly raised, erythematous skin lesion (usually ≥5 cm in diameter) that is round or oval in shape, with central clearing (Fig. 8-55)
- Early disseminated infection usually manifested by multiple erythema migrans skin lesions, by neurologic symptoms such as facial palsy, meningitis, or encephalitis or by symptoms of carditis such as lightheadedness, palpitations, dyspnea, chest pain, or syncope
- Late disease usually manifested by arthritis atrophicans

FIGURE 8-55 Erythema migrans (lyme disease).

ABNORMALITIES

SKIN: CUTANEOUS REACTIONS

Drug Eruptions

Pathophysiology

- Immunologically mediated cutaneous reactions to medications include immunoglobulin E (IgE)–dependent, cytotoxic, immune complex, and cell-mediated hypersensitivity reactions.
- Nonimmunologically mediated reactions include direct release of mast cell mediators and idiosyncratic reactions.

Subjective Data

- Rash appears from 1 to several days after taking a drug
- Pruritus characteristic

Objective Data

- Most common: discrete or confluent erythematous macules and papules on the trunk, face, extremities, palms, or soles of the feet (Fig. 8-56)
- Rash fades in 1 to 3 weeks

FIGURE 8-56 Drug eruption. *(From Zaoutis and Chiang 2007.)*

Acanthosis Nigricans (AN)

A nonspecific reaction pattern associated with obesity, certain endocrine syndromes, or malignancies or as an inherited disorder

Pathophysiology

- Insulin resistance and hyperinsulinism may lead to an activation of insulin-like growth factor receptors, promoting epidermal growth.
- Inherited form: rare, autosomal dominant trait with no obesity or associated endocrinopathies
- Malignant form: results from secretion of tumor products with insulin-like activity or transforming growth factor alpha, which stimulates keratinocytes to proliferate

Subjective Data

- May report history of obesity, endocrine disorders
- With a rise in childhood obesity, this is seen more often in children and adolescents.
- Appearance in older adult associated with malignancy

Objective Data

- Symmetric, brown thickening of the skin with plaques or patches of thickened skin with a velvety or slightly verrucous texture (Fig. 8-57)
- Lesions range in severity from slight discoloration of a small area to extensive involvement of wide areas.
- Most common site of involvement is the axillae, but the changes may be observed in other flexural areas of the neck, groin, and arms.
- Involvement of the dorsal and palmar hands or mucosal surfaces may indicate malignant association.

FIGURE 8-57 Acanthosis nigricans. *(From Lemmi and Lemmi, 2009.)*

SKIN: DISEASE CAUSED BY BIOLOGIC WARFARE

Of the numerous biologic agents that may be used as weapons, a limited number produce skin lesions. The Differential Diagnosis table below describes the cutaneous manifestations from two such pathogens.

DIFFERENTIAL DIAGNOSIS

Cutaneous Manifestations of Two Pathogens That May Be Used in Biologic Warfare

Disease	Pathogen	Communicability	Incubation	Skin Lesions	Accompanying Symptoms
Cutaneous anthrax* Anthrax (Skin Form). A Gram-stained smear of material taken from the lesion will reveal the gram-positive rods of *Bacillus anthracis*. *(From Beeching and Nye, 1996.)*	Spore-forming bacterium *Bacillus anthracis*	Direct person-to-person spread extremely unlikely Anthrax commonly infects herbivorous mammals who can ingest or inhale the spores while grazing. Diseased animals can spread anthrax to humans, either by direct contact (e.g., inoculation of infected blood to broken skin) or by consumption of a diseased animal's flesh.	Up to 12 days following deposition of organism into skin with previous abrasion	Pruritic macule or papule that enlarges into a round ulcer by day 2. Central necrosis develops with a painless ulcer covered by black eschar, which dries and falls off in 1 to 2 weeks. May be accompanied by 1- to 3-mm vesicles that discharge clear or serosanguineous fluid.	Lymphangitis; lymphadenopathy
Smallpox Smallpox. This archival photograph shows eczema vaccinatum acquired from a relative who had recently been vaccinated against smallpox. *(From Beeching and Nye, 1996.)*	Variola virus	Direct transmission by infected saliva droplets. Most infectious during the first week of illness. However, some risk of transmission lasts until all scabs have fallen off. Contaminated clothing or bed linen could also spread the virus.	12 days (range: 7 to 17 days) following exposure	Rash appears 2 to 3 days after systemic symptoms, first on the mucosa of the mouth and pharynx, face and forearms, spreading to the trunk and legs. Starts with flat red lesions that evolve at the same rate (compared with varicella, which matures in crops). Lesions become vesicular, then pustular, and begin to crust early in the second week.	Initial systemic symptoms include high fever, fatigue, headache, and backache.

*Respiratory and gastrointestinal forms of anthrax also exist.

ABNORMALITIES

SKIN: MALIGNANT/NEOPLASTIC ABNORMALITIES

Basal Cell Carcinoma

The most common form of skin cancer

Pathophysiology

- Cancer arises in the basal layer of the epidermis
- Occurs in various clinical forms including nodular, pigmented, cystic, sclerosing, and superficial
- Occurs most frequently on exposed parts of the body—the face, ears, neck, scalp, shoulders

Subjective Data

- Persistent sore or lesion that has not healed
- May have crusting
- May itch

Objective Data

- Shiny nodule that is pearly or translucent; may be pink, red, or white, tan, black, or brown (Fig. 8-58)
- Open sore; may have crusting; may bleed
- Reddish patch or irritated area, frequently occurring on the chest, shoulders, arms, or legs
- Pink growth with a slightly elevated rolled border and a crusted indentation in the center; as the growth slowly enlarges, tiny blood vessels may develop on the surface.
- Scarlike area that is white, yellow or waxy, and often has poorly defined borders; the skin appears shiny and taut.

FIGURE 8-58 Two common presentations of basal cell carcinoma. *(From Lemmi and Lemmi, 2000.)*

Squamous Cell Carcinoma

Second most common form of skin cancer

Pathophysiology

- This malignant tumor arises in the epithelium.
- Lesions occur most commonly in sun-exposed areas, particularly the scalp, back of hands, lower lip, and ear; the rim of the ear and the lower lip are especially vulnerable.

Subjective Data

- Persistent sore or lesion that has not healed or that has grown in size
- May have crusting and/or bleeding

Objective Data

- Elevated growth with a central depression (Fig. 8-59)
- Wartlike growth; may have crusting, may bleed
- Scaly red patch with irregular borders may have crusting, may bleed
- Open sore; may have crusting

FIGURE 8-59 Squamous cell carcinoma. *(From Lemmi and Lemmi, 2009.)*

Malignant Melanoma

Lethal form of skin cancer that develops from melanocytes

Pathophysiology

- Melanocytes migrate into the skin, eye, central nervous system, and mucous membrane during fetal development.
- Less than half of the melanomas develop from nevi; the majority arise de novo from melanocytes.
- The exact cause of malignancy is not known; heredity, hormonal factors, ultraviolet light exposure, or an autoimmunologic effect may contribute to causation.

Subjective Data

- New mole or preexisting mole that has changed or is changing
- New pigmented lesion that has irregularities (Fig. 8-60)
- History of melanoma
- History of dysplastic or atypical nevi
- Family history of melanoma (first-degree relative)

Objective Data

- ABCDE changes in moles (Fig. 8-61)
- *A* Asymmetry of lesion. One-half of a mole or birthmark does not match the other
- *B* Borders. Edges are irregular, ragged, notched, or blurred. Pigment may be streaming from the border.
- *C* Color. The color is not the same all over and may have differing shades of brown or black, sometimes with patches of red, white, or blue.
- *D* Diameter. The diameter is >6 mm (about the size of a pencil eraser) or is growing larger.
- *E* Evolution. Changes in existing pigmented lesions, particularly in a nonuniform, asymmetric manner

FIGURE   8-60 Malignant   melanoma. *(Courtesy Walter Tunnessen, MD, University of Pennsylvania, Philadelphia.)*

| Asymmetry | Border | Color | Diameter |

FIGURE 8-61 ABCD changes in moles. *(Reproduced with permission from the American Academy of Dermatology, 2010. All rights reserved.)*

ABNORMALITIES

Kaposi Sarcoma (KS)

A neoplasm of the endothelium and epithelial layer of the skin

Pathophysiology

- Caused by the Kaposi sarcoma herpes virus 8 (KSHV)
- Individuals infected with KSHV are more likely to develop KS if their immune system is compromised.
- Commonly associated with human immunodeficiency virus (HIV) infection

Subjective Data

- Soft bluish purple and painless skin lesions
- May report peripheral lymphedema
- May be presenting symptom of HIV/acquired immune deficiency syndrome (AIDS)

Objective Data

- Cutaneous lesions are characteristically soft, vascular, bluish purple, and painless.
- Lesions may be either macular or papular and may appear as plaques, keloids, or ecchymotic areas (Fig. 8-62).
- KS lesions may be limited to the skin or involve the mucosa, viscera, and lymph nodes or any organ.

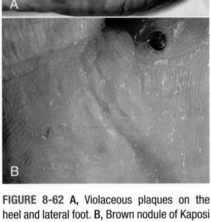

FIGURE 8-62 A, Violaceous plaques on the heel and lateral foot. **B,** Brown nodule of Kaposi sarcoma.

HAIR DISORDERS

Alopecia Areata

Sudden, rapid, patchy loss of hair, usually from the scalp or face

Pathophysiology

- Cause unknown; a genetic–environmental interaction may trigger the disease
- Any hair-bearing surface may be affected.
- Regrowth begins in 1 to 3 months; the prognosis for total regrowth is excellent in cases with limited involvement.

Subjective Data

- Sudden, rapid, patchy hair loss
- May also report nail pitting
- May have family history

Objective Data

- Hair loss is in sharply defined round areas (Fig. 8-63).
- The hair shaft is poorly formed and breaks off at the skin surface.

FIGURE 8-63 Alopecia areata. *(From Lemmi and Lemmi, 2009.)*

Scarring Alopecia

Replacement of hair follicles with scar tissue

Pathophysiology	Subjective Data	Objective Data
• Skin disorders of the scalp or follicles result in scarring and destruction of hair follicles and permanent hair loss.	• May have other concurrent skin or systemic disorders	• Patchy hair loss • Scalp may be inflamed • Hair follicles may be pustular or plugged.

Traction Alopecia

Hair loss that is the result of prolonged, tightly pulled hairstyles

Pathophysiology	Subjective Data	Objective Data
• Prolonged tension of the hair from traction breaks the hair shaft • Follicle is not damaged and the loss is reversible	• History of wearing certain hairstyles such as braids or from using hair rollers and hot combs	• Patchy hair loss that corresponds directly to the area of stress • Scalp may or may not be inflamed

Hirsutism

Growth of terminal hair in women in the male distribution pattern on the face, body, and pubic areas

Pathophysiology	Subjective Data	Objective Data
• Caused by high androgen levels (from ovaries or adrenal glands) or by hair follicles that are more sensitive to normal androgen levels; free testosterone is the androgen that causes hair growth. • Many causes, including genetic, physiologic, endocrine, drug-related, and systemic disorders	• Excessive hair growth on the face or body • Onset, severity, and rate depend on underlying cause	• Presence of thick, dark terminal hairs in androgen-sensitive sites: face, chest, areola, external genitalia, upper and lower back, buttocks, inner thigh, and linea alba (Fig. 8-64) • Hirsutism may or may not be accompanied by other signs of virilization.

FIGURE 8-64 Facial hirsutism. Terminal hair growth is visible on the chin of this 40-year-old woman with idiopathic hirsutism. *(From Lawrence and Cox, 1993.)*

NAILS: INFECTION

Paronychia

Inflammation of the paronychium

Pathophysiology	History	Objective Data
• Invasion of bacteria between the nail fold and the nail plate • Can occur as an acute or chronic process	• Acute: history of nail trauma or manipulation; acute onset • Chronic: history of repeated exposure to moisture, e.g., through hand washing; evolves slowly initially with tenderness and mild swelling	• Redness, swelling, and tenderness at the lateral and proximal nail folds • Purulent drainage often accumulates under the cuticle (Fig. 8-65). • Chronic paronychia can produce rippling of the nails.

FIGURE 8-65 **Paronychia.** *(From Cuppett and Walsh, 2005.)*

Onychomycosis

Fungal infection of the nail

Pathophysiology	Subjective Data	Objective Data
• The fungus grows in the nail plate, causing it to crumble.	• Characteristic nail changes • May report associated discomfort, paresthesia, loss of manual dexterity; may interfere with ability to exercise, or walk	• In the most common form, the distal nail plate turns yellow or white as hyperkeratotic debris accumulates, causing the nail to separate from the nail bed (onycholysis). • Pitting does not occur, distinguishing it from psoriasis (Fig. 8-66).

FIGURE 8-66 **Onychomycosis.** *(From Lemmi and Lemmi, 2009.)*

NAILS: INJURY

Ingrown Nails

Nail pierces the lateral nail fold and grows into the dermis

Pathophysiology	Subjective Data	Objective Data
• Caused by lateral pressure of poorly fitting shoes, improper or excessive trimming of the lateral nail plate, or trauma	• Pain and swelling • History related to cause: tight shoes, excessive trimming, trauma	• Redness and swelling at the area of nail penetration (Fig. 8-67) • Commonly involves the large toe

FIGURE 8-67 **Ingrown toenail.** Swelling and inflammation occur at lateral nail fold. *(From White, 1994.)*

Subungual Hematoma

Trauma to the nail plate severe enough to cause immediate bleeding and pain

Pathophysiology

- Amount of bleeding may be sufficient to cause separation and loss of the nail plate
- Trauma to the proximal nail fold may also cause bleeding that is not apparent for several days.
- Hematoma remains until the nail grows out or is decompressed to release the blood and relieve the pressure.

Subjective Data

- Trauma to the nail
- May be very painful

Objective Data

- Discolored dark nail (Fig. 8-68)

FIGURE 8-68 **Subungual hematoma.** *(From Baren et al, 2008.)*

Onycholysis

Loosening of the nail plate with separation from the nail bed that begins at the distal groove

Pathophysiology

- Associated most commonly with minor trauma to long fingernails
- Other causes include psoriasis, *Candida* or *Pseudomonas* infection, medications, allergic contact dermatitis, and hyperthyroidism.

Subjective Data

- Painless separation of the plate from the bed
- May report history of nail trauma

Objective Data

- Nonadherent portion of the nail opaque with a white, yellow, or green tinge (Fig. 8-69)

FIGURE 8-69 **Onycholysis.** Separation of nail plate starts at distal groove. *(From Scher and Daniel, 2005.)*

ABNORMALITIES

NAILS: CHANGES ASSOCIATED WITH SYSTEMIC DISEASE

Koilonychia (Spoon Nails)

Central depression of the nail with lateral elevation of the nail plate

Pathophysiology

- Associated with iron deficiency anemia, syphilis, fungal dermatoses, and hypothyroidism

Subjective Data

- History consistent with associated disorders

Objective Data

- Concave curvature and spoon appearance (Fig. 8-70; see also Fig. 8-19)

FIGURE 8-70 **Koilonychia.** *(From White, 1994.)*

Beau Lines

Transverse depression in the nail bed

Pathophysiology

- Temporary interruption of nail formation due to systemic disorders
- Associated with coronary occlusion, hypercalcemia, and skin disease

Subjective Data

- History consistent with associated disorders

Objective Data

- Transverse depressions at the bases of the lunulae (crescent-shaped "moon") in all of the nails
- Grooves disappear when the nails grow out (Fig. 8-71).

FIGURE 8-71 **Beau lines following systemic disease.** *(From Lemmi and Lemmi, 2009.)*

White Banding (Terry Nails)

Transverse white bands

Pathophysiology

- Associated with cirrhosis, chronic congestive heart failure, adult-onset diabetes mellitus, and age
- Speculated that it occurs as part of aging and that associated diseases "age" the nail (Habif, 2004)

Subjective Data

- History consistent with associated disorders

Objective Data

- Transverse white bands cover the nail except for a narrow zone at the distal tip (Fig. 8-72).

FIGURE 8-72 **Terry nails; transverse white bands.** *(From Swartz, 2009.)*

Psoriasis

Chronic and recurrent disease of keratin synthesis

Pathophysiology
- Nail involvement usually occurs simultaneously with skin disease but may occur as an isolated finding (see Psoriasis, above, in Skin: Inflammatory and Infectious Conditions)

Subjective Data
- Psoriatic lesions on skin

FIGURE 8-73 Nail pitting. *(From White and Cox, 2000.)*

Objective Data
- Pitting, onycholysis, discoloration, and subungual thickening
- Yellow scaly debris often accumulates, elevating the nail plate
- Severe psoriasis of the matrix and nail bed results in grossly malformed nails and splinter hemorrhages (Fig. 8-73).
- Can be associated with psoriatic arthritis in up to 30% of patients

NAILS: PERIUNGUAL GROWTHS

Warts

Epidermal neoplasms caused by viral infection

Pathophysiology
- Caused by human papilloma virus (HPV)

Subjective Data
- A growth at the nail fold

FIGURE 8-74 Periungual warts. *(From Lawrence and Cox, 1993.)*

Objective Data
- Occur at the nail folds and extend under the nail
- Longitudinal nail groove in the nail may occur from warts located over the nail matrix (Fig. 8-74)

Digital Mucous Cysts

Cystlike structures contain a clear, jelly-like substance

Pathophysiology
- Cysts on the proximal nail fold are not connected to the joint space or tendon sheath; they result from localized fibroblast proliferation; compression of the nail-matrix cells induces a longitudinal nail groove.
- Cysts located on the dorsal-lateral finger at the distal interphalangeal (DIP) joint are probably caused by herniation of tendon sheaths or joint linings and are related to ganglion and synovial cysts.

Subjective Data
- Cyst on the proximal nail fold or dorsal-lateral aspect of distal finger

FIGURE 8-75 Digital mucous cysts causing a groove in the nail plate. *(From White, 1994.)*

Objective Data
- Cyst containing clear substance
- Longitudinal nail groove may occur from cysts located at the proximal nail fold (Fig. 8-75)

ABNORMALITIES

✂ Pregnant Women

Pruritic Urticarial Papules and Plaques of Pregnancy (PUPPP)

A benign dermatosis that usually arises late in the third trimester of a first pregnancy

Pathophysiology	Subjective Data	Objective Data
• Etiology of PUPPP unclear • Immunologic mechanisms, hormonal abnormalities, and abdominal skin distention have been suggested as etiologic mechanisms (Brzoza, 2007) • Relationship between the maternal immune system and fetal cells has been proposed (Tunzi and Gray, 2007) • Eruption usually resolves promptly after delivery and does not usually recur in subsequent pregnancies	• Intensely pruritic rash that began on the abdomen • After a few days, the eruption spreads to the thighs, buttocks, and arms.	• Erythematous, urticaria-like papules and plaques on abdomen, thighs, buttock, arms • Periumbilical area is spared • Usually no lesions on face, palms, or soles • Often halos of blanching surround the papules • Small vesicles may be present but larger bullae do not occur and would suggest the more rare herpes gestationis.

Herpes Gestationis (Pemphigoid Gestationis)

Rare autoimmune disorder of pregnancy

Pathophysiology	Subjective Data	Objective Data
• Condition not related to the herpes virus infection; it was named on the basis of the clinical feature of herpetiform blisters. • Etiology unknown, considered as an autoimmune-mediated dermatosis closely related to the pemphigoid group • Can have severe complications for the pregnant woman; the mother can develop necrosis of affected skin as well as kidney damage.	• Intense unrelenting pruritus • Increased risk of other autoimmune diseases	• Initial clinical manifestations are erythematous urticarial patches and plaques, which typically are periumbilical. • Lesions progress to tense vesicles and blisters. • Palms and soles frequently affected • Infants can be born with this rash, but it usually clears up within a few weeks of birth without treatment.

✂ Infants and Children

Seborrheic Dermatitis

Chronic, recurrent, erythematous scaling eruption localized in areas where sebaceous glands are concentrated (e.g., scalp, back, and intertriginous and diaper areas)

Pathophysiology	Subjective Data	Objective Data
• Little known about cause; however, an overabundance of or an inappropriate immune reaction to a common species of *Malassezia* (formerly *Pityrosporum*) has been suggested (Dattner, 2012). • Condition most commonly occurs in infants within the first 3 months of life	• Parent reports thick greasy scalp scales or body rash • No associated symptoms	• Scalp lesions are scaling, adherent, thick, yellow, and crusted ("cradle cap") and can spread over the ear and down the nape of the neck (Fig. 8-76). • Lesions elsewhere are erythematous, scaling, and fissured.

FIGURE 8-76 Pustular seborrheic dermatitis. *(From Lemmi and Lemmi, 2000.)*

Miliaria Rubra ("Prickly Heat")

Pathophysiology

- Caused by sweat retention from occlusion of sweat ducts during periods of heat and high humidity
- Results from immaturity of skin structures
- Overdressed babies are susceptible to this condition in the summer.

Subjective Data

- Parent reports rash noted when undressing the infant

Objective Data

- Irregular, red, macular rash, usually on covered areas of the skin (Fig. 8-77)

FIGURE 8-77 Miliaria in infant. *(From Habif, 2004.)*

Impetigo

Common, contagious superficial skin infection

Pathophysiology

- Caused by staphylococcal or streptococcal infection and/or infection of the epidermis

Subjective Data

- Lesion, typically on the face, that itches and burns
- Also on other parts of body associated with minor injuries or insect bites

Objective Data

- Initial lesion is a small erythematous macule that changes into a vesicle or bulla with a thin roof.
- Lesion crusts with a characteristic honey color from the exudate as the vesicles or bullae rupture (Fig. 8-78)
- May have regional lymphadenopathy

FIGURE 8-78 Impetigo. Note characteristic crusting. *(From Lemmi and Lemmi, 2009.)*

Acne Vulgaris

Pathophysiology

- Androgens stimulate the pilosebaceous units at the time of puberty to enlarge and produce large amounts of sebum.
- Simultaneously, the keratinization process in the pilosebaceous canal is disrupted with impaction and obstruction of the outflow of sebum resulting in comedo formation—open blackheads and closed whiteheads.
- Wall of the closed comedo may rupture, spilling the follicular contents into the dermis, leading to the development of inflammatory papules.
- The presence of *Propionibacterium acnes* brings in neutrophils, which cause the inflammatory response.

Subjective Data

- Most commonly reported by adolescent
- May occur initially as an adult or continue into the adult years
- Patient reports comedones (plugged follicles—blackheads and whiteheads), papules, and pustules over the forehead, nose, cheeks, lower face, chest, and back that evolve on the face, chest, and back

Objective Data

- Noninflammatory acne: comedones
- Inflammatory acne: papules or nodules (Fig. 8-79)
- Characteristic "ice pick" scarring may be present from previous lesions

FIGURE 8-79 Acne in dolescent. *(From Swartz, 2006.)*

Chickenpox (Varicella)

Acute, highly communicable disease common in children and young adults

Pathophysiology

- Caused by the varicella zoster virus (VZV)
- VZV is communicable by direct contact, droplet transmission, and airborne transmission
- Incubation period 2 to 3 weeks; the period of communicability lasts from 1 or 2 days before onset of the rash until lesions have crusted over.
- Preventable by immunization
- After primary infection, VZV remains dormant in sensory nerve roots for life.

Subjective Data

- Fever, headache, sore throat, mild malaise
- Pruritic rash that started on scalp and then moved to extremities
- Started as maculopapular and in a few hours became vesicular
- Child has not had varicella vaccine.

Objective Data

- Maculopapular and vesicular lesions on trunk, extremities, face, buccal mucosa, palate, or conjunctivae (Fig. 8-80)
- Lesions usually occur in successive outbreaks, with several stages of maturity present at one time.
- Complications include conjunctival involvement, secondary bacterial infection, viral pneumonia, encephalitis, aseptic meningitis, myelitis, Guillain-Barré syndrome, and Reye syndrome.

FIGURE 8-80 Varicella (Chickenpox). Note vesicular lesions. *(From Lemmi and Lemmi, 2000.)*

Measles (Rubeola)

Also called hard measles or red measles

Pathophysiology

- Measles virus infects by invasion of the respiratory epithelium
- Local multiplication at the respiratory mucosa leads to a primary viremia, during which the virus spreads in leukocytes to the reticuloendothelial system.
- Both endothelial and epithelial cells are infected; infected tissues include thymus, spleen, lymph nodes, liver, skin, conjunctiva, and lung.
- Incubation period is commonly 18 days; the period of communicability lasts from a few days before the fever to 4 days after appearance of the rash.
- Disease preventable by immunization

Subjective Data

- Fever, conjunctivitis, stuffy nose, and cough, followed by a red, blotchy rash first on the face and then spreading to trunk and extremities
- Child has not had measles vaccine.
- International travel or exposure to individuals from endemic areas

Objective Data

- Koplik spots (discrete white macular lesions) on the buccal mucosa
- Macular rash develops on the face and neck.
- Maculopapular lesions on trunk and extremities in irregular confluent patches
- Rash lasts 4 to 7 days (Fig. 8-81)
- Symptoms may be mild or severe
- Complications involve infection of the respiratory tract and central nervous system.

FIGURE 8-81 Rubeola. *(From Zitelli and Davis, 1997.)*

German Measles (Rubella)

Mild, febrile, highly communicable viral disease

Pathophysiology

- Spread in droplets that are shed from respiratory secretions of infected persons
- Patients are most contagious while the rash is erupting, but they may shed virus from the throat from 10 days before until 15 days after the onset of the rash.
- Incubation period is 14 to 23 days
- Disease preventable by immunization

Subjective Data

- Low-grade fever, stuffy nose, sore throat, and cough
- This is followed by a macular rash on the face and trunk that rapidly becomes papular.

Objective Data

- Generalized light pink to red maculopapular rash
- By the second day, rash spreads to the upper and lower extremities; it fades within 3 days.
- Reddish spots occur on the soft palate during the prodrome or on the first day of the rash (Forschheimer spots) (Fig. 8-82).
- Infection during the first trimester of pregnancy may lead to infection of the fetus and may produce a variety of congenital anomalies (congenital rubella syndrome).

FIGURE 8-82 **Rubella (German measles). A,** Note the pinkish red, maculopapular eruption. **B,** Red palatal lesions (Forschheimer spots) are seen in some patients on day 1 of the rash. *(Courtesy Dr. Michael Sherlock; from Zitelli and Davis, 1997.)*

Hair-Pulling (Trichotillomania)

Loss of scalp hair can be caused by physical manipulation

Pathophysiology

- Hair is twisted around the finger and pulled or rubbed until it breaks off; the act of manipulation is usually an unconscious habit.

Subjective Data

- May report tension, anxiety, emotional stressors

Objective Data

- Affected area has an irregular border, and hair density is greatly reduced, but the site is not bald (Fig. 8-83)

FIGURE 8-83 **Trichotillomania.** *(From Paller and Mancini, 2011.)*

ABNORMALITIES

Patterns of Injury in Physical Abuse

Physical findings in children who are physically abused include bruises, burns, lacerations, scars, bony deformities, alopecia, retinal hemorrhages, dental trauma, and head and abdominal injuries. Skin and hair abnormalities may be the most visible clues in detecting this problem. It is important to examine the skin that is usually covered by clothing. Some skin and hair findings commonly associated with physical abuse are described in the following paragraphs.

- *Bruises:* These may be patterned consistent with the implement used, such as belt marks (Fig. 8-84), marks from a looped electric cord, and oval or fingertip grab marks. Bruising associated with abuse occurs over soft tissue; toddlers and older children who bruise themselves accidentally do so over bony prominences. Any bruise in an infant who is not yet developmentally able to be mobile should be cause for concern.
- *Lacerations:* Lacerations of the frenulum and lips are associated with forced feeding. Human bites can cause breaks in the skin and leave a characteristic bite mark.
- *Burns:* Patterns that are common include scald burns in stocking and glove distribution (when hands or feet are placed on hot surface or immersed); buttock burns consistent with immersion (Fig. 8-85); and cigarette burns (Fig. 8-86), a characteristic small, round burn, often on areas hidden by clothing. The absence of splash marks or a pattern consistent with spills of hot liquids may be helpful in differentiating accidental from deliberate burns.
- *Hair loss:* Patchy hair loss or bald spots, in the absence of a scalp disorder such as ringworm, may indicate repeated hair-pulling.

FIGURE 8-84 This contusion in the configuration of a closed horseshoe with a central linear abrasion was inflicted with a belt buckle. *(From Zitelli and Davis, 1997.)*

FIGURE 8-85 Burns on the perineum, thighs, legs, and feet. *(Courtesy Dr. Thomas Layton, Mercy Hospital, Pittsburgh; from Zitelli and Davis, 1997.)*

FIGURE 8-86 Cigarette burn. This older burn has begun to granulate. *(From Zitelli and Davis, 1997.)*

✤ Older Adults

Stasis Dermatitis

Pathophysiology

- Occurs on the lower legs in some patients with venous insufficiency
- Incompetent venous valves, inadequate tissue support, and postural hydrostatic pressure contribute to the development of venous stasis.
- Dermatologic changes secondary to the effects of extravasated blood, which induces a mild inflammatory response in the dermis and subcutaneous fat
- Most patients with venous insufficiency do not develop dermatitis, which suggests that genetic or environmental factors may play a role.
- May occur as an allergic response to an epidermal protein antigen created through increased hydrostatic pressure, or because the skin has been compromised and is more susceptible to irritation and trauma (Habif, 2004)

Subjective Data

- Sense of fullness or dull aching in the lower legs and ankles
- Gradual increase in pigmentation and redness
- Area may be itchy and/or painful

FIGURE 8-87 Stasis dermatitis in older adult. *(From Swartz, 2009.)*

Objective Data

- Erythematous, scaling, weeping patches on lower extremity; ulceration may be present (Fig. 8-87).
- Dermatitis may be acute, subacute, or chronic and recurrent.

Solar Keratosis (Actinic Keratosis)

Squamous cell carcinoma confined to the epidermis

Pathophysiology

- Occurs secondary to chronic sun damage
- Most lesions remain superficial; lesions that extend more deeply to involve the papillary and/or reticular dermis are termed *squamous cell carcinoma*.

Subjective Data

- History of chronic sun exposure
- Increasing number of lesions with age

FIGURE 8-88 Actinic keratosis in older adult in area of sun exposure. *(From Busam, 2009.)*

Objective Data

- Slightly raised erythematous lesion that is usually less than 1 cm in diameter with an irregular, rough surface
- Lesion is most common on the dorsal surface of the hands, arms, neck, and face (Fig. 8-88)

Physical Abuse in Older Adults

Abuse in older adults can assume the form of physical abuse, neglect, sexual abuse, psychologic abuse, financial abuse, or violation of rights. Physical neglect is probably the most common type of abuse encountered by health care professionals. However, be aware that when one form of abuse is present, it is typically accompanied by other forms.

Physical abuse and neglect may present with clues that aid in detection. Assessment of general appearance may indicate poor hygiene, emaciation, healed fractures with deformity, and unexplained trauma. Carefully inspect the skin, particularly on hidden areas such as the axillae, inner thighs, soles of the feet, palms, and abdomen; look for bruising, burns, abrasions, or areas of tenderness. Bruising on extensor surfaces is common and usually occurs accidentally; bruising at various stages of resolution located on inner soft surfaces is more likely to indicate abuse.

Careful history taking is essential. When abuse is suspected, it is important to ask direct questions, such as "Is anyone hurting or harming you?" or "Have you been confined against your will?" This questioning should occur in a private setting away from accompanying family members or caregivers. Determination of mental status is also essential (see Chapter 5) because unintended self-neglect or abuse is also possible. If the patient is cognitively impaired, abuse by another may still be present but needs to be corroborated.

CHAPTER 9

Lymphatic System

The lymphatic system is examined region by region during the examination of the other body systems (i.e., head and neck, breast and axillary, genitalia, and extremities) and by palpating the spleen. Sometimes you may perform a comprehensive lymphatic examination, exploring all the areas in which the nodes are accessible. Individual chapters in this book discuss the lymphatic system in specific body areas.

evolve *http://evolve.elsevier.com/Seidel*
- Physical Exam Key Points
- NCLEX Review Questions
- Interactive Activities
- Animations
- Videos
- Student Checklist

Physical Examination Preview

Here is a preview of the steps involved in conducting physical examination of the lymphatic system. ⓔ These procedures are explained in detail in this chapter and are available on Evolve in printable formats.

Lymphatic System

1. Inspect the visible nodes and surrounding area for the following characteristics (p. 172):
   - Edema
   - Erythema
   - Red streaks
2. Palpate the superficial lymph nodes and compare side to side for the following (p. 173):
   - Size
   - Consistency
   - Mobility
   - Discrete borders or matting
   - Tenderness
   - Warmth

If you discover an enlarged node, consider the associated region drained by the node to suggest possible sources for a presenting problem.

ANATOMY AND PHYSIOLOGY

The lymphatic system consists of lymph fluid, the collecting ducts, and various tissues including the lymph nodes, spleen, thymus, tonsils, adenoids, and Peyer patches in the small intestine. Bits of lymph tissue are found in other parts of the body including the mucosa of the stomach and appendix, bone marrow, and lungs (Fig. 9-1). Functions of the lymphatic system include conserving fluid and plasma that leak from capillaries, defending the body against disease as part of the immune system, and absorbing lipids from the intestinal tract.

The immune system protects the body from the antigenic substances of invading organisms, removes damaged cells from the circulation, and provides a partial—but often inefficient—barrier to the maturation of malignant cells within the body. When it functions well, the individual has a competent immune system with a normal immune response to antigen exposure. Tissue rejection of transplanted organs is an unwelcome manifestation of immunocompetence. When the immune system fails, the individual may experience a variety of illnesses, such as an allergic reaction or an immunodeficiency—either congenital or acquired (e.g., infection with human immunodeficiency virus [HIV]), or autoimmune, that is allergy to oneself (e.g., systemic lupus erythematosus). An integral part of the immune system, the lymphatic system supports a network of defenses against microorganisms.

Except for the placenta and the brain, every tissue supplied by blood vessels has lymphatic vessels. This wide-ranging presence is essential to the system's role in immunologic and metabolic processes. That role involves the following:

- Movement of lymph fluid within the cardiovascular system, a major factor in the maintenance of fluid balance. Without lymphatic drainage, fluid would build up in interstitial spaces because more fluid leaves capillaries than veins can absorb.
- Filtration of fluid before it is returned to the bloodstream, filtering out substances that could be harmful to the body, and filtering microorganisms from the blood
- Phagocytosis—the ingestion and digestion by cells of solid substances such as other cells, bacteria, and bits of dead tissue or foreign particles—is a specific function of cells in lymph nodes
- Production of lymphocytes within the lymph nodes, tonsils, adenoids, spleen, and bone marrow
- Production of antibodies
- Absorption of fat and fat-soluble substances from the intestinal tract

In addition, the lymphatic system plays an undesirable role in providing at least one pathway for the spread of malignancy.

Lymph is a clear, sometimes milky-colored or yellow-tinged fluid. It contains a variety of white blood cells (mostly lymphocytes) and, on occasion, red blood cells. The lymphatic and cardiovascular systems are intimately related. The fluids and proteins that constitute lymphatic fluid move from the bloodstream into the interstitial spaces. They are then collected throughout the body by a profusion of microscopic tubules (Fig. 9-2). These tubules unite, forming larger ducts that collect lymph and carry it to the lymph nodes around the body.

The lymph nodes receive lymph from the collecting ducts in the various regions (Figs. 9-3 to 9-11), passing it on through efferent vessels. Ultimately, the large ducts merge into the venous system at the subclavian veins.

The drainage point for the right upper body is a lymphatic trunk that empties into the right subclavian vein. The thoracic duct, the major vessel of the lymphatic system, drains lymph from the rest of the body into the left subclavian vein. It returns the various fluids and proteins to the cardiovascular system, forming a closed but porous circle.

The lymphatic system has no built-in pumping mechanisms of its own. Because it depends on the cardiovascular system for this, the movement of lymph is sluggish compared with that of blood. As lymph fluid volume increases, it flows faster in response to mounting capillary pressure, greater permeability of the capillary walls of the cardiovascular system, increased bodily or metabolic activity, and mechanical compression. Conversely, mechanical obstruction will slow or stop the movement of lymph, dilating the system. The permeability of the lymphatic system is protective; if it is obstructed, lymph may diffuse into the vascular system, or collateral connecting channels may develop.

Lymph Nodes

Lymph nodes are discrete structures surrounded by a capsule composed of connective tissue and a few elastic fibrils. Lymph nodes usually occur in groups. Superficial nodes are located in subcutaneous connective tissues, and deeper nodes lie beneath the

FIGURE 9-1 Lymphatic system (lymphoreticular system).

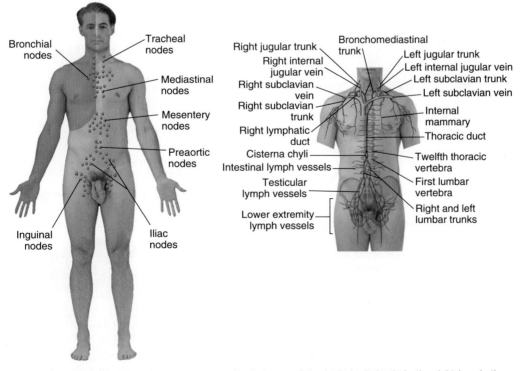

FIGURE 9-2 Lymphatic drainage pathways. Shaded area of the body is drained via the right lymphatic duct, which is formed by the union of three vessels: right jugular trunk, right subclavian trunk, and right bronchomediastinal trunk. Lymph from the remainder of the body enters the venous system by way of the thoracic duct.

ANATOMY AND PHYSIOLOGY

FIGURE 9-3 Lymphatic drainage of lower extremity.

Superior superficial inguinal nodes
Deep sublinguinal node
Inferior superficial inguinal nodes
Great saphenous lymphatic vessels
ANTERIOR VIEW
POSTERIOR VIEW
Popliteal nodes
Small saphenous lymphatic vessels

Preaortic nodes
Common iliac nodes
External iliac nodes
Deep inguinal nodes
Preaortic nodes
Internal iliac nodes
Obturator nodes
Superficial inguinal nodes

FIGURE 9-4 Lymphatic drainage of female genital tract.

Central axillary
Subclavian
Brachial
Mammary (Rotter nodes)
Subscapular
External mammary (anterior pectoral)

FIGURE 9-6 Six groups of lymph nodes may be distinguished in the axillary fossa.

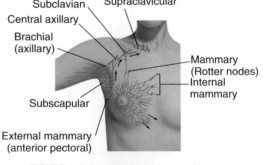

ANTERIOR VIEW
POSTERIOR VIEW
Brachial (axillary) nodes
Epitrochlear nodes
Radial lymphatic vessels
Epitrochlear nodes
Ulnar lymphatic vessels
Median lymphatic vessels
Radial lymphatic vessels

FIGURE 9-5 Systems of Deep and Superficial Collecting Ducts, Carrying Lymph from Upper Extremity to Subclavian Lymphatic Trunk. The only peripheral lymph center is the epitrochlear, which receives some of the collecting ducts from the pathway of the ulnar and radial nerves.

Subclavian
Supraclavicular
Central axillary
Brachial (axillary)
Subscapular
External mammary (anterior pectoral)
Mammary (Rotter nodes)
Internal mammary

FIGURE 9-7 Lymphatic drainage of breast.

fascia of muscles and within the various body cavities. The nodes are numerous and tiny, but some of them may have diameters as large as 0.5 to 1 cm. They defend against the invasion of microorganisms and other particles with filtration and phagocytosis, and they aid in the maturation of lymphocytes and monocytes.

The superficial lymph nodes are the gateway to assessing the health of the entire lymphatic system. Readily accessible to inspection and palpation, they provide some of the earliest clues

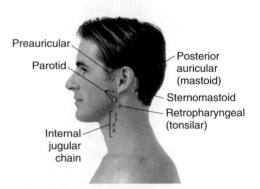

Preauricular
Parotid
Internal jugular chain
Posterior auricular (mastoid)
Sternomastoid
Retropharyngeal (tonsilar)

FIGURE 9-8 Lymph nodes involved with the ear.

Submandibular
Submental
Sublingual
Suprahyoid
Thyrolinguofacial
Internal
jugular chain

FIGURE 9-9 Lymph nodes involved with the tongue.

Preauricular nodes
Parotid
Facial
Submandibular
Submental
Sublingual
Suprahyoid node
Thyrolinguofacial
Anterior deep and superficial cervical
Internal jugular chain

Posterior auricular (mastoid nodes)
Occipital nodes
Sternomastoid nodes
External jugular
Retropharyngeal (tonsillar)
Posterior cervical spinal nerve chain
Posterior superficial cervical chain
Supraclavicular nodes

FIGURE 9-10 Lymphatic drainage system of head and neck. If the group of nodes is commonly referred to by another name, the second name appears in parentheses.

Submandibular
Submental
Suprahyoid
Thyrolinguofacial
Anterior deep and superficial cervical
Posterior superficial cervical
Anterior jugular

Retropharyngeal
Occipital
Posterior cervical spinal nerve chain
Supraclavicular

Internal jugular vein
Sternocleidomastoid muscle

Sternocleidomastoid muscle
Internal jugular chain
Trapezius muscle

FIGURE 9-11 Lymph nodes of neck. Note relationship to the sternocleidomastoid muscle.

to the presence of infection or malignancy (Box 9-1). For example, a palpable supraclavicular node should be suspected as a probable sign of malignancy.

Lymphocytes

Lymphocytes are central to the body's response to antigenic substances. They are not identical in size or function. Some are small, approximately 7 to 8 mm in diameter; others range in size to as much as five times that. They arise from a number of sites in the body, including the lymph nodes, tonsils, adenoids, and spleen, but primarily they are produced in the bone marrow, where early cells (i.e., stem cells) capable of developing in a variety of pathways arise. Lymphocytes that are derived primarily from bone marrow (i.e., B-lymphocytes) produce antibodies and are characterized by the various arrangements of immunoglobulins on their surface.

Marrow-derived cells, which flow first to the thymus, can be further differentiated there as T-lymphocytes. They can sense the difference in cells of the body that have been invaded by foreign substances (e.g., a living virus, bacterium, or parasite; some invasive chemical) or even a malignant change. Found in profusion in the centers of lymph nodes, T-lymphocytes have an important

Box 9-1	The Lymph Nodes Most Accessible to Inspection and Palpation

The more superficial the node, the more accessible it is.

The "Necklace" of Nodes
Parotid and retropharyngeal (tonsillar)
Submandibular
Submental
Sublingual (facial)
Superficial anterior cervical
Superficial posterior cervical
Preauricular and postauricular
Sternocleidomastoid
Occipital
Supraclavicular

The Arms
Axillary
Epitrochlear (cubital)

The Legs
Superficial superior inguinal
Superficial inferior inguinal
Occasionally, popliteal

role in controlling the immune responses brought about by B-lymphocytes. There are two types of immunity: (1) humoral, involving the antibodies produced by B cells; and (2) cellular, involving attacks on "invaders" by the cells themselves. Among lymphocytes, B cells have a relatively short life span of 3 to 4 days. T cells, which are four or five times as numerous as B cells, have a life span of 100 to 200 days. An increased number of lymphocytes in the blood represents a systemic response to most viral infections and to some bacterial infections.

Thymus

The thymus is located in the superior mediastinum, extending upward into the lower neck. In early life, the thymus is essential to the development of the protective immune function (Fig. 9-12). It is the site for production of T-lymphocytes, the cells responsible for cell-mediated immunity reactions and the controlling agent for the humoral immune responses generated by B-lymphocytes. In the adult, however, it has little or no demonstrated function.

Spleen

The spleen is situated in the left upper quadrant of the abdominal cavity between the stomach and the diaphragm. A highly

A Anterior view Lateral view

B Anterior view Lateral view

FIGURE 9-12 Location of thymus gland and its size relative to the rest of the body. **A,** During infancy. **B,** During adult life.

vascular organ, it is composed of two systems: (1) the white pulp, made up of lymphatic nodules and diffuse lymphatic tissue; and (2) the red pulp, made up of venous sinusoids. The spleen has several functions including destroying old red blood cells, producing antibodies, storing red blood cells, and filtering microorganisms from the blood. Its examination, therefore, is essential to the evaluation of the immune system (see Chapter 17).

Tonsils and Adenoids

The palatine tonsils are commonly referred to as "the tonsils." Small and diamond-shaped, they are set between the palatine arches on either side of the pharynx just beyond the base of the tongue. Composed principally of lymphoid tissue, the tonsils are organized as follicles and crypts; both are covered by mucous membrane. The pharyngeal tonsils, or adenoids, are located at the nasopharyngeal border; the lingual tonsils are located near the base of the tongue. Defensive responses to inhaled and intranasal antigens are activated in these tissues. When enlarged, the adenoids and tonsils can obstruct the nasopharyngeal passageway.

Peyer Patches

Peyer patches are small, raised areas of lymph tissue on the mucosa of the small intestine and consist of many clustered lymphoid nodules. Peyer patches are important in immune surveillance in the intestinal tract. They facilitate an immune response when pathogenic microorganisms are detected.

Infants and Children

The immune system and the lymphoid system begin developing at about 20 weeks of gestation The ability to produce antibodies is still immature at birth, increasing the infant's vulnerability to infection during the first few months of life. (see Clinical Pearl, "Umbilical Cord"). The mass of lymphoid tissue is relatively plentiful in infants; increases during childhood, especially between 6 and 9 years of age; then regresses to adult levels by puberty (see Chapter 6, Fig. 6-2).

> **Clinical Pearl**
> *Umbilical Cord*
> The umbilical cord should drop off by 1 to 2 weeks after birth. Delayed umbilical cord separation is associated with leukocyte adhesion defect (LAD), a primary immunodeficiency disorder of phagocytes.

The thymus is at its largest relative to the rest of the body shortly after birth, but reaches its greatest absolute weight at puberty. Then it involutes, replacing much of its tissue with fat and becoming a rudimentary organ in the adult.

The palatine tonsils, like much lymphoid tissue, are much larger during early childhood than after puberty. An enlargement of the tonsils in children is not necessarily an indication of problems.

The lymph nodes have the same distribution in children that they do in adults. The finding of small 2- to 3-mm, discrete, palpable, mobile nodes in the neonate is not unusual. Before 2 years of age, inguinal, occipital, and postauricular nodes are common; after 2 years of age, they are more indicative of a problem. On the other hand, cervical and submandibular nodes are uncommon during the first year and much more common in older children. Supraclavicular nodes are not usually found; their presence, associated with a high incidence of malignancy, is always a cause for concern. Circumcision does not increase the likelihood of inguinal nodes. It is possible that the infant's relatively large mass of lymphoid tissue is needed to compensate for an immature ability to produce antibodies, thus adding to the demand for filtration and phagocytosis.

The lymphatic system gradually reaches adult competency during childhood (Fig. 9-13).

� Pregnant Women

Pregnancy is a state of altered immune function. Implantation and fetal development require changes in the maternal immune system to protect the fetus from maternal immunity yet maintain competence to overcome an infection in the mother. The complex changes are not fully understood, but seem to reflect a balance between enhancement of certain immune mechanisms and suppression of others (Gabbe, 2012).

During pregnancy, the peripheral white blood cell (WBC) count rises progressively from a usual level of about 8000 cells/mm^3 in the first trimester to reach a plateau during the second and third trimesters at a mean level of 8500/mm^3, with a usual range of 5,600 to 12,000/mm^3. This increase is due to circulating segmented neutrophils or granulocytes, possibly due to increased estrogen and cortisol levels. Leukocyte levels return to normal within 1 to 2 weeks of delivery (Gabbe, 2012).

The embryo is an in utero foreign body; however, the mother's hormones and the products of the fetal trophoblast create a unique environment. Uterine contractility decreases and macrophages produce cytokines beneficial to growth of the trophoblast. A balance results. The shift from cell-mediated immunity to antibody production/humoral immunity results in increased maternal susceptibility to certain infectious diseases. However, pregnancy can lead to remission of maternal autoimmune/inflammatory diseases (e.g., rheumatoid arthritis).

✧ Older Adults

The number of lymph nodes may diminish and size may decrease with advanced age; some of the lymphoid structures are lost. The nodes of older patients are more likely to be fibrotic and fatty than those of the young, a contributing factor to impaired ability to resist infection.

REVIEW OF RELATED HISTORY

For each of the symptoms or conditions discussed in this section, targeted topics to include in the history of the present illness are listed. Responses to questions about these topics provide clues for focusing the physical examination and the development of an appropriate diagnostic evaluation. Questions regarding medication use (prescription and over the counter preparations) as well as complementary and alternative therapies are relevant for each.

History of Present Illness

- Enlarged node(s) (lumps, knots, bumps, kernels, swollen glands)
  - Character: onset, location, duration, number, tenderness
  - Associated local symptoms: pain, redness, warmth, red streaks
  - Associated systemic symptoms: malaise, fever, weight loss, night sweats, abdominal pain or fullness, itching (some tumors cause pruritus)
  - Predisposing factors: infection, surgery, trauma
  - Medications: chemotherapy, antibiotics
- Swelling of extremity
  - Unilateral or bilateral, intermittent or constant, duration
  - Predisposing factors: cardiac or renal disorder, surgery, infection, trauma, venous insufficiency
  - Associated symptoms: warmth, redness or discoloration, ulceration
  - Efforts at treatment and their effect: support stockings, elevation

Past Medical History

- Chest imaging; reason and results
- Tuberculosis and other skin testing
- Blood transfusions, use of blood products
- Chronic illness: cardiac, renal, malignancy, HIV infection (see Risk Factors box for HIV infection)
- Surgery: trauma to regional lymph nodes; organ transplant
- Recurrent infections

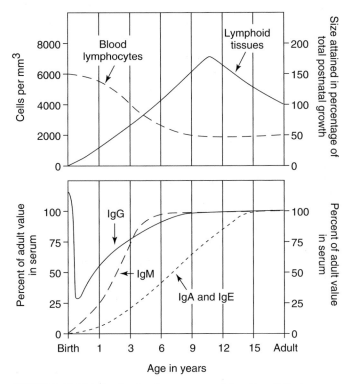

FIGURE 9-13 Relative levels of presence and function of the immune factors.

+ Autoimmune disorder
+ Allergies

Risk Factors

HIV Infection

Adolescents and Adults
Multiple Sexual Contacts
- Prostitution
- Unprotected sexual activity with persons of known history of risk or unknown history
- Sexual activity with intravenous drug users
- Sexual activity with persons infected with HIV
- Sexual activity with homosexual or bisexual men

Intravenous (IV) Drug Use
- Parenteral exposure to HIV blood–contaminated needles and/or syringes
- Sexual activity with IV drug users

Hepatitis, Tuberculosis (TB), or Sexually Transmitted Infection (STI)
- Diagnosis of, or been treated for, hepatitis, TB, or an STI such as syphilis

Blood or Clotting Factor Transfusion
- Transfusion with infected blood or blood concentrates (e.g., factor VIII, factor IX) between 1978 and 1985

Work Related (Rare)
- Puncture of the skin with needles or other sharp objects contaminated with the blood of an HIV-infected patient

Infants and Children
Mother with HIV Infection
- During gestation
- At birth
- During breast-feeding

Sexual Abuse

Family History

+ Malignancy
+ Anemia
+ Recent infectious diseases
+ Tuberculosis
+ Immune disorders
+ Hemophilia

Personal and Social History

+ Travel, especially to Asia, Africa, the Western Pacific, India, Philippines
+ Use of illicit drugs, especially injected
+ Sexual history (risk factors for HIV exposure)

✿ Infants and Children

+ Recurrent infections: tonsillitis, adenoiditis, bacterial infections (e.g., otitis media, cutaneous abscesses, sinus and pulmonary infections), oral candidiasis, chronic diarrhea, chronic severe eczema
+ Present or recent infections, trauma distal to nodes
+ Poor growth, failure to thrive

+ Loss of interest in play or eating
+ Immunization history
+ Maternal HIV infection
+ Hemophilia

✿ Pregnant Women

+ Weeks of gestation
+ Exposure to infections
+ Presence of pets in household (exposure to cat feces or litter)
+ Immunization status: influenza, pneumonia, meningococcal, tetanus/diphtheria/pertussis

✿ Older Adults

+ Presence of an autoimmune disease
+ Present or recent infection or trauma distal to nodes
+ Delayed healing
+ Immunization status: influenza, pneumonia, tetanus/diphtheria/pertussis, shingles (herpes zoster)

EXAMINATION AND FINDINGS

Equipment

+ Centimeter ruler
+ Skin marking pencil

Inspection and Palpation

Disorders of the lymph system present with three physical signs: enlarged lymph nodes (lymphadenopathy), red streaks on the overlying skin (lymphangitis), and lymphedema (Box 9-2). Inspect each area of the body for apparent lymph nodes, edema, erythema, red streaks, and skin lesions. Using the pads of the second, third, and fourth fingers, gently palpate for superficial lymph nodes (see Box 9-1 and Fig. 9-14). Try to detect any hidden enlargement, and note the consistency, mobility, tenderness, size, and warmth of the nodes. In areas where the skin is more mobile, move the skin over the area of the nodes. Press lightly at first, then gradually increase pressure. Heavier pressure

Box 9-2   Terms!

Conditions
Lymphadenopathy (adenopathy)—enlarged lymph node(s)
Lymphadenitis—inflamed and enlarged lymph node(s)
Lymphangitis—inflammation of the lymphatics that drain an area of infection; tender erythematous streaks extend proximally from the infected area; regional nodes may also be tender
Lymphedema—edematous swelling due to excess accumulation of lymph fluid in tissues caused by inadequate lymph drainage
Lymphangioma—congenital malformation of dilated lymphatics

Nodes
Shotty—small non-tender nodes that feel like BBs or buckshot under the skin
Fluctuant—wavelike motion that is felt when the node is palpated
Matted—group of nodes that feel connected and seem to move as a unit

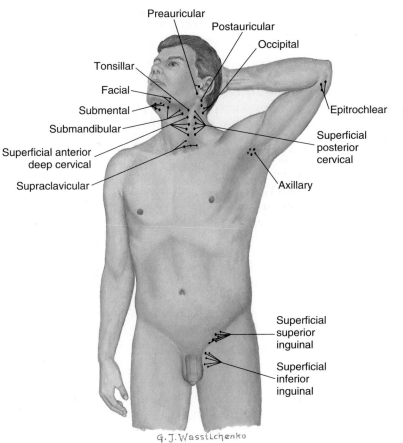

Preauricular
Postauricular
Occipital
Tonsillar
Facial
Submental
Submandibular
Superficial anterior deep cervical
Supraclavicular
Epitrochlear
Superficial posterior cervical
Axillary
Superficial superior inguinal
Superficial inferior inguinal

G. J. Wassilchenko

FIGURE 9-14 Some of the accessible lymph nodes.

alone can push nodes out of the way before you have had a chance to recognize their presence. Easily palpable lymph nodes generally are not found in healthy adults. Superficial nodes that are accessible to palpation but not large or firm enough to be felt are common. You may detect small, movable, discrete, "shotty" nodes (small, multiple nodes that feel like BBs or buckshot under the skin) less than 1 cm in diameter that move under your fingers. Shotty nodes are generally of no clinical consequence and usually represent enlargement of the lymph nodes following viral infection. However, even shotty nodes in the epitrochlear or supraclavicular regions require additional evaluation. A node fixed to surrounding tissues is cause for concern.

When enlarged lymph nodes are encountered, explore the accessible adjacent areas and regions drained by those nodes for signs of possible infection or malignancy. Examine other regions for enlargement. Enlarged lymph nodes in any region should be characterized according to location, size, shape, consistency (fluctuant, soft, firm, hard), tenderness, mobility or fixation to surrounding tissues, and discreteness. Lymph nodes that are enlarged and juxtaposed so that they feel like a large mass rather than discrete nodes are described as "matted." Marking with a skin pencil at the periphery of the node at the 12, 3, 6, and 9 o'clock positions defines the extent of the node and helps guide the assessment of change (see Clinical Pearl, "Reminders about Nodes").

If there is tenderness on touch, note the degree of discoloration or redness and any unusual increase in vascularity, heat, or pulsations. If bruits are audible with the stethoscope, it is a blood vessel, not a lymph node. When you are uncertain of the

Clinical Pearl

Reminders about Nodes

- A hard, fixed, painless node suggests a malignant process.
- The more tender a node, the more likely it is an inflammatory process.
- Nodes do not pulsate; arteries do.
- A palpable supraclavicular node on the left (Virchow node) is a significant clue to thoracic or abdominal malignancy.
- Slow nodal enlargement over weeks and months suggests a benign process; rapid enlargement without signs of inflammation suggests malignancy.

nature of the findings, check whether any large mass transilluminates; as a rule, nodes do not and fluid-filled cysts do.

Lymph nodes that are large, fixed or matted, inflamed, or tender indicate a problem. With bacterial infection, nodes may become warm or tender to the touch, matted, and much less discrete, particularly if the infection persists. It is possible to infer the site of an infection from the pattern of lymph node enlargement. For example, infections of the ear usually drain to the preauricular, retropharyngeal, and deep cervical nodes (see Fig. 9-8).

Lymph nodes to which a malignancy has spread vary greatly in size, from tiny to many centimeters in diameter. They are sometimes discrete, sometimes matted and firmly fixed to underlying tissues; they tend to be harder than expected. Involvement is often asymmetric; contralateral nodes in similar locations may not be palpable.

Fluctuant nodes—nodes that feel like they contain fluid—suggest suppuration from infection. Fixation of the nodes to underlying tissue is most common in metastatic cancer but can also occur with chronic inflammation (see Clinical Pearl, "Not Always Pathology?").

Clinical Pearl

Not Always Pathology

Palpable lymph nodes do not always have a pathologic cause; a submandibular or cervical node less than 1 cm in diameter or an inguinal node less than 2 cm in diameter in an adult may be considered normal. Solitary nodes in other areas are more likely to have a pathologic cause (Armitage, 2012).

Importantly, however, the supraclavicular node that warns of malignancy lies anterior to the sternocleidomastoid muscle.

In tuberculosis, the lymph nodes, often felt in the cervical chains, are usually body temperature, soft, matted, and not tender or painful.

Lymphadenopathy that is widespread, involving several lymph node regions, indicates systemic disease or disorder. Also see Clinical Pearl, "Drugs and Nodes."

Clinical Pearl

Drugs and Nodes

Diphenylhydantoin, particularly, can cause nodal enlargement. So too, on occasion, can aspirin, barbiturates, penicillin, tetracycline, iodide, cephalosporin, sulfonamide, allopurinol, atenolol, captopril, carbamazepine, hydralazine, phenytoin, primidone, pyrimethamine, and quinidine, among others.

The differentiation of an enlarged lymph node from other masses depends on many variables; for example, some sites are incompatible with the distribution of nodes, and some palpable sensations (e.g., thrill, consistency) are not possible with the basic structure of nodes (see the Differential Diagnosis table).

Head and Neck

Lightly palpate the entire neck for nodes. The anterior border of the sternocleidomastoid muscle is the dividing line for the anterior and posterior triangles of the neck and is a useful landmark for describing location. The muscles and bones of the neck together create these "triangles" (Fig. 9-15).

DIFFERENTIAL DIAGNOSIS
Conditions Simulating Lymph Node Enlargement

- Lymphangioma (transilluminates; hemangiomas do not)
- Cystic hygroma (thin-walled, contains clear lymph fluid)
- Hemangioma (tends to feel spongy; appears reddish blue, with color depending on size and extent of blood vessel involvement; Valsalva maneuver may enlarge the mass)
- Branchial cleft cyst (sometimes accompanied by a tiny orifice in the neck along the lower third of the anteromedial border of the sternocleidomastoid muscle between the muscle and the overlying skin; may fluctuate in size when inflamed)
- Thyroglossal duct cyst (midline in the neck; may retract when tongue is protruded)
- Granular cell tumor
- Laryngocele
- Esophageal diverticulum
- Thyroid goiter
- Graves disease
- Hashimoto thyroiditis
- Parotid swelling (e.g., from parotitis or tumor)
- Femoral hernia (below inguinal ligament; protrudes with cough; reducible)

Bending the patient's head slightly forward or to the side will ease taut tissues and allow better accessibility to palpation. Feel for nodes on the head in the following six-step sequence (Fig. 9-16):

1. The occipital nodes at the base of the skull
2. The postauricular nodes located superficially over the mastoid process
3. The preauricular nodes just in front of the ear (Fig. 9-17)
4. The parotid and retropharyngeal (tonsillar) nodes at the angle of the mandible

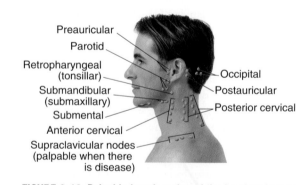

FIGURE 9-16 Palpable lymph nodes of the head and neck.

FIGURE 9-15 The triangles of the neck.

5. The submandibular nodes halfway between the angle and the tip of the mandible
6. The submental nodes in the midline behind the tip of the mandible

Then move down to the neck, palpating in the following four-step sequence:

1. The superficial cervical nodes at the sternocleidomastoid muscle
2. The posterior cervical nodes along the anterior border of the trapezius muscle (Fig. 9-18)
3. The cervical nodes deep to the sternocleidomastoid (the deep cervical nodes may be difficult to feel if you press too vigorously; probe gently with your thumb and fingers around the muscle).
4. The supraclavicular areas, probing deeply in the angle formed by the clavicle and the sternocleidomastoid muscle, the area of Virchow nodes (Fig. 9-19)

On occasion, postauricular nodes associated with ear infection (particularly external otitis) may be surrounded by some cellulitis; this may cause the ears to protrude.

FIGURE 9-17 Palpation of preauricular lymph nodes. Compare the nodes bilaterally.

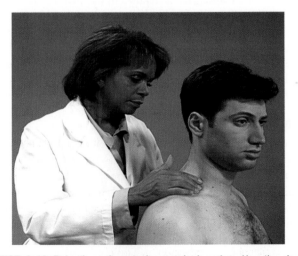

FIGURE 9-18 Palpation of posterior cervical nodes. Use the dorsal surfaces (pads) of the fingertips to palpate along the anterior surface of the trapezius muscle and then move slowly in a circular motion toward the posterior surface of the sternocleidomastoid muscle.

Axillae

Think of the axillary examination by imagining a pentagonal structure: the pectoral muscles anteriorly, the back muscles (i.e., latissimus dorsi and subscapularis) posteriorly, the rib cage medially, the upper arm laterally, and the axilla at the apex. Let the soft tissues roll between your fingers, the chest wall, and muscles as you palpate. A firm, deliberate, yet gentle touch may feel less ticklish to the patient.

On palpation of the axillary lymph nodes, support the patient's forearm with your contralateral arm and bring the palm of your examining hand flat into the axilla; alternatively, let the patient's forearm rest on that of your examining hand (Fig. 9-20). Rotate your fingertips and palm, feeling the nodes; if they are palpable, attempt to glide your fingers beneath the nodes (see Clinical Pearl, "Vaccinations and Nodes"). A more complete examination of the breast, the axilla, and adjacent areas is described in Chapter 16.

Epitrochlear Lymph Nodes

To palpate the epitrochlear nodes, support the arm in one hand as you explore the elbow with the other. Grasp the patient's

FIGURE 9-19 Palpation for supraclavicular lymph nodes. Encourage the patient to relax the musculature of the upper extremities so that the clavicles drop. The examiner's free hand is used to flex the patient's head forward to relax the soft tissues of the anterior neck. The fingers are hooked over the clavicle lateral to the sternocleidomastoid muscle.

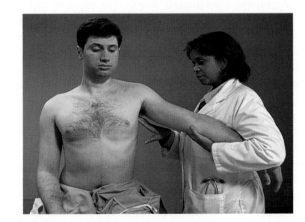

FIGURE 9-20 Soft tissues of axilla are gently rolled against the chest wall and the muscles surrounding the axilla.

FIGURE 9-21 Palpation for epitrochlear lymph nodes is performed in the depression above and posterior to the medial condyle of the humerus.

Clinical Pearl

Vaccinations and Nodes

Immunizations, particularly BCG and smallpox vaccination, administered in the upper arm may cause temporary axillary node enlargement. Rarely, HPV vaccination may cause node enlargement in the head and neck region (Studdiford et al, 2008).

Video: Lymphatic System: Palpating the Inguinal Lymph Nodes

right wrist, palm facing up, with your left hand. The elbow should be in a relaxed position at approximately 90 degrees. Place your right hand under the patient's right elbow and cup your fingers around the elbow to find the area that is proximal and slightly anterior to the medical epicondyle of the humerus. There is a groove between the triceps and biceps muscles. Palpate that groove with your fingers using a circular motion (Fig. 9-21). Repeat using your left hand for the patient's left elbow. An enlarged node can indicate local infection or systemic illness.

Inguinal and Popliteal Lymph Nodes

Use a systematic approach when palpating sites of lymph node clusters. Move the hand in a circular fashion, probing gently without pressing hard. Relieve tension by flexion of the extremity.

To palpate the inguinal and popliteal area, have the patient lie supine with the knee slightly flexed. The superior superficial inguinal (femoral) nodes are close to the surface over the inguinal canals. The inferior superficial inguinal nodes lie deeper in the groin (Fig. 9-22).

The lymphatic drainage of the testes is into the abdomen. Enlarged nodes there are not accessible to inspection and palpation. Nodes in the inguinal area enlarge if there are lesions of the penile and scrotal surfaces. Similarly, the internal female genitalia drain into the pelvic and para-aortic nodes and are not accessible to inspection and palpation; however, the vulva and lower third of the vagina drain into the inguinal nodes. Enlargement of the inguinal nodes suggests infection or metastatic carcinoma in the associated anatomic area. To examine the popliteal nodes, relax the posterior popliteal fossa by flexing the knee. Wrap your hand around the knee and palpate the fossa with your fingers.

FIGURE 9-22 A, Palpation of inferior superficial inguinal (femoral) lymph nodes. **B,** Palpation of superior inguinal lymph nodes.

Staying Well

Hold Back on Invasive Procedures

One way to help patients to keep well is to judiciously limit the number of invasive tests and procedures ordered. Psychologic discomfort and physical discomfort are frequent companions to invasive procedures. The best way to ensure that we avoid the unnecessary discomfort is to perform a knowledgeable and skilled history and physical examination. There are many indications in this chapter for the biopsy of suspicious lymph nodes, but just as importantly—perhaps more so—indications to resist biopsy.

Spleen

Examination of the spleen is detailed in Chapter 17. The spleen is involved in all systemic inflammations, generalized hematopoietic disorders, and many metabolic disturbances. In each of these situations, the spleen enlarges. When sufficiently enlarged, the patient may report a pain or a heavy sensation in the left upper quadrant. Massive splenomegaly may cause early satiety or discomfort after eating.

⚘ Infants and Children

The technique of examination is similar for all ages. You may find small, firm, discrete, and movable nodes that are neither warm nor tender located in the occipital, postauricular, cervical, and inguinal chains. Inguinal nodes may even be readily visible in a very thin child. In children, such nodes are not as worrisome as in the adult. Their shape is usually globular or ovoid, sometimes flatter or more cylindrical.

Lymph node enlargement in children is a more common finding compared to adults. In the well child, they are typically not warm, tender, or fluctuant; do not mat together; are not associated with erythema; and have not been demonstrated to be associated with serious illness. It is not unusual to find enlarged postauricular and occipital nodes in children younger than 2 years of age. Past that age, such enlargement is relatively uncommon and may be significant (see the Differential Diagnosis boxes for mumps and for immune deficiency disease in a child). Conversely, cervical and submandibular nodal enlargement is relatively less common in children younger than 1 year of age and much more common in older children (see Clinical Pearl, "Cervical Nodes"). These age distributions should be considered in your decision to further evaluate lymph node enlargement. The discovery of small lymph nodes in the inguinal, cervical, or axillary chains of neonates may not in itself require further investigation (Box 9-3). In general, laboratory tests are not indicated in otherwise well children who have cervical lymphadenopathy.

DIFFERENTIAL DIAGNOSIS
Mumps Versus Cervical Adenitis

Mumps, epidemic parotitis, is characterized by a somewhat painful swelling of the parotid glands unilaterally or bilaterally and, occasionally, by swelling and tenderness of the other salivary glands along the mandible. The swelling can obscure the angle of the jaw and may appear on inspection as a cervical adenitis. On palpation, however, the two are easily distinguished. A cervical adenitis does not ordinarily obscure the angle of the jaw. Your fingers can separate the node from the angle so that you can feel the hard sharpness of the bone, a finding generally not associated with parotid swelling.

DIFFERENTIAL DIAGNOSIS
How to Discover an Immune Deficiency Disease in a Child

Begin with a thorough history in all regards:

- The family history
- Risk factors for HIV infection
- Illness in siblings
- Previous infections and the age of onset of frequent infection
- Previous hospitalizations
- Serious recurring infections and infections that are uncommon (e.g., infection with *Pneumocystis jirovecii;* other infections, particularly fungal, that do not yield to therapy)

Note unusual findings on the physical examination (e.g., generalized lymphadenopathy and enlargement of the liver and/or spleen).

The child who is not growing well, who has recurrent infection, and in whom unusual findings persist could have an immune deficiency. HIV infection in the young can have a long clinical latency. The least suspicion in a child at risk should lead to testing.

Box 9-3   When Lymphadenopathy Requires Further Investigation

Although the detection of lymphadenopathy is common and the number of associated diseases is great, it is not often necessary to perform a biopsy or other laboratory tests. Yet there are situations that indicate a risk for malignancy and require consideration for further investigation:

- Older patients with localized and persistent lymphadenopathy, without evidence of infection or inflammation, might have cancer unless a biopsy proves otherwise
- Young adults and children with localized supraclavicular lymphadenopathy
- Posterior cervical lymphadenopathy adds a risk for malignancy, more than lymphadenopathy that occurs in the anterior cervical chain
- Any lump that grows rapidly and insistently, at any age

Nodes smaller than 0.5 cm generally are not cause for concern, and nodes with a diameter of 1 cm or less in the cervical and inguinal chains do not always indicate a problem. If nodes have grown rapidly and are suspiciously large (i.e., more than 2 cm), mildly painful, or fixed to contiguous tissues and relatively immovable, investigate further.

The palatine tonsils may be enlarged in children; this in itself is not a problem. Excessive enlargement may obstruct the nasopharynx, increasing the risk of sleep apnea and, on rare occasions, pulmonary hypertension (see Chapter 12, Fig. 12-33).

Clinical Pearl
Cervical Nodes

The childhood diseases of rubella, rubeola, and varicella often present with obvious cervical nodes, usually posterior rather than anterior. Hepatitis A or B and infectious mononucleosis have the same pattern of cervical node involvement.

Sample Documentation
History and Physical Examination

Subjective
A 24-year-old male student reports fatigue, fever, sore throat. and discomfort with swallowing for the past 4 days.

Objective
Tonsils enlarged. On palpation bilateral tender and enlarged anterior cervical, posterior cervical, submandibular, and epitrochlear nodes. No supraclavicular, inguinal, or axillary lymphadenopathy. No splenomegaly.

For additional sample documentation, see Chapter 26, pp. 628-631.

ABNORMALITIES

LYMPHATIC SYSTEM

Acute Lymphangitis

Inflammation of one or more lymphatic vessels

Pathophysiology

- Pathogenic organisms enter the lymphatic vessels directly through a wound or as a complication of infection and produce a local inflammatory response.
- Inflammation or infection then extends proximally toward regional lymph nodes

Subjective Data

- Enlarged lymph node
- Pain, malaise, possibly fever
- Minor trauma to the skin distal to the area of infection

Objective Data

- Red streaks in the skin following the course of the lymphatic collecting duct
- Appears as a tracing of rather fine lines streaking up the extremity
- Sometimes indurated and palpable to gentle touch
- Look distal to the inflammation for sites of infection, particularly between digits.

Acute Suppurative Lymphadenitis

Infection and inflammation of a lymph node; may affect a single or localized group of nodes

Pathophysiology

- Most commonly caused by group A beta-hemolytic streptococci and coagulase-positive staphylococcal infection
- Other pathogens may include actinomycotic adenitis as a result of dental disease; mycobacterial lymphadenitis in the presence of the tuberculosis organism; *Pasteurella multocida* infection at the site of a scratch or bite from a dog or cat
- Lymph nodes enlarged because of the cellular infiltration and edema
- Nodes tender because of distention of the capsule
- Acute lymphadenitis most often seen in the cervical region due to microbial drainage from infections of the teeth or tonsils and in the axillary or inguinal regions secondary to infections in the extremities
- Systemic viral infections (particularly in children) and bacteremia often produce generalized lymphadenopathy.

Subjective Data

- Enlarged lymph nodes
- Pain from enlarged lymph nodes

Objective Data

- Involved node usually firm and tender
- Overlying tissue edematous; skin appears erythematous, usually within 72 hours
- When abscess formation is extensive, nodes fluctuant
- Mycobacterial adenitis characterized by an inflammation without warmth that may or may not be slightly tender

Lymphedema

Edematous swelling due to excess accumulation of lymph fluid in tissues caused by inadequate lymph drainage

Pathophysiology

- Result of protein-rich interstitial volume overload, secondary to lymph drainage failure
- Four major physiologic mechanisms: increased blood capillary hydrostatic pressure, decreased plasma protein concentration, increased blood permeability, and blockage of lymph return
- Primary lymphedema: hypoplasia and maldevelopment of the lymphatic system, more common in females than in males; can manifest in infants or later; termed *praecox* in adolescence and *tarda* in patients approaching 40 years of age
- Secondary: acquired damage to regional lymph nodes—pressure from tumors, scar tissue after radiation, or surgical removal of lymph nodes

Subjective Data

- Painless swelling of a limb can be unilateral or bilateral.
- Onset usually gradual
- History of trauma, surgery, or radiation to a regional area
- Travel to areas where filariasis is common
- Family history of leg swelling

Objective Data

- Swelling and often grotesque distortion of the extremities (Fig. 9-23)
- Lymphedema may or may not pit.
- The overlying skin eventually thickens and feels tougher than usual.
- Primary lymphedema often apparent at birth and most often involves the legs, particularly the dorsum of the foot; the degree varies with the severity and distribution of the abnormality and may not appear until young adulthood.
- See Table 9-1 for grading of lymphedema.

FIGURE 9-23 Lymphedema.

DIFFERENTIAL DIAGNOSIS

Lymphedema or Edema?

- Both can be either pitting or nonpitting.
- Except in early stages, lymphedema does not resolve with elevation of the affected area. Edema secondary to increased capillary filtration (e.g., chronic venous insufficiency) usually improves.
- Diuretics do not help lymphedema. They may help edema from other causes.
- Be aware that some patients may have both edema and lymphedema.

Table 9-1	Grading of Lymphedema by the International Society of Lymphology Criteria
STAGING	**DESCRIPTION**
Stage 0	Latent or subclinical Swelling is not evident despite impaired lymph transport.
Stage I	Pitting may occur. There is early accumulation of fluid relatively high in protein content (e.g., in comparison with "venous" edema), and it subsides with limb elevation.
Stage II	Tissue fibrosis is present. Limb elevation alone rarely reduces tissue swelling. Pitting may be present. Late in stage II, the limb may or may not pit as tissue fibrosis supervenes.
Stage III	Pitting is absent. Trophic skin changes are present (acanthosis nigricans, fat deposits, and warty overgrowths).

From the *International Society of Lymphology Consensus Document*, 2003.Stages refer only to the physical condition of the extremities.

ABNORMALITIES

Lymphangioma/Cystic Hygroma
Congenital malformation of dilated lymphatics

Pathophysiology
- Results from a failure of complete development and subsequent obstruction of the lymphatic system; commonly found in the neck

Subjective Data
- Painless cystic masses
- Usually manifest during the first year of life and often enlarged after an upper respiratory infection
- Asymptomatic when in the posterior triangle of the neck, but if found anteriorly may cause airway or swallowing problems

Objective Data
- Soft, nontender, and easily compressible spongy fluid-containing mass without discrete margins
- Most present at birth and apparent early in life, usually in the neck or axilla, less commonly in the chest or extremities
- May be large enough to distort face and neck
- Diagnosis through physical examination and imaging studies (ultrasound, computed tomography, or magnetic resonance imaging), which show a thin-walled, multiloculated cystic mass

---

Lymphatic Filariasis (Elephantiasis)
Massive accumulation of lymphedema throughout the body; the most common cause of secondary lymphedema worldwide

Pathophysiology
- Results from widespread inflammation and obstruction of the lymphatics by the filarial worms *Wuchereria bancrofti* or *Brugia malayi*; transmitted by mosquitoes
- Adequate drainage is prevented, and the patient becomes more susceptible to infection, cellulitis, and fibrosis
- The term *elephantiasis* often incorrectly used to describe the result of any obstruction, congenital or acquired.
- See Differential Diagnosis table.

Subjective Data
- Swelling of limb or body area
- Travel to infected areas: Asia, Africa, the Western Pacific, India, Philippines
- Many patients asymptomatic, but some may develop fever with lymphangitis and lymphadenitis, chronic pulmonary infection, and progressive lymphedema.

Objective Data
- Lymphedema of the entire arm or leg; the genital regions (vulva, scrotum, breasts)
- Diagnosis can be made by identification of microfilariae microscopically in blood.

ABNORMALITIES

DIFFERENTIAL DIAGNOSIS
When the Body Swells

A significant number of pathologic processes can cause swelling of the extremities and other areas in the body. These can stem from, but are not limited to, the cardiovascular system (e.g., congestive heart failure or constrictive pericarditis), diseases of the liver (e.g., obstruction of the hepatic vein [Chiari syndrome] and portal vein thrombosis), and kidney malfunction. The most common cause, particularly of the feet and the ankles, is stasis; the result of deep venous thrombosis, this may occur in otherwise well men and women who must stand or sit for long periods. The failure to move with some regularity increases orthostatic pressure in the legs. Pregnancy is also a common contributor, even in the absence of venous abnormality in the legs. There can also be a significant disruption of lymphatic circulation in the arms after breast surgery with its disruption of lymph flow. Myxedema, a finding associated with hypothyroidism, is typified by a dry, waxy swelling (see Chapter 10, Fig. 10-10). The edema in this condition can cause a rather typical facies, with swollen lips and a thick nose; it, too, does not pit.

Non-Hodgkin Lymphoma

Malignant neoplasm of the lymphatic system and the reticuloendothelial tissues

Pathophysiology

- Non-Hodgkin lymphomas occur most often in lymph nodes in the chest, neck, abdomen, tonsils, and skin; they may also develop in sites other than lymph nodes such as the digestive tract, central nervous system, and around the tonsils.
- Most arise in B cells; the rest occur in T cells
- Histologically, their cells are often undifferentiated but resemble lymphocytes, histiocytes, or plasma cells.

Subjective Data

- Painless enlarged lymph node(s)
- Fever, weight loss, night sweats, abdominal pain, or fullness
- Family history of non-Hodgkin lymphomas

Objective Data

- Nodes may be localized in the posterior cervical triangle or may become matted, crossing into the anterior triangle.
- Nodes usually well-defined and solid
- Cannot distinguish the findings of these conditions from those in Hodgkin lymphoma through physical examination alone

Hodgkin Lymphoma

Malignant lymphoma

Pathophysiology

- Unknown etiology, several subtypes
- Starts in a single node or chain and spreads to contiguous lymph nodes, spleen, liver, and bone marrow
- Neoplastic giant cells release factors that induce the accumulation of reactive lymphocytes, macrophages, and granulocytes.
- Occurs in all races, generally in late adolescence and young adulthood, although it also occurs in people older than 50 years; males are twice as likely to develop Hodgkin lymphoma as are females.
- Most often, Hodgkin lymphoma starts in B-cell lymphocytes located in lymph nodes in the neck area, although any lymph node may be the site of initial disease.

Subjective Data

- Painless enlarged lymph nodes
- May have abdominal pain, sometimes fever
- May have history of infectious mononucleosis

Objective Data

- Clinical presentation variable
- Most commonly, painless enlargement of the cervical lymph nodes, often in the posterior triangle, that is generally asymmetric and progressive (Fig. 9-24)
- Nodes sometimes matted and firm, almost rubbery
- Usually asymmetric; may occasionally be enlarged in similar patterns on both sides of the body
- Nodal size may fluctuate

FIGURE 9-24 Hodgkin disease.
Note the impressive extent of the enlargement.

Epstein-Barr Virus Mononucleosis

Infectious mononucleosis

Pathophysiology	Subjective Data	Objective Data
• Initially infects oral epithelial cells; after intracellular viral replication and cell lysis with release of new virions, virus spreads to contiguous structures such as the salivary glands, with eventual viremia and infection of the entire lymphoreticular system, including the liver and spleen • Incubation period of infectious mononucleosis in adolescents is 30 to 50 days	• Malaise, fatigue, acute or prolonged (longer than 1 week) fever, headache, sore throat, nausea, abdominal pain, and myalgia • Prodromal period may last 1 to 2 weeks	• Generalized lymphadenopathy most commonly in the anterior and posterior cervical nodes and the submandibular lymph nodes and less commonly in the axillary and inguinal lymph nodes • Epitrochlear lymphadenopathy is particularly suggestive of infectious mononucleosis. • Hepatomegaly; symptomatic hepatitis or jaundice is uncommon, but elevated liver enzymes are common. • Splenomegaly to 2 to 3 cm below the costal margin is typical; massive enlargement is uncommon. • Moderate to severe pharyngitis with tonsillar enlargement, occasionally with exudates • Petechiae at the junction of the hard and soft palate frequently seen • Diagnosis with mononucleosis spot test

Toxoplasmosis

Zoonosis, caused by the parasite *Toxoplasma gondii*

Pathophysiology	Subjective Data	Objective Data
• Ingestion or inhalation of oocysts in soil/fomites, undercooked meat, or raw eggs; cat feces or litter • Infection persists for life without signs of disease. • In immunosuppressed persons, quiescent parasites multiply, resulting in neurologic disease or other organ manifestations. • May cause serious congenital infection if a woman is exposed during pregnancy, particularly in the first trimester; transmitted directly from pregnant mother to fetus	• No significant symptoms • History of eating raw or rare meat or uncooked eggs • History of direct contact with cat feces, cleaning the litter box, gardening in feces-contaminated soil	• Single node, chronically enlarged and nontender • Node is usually in the posterior cervical chain

Roseola Infantum (HHV-6)

Infection by human herpes virus 6

Pathophysiology	Subjective Data	Objective Data
• Common in infancy with peak age of acquisition 2 years • Virus present in the saliva of most adults and is readily transmitted by oral secretions • Latency permits persistence of the virus in the presence of a fully developed immune response and allows lifelong infection of the host. • Through periodic reactivation of latent virus and the production of recurrent infection; virus shedding occurs at intervals throughout life, allowing the virus to be spread to new susceptible hosts	• Fever—usually high grade and persistent over 3 to 4 days • Sometimes associated with a mild respiratory illness and lymphadenopathy	• Adenopathy, discrete and not tender, involves the occipital and postauricular chains and may last a while • When the fever diminishes, a morbilliform fine maculopapular rash occurs, spreading from the trunk to the extremities; the child begins feeling much better.

Herpes Simplex (HSV)

Infection by human herpes virus 1 (HSV-1) or human herpes virus 2 (HSV-2)

Pathophysiology	Subjective Data	Objective Data
• Transmitted by oral secretions, genital secretions, and close contact • HSV causes lytic infection of fibroblasts and epithelial cells, and establishes latent infection in neurons; HSV-1 has predilection for oropharyngeal infection and HSV-2 for genital infection; although both viruses can infect and produce latent infection at either site, reactivation of each is most common at the preferred site.	• Burning, itching lesions • May report enlarged lymph nodes	• Discrete labial and gingival vesicles or ulcers (Fig. 9-25) • May have enlargement of the anterior cervical and submandibular nodes • These nodes tend to be somewhat firm, quite discrete, movable, and tender; the frequency of this condition and the symptoms are generally sufficient to establish the diagnosis; a viral culture can be obtained if necessary.

FIGURE 9-25 Herpes simplex.

Cat Scratch Disease

A common cause of subacute or chronic lymphadenitis in children

Pathophysiology	Subjective Data	Objective Data
• Caused mainly by *Bartonella henselae* and *Bartonella clarridgeiae*; usually follows a bite, scratch, or other penetrating injury from a kitten or cat; the organisms, however, rarely cause illness in the cat	• Bite, scratch, or wound from cat or kitten • Inoculation lesion: a papule or pustule lasts 3 to 5 days and then becomes vesicular and crusts in 2 to 3 days • Painful enlarged lymph nodes	• Inoculation lesion; may be healing • Lymphadenopathy develops in 1 to 2 weeks in the region that drains the primary lesion. • Single lymph node most often, but multiple nodes are involved occasionally • Tender nodes commonly in head, neck, and axillae; the accessible nodal areas in the arms and legs are less often involved. • Nodes can be very large—up to several centimeters; often red and tender and occasionally suppurate • Diagnosis can be made in the presence of a nodal enlargement lasting longer than 3 weeks, accompanied by an inoculation lesion of the skin and following an interaction with a cat, a cat scratch, or cat lick on a break in the skin. • Lymphadenopathy can last for 2 to 4 months or even longer.

Human Immunodeficiency Virus/Acquired Immune Deficiency Syndrome (HIV/AIDS)

Pathophysiology	Subjective Data	Objective Data
• Characterized by the dysfunction of cell-mediated immunity • HIV seropositivity (HIV+): antibodies to HIV present, but sequelae of recurrent infections and neoplastic disease has not yet occurred • AIDS manifested clinically as the development of recurrent, often severe, opportunistic infections • Common life-threatening diseases associated with full-blown AIDS include Kaposi sarcoma, *Pneumocystis jiroveci* pneumonia, pulmonary tuberculosis, recurrent pneumonia, invasive cervical cancer, a parotid enlargement simulating mumps, anemia and thrombocytopenia, chronic diarrhea, and recurrent infections	• Enlarged lymph nodes • Initial symptoms include severe fatigue, malaise, weakness, persistent unexplained weight loss, fevers, arthralgias, and persistent diarrhea.	• Generalized lymphadenopathy • In children there may be a prolonged clinical latent period, but initial signs may include neurodevelopmental problems with loss of developmental milestones. • Progressive infection characterized by decreasing $CD4^+$ T-lymphocyte count and increasing viral load level

Serum Sickness (Type III Hypersensitivity Reaction)

Serum sickness is an immune complex disease.

Pathophysiology	Subjective Data	Objective Data
• Systemic type III hypersensitivity reaction in response to antigens • Mediated by the tissue deposition of circulating immune complexes, the activation of complement, and the ensuing inflammatory response • Patient can react similarly to repeated exposure to the stimuli; subsequent reactions may be even more severe and even fatal	• Enlarged lymph nodes • Pain, pruritus, and erythematous swelling at the injection site • Urticaria, other rashes, lymphadenopathy, joint pain, fever, and at times facial edema • Medications: beta-lactam antibiotics (especially cefaclor), sulfonamide antibiotics, minocycline • Organ transplant	• Findings become apparent about 7 to 10 days following administration of the provoking substance. • Urticaria, maculopapular or purpuric lesions • Lymphadenopathy most prominent in the area draining the injection site; can be generalized • Facial and neck edema • Symptoms subside slowly, recurring at times over several weeks.

Latex Allergy Type IV Dermatitis (Delayed Hypersensitivity)

Pathophysiology
- Allergic contact dermatitis that involves the immune system and is caused by the chemicals used in latex products

Subjective Data
- Exposure to latex
- Allergy to cross-sensitizing foods (e.g., banana, avocado, potato, tomato, kiwi)

Objective Data
- Skin reaction usually begins 24 to 48 hours after contact
- Vesicular lesions, erythema
- Reaction may progress to oozing skin blisters

Latex Allergy Type I Reaction

Pathophysiology
- True allergic reaction caused by protein antibodies (IgE antibodies) that form as a result of interaction between a foreign protein and the body's immune system
- Antigen-antibody reaction causes release of histamine, leukotrienes, prostaglandins, and kinins; these chemicals cause the symptoms of allergic reactions.

Subjective Data
- Exposure to latex
- Allergy to cross-sensitizing foods (e.g., banana, avocado, potato, tomato, kiwi)

Objective Data
- Local urticaria (skin wheals), generalized urticaria with angioedema (tissue swelling), asthma, eye/nose itching and gastrointestinal symptoms, anaphylaxis (cardiovascular collapse)

CHAPTER 10

Head and Neck

The head provides the bony housing and protective cover for the brain, including the organs that provide senses of vision, hearing, smell, and taste. The neck provides stability and support for the head and holds vital vessels, the trachea, esophagus, and spinal cord. A flexible cervical spine is necessary for head movement, balance adaptation, and increasing extent of vision.

evolve *http://evolve.elsevier.com/Seidel*
- Physical Exam Key Points
- NCLEX Review Questions
- Interactive Activities
- Videos
- Student Checklist

ANATOMY AND PHYSIOLOGY

The skull is composed of seven bones (two frontal, two parietal, two temporal, and one occipital) that are fused together and covered by the scalp. Bones of the skull are helpful in identifying landmarks on the head (Fig. 10-1). The bony structure of the face is formed from the fused frontal, nasal, zygomatic, ethmoid, lacrimal, sphenoid, and maxillary bones and the movable mandible. The face has cavities for the eyes, nose, and mouth.

Physical Examination Preview

Here is a preview of the steps involved in conducting a physical examination of the head and neck. ⓔ These procedures are explained in detail in this chapter and are available on Evolve in printable formats.

Head and Neck

Head
1. Observe head position (p. 189):
   - Tilted
   - Tremor
2. Inspect skull and scalp for the following (pp. 189 and 192):
   - Size
   - Shape (molding)
   - Symmetry
   - Lesions
   - Trauma
3. Inspect facial features, including the following (p. 189):
   - Symmetry
   - Shape
   - Unusual features
   - Tics
   - Characteristic facies
   - Pallor or pigmentation variations
4. Palpate head and scalp, noting the following (p. 192):
   - Symmetry
   - Tenderness (particularly over areas of frontal and maxillary sinuses)
   - Scalp movement
   - Sutures/fontanels
   - Hair texture, color, and distribution

5. When appropriate, auscultate the temporal arteries and palpate, noting the following (p. 192):
   - Thickening
   - Hardness
   - Tenderness
6. Inspect and palpate the salivary glands (p. 192).
7. Transilluminate skull of infants with rapidly increasing head circumference.

Neck
1. Inspect the neck for the following (pp. 192-193):
   - Symmetry
   - Alignment of trachea
   - Fullness
   - Masses, webbing, and skinfolds
2. Palpate the neck, noting the following (p. 193):
   - Tracheal position
   - Tracheal tug
   - Movement of hyoid bone and cartilages with swallowing
   - Lymph nodes
   - Paravertebral musculature and spinous processes
3. Palpate the thyroid gland for the following (p. 194):
   - Size
   - Shape
   - Configuration
   - Consistency
   - Tenderness
   - Nodules
   - If gland is enlarged, auscultate for bruits
4. Evaluate range of motion of the neck (p. 193 and Chapter 21, pp. 516 and 518).

FIGURE 10-1 Bones of the skull.

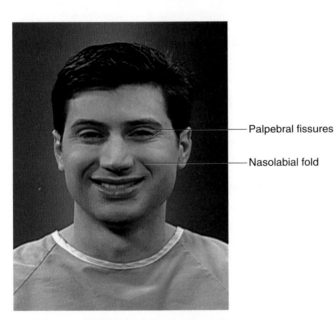

Palpebral fissures

Nasolabial fold

FIGURE 10-2 Landmarks of the face.

Major facial landmarks are the palpebral fissures and the nasolabial folds (Fig. 10-2). Facial muscles are innervated by cranial nerve (CN) V and CN VII. The temporal artery is the major accessible artery of the face, passing just anterior to the ear, over the temporal muscle, and onto the forehead.

The paired parotid, submandibular, and sublingual salivary glands produce saliva, which moistens the mouth, inhibits formation of dental caries, and starts the digestion of carbohydrates. The parotid glands are located anterior to the ear and above the mandible, the submandibular glands are located medial to the mandible at the angle of the jaw, and the sublingual glands are located anteriorly in the floor of the mouth.

The neck is formed by the cervical vertebrae, ligaments, and the sternocleidomastoid and trapezius muscles, which give it support and movement. The neck begins at the clavicles and sternum inferiorly and at the base of the skull superiorly. It contains the trachea, esophagus, internal and external jugular veins, common carotid, internal and external carotid arteries, and thyroid (Fig. 10-3). Horizontal mobility is greatest between cervical vertebrae 4 and 5 or 5 and 6 in adults. The sternocleidomastoid muscle extends from the upper sternum and medial third of the clavicle to the mastoid process (see Fig. 21-2, C). The trapezius muscle extends from the scapula, the lateral third of the clavicle, and the vertebrae to the occipital prominence (see Fig. 21-2, C and D).

The relationship of these muscles to each other and to adjacent bones creates triangles used as anatomic landmarks. The anterior triangle is formed by the medial border of the sternocleidomastoid muscles, the mandible, and the midline (Fig. 10-4). The posterior triangle is formed by the trapezius and sternocleidomastoid muscles and the clavicle (see Fig. 10-4) and contains the posterior cervical lymph nodes (Fig. 10-5). (For a more complete description of the lymph nodes of the head and neck, see Figs. 9-8 through 9-11.)

The hyoid bone, cricoid cartilage, trachea, thyroid, and anterior cervical lymph nodes lie inside these triangles (see Fig. 10-3). The common carotid artery and internal jugular vein are deep and run parallel to the sternocleidomastoid muscle along its medial margin. The external jugular vein crosses the surface of the sternocleidomastoid muscle diagonally. The hyoid bone lies just below the mandible. The thyroid cartilage is shaped like a shield, its notch on the upper edge marking the level of bifurcation of the common carotid artery. The cricoid cartilage is the uppermost ring of the tracheal cartilages.

The thyroid is the largest endocrine gland in the body, producing two hormones, thyroxine (T_4) and triiodothyronine (T_3). Its two lateral lobes are butterfly-shaped and are joined by an isthmus at their lower aspect (see Fig. 10-3). This isthmus lies across the trachea below the cricoid cartilage. A pyramidal lobe, extending upward from the isthmus and slightly to the left of midline, is present in about one third of the population. The lobes curve posteriorly around the cartilages and are in large part covered by the sternocleidomastoid muscles.

FIGURE 10-3 Underlying structures of the neck. A, Anterior view. B, Lateral view.

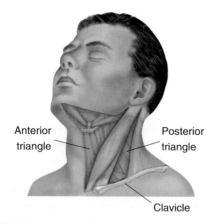

FIGURE 10-4 Anterior and posterior triangles of the neck.

�֍ Infants

In infants, the seven cranial bones are soft and separated by the sagittal, coronal, and lambdoid sutures (Fig. 10-6). The anterior and posterior fontanels are the membranous spaces formed where four cranial bones meet and intersect. Spaces between the cranial bones permit the expansion of the skull to accommodate brain growth. Ossification of the sutures begins after completion of brain growth, at about 6 years of age, and is finished by adulthood. The fontanels ossify earlier, with the posterior fontanel usually closing by 2 months of age and the anterior fontanel closing by 12 to 15 months of age.

The process of birth through the vaginal canal often causes molding of the newborn skull, during which the cranial bones may shift and overlap. Within days, the newborn skull usually resumes its appropriate shape and size.

�֍ Children and Adolescents

Subtle changes in facial appearance occur throughout childhood. In the male adolescent, the nose and thyroid cartilage enlarge, and facial hair develops, emerging first on the upper lip, then the cheeks, lower lip, and chin.

�֍ Pregnant Women

The fetal thyroid gland becomes functional in the second trimester. Before this time the mother is the source of thyroid hormone and pregnant women require increased iodine intake.

As long as adequate iodine intake is maintained, the size of the thyroid will not change on physical examination. A slight enlargement may be detectable on ultrasound (Fig. 10-7).

�֍ Older Adults

The rate of T_4 production and degradation gradually decreases with aging, and the thyroid gland becomes more fibrotic.

REVIEW OF RELATED HISTORY

For each of the symptoms or conditions discussed in this section, targeted topics to include in the history of the present illness are listed. Responses to questions about these topics provide clues for focusing the physical examination and the development of an appropriate diagnostic evaluation. Questions regarding medication use (prescription and over the counter preparations) as well as complementary and alternative therapies are relevant for each.

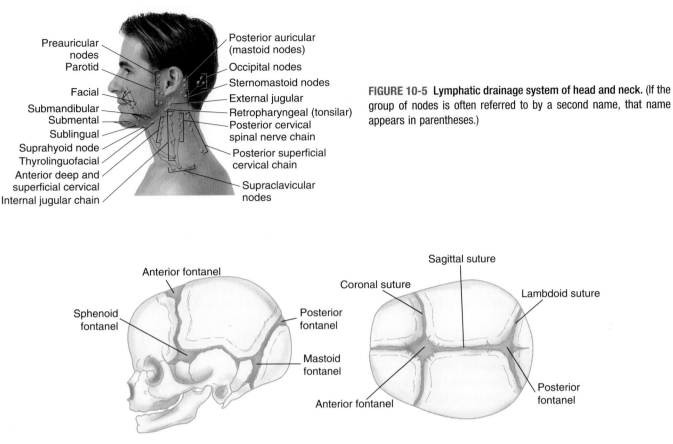

FIGURE 10-5 Lymphatic drainage system of head and neck. (If the group of nodes is often referred to by a second name, that name appears in parentheses.)

FIGURE 10-6 Fontanels and sutures on the infant's skull.

FIGURE 10-7 Thyroid enlargement in pregnancy. Note the large nodule in the patient's left lobe. Thyroid size increases in pregnancy in areas of iodine deficiency but not in those with sufficient iodine. *(From Lemmi and Lemmi, 2009.)*

History of Present Illness

+ Traumatic brain injury
  + Independent observer's description of event
  + State of consciousness after injury: immediately and 5 minutes later; duration of unconsciousness; combative, confused, alert, or dazed (see Chapter 27, page 632)

+ Predisposing factors: seizure disorder, hypoglycemia, poor vision, light-headedness, syncope
+ Associated symptoms: head or neck pain, laceration, local tenderness, change in breathing pattern, blurred or double vision, discharge from nose or ears, nausea or vomiting, urinary or fecal incontinence, ability to move all extremities
+ Headache
  + Onset: early morning, during day, during night; gradual versus abrupt
  + Duration: minutes, hours, days, weeks; relieved by medication or sleep; resolves spontaneously; occurs in clusters; headache-free periods
  + Location: entire head, unilateral, specific site (neck, sinus region, behind eyes, hatband distribution)
  + Character: throbbing, pounding, boring, dull, nagging, constant pressure, aggravated with movement
  + Severity: grade each event severity on a scale from 1 (mild) to 10 (severe)
  + Visual prodrome: scotoma; hemianopia (decreased vision or blindness takes place in half the visual field of one or both eyes); distortion of size, shape, or location
  + Pattern: worse in morning or evening, worse or better as day progresses, awakens patient from or occurs only during sleep
  + Episodes closer together or worsening, lasting longer

- Change in level of consciousness as pain increases
- Associated symptoms: nausea, vomiting, diarrhea, photophobia, visual disturbance, difficulty falling asleep, increased lacrimation, nasal discharge, tinnitus, paresthesias, mobility impairment
- Precipitating factors: fever, fatigue, stress, food additives, prolonged fasting, alcohol, seasonal allergies, menstrual cycle, sexual intercourse, oral contraceptives, amount of caffeine intake
- Efforts to treat: sleep, pain medication, need for daily medications, rebound if pain medications are not taken or if caffeine not consumed
- Medications: anticonvulsants, antiarrhythmics, beta-blockers, calcium channel blockers, oral contraceptives, serotonin antagonists or agonists, selective serotonin reuptake inhibitors, antidepressants, nonsteroidal antiinflammatory drugs, narcotics, caffeine-containing medication
- Stiff neck
  - Neck injury or strain, traumatic brain injury, neck swelling
  - Fever, associated headache, other symptoms of meningitis
  - Character: limitation of movement; pain with movement, pain relieved by movement; continuous or cramping pain; radiation patterns to arms, shoulders, hands, or down the back
  - Predisposing factors: unilateral vision or hearing loss, work position (e.g., long hours in front of a computer)
  - Efforts to treat: heat, physical therapy
  - Medications: analgesics, muscle relaxants
- Thyroid problem
  - Change in temperature preference: more or less clothing than worn by other members of the household
  - Neck swelling; difficulty swallowing; redness; pain with touch, swallowing, or hyperextension of the neck; difficulty buttoning shirt
  - Change in texture of hair, skin, or nails; increased pigmentation of skin at pressure points
  - Change in mood and energy, irritability, nervousness, or lethargy, disinterest
  - Increased prominence of eyes (exophthalmos), periorbital swelling, blurred or double vision
  - Tachycardia, palpitations
  - Change in menses
  - Change in bowel habits
  - Medications: thyroid preparations

Past Medical History

- Traumatic brain injury, subdural hematoma, recent lumbar puncture
- Radiation treatment around head and neck
- Headaches (see Differential Diagnosis, page 198)
- Surgery for tumor, goiter
- Seizure disorder
- Thyroid dysfunction

Family History

- Headaches: type, character, similarity to that of the patient
- Thyroid dysfunction

Personal and Social History

- Employment: type of work, risk of traumatic brain injury, use of helmet or other protective head gear, exposure to toxins or chemicals
- Stress; tension; demands at home, work, or school
- Potential risk of injury: participation in sports, handrails available, use of seat belts, car seats and booster seats, unsafe environment
- Nutrition: recent weight gain or loss, food intolerances, eating habits (e.g., skipping meals)
- Use of illicit drugs
- Sports participation, weight training, use of protective padding and helmet, if necessary

� Infants

- Prenatal history: maternal use of drugs or alcohol, uterine abnormalities, treatment of hyperthyroidism
- Birth history: birth order (firstborn more likely to experience torticollis); vaginal or cesarean section delivery; presentation, difficulty of delivery, use of forceps or other assist device (associated with caput succedaneum, cephalhematoma, Bell palsy, molding)
- Unusual head shape: bulging or flattening (congenital anomaly or positioning in utero), preterm infant, head held at angle, preferred position at rest
- Strength of head control
- Acute illness: diarrhea, vomiting, fever, limited neck movement, irritability (associated with meningitis)
- Congenital anomalies: craniofacial abnormalities (e.g., Pierre-Robin sequence, encephalocele, microcephaly, hydrocephaly)
- Neonatal screening for congenital hypothyroidism

✤ Pregnant Women

- Weeks of gestation or postpartum
- Presence of preexisting disease (e.g., hypothyroidism, hyperthyroidism), ingestion of iodine or use of antithyroid medication
- History of pregnancy-induced hypertension (PIH)
- Alcohol use

✤ Older Adults

- Dizziness or vertigo with head or neck movement
- Weakness or impaired balance, increasing risk of falling and head injury

EXAMINATION AND FINDINGS

Equipment

- Tape measure (primarily for infants)
- Stethoscope

+ Cup of water (for evaluation of thyroid gland)
+ Transilluminator (or flashlight) for infants)

Head and Face

Inspection

Begin examining the head and neck with inspection of head position and facial features; continue to observe throughout the history and physical examination. The patient's head should be upright and still. A horizontal jerking or bobbing motion may be associated with a tremor; a nodding movement may be associated with aortic insufficiency, especially if the nodding is synchronized with the pulse. Holding the head tilted to one side to favor a good eye or ear often occurs with unilateral hearing or vision loss, but is also associated with torticollis (shortening or excessive contraction of the sternocleidomastoid muscle; see Fig. 10-36).

Inspect facial features (i.e., eyelids, eyebrows, palpebral fissures, nasolabial folds, and mouth) for shape and symmetry with rest (some slight asymmetry is common) movement, and expression. By doing this, the integrity of CN V and VII (trigeminal and facial) has been partially tested. Complete evaluation of the cranial nerves is detailed in Chapter 22 pp. 553-556.

Facies is defined as an expression or appearance of the face and features of the head and neck that, when considered together, is characteristic of a clinical condition or syndrome. Once a facies is recognized, the examiner may be able to diagnose the condition or syndrome even before completing the examination. Note any change in the shape of the face or any unusual features, such as edema, bruising, coarsened features, exophthalmos, hirsutism, lack of expression, excessive perspiration, pallor, or pigmentation variations. Facies may develop slowly and the health care provider should be alert to early changes suggestive of a developing facies. For example, a patient with early changes of acromegaly is shown in Fig. 10-14. One way to better appreciate these changes is to ask the patient to provide an old photograph of herself. Figures 10-8 through 10-22 demonstrate some facies and their associated disorders.

When facial asymmetry is present, note whether all features on one side of the face are affected, or only a portion of the face, such as the forehead, lower face, or mouth. Suspect facial nerve paralysis when the entire side of the face is affected, and suspect facial nerve weakness when the lower face is affected (see Fig. 10-13). If only the mouth is involved, suspect a problem with the peripheral trigeminal nerve.

Tics, which are spasmodic muscular contractions of the face, head, or neck, should be noted. They may be associated with pressure on or degenerative changes of the facial nerves, a feature of Tourette syndrome, or possibly psychogenic in origin.

Inspect the skull for size, shape, and symmetry. Examine the scalp by systematically parting the hair from the frontal to occipital region, noting any lesions, scabs, tenderness, nits, or scaliness (Fig. 10-23). Pay special attention to the areas behind the ears, at the hairline, and at the crown of the head. Note any hair loss (alopecia) pattern. In men, it is common to see bitemporal recession of hair or balding over the crown of the head. In young girls and women, hair loss may be associated with tight braiding. In

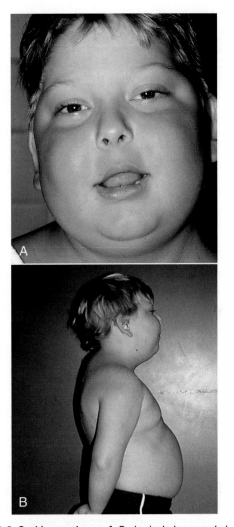

FIGURE 10-8 Cushing syndrome. A, Facies include a rounded or "moon-shaped" face with thin, erythematous skin. **B,** Side view. Shows upper thoracic fat pad (buffalo hump). *(From Zitelli and Davis, 2007.)*

FIGURE 10-9 Hippocratic facies. Note sunken appearance of the eyes, cheeks, and temporal areas; sharp nose; and dry, rough skin seen in this patient in the terminal stages of throat cancer. *(From Lemmi and Lemmi, 2009.)*

FIGURE 10-10 **Myxedema facies.** Note dull, puffy, yellowed skin; coarse, sparse hair; temporal loss of eyebrows; periorbital edema; and prominent tongue. *(From Lemmi and Lemmi, 2009.)*

FIGURE 10-11 **Hyperthyroid facies.** Note fine, moist skin with fine hair, prominent eyes and lid retraction, and staring or startled expression. *(From Lemmi and Lemmi, 2000.)*

FIGURE 10-12 **Butterfly rash of systemic lupus erythematosus.** Note butterfly-shaped rash over malar surfaces and bridge of nose. Either a blush with swelling or scaly, red, maculopapular lesions may be present. *(Courtesy Walter Tunnessen, MD, Chapel Hill, NC.)*

FIGURE 10-13 **Bell palsy.** Left facial palsy (cranial nerve VII). Facies include asymmetry of one side of the face, eyelid not closing completely, drooping lower eyelid and corner of mouth, and loss of nasolabial fold. *(From Lemmi and Lemmi, 2009.)*

FIGURE 10-14 **Early acromegaly.** Note the coarsening of features with broadening of the nasal alae and prominence of the zygomatic arches. *(Courtesy Gary Wand, MD, The Johns Hopkins University and Hospital, Baltimore, MD.)*

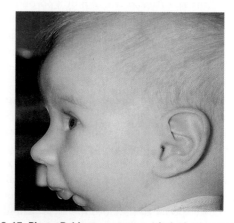

FIGURE 10-15 **Pierre-Robin sequence; a triad of micrognathia, glossoptosis, and palatal clefting.** Shows a lateral view with severe micrognathia and cleft palate. Note the small retruded mandible. *(From Zitelli and Davis, 2007.)*

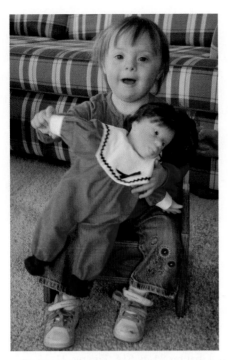

FIGURE 10-16 Down syndrome. Note depressed nasal bridge, epicanthal folds, mongoloid slant of eyes, and low-set ears. *(From Hockenberry and Willson, 2011.)*

FIGURE 10-17 Hurler syndrome. Facies includes enlarged skull with low forehead, corneal clouding, and short neck. *(From Ansell et al, 1992.)*

FIGURE 10-18 Hydrocephalus. A, Coronal view with characteristic enlarged head, thinning of the scalp with dilated scalp veins, and bossing of the skull. **B,** Anteroposterior view demonstrating sclera visible above the iris. In this case, the infant has paresis of upward gaze. This phenomenon is often termed the "sunsetting sign." *(From Zitelli and Davis, 2007.)*

FIGURE 10-19 Fetal alcohol syndrome. This is one of the most common causes of acquired intellectual disability. Note the poorly formed philtrum; widespread eyes, with inner epicanthal folds and mild ptosis; hirsute forehead; short nose; and relatively thin upper lip. *(From Zitelli and Davis, 1997.)*

FIGURE 10-20 Treacher-Collins syndrome. Note the maxillary hypoplasia, micrognathia, and auricular deformity. *(From Zitelli and Davis, 2007.)*

FIGURE 10-21 **Apert syndrome.** Note the severe maxillary and midfacial hypoplasia. *(From Zitelli and Davis, 2007.)*

FIGURE 10-22 **Crouzon syndrome.** Observe the severe maxillary and midfacial hypoplasia with low-set ears. *(From Zitelli and Davis, 2007.)*

FIGURE 10-23 **Inspection of the scalp.**

children, a common cause of hair loss is tinea capitis (fungal infection of the scalp).

Palpation

Palpate the skull in a gentle rotary movement progressing systematically from front to back. The skull should be symmetric and smooth. The bones should be indistinguishable as the sites of fusion are not generally palpable after 6 months of age; however, the ridge of the sagittal suture may be felt on some individuals. The scalp should move freely over the skull, and no tenderness, swelling, or depressions on palpation are expected. An indentation or a depression of the skull may indicate a skull fracture.

Palpate the patient's hair, noting its texture, color, and distribution. Hair should be smooth and symmetrically distributed and have no splitting or cracked ends. Coarse, dry, and brittle hair may be associated with hypothyroidism. Fine, silky hair may be associated with hyperthyroidism or may be familial.

Palpate the temporomandibular joint space bilaterally, as described in Chapter 21, p. 516, Figures 21-26 and 21-27.

Inspect for any asymmetry or enlargement of the salivary glands. If noted, palpate for possible discrete enlargement (see Fig. 10-33), noting whether the gland is fixed or movable, soft or hard, tender or nontender. With the patient's mouth open, try to express material through the salivary ducts as you press on the glands. The parotid duct, also known as the Stensen duct, opens into the mouth next to the maxillary second molar tooth. The submandibular duct (Wharton duct) opens in a small papilla at the sides of the frenulum. An enlarged, tender gland may suggest either viral or bacterial infection or a ductal stone preventing saliva from exiting the gland. A discrete nodule may represent a cyst or tumor, either benign or malignant.

Percussion

Percussion of the head and neck is not routinely performed. One exception is when evaluating for hypocalcemia, percussion on the masseter muscle may produce a hyperactive masseteric reflex, the Chvostek sign.

Auscultation

Auscultation of the skull is not routinely performed. However, intracranial bruits are considered common in childhood, and uncommon in neonates; in individuals who have developed diplopia, a bruit or blowing sound over the orbit rarely may be heard and suggests an expanding cerebral aneurysm. If you suspect a vascular anomaly of the brain, use the bell of the stethoscope and listen over the temporal region, over the eyes, and below the occiput (Fig. 10-24). A bruit is highly suggestive of a vascular anomaly and can be associated with temporal arteritis.

Neck

Inspection

Inspect the neck in the usual anatomic position, in slight hyperextension, and as the patient swallows. Look for bilateral

FIGURE 10-24 Auscultation for a temporal bruit.

FIGURE 10-25 Position of the thumbs to evaluate the midline position of the trachea.

symmetry of the sternocleidomastoid and trapezius muscles, alignment of the trachea, landmarks of the anterior and posterior triangles, and any subtle fullness at the base of the neck. Note any apparent masses, webbing, excess skinfolds, unusual shortness, or asymmetry. Observe for any distention of the jugular vein or prominence of the carotid arteries. Carotid artery and jugular vein examination is described in Chapter 15, pp. 336-337.

Webbing, excessive posterior cervical skin, or an unusually short neck may be associated with chromosomal anomalies (e.g., Turner syndrome). The transverse portion of the omohyoid muscle in the posterior triangle can sometimes be mistaken for a mass. Marked edema of the neck may be associated with local infections (e.g., cervical lymphadenitis). A mass filling the base of the neck or visible thyroid tissue that glides upward when the patient swallows may indicate an enlarged thyroid (see Fig. 10-7).

Evaluate range of motion by asking the patient to flex, extend, rotate, and laterally turn the head and neck (see Chapter 21, pp. 516 and 518). Movement should be smooth and painless and should not cause dizziness. Nuchal rigidity, resistance to flexion of the neck, may be associated with meningeal irritation. CN XI (spinal accessory) may also be examined (see Chapter 22, p. 556 and Table 22-3, p. 553).

Palpation

The ability to palpate and identify structures in the neck varies with the patient's habitus.

Palpate the trachea for midline position. Place a thumb along each side of the trachea in the lower portion of the neck (Fig. 10-25). Compare the space between the trachea and the sternocleidomastoid muscle on each side. An unequal space indicates displacement of the trachea from the midline and may be associated with a mass or pathologic condition in the chest.

Identify the hyoid bone and the thyroid and cricoid cartilages. They should be smooth and nontender and should move under your finger when the patient swallows. On palpation, the cartilaginous rings of the trachea in the lower portion of the neck should be distinct and nontender.

With the patient's neck extended, position the index finger and thumb of one hand on each side of the trachea below the thyroid isthmus (Fig. 10-26). A tugging sensation, synchronous

FIGURE 10-26 Position of the thumb and finger to detect tracheal tugging.

with the pulse, is evidence of tracheal tug sign (Cardarelli sign or Oliver sign), suggesting the presence of an aortic aneurysm (see Clinical Pearl, "Cardarelli Sign and Oliver Sign").

The paravertebral muscles and posterior spinous processes should be palpated for tenderness. This exam coupled with neck range of motion is helpful in evaluation of a stiff neck. See Chapter 21, p. 516.

Lymph Nodes

Inspect and palpate the head and neck for lymph nodes. A description of the sequence is given in Chapter 9, pp. 174-175.

Thyroid Gland

Examination of the thyroid gland involves inspection, palpation, and occasionally auscultation. Begin by asking patients to gently extend their neck. (Hyperextension can actually make the examination more difficult.) Ask them to swallow, which often permits

Clinical Pearl

Cardarelli Sign and Oliver Sign

Cardarelli sign can be felt by pressing on the thyroid cartilage and displacing it to the patient's left. This increases contact between the left bronchus and the aorta, allowing systolic pulsations from the aorta to be felt at the surface if an aneurysm is present. Oliver sign is elicited by gently grasping the cricoid cartilage and applying upward pressure while the patient stands with his or her chin extended upward. Due to the anatomic position of the aortic arch, which overrides the left main bronchus, a downward tug of the trachea may be felt if an aneurysm is present.

FIGURE 10-27 Palpation of the right thyroid lobe and lateral border from in front of the patient.

visualization of the gland's size, symmetry, and contour as it moves with swallowing. An enlarged thyroid gland may be visible only when observing from the lateral aspect. A glass of water is an indispensable aid for proper examination of the thyroid; it helps the patient swallow multiple times.

Palpation of the thyroid gland requires a gentle touch. Nodules and asymmetry will be more difficult to detect while pressing too hard. Palpate the thyroid for size, shape, configuration, consistency, tenderness, and the presence of any nodules. Although the thyroid gland may be palpated from in front or behind the patient, facing the patient facilitates the correlation of inspection with palpation findings. It is also more convenient in examining rooms where the table is against a wall. Choose one approach to use consistently.

Evidence-Based Practice in Physical Examination

Thyroid Examination

Estimates of size tend to be exaggerated when the gland is small and underestimated when the gland is markedly enlarged (more than twice normal size). Evaluations were made by comparing the estimated size on physical examination with the size measured by ultrasound or after surgical excision. The estimation of thyroid size by lateral inspection is the most sensitive test for determining the presence of a goiter; a thyroid that is not visible on lateral inspection rules out a goiter.

For both approaches, position the patient to relax the sternocleidomastoid, with the neck flexed slightly forward and laterally toward the side being examined. Ask the patient to hold a sip of water in the mouth until you have your hands positioned, and then instruct the patient to swallow.

To palpate the thyroid using the frontal approach, have the patient sit on the examining table. First place your thumb over the trachea approximately 3 cm beneath the prominence of the thyroid cartilage during a swallow attempt to identify the isthmus. To examine the right lobe of the thyroid, use your left thumb and press the trachea toward the patient's left with your left thumb. Such pressure helps move the right lobe out of the tracheoesophageal groove for easier palpation with your right hand. Then place the first three fingers of your right hand in the right thyroid bed with your fingertips medial to the margin of the sternocleidomastoid muscle. Leave your fingers still while the

patient again swallows, thus allowing the gland to move beneath your fingers (Fig. 10-27). To examine the left lobe, move your hands to the reverse corresponding positions. By palpating above the cricoid cartilage, you may be able to feel the pyramidal lobe of the thyroid, if present.

For examining the thyroid from behind, have the patient sit with the neck at a comfortable level. Position two fingers of each hand on the sides of the trachea just beneath the cricoid cartilage. Ask the patient to swallow, feeling for movement of the isthmus. Then displace the trachea to the left (using your fingers of your right hand), and with the first three fingers of your left hand medial to the left sternocleidomastoid, palpate the left lobe as the patient again swallows. To palpate the right lobe, again move your hands to the reverse corresponding positions (Fig. 10-28).

Clinical Pearl

Is It the Thyroid Gland?

The thyroid gland moves with swallowing; subcutaneous fat mimicking a goiter does not.

The thyroid lobes, if felt, should be small, smooth, and free of nodules. The gland should rise freely with swallowing. The thyroid at its broadest dimension is approximately 4 cm, and the right lobe is often 25% larger than the left. The consistency of the thyroid tissue should be firm yet pliable. Coarse tissue or a gritty sensation suggests an inflammatory process. If nodules are present, they should be characterized by number, whether they are smooth or irregular, and whether they are soft or hard. An enlarged, tender thyroid may indicate thyroiditis.

If the thyroid gland is enlarged, auscultate for vascular sounds with the bell of the stethoscope. In a hypermetabolic state, the blood supply is dramatically increased and a vascular bruit (a soft rushing sound) may be heard (see Clinical Pearl, "Is It the Thyroid Gland?").

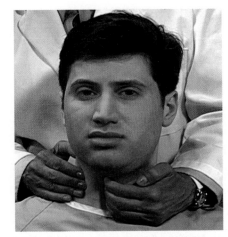

FIGURE 10-28 Palpation of the right thyroid lobe from behind the patient. Displace the trachea to the patient's right and palpate the right lobe as the patient again swallows.

❀ Infants

Inspection

Measure the infant's head circumference and compare it with expected size for age and previous points on the growth chart, as detailed in Chapter 6, pp. 84-85. Inspect the infant's head from all angles for symmetry of shape, noting any prominent bulges or depressions (see Clinical Pearl, "Examining the Head"). Inspect the scalp for scaling and crusting, birthmarks or skin lesions, dilated scalp veins, the presence of excessive hair, or an unusual hairline. Dilated scalp veins and a head circumference increasing faster than expected may indicate increased intracranial pressure (hydrocephalus; see Fig. 10-18).

> **Clinical Pearl**
>
> *Examining the Head*
>
> Examining the head from above is helpful for evaluating head shape

Birth trauma may cause swelling of the scalp. Caput succedaneum is subcutaneous edema over the presenting part of the head at delivery (Fig. 10-29). It is the most common form of birth trauma of the scalp and usually occurs over the occiput and crosses suture lines. The affected part of the scalp feels soft, and the margins are poorly defined. Generally, the edema goes away in a few days.

Cephalhematoma is a subperiosteal collection of blood and is therefore bound by the suture lines. It is commonly found in the parietal region and, unlike caput, may not be immediately obvious at birth. A cephalhematoma is firm, and its edges are well defined; it does not cross suture lines. As it ages, the cephalhematoma may liquefy and become fluctuant on palpation (Fig. 10-30).

Inspect the face for spacing of the features, symmetry, paralysis, skin color, and texture. Uterine positioning can cause some facial asymmetry in the newborn.

FIGURE 10-29 Caput succedaneum. Significant scalp edema as a result of compression during transit through birth canal. Edema does cross suture lines. *(From Zitelli and Davis, 2007.)*

Head shape with an unusual contour may be related to premature or irregular closing of suture lines. Preterm infants often have long, narrow heads (brachiocephaly) because their soft cranial bones become flattened with positioning and the weight of the head. Note any skull asymmetry or a particularly flattened spot on the back or one side of the head (plagiocephaly). Plagiocephaly can result from premature fusion of one of the sutures (craniosynostosis; see Fig. 10-39) or from external deformation (positional plagiocephaly). Positional plagiocephaly is common among infants with torticollis. Bossing (bulging of the skull) of the frontal areas is associated with prematurity, thalassemia, Paget disease, and rickets. Bulging in other areas of the skull may indicate cranial defects or intracranial masses.

Observe the infant's head control, position, and movement. Note any jerking, tremors, or inability to move the head in one direction. Chapter 21, p. 529 and Chapter 22, p. 566 provide further details.

Inspect the infant's neck for symmetry, size, and shape. Note the presence of edema, distended neck veins, pulsations, masses, webbing, or excessive nuchal skin. To observe the newborn's neck, which is usually not easily visible in the supine position, elevate the upper back of the infant and permit the head to fall back into extension. The neck appears short during infancy and lengthens by 3 to 4 years of age. Marked edema may indicate a localized infection. A cystic mass high in the neck may be a thyroglossal duct cyst or a branchial cleft cyst. A mass over the clavicle, changing size with crying or respiration, suggests a cystic hygroma.

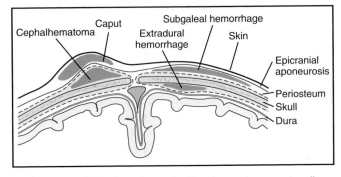

FIGURE 10-30 Cephalhematoma. Swelling does not cross suture lines. *(From Zitelli and Davis, 2007.)*

EXAMINATION AND FINDINGS

Palpation

Palpate the infant's head, identifying suture lines and fontanels. Note any tenderness over the scalp. Suture lines feel ridgelike until about 6 months of age, after which they are usually no longer palpable. Vaginally delivered newborns may have molding with prominent ridges from overriding sutures. Fontanels may be small or not palpable at birth. Molding of the head at delivery can be very distressing for parents. Reassure the parents that the abnormal shape generally disappears relatively quickly; reassurance is necessary (Fig. 10-31). Drawings can help you explain that the infant's cranial bones overlap and that their relative lack of development is a protective device for the brain. Symmetry of the head is usually regained within 1 week of birth, with fontanels and suture line resuming their appropriate shape and size. A third fontanel (the mastoid fontanel), located between the anterior and posterior fontanels, may be an expected variant but is also common in infants with Down syndrome. Any palpable ridges in addition to the expected suture lines may indicate skull fractures.

Measure the size of the anterior and posterior fontanels using two dimensions (anteroposterior and lateral). In infants younger than 6 months, the anterior fontanel diameter should not exceed 4 to 5 cm. It should get progressively smaller beyond that age, closing completely by 12 to 15 months of age.

With the infant in a supported sitting position, palpate the anterior fontanel for bulging or depression. It should feel slightly depressed, and some pulsation is expected. A bulging fontanel protrudes above the level of the bones of the skull when the infant is sitting and feels tense, similar to the fontanel of an infant during the expiratory phase of crying. A bulging fontanel with marked pulsations may indicate increased intracranial pressure from a space-occupying mass or meningitis.

Palpate the scalp firmly above and behind the ears to detect craniotabes (German word *crani* for "skull" and the Latin word *tabes* for "wasting"), a softening of the outer table of the skull. A snapping sensation, similar to the feeling of pressing on a

FIGURE 10-31 Molding of the newborn head. *(From Zitelli and Davis, 2007.)*

ping-pong ball, indicates craniotabes that may be associated with prematurity, rickets, hydrocephalus, marasmus, syphilis, or thalassemia.

Palpate the sternocleidomastoid muscle, noting its tone and the presence of any masses. A mass in the lower third of the muscle may indicate a hematoma. Palpate the trachea. The thyroid is difficult to palpate in an infant unless it is enlarged. The presence of a goiter, which may cause respiratory distress, results from intrauterine deprivation of thyroid hormone. Palpate the clavicles; a crunch is indicative of fracture that occurred at the time of birth in newborns.

Transillumination

You can transilluminate the skull of infants who have suspected intracranial lesions or a rapidly increasing head circumference Although transillumination is performed less often today because of the availability of computed tomography (CT) scans, it is less expensive and still quite helpful. Perform the procedure in a completely darkened room, allowing a few minutes to elapse for your eyes to adjust. The transilluminator is placed firmly against the infant's scalp so that no light escapes (Fig. 10-32). Begin at the midline frontal region and inch the transilluminator over the entire head. Observe the ring of illumination through the scalp

FIGURE 10-32 Transillumination of the infant's scalp.

and skull around the light, noting any asymmetry. A ring of 2 cm or less beyond the rim of the transilluminator is expected on all regions of the head except the occiput, where the ring should be 1 cm or less. Illumination beyond these parameters suggests excess fluid or decreased brain tissue in the skull.

�֎ Children

Direct percussion of the skull with one finger is useful to detect the Macewen sign (percussion of the skull near the junction of the frontal, temporal, and parietal bones producing a stronger resonant sound when either hydrocephalus or a brain abscess is present). The resonant sound is expected when the fontanels are open and may indicate increased intracranial pressure after fontanel closure.

Cranial bruits are common in children up to 5 years of age or in children with anemia. After age 5 years, their presence may suggest vascular anomalies or increased intracranial pressure.

The thyroid of the young child may be palpable. Using techniques described for adults, note the size, shape, position, mobility, and any tenderness. No tenderness should be present. An enlarged, tender thyroid may indicate thyroiditis.

✖ Pregnant Women

Beginning after 16 weeks of gestation, many pregnant women develop blotchy, brownish hyperpigmentation of the face, particularly over the malar prominences and the forehead (see Chapter 8 p. 141, Fig. 8-34. This chloasma, also called "mask of pregnancy," may further darken with sun exposure, but generally it fades after delivery. The thyroid gland may hypertrophy and become palpable (see Fig. 10-7). The hypertrophy is caused by hyperplasia of the glandular tissue and increased vascularity. Because of increased vascularity, a thyroid bruit may be heard. The presence of a goiter is not an expected finding. Pregnancy can make the diagnosis of hyperthyroidism difficult. The presence of weight loss, tachycardia, and bruit over the thyroid are highly suggestive. Confirmation of the diagnosis is made by measuring blood levels of thyroid-stimulating hormone (TSH) and free T_4.

✖ Older Adults

The facies of older adults vary with their nutritional status. The eyes may appear sunken with soft bulges underneath, and the eyelids may appear wrinkled and hang loose.

Use caution when evaluating range of motion in the older adult's neck. Rather than have the patient perform an entire rotational maneuver, go slowly and evaluate each movement separately. Note any pain, crepitus, dizziness, jerkiness, or limitation of movement.

With aging, the thyroid becomes more fibrotic, feeling more nodular or irregular to palpation.

Sample Documentation

History and Physical Examination

Subjective

A 32-year-old woman seeks care for a painless swelling in her neck. No difficulty swallowing or with movement of her neck. Her maternal grandmother and two maternal aunts have goiters. She has lost 5 pounds over the past 2 months without trying. She denies nervousness, palpitations, weakness, or menstrual changes.

Objective

Head: Held erect and midline; skull normocephalic, symmetrical and smooth without deformities; facial features symmetrical; salivary glands nontender; temporal artery pulsations visible bilaterally, soft and nontender to palpation; no bruits.

Neck: Trachea midline; no jugular venous distention (JVD) or carotid artery prominence; thyroid palpable, firm, gritty to palpation and symmetrically enlarged; thyroid and cartilages move with swallowing; no nodules, tenderness, or bruits; full range of motion of the neck without discomfort.

For additional sample documentation, see Chapter 26, pp. 628-631.

DIFFERENTIAL DIAGNOSIS

Comparison of Various Types of Headaches

Characteristic	Migraine	Medication Rebound	Cluster	Hypertensive	Muscular Tension	Temporal Arteritis	Space-occupying Lesion
Age at onset	Childhood		Adulthood	Adulthood	Adulthood	Older adulthood	Any
Location	Unilateral or generalized	Holocranial or diffuse	Unilateral	Bilateral or occipital	Unilateral or bilateral	Unilateral or bilateral	Localized
Duration	Hours to days	Hours to days	½ to 2 hours	Hours	Hours to days	Hours to days	Rapidly increasing frequency
Time of onset	Morning or night	Predictably begins within hours to days of the last dose of the medication	Night	Morning	Anytime, commonly in afternoon or evening	Anytime	Awakening from sleep
Quality of pain	Pulsating or throbbing	Dull or throbbing	Intense burning, boring, searing, knifelike	Throbbing	Bandlike, constricting	Throbbing	

Continued

ABNORMALITIES

DIFFERENTIAL DIAGNOSIS
Comparison of Various Types of Headaches—cont'd

Characteristic	Migraine	Medication Rebound	Cluster	Hypertensive	Muscular Tension	Temporal Arteritis	Space-occupying Lesion
Prodromal event	Vague neurologic changes, personality change, fluid retention, appetite loss to well-defined neurologic event, scotoma, aphasia, hemianopsia, aura	Daily analgesics use and or daily caffeine use	Personality changes, sleep disturbances	None	None	None	Aggravated by coughing or bending forward
Precipitating event	Menstrual period, missing meals, birth control pills, letdown after stress	Abrupt discontinuation of analgesics	Alcohol consumption	None	Stress, anger, bruxism	None	Develops in temporal relation to the neoplasm
Frequency	Twice a week	Gradual increase in headache frequency to daily	Several times nightly for several nights, then none	Daily	Daily	Daily	Progressive
Gender predilection	Females	Female	Males	Equal	Equal	Equal	Equal
Other symptoms	Nausea, vomiting	Alternate or preventive medications fail to control the headache	Increased lacrimation, nasal discharge	Generally remits as day progresses	None	None	Vomiting, confusion, abnormal neurologic findings, gait abnormality, papilledema, nystagmus

ABNORMALITIES

HEAD

Headaches
Pain in the head

Pathophysiology
- Common concern
- Probably one of the most self-medicated

Subjective Data
- Description (i.e., constant, severe, recurrent)
- Associated symptoms (e.g., tearing)
- Exposures (including medications)
- See Differential Diagnosis table on p. 198

Objective Data
- Normal physical exam, in many cases
- Neurologic deficits, in some cases
  - Abnormal gait
  - Papilledema
  - Nystagmus

Salivary Gland Tumor
Tumor in any of the salivary glands, but most commonly in the parotid (Fig. 10-33)

Pathophysiology
- Exact mechanism by which tumor growth occurs is incompletely understood

Subjective Data
- Slow-growing painless lumps, either in front of ear or under jaw
- Difficulty opening the mouth and tongue numbness or weakness

Objective Data
- Benign tumors usually smooth, malignant often irregular
- Facial weakness, fixation of the lump, sensory loss, ulceration

FIGURE 10-33 Malignant right parotid gland tumor. *(From Lemmi and Lemmi, 2000.)*

NECK

Thyroglossal Duct Cyst

Palpable cystic mass in the neck

Pathophysiology

- Remnant of fetal development
- Rises from the foramen cecum at junction of anterior two thirds and posterior third of tongue (Fig. 10-34)
- Any part can persist, causing a sinus, fistula, or cyst.

Subjective Data

- Tenderness, redness, swelling in midline of neck
- Difficulty swallowing or breathing

Objective Data

- Freely movable cystic mass in neck midline
- Moves upward with tongue protrusion and swallowing
- May have small opening in skin, with drainage of mucus

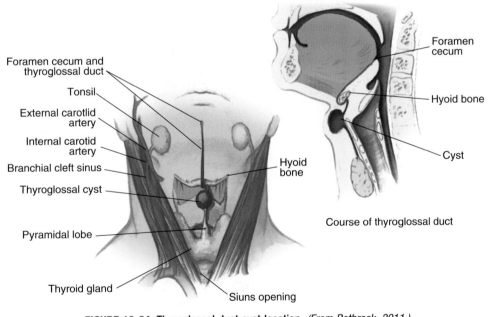

FIGURE 10-34 Thyroglossal duct cyst location. *(From Rothrock, 2011.)*

Branchial Cleft Cyst

Congenital lesion formed by incomplete involution of branchial cleft

Pathophysiology

- Epithelium-lined cyst with or without a sinus tract to overlying skin (Fig. 10-35)

Subjective Data

- Solitary, painless in lateral neck
- May have intermittent swelling and tenderness
- Discharge if associated with a sinus tract

Objective Data

- Oval, moderately movable smooth, nontender, fluctuant mass along anteromedial border of sternocleidomastoid muscle
- Usually asymptomatic
- If infected, tenderness and erythema

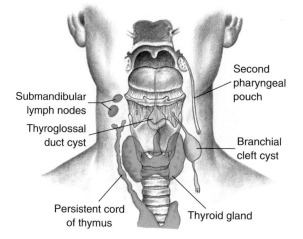

FIGURE 10-35 Branchial cleft cyst location in relation to other neck masses.

Torticollis (Wry Neck)

Shortening or excessive contraction of the sternocleidomastoid muscle

Pathophysiology

- Often result of birth trauma or intrauterine malposition
- Acquired torticollis is result of tumors, trauma, cranial nerve IV palsy, muscle spasms, infection, or drug ingestion.

Subjective Data

- Circumstances surrounding birth, trauma, medications
- Stiff neck, decreased range of motion of neck
- Possible vision problem

Objective Data

- Head tilted and twisted toward the affected sternocleidomastoid muscle with chin elevated and turned toward the opposite side (Fig. 10-36)
- A hematoma may be palpated shortly after birth, and within 2 to 3 weeks.
- Firm, fibrous mass may be felt in the muscle

FIGURE 10-36 Torticollis, or wry neck.
(From Zitelli and Davis, 2007.)

THYROID

Hypothyroidism

Underactive thyroid

Pathophysiology

- Primary: thyroid gland produces insufficient amounts of thyroid hormone.
- Secondary: insufficient thyroid hormone secretion due to inadequate secretion of either thyroid-stimulating hormone (TSH) from the pituitary gland or thyrotropin-releasing hormone (TRH) from the hypothalamus
- More common than hyperthyroidism

Subjective Data

- Weight gain, constipation, fatigue, and cold intolerance (see Table 10-1)

Objective Data

- Normal size thyroid, goiter, or nodule(s)

Table 10-1	Hyperthyroidism Versus Hypothyroidism	
System or Structure Affected	**Hyperthyroidism**	**Hypothyroidism**
Constitutional		
Temperature preference	Cool climate	Warm climate
Weight	Loss	Gain
Emotional state	Nervous, easily irritated, highly energetic	Lethargic, complacent, disinterested
Hair	Fine, with hair loss; failure to hold a permanent wave	Coarse, with tendency to break
Skin	Warm, fine, hyperpigmentation at pressure points	Coarse, scaling, dry
Fingernails	Thin, with tendency to break; may show onycholysis	Thick
Eyes	Bilateral or unilateral proptosis, lid retraction, double vision	Puffiness in periorbital region
Neck	Goiter, change in shirt neck size, pain over the thyroid	No goiter
Cardiac	Tachycardia, dysrhythmia, palpitations	No change noted
Gastrointestinal	Increased frequency of bowel movements; diarrhea rare	Constipation
Menstrual	Scant flow, amenorrhea	Menorrhagia
Neuromuscular	Increasing weakness, especially of proximal muscles	Lethargic, but good muscular strength

Hyperthyroidism

Overactive thyroid

Pathophysiology

- Excess thyroid hormone causes an increase in the metabolic rate.
- Associated with increased total body heat production and increased heart contractility, heart rate, and vasodilation
- Multinodular goiter (Plummer disease)

Subjective Data

- Weight loss, tachycardia, diarrhea, and heat sensitivity (see Table 10-1)

Objective Data

- Normal size thyroid, goiter, or nodule(s)
- Fine hair, bridle nails, proptosis, tachycardia

Myxedema

Skin and tissue disorder usually due to severe prolonged hypothyroidism (see Fig. 10-10)

Pathophysiology

- Decrease in metabolic rate, resulting in accumulation of hyaluronic acid and chondroitin sulfate in the dermis
- Deposition of glycosaminoglycan in all organ systems leads to mucinous edema of facial features.

Subjective Data

- Cognitive impairment, slowed mentation, poor concentration, decreased short-term memory, social withdrawal, psychomotor retardation, depressed mood, and apathy
- Constipation
- Muscle pains
- Hearing problems, deafness

Objective Data

- Coarse thick skin, thickening nose, swollen lips, puffiness around eyes
- Slow speech
- Mental dullness, lethargy, mental problems
- Weight gain
- Thin brittle hair, with bald patches

Graves Disease

Autoimmune antibodies to thyroid-stimulating hormone receptor leading to overactive thyroid

Pathophysiology

- More common in women during third and fourth decades

Subjective Data

- Symptoms of hyperthyroidism (palpitations, heat intolerance, weight loss, fatigue, increased appetite, tachycardia) (see Table 10-1)

Objective Data

- Diffuse thyroid enlargement; most commonly with prominent eyes (exophthalmos) (see Fig. 10-11)
- Dermatologic, constitutional, menstrual, and musculoskeletal abnormalities, nonpitting edema (pretibial myxedema)

Hashimoto Disease

Autoimmune antibodies against thyroid gland

Pathophysiology

- Often causes hypothyroidism
- More common in children and women between 30 and 50 years

Subjective Data

- Progresses slowly over a number of years
- Signs and symptoms of hypothyroidism; weight gain, nausea, fatigue (see Table 10-1)

Objective Data

- Enlarged nontender smooth thyroid

ABNORMALITIES

✣ Infants

Encephalocele

Neural tube defect with protrusions of brain and membranes that cover it through openings in the skull

Pathophysiology

- Failure of the neural tube to close completely during fetal development can occur any place on the scalp (Fig. 10-37).
- Genetic component; often occurs in families with a history of spina bifida and anencephaly

Subjective Data

- Prior to birth are visible only by intrauterine ultrasound or seen immediately after birth

Objective Data

- Visible sac of tissue protruding through skull
- Craniofacial abnormalities or other brain malformations, hydrocephalus

FIGURE 10-37 Encephalocele. *(From Zitelli and Davis, 2007.)*

Hydrocephalus

A problem in the formation, flow, or absorption of cerebrospinal fluid (CSF) that leads to an increase in volume of the CSF

Pathophysiology

- Normal flow of CSF is from the choroid plexus, to the lateral ventricle, then to the interventricular foramen of Monro, the third ventricle, the aqueduct of Sylvius, the fourth ventricle, the 2 lateral foramina of Luschka and the medial foramen of Magendie, the subarachnoid space, the arachnoid granulations, the dural sinus, and finally into venous circulation
- Abnormalities in the CSF circulation can arise from:
  - Congenital malformations, congenital infections, e.g., toxoplasmosis
  - Acquired abnormalities, e.g., intracranial mass, intracranial hemorrhage, meningitis, and trauma

Subjective Data

- Poor feeding
- Irritability
- Decreased activity
- Vomiting

Objective Data

- Head enlargement (see Fig. 10-18)
- Separation of cranial sutures
- Dilated scalp veins
- Tense anterior fontanelle
- Sunsetting sign (see Fig. 10-18)
- Increased tone (spasticity)
- Macewen sign (percussion of the skull near the junction of the frontal, temporal, and parietal bones will be more resonant or have a "cracked pot" sound.

Microcephaly

Circumference of head is smaller than normal because the brain has not developed properly or has stopped growing (Fig. 10-38).

Pathophysiology

- Present at birth or may develop in first few years of life
- Multiple causes including congenital infections and neuroanatomic abnormalities (e.g., cerebral dysgenesis or craniostenosis)

Subjective Data

- Associated with intellectual disability and failure of brain to develop normally

Objective Data

- Head circumference is 2 to 3 standard deviations below mean for age.

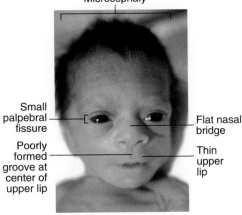

FIGURE 10-38 Primary familial microcephaly. The facial features of an infant with fetal alcohol syndrome (FAS) include short palpebral (eye) fissures; a flat nasal bridge; a thin, flat upper lip; a poorly formed groove at the center of the upper lip; and a small head (microcephaly). *(From Leifer, 2011.)*

Craniosynostosis

Premature closure of one or more cranial sutures before brain growth complete

Pathophysiology

- Leads to misshapen skull (Fig. 10-39)
- Involved sutures determine shape of the head.

Subjective Data

- Abnormally shaped skull, usually not accompanied by mental retardation

Objective Data

- Skull growth restricted perpendicular to fused suture
- If multiple sutures fuse while brain is still growing, intracranial pressure can increase (see signs of increased cranial pressure in Chapter 27 p. 643)

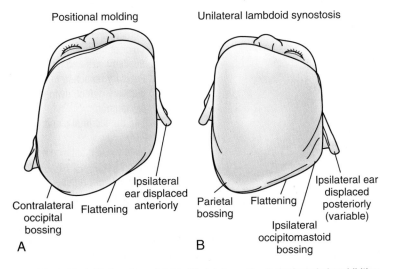

FIGURE 10-39 A, Vertex view of right-sided deformational plagiocephaly exhibiting a parallelogram head shape. **B,** Vertex view of right-sided lambdoid craniosynostosis exhibiting a trapezoid-like head shape. *(From Zitelli and Davis, 2007.)*

CHAPTER 11

Eyes

The comprehensive eye examination involves a series of tests evaluating vision as well as the general health of the eyes and includes screening for ophthalmologic diseases or ocular manifestation of systemic diseases.

ANATOMY AND PHYSIOLOGY

The eye is the sensory organ that transmits visual stimuli to the brain for interpretation (Fig. 11-1). It occupies the orbital cavity; only its anterior aspect exposed. The eye itself is a direct embryologic extension of the brain.

There are four rectus and two oblique muscles attached to the eye (Fig. 11-2). The eye itself is connected to the brain by cranial nerve (CN) II, the optic nerve.

Physical Examination Preview

Here is a preview of the steps involved in conducting physical examination of the eyes. ⊜ These procedures are explained in detail in this chapter and are available on Evolve in printable formats.

Eyes
1. Measure visual acuity, noting the following (pp. 208-209):
   - Near vision
   - Distant vision
   - Peripheral vision
2. Inspect the eyebrows for the following (p. 210):
   - Hair texture
   - Size
   - Extension to temporal canthus
3. Inspect the orbital area for the following (p. 210):
   - Edema
   - Redundant tissues or edema
   - Lesions
4. Inspect the eyelids for the following (pp. 210-211):
   - Ability to open wide and close completely
   - Eyelash position
   - Ptosis
   - Fasciculations or tremors
   - Flakiness
   - Redness
   - Swelling
5. Palpate the eyelids for nodules (p. 211).
6. Inspect the orbits (p. 210).
7. Pull down the lower lids and inspect palpebral conjunctivae, bulbar conjunctiva, and sclerae for the following (pp. 211-212):
   - Color
   - Discharge
   - Lacrimal gland punctum
   - Pterygium
8. Inspect the external eyes for the following (pp. 212-214):
   - Corneal clarity
   - Corneal sensitivity
   - Corneal arcus
   - Color of irides
   - Pupillary size and shape
   - Pupillary response to light and accommodation, afferent pupillary defect, swinging flashlight test
   - Nystagmus
9. Palpate the lacrimal gland in the superior temporal orbital rim (p. 214).
10. Evaluate muscle balance and movement of eyes with the following (pp. 214-216):
    - Corneal light reflex
    - Cover-uncover test
    - Six cardinal fields of gaze
11. Ophthalmoscopic examination (pp. 216-218):
    - Lens clarity
    - Red reflex
    - Retinal color and lesions
    - Characteristics of blood vessels
    - Disc characteristics
    - Macula characteristics
    - Depth of anterior chamber

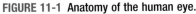

FIGURE 11-1 Anatomy of the human eye.

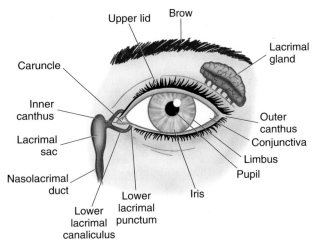

FIGURE 11-3 Important landmarks of the left external eye. *(From Thompson et al, 1997.)*

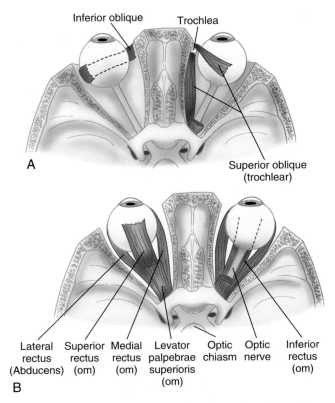

FIGURE 11-2 Extraocular muscles of the eye as viewed from above. **A,** The oblique muscles. **B,** The recti muscles (*om*, oculomotor). The cranial nerves, which innervate the muscles, are listed in Figure 11-22.

External Eye

The external eye is composed of the eyelid, conjunctiva, lacrimal gland, eye muscles, and the bony orbit. The orbit also contains fat, blood vessels, nerves, and supporting connective tissue (see Fig. 11-1).

Eyelid

The eyelid is composed of skin, striated muscle, the tarsal plate, and conjunctivae. Meibomian glands in the eyelid provide oils to the tear film. The tarsus provides a skeleton to the lid. The eyelid distributes tears over the surface of the eye, limits the amount of light entering it, and protects the eye from foreign bodies. Eyelashes extend from the anterior border of each lid.

Conjunctiva

The conjunctiva is a clear, thin mucous membrane. The palpebral conjunctiva is the part of the conjunctiva that coats the inside of the eyelids. The bulbar (or ocular) conjunctiva is the part of the conjunctiva that covers the outer surface of the eye. The bulbar conjunctiva protects the anterior surface of the eye with the exception of the cornea and the surface of the eyelid in contact with the globe.

Lacrimal Gland

The lacrimal gland is located in the temporal region of the superior eyelid and produces tears that moisten the eye (Fig. 11-3). Tears flow over the cornea and drain via the canaliculi to the lacrimal sac and duct and then into the nasal meatus.

Eye Muscles

Each eye is moved by six muscles—the superior, inferior, medial, and lateral rectus muscles and the superior and inferior oblique muscles (see Figs. 11-2 and 11-22). They are innervated by CNs III (oculomotor), IV (trochlear), and VI (abducens). The oculomotor nerve controls the levator palpebrae superioris (which elevates and retracts the upper eyelid) and all extraocular muscles except for the superior oblique muscle and the lateral rectus muscle. The superior oblique is the only muscle innervated by the trochlear nerve and the lateral rectus muscle is the only muscle innervated by the abducens nerve.

Internal Eye

The internal structures of the eye are composed of three separate layers. The outer wall of the eye is composed of the sclera posteriorly and the cornea anteriorly. The middle layer or uvea consists

ANATOMY AND PHYSIOLOGY

of the choroid posteriorly and the ciliary body and iris anteriorly. The inner layer of nerve fibers is the retina (see Fig. 11-1).

Sclera

The sclera is the dense, avascular structure that appears anteriorly as the white of the eye. It physically supports the internal structure of the eye.

Cornea

The cornea constitutes the anterior sixth of the globe and is continuous with the sclera. It is optically clear, has rich sensory innervation, and is avascular. It is a major part of the refractive power of the eye.

Uvea

The iris, ciliary body, and choroids comprise the uveal tract (see Fig. 11-1). The iris is a circular, contractile muscular disc containing pigment cells that produce the color of the eye. The central aperture of the iris is the pupil, through which light travels to the retina. By dilating and contracting, the iris controls the amount of light reaching the retina. The ciliary body produces the aqueous humor (fluid that circulates between the lens and cornea) and contains the muscles controlling accommodation. The choroid is a pigmented, richly vascular layer that supplies oxygen to the outer layer of the retina.

Lens

The lens is a biconvex, transparent structure located immediately behind the iris (see Fig. 11-1). It is supported circumferentially by fibers arising from the ciliary body. The lens is highly elastic, and contraction or relaxation of the ciliary body changes its thickness, thereby permitting images from varied distances to be focused on the retina.

Retina

The retina is the sensory network of the eye. It transforms light impulses into electrical impulses, which are transmitted through the optic nerve, optic tract, and optic radiation to the visual cortex in the brain and then to interpretation in the cerebral cortex. The optic nerve passes through the optic foramen along with the ophthalmic artery and vein. The optic nerve communicates with the brain and the autonomic nervous system of the eye. Accurate binocular vision is achieved when an image is fused on the retina by the cornea and the lens. An object may be perceived in each visual cortex, even when one eye is covered, if the light impulse is cast on both the temporal and the nasal retina. Fibers located on the nasal retina decussate in the optic chiasm (Fig. 11-4). Accurate binocular vision also requires the synchronous functioning of the extraocular muscles.

Major landmarks of the retina include the optic disc, from which the optic nerve originates, together with the central retinal artery and vein. The macula, or fovea, is the site of central vision (see Fig. 11-1).

✿ Infants and Children

The eyes develop during the first 8 weeks of gestation and may become malformed due to maternal drug ingestion or infection

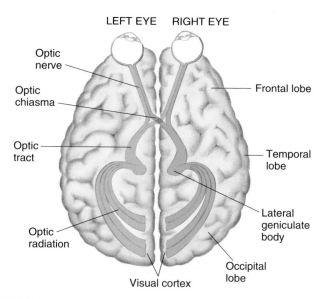

FIGURE 11-4 The optic chiasm. *(Modified from Thompson et al, 1997.)*

during this time. The development of vision, which is dependent on maturation of the nervous system, occurs over a longer period (Table 11-1). Term infants are hyperopic, with a visual acuity of less than 20/400 (see Visual Acuity Testing, pp. 208-209). Although peripheral vision is fully developed at birth, central vision matures later. One of the earliest visual responses is the infant's regard for the mother's face. By 2 to 3 weeks of age, the lacrimal gland begins producing a full volume of tears and many infants will show an interest in large objects. Lacrimal drainage is complete at the time of term birth. By 3 to 4 months of age, binocular vision development is complete. By 6 months, vision has developed sufficiently so that the infant can differentiate colors.

Young children become less hyperopic with growth. The globe of the eye grows as the child's head and brain grow, and adult visual acuity is achieved at about 4 years of age.

✿ Pregnant Women

The eyes undergo several changes during pregnancy because of physiologic and hormonal adaptations. These changes can result in hypersensitivity and can change the refractory power of the eye. Tears contain an increased level of lysozyme, resulting in a greasy sensation and perhaps blurred vision for contact lens wearers. Diabetic retinopathy may worsen significantly. Mild corneal edema and thickening associated with blurred vision may occur, especially in the third trimester.

Intraocular pressure falls most notably during the latter half of pregnancy.

✿ Older Adults

The major physiologic eye change that occurs with aging is a progressive weakening of accommodation (focusing power) known as presbyopia. In general, by 45 years of age, the lens becomes more rigid and the ciliary muscle becomes weaker. The lens also continues to form fibers throughout life. Old fibers are compressed centrally, forming a denser central region that

Table 11-1	Chronology of Visual Development
Age	**Levels of Development**
Birth	Awareness of light and dark; infant closes eyelids in bright light
Neonatal	Visual acuity 20/400 (6/120) Rudimentary fixation on near objects, able to regard mother's face
2 weeks	Transitory fixation, usually monocular at a distance of roughly 3 feet Follows large, conspicuously moving objects
4 weeks	Visual acuity 20/300 (6/90) Moving objects evoke binocular fixation briefly
6 weeks	Follows moving objects with jerky eye movements
8 weeks	Visual following now achieved by a combination of head and eye movements
12 weeks	Enjoys light objects and bright colors Beginning of depth perception Fusion of images begins to appear
16 weeks	Visual acuity 20/300 to 20/200 (6/90 to 6/60) Fixates immediately on moving target, visually pursues dropped toy
20 weeks	Shows interest in stimuli more than 3 feet away Retrieves a dropped 1-inch cube Can maintain voluntary fixation of stationary object even in the presence of competing moving stimulus
24 weeks	Visual acuity 20/50 (6/15) to 20/200 (6/60) Can maintain voluntary fixation of stationary object even in the presence of competing moving stimulus Hand-eye coordination appearing Will fixate on a string Binocular fixation clearly established
26 weeks	Marked interest in tiny objects
28 weeks	Tilts head backward to gaze up
40 weeks	Visual acuity 20/200 (6/70) Discriminates simple geometric forms (squares and circles)
52 weeks	Looks at pictures with interest Convergence well established
12-18 months	Localization in distance crude—runs into large objects
18 months	Accommodation well developed Visual acuity 20/40 (6/12)
2 years	Visual acuity 20/30 (6/9) Convergence smooth
3 years	Visual acuity 20/20 (6/6)

American Optometric Association, 2002.

may cause loss of clarity of the lens and contribute to cataract formation (clouding of the lens that can become partially or totally opaque) (see Fig. 11-43, p. 225).

Risk Factors

Cataract Formation

- Family history of cataracts
- Steroid medication use
- Exposure to ultraviolet light
- Cigarette smoking
- Diabetes mellitus
- Aging

REVIEW OF RELATED HISTORY

For each of the symptoms or conditions discussed in this section, targeted topics to include in the history of the present illness are listed. Responses to questions about these topics provide clues for focusing the physical examination and the development of an appropriate diagnostic evaluation. Questions regarding medication use (prescription and over the counter preparations) as well as complementary and alternative therapies are relevant for each.

History of Present Illness

- Red eye (presence of conjunctival injection or redness)
  - Difficulty with vision: one or both eyes, corrected by lenses
  - Recent injury or foreign bodies; sleeping in contact lenses
  - Pain: with or without loss of vision, in or around the eye, superficial or deep, insidious or abrupt in onset; burning, itching, or nonspecific uncomfortable or gritty sensation
  - History of swelling, infections, or eye surgery
  - History of recent illness or similar symptoms in the household
  - Allergies: type, seasonal, associated symptoms
  - Eye secretions: color (clear or yellow), consistency (watery or purulent), duration, tears that run down the face, decreased tear formation with sensation of gritty eyes
  - Medications: eye drops or ointments, antibiotics, artificial tears, mydriatics; glaucoma medications, antioxidant vitamins (to prevent macular degeneration), steroids (which promote cataract formation)
- Vision problem
  - Eyelids: recurrent hordeola (stye; acute infection of sebaceous glands of Zeis), chalazion (chronic blockage of meibomian gland), ptosis of the lids so that they interfere with vision (unilateral or bilateral), growths or masses, itching
  - Involves one or both eyes, corrected by lenses, involving near or distant vision, primarily central or peripheral, transient or sustained
  - Cataracts (bilateral or unilateral), types (e.g., infantile, senile, diabetic, traumatic, surgical treatment)
  - Adequacy of color vision
  - Presence of halos around lights, floaters, or diplopia (when one eye is covered or when both eyes are open)

+ Trauma: to the eye as a whole or a specific structure (e.g., cornea) or supporting structures (e.g., the floor of the orbit); events surrounding the trauma; efforts at correction and degree of success

Past Medical History

+ Eye surgery: condition requiring surgery, laser vision correction, date of surgery, outcome
+ Chronic illness that may affect eyes or vision: glaucoma, diabetes, atherosclerotic cardiovascular disease (ASCVD), hypertension, thyroid dysfunction, autoimmune diseases, human immunodeficiency virus (HIV), inflammatory bowel diseases
+ Medications: steroids, hydroxychloroquine, antihistamines, antidepressants, antipsychotics, antiarrhythmics, beta-blockers

Family History

+ Retinoblastoma (often an autosomal dominant disorder)
+ Glaucoma, macular degeneration, diabetes, hypertension, or other diseases that may have an impact on vision or eye health
+ Cataracts
+ Color blindness, retinal detachment, retinitis pigmentosa, or allergies affecting the eye
+ Nearsightedness, farsightedness, strabismus, or amblyopia

Personal and Social History

+ Employment: exposure to irritating gases, chemicals, foreign bodies, or high-speed machinery
+ Activities: participation in sporting activities that might endanger the eye (e.g., boxing, lacrosse, hockey, basketball, football, paintball, martial arts, rifle shooting, racquetball, fencing, motorcycle riding)
+ Use of protective devices during work or activities that might endanger the eye
+ Corrective lenses: when last changed, how long worn, type (glasses or contact lenses), adequacy of corrected vision; methods of cleaning and storage, insertion and removal procedures of contact lenses; date of last eye examination
+ History of cigarette smoking (a risk factor for cataract formation, glaucoma, macular degeneration, thyroid eye disease)

❀ Infants and Children

+ Preterm: resuscitative efforts, mechanical ventilation or oxygen used, retinopathy of prematurity, birth weight, gestational age, sepsis, intracranial hemorrhage
+ Maternal history of sexually transmitted infections
+ Congenital abnormalities of the eye
+ Symptoms of congenital abnormalities including failure of infant to gaze at mother's face or other objects; failure of infant to blink when bright lights or threatening movements are directed at the face

+ White area in the pupil on a photograph or on examination (leukocoria); inability of one eye to reflect light properly (may indicate retinoblastoma or other serious intraocular problem)
+ Excessive tearing or discharge, erythema
+ Strabismus some or all of the time; frequency; when first noted; occurring when fatigued, sick, or otherwise stressed; associated with frequent blinking or squinting, nystagmus
+ Young children: excessive rubbing of the eyes, frequent hordeola, inability to reach for and pick up small objects, night vision difficulties
+ School-age children: necessity of sitting near the front of the classroom to see the teacher's work; poor school performance not explained by intellectual ability

❀ Pregnant Women

+ Presence of disorders that can cause ocular complications such as pregnancy-induced hypertension (PIH) or gestational diabetes. Symptoms indicative of PIH: diplopia, scotomata, blurred vision, or amaurosis
+ Use of topical eye medications (may cross the placental barrier)

❀ Older Adults

+ Visual acuity: decrease in central vision, distortion of central vision, use of dim or bright light to increase visual acuity, difficulty with glare. Difficulty in performing near work without lenses
+ Excess tearing
+ Dry eyes
+ Nocturnal eye pain (sign of subacute angle closure and a symptom of glaucoma)
+ Difficulty with depth perception

EXAMINATION AND FINDINGS

Equipment

+ Snellen chart or Lea Cards, Landolt C, or HOTV chart (see Chapter 3 pp. 43-44 and Fig. 3-17 A, B)
+ Rosenbaum or Jaeger near vision card (see Chapter 3, p. 44)
+ Penlight
+ Cotton wisp
+ Ophthalmoscope (see Chapter 3, pp. 42-43 and Figs. 3-13 and 3-15)
+ Eye cover, gauze, or opaque card

Visual Acuity Testing

Measurement of visual acuity—the discrimination of small visual details—tests CN II (optic nerve) and is essentially a measurement of central vision. This important assessment is often inappropriately neglected by examiners who are not ophthalmologists. Position the patient 20 feet (6 m) away from the Snellen chart (see Fig. 3-17, p. 44). Make sure the chart is well lighted. Alternatively, special charts for use 10 feet (3 m) away from the patient are available. Test each eye individually by covering one eye with an opaque card or gauze, being careful to avoid applying pressure to the eye. If you test the patient with and without corrective lenses, record the readings separately. Always test vision without glasses first.

Ask the patient to identify all of the letters, beginning at any line. Determine the smallest line in which the patient can identify all of the letters and record the visual acuity designated by that line. (For more information, see Chapter 3, pp. 43-44.) When testing the second eye, you may want to ask the patient to read the line from right to left to reduce the chance of recall influencing the response. Conduct the test rapidly enough to prevent the patient from memorizing the chart. However, avoid going too quickly when asking that the lines on the chart be read or that other judgments must be made. It is wise to pace the assessment slowly for patient comfort and to allow time for the patient to reason out a response. Visual acuity is recorded as a fraction in which the numerator indicates the distance of the patient from the chart (e.g., 20 feet or 6 m), and the denominator indicates the distance at which the average eye can read the line. Thus, 20/200 (6/60) means that the patient can read at 20 feet (6 m) what the average person can read at 200 feet (6 m). The smaller the fraction, the worse is the vision. Vision not correctable to better than 20/200 is considered legal blindness (see Clinical Pearl, "Is It Blurry or Is It Double?").

Perform a pinhole test if the visual acuity is recorded at a fraction less than 20/20 (or 6/6), to see if the observed decrease in acuity was caused by a refractive error. Ask the patient to hold a pinhole occluder (or a piece of paper with a small hole in it) over the uncovered eye. This maneuver permits light to enter only the central portion of the lens. Expect an improvement in visual acuity by at least one line on the chart if refractive error is responsible for the diminished acuity (see Clinical Pearl, "Factors that Affect Visual Acuity Testing").

> ### Clinical Pearl
>
> *Is It Blurry or Is It Double?*
>
> Blurred vision and diplopia are sometimes confused by the patient. Blurred vision represents a problem with visual acuity and there are many causes. Diplopia is the perception of two images and may be monocular or binocular. Monocular diplopia is an optical problem; binocular diplopia is an alignment problem.

> ### Clinical Pearl
>
> *Factors That Affect Visual Acuity Testing*
>
> Testing of visual acuity involves many complex factors not necessarily related to the ability to see the test object. Motivation and interest (including malingering), as well as literacy, intelligence, and attention span, can modify the results of sensory testing.

Measurement of near vision should also be tested in each eye separately with a handheld card such as the Rosenbaum Pocket Vision Screener. Have the patient hold the card at a comfortable distance (about 35 cm, or 14 inches) from the eyes and read the smallest line possible.

FIGURE 11-5 Evaluation of peripheral fields of vision. A, Temporal field. B, Nasal field.

Peripheral vision can be accurately measured with sophisticated instruments, but is generally estimated by the confrontation test. Sit or stand opposite the patient at eye level at a distance of about 1 m (3 feet). Ask the patient to cover the right eye while you cover your left eye, so the open eyes are directly opposite each other (Fig. 11-5). Both you and the patient should be looking at each other's eye. Fully extend your arm midway between the patient and yourself and then move your arm slowly centrally. Have the patient tell you when the fingers are first seen. Compare the patient's response to the time you first note the fingers. Test the nasal, temporal, superior, and inferior fields. Remember that the nose itself interferes with the nasal portion of the visual field. Unless you are aware of a problem with your vision, you can feel comfortable that the fields are full if they correspond with yours. The confrontation test is imprecise and can be considered significant only when it is abnormal. Lesions most likely to produce confrontation abnormalities include stroke, retinal detachment, optic neuropathy, pituitary tumor compression at the optic chiasm, and central retinal vascular occlusion.

Color vision is rarely tested in the routine physical examination. Color plates are available in which numerals are produced in primary colors and surrounded by confusing colors. The patient is asked to read the numbers. The tests vary in degree of difficulty. For routine testing, check the patient's ability to appreciate primary colors. Red testing may be particularly helpful in determining subtle optic nerve disease, even when visual acuity remains nearly normal. An afferent pupillary defect (see p. 213) often coexists with a red defect.

External Examination

Carry out examination of the eyes in a systematic manner, beginning with the appendages (i.e., the eyebrows and surrounding tissues) and moving inward.

EXAMINATION AND FINDINGS

FIGURE 11-6 **Xanthelasma.** *(Courtesy John W. Payne, MD, The Wilmer Ophthalmological Institute, The Johns Hopkins University and Hospital, Baltimore, MD.)*

FIGURE 11-7 **Ptosis, a drooping of the upper eyelid.** *(From Patzelt, 2009.)*

Surrounding Structures

Inspect the eyebrows for size, extension, and texture of the hair. Note whether the eyebrows extend beyond the eye itself or end short of it. If the patient's eyebrows are coarse or do not extend beyond the temporal canthus, the patient may have hypothyroidism. If the brows appear unusually thin, ask if the patient waxes or plucks them.

Inspect the orbital and periorbital area for edema, puffiness, or redundant tissue below the orbit. Although puffiness may represent the loss of elastic tissue that occurs with aging, periorbital edema is always abnormal; the significance varies directly with the amount. It may represent the presence of thyroid eye disease, allergies, or (especially in youth) the presence of renal disease (nephrotic syndrome). You may see flat to slightly raised, oval, irregularly shaped, yellow-tinted lesions on the periorbital tissues that represent depositions of lipids and may suggest that the patient has an abnormality of lipid metabolism. These lesions are called *xanthelasma* (Fig. 11-6), an elevated plaque of cholesterol deposited in macrophages, most commonly in the nasal portion of the upper or lower lid.

Eyelids

Examine the patient's lightly closed eyes for fasciculations or tremors of the lids, a sign of hyperthyroidism. Inspect the eyelids for their ability to close completely and open widely. Observe for flakiness, redness, or swelling on the eyelid margin. Eyelashes should be present on both lids and should curve away from the globe.

When the eye is open, the superior eyelid should cover a portion of the iris but not the pupil itself. If one superior eyelid covers more of the iris than the other or extends over the pupil, then ptosis of that lid is present. Ptosis indicates a congenital or acquired weakness of the levator muscle or a paresis of a branch of the third cranial nerve (Fig. 11-7). Record the difference between the two lids in millimeters. The average upper lid position is 2 mm below the limbus (the border of the cornea and the sclera), and the average lower lid position is at the lower limbus.

You should also note whether the lids evert or invert. When the lower lid is turned away from the eye, it is called *ectropion* and may result in excessive tearing (Fig. 11-8). The inferior punctum, which serves as the tear-collecting system, is pulled outward and cannot collect the secretions of the lacrimal gland.

FIGURE 11-8 **Ectropion.** *(From Stein et al, 1988.)*

FIGURE 11-9 **Entropion.** Note that this patient has undergone corneal transplantation. *(From Palay and Krachmer, 1997.)*

When the lid is turned inward toward the globe, a condition known as entropion (Fig. 11-9), the lid's eyelashes may cause corneal and conjunctival irritation, increasing the risk of a secondary infection. The patient often reports a foreign body sensation.

An acute suppurative inflammation of the follicle of an eyelash can cause an erythematous or yellow lump. This hordeolum or stye is generally caused by a staphylococcal infection (Fig. 11-10).

Crusting along the eyelashes may represent blepharitis caused by bacterial infection, seborrhea, psoriasis, a manifestation of rosacea, or an allergic response (Fig. 11-11).

Ask the patient to close the eyes, and note whether the eyelids meet completely. If the closed lids do not completely cover the globe (a condition called *lagophthalmos*), the cornea may become dried and be at increased risk of infection. Thyroid eye disease,

FIGURE 11-10 **Acute hordeolum of upper eyelid.** *(From Palay and Krachmer, 1997.)*

FIGURE 11-12 **Pulling lower eyelid down to inspect the conjunctiva.**

FIGURE 11-11 **Blepharitis.** *(From Zitelli and Davis, 1997.)*

seventh nerve palsy (Bell palsy), and overaggressive ptosis or blepharoplasty surgical repair are common causes.

Palpation

Palpate the eyelids for nodules. Palpation of the orbit is one of the simplest methods for intraocular pressure assessment. Gentle palpation through closed lids (digital palpation tonometry) can confirm that the involved eye is much harder than the uninvolved eye. Determine whether the orbit can be gently pushed into the orbit without discomfort. Pain on palpation is consistent with scleritis, orbital cellulitis, and cavernous sinus thrombosis. An eye that feels very firm and resists palpation may indicate severe glaucoma or retrobulbar tumor.

Conjunctiva

The conjunctivae are usually translucent and free of erythema. Inspect the palpebral conjunctiva by having the patient look upward while you draw the lower lid downward noting translucency and vascular pattern (Fig. 11-12).

Inspect the upper tarsal conjunctiva only when there is a suggestion that a foreign body may be present. Ask the patient to look down while you pull the eyelashes gently downward and forward to break the suction between the lid and globe. Next, evert the lid on a small cotton-covered applicator (Fig. 11-13). After you inspect and remove any foreign body that may be present, return the eyelid to its regular position by asking the patient to look up while you apply downward pressure against the eyelid.

FIGURE 11-13 **Everting upper eyelid.** *A*, Placing applicator above the globe. *B*, Withdrawing the lid from the globe.

Observe the conjunctiva for erythema or exudate. An erythematous or cobblestone appearance, especially on the tarsal conjunctiva, may indicate an allergic (Fig. 11-14) or infectious conjunctivitis (Fig. 11-15). Bright red blood in a sharply defined area surrounded by healthy-appearing conjunctiva indicates subconjunctival hemorrhage (Fig. 11-16). The blood stays red because of direct diffusion of oxygen through the conjunctiva. Subconjunctival hemorrhages may occur spontaneously in pregnancy or during labor; these resolve spontaneously.

FIGURE 11-14 Erythematous eye from a chemical allergy. *(From Lemmi and Lemmi, 2009.)*

FIGURE 11-15 Acute purulent conjunctivitis. *(From Newell, 1996.)*

FIGURE 11-16 Subconjunctival hemorrhage. *(From Lemmi and Lemmi, 2009.)*

FIGURE 11-17 Pterygium. *(Courtesy John W. Payne, MD, The Wilmer Ophthalmological Institute, The Johns Hopkins University and Hospital, Baltimore, MD.)*

FIGURE 11-18 Testing corneal sensitivity.

FIGURE 11-19 Corneal arcus senilis. *(From Palay and Krachmer, 1997.)*

A pterygium is an abnormal growth of conjunctiva that extends over the cornea from the limbus. It occurs more commonly on the nasal side (Fig. 11-17) but may arise temporally as well. A pterygium is more common in people heavily exposed to ultraviolet light. It can interfere with vision if it advances over the pupil.

Cornea

Examine the cornea for clarity by shining a light tangentially on it. Because the cornea is normally avascular, blood vessels should not be present. Corneal sensitivity, controlled by CN V (trigeminal nerve), is tested by touching a wisp of cotton to the cornea (Fig. 11-18). The expected response is a blink, which indicates intact sensory fibers of CN V and motor fibers of CN VII (facial nerve). Decreased corneal sensation is often associated with diabetes, herpes simplex and herpes zoster viral infections, and after trigeminal neuralgia surgery.

You may note a corneal arcus (arcus senilis), which is composed of lipids deposited in the periphery of the cornea. It may in time form a complete circle (circus senilis) (Fig. 11-19). Note the subtle clear area between the limbus and the arcus. An arcus is seen in many individuals older than 60 years. If present before age 40, arcus senilis may indicate a lipid disorder. It is possible to have more than one process; Figure 11-20 demonstrates both corneal circus senilis and a pterygium.

Iris and Pupil

The iris pattern should be clearly visible. In general, the irides are the same color. Note any irregularity in the shape of the pupils. Expect them to be round, regular, and equal in size. Bilateral and unilateral pupil abnormalities are listed in Table 11-2.

EXAMINATION AND FINDINGS

Estimate the pupillary sizes and compare them for equality. Pupils may show size variation in a number of ways. Miosis is pupillary constriction to less than 2 mm. The miotic pupil fails to dilate in the dark. It is commonly caused by ingestion of narcotics such as morphine, but drugs that control glaucoma may also cause miosis. Pupillary dilation of more than 6 mm and failure of the pupils to constrict with light characterize mydriasis. Mydriasis is an accompaniment of coma (e.g., due to diabetes, alcohol, uremia, epilepsy, or brain trauma), or may be caused by some eye drops (e.g., some glaucoma medications, atropine, or strabismus management in children). Anisocoria, inequality of pupillary size, is a common variation but may also occur in a large range of disease states.

Test the pupils for response to light both directly and consensually. Dim the lights in the room so that the pupils dilate. Shine a penlight directly into one eye and note whether the pupil constricts. Expect the consensual response of the opposite pupil constricting simultaneously with the tested pupil. Repeat the test by shining the light in the other eye.

To evaluate the health of the optic nerve, look for an afferent pupillary defect by performing the swinging flashlight test. Shine the light in one eye and then rapidly swing to the other. There should be a slight dilation in the second eye while the light is crossing the bridge of the nose but it should constrict equally to the first eye as the light enters the pupil. Repeat going in the other direction. If the pupil continues to dilate rather than constrict, an afferent pupillary defect is present; also called a *Marcus-Gunn pupil*. This is an important sign of optic nerve disease and can be present in any eye with poor vision from severe retinal disease. There are many causes of afferent papillary defect including optic neuritis, glaucoma and optic nerve tumor, and multiple sclerosis. It is possible for an eye to have good visual acuity and an afferent defect. The eye, however, is not normal and the cause must be investigated.

Test the pupils for constriction to accommodation as well. Ask the patient to look at a distant object and then at a test object (either a pencil or your finger) held 10 cm from the bridge of the nose. Expect the pupils to constrict when the eyes focus on the near object. With some patients, especially those with dark irides, it may be easier to observe pupillary dilation when the patient looks from near to far. Testing for pupillary response to accommodation is of diagnostic importance only if there is a defect in

FIGURE 11-20 Arcus senilis and pterygium. *(From Lemmi and Lemmi, 2009.)*

Table 11-2   Descriptions of Various Pupil Abnormalities

Abnormality	Contributing Factors	Appearance
Bilateral		
Miosis (pupillary constriction; usually less than 2 mm in diameter)	Iridocyclitis; miotic eye drops (e.g., pilocarpine given for glaucoma); drug abuse	
Mydriasis (pupillary dilation; usually more than 6 mm in diameter)	Iridocyclitis; mydriatic or cycloplegic drops (e.g., atropine); midbrain (reflex arc) lesions or hypoxia; oculomotor (cranial nerve [CN] III) damage; acute-angle glaucoma (slight dilation); drug abuse	
Failure to respond (constrict) with increased light stimulus	Iridocyclitis; retinal degeneration; optic nerve (CN II) destruction; midbrain synapses involving afferent papillae fibers or oculomotor nerve (CN III) (consensual response is also lost); impairment of efferent fibers (parasympathetic) that innervate sphincter pupillae muscle; mydriatics	
Argyll Robertson pupil	Bilateral, miotic, irregularly shaped pupils that fail to constrict with light but retain constriction with convergence; pupils may or may not be equal in size; commonly caused by neurosyphilis or lesions in midbrain where afferent pupillary fibers synapse	

Continued

Table 11-2   Descriptions of Various Pupil Abnormalities—cont'd

Abnormality	Contributing Factors	Appearance
Unilateral Anisocoria (unequal size of pupils)	Congenital (approximately 20% of healthy people have minor or noticeable differences in pupil size, but reflexes are normal) or caused by local eye medications (constrictors or dilators), or unilateral sympathetic or parasympathetic pupillary pathway destruction (NOTE: Examiner should test whether pupils react equally to light; if response is unequal, examiner should note whether larger or smaller eye reacts more slowly [or not at all], because either pupil could represent the abnormal size.)	
Iritis constrictive response	Acute uveitis is commonly unilateral; constriction of pupil accompanied by pain and reddened eye, especially adjacent to the iris	
Oculomotor nerve (CN III) damage	Pupil dilated and fixed; eye deviated laterally and downward; ptosis	
Adie pupil (tonic pupil)	Affected pupil dilated and reacts slowly or fails to react to light; responds to convergence; caused by impairment of postganglionic parasympathetic innervation to sphincter pupillae muscle or ciliary malfunction; often accompanied by diminished tendon reflexes (as with diabetic neuropathy or alcoholism)	

the pupillary response to light. A failure to respond to direct light but retaining constriction during accommodation is sometimes seen in patients with diabetes or syphilis.

Lens

Inspect the lens, which should be transparent. Shining a light on the lens may cause it to appear gray or yellow, but should still be able to allow the light to pass through. Later examination of the lens with the ophthalmoscope will help judge the clarity.

Sclera

The sclera should be examined primarily to ensure that it is white. The sclera should be visible above the iris only when the eyelids are wide open. If liver or a hemolytic disease is present, the sclera may become pigmented and appear either yellow or green. Senile hyaline plaque appears as a dark, slate gray pigment just anterior to the insertion of the medial rectus muscle (Fig. 11-21). Its presence does not imply disease but should be noted.

Lacrimal Apparatus

Inspect the region of the lacrimal gland and palpate the lower orbital rim near the inner canthus. The puncta should be seen as slight elevations with a central depression on both the upper and lower lid margins nasally. If the temporal aspect of the upper lid

FIGURE 11-21 Senile hyaline plaque. *(From Newell, 1996.)*

feels full, evert the lid and inspect the gland. The lacrimal glands are rarely enlarged but may become enlarged in some conditions such as tumors, lymphoid infiltration, sarcoid disease, and Sjögren syndrome. Despite the enlargement, the patient may report dry eyes because the glands produce inadequate tears.

Extraocular Muscles

Full movement of the eyes is controlled by the integrated function of the CNs III (oculomotor), IV (trochlear), and VI (abducens) and the six extraocular muscles. You may hold the patient's

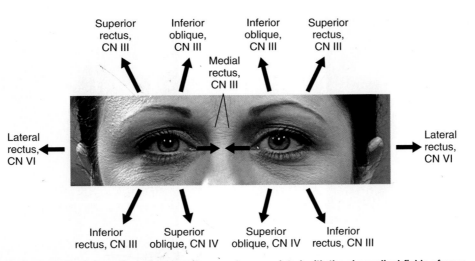

FIGURE 11-22 Cranial nerves and extraocular muscles associated with the six cardinal fields of gaze.

Physical Variations

Eye Protrusion

The mean protrusion of the eye for black males exceeds that of white males by 2 to 4 mm. Anthropometric studies showed that blacks have a rectangular, shallower orbit, Asians have a rounder orbit, and whites are somewhere between the two. There is also a reduction in ocular protrusion with increasing age.

Data from Ahmadi et al, 2007; Barretto, and Mathog, 1999; Quant and Woo, 1992.

chin to prevent movement of the head and ask him or her to watch your finger as it moves through the six cardinal fields of gaze (Fig. 11-22). Then ask the patient to look to the extreme lateral (temporal) positions. Do not be surprised to observe a few horizontal rhythmic movements (nystagmic beats).

Occasionally, you may note sustained nystagmus, involuntary rhythmic movements of the eyes that can occur in a horizontal, vertical, rotary, or mixed pattern. Jerking nystagmus, characterized by faster movements in one direction, is defined by its rapid movement phase. For example, if the eye moves rapidly to the right and then slowly drifts leftward, the patient is said to have nystagmus to the right.

Finally, have the patient follow your finger in the vertical plane, going from ceiling to floor. Observe the coordinated movement of the globes and the superior lids. The movement should be accomplished smoothly and without exposure of the sclera. Full movements indicate integrity of muscle strength and cranial nerves. Lid lag, the exposure of the sclera above the iris when the patient is asked to follow your finger as you direct the eye in a smooth movement from ceiling to floor, may indicate thyroid eye disease.

Use the corneal light reflex to test the balance of the extraocular muscles. Direct a light source at the nasal bridge from a distance of about 30 cm. Ask the patient to look at a nearby object (but not the light source). This will encourage the effort of both eyes to converge. The light should be reflected symmetrically from both eyes. If you find an imbalance with the corneal light reflex test, perform the cover-uncover test (Fig. 11-23) or

FIGURE 11-23 Evaluating eye fixation by the cover-uncover test. **A,** Patient focuses on near object. **B,** Examiner evaluates movement of covered eye as cover is removed.

use StrabismoScope or photoscreening (see Chapter 3, p. 43, Fig. 3-16) to evaluate. To perform the cover-uncover test, ask the patient to stare straight ahead at a near fixed point. Cover one eye and observe uncovered eye for movement as it focuses on the designated point. Remove the cover and watch for movement of the newly uncovered eye as it fixes on the object. Repeat the process, covering the other eye. If the eye being tested is the strabismic eye (crossed eye; both eyes not looking at the same place at the same time), then it will fixate on the object by moving

EXAMINATION AND FINDINGS

FIGURE 11-24 **Strabismus.** *(Courtesy Freda Lemmi, 2009.)*

FIGURE 11-25 **A,** Visualization of the red reflex. **B,** Examination of the optic fundus.

after the "straight" eye is covered as long as the vision in this eye is good enough (Fig. 11-24). If the "straight" eye is being tested, there will be no movement, as it is already fixated. Depending on the direction that the strabismic eye deviates, the direction of deviation may be assessed. *Exotropic* is outward (away from the midline) and *esotropic* is inward (toward the nose). Movement of the covered or uncovered eye mandates referral to an ophthalmologist.

Ophthalmoscopic Examination

The ophthalmoscopic (funduscopic) examination of the eyes can be a tiring process for the patient. Give the patient brief intervals of rest from the bright light to reduce fatigue and improve comfort.

Inspection of the interior of the eye permits visualization of the optic disc, arteries, veins, and retina. Adequate pupillary dilation is necessary and can often be achieved by dimming the lights in the examining room. Instillation of medications that cause mydriasis is used in some cases (Box 11-1).

Examine the patient's right eye with your right eye and the patient's left eye with your left. Hold the ophthalmoscope in the hand that corresponds to the examining eye. (The structure of the ophthalmoscope is detailed in Chapter 3, pp. 42-43.) Change the lens of the ophthalmoscope with your index finger. Start with the lens on the 0 setting, and stabilize yourself and the patient by placing your free hand on the patient's shoulder or head (Fig. 11-25). If using a PanOptic ophthalmoscope (see Chapter 3, p. 43, Fig. 3-15 you can use your dominant eye to examine both of the patient's eyes due to the increased distance between the patient and examiner. The focus wheel is adjusted with your thumb.

With the patient looking at a distant fixation point, direct the light of the ophthalmoscope at the pupil from about 30 cm (12 inches) away. If using a PanOptic ophthalmoscope focus on an object 15 to 20 feet away, then slowly position the eye cup over the patient's eye. With either scope, visualize a red reflex first. The red reflex is caused by the light illuminating the retina. Any opacities in the path of the light will stand out as black densities. Absence of the red reflex is often the result of an improperly

---

Box 11-1   Test for Applying Mydriatics

Before instillation of a mydriatic, inspect the patient's anterior chamber by shining a focused light tangentially at the limbus (the union of the conjunctiva and the sclera). Note the illumination of the iris nasally. This portion of the iris is not lighted when the patient has a shallow anterior chamber, indicating a risk of acute-angle glaucoma. Mydriatics should be avoided in these patients.

Evaluation of depth of anterior chambers. **A,** Usual anterior chamber. **B,** Shallow anterior chamber.

FIGURE 11-28 **Fundus of a black patient.** *(From Medcom, 1983.)*

Superior nasal arteries and veins

Superior temporal arteries and veins

Optic disc

Fovea centralis

Inferior nasal arteries and veins

Inferior temporal arteries and veins

FIGURE 11-26 **Retinal structures of the left eye.**

FIGURE 11-27 **A,** Normal right fundus in a white patient. **B,** Normal left fundus. *(From Lemmi and Lemmi, 2009.)*

positioned ophthalmoscope, but it may also indicate total opacity of the pupil by a cataract or by hemorrhage into the vitreous humor. If you locate the red reflex and then lose it as you approach the patient, simply move back and start again.

No discrete areas of lighter or darker pigmentation are expected when viewing the fundus except for crescents or dots at the disc margin, most commonly along the temporal edge.

As you approach the eye gradually, the retinal details should become apparent (Figs. 11-26 and 11-27, *A,B*). At any one time, you will see only a small portion of the retina. A blood vessel will probably be the first structure seen when you are about 3 to 5 cm from the patient. You may have to adjust the ophthalmoscope

lens to be able to see the retinal details. If your patient is myopic, you will need to use a minus (red) lens; if the patient is hyperopic or lacks a lens (aphakic), you will need a plus lens (see Chapter 3, p. 42). When fundus details come into focus, you will note the branching of blood vessels. Because they always branch away from the optic disc, you can use these landmarks to find the optic disc. The optic disk is where the retina converges to the optic nerve and because there are no photoreceptors (rods and cones) in this part of the retina and it cannot respond to light stimulation, it is called a "blind spot."

Next, look at the vascular supply of the retina. The blood vessels on the disc divide into superior and inferior branches and then into nasal and temporal ones. Venous pulsation may be seen on the disc and should be noted. Arterioles are smaller than venules, generally by a ratio of 3:5 to 2:3. The light reflected from arterioles is brighter than that from venules, and the oxygenated blood is a brighter red. Follow the blood vessels distally as far as you can in each of the four quadrants. Note especially the sites of crossing of the arterioles and venules, because their characteristics may change when hypertension is present. Expected characteristics found on ophthalmologic examination in a patient with hypertension include narrowing of vessels, increased vascular tortuosity, copper wiring (diffuse red-brown reflex), arteriovenous nicking, and retinal hemorrhages.

Finally, examine the optic disc itself. The disc margin should be sharp and well defined, especially in the temporal region. The disc is generally yellow to creamy pink, but the color varies with race, being darker in individuals whose skin is dark (Fig. 11-28; see Clinical Pearl, "Fundus Pigmentation"). It is about 1.5 mm in diameter and is the unit of measurement in describing lesion size and location on the fundus. For example, an abnormality of a blood vessel may occur 2 disc diameters from the optic nerve at the 2 o'clock position (Fig. 11-29).

Clinical Pearl

Fundus Pigmentation

The fundus, or retina, appears as a yellow or reddish pink background, depending on the amount of melanin in the pigment epithelium. The pigment generally varies with the skin color of the patient (see Fig. 11-28).

FIGURE 11-29 Method of describing the position and dimension of a lesion in terms of disc diameter. The lesion in this illustration is described as being 2 disc diameters (DD) from the optic disc at the 2 o'clock position. The lesion is ⅔ DD long and ⅓ DD wide.

FIGURE 11-30 Myelinated retinal nerve fibers. *(Courtesy Andrew P. Schachat, MD, The Wilmer Ophthalmological Institute, The Johns Hopkins University and Hospital, Baltimore, MD.)*

FIGURE 11-31 Severe papilledema. *(Courtesy John W. Payne, MD, The Wilmer Ophthalmological Institute, The Johns Hopkins University and Hospital, Baltimore, MD.)*

Next examine the macula, also called the *fovea centralis* or *macula lutea*. The site of central vision, it is located approximately 2 disc diameters temporal to the optic disc. It may be impossible to examine when the pupil is not dilated, because shining light on it induces strong pupillary constriction. To bring it into your field of vision, ask the patient to look directly at the light of the ophthalmoscope. No blood vessels enter the fovea, and it appears as a lighter dot surrounded by an avascular area.

FIGURE 11-32 Marked glaucomatous optic nerve head cupping. Compare the disappearance of blood vessels here with the blood vessels of the optic disc in Figures 11-26 and 11-27. *(Courtesy Andrew P. Schachat, MD, The Wilmer Ophthalmological Institute, The Johns Hopkins University and Hospital, Baltimore, MD.)*

Unexpected Findings

Occasionally, you may see unexpected findings such as myelinated nerve fibers, papilledema, glaucomatous cupping, drusen bodies, cotton wool bodies, or hemorrhages (Table 11-3).

Drusen bodies can appear as small, discrete spots that are slightly more yellow than the retina. With time the spots enlarge. Similar appearing lesions may occur in many conditions that affect the pigment layers of the retina, but most commonly they are a consequence of the aging process and, depending on size and number, are a precursor of senile macular degeneration (Fig. 11-33, *A*).

When drusen bodies are noted to be increasing in number or in intensity of color, use an Amsler grid to evaluate the patient's central vision. Instruct the patient to observe the grid with each eye, using reading glasses if needed, and to note any distortion of the grid pattern. Distortion could represent macular degeneration (see Abnormalities, p. 230). Figure 11-33, *B*, shows the grid of an individual with drusen bodies who has developed fluid leakage in the area of the macula.

Hemorrhages in the retina vary in color and shape, depending on the cause and location. A hemorrhage at the disc margin often indicates poorly controlled glaucoma or undiagnosed glaucoma (Fig. 11-34, *A*). Also note the loss of the vessels at the inferior margin of the disc. Flame-shaped hemorrhages occur in the nerve fiber layers, and the blood spreads parallel to the nerve fibers (Fig. 11-34, *B*). Round hemorrhages tend to occur in the deeper layers and may appear as a dark color instead of the bright red that is characteristic of flame hemorrhages. Dot hemorrhages may actually represent microaneurysms, which are common in diabetic retinopathy. The direct ophthalmoscope does not permit the distinction between dot hemorrhages and microaneurysms. Vascular changes that suggest systemic hypertension may be observed in the retina and are described in Box 11-2.

⚘ Infants

Infants often shut their eyes tightly when eye examination is attempted. It is difficult to separate the eyelids, and often the lids evert when too much effort is exerted. If a parent is present, have the parent hold the infant over a shoulder, and position yourself behind the parent. Turning off the overhead lights can be helpful too (see Clinical Pearl, "Examining an Infant's Eyes").

Table 11-3 Unexpected Retinal Findings

Unexpected Finding	Description	Significance
Myelinated retinal nerve fibers (see Fig. 11-30)	White area with soft, ill-defined peripheral margins usually continuous with the optic disc Absence of pigment, feathery margins, and full visual fields help distinguish this benign condition from chorioretinitis. Contrast with Fig. 11-48, page 228. Nerve fiber layer is the innermost retinal surface; the vessels lie deeper in the retina. Note how the myelinated nerve fibers obscure areas of the retinal blood vessels, particularly inferiorly.	No physiologic significance
Papilledema (see Fig. 11-31)	Loss of definition of optic disc margin, initially occurs superiorly and inferiorly, then nasally and temporally central vessels pushed forward, and veins are markedly dilated. Venous pulsations are not visible and cannot be induced by pressure applied to the globe. Venous hemorrhages may occur.	Caused by increased intracranial pressure transmitted along the optic nerve. Initially, vision is not altered.
Glaucomatous optic nerve head cupping (see Fig. 11-32)	Physiologic disc margins are raised with a lowered central area. Blood vessels may disappear over the edge of the physiologic disc and be seen again deep within the disc. Occasionally atrophy occurs unilaterally; always compare cupping on the two retina. Compare with healthy vessels as seen in Figures 11-26 and 11-27. Impairment of blood supply may lead to optic atrophy, causing the disc to appear much whiter than usual. The cup is usually not particularly enlarged in contrast to glaucomatous atrophy.	Result of increased intraocular pressure with loss of nerve fibers and death of ganglion cells Peripheral visual fields are constricted.
Cotton wool spot (see Fig. 11-44)	Ill-defined, yellow areas caused by infarction of nerve layer of the retina	Vascular disease secondary to hypertension or diabetes mellitus is a common cause.

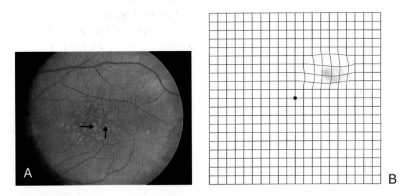

FIGURE 11-33 **A,** Drusen bodies. **B,** Amsler grid showing visual changes seen caused by fluid leakage under the retina. *(A, Courtesy Robert P. Murphy, MD, Glaser Murphy Retina Treatment Center, Baltimore, MD. B, Courtesy Brent A. Bauer, MFA, The Wilmer Ophthalmological Institute, The Johns Hopkins University and Hospital, Baltimore, MD.)*

Clinical Pearl

Examining an Infant's Eyes

Even when the infant is crying, there is often a moment when the infant's eyes open. This gives you an opportunity to learn something about the eyes, including their symmetry, extraocular muscular balance, and whether there is a light reflex.

FIGURE 11-34 **A,** Hemorrhage at the disc margin. **B,** Flame hemorrhages. *(A, Courtesy John W. Payne, MD, The Wilmer Ophthalmological Institute, The Johns Hopkins University and Hospital, Baltimore, MD. B, Courtesy Robert P. Murphy, MD, Glaser Murphy Retina Treatment Center, Baltimore, MD.)*

Begin by inspecting the infant's external eye structures. Note the size of the eyes, paying particular attention to small or differently sized eyes. Inspect the eyelids for swelling, epicanthal folds, and position. To detect epicanthal folds, look for a vertical fold of skin nasally that covers the lacrimal caruncle (Fig. 11-35). Prominent epicanthal folds are an expected variant in Asian infants, and may be seen in infants of other racial and ethnic backgrounds, but they may also be suggestive of Down syndrome or other congenital anomalies. Observe the alignment and slant of the palpebral fissures of the infant's eyes. Draw an imaginary line through the medial canthi and extend the line past the outer canthi of the eyes. The medial and lateral canthi are usually horizontal. When the outer canthi are above the line, an upward slant is present. When the outer canthi are below the line, a downward slant is present (Fig. 11-36).

Inspect the level of the eyelid covering the eye. To detect the sunsetting sign, rapidly lower the infant from upright to supine position. Look for sclera above the iris (see Fig. 6-16, p. 93). This sign may be an expected variant in newborns; however, it also may be observed in infants with hydrocephalus and brainstem lesions.

FIGURE 11-35 Epicanthal folds. *(From Zitelli and Davis, 2007.)*

Box 11-2   Hypertensive Retinopathy

- Retinal changes associated with hypertension have historically been classified according to the Keith-Wagner-Barker (KWB) system of four groups of increasing severity (Keith et al, 1939). They described changes in the vascular supply, the retina itself, and the optic disc. Criticism of this system argues that the retinopathy grades are not closely correlated with severity of hypertension (Wong and Mitchell, 2004).
- The arteriole-venule size ratio is usually 3:5. That ratio decreases as arterioles become smaller because of smooth muscle contraction, hyperplasia, or fibrosis. Venules do not have a smooth muscle coat but share the adventitia of the arteriole where the

arteriole and venule cross. Thickening of the arteriolar coat results in apparent nicking of the venule where the venule passes beneath the arteriole, or the venule may appear elevated when it passes over the arteriole.
- Classically, the KWB system is divided into four degrees and their morphologic classification has been widely used. However, a more pathophysiologic division has been adopted. This three-degree classification includes mild, moderate, and severe (Wong and Mitchell, 2004). In this classification scale, groups 1 and 2 of the KWB system have been combined.

Grade of Retinopathy	Retinal Signs	Systemic Associations
None	No detectable changes	None
Mild	Retinal arteriolar narrowing, arteriovenous nicking, opacity (copper wiring) of arteriolar wall	Modest association with risk of clinically significant stroke, subclinical stroke, coronary heart disease and death
Moderate	Hemorrhage (blot, dot, or flame-shaped), cotton-wool spots, hard exudates, and microaneurysms	Strong association with clinically significant stroke, cognitive decline, and death from cardiovascular causes
Malignant	Some or all of the above, plus optic disc edema (papilledema)	Strong association with death, presence of papilledema mandates rapid lowering of blood pressure

FIGURE 11-36 Drawing a line between the two medial canthi and extending it temporally to determine whether a Mongolian or anti-Mongolian slant is present. *(Courtesy Matthew Watson.)*

FIGURE 11-37 Swollen eyelids in a newborn.

Observe the distance between the eyes, looking for a wide spacing, or hypertelorism, which may be associated with craniofacial defects including some with intellectual disability. Pseudostrabismus, the false appearance of strabismus caused by a flattened nasal bridge or epicanthal folds, is an expected variant in Asian and Native American/American Indian infants, as well as in some whites. Pseudostrabismus generally disappears by about 1 year of age. Use the corneal light reflex to distinguish pseudostrabismus from strabismus. An asymmetric light reflex may indicate a true strabismus or hypertelorism.

Inspect the sclera, conjunctiva, pupil, and iris of each eye. Inspect and compare corneal sizes. Enlarged corneas may be a sign of congenital glaucoma. The newborn's eyelids may be swollen or edematous from birth trauma (Fig. 11-37) but, if accompanied by conjunctival inflammation and drainage, may represent ophthalmia neonatorum (neonatal bacterial conjunctivitis). Any redness, hemorrhages, discharge, or granular appearance beyond the newborn period may indicate infection, allergy, or trauma. Inspect each iris and pupil for any irregularity in shape. A coloboma, or keyhole pupil, is often associated with other congenital anomalies. White specks scattered in a linear pattern around the entire circumference of the iris, called *Brushfield spots*, strongly suggest Down syndrome (trisomy 13).

Test CNs II, III, IV, and VI in the following manner:

- Examine vision grossly by observing the infant's preference for looking at certain objects. Expect the infant to focus on and track a light or face through 60 degrees.
- Elicit the optical blink reflex by shining a bright light at the infant's eyes, noting the quick closure of the eyes and dorsiflexion of the head.
- Perform the corneal reflex as in adults.

Assess the red reflex bilaterally in every newborn. Observe for any opacities, dark spots, or white spots. Opacities or interruption of the red reflex may indicate congenital cataracts or retinoblastoma or other serious intraocular pathology (Table 11-4).

A funduscopic examination is difficult to conduct on a newborn or young infant and is generally deferred until the infant is 2 to 6 months of age unless there is concern about a congenital eye abnormality, suspicion of physical abuse (shaken baby syndrome), trauma, or need for an assessment for retinopathy of prematurity.

✿ Children

Perform the inspection of the young child's external eye structures as described for the infant.

Test visual acuity (when the child is cooperative) with the Snellen E game or other standardized vision chart for children such as the HOTV, usually beginning at about 3 years of age (see Fig. 3-17*A*, *B* on p. 44). Have one examiner point to the line on the chart and another assist the child with covering one eye. As with adults, have the child stand 20 feet (6 m) away. Allow the child to practice following the instructions before you administer the test. Instruct the child to point his or her arm or finger in the direction of the legs of the "E" or point to the correct letter or direction of the E on a card held in front of him or her. Test each eye separately. If the child wears glasses, vision should be tested both with and without corrective lenses and recorded separately.

Examine visual acuity of younger children by observing their activities. Provide an opportunity for the child to play with toys in the examining room. Watch the child stacking, building, or placing objects inside of others. Children usually have no visual difficulties in one eye if these tasks are performed well. The anticipated visual acuity for children aged 3 to 5 years should be 20/40 or better, and a 6-year-old's visual acuity should be 20/30 or better. A child with vision that falls outside this range should be referred to a specialist for evaluation. Photoscreening is recommended as an alternative to visual acuity screening with vision charts from 3 through 5 years of age, after age 5 years visual acuity screening with vision charts becomes more efficient and less costly (American Academy of Ophthalmology, 2007; American Academy of Pediatrics, 2012; U.S. Preventive Services Task Force, 2011).

When you are testing visual acuity in the child, any difference in the scores between the eyes should be noted. A child with a two-line difference between the eyes even within the passing range (e.g., 20/25 and 20/40) should also be referred to a specialist.

Examine extraocular movements and CNs III, IV, and VI as performed with adults. You may need to hold the child's head

Table 11-4 Pediatric Eye Evaluation Screening Recommendations for Health Care Providers

Recommended Age for Screening	Screening Method	Criteria for Referral to An Ophthalmologist
Newborn to 3 months	Red reflex Inspection for constant strabismus	Abnormal or asymmetric Structural abnormality
6 months to 1 year	Fix and follow with each eye Alternate occlusion Corneal light reflex Red reflex Inspection for strabismus	Failure to fix and follow in cooperative infant Failure to object equally to the covering of each eye Asymmetric Abnormal or asymmetric Structural abnormality
3 to 5 years	Visual acuity* Corneal light reflex/cover-uncover Stereoacuity† Red reflex Inspection	20/40 or worse, or 2 lines of difference between the eyes Asymmetric/ocular fixation movements Failure to appreciate asymmetric random dot or Titmus stereogram Abnormal or asymmetric Structural abnormality
6 years and older	Visual acuity* Corneal light reflex/cover-uncover Stereoacuity† Red reflex Inspection	20/30 or worse, or 2 lines of difference between the eyes Asymmetric/ocular fixation movements Failure to appreciate stereopsis Abnormal or asymmetric Structural abnormality

Copyright American Academy of Ophthalmology: Preferred Practice Pattern: Pediatric Eye Evaluations, 2003.
NOTE: These recommendations are based on expert opinion.
*Figures, letters, "tumbling E," or optotypes.
†Optional: Random Dot E Game (RDE), Titmus Stereograms (Titmus Optical, Inc, Petersburg, VA), Randot Stereograms (Stereo Optical Company, Inc, Chicago, IL).

still and use an appealing toy or object for the child to follow through the six cardinal fields of gaze. Peripheral vision can be tested in cooperative children; the young child may prefer to sit on the parent's lap while these tests are performed.

Patience is often needed to gain the child's cooperation for the funduscopic examination. The young child is often unable to keep the eyes still and focused on a distant object. Do not hold the child's eyelids open forcibly because that may lead to some resistance. Rather than move the ophthalmoscope to visualize all retinal fields, inspect the optic disc, the fovea, and the vessels as they pass by. Often the results are better when the child sits on the parent's lap. If this position is used, examine the child as you would an adult.

⚘ Pregnant Women

Retinal examination in the pregnant woman can help differentiate between chronic hypertension and PIH. Vascular tortuosity, angiosclerosis, hemorrhage, and exudates may be seen in patients with a long-standing history of hypertension. In the patient with PIH, however, there is segmental arteriolar narrowing with a wet, glistening appearance indicative of edema. This finding is not exclusive to pregnant women. Hemorrhages and exudates are rare. Detachment of the retina may occur with spontaneous reattachment after hypertension is successfully controlled.

Because of systemic absorption, cycloplegic and mydriatic agents should be avoided unless there is a need to evaluate for retinal disease. Use of nasolacrimal duct occlusion after instillation of topical eye medications may reduce systemic absorption.

⚘ Older Adults

Lacrimal glands begin to involute and tear production decreases. The most common causes of decreased visual function include glaucoma, cataracts, and macular degeneration.

Sample Documentation

Eyes

Subjective

A 37-year-old man reports sudden loss of vision in his right eye, no pain. Has had diabetes mellitus since age 12. Received laser therapy 2 years ago for retinopathy.

Objective

Visual acuity 20/40 left eye, by Snellen measurement; right eye, sees light only. Visual field is full by confrontation, left eye. Extraocular movements intact and full; no nystagmus. Lids and globes are symmetric. No ptosis. Eyebrows full; no edema or lesions evident. Conjunctivae clear. Sclerae white, anicteric (without jaundice). No discharge. Cornea clear; corneal reflex intact bilaterally. Irides blue. Pupils equal and round. Both pupils are reactive to light directly and consensually. Ophthalmologic examination reveals a red reflex, left eye. The left disc is well defined and cream-colored. No venous pulsations evident at the disc. Arteriole-venule ratio is 3:5; no nicking or crossing changes seen. Multiple blackened laser scars in the periphery circumferentially. Dot hemorrhages and hard exudates also noted. Macula yellow and free of lesions. No red reflex or retina can be seen, right eye and there is blood in the vitreous.

For additional sample documentation, see Chapter 26, pp. 628-631.

ABNORMALITIES

EXTERNAL EYE

Exophthalmos

Bulging of eye anteriorly out of orbit (Fig. 11-38)

Pathophysiology

- Can be from an increase in volume of orbital contents
- Most common cause is Graves disease
- In Graves disease, it is due to abnormal connective tissue deposition in orbit and extraocular muscles
- Bilateral or unilateral
- When unilateral, a retro-orbital tumor must be considered

Subjective Data

- Trauma that can cause complete or partial dislocation of the eye

FIGURE 11-38 Thyroid exophthalmos. See also Figure 10-11. *(From Stein et al, 1994.)*

Objective Data

- Apparent eye protrusion, lids do not reach the iris
- Measurement of degree of exophthalmos is performed using an exophthalmometer, usually by an ophthalmologist

Episcleritis

Inflammation of the superficial layers of the sclera anterior to the insertion of the rectus muscles (Fig. 11-39)

Pathophysiology

Pathophysiology is poorly understood. There are two kinds:
- Simple
  - Intermittent episodes of moderate-to-severe inflammation
  - Often recur at 1- to 3-month intervals
  - Lasting 7-10 days, and resolving after 2-3 weeks
- Nodular
  - Prolonged attacks of inflammation that are typically more painful than simple episcleritis

Most cases are idiopathic; may have an underlying systemic condition such as autoimmune disorders, including Crohn disease, rheumatoid arthritis, systemic lupus erythematosus, polyarteritis nodosa, psoriatic arthritis, gout, atopy, foreign bodies, chemical exposure, or infection

Subjective Data

- Acute onset of mild-to-moderate discomfort or photophobia
- Painless injection (redness) and/or watery discharge without crusting

FIGURE 11-39 Episcleritis. *(From Lemmi and Lemmi, 2009.)*

Objective Data

- Diffuse or localized injection of the bulbar conjunctiva
- Purplish elevation of a few millimeters
- Watery discharge

Band Keratopathy

Deposition of calcium in the superficial cornea (Fig. 11-40)

Pathophysiology

- Most commonly in patients with chronic corneal disease
- May occur in patients with hypercalcemia, hyperparathyroidism, and occasionally in individuals with trauma, renal failure sarcoidosis, or syphilis

Subjective Data

- Decrease in vision as deposition progresses
- Foreign body sensation and irritation

Objective Data

- Line just below the pupil; passes over the cornea rather than around the iris as arcus senilis does
- Horizontal grayish bands interspersed with dark areas that look like holes

ABNORMALITIES

FIGURE 11-40 Band keratopathy. *(Courtesy John W. Payne, MD, The Wilmer Ophthalmological Institute, The Johns Hopkins University and Hospital, Baltimore, MD.)*

Corneal Ulcer

Disruption of the corneal epithelium and stroma (Fig. 11-41)

Pathophysiology	Subjective Data	Objective Data

Causes:
• Rheumatologic disorder
   • Connective tissue disease, such as rheumatoid arthritis, Sjögren syndrome, or a systemic vasculitic disorder (e.g., systemic lupus erythematosus, Wegener granulomatosis, polyarteritis nodosa)
   • Infection: Viral infection (e.g., herpes simplex virus), bacterial infection
   • Extreme dryness: Incomplete lid closure or poor lacrimal gland function
	• Pain
	• Photophobia
	• History of wearing contact lenses
	• Blurry vision
	• Feeling that something is in the eye
		• Visual acuity affected variably, depending on ulcer location
		• Inflammation and erythema of the lids and conjunctiva
		• Purulent exudates
		• Ulcer often round or oval, and the border sharply demarcated, with the base appearing ragged and gray

FIGURE 11-41 Corneal ulcer in the lower temporal quadrant of the left cornea stained with rose bengal. *(Courtesy John W. Payne, MD, The Wilmer Ophthalmological Institute, The Johns Hopkins University and Hospital, Baltimore.)*

EXTRAOCULAR MUSCLES

Strabismus

Both eyes do not focus on an object simultaneously, but can focus with either eye (see Fig. 11-24)

Pathophysiology	Subjective Data	Objective Data
• Paralytic, caused by impairment of one or more extraocular muscles • Nonparalytic with no primary muscle weakness • May be a sign of increased intracranial pressure • Cranial nerve III is particularly vulnerable to damage from brain swelling	• Poor vision • May have sudden onset of double vision • Report of eye deviation	• If an extraocular muscle has become impaired, the eye will not move in the direction controlled by that muscle; for example, if the right sixth nerve is damaged, the right eye does not move temporally • Detected by the cover-uncover test (see Fig. 11-24) or in children with use of StrabismoScope or photoscreening

INTERNAL EYE

Horner Syndrome

Interruption of sympathetic nerve innervation to the eye

Pathophysiology

- Can be congenital, acquired, or hereditary (autosomal dominant)
- May result from lesion of the primary neuron, stroke, trauma to the brachial plexus, tumors, dissecting carotid aneurysm, or operative trauma
- Results in triad of ipsilateral miosis, mild ptosis, and loss of hemifacial sweating (Fig. 11-42)

Subjective Data

- Symptoms depend on the underlying cause

FIGURE 11-42 Horner syndrome (right eye). *(From Patzelt, 2009.)*

Objective Data

- The ptosis is subtle and appreciated by noting the amount of iris seen superiorly in opposite eye is greater
- Pupil on affected side may be round and constricted
- Anisocoria (difference in pupil size) is greater in darkness
- Affected pupil dilates more slowly than the normal pupil (dilation lag)
- Dry skin is on the same side of their face as the affected pupil

Cataracts

Opacity in lens (Fig. 11-43)

Pathophysiology

- Most commonly from denaturation of lens protein caused by aging
- With aging, cataracts are generally central
- Peripheral cataracts may occur in hypoparathyroidism
- Medications such as steroids can cause cataracts
- Congenital cataracts can result from a number of genetic defects, maternal infections such as rubella, or other fetal insults during the first trimester of pregnancy

Subjective Data

- Cloudy or blurry vision
- Faded colors
- Headlights, lamps, or sunlight may appear too bright
- Halo may appear around lights
- Poor night vision or double vision
- Frequent prescription changes

Objective Data

- Cloudiness of the lens, often obvious without special viewing equipment

FIGURE 11-43 **A,** Snowflake cataract of diabetes. **B,** Senile cataract. *(From Donaldson, 1976.)*

Diabetic Retinopathy (Background or Non-Proliferative)

Dot hemorrhages or microaneurysms and the presence of hard and soft exudates

Pathophysiology

- Hard exudates are the result of lipid transudation through incompetent capillaries
- Soft exudates (also called cotton-wool spots) are caused by infarction of the nerve layer (Fig. 11-44)

Subjective Data

- In the initial stages, patients asymptomatic
- Blurred vision, distortion, or visual acuity loss in more advanced stages

Objective Data

- On ophthalmoscopic exam, blood vessels with balloon-like sacs (microaneurysms)
- Blots of hemorrhages on the retina itself
- Tiny yellow patches of hard exudates

ABNORMALITIES

ABNORMALITIES

Cotton-wool spot
(soft exudates)

FIGURE 11-44 Background diabetic retinopathy. Note flame-shaped and dot-blot hemorrhages, cotton-wool spots, and microaneurysms. *(From Yannuzzi et al, 1995; courtesy of Drs. George Blankenship and Everett Ai and the Diabetes 2000 Program, St. Louis, MO.)*

Hemorrhage

Diabetic Retinopathy (Proliferative)

Development of new vessels as result of anoxic stimulation (Fig. 11-45)

Pathophysiology

- Vessels grow out of the retina toward the vitreous humor
- May occur in peripheral retina or on optic nerve itself
- New vessels lack supporting structure of healthy vessels and are likely to hemorrhage
- Bleeding from these vessels is a major cause of blindness in patients with diabetes
- Laser therapy can often control this neovascularization and prevent blindness

Subjective Data

- Generally asymptomatic
- Floaters, blurred vision, or progressive visual acuity loss in advanced stages

Objective Data

- Visualization of these vessels may require change in the lens setting of the ophthalmoscope
- Vitreous hemorrhage may also be seen, which can obstruct the view of the retina

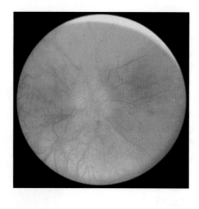

FIGURE 11-45 Proliferative diabetic retinopathy. *(Courtesy John W. Payne, MD, The Wilmer Ophthalmological Institute, The Johns Hopkins University and Hospital, Baltimore, MD.)*

Lipemia Retinalis

Creamy white appearance of retinal vessels that occurs with excessively high serum triglyceride levels

Pathophysiology

- Occurs when the serum triglyceride level exceeds 2000 mg/dL (Fig. 11-46)
- Seen in some of the hyperlipidemic states

Subjective Data

- Elevated serum triglyceride levels
- No vision symptoms

Objective Data

- Peripheral fundus changes in early stages
- Initially, vessels appear salmon pink; as triglyceride level rises, they become whitish
- Abnormalities resolve as the triglyceride levels return to normal

FIGURE 11-46 Lipemia retinalis. *(From Newell, 1996.)*

Retinitis Pigmentosa

Autosomal recessive disorder in which the genetic defects cause cell death, predominantly in the rod photoreceptors

Pathophysiology

Genetic defect causes cell death (apoptosis) in the photoreceptors. The associated conditions are:

- Deafness (Usher syndrome)
- Paralysis of one or more extraocular muscles (ophthalmoplegia), dysphasia, ataxia, and cardiac conduction defects are seen in the mitochondrial DNA disorder (Kearns-Sayre syndrome)
  - Intellectual delay, peripheral neuropathy, acanthotic (spiked) red blood cells, ataxia, steatorrhea, absence of very-low-density lipoprotein (VLDL) (abetalipoproteinemia is absence of VLDL)

Subjective Data

- Earliest symptom is night blindness
- Tunnel vision or reports of bumping into furniture
- Loss of vision is painless and progresses over years to decades

Objective Data

- Normal exam in the early stages
- Optic atrophy with a waxy pallor, narrowing of the arterioles, and peripheral "bone spicule" pigmentation are hallmarks of advanced disease (Fig. 11-47)

FIGURE 11-47 Retinitis pigmentosa. **A,** Optic atrophy and narrowing of the arterioles. **B,** Classic "bone spicule" pigmentation in the retinal periphery. *(Courtesy John W. Payne, MD, The Wilmer Ophthalmological Institute, The Johns Hopkins University and Hospital, Baltimore, MD.)*

Glaucoma

Disease of the optic nerve wherein the nerve cells die, usually due to excessively high intraocular pressure

Pathophysiology

- Acute angle may occur acutely with dramatically elevated intraocular pressure if the iris blocks the exit of aqueous humor from the anterior chamber
- Open angle caused by decreasing aqueous humor absorption leads to increased resistance and painless buildup of pressure in the eye
- May also be congenital as a result of improper development of the eye's aqueous outflow system

Subjective Data

- In chronic glaucoma, which is more common, symptoms are absent except for gradual loss of peripheral vision over a period of years
- Acute glaucoma is accompanied by intense ocular pain, blurred vision, halos around lights, a red eye, and a dilated pupil
- Occasionally, patients report stomach pain, nausea, and vomiting

Objective Data

- Optic nerve damage can clearly be seen during a dilated eye examination and produces a characteristic appearance of the optic nerve (increased cupping) (see Fig. 11-32)
- Visual field tests may show loss of peripheral vision.

Chorioretinitis (Chorioretinal Inflammation)

Inflammatory process involving both the choroid and the retina

Pathophysiology

- Most common cause is laser therapy for diabetic retinopathy but may also be seen in histoplasmosis, cytomegalovirus, toxoplasmosis, or congenital rubella infections

Subjective Data

- History of cleaning cat litter box, laser surgery, or other causal agents
- Pain
- Reduced visual acuity
- Floaters
- Photophobia

Objective Data

- Sharply defined lesion; generally whitish yellow and becomes stippled with dark pigment in later stages ending with a chorioretinal scar (Fig. 11-48)
- Visual field defect can be detected in individuals with a large lesion
- Chorioretinal scar appears; whitish lesions with well demarcated borders
- May be single or multiple
- Feathery martins contrast with myelinated retinal nerve fibers, page 218, Fig. 11-30

ABNORMALITIES

FIGURE 11-48 Patches of chorio-retinitis adjacent to the optic disc. *(From Stein et al, 1994.)*

VISUAL FIELDS

Visual Field Defects

Defective vision or blindness

Pathophysiology

- May be consequence of degenerative changes within the eye (e.g., cataract) or from a lesion of the optic nerve anterior to its decussation (Figs. 11-49, *1* and 11-50, *A*)
- Most common cause is interruption of the vascular supply to the optic nerve (Figs. 11-49, *1* and 11-50, *A*)
- Bitemporal hemianopia (Figs. 11-49, *2* and 11-50, *B*) is caused by a lesion—most commonly a pituitary tumor—interrupting the optic chiasm
- Homonymous hemianopia can be caused by lesions of the optic nerve radiation on either side of the brain occurring after the optic chiasm (Figs. 11-49, *3* and 11-50, *C*)

Subjective Data

- Defective vision or blindness

Objective Data

- Visual field defects (see Fig. 11-50)

FIGURE 11-49 Site of lesions causing visual loss. *1,* Total blindness left eye. *2,* Bitemporal hemianopia. *3,* Left homonymous hemianopia.

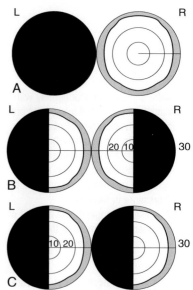

FIGURE 11-50 Visual fields corresponding to lesions shown in Figure 11-49. **A,** Total blindness left eye. **B,** Bitemporal hemianopia. **C,** Left homonymous hemianopia. *(Modified from Stein et al, 1994.)*

✿ Children and Infants

Retinoblastoma

Embryonic malignant tumor arising from the retina

Pathophysiology

- Usually develops during the first 2 years of life
- Transmitted either by autosomal dominant trait or by chromosomal mutation (*RB1* gene on chromosome 13)
- Most common retinal tumor in children

Subjective Data

- Family history of retinoblastoma
- White reflex on photographs

FIGURE 11-51 Retinoblastoma. *(From Stein et al, 1994.)*

Objective Data

- Initial sign is leukocoria, a white reflex (also called a *cat's eye reflex*) rather than the usual red reflex
- Ill-defined mass arising from retina on funduscopic examination; chalky white areas of calcification can be seen (Fig. 11-51)

Retinopathy of Prematurity (ROP)

Disruption of normal progression of retinal vascular development in preterm infant

Pathophysiology

- Results in abnormal proliferation of blood vessels (neovascularization)
- More common in infants with a birth weight of ≤1500 g or gestational age of 30 weeks or less

Subjective Data

- Prematurity
- High oxygen concentration, blood transfusions, respiratory distress, breathing difficulties

FIGURE 11-52 **Retinopathy of prematurity.** Changes found in posterior pole of the left eye in the cicatricial (scar forming) stage of the disease with traction on the retina in the posterior pole. *(Courtesy John W. Payne, MD, The Wilmer Ophthalmological Institute, The Johns Hopkins University and Hospital, Baltimore, MD.)*

Objective Data

- Straight, temporally diverted blood vessels on funduscopic examination (Fig. 11-52)
- Can be mild with no visual defects, or refractive error, amblyopia, or progress to retinal detachment and blindness

ABNORMALITIES

Retinal Hemorrhages in Infancy

Abnormal bleeding of the blood vessels in the retina

Pathophysiology

- Results from acceleration-deceleration abuse impact head injury in shaken baby syndrome
- Usually bilaterally
- Other causes:
  - Hypertension
  - Bleeding problems/leukemia
  - Meningitis/sepsis/endocarditis
  - Vasculitis
  - Retinal diseases (e.g., infection, hemangioma)
  - Anemia
  - Hypoxia/hypotension

Subjective Data

- Altered responsiveness without good explanation (suspicion of physical abuse)

Objective Data

- Dilated funduscopic exam shows retinal hemorrhages (Fig. 11-53)

FIGURE 11-53 Multiple retinal hemorrhages are seen on funduscopic examination of this infant who was a victim of the shaken baby syndrome. *(Courtesy Daniel Garibaldi, MD, The Wilmer Ophthalmological Institute, The Johns Hopkins University and Hospital, Baltimore, MD.)*

✣ Older Adult

Macular Degeneration

Macular degeneration, also called *age-related macular degeneration* (AMD or ARMD), is caused when part of the retina deteriorates.

Pathophysiology

Two types:

- Dry (atrophic)
  - From the gradual breakdown of cells in the macula
  - Results in a gradual blurring of central vision
- Wet (exudative or neovascular)
  - New abnormal blood vessels grow under the center of the retina.
  - The blood vessels leak, bleed, and scar the retina, distorting or destroying central vision.
  - In contrast to the dry type, vision loss may be rapid.
  - Leading cause of legal blindness in people older than 55 years in the United States

Subjective Data

- Blurred or decreased central vision
- Blind spots, or scotomas
- Straight lines looking irregular or bent (metamorphopsia)
- Objects appearing a different color or shape in each eye
- Objects appearing smaller in one eye (micropsia)

Objective Data

- Dry form
  - Drusen (multiple spots in the macular region); see Figure 11-33.
  - Thinning and loss of the retina, and the choroid
- Wet form
  - Exudates, blood, scarring, and new blood vessel membranes below the retina

CHAPTER 12

Ears, Nose, and Throat

Examination of the ears, nose, and throat provides information about their integrity and function, as well as the associated respiratory and digestive tracts. The special senses of smell, hearing, equilibrium, and taste are also associated with the ears, nose, and mouth.

evolve http://evolve.elsevier.com/Seidel
- Physical Exam Key Points
- NCLEX Review Questions
- Interactive Activities
- Animations
- Videos
- Student Checklist

Physical Examination Preview

Here is a preview of the steps involved in conducting physical examination of the ears, nose, and throat. ⓔ These procedures are explained in detail in this chapter and are available on Evolve in printable formats.

Ears

1. Inspect the auricles and surrounding area for the following (see p. 239):
   - Size, shape, and symmetry
   - Landmarks
   - Color
   - Position
   - Deformities or lesions
2. Palpate the auricles and mastoid area for tenderness, swelling, and nodules (see pp. 239-240).
3. Inspect the auditory canal with an otoscope, noting the following (see p. 240):
   - Cerumen
   - Color
   - Lesions
   - Discharge
   - Foreign bodies
4. Inspect the tympanic membrane for the following (see pp. 240-241):
   - Landmarks
   - Color
   - Contour
   - Perforations
   - Mobility
5. Assess hearing through the following (see pp. 240-242):
   - Response to questions during history
   - Response to a whispered voice
   - Response to tuning fork for air and bone conduction

Nose and Sinuses

1. Inspect the external nose, noting the shape, size, color, and nares (see p. 242).

2. Palpate the bridge and soft tissues of the nose, noting the following (see p. 242):
   - Tenderness
   - Displacement of cartilage and bone
   - Masses
3. Evaluate the patency of the nares (see pp. 242-243).
4. Inspect the nasal mucosa and nasal septum for the following (see pp. 243-244):
   - Color
   - Alignment
   - Discharge
   - Selling of turbinates
   - Perforation
5. Inspect the frontal and maxillary sinus area for swelling (see p. 244).
6. Palpate the frontal and maxillary sinuses for the tenderness or pain, and swelling (see p. 244).

Mouth

1. Inspect and palpate the lips for symmetry, color, and edema (see p. 245).
2. Inspect the teeth for the following (see pp. 245-247):
   - Occlusion
   - Caries
   - Loose or missing teeth
   - Surface abnormalities
3. Inspect and palpate the gingivae and buccal mucosa for color, lesions, and tenderness (see pp. 246-247).
4. Inspect the tongue for color, symmetry, swelling, and ulcerations (see p. 247).
5. Assess the function of cranial nerve XII (hypoglossal) (see p. 247).
6. Palpate the tongue (see p. 247).
7. Inspect the palate and uvula (see pp. 247-248).
8. Elicit gag reflex (cranial nerves IX and X) (see p. 248).
9. Inspect the oropharyngeal characteristics of the tonsils and posterior wall of pharynx (see pp. 248-249).

ANATOMY AND PHYSIOLOGY

ANATOMY AND PHYSIOLOGY

Ears and Hearing

The ear is a sensory organ that identifies, localizes, and interprets sound and helps to maintain balance. It is divided into the external, middle, and inner ear (Figs. 12-1 and 12-2).

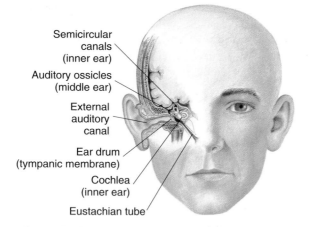

FIGURE 12-1 **Cross section of the external, middle, and inner ear in relation to other structures of the head and face.**

The external ear, including the auricle (or pinna) and external auditory canal, is cartilage-covered skin. The auricle, extending slightly outward from the skull, is positioned on a nearly vertical plane. Note its structural landmarks in Figure 12-3.

The external auditory canal, an S-shaped pathway leading to the middle ear, is approximately 2½ cm (1 in) long in adults. Its skeleton of bone and cartilage is covered with thin, sensitive skin. This canal lining is protected and lubricated with cerumen, secreted by the apocrine glands in the distal third of the canal. Cerumen provides an acidic pH environment that inhibits the growth of microorganisms.

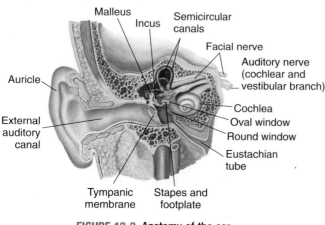

FIGURE 12-2 **Anatomy of the ear.**

The middle ear is an air-filled cavity in the temporal bone. It contains the ossicles, three small connected bones (malleus, incus, and stapes) that transmit sound from the tympanic membrane to the oval window of the inner ear. The air-filled cells of

the mastoid area of the temporal bone are continuous with the middle ear. The tympanic membrane, surrounded by a dense fibrous ring (annulus), separates the external ear from the middle ear. It is concave, being pulled in at the center (umbo) by the malleus. The tympanic membrane is translucent, permitting the middle ear cavity and malleus to be visualized. Its oblique position to the auditory canal and conical shape account for the triangular light reflex. Most of the tympanic membrane is tense (the pars tensa), but the superior portion (pars flaccida) is more flaccid (Fig. 12-4).

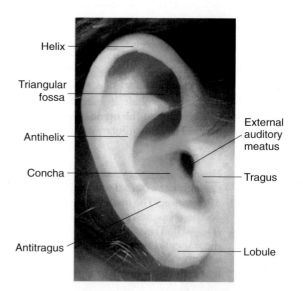

FIGURE 12-3 **Anatomic structures of the auricle.** The helix is the prominent outer rim, whereas the antihelix is the area parallel and anterior to the helix. The concha is the deep cavity containing the auditory canal meatus. The tragus is the protuberance lying anterior to the auditory canal meatus, and the antitragus is the protuberance on the antihelix opposite the tragus. The lobule is the soft lobe on the bottom of the auricle.

FIGURE 12-4 **Structural landmarks of the right tympanic membrane in relation to a clock face.**

The middle ear mucosa produces a small amount of mucus that is rapidly cleared by the ciliary action of the eustachian tube, a cartilaginous, fibrous, and bony passageway between the nasopharynx and the middle ear. The eustachian tube drains into the posterior aspect of the inferior turbinate of the nose. Muscles briefly open this passage (during swallowing, yawning, or sneezing) to clear middle ear secretions and to equalize the middle ear pressure with atmospheric pressure. The equalized pressure in the middle ear permits the tympanic membrane to vibrate freely.

The inner ear is a membranous, curved cavity inside a bony labyrinth consisting of the vestibule, semicircular canals, and cochlea. The cochlea, a coiled structure containing the organ of Corti, transmits sound impulses to the eighth cranial nerve. The semicircular canals contain the end organs for vestibular function. Equilibrium receptors in the semicircular canals and vestibule of the inner ear respond to changes in direction of movement and send signals to the cerebellum to maintain balance.

Hearing is the interpretation of sound waves by the brain. Sound waves travel through the external auditory canal, strike the tympanic membrane, and cause it to vibrate. The malleus, attached to the tympanic membrane, and the serially connected incus and stapes begin vibrating. The vibrations are passed from the stapes to the oval window of the inner ear (see Fig. 12-2). Oval window movement causes cochlear endolymph fluid motion to be transmitted to the round window, where it is dissipated. Hair cells in the organ of Corti detect sound vibrations and send the information to the auditory division of the eighth cranial nerve. These impulses are transmitted to the temporal lobe of the brain for interpretation. Sound vibrations may also be transmitted by bone directly to the inner ear.

Nose, Nasopharynx, and Sinuses

The nose and nasopharynx provide a passage for inspired and expired air; humidify, filter, and warm inspired air; identify odors; and provide resonance of laryngeal sound. The external nose is formed by skin-covered bone and cartilage. The nares, anterior openings of the nose, are surrounded by the cartilaginous ala nasi and columella. The frontal and maxillary bones form the nasal bridge (Fig. 12-5).

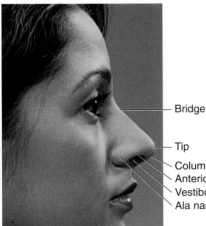

— Bridge

— Tip

— Columella
— Anterior naris (nostril)
— Vestibule
— Ala nasi

FIGURE 12-5 Anatomic structures of the external nose.

The nasal floor is formed by the hard and soft palate, whereas the roof is formed by the frontal and sphenoid bone. The internal nose is covered by a vascular mucous membrane thickly lined with small hairs and mucous secretions. These hairs and

mucus collect and carry debris and bacteria from the inspired air to the nasopharynx for swallowing or expectoration. The mucus contains immunoglobulins and enzymes that serve as a defense against infection. Receptors for smell are located in the olfactory epithelium.

The internal nose is divided by the septum into two anterior cavities: the vestibules. Inspired air enters the nose through the nares and passes through the vestibules to the choanae, posterior openings leading to the nasopharynx. The cribriform plate, housing the sensory endings of the olfactory nerve, lies on the roof of the nose. The Kiesselbach plexus, a convergence of small fragile arteries and veins, is located on the anterior-superior portion of the septum. The adenoids lie on the posterior wall of the nasopharynx (Fig. 12-6).

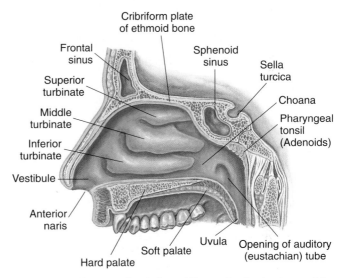

Cribriform plate of ethmoid bone

Frontal sinus

Sphenoid sinus

Sella turcica

Superior turbinate

Middle turbinate

Inferior turbinate

Choana

Pharyngeal tonsil (Adenoids)

Vestibule

Anterior naris

Hard palate

Soft palate

Uvula

Opening of auditory (eustachian) tube

FIGURE 12-6 Cross-sectional view of the anatomic structures of the nose and nasopharynx.

Turbinates, parallel curved bony structures covered by vascular mucous membrane, form the lateral walls of the nose and protrude into the nasal cavity. They increase the nasal surface area to warm, humidify, and filter inspired air. A meatus below each turbinate is named for the turbinate above it. The inferior meatus drains the nasolacrimal duct, the medial meatus drains the paranasal sinuses, and the superior meatus drains the posterior ethmoid sinus.

The paranasal sinuses are air-filled, paired extensions of the nasal cavities within the bones of the skull. They are lined with mucous membranes and cilia that move secretions along excretory pathways. Their openings into the medial meatus of the nasal cavity are easily obstructed.

Only the maxillary and frontal sinuses are accessible for physical examination. The maxillary sinuses lie along the lateral wall of the nasal cavity in the maxillary bone. The frontal sinuses are in the frontal bone superior to the nasal cavities. The ethmoid sinuses lie behind the frontal sinuses and near the superior portion of the nasal cavity. The sphenoid sinuses are deep in the skull behind the ethmoid sinuses (Fig. 12-7).

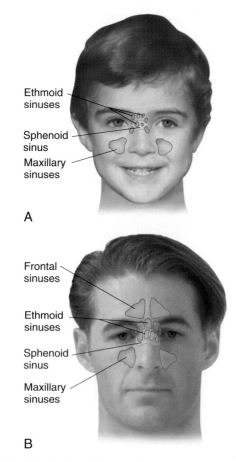

FIGURE 12-7 **Anterior view of the cranial sinuses. A, Six-year-old child. B, Adult.**

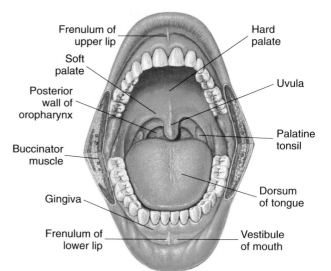

FIGURE 12-8 **Anatomic structures of the oral cavity.**

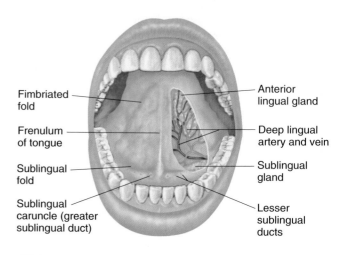

FIGURE 12-9 **Landmarks of the ventral surface of the tongue.**

Mouth and Oropharynx

The mouth and oropharynx release air for vocalization and for expiration. They also provide passage for food, liquid, and saliva (either swallowed or vomited); initiate digestion by solid food mastication and salivary gland secretion; and identify taste. The oral cavity is divided into the mouth and the vestibule, the space between the buccal mucosa and the outer surface of the teeth and gums. The mouth, housing the tongue, teeth, and gums, is the anterior opening of the oropharynx. The bony arch of the hard palate and the fibrous soft palate form the roof of the mouth. The uvula hangs from the posterior margin of the soft palate (Fig. 12-8).

Loose, mobile tissue covering the mandibular bone forms the floor of the mouth. The tongue is anchored to the back of the oral cavity at its base and to the floor of the mouth by the frenulum. The dorsal surface of the tongue is covered with thick mucous membrane supporting the filiform papillae. Fungiform papillae (taste receptors) are scattered throughout the filiform papillae of the tongue, and specific areas are sensitive to the five basic taste sensations of sour, sweet, salty, bitter, and umami (savory). The ventral surface of the tongue has visible veins and fimbriated folds (fringelike projections of thin mucous membrane) (Fig. 12-9).

The parotid, submandibular, and sublingual salivary glands are located in tissues surrounding the oral cavity. The secreted saliva initiates digestion and moistens the mucosa. Stensen ducts are parotid gland outlets that open on the buccal mucosa opposite the second molar on each side of the upper jaw. Wharton ducts, outlets of the submandibular glands, open on each side of the frenulum under the tongue. The sublingual glands have many ducts opening along the sublingual fold.

The gingivae, fibrous tissue covered by mucous membrane, are attached directly to the teeth and the maxilla and mandible. The roots of the teeth are anchored to the alveolar ridges of the maxilla and mandible. The enamel-covered crown is visible to examination. Adults generally have 32 permanent teeth (Fig. 12-10).

The oropharynx, continuous with but inferior to the nasopharynx, is separated from the mouth by bilateral anterior and posterior tonsillar pillars. The tonsils, lying in the cavity between these pillars, have crypts that collect cell debris and food particles.

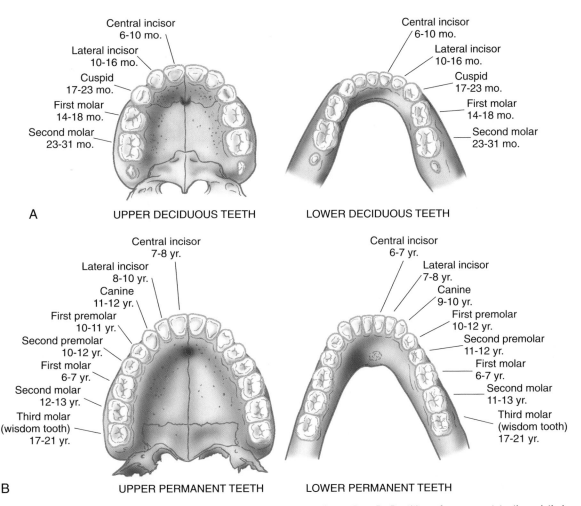

Central incisor
6-10 mo.
Lateral incisor
10-16 mo.
Cuspid
17-23 mo.
First molar
14-18 mo.
Second molar
23-31 mo.

Central incisor
6-10 mo.
Lateral incisor
10-16 mo.
Cuspid
17-23 mo.
First molar
14-18 mo.
Second molar
23-31 mo.

A   UPPER DECIDUOUS TEETH   LOWER DECIDUOUS TEETH

Central incisor
7-8 yr.
Lateral incisor
8-10 yr.
Canine
11-12 yr.
First premolar
10-11 yr.
Second premolar
10-12 yr.
First molar
6-7 yr.
Second molar
12-13 yr.
Third molar
(wisdom tooth)
17-21 yr.

Central incisor
6-7 yr.
Lateral incisor
7-8 yr.
Canine
9-10 yr.
First premolar
10-12 yr.
Second premolar
11-12 yr.
First molar
6-7 yr.
Second molar
11-13 yr.
Third molar
(wisdom tooth)
17-21 yr.

B   UPPER PERMANENT TEETH   LOWER PERMANENT TEETH

FIGURE 12-10 A, Dentition of deciduous teeth and their sequence of eruption. **B,** Dentition of permanent teeth and their sequence of eruption.

Swallowing is initiated when food is forced by the tongue toward the pharynx. Muscles in the pharynx contract and prevent movement of the food into the nasopharynx while respiration is inhibited as the epiglottis closes. Food is then propelled into the esophagus.

⚜ Infants and Children

Because development of the inner ear occurs during the first trimester of pregnancy, an insult to the fetus during that time may impair hearing. The infant's external auditory canal is shorter than the adult's and has an upward curve. The infant's eustachian tube is wider, shorter, and more horizontal than the adult's, which allows easier reflux of nasopharyngeal secretions. As the child grows, the eustachian tube lengthens and its pharyngeal orifice moves inferiorly. Growth of lymphatic tissue, specifically the adenoids, may occlude the eustachian tube and interfere with aeration of the middle ear, predisposing young children to middle ear effusion.

Although the maxillary and ethmoid sinuses are present at birth, they are very small. The sphenoid sinuses are present by 5 years of age. The frontal sinuses begin to develop at about 7 to 8 years of age and complete development during adolescence. Infections of the paranasal sinuses can occur during childhood.

Salivation increases by the time the infant is 3 months old, and the infant drools until swallowing is learned. The 20 deciduous teeth usually erupt between 6 and 24 months of age (see Fig. 12-10). The permanent teeth begin forming in the jaw by 6 months of age. Pressure from these teeth causes resorption of the deciduous teeth roots until the crown is shed. Eruption of the permanent teeth begins about 6 years of age and is completed around 14 or 15 years of age in most races/ethnicities. Tooth eruption timing may be delayed in cases of poor nutritional status and chronic conditions.

⚜ Pregnant Women

Elevated levels of estrogen cause increased vascularity of the upper respiratory tract. The capillaries of the nose, pharynx, and eustachian tubes become engorged, leading to symptoms of nasal stuffiness, decreased sense of smell, epistaxis, a sense of fullness in the ears, and impaired hearing. Increased vascularity and proliferation of connective tissue of the gums also may occur. Hormone-induced laryngeal changes may lead to hoarseness, deepening or cracking of the voice, vocal changes, or persistent cough.

✤ Older Adults

Nearly a third of adults older than 65 years have hearing loss (Huether, 2010). Age-related hearing loss is associated with degeneration of hair cells in the organ of Corti, loss of cortical and organ of Corti auditory neurons, degeneration of the cochlear conductive membrane, and decreased vascularity in the cochlea. Sensorineural hearing loss first occurs with high-frequency sounds and then progresses to tones of lower frequency. Loss of high-frequency sounds usually interferes with the understanding of speech and localization of sound. Conductive hearing loss may result from an excess deposition of bone cells along the ossicle chain, causing fixation of the stapes in the oval window, cerumen impaction, or a sclerotic tympanic membrane.

Deterioration of the sense of smell results from loss of olfactory sensory neurons beginning at about 60 years of age. The sense of taste begins deteriorating at about 50 years of age as the number of papillae on the tongue and salivary gland secretion decrease, reducing the perception of sweet sensations (Huether, 2010). However, a wide variation in rate of smell and taste deterioration occurs.

Cartilage formation continues in the ears and nose, making the auricle and nose larger and more prominent. The soft tissues of the mouth change as the granular lining on the lips and cheeks becomes more prominent. The gingival tissue may recede and be more vulnerable to trauma, allowing teeth to erode more easily at the gum line. The tongue becomes more fissured. The older adult may have altered motor function of the tongue, leading to problems with swallowing. Saliva production may decrease as a result of disease or medications taken (e.g., anticholinergics and diuretics). Lost teeth may contribute to diet changes or malocclusion and difficulty chewing. Sensitivity to odors and taste declines.

REVIEW OF RELATED HISTORY

For each of the conditions discussed in this section, selected topics to include in the history of the present illness are listed. Responses to questions about these topics help fully assess the patient's condition and provide clues for focusing the physical examination. Questions regarding medication use (prescription and over the counter) as well as complementary and alternative therapies are relevant for each area.

History of Present Illness

- ✦ Ear pain
  - ✦ Onset, duration, and course
  - ✦ Concurrent upper respiratory infection, frequent swimming, trauma to the head; related complaints in the mouth, teeth, sinuses, throat, or temporomandibular joint
  - ✦ Associated symptoms: pain, fever, discharge (e.g., waxy, serous, mucoid, purulent, sanguinous); itchiness; reduced hearing, ringing in ear, vertigo; association with diving or flying

- ✦ Method of ear canal cleaning; problems with impacted cerumen
- ✦ Medications: antibiotics, ear drops (e.g., acetic acid, anesthetic, topical steroids, cerumen softeners)
- ✦ Hearing loss: one or both ears
  - ✦ Onset: instant (may indicate vascular or autoimmune process), over a few hours or days (may indicate viral infection), slow or gradual
  - ✦ Hears best: on telephone, in quiet or noisy environment; all sounds reduced or some sounds garbled; inability to discriminate words; complains about people mumbling
  - ✦ Speech: soft or loud, articulation of speech sounds
  - ✦ Associated symptoms: tinnitus, ear pain, foreign body, prior cerumen impactions
  - ✦ Management: hearing aid, when worn, battery change frequency; lip reading, sign language used
  - ✦ Ototoxic medications: aminoglycosides, gentamicin, streptomycin, quinine, cisplatin, salicylates, and furosemide

---

Risk Factors

Hearing Loss

Adults
- Exposure to industrial or recreational noise
- Genetic disease: Ménière disease
- Neurodegenerative and autoimmune disorders
- Syphilis
- Ototoxic medication use

Infants and Children
- Prenatal factors: perinatal infection, irradiation, drug abuse
- Neonatal intensive care unit stay of 5 days or longer that may involve assisted ventilation, hyperbilirubinemia requiring transfusion, or extracorporeal membranous oxygenation (Katbamna et al, 2008)
- Infection: bacterial meningitis, recurrent episodes of acute otitis media or otitis media with effusion
- Cleft palate, craniofacial abnormalities
- Ototoxic medication
- Head trauma
- Hypoxic episode
- Family history of child with permanent hearing loss

- ✦ Vertigo (a false sense of motion)
  - ✦ Time of vertigo onset, time of day, duration, circumstances, past episodes
  - ✦ Description of sensation (to and fro movement or rotary motion—room moving around patient or patient spinning), change of sensation with turning over in bed or head turning, any position better than others
  - ✦ Associated symptoms: nausea, vomiting, tinnitus, hearing loss or change, headache, double vision, ear fullness
  - ✦ Unsteadiness, loss of balance, falling
  - ✦ Medications: ototoxic medications such as aminoglycosides, gentamicin, streptomycin, quinine, cisplatin,

salicylates, furosemide; salt-retaining medications such as corticosteroids
+ Nasal discharge
  + Character (e.g., watery, mucoid, purulent, crusty, bloody); odor, amount, duration, unilateral or bilateral
  + Associated symptoms: sneezing, nasal congestion or stuffiness, itching, habitual sniffling, nasal obstruction, mouth breathing, malodorous breath, sore throat, eye burning or itching, cough
  + Seasonality of symptoms; allergies or concurrent upper respiratory infection; frequency of occurrence
  + Tenderness over face and sinuses, postnasal drip, daytime cough, face pain, headache, recent injury
+ Snoring
  + Change in snoring pattern, complaints of snoring loudness by partner, periods of apnea
  + Daytime sleepiness (associated with obstructive sleep apnea)
+ Nosebleed
  + Frequency, duration, amount of bleeding, nasal obstruction, treatment, difficulty stopping the bleeding
  + Predisposing factors: concurrent upper respiratory infection, dry heat, nose picking, forceful nose blowing, trauma, allergies, dry air or climate
  + Site of bleeding: unilateral or bilateral, alternating sides
+ Sinus pain
  + Fever, malaise, cough, headache, maxillary toothache, eye pain
  + Nasal congestion, colored nasal discharge
  + Pain: tenderness or pressure over sinuses, pain increases when bending forward
  + Medications: change in symptoms with decongestants
+ Dental problems
  + Pain: with chewing, localized to tooth or entire jaw, severity, interference with eating, foods no longer eaten; tooth grinding; associated with temporomandibular joint problems
  + Swollen or bleeding gums, mouth ulcers or masses, tooth loss
  + Dentures or dental appliances (e.g., braces, retainers): snugness of fit, areas of irritation, length of time dentures or appliances worn daily
  + Malocclusion: difficulty chewing, tooth extractions, previous orthodontic work
  + Medications: phenytoin, cyclosporine, calcium channel blockers, mouth rinses
+ Mouth lesions
  + Intermittent or constantly present, duration, painful or painless; excessive dryness of mouth; halitosis
  + Associated with stress, foods, seasons, fatigue, tobacco use, alcohol use, dentures
  + Variations in tongue character: swelling, size change, color, coating, ulceration, difficulty moving tongue
  + Lesions any place else on the body (e.g., vagina, urethra, anus)
  + Medications: mouth rinses

Risk Factors

Oral Cavity and Oropharyngeal Cancer

- Tobacco use: cigarettes, cigars, pipes, chewing tobacco, snuff; risk increases with frequency and duration of tobacco use
- Alcohol use: heavy consumption has higher risk, especially when combined with tobacco use
- Oral infection with human papilloma virus (type HPV 16)
- Older than 55 years
- Gender: higher rate in men than women
- UV light exposure associated with cancer of the lip
- Weakened immune system: HIV infection, previous malignancy, graft versus host disease
- Inherited genetic syndromes: Fanconi anemia, dyskeratosis congenita

American Cancer Society, 2012; National Cancer Institute, 2012.

+ Sore throat
  + Pain with swallowing, associated with upper respiratory infection, exposure to streptococci or gonorrhea, postnasal drip, mouth breathing, fever
  + Exposure to dry heat, smoke, or fumes
  + Medications: antibiotics, nonprescription lozenges or sprays
+ Hoarseness
  + Onset: acute, chronic
  + Change in voice quality (e.g., breathy, pitch alteration); need to clear throat frequently
  + Associated problems: overuse of voice, allergies, inhalation of smoke or other irritants, gastroesophageal reflux, recent surgery requiring intubation or intensive care treatment
+ Difficulty swallowing
  + Solids, liquids, or both; progressive difficulty
  + Feeling of food in throat, tightness, or substernal fullness
  + Drooling, swallowed liquids coming out of nose, coughing or choking when swallowing

Past Medical History

+ Systemic disease: hypertension, cardiovascular disease, diabetes mellitus, nephritis, bleeding disorder, gastrointestinal disease, reflux esophagitis, asthma
+ Ear: frequent ear infections during childhood; surgery; labyrinthitis; antibiotic use, dosage, and duration
+ Nose: trauma, surgery, chronic nosebleeds
+ Sinuses: chronic postnasal drip, recurrent or chronic sinusitis, allergies
+ Throat: frequent documented streptococcal infections, tonsillectomy, adenoidectomy

Family History

+ Hearing problems or hearing loss, Ménière disease
+ Allergies
+ Hereditary renal disease

EXAMINATION AND FINDINGS

Personal and Social History

+ Environmental hazards: exposure to loud, continuous noises (factory, airport, music through headphones—associated with hearing loss); use of protective hearing devices
+ Nutrition: excessive sugar intake, foods eaten (associated with caries)
+ Oral care patterns: tooth brushing and flossing; last visit to dentist; current condition of teeth; braces, dentures, bridges, crowns, mouth guard use
+ Tobacco use: pipe, cigarettes, cigars, smokeless; amount, number of pack-years (associated with oral cancer)
+ Alcohol use
+ Intranasal cocaine use

� Infants and Children

+ Prenatal: perinatal infection (e.g., toxoplasmosis, cytomegalovirus, syphilis), irradiation, alcohol and drug abuse, hypertension, Rh incompatibility, diabetes
+ Prematurity: birth weight less than 1500 g, prolonged mechanical ventilation, anoxia, ototoxic medication use
+ Serum bilirubin greater than 20 mg/100 mL
+ Infection: meningitis, encephalitis, recurrent episodes of acute otitis media with or without tympanostomy tube placement, prolonged episodes of otitis media with effusion, unilateral mumps
+ Secondary tobacco smoke exposure, out-of-home childcare (associated with occurrence of otitis media), siblings in the home
+ Congenital defect: cleft palate, choanal atresia or stenosis, other craniofacial abnormality, snoring
+ Playing with small objects (easily placed in nose or ears)
+ Behaviors indicating hearing loss: no reaction to calling name or caregiver's voice, language delay such as no babbling after 6 months of age, no communicative speech and reliance on gestures after 15 months of age, inattention compared with children of the same age
+ Failure on language domain of developmental screening tool; failure on hearing screen
+ Dental care: fluoride supplementation or fluoridated water; goes to sleep with bottle of milk or juice; when first tooth erupted; number of teeth present; thumb sucking, pacifier use

✻ Pregnant Women

+ Weeks of gestation or postpartum
+ Presence of symptoms before pregnancy
+ Pattern of dental care
+ Exposure to infection

✻ Older Adults

+ Hearing loss causing any interference with daily life
+ Any physical disability: interference with oral care or denture care, problems operating hearing aid
+ Deterioration of teeth, extractions, difficulty chewing
+ Dry mouth (xerostomia)
+ Medications decreasing salivation: anticholinergics, diuretics, antihypertensives, antihistamines, antispasmodics, antidepressants, tranquilizers; ototoxic drugs

---

Evidence-Based Practice in Physical Examination

Detection of Hearing Loss

Asking patients if they have a hearing problem or if they think that they have a hearing loss is associated with detecting a mild to moderate hearing impairment with audiometric assessment (sensitivity of 71% to 93% and specificity of 56% to 71%) (Gates et al, 2003).

EXAMINATION AND FINDINGS

Equipment

+ Otoscope with pneumatic attachment
+ Nasal speculum
+ Tongue blades
+ Tuning fork (512 Hz and 1024 Hz approximate vocal frequencies)
+ Gauze
+ Gloves
+ Penlight, sinus transilluminator, or light from otoscope

Ears and Hearing

External Ear

Inspect the auricles for size, shape, symmetry, landmarks, color, and position on the head. Examine the lateral and medial surfaces and surrounding tissue, noting color, presence of deformities, lesions, and nodules. The auricle should have the same color as the facial skin, without moles, cysts or other lesions, deformities, or nodules. No skin tags, openings, or discharge should be present in the preauricular area. A Darwin tubercle, a thickening along the upper ridge of the helix, is an expected variation. Preauricular skin tags and preauricular pits, found in front of the ear where the upper auricle originates, are other expected variations (Fig. 12-11, *A-C*).

The auricle color may vary with certain conditions. Blueness may indicate some degree of cyanosis. Pallor or excessive redness may result from vasomotor instability. Frostbite can cause extreme pallor.

An unusual size or shape of the auricle may be a familial trait or indicate abnormality. A cauliflower ear results from blunt trauma and necrosis of the underlying cartilage. Tophi—small, whitish uric acid crystals along the peripheral margins of the auricles—may indicate gout. Sebaceous cysts, elevations in the skin with a punctum indicating a blocked sebaceous gland, are common (Fig. 12-11, *D-F*).

To check the auricle's position, draw an imaginary line between the inner canthus of the eye and the most prominent protuberance of the occiput (Fig. 12-12). The top of the auricle should be at or above this line. Draw a vertical imaginary line perpendicular to the previous line just anterior to the auricle. The auricle's position should be almost vertical, with no more than a 10-degree lateral posterior angle. A low-set position or unusual angle may indicate chromosomal aberrations or renal disorders.

Inspect the external auditory canal for discharge and note any odor. A purulent, foul-smelling discharge is associated with otitis externa, perforated acute otitis media, or a foreign body. In cases

FIGURE 12-11 A, Preauricular skin tag. **B,** Auricular sinus. **C,** Darwin tubercle. **D,** Cauliflower ear. **E,** Tophi. **F,** Sebaceous cysts. *(A, B, From Zitelli and Davis, 1997; C, D, F, from Bingham et al, 1992; E, from American College of Rheumatology, 2009.)*

FIGURE 12-12 Assessment of auricle alignment showing expected position. Imaginary line extends from inner eye canthus to occiput.

of head trauma, a bloody or serous discharge is suggestive of a skull fracture.

Palpate the auricles and mastoid area for tenderness, swelling, or nodules. The consistency of the auricle should be firm, mobile, and without nodules. If folded forward, it should readily recoil to its usual position. Pull gently on the lobule; if pain is present, the external auditory canal may be inflamed. Tenderness or swelling in the mastoid area may indicate mastoiditis.

Otoscopic Examination

The otoscope is used to inspect the external auditory canal and middle ear (see Fig. 3-18). Select the largest speculum that will fit comfortably in the patient's ear. Hold the handle of the otoscope between your thumb and index finger, supported on the

middle finger (many examiners use the right hand for the right ear and the left hand for the left ear). Depending on your preference, the bottom of the handle may rest against the palm of the hand or space between the thumb and index finger. Use the ulnar side of your hand to rest against the patient's head, stabilizing the otoscope as it is inserted into the canal. Examination of the tympanic membrane with the otoscope requires manipulation of the auricle. Use a firm but gentle grasp to avoid causing discomfort. Tilt the patient's head toward the opposite shoulder and as the speculum is inserted, pull the patient's auricle upward and back to straighten the auditory canal for the best view (Fig. 12-13).

FIGURE 12-13 To examine the adult's ear with the otoscope, straighten the external auditory canal by pulling the auricle up and back.

EXAMINATION AND FINDINGS

Slowly insert the speculum to a depth of 1 or 1½ cm (½ inch) and inspect the auditory canal from the meatus to the tympanic membrane, noting discharge, scaling, excessive redness, lesions, foreign bodies, and cerumen. Avoid touching the bony walls of the auditory canal (the inner two thirds) with the speculum because this will cause pain. Expect to see minimal cerumen, a uniformly pink color, and hairs in the outer third of the canal. Cerumen may vary in color and texture but should have no odor (see Physical Variations, "Types of Cerumen"). No lesions, discharge, or foreign body should be present (see Clinical Pearl, "Cleaning an Obstructed Auditory Canal").

Inspect the tympanic membrane for landmarks, color, contour, and perforations. Gently move the otoscope to see the entire tympanic membrane and the annulus. The tympanic membrane should be a translucent, pearly gray color, with visible landmarks (umbo, handle of malleus, and light reflex) and no perforations (Fig. 12-14, *A*). Its contour should be slightly conical with a concavity at the umbo. A bulging tympanic membrane is more conical, usually with a loss of bony landmarks and a distorted light reflex. A retracted tympanic membrane is more concave, usually with accentuated bony landmarks and a distorted light reflex. Figure 12-14, *B-F*, shows the tympanic membrane associated with various conditions, and Table 12-1 shows tympanic membrane characteristics associated with middle ear disorders.

The pneumatic attachment of the otoscope is used to provide information about tympanic membrane mobility and the middle ear space, such as the presence of middle ear effusion. The otoscope should have no air leaks. Make sure the speculum inserted

Physical Variations

Types of Cerumen

Cerumen comes in two main varieties—wet and dry—and it is a genetic trait. Wet cerumen is dark and sticky and is found predominantly in whites and blacks. Dry cerumen is light brown to gray, flaky, and sparse; it can lie in the ear canal as a thin flake. Dry cerumen occurs predominantly in Asians and Native Americans.

Data from Yoshiura et al, 2006.

Clinical Pearl

Cleaning an Obstructed Auditory Canal

If the patient with an ear or hearing concern has a tympanic membrane obscured by cerumen, the canal can be cleaned by warm water irrigation or by a cerumen spoon. Take care when using a cerumen spoon as the auditory canal is easily abraded, causing pain and bleeding. Irrigation with water at body temperature is preferable in young patients. Do not perform water irrigation in the presence of otitis externa, a perforated tympanic membrane, pressure-equalizing tubes, or an opening into the mastoid bone.

into the canal seals it from the outside air. Specula that come with the otoscope are sized better for sealing, and they can be cleaned with alcohol swabs between patients. Disposable specula may not be large enough for a tight fit. A piece of rubber tubing around the end of the speculum tip may help achieve a seal in a

FIGURE 12-14 A, Healthy tympanic membrane. **B,** Tympanic membrane partially obscured by cerumen. **C,** Bulging tympanic membrane with loss of bony landmarks. **D,** Perforated tympanic membrane. **E,** Perforated tympanic membrane that has healed. **F,** Tympanostomy tube protruding from the right tympanic membrane. *(A-E, Courtesy Richard A. Buckingham, MD, Clinical Professor, Otolaryngology, Abraham Lincoln School of Medicine, University of Illinois, Chicago; F, from Bingham et al, 1992.)*

Table 12-1	Tympanic Membrane Signs and Associated Conditions
Signs	**Associated Conditions/Causes**
Mobility	
Bulging with no mobility	Middle ear effusion due to pus or fluid
Retracted with no mobility	Obstruction of eustachian tube with or without middle ear effusion
Mobility with negative pressure only	Obstruction of eustachian tube with or without middle ear effusion
Excess mobility in small areas	Healed perforation, atrophic tympanic membrane
Color	
Amber or yellow	Serous fluid in middle ear (otitis media with effusion)
Blue or deep red	Blood in middle ear
Chalky white	Infection in middle ear (acute otitis media)
Redness	Infection in middle ear (acute otitis media), prolonged crying
Dullness	Fibrosis, otitis media with effusion
White flecks, dense white plaques	Healed inflammation
Air Bubbles	Serous fluid in middle ear

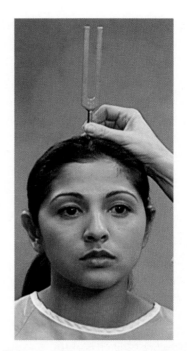

FIGURE 12-15 Weber Test. Touching only the handle, place the base of the tuning fork on the midline of the skull. Avoid touching the vibrating tines.

large auditory canal. Gently apply positive pressure (slight bulb compression) to make the membrane move toward the middle ear. Keep the bulb compressed, unseal and then reseal the speculum, and then apply negative pressure (release compressed bulb) to make the membrane move toward your eye. Movement to positive and negative pressure is expected and is indicated by a change in the cone of light appearance. No movement is expected when the tympanic membrane is perforated or a pressure-equalizing tube is in place. No movement with positive and negative pressure may be a sign of acute otitis media or otitis media with effusion.

Hearing Evaluation

Cranial nerve VIII is tested by evaluating hearing. Hearing screening begins when the patient responds to your questions and directions. Note any behaviors such as cupping a hand behind the ear or tilting an ear toward you when listening. The patient should respond without excessive requests for repetition. Speech with a monotonous tone and erratic volume may indicate hearing loss.

Whispered Voice. Check the patient's response to your whispered voice, one ear at a time. Mask the hearing in the untested ear by having the patient insert a finger in the ear canal. Stand to the side of the patient at a consistent distance best for you, about 30 to 60 cm (1 to 2 feet) away from the ear being tested, and out of the patient's line of vision. To soften the whisper, exhale fully before whispering a random combination of three to six letters and numbers (e.g., 3, T, 9). Ask the patient to repeat what was heard. The patient should correctly repeat 50% of the sounds. Repeat the process with different numbers and letters with the other ear (Kerber and Baloh, 2012).

Weber and Rinne Tests. The tuning fork is used to compare hearing by bone conduction with that by air conduction. Hold the stem of the tuning fork without touching the tines, and stroke or tap the tines gently to make them vibrate.

The Weber test helps assess unilateral hearing loss. Place the base of the vibrating tuning fork on the midline of the patient's head (Fig. 12-15). Ask the patient if the sound is heard equally in both ears or is better in one ear (lateralization of sound). Avoid giving the patient a cue as to the best response. The patient should hear the sound equally in both ears. If the sound is lateralized, have the patient identify which ear hears the sound better. To test the reliability of the patient's response, repeat the procedure while occluding one ear, and ask which ear hears the sound better. It should be heard best in the occluded ear.

The Rinne test helps distinguish whether the patient hears better by air or bone conduction. Place the base of the vibrating tuning fork against the patient's mastoid bone and ask the patient to tell you when the sound is no longer heard. Time this interval of bone conduction, noting the number of seconds. Quickly position the still vibrating tines 1 to 2 cm (½ to 1 in) from the auditory canal, and again ask the patient to tell you when the sound is no longer heard. Continue timing the interval of sound due to air conduction heard by the patient (Fig. 12-16). Compare the number of seconds sound is heard by bone conduction versus air conduction. Air-conducted sound should be heard twice as long as bone-conducted sound (e.g., if bone-conducted sound is heard

Video: Ears, Nose, and Throat: Inspecting the Nasal Cavity

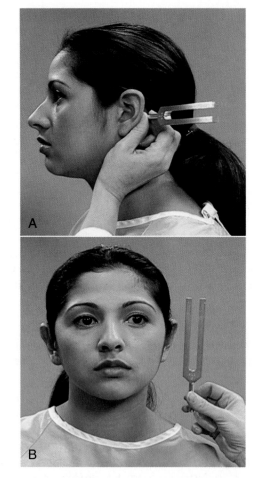

FIGURE 12-16 Rinne test. **A,** Place the tuning fork on the mastoid bone for bone conduction. **B,** To test for air conduction hold the tuning fork 1 to 2 cm ($\frac{1}{2}$ to 1 inch) from the ear with the tines facing forward.

Table 12-2	Interpretation of Tuning Fork Tests		
Test	Expected Findings	Conductive Hearing Loss	Sensorineural Hearing Loss
Weber	No lateralization, but will lateralize to ear occluded by patient	Sound heard better in affected ear unless sensorineural loss	Sound lateralizes to better ear unless conductive loss
Rinne	Air conduction heard longer than bone conduction by 2:1 ratio (Rinne positive)	Bone conduction heard longer than air conduction in affected ear (Rinne negative)	Air conduction heard longer than bone conduction in affected ear, but less than 2:1 ratio

for 15 seconds, air-conducted sound should be heard for an additional 15 seconds).

Table 12-2 provides guidelines to help distinguish between conductive and sensorineural hearing loss using the Weber and Rinne tests. Refer all patients with unexpected findings during the hearing screening for a thorough auditory evaluation (see Clinical Pearl, "Ménière Disease").

Clinical Pearl

Ménière Disease

The triad of hearing loss, tinnitus, and vertigo constitutes Ménière syndrome and if another cause cannot be determined, it is defined as Ménière disease (Crane et al, 2010). See p. 257.

Nose, Nasopharynx, and Sinuses

External Nose

Inspect the nose for deviations in shape, size, and color. Observe the nares for discharge and for flaring or narrowing. The skin should be smooth without swelling and conform to the color of the face. The columella should be directly midline, and its width should not exceed the diameter of a naris. The nares are usually oval in shape and symmetrically positioned. A depression of the nasal bridge or saddle-nose deformity can result from a fractured nasal bone or previous nasal cartilage inflammation. Nasal flaring is associated with respiratory distress, whereas narrowing of the nares on inspiration may be indicative of chronic nasal obstruction and mouth breathing. A transverse crease at the junction between the cartilage and bone of the nose may indicate chronic nasal itching and allergies.

If discharge is present, describe its character (e.g., watery, mucoid, purulent, crusty, or bloody); amount and color; and whether unilateral or bilateral. Potential conditions associated with nasal discharge characteristics include the following:

+ Allergy—bilateral watery discharge and associated sneezing and nasal congestion
+ Epistaxis or trauma—bloody discharge
+ Rhinitis or upper respiratory infection—bilateral mucoid or purulent discharge
+ Foreign body—unilateral, purulent, thick, greenish, malodorous discharge
+ Cerebrospinal fluid leakage—unilateral watery discharge occurring after head trauma

Palpate the bridge and soft tissues of the nose. Note any displacement of bone and cartilage, tenderness, or masses. Place one finger on each side of the nasal arch and gently palpate, moving the fingers from the nasal bridge to the tip. The nasal structures should feel firm and stable to palpation without crepitus. No tenderness or masses should be present.

Evaluate the patency of the nares. Occlude one naris by placing a finger on the side of the nose, and ask the patient to breathe in and out with the mouth closed. Repeat the procedure with the other naris. Nasal breathing should be noiseless and easy through the open naris.

Nasal Cavity

Use a nasal speculum and good light source to inspect the nasal cavity. Hold the speculum in the palm of one hand. Use your other hand to change the patient's head position. Insert the speculum slowly and cautiously. Do not overdilate the naris or touch the nasal septum to avoid causing pain (Fig. 12-17). Inspect the nasal mucosa for color, discharge, masses, lesions, and swelling of the turbinates (see Clinical Pearl, "Cocaine Abuse"). Inspect the nasal septum for alignment, perforation, bleeding, and crusting. Keep the patient's head erect to examine the vestibule and inferior nasal turbinate. Tilt the patient's head back to visualize the middle meatus and middle turbinate; then cautiously move the speculum tip toward the midline to examine the septum. Only the inferior and middle turbinates will be visible. Repeat in the other naris.

Clinical Pearl

Cocaine Abuse

When individuals nasally insufflate ("snort," "sniff") cocaine, signs of recent use include rhinorrhea, hyperemia, and edema of the nasal mucosa. White powder may still be present on the nasal hairs. Signs of chronic use include scabs on the nasal mucosa, decreased perception of taste and smell, and perforation of the nasal septum.

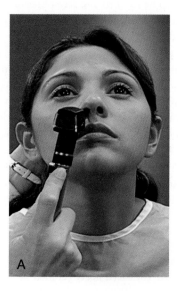

Middle turbinate
Nasal airway
Middle meatus
Nasal septum
Inferior turbinate
Floor of nose
Inferior meatus
B

FIGURE 12-17 A, Use of the nasal speculum. Avoid touching the nasal septum. **B,** View of the nasal mucosa through the nasal speculum.

Expect the nasal mucosa to glisten and appear deep pink (pinker than the buccal mucosa). A film of clear discharge is often apparent on the nasal septum. Purulent discharge may be associated with an upper respiratory infection, sinusitis, or a foreign body. Hairs may be present in the vestibule. Increased redness of the mucosa may occur with an infection, whereas localized redness and swelling in the vestibule may indicate a furuncle. Expect the turbinates to be firm and the same color as the surrounding area. Turbinates that appear bluish gray or pale pink with a swollen, boggy consistency may indicate allergies. A rounded, elongated mass projecting into the nasal cavity from boggy mucosa may be a polyp (Fig. 12-18, *A*).

Expect the nasal septum to be close to midline and fairly straight with the anterior septum thicker than the posterior septum. A nasal septum deviation may be indicated by asymmetric size of the posterior nasal cavities (see Fig 12-18, *B*). No perforations, bleeding, or crusting should be apparent. Crusting over the anterior portion of the nasal septum (Kiesselbach plexus) may occur at the site of epistaxis.

The sense of smell (cranial nerve I) is often tested with recognition of different odors. This procedure is described in Chapter 22.

Sinuses

Inspect the frontal and maxillary sinus areas for swelling. To palpate the frontal sinuses, use your thumbs to press up under the bony brow on each side of the nose. Then press up under the zygomatic processes, using either your thumbs or index and middle fingers to palpate the maxillary sinuses. Expect no tenderness or swelling over the soft tissue. Swelling, tenderness, and pain over the sinuses may indicate infection or obstruction.

FIGURE 12-18 Unexpected findings on nasal examination. A, Nasal polyp (allergic). **B,** Deviation of the nasal septum. *(A, From Goldman, 2008; B, from Cummings et al, 2010.)*

A   B

FIGURE 12-19 Transillumination of the sinuses: placement of the light source and expected area of transillumination. **A,** For the maxillary sinus. **B,** For the frontal sinus.

Transillumination of the frontal and maxillary sinuses may be performed if sinus tenderness is present or infection is suspected. A sinus transilluminator or small, bright light is used. To transilluminate the maxillary sinuses, darken the room completely and place the light source lateral to the nose, just beneath the medial aspect of the eye. Look through the patient's open mouth for illumination of the hard palate. To transilluminate the frontal sinuses, place the light source against the medial aspect of each supraorbital rim. Look for a dim red glow just above the eyebrow (Fig. 12-19). Bilateral findings may vary because the frontal sinuses develop differently. The sinuses may show differing degrees of illumination, opaque (no transillumination), dull (reduced transillumination), or a glow (expected transillumination). An opaque response may indicate that either the sinus is filled with secretions or it never developed. Asymmetry of transillumination is a significant finding.

Evidence-Based Practice in Physical Examination

Predictors of Sinusitis

The most important clinical signs for sinusitis in adults include a maxillary toothache, purulent nasal secretion, poor response to decongestants, abnormal transillumination, and patient report of colored nasal secretions. The likelihood ratio of sinusitis is 6:4 when four or more clinical signs are present, and the absence of any of these findings makes the diagnosis of sinusitis less likely (Simel and Williams, 2009).

Mouth and Oropharynx

Lips

With the patient's mouth closed, inspect and palpate the lips for symmetry, color, edema, and surface abnormalities. The lip color should be pink in whites and more bluish in individuals with darker skin. Lip symmetry, both at rest and with movement, is expected. No lesions should interrupt the distinct vermillion border between the lips and the facial skin. The lip surface characteristics are expected to be smooth and free of lesions.

Dry, cracked lips (cheilitis) may be caused by dehydration from wind chapping, dentures, braces, or excessive lip licking. Deep fissures at the corners of the mouth (cheilosis) may indicate riboflavin deficiency or overclosure of the mouth, allowing saliva to macerate the tissue. Swelling of the lips may be caused by infection or allergy (angioedema). Lip pallor is associated with anemia, whereas circumoral pallor is associated with scarlet fever. Cyanosis (bluish purple lips) results from hypoxia associated with a respiratory or cardiovascular condition. Round, oval, or irregular bluish gray macules on the lips and buccal mucosa are associated with Peutz-Jeghers syndrome. Lesions, plaques, vesicles, nodules, and ulcerations may be signs of infections, irritations, or skin cancer (Fig. 12-20, *A-F*).

Buccal Mucosa, Teeth, and Gums

Ask the patient to clench his or her teeth and smile to observe the occlusion of the teeth. The facial nerve (cranial nerve VII) is also tested with this maneuver. Proper tooth occlusion is apparent when the upper molars fit into the groove on the lower molars and the premolars and canines interlock fully. Indications of malocclusion and problems with the bite include protrusion of the upper incisors (overbite), protrusion of lower incisors or failure of the upper incisors to overlap with the lower incisors (crossbite), and failure of back teeth to meet (open bite) (Fig. 12-21). Three classes of malocclusion are listed in Table 12-3.

Have the patient remove any dental appliances and open the mouth partially. Using a tongue blade and bright light, inspect the buccal mucosa, gums, and teeth. Expect the mucous membranes to be pinkish red, smooth, and moist. The Stensen duct is a whitish yellow or whitish pink protrusion in approximate alignment with the second upper molar. When swelling is noted around the Stensen duct, use gloved hands to milk the tissue toward the Stensen duct. A small amount of clear saliva is expected. Small stones or exudate coming from the Stensen duct is unexpected.

Fordyce spots, an expected variant, are ectopic sebaceous glands that appear on the buccal mucosa and lips as numerous

FIGURE 12-20 **Unexpected findings on the lips. A,** Angular cheilitis. **B,** Actinic cheilitis. **C,** Angioedema. **D,** Herpes simplex lesions (cold sores). **E,** Squamous cell carcinoma of the lip. **F,** Peutz-Jeghers syndrome. (*A-C, From Habif, 2004; D, from Goldman, 2008; E, from Stewart et al, 1978; F, from Chessell et al, 1984.*)

FIGURE 12-21 **A,** Class I malocclusion. **B,** Class III malocclusion. (*Courtesy Drs. Abelson and Cameron, Lutherville, MD.*)

Table 12-3 Classification of Malocclusion

Classification	Characteristics
Class I	Molars have customary relationship, but the line of occlusion is incorrect because of rotated or malpositioned teeth.
Class II	Lower molars are distally positioned in relation to the upper molars; the line of occlusion may or may not be correct.
Class III	Lower molars are medially positioned in relation to the upper molars; the line of occlusion may or may not be correct.

small, yellow-white, raised lesions (see Fig. 12-22, *A*). Patchy pigmented mucosa is often found in individuals with dark skin (see Fig. 12-22, *B*). Whitish or pinkish scars are a common result of trauma from poor tooth alignment. A red spot on the buccal mucosa at the opening of the Stensen duct is associated with parotitis (mumps). Aphthous ulcers on the buccal mucosa appear as white, round, or oval ulcerative lesions with a red halo (see Fig. 12-22, *C*). A thickened white patch lesion that cannot be wiped away may be leukoplakia, a premalignant oral lesion (see Fig. 12-22, *D*). See Physical Variations, "Buccal Mucosa, Teeth, and Gums".

Physical Variations
Buccal Mucosa, Teeth, and Gums

Leukoedema is a diffuse filmy grayish surface with white streaks, wrinkles, or milky alteration. This asymptomatic benign lesion of the buccal mucosa is considered a normal variant. It is found in 90% of black adults and nearly 50% of black adolescents. This lesion may be seen in white adults, but with much lower frequency than in black adults (Bhattacharyya and Chehal, 2011).

The gingivae are expected to be coral pink in whites and may be more hyperpigmented in other races. Gingiva usually have a slightly stippled or dotted pink appearance with a clearly defined, tight margin at each tooth. The gum surface beneath dentures should have no inflammation, swelling, or bleeding.

Using gloves, palpate the gums for any lesions, induration, thickening, or masses. Expect the gingiva to feel firm and tightly bound to the underlying bone. No tenderness should be elicited. Epulis, a localized gingival enlargement or granuloma, is usually an inflammatory rather than neoplastic change. Gingival enlargement occurs with pregnancy, puberty, vitamin C deficiency, with certain medications (e.g., phenytoin, cyclosporine, and calcium

FIGURE 12-22 Findings on the buccal mucosa. A, Fordyce spots. B, Patchy coloration of mucous membranes in individual of dark skin color. C, Aphthous ulcer. D, Leukoplakia. *(A, From Wood and Goaz, 1991; B, courtesy Antoinette Hood, MD, Indiana University School of Medicine, Indianapolis; C, from Kumar, 2006; D, from Cummings, 2010.)*

FIGURE 12-23 Unexpected findings of the gingiva. A, Plasma cell gingivitis. B, Phenytoin-related hyperplasia of the gingival. *(A, from Wood and Goaz, 1991; B, from Goldman, 2008.)*

channel blockers), and in leukemia (Khera et al, 2005). Easily bleeding, swollen gums with enlarged crevices between the teeth and gum margins, or pockets containing debris at tooth margins, are associated with gingivitis or periodontal disease (Fig. 12-23).

Inspect and count the teeth, noting wear, notches, caries, and missing teeth. If you are concerned about loose teeth, probe each with a tongue blade to identify those that are not firmly anchored. Loose teeth can be the result of periodontal disease or trauma. The teeth generally have an ivory color but may be stained yellow from tobacco or brown from coffee or tea. Suspect caries when discolorations are seen on the crown of a tooth.

Oral Cavity

Inspect the dorsum of the tongue, noting any swelling, variation in size or color, coating, or ulcerations. Ask the patient to extend the tongue while you inspect for deviation, tremor, and limitation of movement. The procedure also tests the hypoglossal nerve (cranial nerve XII). Expect the protruded tongue to be maintained at the midline. No atrophy or fasciculations should be present. Deviation to one side indicates tongue atrophy and hypoglossal nerve impairment (Fig. 12-24, *A*).

The tongue appears dull red, moist, and glistening. A smooth, yet roughened surface with papillae and small fissures is seen on its anterior portion. The posterior portion should have rugae or a smooth, slightly uneven surface with a thinner mucosa than the anterior portion. The geographic tongue, an expected variant, has superficial denuded circles or irregular areas exposing the tips of papillae. A smooth red tongue with a slick appearance (glossitis) may indicate a vitamin B_{12} deficiency. The hairy tongue with yellow-brown to black elongated papillae on the dorsum sometimes follows antibiotic therapy (see Fig. 12-24, *B-D*).

Ask the patient to touch the tongue tip to the palate area directly behind the upper incisors. Inspect the floor of the mouth and the ventral surface of the tongue for swelling and varicosities, also observing the frenulum, sublingual ridge, and Wharton ducts. Expect the ventral surface of the tongue to be pink and smooth with large veins between the frenulum and fimbriated folds. Wharton ducts are apparent on each side of the frenulum. A ranula (mucocele) may be seen on the floor of the mouth when the duct of a sublingual salivary gland is obstructed (see Fig. 12-24, *E*). Lesions on the tongue may be due to an infectious process (see Fig. 12-24, *F*).

Wrap the tongue with a piece of gauze and gently pull it to each side while inspecting the lateral borders (Fig. 12-25). Scape any white or red margins to distinguish between food particles and leukoplakia or another fixed abnormality.

Palpate the tongue and the floor of the mouth for lumps, nodules, or ulceration. Expect the tongue to have a smooth, even

FIGURE 12-24 Findings on the tongue and mouth floor. A, Left hypoglossal paralysis. The tongue deviates to the weak side. Note atrophy on the tongue's right side. **B,** Geographic tongue. **C,** Glossitis, smooth tongue resulting from vitamin deficiency. **D,** Black hairy tongue. **E,** Ranula (obstructed sublingual salivary gland). **F,** Primary gingivostomatitis showing lesions on the tongue. *(A, Courtesy Daniel M. Laskin, DDS, MS, Medical College of Virginia, Virginia Commonwealth University, Richmond, VA; B, C, courtesy Antoinette Hood, MD, Indiana University School of Medicine, Indianapolis; D, from Wood and Goaz, 1991; E, from Zitelli and Davis, 2007; F, reproduced with permission of the Wellcome Foundation Ltd.)*

FIGURE 12-25 Inspection of lateral borders of the tongue.

Staying Well

Screening for Oral Cancer

Carefully examine each of the following areas of the oral cavity, face, and neck to detect signs of oral cancer:

• Inspect the vermilion border of the lips (a high-risk site), the labial mucosa, the attached gingival tissues, alveolar gingival mucosa, and vestibule by raising and lowering the lips.
• Inspect the buccal mucosa and hard palate.
• Inspect the dorsal surface of the tongue. With the tongue extended right, inspect the left lateral and ventral surfaces of the tongue and lateral floor of the mouth. Extend the tongue to the left to inspect the right tongue surfaces.
• Inspect the anterior floor of the mouth.
• Place a gloved finger on the floor of the mouth and a finger of the other hand on the tissue behind the mandible. Compress the tissue between the fingers to palpate the floor of the mouth.
• Inspect and palpate the throat, neck, and temporomandibular areas.

Physical Variations

Mandible and Uvula

A bony protuberance, the mandibular torus, occurs bilaterally on the lingual surface of the mandible, near the canine and premolar teeth, and is an expected variant. It occurs in 7% to 10% of the population. A torus in the palate is a symmetric bony protuberance from the midline of the hard palate. It is an expected variant in 20% to 35% of the population (Gonsalves et al, 2007).

texture without nodules, ulcerations, or areas of induration. Any ulcer, nodule, or thickened white patch on the lateral or ventral surface of the tongue may be suggestive of malignancy. Table 12-4 presents the oral manifestations of human immunodeficiency virus (HIV) infection, and Figure 12-26 shows oral Kaposi sarcoma.

Ask the patient to tilt the head back for inspection of the palate and uvula. The whitish hard palate should be dome-shaped with transverse rugae. The pinker soft palate is contiguous with the hard palate. The uvula, a midline continuation of the soft palate, varies in length and thickness. The hard palate may have a bony protuberance at the midline, called torus palatinus, an expected variant (Fig. 12-27, *A*). A nodule on the palate that is not at the midline may indicate a tumor. See Physical Variations, "Mandible and Uvula".

Movement of the soft palate is evaluated by asking the patient to say "ah." Depressing the tongue may be necessary for this maneuver. As the patient vocalizes, observe the soft palate rise symmetrically with the uvula remaining in the midline. This maneuver also tests the glossopharyngeal and vagus nerves (cranial nerves IX and X). Deviation of the uvula to one side may indicate vagus nerve paralysis or peritonsillar abscess. The uvula deviates to the unaffected side in both instances. A bifid

EXAMINATION AND FINDINGS

Table 12-4   Oral Manifestations of HIV Infection

Lesion	Characteristics
Oral hairy leukoplakia	White, irregular lesions on lateral side of tongue or buccal mucosa; may have prominent folds or "hairy" projections
Angular cheilitis	Red, unilateral or bilateral fissures at corners of mouth
Candidiasis	Creamy white plaques on oral mucosa that bleed when scraped
Herpes simplex	Recurrent vesicular, crusting lesions on the vermilion border of the lip
Herpes zoster	Vesicular and ulcerative oral lesions in the distribution of the trigeminal nerve; may also be on gingiva
Human papillomavirus	Single or multiple, sessile or pedunculated nodules in the oral cavity
Aphthous ulcers	Recurrent circumscribed ulcers with an erythematous margin
Periodontal disease	In a mouth with little plaque or calculus, gingivitis with bone and soft tissue degeneration accompanied by severe pain
Kaposi sarcoma	In the mouth, incompletely formed blood vessels proliferate, forming lesions of various shades and size as blood extravasates in response to the malignant tumor of the epithelium

FIGURE 12-26 Oral Kaposi sarcoma. A, Moderately advanced. **B,** Advanced lesion. *(From Grimes, 1991; courtesy Sol Silverman Jr., DDS, University of California, San Francisco.)*

FIGURE 12-27 A, Torus palatinus. **B,** Bifid uvula. *(A, Courtesy Drs. Abelson and Cameron, Lutherville, MD; B, from Hawke, 1997.)*

uvula is often a benign condition and may be a normal variant in some Native Americans; however, it may indicate a submucous cleft palate (Fig. 12-27, *B*). A bifid uvula has recently been associated with Loeys-Dietz syndrome, a disorder in which aortic root dilation and aortic dissection may occur (Aalberts, 2008).

Oropharynx

Inspect the oropharynx using a tongue blade to depress the tongue (see Clinical Pearl, "Use of a Tongue Blade"). Observe the tonsillar pillars, noting the size of tonsils, if present, and the integrity of the retropharyngeal wall. The tonsils, usually the same pink color of the pharynx, are expected to fit within the tonsillar pillars. Tonsils may have crypts where cellular debris and food particles collect. If the tonsils are reddened, hypertrophied, and covered with exudate, an infection may be present (Fig. 12-28).

Clinical Pearl

Use of a Tongue Blade

Most patients dislike the gag reflex associated with use of a tongue blade. Moisten the tongue blade with warm water to help reduce triggering of the gag reflex.

Evidence-Based Practice in Physical Examination

Predictors of Streptococcal Pharyngitis

The Centor clinical prediction rule can help to distinguish between adults who may or may not have streptococcal pharyngitis. Four clinical signs assessed include enlargement of the tonsils, exudates on the tonsils, tender and enlarged anterior cervical nodes, and absence of cough. The presence of three to four clinical signs increases the probability of streptococcal pharyngitis, which should be confirmed by a rapid strep screen or throat culture. The presence of a measured temperature greater than 38.0° C is another important finding. The Centor clinical prediction rule has not been validated in the pediatric population (Ebell et al, 2009). A rapid strep test or throat culture is still important for an accurate diagnosis.

FIGURE 12-28 Findings of the oropharynx. A, Tonsillitis and pharyngitis. **B,** Acute viral pharyngitis. **C,** Postnasal drip. *(A, B, Courtesy Edward L. Applebaum, MD, Head, Department of Otolaryngology, University of Illinois Medical Center, Chicago.)*

The posterior wall of the pharynx should be smooth, glistening, pink mucosa with some small, irregular spots of lymphatic tissue and small blood vessels. A red bulge adjacent to the tonsil and extending beyond the midline may indicate a peritonsillar abscess. A yellowish mucoid film in the pharynx is typical of postnasal drip.

After preparing the patient for a gag response, touch the posterior wall of the pharynx. Elicitation of the gag reflex tests the glossopharyngeal and vagus nerves (cranial nerves IX and X). Expect a bilateral response. See Chapter 5 for assessment of voice quality.

✤ Infants

Ears. The ears, nose, mouth, and throat are common sites of congenital malformations in the newborn and require a thorough examination.

The auricle should be well formed with all landmarks present on inspection. The newborn's auricle is very flexible and instantly recoils after bending. The premature infant's auricles may appear flattened with limited incurving of the upper auricle, and ear recoil is slower.

The tip of the auricle should cross the imaginary line between the inner canthus of the eye and the prominent portion of the occiput, varying no more than 10 degrees from vertical. Auricles either poorly shaped or positioned too low are associated with renal disorders and congenital anomalies.

To perform the otoscopic examination place the infant in a supine or prone position so the head can be turned side to side. Many examiners prefer to hold the otoscope in the right hand for the right ear and left hand for the left ear. Hold the otoscope so that the ulnar surface of your hand rests against the infant's head. The otoscope will move as the infant's head moves, reducing the risk for trauma to the auditory canal. Use your other hand to stabilize the infant's head as the thumb and index finger pull the auricle down to straighten the upward curvature of the canal. The tympanic membrane is usually in an extremely oblique position in the newborn. Because the tympanic membrane does not become conical for several months, the light reflex may appear diffuse. Limited mobility, dullness, and opacity of a pink or red tympanic membrane may be noted in neonates. As the middle ear matures during early infancy, the tympanic membrane takes on the expected appearance.

Hearing screening is recommended for all newborns. Hearing screening and audiometry should also be performed at regular intervals for all infants and children. Knowledge of the sequence of hearing development is necessary to evaluate the infant's hearing (Table 12-5). To conduct a hearing screening, use a bell, whisper, or rub your fingers together as a sound stimulus, taking care that the infant responds to sound rather than to the air movement generated. Remember that responses to repeated sound stimuli will decrease as the infant tunes out the stimulus.

Nose and Sinuses. Expect the external nose to have a symmetric appearance and be positioned midline on the face. Minimal movement of the nares with breathing should be apparent. Deviation of the nose from midline may be related to fetal position.

Table 12-5	The Sequence of Expected Hearing and Speech Response
Age	**Response**
Birth to 3 months	Startles, wakes, or cries when hearing a loud sound; quiets to parent's voice; makes vowel sounds "oh" or "ah"
4 to 6 months	Turns head toward an interesting sound, localizes sound on a horizontal plane; responds to parent's voice; listens and enjoys sound-producing toys; starts babbling and cooing
7 to 12 months	Responds to own name, telephone ringing, and person's voice, even if not loud; listens when spoken to; localizes sounds on all planes by turning eyes and head toward sound; babbles with short and long strings of sounds; begins to imitate speech sounds

Modified from American Speech Language and Hearing Association: *How does your child hear and talk?*, 2012. Retrieved from www.asha.org/public/speech/development/01.htm.

A saddle-shaped nose with a low bridge and broad base, a short small nose, or a large nose may suggest a chromosomal disorder or congenital anomaly.

Inspect the internal nose by gently tilting the nose tip upward with your thumb and shining a light inside. Small amounts of clear fluid discharge may be seen in crying infants.

Newborns are obligatory nose breathers, so assess nasal patency at birth. With the infant's mouth closed, occlude one naris and then the other, observing the breathing pattern. When obstructed, the infant will be unable to breathe through the open naris. With any breathing difficulty, a small catheter is passed through each naris to the choana, the posterior nasal opening to assess patency. An obstruction may indicate choanal atresia or stenosis, or septal deviation resulting from delivery trauma.

The paranasal sinuses are poorly developed during infancy, and examination is generally unnecessary.

Mouth. The lips should be well formed with no cleft (see Physical Variations, "Cleft Lip and Palate"). The newborn may have sucking calluses on the upper lips, appearing as plaques or crusts, for the first few weeks of life. An absent philtrum suggests a congenital abnormality.

Physical Variations

Cleft Lip and Palate

The incidence of cleft lip and palate is higher in northern Europeans, Asians, Native Americans, and Australian aborigines. Africans and populations of African descent are more likely to have cleft lip only (Vieira, 2008).

The crying infant provides an opportunity to examine the mouth. Avoid depressing the tongue because this stimulates a strong reflex protrusion of the tongue, making visualization of the mouth difficult.

The buccal mucosa should be pink and moist with sucking pads but with no other lesions. Scrape any white patches on the tongue or buccal mucosa with a tongue blade. Nonadherent patches are usually milk deposits, but adherent patches may indicate candidiasis infection (thrush) (Fig. 12-29, *A*). Secretions that accumulate in the newborn's mouth that require frequent suctioning may indicate esophageal atresia.

Drooling is common between 6 weeks and 6 months of age until infants learn to swallow saliva. Drooling after that age is often attributed to teething and usually disappears by 2 years of age. If drooling persists, be concerned about a potential neurologic or oral motor disorder or an anomaly of the teeth or the upper gastrointestinal tract.

The newborn's gums should have no teeth and be smooth with a serrated edge of tissue along the buccal margins. Pearl-like retention cysts along the buccal margin are an expected variant and disappear in 1 to 2 months. If natal teeth are found in a newborn, determine if they are loose and could be aspirated (Fig. 12-29, *B*). Such teeth are not usually firmly fixed and may need to be removed, but seek parental permission. In older infants, count the deciduous teeth, noting any unusual sequence of eruption (see Fig. 12-10, *A*).

Expect the tongue to fit well in the floor of the mouth. The frenulum of the tongue usually attaches at a point midway between the ventral surface of the tongue and its tip. If the tongue does not protrude beyond the alveolar ridge (tongue tie),

FIGURE 12-29 Findings in the infant's mouth. A, Candidiasis infection (thrush). **B,** Natal teeth. **C,** Short frenulum. **D,** Macroglossia. **E,** Epstein pearls. *(A, B, D, Courtesy Mead Johnson and Co., Evansville, IN; C, E, from Zitelli and Davis, 2007.)*

feeding difficulties may occur (Fig. 12-29, *C*). Macroglossia is associated with congenital anomalies such as congenital hypothyroidism (Fig. 12-29, *D*).

The palatal arch should be dome-shaped with no clefts in either the hard or soft palate. A narrow, flat palate or a high, arched palate (associated with congenital anomalies) will affect the tongue's placement and lead to feeding and speech problems. Petechiae are often seen on the newborn's soft palate. Epstein pearls—small, whitish yellow masses at the juncture between the hard and soft palate—are common and disappear within a few weeks after birth (Fig. 12-29, *E*). The soft palate is expected to rise symmetrically when the infant cries.

Insert your gloved index finger into the infant's mouth, with the fingerpad to the roof of the mouth. Simultaneously evaluate the infant's suck and palpate the hard and soft palates. (This maneuver may be performed when quieting the infant to auscultate the heart and lungs.) The infant, unless recently fed, is expected to have a strong suck, with the tongue pushing vigorously upward against the finger. Further investigate the absence of a strong suck reflex or disinterest in sucking. Neither the hard nor soft palate should have palpable clefts. Stimulate the gag reflex by touching the tonsillar pillars. A bilateral gag reflex should be present.

�֍ Children

Because the young child often resists otoscopic and oral examinations, it may be wise to postpone these procedures until the end. Be prepared to immobilize if encouraging the child to cooperate fails. Another person, usually the parent, may be needed to effectively hold the child. Positioning the child on a parent's lap rather than prone or supine on the examining table makes the child feel more secure. One option is to seat the baby or toddler in the parent's lap, with the back to the parent's chest and legs between the adult's legs. The parent can then restrain the child's arms with one arm and control the child's head with the other (Fig. 12-30, *A*).

To perform the otoscopic examination on an older toddler, face the child sideways with one arm placed around the parent's waist. The parent holds the child firmly against his or her trunk, using one arm to restrain the child's head and the other arm to restrain the child's arm and body. You further stabilize the child's head as you insert the otoscope. For the oral examination, face the child forward.

When the child actively resists the examination in other positions, place him or her in supine position on the examining table. The parent holds the child's arms extended above the head and assists in immobilizing the head. Lie across the child's trunk and stabilize the child's head with your hands as you insert the otoscope or tongue blade. A third person may need to hold the child's legs (Fig. 12-30, *B*).

Ears. When performing the otoscopic examination, pull the auricle either downward and back or upward and back to gain the best view of the tympanic membrane. As the child grows, the shape of the auditory canal changes to the S-shaped curve of the adult. If the child is or has been crying, dilation of blood vessels in the tympanic membrane can cause redness. The pneumatic otoscope is especially important for distinguishing a red

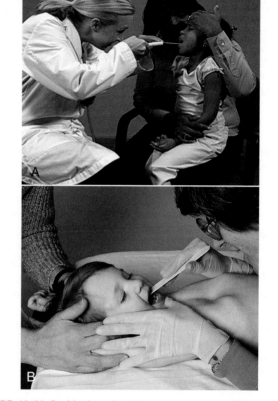

FIGURE 12-30 **Positioning of toddler for oral examination. A,** Sitting position. **B,** Supine position.

1. Normal middle ear system
2. Stages of middle ear effusion with retraction
3. and mobility only with negative pressure
4. Stiffened middle ear system as a consequence of otosclerosis, adhesive otitis media, or thickened tympanic membrane
5. Flaccid tympanic membrane or ossicle discontinuity

FIGURE 12-31 **Tympanometer wave pattern associated with middle ear conditions.**

tympanic membrane caused by crying (the membrane is mobile) from that resulting from disease (no mobility). See Differential Diagnosis on p. 254. Tympanometry provides an accurate way to identify middle ear effusion (Fig. 12-31) (also see Chapter 3). See Physical Variations, "Acute Otitis Media".

EXAMINATION AND FINDINGS

FIGURE 12-32 Early childhood caries. *(From Zitelli and Davis, 2007.)*

Screen the toddler's hearing by observing the response to a whispered voice and various noisemakers (e.g., rattle, bell, or tissue paper). Position yourself behind the child while the parent distracts the child. Whisper or use a noisemaker. Expect the child to turn toward the sound consistently. Development of speech provides another indication of hearing acuity.

When testing the hearing of a young child, whisper words that will have more meaning for them (e.g., "Big Bird," "Mickey Mouse," "Sponge Bob," "Spider Man"). Another way to evaluate the young child's hearing is by asking the child to perform tasks, using a soft voice. Avoid giving visual cues. The Weber and Rinne tests are used when the child understands directions and can cooperate with the examiner, usually between 3 and 4 years of age. Audiometry should be performed in all young children at regular intervals.

Nose and Sinuses. To inspect the internal nose, shine a light while tilting the nose tip upward with your thumb. If a larger area needs to be visualized, the largest otoscope speculum may be used.

Palpate the paranasal sinuses after they have developed (maxillary sinuses at 4 years of age and frontal sinuses at 7 to 8 years of age). Note any periorbital edema or tenderness in the sinus areas. The child with nasal discharge, nasal congestion, and/or cough that has not improved after 10 days following an upper respiratory infection may have a sinus infection if either of these signs is present (DeMuri and Wald, 2010).

Mouth. Encourage the child to cooperate with the oral examination. Letting the child hold and manipulate the tongue blade and light may reduce the fear of the procedure. Begin with a nonthreatening request, such as "please show me your teeth." Flattened edges on the teeth may indicate bruxism (compulsive, unconscious grinding of the teeth). Multiple brown areas or caries on the upper and lower incisors may be the result of a bedtime bottle of juice or milk, commonly called "early childhood caries" (Fig. 12-32). Teeth with a black or gray color may indicate pulp decay or oral iron therapy. Mottled or pitted teeth are often the result of tetracycline treatment during tooth development or enamel dysplasia. Chalky white lines or speckles on the cutting edges of permanent incisors may result from excessive fluoride intake.

If the child will protrude the tongue and say "ah," the tongue blade is often unnecessary for the oral examination. Ask the child to "pant like a puppy" to raise the palate. When the child refuses to open the mouth, insert a moistened tongue blade through the lips to the back molars. Gently but firmly insert the tongue blade between the back molars and press the tongue blade to the tongue. This maneuver will stimulate the gag reflex and provide a brief view of the mouth and oropharynx.

Koplik spots, white specks with a red base on the buccal mucosa opposite the first and second molars, occur in the prodromal phase of rubeola (measles).

The tonsils, lying deep in the oral cavity, should match the color of the pharynx. They gradually enlarge to their peak size by about 6 years of age, but the oropharynx should retain an unobstructed passage. Enlarged tonsils are graded to describe their size and potential for airway obstruction (Fig. 12-33). A tonsil pushed backward or forward, possibly displacing the uvula, suggests a peritonsillar abscess or other mass (see p. 258). When the tongue is depressed, the epiglottis is visible as a glistening pink structure behind the base of the tongue.

Pregnant Women

Pregnant women have increased vascularity of the respiratory tract, resulting in edema and erythema of the nose and pharynx and nasal congestion. Higher estrogen production leads to increased nasal mucous secretions, and often cold symptoms occur throughout pregnancy. Nosebleeds may occur. Tympanic membranes may have increased vascularity and be retracted or bulging with serous fluid. The gums may appear reddened, swollen, and spongy, with the hypertrophy resolving within 2 months of delivery.

Older Adults

Ears and Hearing. Inspect the auditory canal of the patient who wears a hearing aid for areas of irritation from the ear mold. Coarse, wirelike hairs are often present along the periphery of the auricle. On otoscopic examination, the tympanic membrane landmarks may appear slightly more pronounced from sclerotic changes.

Some degree of sensorineural hearing loss with advancing age (presbycusis) may be noted (see p. 256). Conductive hearing loss from otosclerosis and cerumen impaction may also occur.

Nose. The nasal mucosa may appear dryer, less glistening. An increased number of bristly hairs in the vestibule is common, especially in men.

FUNCTIONAL ASSESSMENT

Ears, Nose, and Throat

The ability to perform activities of daily living is often dependent on the ability to hear, speak, chew food, and swallow. Hearing is important for the personal social components of the functional assessment. The ability to chew and swallow food is important for adequate nutrition. When the patient has dentures, a hearing aid, or other assistive device, evaluate how effectively the patient uses these devices and is able to care for them.

Mouth. The lips have increased vertical markings and appear dryer when salivary flow is reduced. The buccal mucosa is thinner, less vascular, and less shiny than that of the younger adult. The tongue may appear more fissured, and veins on its ventral surface may appear varicose (Fig. 12-34, *A,B*).

The oral tissues may be dryer (xerostomia) when prescribed medications (e.g., anticholinergic or antidepressant drugs) diminish salivary gland secretions or when Sjögren syndrome, a chronic inflammatory condition of the exocrine glands, is present. Decreased saliva may cause an increase in dental caries and oral discomfort.

Natural teeth may be worn down, shortening the crown and altering enamel thickness. Dental caries may be present, and dental restorations may have deteriorated. The teeth may appear longer as resorption of the gum and bone progresses, revealing the teeth roots (Fig. 12-34, *C*). Many adults older than 65 years have missing teeth. Dental malocclusion may be caused by the migration of remaining teeth after extractions.

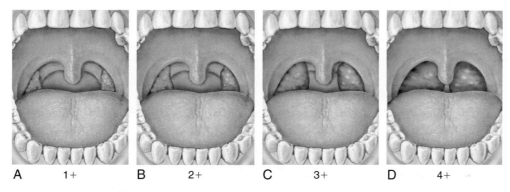

A   1+   B   2+   C   3+   D   4+

FIGURE 12-33 Enlarged tonsils are graded to describe their size: **A,** 1+, visible; **B,** 2+, halfway between tonsillar pillars and the uvula; **C,** 3+, nearly touching the uvula; **D,** 4+, touching each other.

FIGURE 12-34 Common findings in the older adult's mouth. A, Fissured tongue. **B,** Varicose veins on tongue. **C,** Attrition of teeth and resorption of gums. *(A, B, Courtesy Drs. Abelson and Cameron, Lutherville, MD; C, courtesy Daniel M. Laskin, DDS, MS, Medical College of Virginia, Virginia Commonwealth University, Richmond, VA.)*

Sample Documentation

History and Physical Examination

Subjective

A 55-year-old man concerned about hearing loss for the past few months, particularly difficult to hear people talking. Has difficulty hearing on the phone and in conversations when multiple people are talking. Hears noise in both ears when trying to go to sleep at night. No ear pain. No nasal discharge or sinus pain. No mouth lesions or masses, no recent dental problems, no sore throat. No head trauma or exposure to ototoxic medications.

Objective

Ears: Auricles in alignment, lobes without masses, lesions, or tenderness. Canals completely obstructed by cerumen. After irrigation, tympanic membranes are pearly gray, intact, with bony landmarks and light reflex visualized bilaterally. No evidence of fluid behind tympanic membrane or retraction. Conversational hearing appropriate. Able to hear whispered voice. Weber—sound heard equally in both ears; Rinne—air conduction greater than bone conduction bilaterally (30 sec/15 sec).

Nose: No discharge or polyps, mucosa pink and moist, septum midline, patent bilaterally. No edema over frontal or maxillary sinuses. No sinus tenderness to palpation.

Mouth: Buccal mucosa pink and moist without lesions. Twenty-six teeth present in various states of repair. Lower second molars (18, 30) absent bilaterally. Gingiva pink and firm. Tongue midline with no tremors, fasciculation, or lesions.

Pharynx: Clear without erythema, tonsils 1+ without exudate. Uvula rises evenly and gag reflex is intact. No hoarseness.

For additional sample documentation, see Chapter 26, pp. 628-631.

ABNORMALITIES

EAR

Otitis Media with Effusion and Acute Otitis Media

An inflammation of the middle ear resulting in the collection of serous, mucoid, or purulent fluid (effusion) when the tympanic membrane is intact

Pathophysiology

- The eustachian tube may be dysfunctional or obstructed by enlarged lymphoid tissue in the nasopharynx; the middle ear absorbs the air and creates a vacuum; the middle ear mucosa then secretes a transudate.
- Acute otitis media occurs when the effusion in the middle ear becomes infected with bacterial organisms.

Subjective Data

- See the Differential Diagnosis table below (Fig. 12-35 *A, B, C*)

Objective Data

- See the Differential Diagnosis table.

DIFFERENTIAL DIAGNOSIS

Otitis Externa, Otitis Media with Effusion, and Acute Otitis Media

Signs and Symptoms	Otitis Externa	Otitis Media with Effusion	Acute Otitis Media
Initial symptoms	Itching in ear canal; typically occurs after swimming	Sticking or cracking sound on yawning or swallowing; no signs of dizziness	Abrupt onset, fever, feeling of blockage, anorexia, irritability
Pain	Intense with movement of pinna, chewing	Discomfort, feeling of fullness	Deep-seated earache that interferes with activity or sleep, pulling at ear
Discharge	Watery, then purulent and thick, mixed with pus and epithelial cells; musty, foul-smelling	None	Only if tympanic membrane ruptures or through tympanostomy tubes; foul-smelling
Hearing	Conductive loss caused by exudate and swelling of ear canal	Conductive loss as middle ear fills with fluid	Conductive loss as middle ear fills with pus
Inspection	Canal is red, edematous; tympanic membrane obscured	Tympanic membrane retracted or bulging, impaired mobility, yellowish; air–fluid level and/or bubbles	Tympanic membrane with distinct erythema, thickened or clouding; bulging; limited or absent movement to positive or negative pressure, air–fluid level and/or bubbles

FIGURE 12-35 **Otitis media with effusion. A,** The middle ear filled with serous fluid; note the bulging appearance and distorted light reflex. **B,** Air-fluid levels in upper middle ear. **C,** Acute otitis media. Note the red bulging tympanic membrane with obscured bony landmarks and distorted light reflex. *(Courtesy Richard A. Buckingham, MD, Clinical Professor, Otolaryngology, Abraham Lincoln School of Medicine, University of Illinois, Chicago.)*

Otitis Externa

An inflammation of the auditory canal and external surface of the tympanic membrane

Pathophysiology	Subjective Data	Objective Data
• Water retained in the ear canal causes tissue maceration, desquamation, and microfissures that favor bacterial or fungal growth.	• See the Differential Diagnosis table on p. 254. (Fig. 12-36)	• See the Differential Diagnosis table.

FIGURE 12-36 **Otitis externa.** The inflammation in the auditory canal often extends with inflammation of the pinna. *(From Lemmi and Lemmi, 2009.)*

Cholesteatoma

Trapped epithelial tissue behind the tympanic membrane that is often the result of untreated or chronic recurrent otitis media

Pathophysiology	Subjective Data	Objective Data
• As the epithelial tissue enlarges, it can perforate the tympanic membrane, erode the ossicles and temporal bone, and invade the inner ear structures.	• History of acute otitis media • Unilateral hearing loss • Fullness in the ear • Tinnitus, mild vertigo • Discharge from the ear canal (Fig. 12-37)	• Spherical white cyst behind intact tympanic membrane • Tympanic membrane may bulge. • Foul-smelling discharge if the tympanic membrane is perforated • Conductive hearing loss

ABNORMALITIES

FIGURE 12-37 Cholesteatoma.
(Courtesy Richard A. Buckingham, MD, Clinical Professor, Otolaryngology, Abraham Lincoln School of Medicine, University of Illinois, Chicago.)

HEARING LOSS

Conductive Hearing Loss

Reduced transmission of sound to the middle ear

Pathophysiology

- Causes include cerumen impaction, otitis media with effusion, infection, foreign body, cholesteatoma, stiffening of the ossicles, and otosclerosis (bone deposition immobilizing the stapes).

Subjective Data

- Turns sound controls louder on TV, radio, music players
- Hears better in noisy environment
- Asks to have information repeated
- Speaks softly (hears own voice by bone conduction)

Objective Data

- Bone conduction heard longer than air conduction with Rinne test
- Lateralization to affected ear with Weber test
- Loss of low-frequency sounds
- Loss of 11 to 30 decibels (dB) on audiometry with cerumen impaction (Subha and Raman, 2006)

Sensorineural Hearing Loss

Reduced transmission of sound in the inner ear

Pathophysiology

- A disorder of the inner ear, damage to cranial nerve VIII, genetic disorders, systemic disease, ototoxic medication, trauma, tumors, or prolonged exposure to loud noise
- Presbycusis in older adults results from degenerative changes in the inner ear or vestibular nerve.

Subjective Data

- Complains that people mumble
- Has difficulty understanding speech
- Speaks more loudly
- Unable to hear in a crowded room

Objective Data

- Air conduction heard longer than bone conduction with Rinne test
- Lateralization to unaffected ear
- Loss of high-frequency sounds (consonants, e.g., *t, p, s*)

Ménière Disease (Endolymphatic Hydrops)

A disorder of progressive hearing loss that in some cases is hereditary

Pathophysiology

- May be caused by inadequate absorption of endolymph fluid by the endolymph sac or an abnormal endolymph drainage system; this allows endolymph fluid to flow into the perilymphatic fluid space, leading to depolarization of the hearing and balance nerves.

Subjective Data

- Sudden onset of severe vertigo (related to moving the head) lasting minutes to several hours
- Hearing loss
- Whistling or roaring sounds in affected ear (tinnitus); may be continuous or intermittent
- Sensitivity to sound
- Fullness or pressure in ears
- Nausea and vomiting
- Episodes in clusters with periods of remission

Objective Data

- Hearing loss to low tones initially with fluctuating progression to profound sensorineural hearing loss
- Imbalance
- Nystagmus

ABNORMALITIES

Vertigo

The illusion of rotational movement by a patient, often due to a disorder of the inner ear (see also Ménière disease)

Pathophysiology	Subjective Data	Objective Data
• Acute vestibular neuronitis—inflammation of the vestibular nerve following an acute viral upper respiratory infection • Benign paroxysmal positional vertigo—otolith fragments gravitate into the semicircular canal, and nerve sensors in the canal cause vertigo with head movements.	Acute vestibular neuronitis: • Spontaneous episodes of vertigo that is severe initially and lessens over a few days • Difficulty walking • Nausea and vomiting Benign paroxysmal positional vertigo: • Episode of vertigo with head or body movements • Lasts less than a minute	Acute vestibular neuronitis: • Spontaneous horizontal nystagmus with or without rotary nystagmus • Staggering gait Benign paroxysmal positional vertigo: • May have no physical findings • Rotary nystagmus with Dix-Hallpike maneuver

SINUSES

Sinusitis

A bacterial infection of one or more of the paranasal sinuses

Pathophysiology	Subjective Data	Objective Data
• Inflammation, allergies, or structural defect of the nose may block the sinus meatus and prevent the sinus cavity from draining, creating an environment for infection; overproduction of mucus may result from inflammation and increase susceptibility to infection.	• Upper respiratory infection that worsens or persists after 7 to 10 days (Leung and Katial, 2008) • Frontal headache, facial pain or pressure, or pain in a maxillary tooth • Purulent nasal discharge or nasal congestion • Persistent cough, may be worse at night	• May have no physical findings • Purulent nasal discharge from middle meatus, may be unilateral • Tenderness over frontal or maxillary sinuses • Swelling over orbital or involved sinus • Sinus does not transilluminate • Sinus radiograph indicates filled sinus cavity (Simel and Williams, 2009) • Preadolescent children may have daytime and nighttime cough, halitosis, and fever (DeMuri and Wald, 2010).

MOUTH AND OROPHARYNX

Acute Pharyngitis

Infection of tonsils or posterior pharynx by microorganisms

Pathophysiology	Subjective Data	Objective Data
• Microorganisms causing infection often include group A beta-hemolytic streptococci, other streptococcal species, *Neisseria gonorrhea, Mycoplasma pneumoniae*	• Sore throat, may be referred to pain in ears, dysphagia • Fever and malaise • Fetid breath • May have associated abdominal pain and headache (Fig. 12-38)	• Red and swollen tonsils • Crypts filled with purulent exudate • Enlarged anterior cervical lymph nodes • Palatal petechiae

FIGURE 12-38 Tonsillitis and pharyngitis. Notice the erythema and exudate in crypts of the tonsils. *(Courtesy Edward L. Applebaum, MD, Head, Department of Otolaryngology, University of Illinois Medical Center, Chicago.)*

ABNORMALITIES

Peritonsillar Abscess

A deep infection in the space between the soft palate and tonsil

Pathophysiology

- When Weber glands (mucous salivary glands in the space superior to the tonsil in the soft palate with a duct on the surface of the tonsil) become inflamed, the duct is obstructed, leading to cellulitis of the soft palate (Galioto, 2008).

Subjective Data

- Dysphagia and drooling
- Severe sore throat with pain radiating to the ear; pain is worse on one side
- Malaise and fever (Fig.12-39]

Objective Data

- Unilateral red and swollen tonsil and adjacent soft palate
- Tonsil may be pushed forward or backward; may displace the uvula to contralateral side
- Trismus (spasm of masticator muscles)
- Muffled voice
- Fetid breath
- Cervical lymphadenopathy

FIGURE 12-39 Swelling of peritonsillar abscess. *(Courtesy Daniel M. Laskin, DDS, MS, Medical College of Virginia, Virginia Commonwealth University, Richmond, VA.)*

Retropharyngeal Abscess

A life-threatening infection in the lateral pharyngeal space that has the potential to occlude the airway; most commonly occurs in children

Pathophysiology

- May result from trauma to the posterior pharyngeal wall, dental infection, or other pharyngeal infection (e.g., peritonsillar abscess) that extends to the retropharyngeal lymph nodes
- Group A streptococci and *Staphylococcus aureus* are common causative organisms.

Subjective Data

- Recent upper respiratory infection
- Acutely ill, fever
- Drooling
- Anorexia
- Irritable and anxious
- Pain in the neck and jaw with referral to ear
- Will not move neck (Fig. 12-40)

Objective Data

- Fever
- Lateral neck movement increases pain; torticollis
- Restlessness
- Lateral pharyngeal wall is distorted medially
- Trismus
- Respiratory distress
- Muffled voice

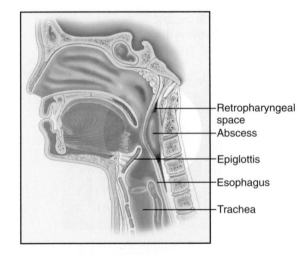

Retropharyngeal space
Abscess
Epiglottis
Esophagus
Trachea

FIGURE 12-40 Retropharyngeal abscess. Note the reduced airway size next to the epiglottis.

ABNORMALITIES

Oral Cancer

A cancer involving the oral cavity or related structures

Pathophysiology

- Most often, squamous cell carcinoma that originates in the basal cell layer of the oral mucosa
- May occur as a primary lesion or metastasis from a distant site to the jaw or related structure (McDowell, 2006)

Subjective Data

- Uses of tobacco products; alcohol abuse
- Painless sore in mouth that does not heal
- Pain with later-stage lesions (Fig. 12-41)

FIGURE 12-41 Squamous cell cancer on the tongue. *(Courtesy Daniel M. Laskin, DDS, MS, Medical College of Virginia, Virginia Commonwealth University, Richmond, VA.)*

Objective Data

- Ulcerative lesion (red or white) appearing as piled-up edges around a core on the lateral border or floor of the mouth
- A red or white patch on the gums, tongue, tonsil, hard or soft palate, or buccal mucosa
- Firm, nonmobile mass
- Tooth mobility when no periodontal disease is present
- Cervical lymphadenopathy

Periodontal Disease

A chronic infection of the gums, bones, and other tissues that surround and support the teeth

Pathophysiology

- Often results from poor dental hygiene (calculus not removed below the gum line) leading to chronic inflammation and infection of the gingiva and periodontal tissue; underlying bone is reabsorbed and teeth loosen.

Subjective Data

- Red and swollen gums that bleed easily with brushing
- Tender gums and loose teeth
- Teeth sensitive to temperature or hurt when eating

Objective Data

- Plaque and tartar buildup on teeth; teeth appear long
- Deep pockets between the teeth and gingiva
- Loose or missing teeth
- Halitosis

Cleft Lip and Palate

This most common craniofacial congenital malformation is the result of the lip or palate failing to fuse during embryonic development prior to the 12th week of gestation.

Pathophysiology

- Believed to have multifactorial causes that can include genetic disorders, fetal exposure to teratogens (e.g., anticonvulsants, alcohol) and conditions present in the mother (e.g., diabetes, folate deficiency, and maternal smoking) (Arosarena, 2007)

Subjective Data

- Difficulty sucking
- Failure to gain weight (Fig. 12-42)

Objective Data

- Apparent at birth
- Cleft may be unilateral or bilateral; may involve the lip, hard palate, or soft palate, or all three; a partial cleft in any of these tissues may be seen.

FIGURE 12-42 Unilateral cleft lip and palate. *(From Zitelli and Davis, 1997.)*

CHAPTER 13

Chest and Lungs

The chest and lungs allow for respiration. The purpose of respiration is to keep the body adequately supplied with oxygen and protected from excess accumulation of carbon dioxide. It involves the movement of air back and forth from the alveoli to the outside environment, gas exchange across the alveolar-pulmonary capillary membranes, and circulatory system transport of oxygen to, and carbon dioxide from, the peripheral tissues. This chapter focuses on the examination of the chest and lungs.

evolve *http://evolve.elsevier.com/Seidel*
- Physical Exam Key Points
- NCLEX Review Questions
- Interactive Activities
- Animations
- Audio Clips
- Videos
- Student Checklist

ANATOMY AND PHYSIOLOGY

The chest, or thorax, is a structure of bone, cartilage, and muscle capable of movement as the lungs expand. It consists anteriorly of the sternum, manubrium, xiphoid process, and costal cartilages; laterally, of the 12 pairs of ribs; and posteriorly, of the 12 thoracic vertebrae (Figs. 13-1 and 13-2). All the ribs are connected to the thoracic vertebrae; the upper seven are attached anteriorly to the sternum by the costal cartilages, and ribs 8, 9, and 10 join with the costal cartilages just above them. Ribs 11 and 12, sometimes referred to as floating ribs, attach posteriorly but not anteriorly. The lateral diameter of the chest generally exceeds the anterior-posterior (AP) diameter in adults.

The primary muscles of respiration are the diaphragm and the intercostal muscles. The diaphragm is the dominant muscle. It contracts and moves downward during inspiration, lowering the abdominal contents to increase the intrathoracic space. The external intercostal muscles increase the AP chest diameter during inspiration, and the internal intercostals decrease the lateral diameter during expiration. The sternocleidomastoid and trapezius muscles may also contribute to respiratory movements. These "accessory" muscles are used during exercise or when there is pulmonary compromise (Fig. 13-3).

Physical Examination Preview

Here is a preview of the steps involved in conducting physical examination of the chest and lungs. Ⓔ These procedures are explained in detail in this chapter and are available on Evolve in printable formats.
1. Inspect the chest; front and back, noting thoracic landmarks, for the following (p. 268):
   - Size and shape (anteroposterior [AP] diameter compared with the lateral diameter)
   - Symmetry
   - Color
   - Superficial venous patterns
   - Prominence of ribs
2. Evaluate respirations for the following (p. 270):
   - Rate
   - Rhythm or pattern
3. Inspect chest movement with breathing for symmetry and use of accessory muscles (p. 271).
4. Note any audible sounds with respiration (e.g., stridor or wheezes) (p. 272).
5. Palpate the chest for the following (p. 273):
   - Thoracic expansion
   - Sensations such as crepitus, grating vibrations
   - Tactile fremitus
6. Perform direct or indirect percussion on the chest, comparing sides, for the following (p. 274):
   - Diaphragmatic excursion
   - Percussion tone intensity, pitch, duration, and quality
7. Auscultate the chest with the stethoscope diaphragm, from apex to base, comparing sides for the following (p. 276):
   - Intensity, pitch, duration, and quality of breath sounds
   - Unexpected breath sounds (crackles, rhonchi, wheezes, friction rubs)
   - Vocal resonance

The interior of the chest is divided into three major spaces: the right and left pleural cavities and the mediastinum. The mediastinum, situated between the lungs, contains the heart and major blood vessels. The pleural cavities are lined with serous membranes (parietal and visceral pleurae) that enclose the lungs. The spongy and highly elastic lungs are paired but not symmetric, the right having three lobes and the left having two

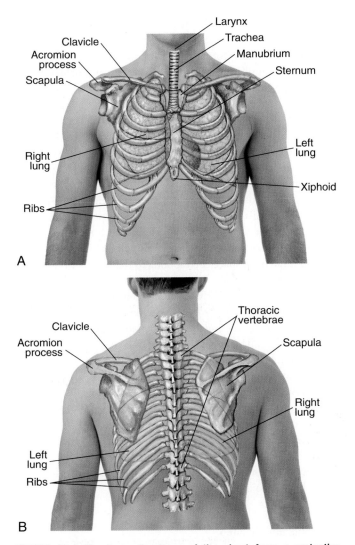

A

B

FIGURE 13-1 The bony structures of the chest form a protective expandable cage around the lungs and heart. A, Anterior view. **B,** Posterior view. *(From Thompson and Wilson, 1996.)*

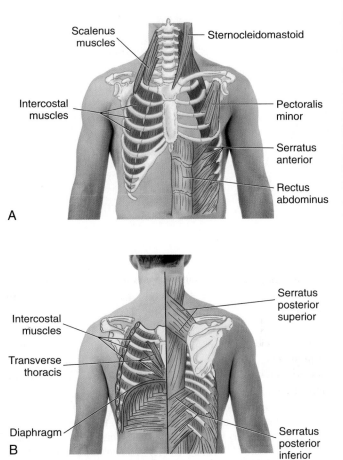

A

B

FIGURE 13-3 Muscles of ventilation. A, Anterior view. **B,** Posterior view.

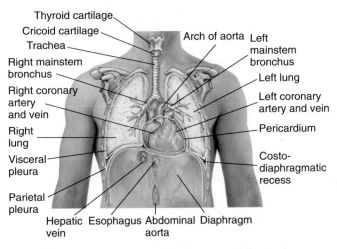

FIGURE 13-2 Chest cavity and related anatomic structures.

(Fig. 13-4). The left upper lobe has an inferior tonguelike projection, the lingula, which is a counterpart of the right middle lobe. Each lung has a major fissure—the oblique—that divides the upper and lower portions. In addition, a lesser horizontal fissure divides the upper portion of the right lung into the upper and middle lobes at the level of the fifth rib in the axilla and the fourth rib anteriorly. The lung is not fully grown at birth. The number of alveoli increases at a very rapid rate in the first 2 years of life. This slows down by the age of 8 years. Each lobe consists of blood vessels, lymphatics, nerves, and an alveolar duct connecting with the alveoli (as many as 300 million in an adult). The entire lung is shaped by an elastic subpleural tissue that limits its expansion. Each lung apex is rounded and extends anteriorly about 4 cm above the first rib into the base of the neck in adults. Posteriorly, the apices of the lungs rise to about the level of T1. The lower borders descend on deep inspiration to about T12 and rise on forced expiration to about T9. The base of each lung is broad and concave, resting on the convex surface of the diaphragm. The medial surfaces of the lung are to some extent concave, providing a cradle for the heart.

The tracheobronchial tree is a tubular system that provides a pathway along which air is filtered, humidified, and warmed as it moves from the upper airway to the alveoli. The trachea is 10 to 11 cm long and about 2 cm in diameter. It lies anterior to the

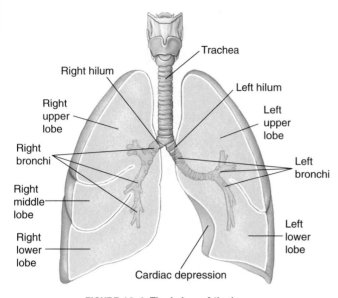

FIGURE 13-4 The Lobes of the lungs.

Box 13-1   Visualizing the Lungs from the Surface

Anteriorly

The right lung may ride higher because of the fullness of the dome of the liver. Except for an inferior lateral triangle, the anterior view on the right is primarily the upper and middle lobes, separated by the horizontal fissure at about the fifth rib in the midaxilla to about the fourth at the sternum; on the left as on the right, the lower lobe is set off by a diagonal fissure stretching from the fifth rib at the axilla to the sixth at the midclavicular line.

Posteriorly

Except for the apices, the posterior view is primarily the lower lobe, which extends from about T3 to T10 or T12 during the respiratory cycle.

Right Lateral

The lung underlies the area extending from the peak of the axilla to the seventh or eighth rib. The upper lobe is demarcated at about the level of the fifth rib in the midaxillary line and the sixth rib more anteriorly.

Left Lateral

The lung underlies the area extending from the peak of the axilla to the seventh or eighth rib. The entire expanse is virtually bisected by the oblique fissure from about the level of the third rib medially to the sixth rib anteriorly.

esophagus and posterior to the isthmus of the thyroid. The trachea divides into the right and left main bronchi at about the level of T4 or T5 and just below the manubriosternal joint (Box 13-1).

The right bronchus is wider, shorter, and more vertically placed than the left bronchus (and therefore more susceptible to aspiration of foreign bodies). The main bronchi are divided into three branches on the right and two on the left, each branch supplying one lobe of the lungs. The branches then begin to subdivide into terminal bronchioles and ultimately into respiratory bronchioles.

The bronchial arteries branch from the anterior thoracic aorta and the intercostal arteries, supplying blood to the lung tissue. The bronchial vein is formed at the hilum of the lung, but most of the blood supplied by the bronchial arteries is returned by the pulmonary veins (Fig. 13-5).

Anatomic Landmarks

The following topographic markers on the chest are used to describe findings (Fig. 13-6):

1. The nipples
2. The manubriosternal junction (angle of Louis). A visible and palpable angulation of the sternum and the point at which the second rib articulates with the sternum. One can count the ribs and intercostal spaces from this point. The number of each intercostal space corresponds to that of the rib immediately above it.
3. The suprasternal notch. A depression, easily palpable and most often visible at the base of the ventral aspect of the neck, just superior to the manubriosternal junction.
4. Costal angle. The angle formed by the costal margins at the sternum. It is usually no more than 90 degrees, with the ribs inserted at approximately 45-degree angles.
5. Vertebra prominens. The spinous process of C7. It can be more readily seen and felt with the patient's head bent forward. If two prominences are felt, the upper is that of the spinous process of C7, and the lower is that of T1. It is difficult to use this as a guide to counting ribs posteriorly because the spinous processes from T4 down project obliquely, thus overlying the rib below the number of its vertebra.
6. The clavicles

✥ Infants and Children

Prior to birth the lungs contain no air, and the alveoli are collapsed. Fetal gas exchange is mediated by the placenta. Relatively passive respiratory movements occur throughout gestation; they do not open the alveoli or move the lung fields.

At birth the change in respiratory function is rapid and dramatic. After the infant's initial gasp and cry, the lungs fill with air for the first time. When the umbilical cord is cut shortly thereafter, maternal blood is no longer coming through the placenta. At this point blood flows through the infant lungs more vigorously. The pulmonary arteries expand and relax, offering much less resistance than the systemic circulation. This relative decrease in pulmonary pressure most often leads to closure of the foramen ovale within minutes after birth, and the increased oxygen tension in the arterial blood usually stimulates contraction and closure of the ductus arteriosus (see Clinical Pearl, "Patent Ductus Arteriosus [PDA]"). The pulmonary and systemic circulations adopt their mature configurations, and the lungs are fully integrated for postnatal function.

The chest of the newborn is generally round, the AP diameter approximating the lateral diameter, and the circumference is roughly equal to that of the head until the child is about 2 years old (Fig. 13-7). With growth, the chest assumes adult proportions, with the lateral diameter exceeding the AP diameter.

FIGURE 13-5 Pulmonary circulation.

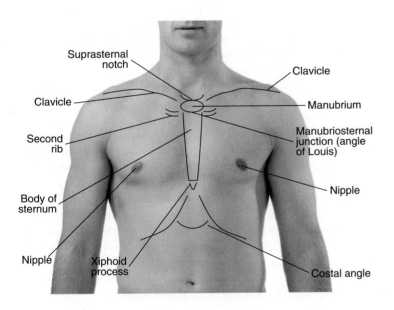

FIGURE 13-6 Topographic landmarks of the chest.

ribs flare include an increase in the lateral diameter of about 2 cm and an increase in the circumference of 5 to 7 cm. The costal angle progressively increases from about 68.5 degrees to approximately 103.5 degrees in later pregnancy. The diaphragm at rest rises as much as 4 cm above its usual resting position, yet diaphragmatic movement increases so that the major work of breathing is done by the diaphragm. Minute ventilation increases due to increased tidal volume, though the respiratory rate remains unchanged.

✤ Older Adults

The barrel chest that is seen in many older adults results from loss of muscle strength in the thorax and diaphragm (see Fig. 13-9), coupled with the loss of lung resiliency. In addition, skeletal changes of aging tend to emphasize the dorsal curve of the thoracic spine, resulting in an increased AP chest diameter. There may also be stiffening and decreased expansion of the chest wall.

Clinical Pearl

Patent Ductus Arteriosus (PDA)

The foramen ovale and the ductus arteriosus do not always close so readily. This failure to close is more common in premature infants born before 30 weeks of gestation. A large PDA can lead to left ventricular overload and heart failure.

The relatively thin chest wall of the infant and young child makes the bony structure more prominent than in the adult. It is more cartilaginous and yielding, and the xiphoid process is often more prominent and more movable.

✤ Pregnant Women

Mechanical and biochemical factors, including the enlarged uterus and an increased level of circulating progesterone, interact to create changes in the respiratory function of the pregnant woman. Anatomic changes that occur in the chest as the lower

FIGURE 13-7 Chest of healthy infant. Note that the anteroposterior diameter is approximately the same as the lateral diameter.

The alveoli become less elastic and relatively more fibrous. The associated loss of some of the interalveolar folds decreases the alveolar surface available for gas exchange. This and the loss of strength in the muscles of respiration result in underventilation of the alveoli in the lower lung fields and a decreased tolerance for exertion. The net result of these changes is a decrease in vital capacity and an increase in residual volume.

Aging mucous membranes tend to become drier and older adults are less able to clear mucus. Retained mucus encourages bacterial growth and predisposes the older adult to respiratory infection.

REVIEW OF RELATED HISTORY

For each of the symptoms or conditions discussed in this section, targeted topics to include in the history of the present illness are listed. Responses to questions about these topics provide clues for focusing the physical examination and the development of an appropriate diagnostic evaluation. Questions regarding medication use (prescription and over the counter preparations) as well as complementary and alternative therapies are relevant for each.

History of Present Illness

- Cough
  - Onset: sudden, gradual; duration
  - Nature of cough: dry, moist, wet, hacking, hoarse, barking, whooping, bubbling, productive, nonproductive
  - Sputum production: duration, frequency, with activity, at certain times of day
  - Sputum characteristics: amount, color (clear, purulent, blood-tinged, mostly blood), foul odor
  - Pattern: occasional, regular, paroxysmal; related to time of day, weather, activities (e.g., exercise), talking, deep breaths; change over time
  - Severity: tires patient, disrupts sleep or conversation, causes chest pain

- Associated symptoms: shortness of breath, chest pain or tightness with breathing, fever, nasal congestion, noisy respirations, hoarseness, gagging
- Efforts to treat: prescription or nonprescription drugs, vaporizers

Coughs

Coughs are a common symptom of a respiratory problem. They are usually preceded by a deep inspiration; this is followed by closure of the glottis and contraction of the chest, abdominal, and even the pelvic muscles, and then a sudden, spasmodic expiration, forcing a sudden opening of the glottis. Air and secretions are exhaled. The causes may be related to localized or more general insults at any point in the respiratory tract. Coughs may be voluntary, but they are usually reflexive responses to an irritant such as a foreign body (microscopic or larger), an infectious agent, or a mass of any sort compressing the respiratory tree. They may also be a clue to an anxiety state.

Staying Well

Discuss Cigarette Use

Chronic obstructive pulmonary disease is the third leading cause of death in the United States. The major risk factor is cigarette smoking. Although as many as 20% of people who die from the disease have never smoked, the vital key to prevention is the cessation of smoking or, better yet, never starting. A major risk to the preservation of pulmonary health during late childhood and adolescence is the first experiment with any tobacco product. It is our responsibility as care providers to work with patients to help them recognize the health risks of smoking and develop action steps toward quitting.

Describe a cough according to its moisture, frequency, regularity, pitch and loudness, quality, and circumstances. The type of cough may offer some clue to the cause. Although a cough may not have a serious cause, do not ignore it.

Dry or Moist. A moist or productive cough may be caused by infection and can be accompanied by sputum production. A dry or nonproductive cough can have a variety of causes (e.g., cardiac problems, allergies, gastroesophageal reflux with pharyngeal irritation), which may be indicated by the quality of its sound.

Onset. An acute onset, particularly with fever, suggests infection; in the absence of fever, a foreign body or inhaled irritants are additional possible causes.

Frequency of Occurrence. Note whether the cough is seldom or often present. An infrequent cough may result from allergens or environmental insults.

Regularity. A regular, paroxysmal cough is heard in pertussis. An irregularly occurring cough may have a variety of causes (e.g., smoking, early congestive heart failure, an inspired foreign body or irritant, or a tumor within or compressing the bronchial tree).

Pitch and Loudness. A cough may be loud and high-pitched or quiet and relatively low-pitched.

Postural Influences. A cough may occur soon after a person has reclined or assumed an erect position (e.g., with a nasal drip or pooling of secretions in the upper airway).

Quality. A dry cough may sound loud and harsh if it is caused by compression of the respiratory tree (as by a tumor) or hoarse if it is caused by croup. Pertussis produces an inspiratory whoop at the end of a paroxysm of coughing in older children and adults.

Sputum

The production of sputum is generally associated with cough. Sputum in more than small amounts and with any degree of consistency always suggests the presence of disease. If the onset is acute, infection is most probable. Once there is some chronicity, the possibility of a significant anatomic change (e.g., tumor, cavitation, or bronchiectasis) becomes apparent. The Differential Diagnosis table below delineates possible pathologic conditions and their accompanying sputum findings.

+ Shortness of breath (Box 13-2)
  + Onset: sudden or gradual; duration; gagging or choking event before onset
  + Pattern
  + Position most comfortable, number of pillows used to sleep comfortably
  + Related to extent of exercise, certain activities, time of day, eating, environmental exposure
  + Harder to inhale or exhale
  + Severity: extent of activity limitation, fatigue with breathing, anxiety about getting air
  + Associated symptoms: pain or discomfort (relationship to specific point in respiratory exertion, location), cough, diaphoresis, ankle edema
  + Efforts to treat: oxygen use

DIFFERENTIAL DIAGNOSIS
Some Causes of Sputum

Cause	Possible Sputum Characteristics
Bacterial infection	Yellow, green, rust (blood mixed with yellow sputum), clear, or transparent; purulent; blood streaked; sticky
Viral infection	Blood-streaked (not common)
Chronic infectious disease	All of the above; particularly abundant in the early morning; slight, intermittent blood streaking; occasionally, large amounts of blood*
Cancer	Slight, persistent, intermittent blood streaking
Infarction	Blood clotted; large amounts of blood
Tuberculous cavity	Occasional large amounts of blood*

*Ascertain that the blood is not swallowed from a nosebleed.

Box 13-2 Descriptors of Respiration

Dyspnea, difficult and labored breathing with shortness of breath, is commonly observed with pulmonary or cardiac compromise. A sedentary lifestyle and obesity can cause it in an otherwise well person. In general, dyspnea increases with the severity of the underlying condition. It is important to establish the amount and kind of effort that produces dyspnea:

- Is it present even when the patient is resting?
- How much walking? On a level surface? Upstairs?
- Is it necessary to stop and rest when climbing stairs?
- With what other activities of daily life does dyspnea begin? With what level of physical demand?

Other manifestations of respiratory difficulty include the following:

Orthopnea—shortness of breath that begins or increases when the patient lies down; ask whether the patient needs to sleep on more than one pillow and whether that helps.

Paroxysmal nocturnal dyspnea—a sudden onset of shortness of breath after a period of sleep; sitting upright is helpful.

Platypnea—dyspnea increases in the upright posture.

+ Chest pain (see Clinical Pearl, "Chest Pain")
  + Onset and duration; associated with trauma, coughing, lower respiratory infection, recent anesthesia, history of thrombosis
  + Associated symptoms: shallow breathing, fever, coughing, anxiety about getting air, radiation of pain to neck or arms
  + Efforts to treat: heat, splinting, pain medication
  + Other medications: illicit drug use (e.g., cocaine)

Past Medical History

+ Thoracic, nasal, and/or pharyngotracheal trauma or surgery, hospitalizations for pulmonary disorders, dates

> **Clinical Pearl**
>
> *Chest Pain*
>
> Chest pain does not generally originate in the heart when:
> - There is a constant achiness that lasts all day.
> - It does not radiate.
> - It is made worse by pressing on the chest wall.
> - It is a fleeting, needle-like jab that lasts only a few seconds.
> - It is situated in the shoulders or between the shoulder blades in the back.
>
>   Think of the heart but, importantly, in such circumstances, also think of other possibilities in the chest.

- Use of oxygen or ventilation-assisting devices including continuous or bilevel positive airway pressure machines (CPAP or BiPAP, respectively)
- Chronic pulmonary diseases: tuberculosis (date, treatment, compliance), bronchitis, emphysema, bronchiectasis, asthma, cystic fibrosis
- Other chronic disorders: cardiac, cancer, blood clotting disorders
- Testing: allergy, pulmonary function tests, tuberculin skin tests, chest imaging
- Immunization against *Streptococcus pneumoniae*, influenza

Family History

- Tuberculosis
- Cystic fibrosis
- Emphysema
- Allergy, asthma, atopic dermatitis
- Malignancy
- Bronchiectasis
- Bronchitis
- Clotting disorders (risk of pulmonary embolism)

Personal and Social History

- Employment: nature of work, extent of physical and emotional effort and stress, environmental hazards, exposure to chemicals, animals, vapors, dust, pulmonary irritants (e.g., asbestos), allergens, use of protective masks
- Home environment: location, possible allergens, type of heating, use of air conditioning, humidifier, ventilation, use of smoke and carbon monoxide detectors in the home
- Tobacco use: type of tobacco (cigarettes, cigars, pipe, smokeless), duration and amount (Pack years = Number of years of smoking × Number of packs smoked per day), age started, efforts to quit smoking with factors influencing success or failure, the extent of smoking by others at home or at work (second-hand smoking)
- Exposure to respiratory infections, influenza, tuberculosis
- Nutritional status: weight loss or obesity
- Use of complementary and alternative therapies
- Regional or travel exposures (e.g., tuberculosis [TB] infection in India, China, Indonesia, South Africa, and Nigeria;

histoplasmosis in southeastern and midwestern United States; coccidioidomycosis [valley fever] in southwestern United States, Mexico, Central and South America; schistosomiasis in east and southwest Asia, Africa, and the Caribbean)
- Hobbies: owning birds or other animals, woodworking or welding
- Use of alcohol or illicit drugs (e.g., cocaine, inhaled methamphetamine); see Clinical Pearl, "Pain from Cocaine"
- Exercise tolerance: amount of exercise, diminished ability to perform up to expectations

> **Clinical Pearl**
>
> *Pain from Cocaine*
>
> If an adult—especially a young adult—or an adolescent describes severe, acute chest pain, ask about drug use, particularly cocaine. Cocaine can cause tachycardia, hypertension, coronary arterial spasm (with infarction), and pneumothorax (lung collapse) with severe acute chest pain being the common result.

⚘ Infants and Children

- Low birth weight: prematurity, history of intubation, duration of ventilation assistance, respiratory distress syndrome, bronchopulmonary dysplasia (chronic lung disease), transient tachypnea of the newborn
- Coughing or difficulty breathing of sudden onset, possible aspiration of small object, toy, or food
- Possible ingestion of kerosene, antifreeze, or hydrocarbons in household cleaners
- Apneic episodes: associated perioral cyanosis, breath-holding, posttussive emesis, history of sudden infant death in sibling
- Swallowing dysfunction or other neuromuscular disorders, recurrent spitting up and gagging, recurrent pneumonia (possible gastroesophageal reflux)
- Immunization status—especially pneumococcal and influenza vaccines

⚘ Pregnant Women

- Weeks of gestation or estimated date of delivery
- Presence of multiple fetuses, polyhydramnios, or other conditions in which a larger uterus displaces the diaphragm upward
- Exercise type and energy expenditure
- Exposure to and frequency of respiratory infections, status of influenza immunization

⚘ Older Adults

- Exposure to and frequency of respiratory infections, status of pneumococcal vaccination and influenza immunization
- Need for supplemental oxygen
- Effects of weather on respiratory efforts and occurrence of infections
- Immobilization or marked sedentary habits
- Difficulty swallowing

- Alteration in daily living habits or activities as a result of respiratory symptoms
- Because older adults are at risk for chronic respiratory diseases (lung cancer, chronic bronchitis, emphysema, and tuberculosis), reemphasize the following:
  - Smoking history
  - Cough, dyspnea on exertion, or breathlessness
  - Blood-tinged or yellowish/greenish sputum
  - Fatigue
  - Significant weight changes
  - Fever, night sweats

Equipment

- Marking pen
- Centimeter ruler and tape measure
- Stethoscope with bell and diaphragm (for infants, you need a smaller stethoscope)
- Drapes

Clinical Pearl

The Sequence of Steps

The sequence of steps in examination of the chest and lungs is inspection, palpation, percussion, and auscultation. The integration of all four, together with the history, will often provide adequate information regarding the pathologic process. Listening to the lungs without also inspecting and palpating the chest will deny you the chance to interpret your findings in the most accurate way. Dullness on percussion, for example, is present in both pleural effusion and lobar pneumonia. Breath sounds are absent in the former and may be bronchial in the latter. On palpation you will often find that tactile fremitus is absent when an effusion exists and is increased with lobar pneumonia.

EXAMINATION AND FINDINGS

Inspection

Have the patient sit upright, if possible without support, unclothed to the waist. Clothing of any kind is a barrier for inspection, palpation, percussion, and auscultation. A drape should cover the patient when full exposure is not necessary. The room and stethoscope should be comfortably warm, and a bright tangential light is needed to highlight chest movement. Position the patient so that the light source comes at different angles to accentuate findings that are more subtle and otherwise difficult to detect, such as retractions, or the presence of deformity (e.g., minimal pectus excavatum). If the patient is in bed and mobility is limited, you should have access to both sides of the bed. After informing the patient, do not hesitate to raise and lower the bed as needed.

Note the shape and symmetry of the chest from both the back and the front, the costal angle, the angle of the ribs, and the intercostal spaces. The bony framework is obvious, the clavicles prominent superiorly, the sternum usually rather flat and free of an abundance of overlying tissue. (Box 13-3 lists thoracic landmarks to use as you record findings.) The chest will not be absolutely symmetric, but one side can be used as a comparison for the other. The AP diameter of the chest is ordinarily less than the lateral diameter (Fig. 13-8). The relationship is expressed as the thoracic ratio and is expected to be about 0.70 to 0.75. It does increase with age; however, when the AP diameter approaches or equals the lateral diameter (a ratio of 1.0 or even greater), there is most often a chronic condition present. Barrel chest (Fig. 13-9) results from compromised respiration as in, for example, chronic asthma, emphysema, or cystic fibrosis. The ribs are more horizontal, the spine is somewhat kyphotic, and the sternal angle is more prominent. The trachea may be posteriorly displaced.

Other changes in chest wall contour may be the result of structural problems in the spine, rib cage, or sternum. The spine may be deviated either posteriorly (kyphosis) or laterally (scoliosis) (see Figs. 21-31, *B*, and 21-72). Two common structural findings are pigeon chest (pectus carinatum), which is a prominent sternal protrusion, and funnel chest (pectus excavatum), which is an indentation of the lower sternum above the xiphoid process (Fig. 13-12). See Clinical Pearl, "The Sequence of Steps."

Observing Respiration

Determine the respiratory rate. The rate should be 12 to 20 respirations per minute; the ratio of respirations to heartbeats is approximately 1:4. Do not tell the patient that you are going to

FIGURE 13-8 Thorax of healthy adult male. Note that the anteroposterior diameter is less than the lateral diameter.

EXAMINATION AND FINDINGS

FIGURE 13-9 **Barrel chest.** Note increase in the anteroposterior diameter.

count the respirations to prevent the patient from varying the rate. Count the respiratory rate after palpating the pulse, just as if you were counting the pulse rate for a longer time. Respiratory rates can vary in the different waking and sleep states. The expected rate of respirations (breaths per minute) depends on a number of factors, including the age of the individual and the degree of exertion. Noting the behavior of the patient relative to the rate is often helpful.

Note the pattern (or rhythm) of respiration and the way in which the chest moves (Fig. 13-13). Expect the patient to breathe easily, regularly, and without apparent distress. The pattern of breathing should be even, neither too shallow nor too deep. Note any variations in respiratory rate.

The normal resting adult respiratory rate is 12 to 20 breaths/min. Tachypnea is a persistent respiratory rate above this in an adult. Confirm that the respiratory rate is persistent. Rapid breathing may occur during hyperventilation or simply as a self-conscious response to your observation. It is often a symptom of protective splinting from the pain of a broken rib or pleurisy. Massive liver enlargement or abdominal ascites may prevent descent of the diaphragm and produce a similar pattern. Bradypnea, a rate slower than 12 respirations per minute, may indicate neurologic or electrolyte disturbance, infection, or a conscious response to protect against the pain of pleurisy or other irritative phenomena. It may also indicate an excellent level of cardiorespiratory fitness.

Note any variations in respiratory rhythm. It may be difficult to discern abnormalities unless they are quite obvious

(Box 13-4). Hyperventilation can be due to breathing rapidly (tachypnea), breathing deeply (hyperpnea), or both. Exercise and anxiety can cause hyperpnea, but so can central nervous system and metabolic disease. Kussmaul breathing, always deep and most often rapid, is the eponym applied to the respiratory effort associated with metabolic acidosis. Hypopnea, on the other hand, refers to abnormally shallow respirations (e.g., when pleuritic pain limits excursion).

A regular periodic pattern of breathing with intervals of apnea followed by a crescendo/decrescendo sequence of respiration is called periodic breathing or Cheyne-Stokes respiration (see Fig. 13-13). Children and older adults may exhibit this pattern during sleep, but otherwise it occurs in patients who are seriously ill, particularly those with brain damage at the cerebral level or with drug-associated respiratory compromise (Box 13-5).

An occasional deep, audible sigh that punctuates an otherwise regular respiratory pattern is associated with emotional distress or an incipient episode of more severe hyperventilation. Sighs also occur in normal respiration.

If the pulmonary tree is seriously obstructed for any reason, inspired air has difficulty overcoming the resistance and getting out. Air trapping is the result of a prolonged but inefficient expiratory effort. The rate of respiration increases in order to compensate; as this happens, the effort becomes more shallow, the amount of trapped air increases, and the lungs inflate. This can lead to a barrel chest.

Biot or ataxic respiration consists of irregular respirations varying in depth and interrupted by intervals of apnea, but lacking the repetitive pattern of periodic respiration. On occasion, the respirations may be regular, but the apneic periods may occur in an irregular pattern. Biot respiration usually is associated with severe and persistent increased intracranial pressure, respiratory compromise resulting from drug poisoning, or brain damage at the level of the medulla and generally indicates a poor prognosis.

Inspect the chest wall movement during respiration. Again, different angles of illumination will aid inspection and help delineate chest wall movement and possible deformities. Expansion should be symmetric, without apparent use of accessory

EXAMINATION AND FINDINGS

Box 13-3	**Thoracic Landmarks**

In conjunction with the anatomic landmarks of the chest, the following imaginary lines on the surface will help localize the findings on physical examination (Fig. 13-10):

Midsternal line: vertically down the midline of the sternum

Right and left midclavicular lines: parallel to the midsternal line, beginning at midclavicle; the inferior borders of the lungs generally cross the sixth rib at the midclavicular line

Right and left anterior axillary lines: parallel to the midsternal line, beginning at the anterior axillary folds

Right and left midaxillary lines: parallel to the midsternal line, beginning at the midaxilla

Right and left posterior axillary lines: parallel to the midsternal line, beginning at the posterior axillary folds

Vertebral line: vertically down the spinal processes

Right and left scapular lines: parallel to the vertebral line, through the inferior angle of the scapula when the patient is erect

The spinous process of the seventh cervical vertebra is readily palpated. The thoracic vertebrae can then be counted down from that point (Fig. 13-11).

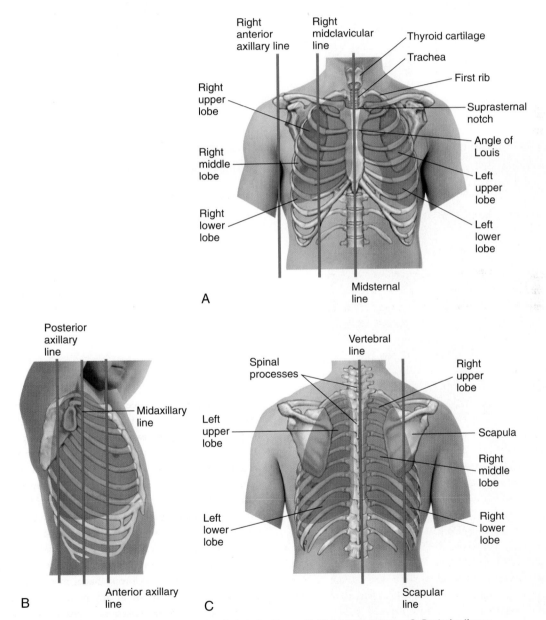

FIGURE 13-10 **Thoracic landmarks. A,** Anterior thorax. **B,** Right lateral thorax. **C,** Posterior thorax.

Continued

Box 13-3 | Thoracic Landmarks—cont'd

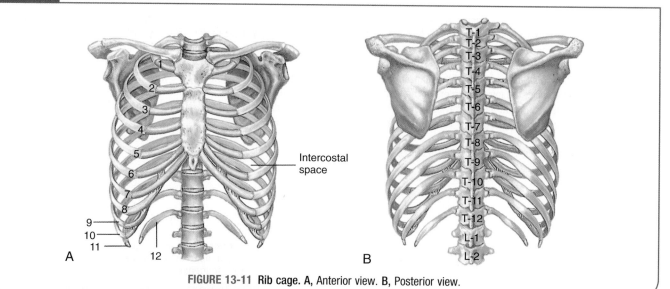

Intercostal space

FIGURE 13-11 Rib cage. **A**, Anterior view. **B**, Posterior view.

FIGURE 13-12 **A**, Pectus excavatum. **B**, Pectus carinatum. *(From Townsend et al, 2008.)*

Box 13-4 | Influences on the Rate and Depth of Breathing

The rate and depth of breathing will:

Increase With	Decrease With
Acidosis (metabolic)	Alkalosis (metabolic)
Central nervous system lesions (pons)	Central nervous system lesions (cerebrum)
Anxiety	Myasthenia gravis
Aspirin poisoning	Narcotic overdoses
Oxygen need (hypoxemia)	Obesity (extreme)
Pain	

muscles. Chest asymmetry can be associated with unequal expansion and respiratory compromise caused by a collapsed lung or limitation of expansion by extrapleural air, fluid, or a mass. Unilateral or bilateral bulging can be a reaction of the ribs and interspaces to respiratory obstruction. A prolonged expiration and bulging on expiration are probably caused by airway outflow obstruction or the valvelike action of compression by a tumor, aneurysm, or enlarged heart. When this happens, the costal angle widens beyond 90 degrees.

Retractions are seen when the chest wall seems to cave in at the sternum, between the ribs, at the suprasternal notch, above the clavicles, and at the lowest costal margins. This suggests an obstruction to inspiration at any point in the respiratory tract. As intrapleural pressure becomes increasingly negative, the musculature "pulls back" in an effort to overcome blockage. Any significant obstruction makes the retraction observable with each inspiratory effort. The degree and level of retraction depend on the extent and level of obstruction (Box 13-6). When the obstruction is high in the respiratory tree (e.g., with tracheal or laryngeal involvement), breathing is characterized by stridor. With

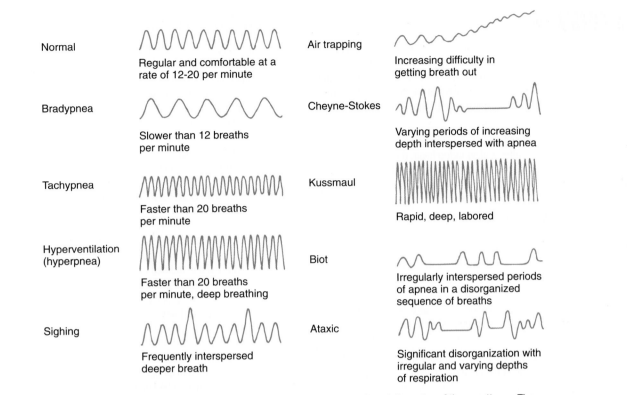

Normal	Regular and comfortable at a rate of 12-20 per minute	Air trapping	Increasing difficulty in getting breath out
Bradypnea	Slower than 12 breaths per minute	Cheyne-Stokes	Varying periods of increasing depth interspersed with apnea
Tachypnea	Faster than 20 breaths per minute	Kussmaul	Rapid, deep, labored
Hyperventilation (hyperpnea)	Faster than 20 breaths per minute, deep breathing	Biot	Irregularly interspersed periods of apnea in a disorganized sequence of breaths
Sighing	Frequently interspersed deeper breath	Ataxic	Significant disorganization with irregular and varying depths of respiration

FIGURE 13-13 Patterns of respiration. The horizontal axis indicates the relative rates of these patterns. The vertical swings of the lines indicate the relative depth of respiration.

paradoxic breathing, on inspiration the lower thorax is drawn in, and on expiration, the opposite occurs. This develops when negative intrathoracic pressure is transmitted to the abdomen by a weakened, poorly functioning diaphragm; obstructive airway disease; or during sleep, in the event of upper airway obstruction.

A foreign body in a bronchus (usually the right because of its larger diameter and more vertical placement) causes unilateral retraction, but the suprasternal notch is not involved. Retraction of the lower chest occurs with asthma and bronchiolitis.

Looking for Clues at the Periphery

Observe the lips and nails for cyanosis, the lips for pursing, the fingers for clubbing, and the alae nasi for flaring. Any of these peripheral clues suggests pulmonary or cardiac difficulty. Pursing of the lips can occur with an increased expiratory effort. Patients learn without being taught that it reduces the effort of dyspnea. Clubbing—enlargement of the terminal phalanges of the fingers and/or toes—is associated with emphysema, lung cancer, the cyanosis of congenital heart disease, or cystic fibrosis (see Figs. 8-20, 8-21 and 8-22). Flaring of the alae nasi during inspiration is a sign of air hunger. Smell the breath; pulmonary infection may make it malodorous. Note whether there are supernumerary nipples; these may be a clue to other congenital abnormalities. Look for any superficial venous patterns over the chest, which may be a sign of heart disorders or vascular obstruction. The underlying fat and relative prominence of the ribs give some clue to general nutrition.

Palpation

Palpate the thoracic muscles and skeleton, feeling for pulsations, areas of tenderness, bulges, depressions, masses, and unusual movement. Expect bilateral symmetry and some elasticity of the rib cage, but the sternum and xiphoid should be relatively inflexible and the thoracic spine rigid.

Crepitus, a crackly or crinkly sensation, can be both palpated and heard—a gentle, bubbly feeling. It indicates air in the subcutaneous tissue from a rupture somewhere in the respiratory system or by infection with a gas-producing organism. It may be localized (e.g., over the suprasternal notch and base of the neck) or cover a wider area, potentially involving the arms and face with the associated swelling mimicking an allergic reaction. Crepitus always results from an underlying pathologic process.

A palpable, coarse, grating vibration, usually on inspiration, suggests a pleural friction rub caused by inflammation of the pleural surfaces. Think of it as the feel of leather rubbing on leather.

To evaluate thoracic expansion during respiration, stand behind the patient and place your thumbs along the spinal processes at the level of the tenth rib, with your palms lightly in contact with the posterolateral surfaces (Fig. 13-14). Watch your thumbs diverge during quiet and deep breathing. A loss of symmetry in the movement of the thumbs suggests a problem on one or both sides. A patient who is barrel-chested with chronic obstructive pulmonary disease may not demonstrate this. The chest is so inflated that it cannot expand further and your hands may even come together a bit.

Box 13-5 | Apnea

Apnea, the absence of spontaneous respiration, may have its origin in the respiratory system and in a variety of central nervous system and cardiac abnormalities. Common contributors include seizures, central nervous system trauma or hypoperfusion, a variety of infections of the respiratory passageway, drug ingestions, and obstructive sleep disorders.

Primary apnea	A self-limited condition, and not uncommon after a blow to the head. It is especially noted immediately after the birth of a newborn, who will breathe spontaneously when sufficient carbon dioxide accumulates in the circulation.
Secondary apnea	Breathing stops and will not begin spontaneously unless resuscitative measures are immediately instituted. Any event that severely limits the absorption of oxygen into the bloodstream will lead to secondary apnea.
Reflex apnea	When irritating and nausea-provoking vapors or gases are inhaled, there can be an involuntary, temporary halt to respiration.
Sleep apnea	Characterized by periods of an absence of breathing and oxygenation during sleep. With obstruction, airflow is not maintained through the nose and mouth.
Apneustic breathing	Characterized by a long inspiration and what amounts to expiration apnea. The neural center for control is in the pons. When it is affected, breathing can become gasping because inspirations are prolonged and expiration constrained.
Periodic apnea of the newborn	A normal condition characterized by an irregular pattern of rapid breathing interspersed with brief periods of apnea that one usually associates with rapid eye movement sleep.

Box 13-6   Is the Airway Patent or Obstructed?

Determining the patency of the upper airway is essential to a complete evaluation of pulmonary status. When is the upper airway obstructed?
- When there is:
    - Inspiratory stridor (with an I/E ratio of more than 2:1)
    - A hoarse cough or cry
    - Flaring of the alae nasi
    - Retraction at the suprasternal notch
- Severely so, when:
    - Stridor is inspiratory and expiratory
    - Cough is barking
    - Retractions also involve the subcostal and intercostal spaces
    - Cyanosis is obvious even with supplemental oxygen
- When the obstruction is above the glottis:
    - Stridor tends to be quieter
    - The voice is muffled
    - Swallowing is more difficult
    - Cough is not a factor.
    - The head and neck may be awkwardly positioned to preserve the airway (e.g., extended with retropharyngeal abscess; head to the affected side with peritonsillar abscess)
- When the obstruction is below the glottis:
    - Stridor tends to be louder, more rasping
    - The voice is hoarse
    - Swallowing is not affected
    - Cough is harsh, barking
    - Positioning of the head is not a factor

Tactile Fremitus

Note the quality of the tactile fremitus, the palpable vibration of the chest wall that results from speech or other verbalizations. Fremitus is best felt posteriorly and laterally at the level of the bifurcation of the bronchi. There is great variability depending on the intensity and pitch of the voice and the structure and thickness of the chest wall. In addition, the scapulae obscure fremitus.

Evidence-Based Practice in Physical Examination

Is There a Pleural Effusion?

Based on the review of a number of studies, dullness to percussion and tactile fremitus are the most useful findings for pleural effusion. Dullness to chest percussion makes the probability of a pleural effusion more likely. The absence of reduced tactile vocal fremitus makes pleural effusion less likely.

From Hockenberry, 2009.

FIGURE 13-14 Palpating thoracic expansion. The thumbs are at the level of the tenth rib.

Ask the patient to recite a few numbers or say a few words ("99" is a favorite, as is "Mickey Mouse," depending perhaps on the age) while you systematically palpate the chest with the palmar surfaces of the fingers or with the ulnar aspects of the hand. Use a firm, light touch, establishing even contact. For comparison, palpate both sides simultaneously and symmetrically;

FIGURE 13-15 Two methods for evaluating tactile fremitus. **A,** With palmar surface of both hands. **B,** With ulnar aspect.

or use one hand, alternating between the two sides. Move about the patient, palpating each area carefully, right side to left side (Fig. 13-15). Some examiners prefer to use their dominant hand, moving it back and forth to make comparisons.

Decreased or absent fremitus may be caused by excess air in the lungs or may indicate emphysema, pleural thickening or effusion, massive pulmonary edema, or bronchial obstruction. Increased fremitus, often coarser or rougher in feel, occurs in the presence of fluids or a solid mass within the lungs and may be caused by lung consolidation, heavy but nonobstructive bronchial secretions, compressed lung, or tumor. Gentle, more tremulous fremitus than expected occurs with some lung consolidations and some inflammatory and infectious processes.

Examining the Trachea

Note the position of the trachea. Place an index finger in the suprasternal notch and move it gently, side to side, along the upper edges of each clavicle and in the spaces above to the inner borders of the sternocleidomastoid muscles. These spaces should be equal on both sides, and the trachea should be in the midline directly above the suprasternal notch. This can also be determined by palpating with both thumbs simultaneously (Fig. 13-16). A slight, barely noticeable deviation to the right is not unusual.

The trachea may be deviated because of problems within the chest and may, on occasion, seem to pulsate. Volume loss (from fibrosis or atelectasis such as due to tumor or adenopathy) pulls the trachea toward the affected lung. Thyroid enlargement or pleural effusion may cause the trachea to deviate away from the affected side. Pneumothorax can make the trachea go either way, depending on whether there is a tension pneumothorax. In this case pressure builds up on the side of the collapsed lung, and the deviation is away from the affected side. In contrast to a simple collapsed lung, the trachea deviates to the affected side. Anterior mediastinal tumors may push it posteriorly; with inflammation of the mediastinum (mediastinitis), the trachea may be pushed forward (see Clinical Pearl, "Clue to a Mediastinal Mass").

Clinical Pearl

Clue to a Mediastinal Mass

An anterior mediastinal mass may compress the trachea and compromise respiration. Patients may develop the harsh sound of stridor with more difficulty breathing. Instinctively, the patient may sit up and lean forward in an attempt to relieve the compression—that action is a clue to the possibility of such a mass.

FIGURE 13-16 Palpating to evaluate midline position of the trachea.

Percussion

Percussion tones heard over the chest, as elsewhere, are described in Chapter 3 and summarized in Figure 13-17 and Table 13-1. You can percuss directly or indirectly, as described in Chapter 3. Remember that the heavier the stroke you use, the more likely you are to miss a transitional area from resonance to dullness. Tap sharply and consistently from the wrist without excessive force.

Compare all areas bilaterally, using one side as a control for the other. The following sequence serves as one model. First, examine the back with the patient sitting with head bent forward and arms folded in front. This moves the scapulae

EXAMINATION AND FINDINGS

Video: Chest and Lungs: Following the Percussion and Auscultation Sequence

Video: Atelectasis

Video: Chest and Lungs: Performing Diaphragmatic Excursion

Table 13-1	Percussion Tones Heard over the Chest			
Type of Tone	**Intensity**	**Pitch**	**Duration**	**Quality**
Resonant	Loud	Low	Long	Hollow
Flat	Soft	High	Short	Very dull
Dull	Medium	Medium to high	Medium	Dull thud
Tympanic	Loud	High	Medium	Drumlike
Hyperresonant*	Very loud	Very low	Longer	Booming

See Chapter 3, Table 3-3 on page. 34, for definitions and a more complete discussion of these tones.

*Hyperresonance is an abnormal sound, the result of air trapping (e.g., in obstructive lung disease).

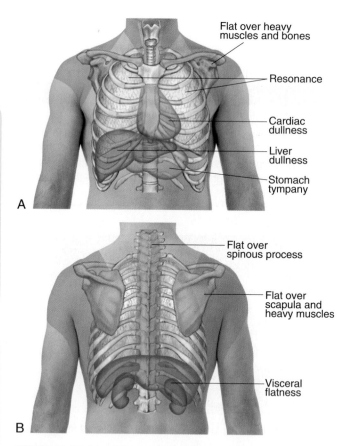

FIGURE 13-17 Percussion tones throughout chest. **A,** Anterior view. **B,** Posterior view.

laterally, exposing more of the lung. Then ask the patient to raise the arms overhead while you percuss the lateral and anterior chest. For all positions, percuss at 4- to 5-cm intervals over the intercostal spaces, moving systematically from superior to inferior and medial to lateral (Figs. 13-18 and 13-19). This sequence is one of many that you may follow. Adopt the one most comfortable for you and use it consistently. Resonance, the expected sound, can usually be heard over all areas of the lungs. Hyperresonance associated with hyperinflation may indicate emphysema, pneumothorax, or asthma. Dullness or flatness

---

Box 13-7	Bad Breath: a Possible Sign of Infection

Smell the Breath

Auscultation of the lungs makes it possible (occasionally, even uncomfortably so) to become aware of a patient's breath odor. Bad breath, even when it is not too distinct, is easily noticed. Infection, either acute or chronic, somewhere in the nasal or oral cavity or deep in the lung, can be the source. An especially foul or putrid odor of breath and/or sputum suggests anaerobic respiratory infections, empyema, bronchiectasis, lung abscess, or a particularly insistent bronchitis. Your nose may provide a significant clue:

Sweet, fruity	Diabetic ketoacidosis; starvation ketosis
Fishy, stale	Uremia (trimethylamines)
Ammonia-like	Uremia (ammonia)
Musty fish, clover	Fetor hepaticus: hepatic failure, portal vein thrombosis, portacaval shunts
Foul, feculent	Intestinal obstruction
Foul, putrid	Nasal/sinus pathology: infection, foreign body, cancer; respiratory infections: empyema, lung abscess, bronchiectasis
Halitosis	Tonsillitis, gingivitis, respiratory infections, Vincent angina, gastroesophageal reflux
Cinnamon	Pulmonary tuberculosis

suggests pneumonia, atelectasis, pleural effusion, pneumothorax, or asthma.

Diaphragmatic Excursion

Measure the diaphragmatic excursion, the movement of the thoracic diaphragm that occurs with inhalation and exhalation.

The following steps suggest one approach to measuring the diaphragmatic excursion:

- Ask the patient to take a deep breath and hold it.
- Percuss along the scapular line until you locate the lower border, the point marked by a change in note from resonance to dullness.
- Mark the point with a marking pen at the scapular line. Allow the patient to breathe, and then repeat the procedure on the other side.
- Ask the patient to take several breaths, to exhale as much as possible, and then to hold (Box 13-7).
- Percuss up from the marked point and make a mark at the change from dullness to resonance. Remind the patient to start breathing. Repeat on the other side.
- Measure and record the distance in centimeters between the marks on each side. The excursion distance is usually 3 to 5 cm (Fig. 13-20).

Alternatively, you might use strips of tape, or use one hand as a stationary landmark, percussing directly with the other and estimating the distance. The diaphragm is usually higher on the right than on the left because it sits over the bulk of the liver. Its descent may be limited by several types of pathologic processes: pulmonary (e.g., as a result of emphysema), abdominal (e.g., massive ascites, tumor), or superficial pain (e.g., fractured rib).

FIGURE 13-18 **A,** Direct percussion using ulnar aspect of fist. **B,** Indirect percussion.

FIGURE 13-19 **Suggested sequence for systematic percussion and auscultation of the thorax. A,** Posterior thorax. **B,** Right lateral thorax. **C,** Left lateral thorax. **D,** Anterior thorax. The pleximeter finger or the stethoscope is moved in the numeric sequence suggested; however, other sequences are possible. It is beneficial to be systematic.

FIGURE 13-20 Measuring diaphragmatic excursion. Excursion distance is usually 3 to 5 cm.

FIGURE 13-21 Auscultation with a stethoscope.

Auscultation

Auscultation with a stethoscope provides important clues to the condition of the lungs and pleura. All sounds can be characterized in the same manner as the percussion notes: intensity, pitch, quality, and duration.

Have the patient sit upright, if possible, and breathe slowly and deeply through the mouth, exaggerating normal respiration. Demonstrate this yourself. Caution the patient to keep a pace consistent with comfort; hyperventilation, which occurs more easily than one might think, may cause faintness, and exaggerated breathing can be tiring, especially for frail patients. Because most pulmonary pathologic conditions patients occur at the lung bases, it is a good idea to examine these first, before fatigue sets in.

The diaphragm of the stethoscope is usually preferable to the bell for listening to the lungs because it transmits the ordinarily high-pitched sounds better and because it provides a broader area of sound. Place the stethoscope firmly on the skin. When the individual breath sound is being evaluated, there should be no movement of the patient or stethoscope except for the respiratory excursion (see Clinical Pearl, "Congestive Heart Failure").

Clinical Pearl

Congestive Heart Failure

If the patient may have congestive heart failure, you should begin auscultation at the base of the lungs to detect crackles that may disappear with continued exaggerated respiration.

To auscultate the back, ask the patient to sit as for percussion, with the head bent forward and arms folded in front to enlarge the listening area (Fig. 13-21). Then have the patient sit more erect with the arms overhead for auscultating the lateral chest. Finally, ask the patient to sit erect with the shoulders back for auscultation of the anterior chest. As with so much else, the exact sequence you adopt is not as important as using the same sequence each time to ensure that the examination is thorough.

Listen systematically at each position throughout inspiration and expiration, taking advantage of a side-to-side comparison as you move downward from apex to base at intervals of several centimeters. The sounds of the middle lobe of the right lung and the lingula on the left are best heard in the respective axillae.

Breath Sounds

Breath sounds are made by the flow of air through the respiratory tree. They are characterized by pitch, intensity, quality, and relative duration of their inspiratory and expiratory phases and are classified as vesicular, bronchovesicular, and bronchial (tubular) (Fig. 13-22 and Table 13-2).

Vesicular breath sounds are low-pitched, low-intensity sounds heard over healthy lung tissue. Bronchovesicular sounds are heard over the major bronchi and are typically moderate in pitch and intensity. The sounds highest in pitch and intensity are the bronchial breath sounds, which are ordinarily heard only over the trachea. Both bronchovesicular and bronchial breath sounds are abnormal if they are heard over the peripheral lung tissue.

Breathing that resembles the noise made by blowing across the mouth of a bottle is defined as amphoric and is most often heard with a large, relatively stiff-walled pulmonary cavity or a tension pneumothorax with bronchopleural fistula. Cavernous breathing, sounding as if coming from a cavern, is commonly heard over a pulmonary cavity in which the wall is rigid (see Clinical Pearl, "Sickle Cell Disease").

Clinical Pearl

Sickle Cell Disease

Persons with sickle cell disease may have frequent pulmonary problems. The acute chest syndrome is the most common form of this. It is typically manifested by chest pain, fever, and tachypnea. A new pulmonary infiltrate is frequently present.

The volume of breath sounds is largely dependent on the speed with which air enters and leaves the mouth. These sounds are relatively more difficult to hear or can be absent in the following situations: fluid or pus has accumulated in the pleural

KEY:

■ Bronchovesicular over main bronchi

■ Vesicular over lesser bronchi, bronchioles, and lobes

■ Bronchial over trachea

FIGURE 13-22 **Expected auscultatory sounds. A,** Anterior view. **B,** Posterior view.

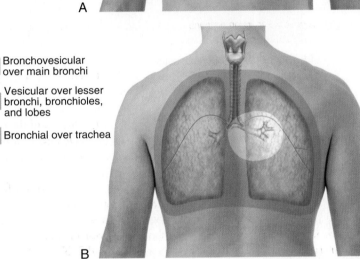

Table 13-2 Characteristics of Normal Breath Sounds

Sound	Characteristics	Findings
Vesicular	Heard over most of lung fields; low pitch; soft and short expirations (see Figs. 13-22 and 13-23); more prominent in a thin person or a child, diminished in the overweight or very muscular patient	
Bronchovesicular	Heard over main bronchus area and over upper right posterior lung field; medium pitch; expiration equals inspiration	
Bronchial/tracheal (tubular)	Heard only over trachea; high pitch; loud and long expirations, sometimes a bit longer than inspiration	

space, secretions or a foreign body obstructs the bronchi, the lungs are hyperinflated, or breathing is shallow from splinting due to pain. Breath sounds are easier to hear when the lungs are consolidated; the mass surrounding the tube of the respiratory tree promotes sound transmission better than air-filled alveoli.

Most of the abnormal sounds heard during lung auscultation are superimposed on the breath sounds. Extraneous sounds such as the crinkling of chest or back hair must be carefully distinguished from far more significant adventitious sounds. Sometimes it helps to moisten chest hair to minimize this problem. Listening through clothing or patient gowns produces extraneous sounds. Avoid this by having your patients bare their skin. The common terms used to describe adventitious sounds are *crackles* (formerly called rales), *rhonchi, wheezes,* and *friction rub* (Fig. 13-23). Crackles are discontinuous; rhonchi and wheezes

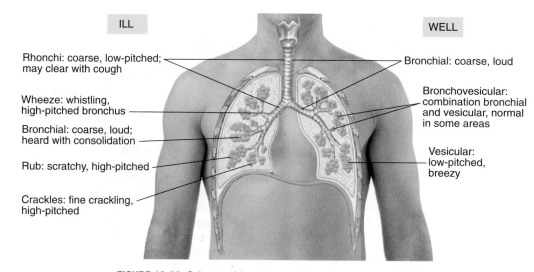

ILL

WELL

Rhonchi: coarse, low-pitched; may clear with cough

Wheeze: whistling, high-pitched bronchus

Bronchial: coarse, loud; heard with consolidation

Rub: scratchy, high-pitched

Crackles: fine crackling, high-pitched

Bronchial: coarse, loud

Bronchovesicular: combination bronchial and vesicular, normal in some areas

Vesicular: low-pitched, breezy

FIGURE 13-23 Schema of breath sounds in the ill and well patient.

Box 13-8 | **Adventitious Breath Sounds**

Fine crackles: high-pitched, discrete, discontinuous crackling sounds heard during the end of inspiration; not cleared by a cough

Medium crackles: lower, more moist sound heard during the midstage of inspiration; not cleared by a cough

Coarse crackles: loud, bubbly noise heard during inspiration; not cleared by a cough

Rhonchi (sonorous wheeze): loud, low, coarse sounds like a snore most often heard continuously during inspiration or expiration; coughing may clear sound (usually means mucus accumulation in trachea or large bronchi)

Wheeze (sibilant wheeze): musical noise sounding like a squeak; most often heard continuously during inspiration or expiration; usually louder during expiration

Pleural friction rub: dry, rubbing, or grating sound, usually caused by inflammation of pleural surfaces; heard during inspiration or expiration; loudest over lower lateral anterior surface

---

are continuous. Box 13-8 gives a detailed description of adventitious breath sounds.

Crackles. A crackle is an abnormal respiratory sound heard more often during inspiration and characterized by discrete discontinuous sounds, each lasting just a few milliseconds. The individual noise tends to be brief and the interval to the next one similarly brief.

Crackles may be fine, high-pitched, and relatively short in duration or coarse, low-pitched, and relatively longer in duration. They are caused by the disruptive passage of air through the small airways in the respiratory tree. High-pitched crackles are described as sibilant; the more low-pitched crackles are termed-*sonorous.* Crackles with a dry quality, more crisp than gurgling, are apt to occur higher in the respiratory tree. You might listen for crackles at the open mouth. If their origin is in the upper airways, they will be easily heard; if in the lower, not so easily.

Rhonchi. Rhonchi (sonorous wheezes) are deeper, more rumbling, more pronounced during expiration, more likely to be prolonged and continuous, and less discrete than crackles. They are caused by the passage of air through an airway obstructed by thick secretions, muscular spasm, new growth, or external pressure. The more sibilant, higher-pitched rhonchi arise from the smaller bronchi, as in asthma; the more sonorous, lower-pitched rhonchi arise from larger bronchi, as in tracheobronchitis. All rhonchi may at times be palpable.

It may be difficult to distinguish between crackles and rhonchi. In general, rhonchi tend to disappear after coughing, whereas crackles do not. If such sounds are present, listen to several respiratory excursions: a few with the patient's accustomed effort, a few with deeper breathing, a few before coughing, and a few after.

Wheezes. A wheeze (sibilant wheeze) is sometimes thought of as a form of rhonchus. It is a continuous, high-pitched, musical sound (almost a whistle) heard during inspiration or expiration. It is caused by a relatively high-velocity airflow through a narrowed or obstructed airway. The longer the wheeze and the higher the pitch, the worse the obstruction. Wheezes may be composed of complex combinations of a variety of pitches or of a single pitch, and they may vary from area to area and minute to minute. If a wheeze is heard bilaterally, it may be caused by the bronchospasm of asthma (reactive airway disease) or acute or chronic bronchitis. Unilateral or more sharply localized wheezing or stridor may occur with a foreign body. A tumor compressing a part of the bronchial tree can create a consistent wheeze or whistle of a single pitch at the site of compression.

Other Sounds. A friction rub occurs outside the respiratory tree. It has a dry, crackly, grating, low-pitched sound and is heard in both expiration and inspiration. It may have a machine-like quality. It may have no significance if heard over the liver or spleen; however, a friction rub heard over the heart or lungs is caused by inflamed, roughened surfaces rubbing together. Over the pericardium, this sound suggests pericarditis; over the lungs, pleurisy. The respiratory rub disappears when the breath is held; the cardiac rub does not.

Mediastinal crunch (Hamman sign) is found with mediastinal emphysema. A great variety of sounds (loud crackles, clicking, and gurgling sounds) are heard over the precordium. They are synchronous with the heartbeat and not particularly so with respiration. These sounds can be more pronounced toward the end of expiration and are easiest to hear when the patient leans to the left or lies down on the left side.

Vocal Resonance

The spoken voice transmits sounds through the lung fields that may be heard with the stethoscope. Ask the patient to recite numbers, names, or other words. These transmitted sounds are usually muffled and indistinct and are best heard medially. Pay particular attention to vocal resonance if there are other unexpected findings during any part of the examination of the lungs, such as dullness on percussion or changes in tactile fremitus. The factors that influence tactile fremitus similarly influence vocal resonance (see Clinical Pearl, "Vocal Resonance").

Clinical Pearl

Vocal Resonance

The generally lower-pitched voices of men lend an intensity to vocal fremitus that is often greater than that in women.

Greater clarity and increased loudness of spoken sounds are defined as bronchophony. If bronchophony is extreme (e.g., in the presence of consolidation of the lungs), even a whisper can be heard clearly and intelligibly through the stethoscope (whispered pectoriloquy). When the intensity of the spoken voice is increased and there is a nasal quality (e.g., e becomes a stuffy broad a), the auditory quality is called egophony. These auditory changes may be present in any condition that consolidates lung tissue. Conversely, vocal resonance diminishes and loses intensity when there is loss of tissue within the respiratory tree (e.g., with the barrel chest of emphysema). See Box 13-9 for a summary of expected findings of a healthy chest and lungs.

❧ Infants

The examination of the chest and lungs of the newborn follows a sequence similar to that for adults. Inspecting without disturbing the baby is key, and for this reason auscultation often occurs at the same time as inspection. Percussion may be unreliable and is typically not performed on infants. The examiner's fingers may be too large for a baby's chest and particularly so for the premature infant.

A newborn's Apgar scores at 1 and 5 minutes after birth tell you a great deal about the infant's condition. An infant whose respirations are inadequate but who is otherwise well may initially score 1 or even 0 on heart rate, muscle tone, response to a

Box 13-9 Summary of Expected Findings of the Chest and Lungs

When the lungs are healthy, the respiratory tree clear, the pleurae unaffected by disease, and the chest wall symmetrically and appropriately structured and mobile, the following characteristics will be found:

- On inspection
  - Symmetry of movement on expansion
  - Absence of retractions
- On palpation
  - Midline trachea without a tug
  - Symmetric, unaccentuated tactile fremitus
- On percussion
  - Range of 3 to 5 cm in the descent of diaphragm
  - Resonant and symmetric percussion notes
- On auscultation
  - Absence of adventitious sounds
  - Vesicular breath sounds, except for bronchovesicular sounds beside the sternum and the more prominent bronchial components in the area of the larger bronchi

Table 13-3 Infant Evaluation at Birth: Apgar Scoring System

	0	1	2
Heart rate	Absent	Slow (below 100 beats/min)	Over 100 beats/min
Respiratory effort	Absent	Slow or irregular	Good crying
Muscle tone	Limp	Some flexion of extremities	Active motion
Response to catheter in nostril (tested after oropharynx is clear)	No response	Grimace	Cough or sneeze
Color	Blue or pale	Body pink, extremities blue	Completely pink

Add the scores of the five individual observations to get the full Apgar score. The lower the total, the more likely it is that there is a problem.

catheter, or color. Depressed respiration often has its origins in the maternal environment during labor, such as sedatives or compromised blood supply to the newborn, or it may result from mechanical obstruction by mucus. Table 13-3 explains the Apgar scoring system. This score requires some subjective judgment and cannot be considered absolute.

Inspect the thoracic cage, noting size and shape; measure the chest circumference, which in the healthy full-term infant is usually about 30 to 36 cm, usually 2 to 3 cm smaller than the head circumference. This difference between the two increases with prematurity. An infant with intrauterine growth retardation will have a relatively smaller chest circumference compared to the head, whereas the infant of a poorly controlled diabetic mother will have a relatively larger chest circumference.

The newborn's lung function is particularly susceptible to a number of environmental factors. The pattern of respirations will vary with feeding and sleep. In the first few hours after birth, the respiratory effort can be depressed by the passive transfer of drugs given to the mother before delivery. Count the respiratory rate for 1 minute. The expected rate varies from 40 to 60 respirations per minute, although a rate of 80 is not uncommon. Babies delivered by cesarean section generally have a more rapid rate than babies delivered vaginally. Note the regularity of respiration. Babies are obligate nose breathers and, at this age, nasal breathing is common. The more premature an infant at birth, the more likely some irregularity in the respiratory pattern will be present. Periodic breathing—a sequence of relatively vigorous respiratory efforts followed by a pause of as long as 10 to 15 seconds—is common. It is cause for concern if the pauses tend to be prolonged and the baby becomes centrally cyanotic (i.e., cyanotic about the mouth, face, and torso). The persistence of periodic breathing episodes in preterm infants is relative to the gestational age of the baby, with the period of breathing cessation diminishing in frequency as the baby approaches term status. In the term infant, periodic breathing should wane in the first days to weeks after birth.

Coughing is rare in the newborn and should be considered a problem. Sneezing, on the other hand, is frequent and expected—it clears the nose. Hiccups are also frequent, although usually silent, particularly after meals. Frequent hiccupping, however, may suggest seizures, drug withdrawal, or encephalopathy, among other possibilities.

Newborns rely primarily on the diaphragm for their respiratory effort, only gradually adding the intercostal muscles. Infants quite commonly also use the abdominal muscles. Paradoxic breathing (the chest wall collapses as the abdomen distends on inspiration) is common, particularly during sleep.

If the chest expansion is asymmetric, suspect some compromise of the baby's ability to fill one of the lungs (e.g., pneumothorax, atelectasis, or diaphragmatic hernia) (Fig. 13-24).

Intestine protruding through hole in diaphragm

FIGURE 13-24 **Diaphragmatic hernia.** *(From Phillips, 2007.)*

Palpate the clavicle, rib cage, and sternum, noting loss of symmetry, unusual masses, or crepitus. Crepitus around a fractured clavicle (with no evidence of pain) is common after a difficult forceps delivery. The newborn's xiphoid process is more mobile and prominent than that of the older child or adult. It has a sharp inferior tip that moves slightly back and forth under your finger.

Auscultate the chest. If the baby is crying and restless, it pays to wait for a quieter moment (see Clinical Pearl, "The Sobbing Baby"). Localization of breath sounds is difficult, particularly in the very small chest of the preterm infant. Breath sounds are easily transmitted from one segment of the auscultatory area to another; therefore, the absence of sounds in any given area may be difficult to detect. Crackles and rhonchi are commonly heard immediately after birth because fetal fluid has not been completely cleared. Whenever auscultatory findings are asymmetric, suspect a problem—for example, with meconium aspiration. Gurgling from the intestinal tract, slight movement, and mucus in the upper airway may all contribute to adventitious sounds, making evaluation difficult. If gastrointestinal gurgling sounds are persistently heard in the chest, one must suspect diaphragmatic hernia, but wide transmission of these sounds can sometimes be deceptive.

Clinical Pearl

The Sobbing Baby

Seize the opportunity that a crying child presents. A sob is often followed by a deep breath. The sob itself allows the evaluation of vocal resonance. The crying child may pause occasionally, and the heart sounds may be heard. These pauses may be a bit prolonged as the breath is held, giving the chance to distinguish a murmur from a breath sound.

Stridor is a high-pitched, piercing sound most often heard during inspiration. It is the result of an obstruction high in the respiratory tree. A compelling sound at any age, it cannot be dismissed as inconsequential, particularly when inspiration (I) may be three to four times longer than expiration (E), giving an I/E ratio of 3:1 or 4:1. When accompanied by a cough, hoarseness, and retraction, stridor signifies a serious problem in the trachea or larynx (e.g., a floppy epiglottis; congenital defects; croup; or an edematous response to an infection, allergen, smoke, chemicals, or aspirated foreign body). Infants who have a narrow tracheal lumen from compression by a congenital malformation, tumor, abscess, or double aortic arch can develop stridor. Retraction at the supraclavicular notch and contraction of the sternocleidomastoid muscles indicate significant respiratory distress.

Respiratory grunting is a mechanism by which the infant tries to expel trapped air or fetal lung fluid while trying to retain air and increase oxygen levels. When persistent, it is cause for concern. Flaring of the alae nasi is another indicator of respiratory distress at this, or any, age.

❀ Children

Children use the thoracic (intercostal) musculature for respiration by the age of 6 or 7 years. In young children, obvious

Box 13-10   Assessment of Respiratory Distress

Important observations to be made of the respiratory effort include the following:

Does a loss of synchrony between left and right occur during the respiratory effort? Is there a lag in movement of the chest on one side? If so, consider atelectasis or diaphragmatic hernia.

Is there stridor? If so, consider croup or epiglottitis.

Is there retraction at the suprasternal notch intercostally or at the xiphoid process? Do the nares dilate and flare with respiratory effort? If so, consider respiratory distress.

Is there an audible expiratory grunt? Is it audible with the stethoscope only or without the stethoscope? If so, consider lower airway obstruction or focal atelectasis.

intercostal exertion (retractions) on breathing suggests an airway problem (e.g., asthma). Usual respiratory rates for children are listed below. Rates decrease with age with a greater variation in the first 2 years of life and without significant gender difference. Sustained rates that exceed the indicated limits should suggest difficulty (Box 13-10).

Age	Respirations per Minute
Newborn	30 to 80
1 year	20 to 40
3 years	20 to 30
6 years	16 to 22
10 years	16 to 20
17 years	12 to 20

If the roundness of the young child's chest persists past the second year of life, be concerned about the possibility of a chronic obstructive pulmonary problem such as cystic fibrosis. The persistence of a barrel chest at the age of 5 or 6 years can be ominous.

Clinical Pearl

Foreign Body

Think about the possibility of a foreign body when a patient, particularly a child, presents with wheezing for the first time, especially if asymmetric. The history may not at first offer a clue.

Children younger than 5 or 6 years may not be able to give enough of an expiration to satisfy you, particularly when you suspect subtle wheezing. Asking them to "blow out" your flashlight or pretend birthday candles or to blow away a bit of tissue in your hand may help bring out otherwise difficult-to-hear end expiratory sounds. It is also easier to hear the breath sounds when the child breathes more deeply after running up and down the hallway (see Clinical Pearl, "Foreign Body").

The child's chest is thinner and ordinarily more resonant than the adult's chest; the intrathoracic sounds are easier to hear, and hyperresonance is common in the young child. With either direct or indirect percussion, it is easy to miss the dullness of an underlying consolidation. If you sense some loss of resonance, give it

as much importance as you would give frank dullness in the adolescent or adult. Also, with percussion, your finger can learn to feel the dull areas, a tactile sense that comes in handy at times with a crying child. The dull areas are sensed as having more resistance than resonant areas because they move less.

Because of the thin chest wall, the breath sounds of the young child may sound louder, harsher, and more bronchial than those of the adult. Bronchovesicular breath sounds may be heard throughout the chest.

Pregnant Women

Pregnant women experience both structural and ventilatory changes. Dyspnea (shortness of breath) is common in pregnancy and is usually a result of normal physiologic changes. Overall, the pregnant woman increases her ventilation by breathing more deeply, not more frequently. Asthma can have a varied course, getting worse, getting better, or being unaffected by the pregnancy with about equal frequency.

Older Adults

The examination procedure for older adults is the same as that for younger adults, although there may be variations in some expected findings. Chest expansion is often decreased. The patient may be less able to use the respiratory muscles because of muscle weakness, general physical disability, or a sedentary lifestyle. Calcification of rib articulations may also interfere with chest expansion, requiring the use of accessory muscles. Bony prominences are marked, and there is loss of subcutaneous tissue. The dorsal curve of the thoracic spine is prominent (kyphosis) with flattening of the lumbar curve (Fig. 13-25). The AP diameter of the chest is increased in relation to the lateral diameter.

Older patients may have more difficulty breathing deeply and holding their breath than younger patients, and they may tire more quickly, even when well. Adapt the pace and demands of the examination to individual needs.

Sample Documentation

History and Physical Examination

Subjective

A 47-year-old woman with a nonproductive cough for past several days. Persistent, worse when lies down. Feels ill. Chest feels "heavy." Feels short of breath when walking up one flight of stairs. Fever up to 101° F. Taking a nonprescription cough syrup without relief.

Objective

Pulse 98, respiratory rate 24, temperature 38.2°C, blood pressure 110/72

Chest, without kyphosis or other distortion. Thoracic expansion symmetric. Respirations rapid and somewhat labored, not accompanied by retractions or stridor. On palpation, no friction rubs or tenderness over the ribs or other bony prominences. Over the left base posteriorly, tactile fremitus increased; percussion note dull; on auscultation, crackles were heard on inspiration and expiration and did not clear with cough; breath sounds diminished. Remainder of lung fields clear and free of adventitious sounds, with resonant percussion tones. Diaphragmatic excursion 3 cm bilaterally.

For additional sample documentation, see Chapter 26, pp. 628-631.

FIGURE 13-25 Pronounced dorsal curvature in older adult. *(A. From Hochber et al, 2008. B, From Errico et al, 2009.)*

ABNORMALITIES

Physical findings associated with many common conditions are listed in Table 13-4.

Table 13-4	Physical Findings Associated with Common Respiratory Conditions*			
Condition	**Inspection**	**Palpation**	**Percussion**	**Auscultation**
Asthma	Tachypnea Nasal flaring Intercostal retractions	Tachycardia Diminished fremitus	Occasional hyperresonance Occasional limited diaphragmatic descent; diaphragmatic level lower	Prolonged expiration Wheezes Diminished lung sounds
Atelectasis	Delayed and/or diminished chest wall movement (respiratory lag), narrowed intercostal spaces on affected side Tachypnea	Diminished fremitus Apical cardiac impulse deviated ipsilaterally Trachea deviated ipsilaterally	Dullness over affected lung	In upper lobe, bronchial breathing, egophony, whispered pectoriloquy In lower lobe, diminished or absent breath sounds Wheezes, rhonchi, and crackles in varying amounts depending on extent of collapse
Bronchiectasis	Tachypnea Respiratory distress Hyperinflation Clubbing (esp. cystic fibrosis)	Few, if any, consistent findings	No unusual findings if there are no accompanying pulmonary disorders	A variety of crackles, usually coarse, and rhonchi, sometimes disappearing after cough
Bronchitis	Occasional tachypnea Occasional shallow breathing Often no deviation from expected findings	Tactile fremitus undiminished	Resonance	Breath sounds may be prolonged. Occasional crackles, expiratory wheezes and rhonchi
Chronic obstructive pulmonary disease	Respiratory distress Audible wheezing Cyanosis Distention of neck veins, peripheral edema (in presence of right-sided heart failure) Clubbing, rarely	Somewhat limited mobility of diaphragm Somewhat diminished vocal fremitus	Occasional hyperresonance	Postpertussive rhonchi (sonorous wheezes) and sibilant wheezing Inspirational crackles (best heard with stethoscope held over open mouth) Breath sounds somewhat diminished
Emphysema	Tachypnea Deep breathing Pursed lips Barrel chest Thin, underweight	Apical impulse may not be felt Liver edge displaced downward Diminished fremitus	Hyperresonance Limited descent of diaphragm on inspiration Upper border of liver dullness pushed downward	Diminished breath and voice sounds with occasional prolonged expiration Diminished audibility of heart sounds Only occasional adventitious sounds
Pleural effusion and/or thickening	Diminished and delayed respiratory movement (lag) on affected side	Cardiac apical impulse shifted contralaterally Trachea shifted contralaterally Diminished fremitus Tachycardia	Dullness to flatness Hyperresonant note in area superior to effusion	Diminished to absent breath sounds Bronchophony, whispered pectoriloquy Egophony and/or crackles in area superior to effusion Occasional friction rub
Pneumonia consolidation	Tachypnea Shallow breathing Flaring of alae nasi Occasional cyanosis Limited movement at times on involved side; splinting	Increased fremitus in presence of consolidation Decreased fremitus in presence of a concomitant empyema or pleural effusion Tachypnea	Dullness if consolidation is great	A variety of crackles with lobar and occasional rhonchi Bronchial breath sounds Egophony, bronchophony, whispered pectoriloquy

Continued

ABNORMALITIES

Table 13-4	Physical Findings Associated with Common Respiratory Conditions*—cont'd			
Condition	**Inspection**	**Palpation**	**Percussion**	**Auscultation**
Pneumothorax	Tachycardia Cyanosis Respiratory distress Bulging intercostal spaces Respiratory lag on affected side Tracheal deviation with tension pneumothorax	Diminished to absent fremitus Cardiac apical impulse, trachea, and mediastinum shifted contralaterally Diminished to absent tactile fremitus Tachycardia Subcutaneous crepitance from air leaking	Hyperresonance	Diminished to absent breath sounds Succussion splash audible if air and fluid mix Sternal and precordial clicks and crackling (Hamman sign) if air underlies that area Diminished to absent whispered voice sounds

*Physical findings will vary in intensity depending on the severity of the underlying problem and on occasion may not be present in the early stages.

Asthma (Reactive Airway Disease)

Small airway obstruction due to inflammation and hyperreactive airways

Pathophysiology
- Acute episodes triggered by allergens, anxiety, cold air, exercise, upper respiratory infections, cigarette smoke, or other environmental agents
- Results in mucosal edema, increased secretions, and bronchoconstriction with increased airway resistance and impeded respiratory flow

Subjective Data
- Episodes of paroxysmal dyspnea
- Chest pain is common and, with it, a feeling of tightness
- Episodes may last for minutes, hours, or days.
- May be asymptomatic between episodes

Objective Data
- Tachypnea and paroxysmal coughing with wheezing on expiration and inspiration
- Expiration becomes more prolonged with labored breathing, fatigue, and anxious expression as airway resistance increases.
- Hypoxemia by pulse oximetry
- Decreased peak expiratory flow rate

Atelectasis

Incomplete expansion of the lung at birth or the collapse of the lung at any age (Fig. 13-26)

Pathophysiology
- Collapse caused by compression from outside (e.g., exudates, tumors) or resorption of gas from the alveoli in the presence of airway obstruction
- Loss of elastic recoil of the lung may be due to thoracic or abdominal surgery, plugging, exudates, or foreign body.

Subjective Data
- Frequently seen in the postoperative setting
- Symptoms of postobstructive pneumonia may develop in the setting of airway obstruction from a foreign body or tumor.

Objective Data
- Auscultation dampened or muted in the involved area because the affected area of the lung is airless
- Radiograph may show consolidation associated with a postobstructive pneumonia.

FIGURE 13-26 Atelectasis. *(From LaFleur Brooks, 2009.)*

Bronchitis

Inflammation of the large airways

Pathophysiology
- Inflammation of the bronchial tubes leads to increased mucus secretions (Fig. 13-27).
- Acute bronchitis is usually due to an infection, whereas chronic bronchitis is usually due to irritant exposure.

Subjective Data
- Acute bronchitis may be accompanied by fever and chest pain.
- In chronic bronchitis, the cough may be productive.

Objective Data
- May have hacking nonproductive cough with minimal auscultation findings with no respiratory distress
- Greater involvement may lead to wheezing or dampened auscultation in the involved areas.

FIGURE 13-27 **Acute bronchitis.** *(Wilson and Giddens, 2013.)*

Pleurisy

Inflammatory process involving the visceral and parietal pleura (Fig. 13-28)

Pathophysiology

- Often the result of pulmonary infection (bacterial or viral) or connective tissue disease (e.g., lupus)
- Sometimes associated with neoplasm or asbestosis

Subjective Data

- Usually sudden onset with chest pain when taking a breath (pleuritic)
- Rubbing of the pleural surfaces can be felt by the patient.
- Pain can be referred to the ipsilateral shoulder if the pleural inflammation is close to the diaphragm.

Objective Data

- Respirations are rapid and shallow with diminished breath sounds.
- A pleural friction rub can be auscultated.
- Fever may be present.

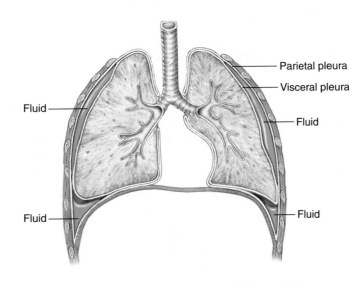

FIGURE 13-28 **Pleurisy.** *(Wilson and Giddens, 2013.)*

Pleural Effusion

Excessive non-purulent fluid in the pleural space (Fig. 13-29)

Pathophysiology

- Sources of fluid vary and include infection, heart failure, renal insufficiency, connective tissue disease, neoplasm, and trauma.

Subjective Data

- Cough with progressive dyspnea is the typical presenting concern.
- Pleuritic chest pain will occur with an inflammatory effusion.

Objective Data

- The findings on auscultation and percussion vary with the amount of fluid present and also with the position of the patient.
- Dullness to percussion and tactile fremitus are the most useful findings for pleural effusion.
- When the fluid is mobile, it will gravitate to the most dependent position.
- In the affected areas, the breath sounds are muted and the percussion note is often hyperresonant in the area above the perfusion.

FIGURE 13-29 Pleural effusion. *(Wilson and Giddens, 2013.)*

Empyema

Purulent exudative fluid collected in the pleural space (Fig. 13-30)

Pathophysiology	Subjective Data	Objective Data
• Non–free-flowing purulent fluid collection develops most commonly from adjacent infected or traumatized tissues. • May be complicated by pneumonia, simultaneous pneumothorax, or a bronchopleural fistula	• Often febrile and tachypneic, with cough and chest pain, and patient appears ill. • Progressive dyspnea develops. • Cough may produce blood or sputum.	• Breath sounds are distant or absent in the affected area. • Percussion note is dull and vocal fremitus is absent. • Chest radiograph with pleural opacity that does not flow freely on lateral decubitus views

FIGURE 13-30 Empyema. *(Wilson and Giddens, 2013.)*

Lung Abscess

Well-defined, circumscribed, inflammatory, and purulent mass that can develop central necrosis (Fig. 13-31)

Pathophysiology	Subjective Data	Objective Data
• Aspiration of food or infected material from upper respiratory or dental sources of infection are most common causes • It may elude diagnosis for some time.	• Malaise, fever, and shortness of breath	• Percussion note is dull and the breath sounds are distant or absent over the affected area • Pleural friction rub may be auscultated. • Cough may produce purulent, foul-smelling sputum.

FIGURE 13-31 Lung abscess. *(Wilson and Giddens, 2013.)*

Pneumonia

Inflammatory response of the bronchioles and alveoli to an infective agent (bacterial, fungal, or viral) (Fig. 13-32)

Pathophysiology

- Acute infection of the pulmonary parenchyma may be due to different organisms that may be acquired in the community or hospital setting.
- Concomitant inflammatory exudates lead to lung consolidation.

Subjective Data

- Rapid onset (hours to days) of cough, pleuritic chest pain, and dyspnea
- Sputum production is common with bacterial infection.
- Chills, fever, rigors, and nonspecific abdominal symptoms of nausea and vomiting may be present.
- Involvement of the right lower lobe can stimulate the tenth and eleventh thoracic nerves to cause right lower quadrant pain and simulate an abdominal process.

Objective Data

- Febrile, tachypneic, and tachycardic
- Crackles and rhonchi are common with diminished breath sounds.
- Egophony, bronchophony, and whisper pectoriloquy
- Dullness to percussion occurs over the area of consolidation.
- In children particularly, but also in adults, audible crackles are not always seen.

FIGURE 13-32 Lobar pneumonia and lobular or bronchopneumonia. *(Wilson and Giddens, 2013.)*

Influenza

Viral infection of the lung. Although this is normally an upper respiratory infection, due to alterations in the epithelial barrier, the infected host is more susceptible to secondary bacterial infection (Fig. 13-33).

Pathophysiology

- Entire respiratory tract may be overwhelmed by interstitial inflammation and necrosis extending throughout the bronchiolar and alveolar tissue
- When mild, it may seem to be just a cold; however, older adults, the very young, and the chronically ill are particularly susceptible.

Subjective Data

- Characterized by cough, fever, malaise, headache, coryza, and mild sore throat, typical of the common cold
- Significant respiratory distress can develop, leading to high morbidity and mortality, especially in the very young, very old, and immunocompromised patients.

Objective Data

- Crackles, rhonchi, and tachypnea are common.

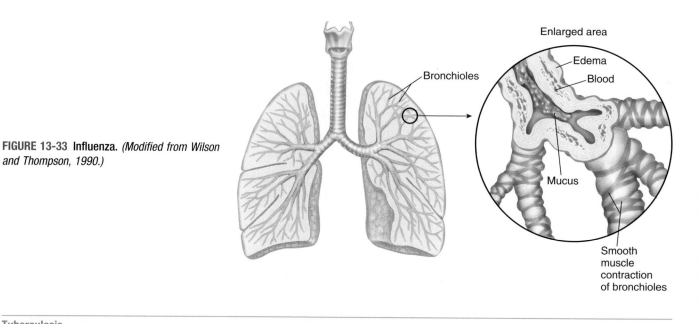

FIGURE 13-33 **Influenza.** *(Modified from Wilson and Thompson, 1990.)*

Tuberculosis

Chronic infectious disease that most often begins in the lung but may then have widespread manifestations (Fig. 13-34)

Pathophysiology	Subjective Data	Objective Data
• The tubercle bacillus is inhaled from the airborne moisture of the coughs and sneezes of infected persons, infecting the recipient's lung. • Potential for a postprimary spread locally or throughout the body	• Latent period: asymptomatic, some regional lymph nodes may be involved • Active infection: fever, cough, weight loss, night sweats • History of travel to region with endemic tuberculosis or close contact with infected person	• Latent disease: no pulmonary findings • Active disease: consolidation and/or pleural effusion may develop with corresponding findings and cough with blood-streaked sputum. • Positive tuberculin skin test and interferon-gamma release assays

FIGURE 13-34 **Tuberculosis.** *(Wilson and Giddens, 2013.)*

Pneumothorax

Presence of air or gas in the pleural cavity (Fig. 13-35)

Pathophysiology	Subjective Data	Objective Data
• May result from trauma or may occur spontaneously, perhaps because of rupture of a congenital or acquired bleb • In *tension pneumothorax*, air leaks continually into the pleural space, resulting in a potentially life-threatening emergency from increasing pressure in the pleural space.	• Minimal collections of air may easily be without symptoms at first, particularly because spontaneous pneumothorax paradoxically has its onset most often when the patient is at rest. • Larger collections provoke dyspnea and chest pain.	• The breath sounds over the pneumothorax are distant. • A mediastinal shift with tracheal deviation away from the involved side can be seen with a tension pneumothorax. • An unexplained but persistent tachycardia may be a clue to a minimal pneumothorax.

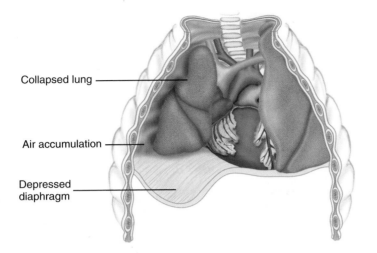

FIGURE 13-35 Pneumothorax.

Hemothorax

Presence of blood in the pleural cavity (Fig. 13-36)

Pathophysiology

- May be the result of trauma or invasive medical procedures (e.g., thoracentesis, central line placement or attempt, pleural biopsy)
- When air is present with the blood, this is called a *hemopneumothorax.*

Subjective Data

- Dyspnea and lightheadedness may develop depending on the degree and acuity of blood loss and decreased pulmonary function.

Objective Data

- Breath sounds will be distant or absent if blood predominates.
- Percussion note will be dull
- Tachycardia and hypotension with excessive blood loss

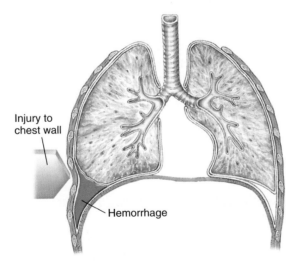

FIGURE 13-36 Hemothorax. *(Wilson and Giddens, 2013.)*

Lung Cancer

Generally refers to bronchogenic carcinoma, a malignant tumor that evolves from bronchial epithelial structures (Fig. 13-37)

Pathophysiology

- Etiologic agents include tobacco smoke, asbestos, ionizing radiation, and other inhaled carcinogenic agents.

Subjective Data

- May cause cough, wheezing, a variety of patterns of emphysema and atelectasis, pneumonitis, and hemoptysis
- Peripheral tumors without airway obstruction may be asymptomatic.

Objective Data

- Findings are based on the extent of the tumor and the patterns of its invasion and metastasis.
- With airway obstruction, a postobstructive pneumonia can develop with consolidation.
- A malignant pleural effusion may develop.

FIGURE 13-37 **Cancer of the lung. A,** Squamous (epidermoid) cell carcinoma. **B,** Small cell (oat cell) carcinoma. **C,** Adenocarcinoma. **D,** Large cell carcinoma.

Pulmonary Embolism

The embolic occlusion of pulmonary arteries is a relatively common condition that is very difficult to diagnose.

Pathophysiology	Subjective Data	Objective Data
• Risk factors include, among others, age older than 40 years, a history of venous thromboembolism, surgery with anesthesia longer than 30 minutes, heart disease, cancer, fracture of the pelvis and leg bones, obesity, and acquired or genetic thrombophilia.	• Pleuritic chest pain with or without dyspnea is a major clue to embolism.	• There may be a low-grade fever or an isolated tachycardia. • Hypoxia by pulse oximetry may be evident.

✿ Infants, Children, and Adolescents

Diaphragmatic Hernia

Result of an imperfectly structured diaphragm, occurs once in slightly more than 2000 live births (see Fig. 13-24)

Pathophysiology	Subjective Data	Objective Data
• On the left side, at least 90% of the time, the liver is not there to get in the way.	• The degree of respiratory distress can be slight or very severe depending on the extent to which the bowel has invaded the chest through the defect.	• Bowel sounds are heard in the chest with a flat or scaphoid abdomen. • The heart is usually displaced to the right. • Tachypnea, retraction, and grunting

Cystic Fibrosis

Autosomal recessive disorder of exocrine glands involving the lungs, pancreas, and sweat glands (Fig. 13-38)

Pathophysiology	Subjective Data	Objective Data
• Thick mucus causes progressive clogging of the bronchi and bronchioles. • Bronchiectasis results with cyst formation and subsequent pulmonary infection. • Many states now screen for this autosomal recessive caused by mutations of *CFTR* (cystic fibrosis transmembrane conductance regulator).	• Cough with sputum is a hallmark in children younger than 5 years. • Salt loss in sweat is distinctive such that a parent may notice that the child's skin tastes unusually salty. • There may be a history of malabsorption, large, bulky stools, constipation, poor weight gain, frequent infection, meconium ileus, or intestinal obstruction.	• Bronchiectasis with the associated findings • Barrel chest • Nasal polyps • Low body mass due to malabsorption • Pulmonary dysfunction leads to clubbing, pulmonary hypertension, and cor pulmonale.

FIGURE 13-38 Cystic fibrosis. *(Wilson and Giddens, 2013.)*

Epiglottitis

Acute, life-threatening infection involving the epiglottis and surrounding tissues (Fig. 13-39, *A*)

Pathophysiology

- Acute inflammation of the epiglottis due to bacterial invasion, leading to life-threatening airway obstruction, may cause death
- Immunization against *Haemophilus influenzae* type B has greatly reduced the incidence in the United States.
- Most common in children between 3 and 7 years old

Subjective Data

- Begins suddenly and progresses rapidly without cough
- Painful sore throat with difficulty swallowing
- Muffled voice

Objective Data

- Child sits straight up with neck extended and head held forward, appearing very anxious and ill, unable to swallow and drools from an open mouth
- High fever
- Beefy red epiglottis

FIGURE 13-39 Croup syndrome. **A,** Acute epiglottitis. **B,** Laryngotracheobronchitis.

Croup (Laryngotracheal Bronchitis)

Syndrome that generally results from infection with a variety of viral agents, particularly the parainfluenza viruses, occurring most often in children from about 1½ to 3 years of age

Pathophysiology

- The inflammation is subglottic and may involve areas beyond the larynx (laryngotracheobronchitis) (see Fig. 13-39, *B*).
- An aspirated foreign body may mimic croup on occasion.

Subjective Data

- An episode begins with upper respiratory symptoms, mild fever
- The child often awakens suddenly after going to bed, often very frightened, with a harsh, barking cough.

Objective Data

- Labored breathing, retraction, hoarseness, barking cough, and inspiratory stridor are characteristic.
- Restless, irritable
- Fever does not always accompany croup; the child does not have the toxic, drooling facies of persons with epiglottitis.

ABNORMALITIES

Tracheomalacia

Lack of rigidity or a floppiness of the trachea or airway

Pathophysiology	Subjective Data	Objective Data
• Trachea narrows in response to the varying pressures of inspiration and expiration. • Tends to be benign and self-limited with increasing age • Need to eliminate the possibilities of fixed lesions (e.g., a vascular lesion), tracheal stenosis, or even a foreign body	• "Noisy breathing" or wheezing in infancy is often inspiratory stridor.	• Stridor, wheezing, and findings of respiratory distress develop with airway collapse or severe compromise.

Bronchiolitis

Bronchiolar (small airway) inflammation leading to hyperinflation of the lungs, occurring most often in infants younger than 6 months

Pathophysiology	Subjective Data	Objective Data
• Usual cause is respiratory syncytial virus; other viral organisms include adenovirus, parainfluenza virus, and human metapneumovirus. • The virus acts as a parasite invading small bronchioles. The virus bursts and invades other cells that die and obstruct and irritate the airway.	• Begins with upper respiratory symptoms • Poor feeding, vomiting and diarrhea, • Lethargy • Expiration becomes difficult, and the infant appears anxious.	• Breaths are rapid and short with generalized retractions and perioral cyanosis developing. • Wheezing, grunting, diminished breath sounds • Altered mental status • Lung hyperinflation leads to an increased AP diameter of the thoracic cage and abdomen. • Hyperresonant percussion

✻ Older Adults

CHRONIC OBSTRUCTIVE PULMONARY DISEASE

COPD is a nonspecific designation that includes a group of respiratory problems in which coughs, chronic and often excessive sputum production, and dyspnea are prominent features. Ultimately, an irreversible expiratory airflow obstruction occurs. Chronic bronchitis, bronchiectasis, and emphysema are the main conditions that are included in this group.

Emphysema

Condition in which the lungs lose elasticity and alveoli enlarge in a way that disrupts function (Fig. 13-40)

Pathophysiology	Subjective Data	Objective Data
• Most patients have an extensive smoking history. • Chronic bronchitis is a common precursor leading to dilation of the air spaces beyond the terminal bronchioles and rupture of alveolar walls, permanently hyperinflating the lung. • Alveolar gas is trapped, in expiration, and gas exchange is seriously compromised.	• Dyspnea is common even at rest, requiring supplemental oxygen when severe. • Cough is infrequent without much production of sputum.	• Chest may be barrel-shaped, and scattered crackles or wheezes may be heard. • Overinflated lungs are hyperresonant on percussion. • Inspiration is limited with a prolonged expiratory effort (i.e., longer than 4 or 5 seconds) to expel air.

FIGURE 13-40 Chronic obstructive pulmonary disease with lobar emphysema. *(Wilson and Giddens, 2013.)*

Bronchiectasis

Chronic dilation of the bronchi or bronchioles caused by repeated pulmonary infections and bronchial obstruction (Fig. 13-41)

Pathophysiology

- Frequently seen in cystic fibrosis
- Malfunction of bronchial muscle tone and loss of elasticity

Subjective Data

- The cough with expectoration of large amounts of sputum is most often the major clue.
- Severe hemoptysis may occur.

Objective Data

- Tachypnea and clubbing
- Crackles and rhonchi, sometimes disappearing after cough

FIGURE 13-41 Bronchiectasis. *(Wilson and Giddens, 2013.)*

Chronic Bronchitis

Large airway inflammation, usually a result of chronic irritant exposure; more commonly a problem for patients older than 40

Pathophysiology

- Large airways are chronically inflamed, leading to mucus production.
- Smoking is prominent in the history with many of these patients being emphysematous.
- Recurrent bacterial infections are common.

Subjective Data

- Dyspnea may be present although not severe.
- Cough and sputum production are impressive.

Objective Data

- Wheezing and crackles
- Hyperinflation with decreased breath sounds and a flattened diaphragm
- Severe chronic bronchitis may result in right ventricular failure with dependent edema.

CHAPTER 14

Heart

The main heart function is to circulate blood through the body and lungs in two separate circulations (one circuit being the body, the second being the lungs). It lies in the mediastinum, to the left of the midline, just above the diaphragm, cradled between the medial and lower borders of the lungs. The cardiac examination is performed as part of the comprehensive physical examination or when a patient presents with signs or symptoms of a cardiac disease process.

evolve *http://evolve.elsevier.com/Seidel*

- Physical Exam Key Points
- NCLEX Review Questions
- Interactive Activities
- Animations
- Videos
- Audio Clips
- Student Checklist

ANATOMY AND PHYSIOLOGY

The heart is positioned behind the sternum and the contiguous parts of the third to the sixth costal cartilages. The area of the chest overlying the heart is the precordium. Because of the heart's conelike shape, the broader upper portion is called the base, and the narrower lower tip of the heart is the apex (Fig. 14-1).

The position of the heart can vary considerably depending on body build, configuration of the chest, and level of the diaphragm. In a tall slender person, the heart tends to hang vertically and to be positioned centrally. With a shorter person, it tends to lie more to the left and more horizontally. Occasionally, the heart may be positioned to the right, either rotated or displaced, or as a mirror image (*dextrocardia*). *Situs inversus* is when the heart and stomach are placed to the right and the liver to the left.

Physical Examination Preview

Here is a preview of the steps involved in conducting a physical examination of the heart. ⊖ These procedures are explained in detail in this chapter and are available on Evolve in printable formats.

Heart

The following steps are performed with the patient sitting, supine, and in the left lateral recumbent positions; these positions are all used to compare findings or enhance the assessment. Having the patient lean forward while in the seated position can bring the heart closer to the chest wall and accentuate findings.

1. Inspect the precordium for the following (p. 305):
   - Apical impulse
   - Pulsations
   - Heaves or lifts
2. Palpate the precordium to detect the following (pp. 305-306):
   - Apical impulse
   - Thrills, heaves, or lifts
3. Percussion to estimate the heart size (optional) (pp. 306-307):
4. Systematically auscultate in each of the five areas while the patient is breathing regularly and holding breath for the following (pp. 307-311):
   - Rate
   - Rhythm

   - S_1
   - S_2
   - Splitting
   - S_3 and/or S_4
   - Extra heart sounds (snaps, clicks, friction rubs, or murmurs)
5. Assess the following characteristics of murmurs (pp. 312-318):
   - Timing and duration
   - Pitch
   - Intensity
   - Pattern
   - Quality
   - Location
   - Radiation
   - Variation with respiratory phase

FIGURE 14-1 Frontal section of the heart.

FIGURE 14-2 Heart within the pericardium.

Structure

The pericardium is a tough, double-walled, fibrous sac encasing and protecting the heart. Several milliliters of fluid are present between the inner and outer layers of the pericardium, providing for low-friction movement (Fig. 14-2).

The epicardium, the thin outermost muscle layer, covers the surface of the heart and extends onto the great vessels. The myocardium, the thick muscular middle layer, is responsible for the pumping action of the heart. The endocardium, the innermost layer, lines the chambers of the heart and covers the heart valves and the small muscles associated with the opening and closing of these valves (Fig. 14-3).

The heart is divided into four chambers. The two upper chambers are the right and left atria (or auricles, because of their earlike shape), and the bottom chambers are the right and left ventricles. The left atrium and left ventricle together are referred to as the *left heart*; the right atrium and right ventricle together are referred to as the *right heart*. The left heart and right heart are divided by a blood-tight partition called the *interventricular septum* (see Fig. 14-1). On the anterior external surface of the heart, the coronary sulcus separates the atria from the ventricles (Fig. 14-4).

The atria are small, thin-walled structures acting primarily as reservoirs for blood returning to the heart from the veins throughout the body. The ventricles are large, thick-walled chambers that pump blood to the lungs and throughout the body. The right and left ventricles together form the primary muscle mass of the heart. In the adult heart, the left ventricle mass is greater than that of the right ventricle because the higher pressure in the systemic circulation requires a greater force of contraction (and more muscle mass) in order for blood to be

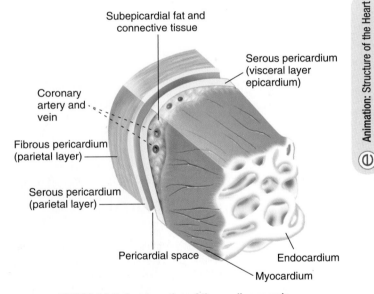

FIGURE 14-3 Cross section of the cardiac muscle.

successfully pumped throughout the body. The adult heart is about 12 cm long, 8 cm wide at the widest point, and 6 cm in its anteroposterior diameter.

Most of the anterior surface of the heart is formed by the right ventricle. The left ventricle is positioned behind the right but extends anteriorly, forming the left border of the heart (see Fig. 14-4). The left atrium is above the left ventricle, forming the more posterior aspect of the heart. The heart is, in effect, turned ventrally on its axis, putting its right side more forward. The left ventricle's contraction and thrust result in the apical impulse

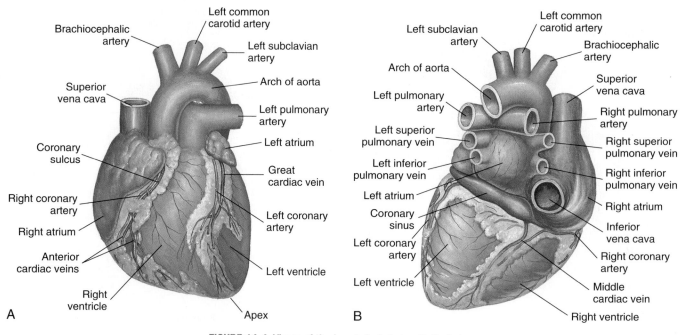

FIGURE 14-4 Views of the heart. **A,** Anterior. **B,** Posterior.

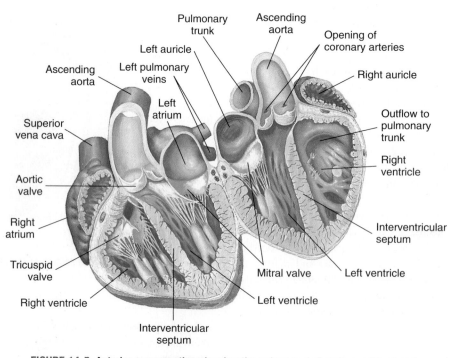

FIGURE 14-5 Anterior cross section showing the valves and chambers of the heart.

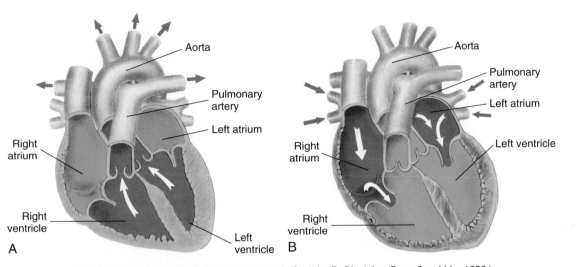

FIGURE 14-6 Blood flow through the heart. **A,** Systole. **B,** Diastole. *(From Canobbio, 1990.)*

usually felt in the fifth left intercostal space at the midclavicular line. The right atrium lies above and slightly to the right of the right ventricle, participating in the formation of the right border of the heart.

The four chambers of the heart are connected by two sets of valves, the atrioventricular and semilunar valves. In the fully formed heart that is free of defect, these are the only intracardiac pathways and permit the flow of blood in only one direction (Fig. 14-5).

The atrioventricular valves, situated between the atria and the ventricles, include the tricuspid and mitral valves. The tricuspid valve, which has three cusps (or leaflets), separates the right atrium from the right ventricle. The mitral valve, which has two cusps, separates the left atrium from the left ventricle. When the atria contract (diastole), the atrioventricular valves open, allowing blood to flow into the ventricles. When the ventricles contract (systole), these valves snap shut, preventing blood from flowing back into the atria (Fig. 14-6). See Clinical Pearl, "Order of Valves."

> ## Clinical Pearl
>
> ### Order of Valves
> The order of the cardiac valves can be remembered by using the sentence "Try Pulling My Arm" for *t*ricuspid, *p*ulmonic, *m*itral, and *a*ortic.

The two semilunar valves each have three cusps. The pulmonic valve separates the right ventricle from the pulmonary artery. The aortic valve lies between the left ventricle and the aorta. Contraction of the ventricles (systole) opens the semilunar valves, causing blood to rush into the pulmonary artery and aorta. When the ventricles relax (diastole), the valves close, shutting off any backward flow into the ventricles (see Fig. 14-6).

Cardiac Cycle

The heart contracts and relaxes rhythmically, creating a two-phase cardiac cycle. During systole, the ventricles contract, ejecting blood from the left ventricle into the aorta and simultaneously from the right ventricle into the pulmonary artery. During diastole, the ventricles dilate, drawing blood into the ventricles as the atria contract, thereby moving blood from the atria to the ventricles (see Fig. 14-6). The volume of blood and the pressure under which it is returned to the heart vary with the degree of body activity, physical and metabolic (e.g., with exercise or fever).

As systole begins, ventricular contraction raises the pressure in the ventricles and forces the mitral and tricuspid valves closed, preventing backflow. This valve closure produces the first heart sound (S_1), the characteristic "lub." The intraventricular pressure rises until it exceeds that in the aorta and pulmonary artery. Then the aortic and pulmonic valves are forced open, and ejection of blood into the arteries begins. Valve opening is usually a silent event (Fig. 14-7).

When the ventricles are almost empty, the pressure in the ventricles falls below that in the aorta and pulmonary artery, allowing the aortic and pulmonic valves to close. Closure of these valves causes the second heart sound (S_2), the "dub." The second heart sound has two components: A_2 is produced by aortic valve closure, and P_2 is produced by pulmonic valve closure. As ventricular pressure falls below atrial pressure, the mitral and tricuspid valves open to allow the blood collected in the atria to refill the relaxed ventricles. Diastole is a relatively passive interval until ventricular filling is almost complete. This filling sometimes produces a third heart sound (S_3). Then the atria contract to ensure the ejection of any remaining blood. This can sometimes be heard as a fourth heart sound (S_4). The cycle begins anew, with ventricular contraction and atrial refilling occurring at about the same time. The cardiac cycle continues without resting and constantly adjusts to the variable demands of work, rest, digestion, and illness.

ANATOMY AND PHYSIOLOGY

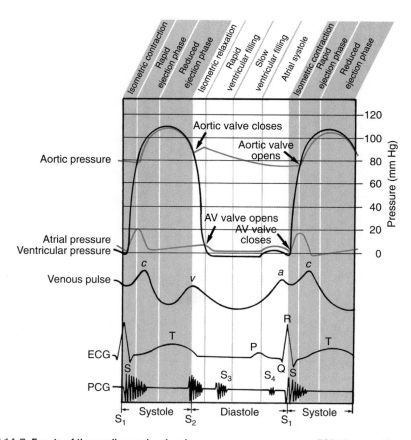

FIGURE 14-7 Events of the cardiac cycle, showing venous pressure waves, ECG (the graphic representing the electrical activity during the cardiac cycle), and heart sounds in systole and diastole. *PCG,* Phonocardiogram. *(Modified from Guzzetta and Dossey, 1992.)*

The events of the cardiac cycle are not exactly identical on both sides of the heart. In fact, pressures in the right ventricle, right atrium, and pulmonary artery are lower than in the left side of the heart, and the same events occur slightly later on the right side than on the left. The effect is that heart sounds sometimes have two distinct components, the first produced by the left side and the second by the right side. For example, the aortic valve closes slightly before the pulmonic, so that S_2 is often heard as two distinct components, referred to as a "split S_2" (A_2, then P_2).

Closure of the heart valves during the cardiac cycle produces heart sounds in rapid succession. Although the valves are anatomically close to each other, their sounds are best heard in an area away from the anatomic site because the sound is transmitted in the direction of blood flow (see Fig. 14-15).

Electrical Activity

An intrinsic electrical conduction system enables the heart to contract and coordinates the sequence of muscular contractions taking place during the cardiac cycle. An electrical impulse stimulates each myocardial contraction. The impulse originates in and is paced by the sinoatrial node (SA node), located in the wall of the right atrium. The impulse then travels through both atria to the atrioventricular node (AV node), located in the atrial septum.

In the AV node the impulse is delayed but then passes down the bundle of His to the Purkinje fibers (heart muscle cells specialized for electrical conduction), located in the ventricular myocardium. Ventricular contraction is initiated at the apex and proceeds toward the base of the heart (Fig. 14-8).

An electrocardiogram (ECG) is a graphic recording of electrical activity during the cardiac cycle. The ECG records electrical current generated by the movement of ions in and out of the myocardial cell membranes. The ECG records two basic events: depolarization, which is the spread of a stimulus through the heart muscle, and repolarization, which is the return of the stimulated heart muscle to a resting state. The ECG records electrical activity as specific waves (Fig. 14-9):

+ P wave—the spread of a stimulus through the atria (atrial depolarization)
+ PR interval—the time from initial stimulation of the atria to initial stimulation of the ventricles, usually 0.12 to 0.20 second
+ QRS complex—the spread of a stimulus through the ventricles (ventricular depolarization), less than 0.10 second
+ ST segment and T wave—the return of stimulated ventricular muscle to a resting state (ventricular repolarization)
+ U wave—a small deflection rarely seen just after the T wave, thought to be related to repolarization of the Purkinje fibers. This is also seen sometimes with electrolyte abnormalities.

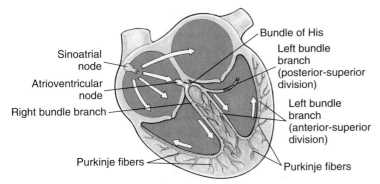

FIGURE 14-8 **Cardiac conduction.** *(From Canobbio, 1990.)*

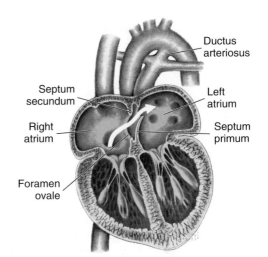

FIGURE 14-10 **Anatomy of the fetal heart.** *(From Thompson et al, 1997.)*

FIGURE 14-9 **Usual electrocardiogram waveform.** *(From Berne and Levy, 1996.)*

+ QT interval—the time elapsed from the onset of ventricular depolarization until the completion of ventricular repolarization. The interval varies with the cardiac rate.

Because the electrical stimulus starts the cycle, it precedes the mechanical response by a brief moment. The sequence of myocardial depolarization is the cause of events on the left side of the heart occurring slightly before those on the right. When the heart is beating at a rate of 68 to 72 beats/min ventricular systole is shorter than diastole. As the rate increases to about 120 beats/min, because of stress or pathologic factors, the two phases of the cardiac cycle tend to approximate each other in length.

⚘ Infants and Children

Fetal circulation, including the umbilical vessels, compensates for the nonfunctional fetal lungs. Blood flows from the right atrium into the left atrium via the foramen ovale (Fig. 14-10). The right ventricle pumps blood through the patent ductus arteriosus rather than into the lungs. The right and left ventricles are equal in weight and muscle mass because they both pump blood into the systemic circulation, unlike the adult heart (Figs. 14-10 and 14-11).

The changes at birth include closure of the ductus arteriosus, usually within 24 to 48 hours, and the functional closure of the interatrial foramen ovale as pressure rises in the left atrium. The mass of the left ventricle increases after birth in response to the left ventricle assuming total responsibility for systemic circulation. By 1 year of age, the relative sizes of the left and right ventricles approximate the adult ratio of 2:1.

The heart lies more horizontally in the chest in infants and young children compared to adults. As a result, the apex of the heart rides higher, sometimes well out into the fourth left intercostal space. In most cases, the adult heart position is reached by the age of 7 years.

⚘ Pregnant Women

The maternal blood volume increases 40% to 50% over the prepregnancy level. The rise is mainly due to an increase in plasma volume, which begins in the first trimester and reaches a maximum after the 30th week. On average, plasma volume increases 50% with a single pregnancy and as much as 70% with a twin pregnancy. The heart works harder to accommodate the increased heart rate and stroke volume required for the expanded blood volume. The left ventricle increases in both wall thickness and mass. The blood volume returns to prepregnancy levels within 3 to 4 weeks after delivery (Table 14-1).

ANATOMY AND PHYSIOLOGY

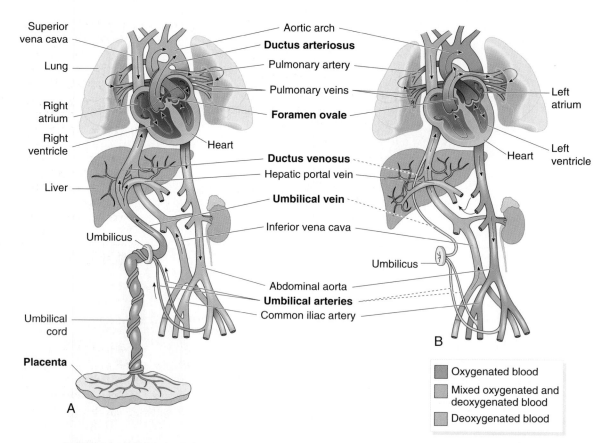

FIGURE 14-11 **Fetal circulation. A,** In utero. **B,** After delivery. *(From Ross and Wilson, Anatomy and Physiology in Health and Illness, 2011.)*

Table 14-1	Hemodynamic Changes during Pregnancy				
	Stage				
Hemodynamic Variable	**First Trimester**	**Second Trimester**	**Third Trimester**	**Labor And Delivery**	**Postpartum Period**
Heart rate	Increased	Peaks at 28th week	Slightly decreased	Increased; bradycardia at delivery	Prepregnancy level within 2 to 6 weeks
Blood pressure	Prepregnancy level	Slightly decreased	Prepregnancy level	Prepregnancy level	Prepregnancy level
Blood volume	Increased	Peaks at 20th week	Gradually decreased	Rises sharply	Prepregnancy level within 2 to 6 weeks
Stroke volume	Increased	Peaks at 28th week	Gradually decreased	Decreased	Prepregnancy level within 2 to 6 weeks
Cardiac output	Increased	Peaks at 20th week	Slightly decreased	Increased	Prepregnancy level within 2 to 6 weeks
Systemic vascular resistance	Decreased	Decreased	Decreased	Sharply decreased at delivery	Prepregnancy level within 2 to 6 weeks

The cardiac output increases approximately 30% to 40% over that of the nonpregnant state and reaches its highest level by about 25 to 32 weeks of gestation. This level is maintained until term. Cardiac output returns to prepregnancy levels about 2 weeks after delivery. As the uterus enlarges and the diaphragm moves upward in pregnancy, the position of the heart is shifted toward a horizontal position, with slight axis rotation.

✤ Older Adults

Heart size may decrease with age unless hypertension or heart disease causes enlargement. The left ventricular wall thickens and the valves tend to fibrose and calcify. Stroke volume decreases, and cardiac output during exercise declines by 30% to 40%. The endocardium thickens. The myocardium becomes less elastic and more rigid so that recovery of myocardial contractility is delayed. The response to stress and increased oxygen demand is less efficient. Tachycardia is poorly tolerated, and after any type of stress, the return to an expected heart rate takes longer. Despite these age-associated changes in heart architecture and contractile properties, the aged heart continues to function reasonably well at rest. Long-standing hypertensive disease, infarcts, and/or other insults and loss of physical conditioning may lead to severe compromise of the heart and to increasingly significant decline in cardiac output.

Cardiac function is further compromised by fibrosis and sclerosis in the region of the SA node and in the heart valves (particularly the mitral valve and aortic cusps) and by increased vagal tone. ECG changes occur secondary to cellular alteration, to fibrosis within the conduction system, and to neurogenic changes.

REVIEW OF RELATED HISTORY

For each of the symptoms or conditions discussed in this section, particular topics to include in the history of the present illness are listed. Responses to questions about these topics provide clues for individualizing the physical examination and the development of a diagnostic evaluation appropriate for the particular patient. Questions regarding medication use (prescription and over the counter preparations) as well as complementary and alternative therapies are relevant for each area.

History of Present Illness

- Chest pain (Boxes 14-1 and 14-2)
  - Onset and duration: sudden, gradual, or vague onset, length of episode; cyclic nature; related to physical exertion, rest, emotional experience, eating, coughing, cold temperatures, trauma, awakens from sleep

---

Box 14-1	Chest Pain

The presence of chest pain suggests heart disease, and it has many causes. *Angina pectoris* is traditionally described as a pressure or choking sensation, substernal or into the neck. The discomfort, which can be intense, may radiate to the jaw and down the left (and sometimes the right) arm. It often begins during strenuous physical activity, eating, exposure to intense cold, windy weather, or exposure to emotional stress. Relief may occur in minutes if the activity can be stopped. Signs of angina pectoris may vary in location, intensity, and radiation, and often arise from sources other than the heart. In women it may vary from the classic signs in men. The "precordial catch," for example, is a sudden, sharp, relatively brief pain that does not radiate, occurs most often at rest, is unrelated to exertion, and may not have a discoverable cause.

Some Possible Causes of Chest Pain
Cardiac
Angina
Acute myocardial infarction
Coronary insufficiency
Myocardial infarction
Nonobstructive, nonspastic angina
Mitral valve prolapse
Aortic
Dissection of the aorta
Pleuropericardial Pain
Pericarditis
Pleurisy
Pneumothorax
Mediastinal emphysema

Gastrointestinal Disease
Hiatus hernia
Reflux esophagitis
Esophageal rupture
Esophageal spasm
Cholecystitis
Peptic ulcer disease
Pancreatitis
Pulmonary Disease
Pulmonary hypertension
Pneumonia
Pulmonary embolus
Bronchial hyperreactivity
Tension pneumothorax
Musculoskeletal
Cervical radiculopathy
Shoulder disorder or dysfunction (e.g., arthritis, bursitis, rotator cuff injury, biceps tendonitis)
Costochondral disorder
Xiphodynia
Psychoneurotic
Illicit drug use (e.g., cocaine)
Herpes zoster: when lesions occur in thoracic region
  Unlike in adults, chest pain in children and adolescents is seldom due to a cardiac problem. It is often difficult to find a cause, but trauma, exercise-induced asthma, and even in a somewhat younger child, the use of cocaine should be among the considerations.

Box 14-2 | Characteristics of Chest Pain

Type	Characteristics
Cardiac	Substernal; provoked by effort, emotion, eating; relieved by rest and/or nitroglycerin; often accompanied by diaphoresis, occasionally by nausea
Pleural	Precipitated by breathing or coughing; usually described as sharp; present during respiration; absent when breath held
Esophageal	Burning, substernal, occasional radiation to the shoulder; nocturnal occurrence, usually when lying flat; relief with food, antacids, sometimes nitroglycerin
From a peptic ulcer	Almost always infradiaphragmatic and epigastric; nocturnal occurrence and daytime attacks relieved by food; unrelated to activity
Biliary	Usually under right scapula, prolonged in duration; often occurring after eating; will trigger angina more often than mimic it
Arthritis/bursitis	Usually lasts for hours; local tenderness and/or pain with movement
Cervical	Associated with injury; provoked by activity, persists after activity; painful on palpation and/or movement
Musculoskeletal (chest)	Intensified or provoked by movement, particularly twisting or costochondral bending; long-lasting; often associated with focal tenderness
Psychoneurotic	Associated with/after anxiety; poorly described; located in intramammary region

DIFFERENTIAL DIAGNOSIS
Comparison of Some Types of Chest Pain

Cardiac	Musculoskeletal	Gastrointestinal
Presence of cardiac risk factors	History of trauma	History of indigestion
Specifically noted time of onset	Vague onset	Vague onset
Related to physical effort or emotional	Related to physical effort	Related to food consumption or psychosocial stress
Disappears if stimulating cause can be terminated	Continues after cessation of effort	May go on for several hours; unrelated to effort
Commonly forces patients to stop effort	Patients often can continue activity	Patients often can continue activity
Patient may awaken from sleep	Delays falling asleep	Patient may awaken from sleep, particularly during early morning
Relief at times with nitroglycerin	Relief at times with heat, nonsteroidal antiinflammatory drugs, or rest	Relief at times with antacids
Pain often in early morning or after washing and eating	Worse in evening after a day of physical effort	No particular relationship to time of day; related to food, tension
Greater likelihood in cold weather	Greater likelihood in cold, damp weather	Anytime

- Character: aching, sharp, tingling, burning, pressure, stabbing, crushing, or clenched fist (Levine) sign
- Location: radiating down arms, to neck, jaws, teeth, scapula; relief with rest or position change
- Severity: interference with activity, need to stop all activity until it subsides, disrupts sleep, severity on a scale of 0 to 10
- Associated symptoms: anxiety; dyspnea (shortness of breath); diaphoresis (sweating); dizziness; nausea or vomiting; faintness; cold, clammy skin; cyanosis; pallor; swelling or edema (noted anywhere, constant or at certain times during day)
- Treatment: rest, position change, exercise, nitroglycerin
- Medications: digoxin, diuretics, beta-blockers, angiotensin-converting enzyme (ACE) inhibitors, calcium channel blockers, nonsteroidal antiinflammatory drugs, antihypertensives

Past Medical History

- Cardiac surgery or hospitalization for cardiac evaluation or disorder
- Congenital heart disease
- Rhythm disorder

Risk Factors
Cardiac Disease

- Gender (men more at risk than women; women's risk is increased in the postmenopausal years and with oral contraceptive use)
- Hyperlipidemia
- Elevated homocysteine level
- Smoking
- Family history of cardiovascular disease, diabetes, hyperlipidemia, hypertension, or sudden death in young adults
- Diabetes mellitus
- Obesity: dietary habits, including an excessively fatty diet
- Sedentary lifestyle without exercise
- Fatigue: unusual or persistent, inability to keep up with contemporaries, inability to maintain usual activities, bedtime earlier
- Associated symptoms: dyspnea on exertion, chest pain, palpitations, orthopnea (shortness of breath [dyspnea] when lying flat), paroxysmal nocturnal dyspnea (dyspnea that awakens someone from sleep), anorexia, nausea, vomiting
- Medications: beta-blockers

- Cough:
  - Onset and duration
  - Character: dry, wet, nighttime, aggravated by lying down
  - Medications: ACE inhibitors
- Difficulty breathing (dyspnea, orthopnea)
- Worsening or remaining stable
- At rest or aggravated by exertion (how much?) (see Box 14-3); on level ground, climbing stairs
- Position: lying down or eased by resting on pillows (how many? or sleep in a recliner?)
- Paroxysmal nocturnal dyspnea (recurring attacks of shortness of breath that wake you up at night gasping for air, coughing, wheezing and feeling like you're suffocating)
- Loss of consciousness (transient syncope)
- Associated symptoms: palpitation, dysrhythmia
- When occurs: unusual exertion, sudden turning of neck (carotid sinus effect), looking upward (vertebral artery occlusion), change in posture

---

- Acute rheumatic fever, characterized by unexplained fever, swollen joints, Sydenham chorea (St. Vitus dance), abdominal pain, skin rash (erythema marginatum) or nodules
- Kawasaki disease (see Chapter 15, p. 349)
- Chronic illness: hypertension, bleeding disorder, hyperlipidemia, diabetes, thyroid dysfunction, coronary artery disease, obesity, congenital heart defect

Family History

- Long QT syndrome
- Marfan syndrome (a genetic disorder of the connective tissue associated with mitral valve prolapse/regurgitation, aortic regurgitation, and aortic dissection)
- Diabetes
- Heart disease
- Dyslipidemia
- Hypertension
- Obesity
- Congenital heart disease, once it occurs in a family, the likelihood of its recurring increases
- Family members with risk factor: morbidity, mortality related to cardiovascular system; ages at time of illness or death; sudden death, particularly in young and middle-aged relatives

Personal and Social History

- Employment: physical demands, environmental hazards such as heat, chemicals, dust, sources of emotional stress
- Tobacco use: type (cigarettes, cigars, pipe, chewing tobacco, snuff), duration of use, amount, age started and stopped; pack-years (number of years smoking times number of packs per day)

Box 14-3	Exercise Intensity

Light: walking 10 to 15 steps, preparing a simple meal for one, retrieving a newspaper from just outside the door, pulling down a bedspread, brushing teeth

Moderate: making the bed, dusting and sweeping, walking a level short block, office filing

Moderately heavy: climbing one or two flights of stairs, lifting full cartons, long walks, sexual intercourse

Heavy: jogging, vigorous athletics of any kind, cleaning the entire house in less than a day, raking a large number of leaves, mowing a large lawn with a hand mower, shoveling deep snow

Adapted from *2008 Physical activity guidelines for Americans*.

- Nutritional status
- Usual diet: proportion of fat, use of salt, food preferences, history of dieting
- Weight: loss or gain, amount and rate
- Alcohol consumption: amount, frequency, duration of current intake
- Known hypercholesterolemia and/or elevated triglycerides (see Risk Factors box)
- Relaxation/hobbies
- Exercise: type, amount, frequency, intensity (Box 14-3)
- Use of illicit drugs: amyl nitrate, cocaine, injection drug use

✂ Infants

- Tiring easily and/or sweating with feeding
- Breathing changes: more heavily or more rapidly than expected during feeding or defecation
- Cyanosis: perioral during eating, more widespread and more persistent, related to crying
- Excessive weight gain compared to caloric intake

EXAMINATION AND FINDINGS

+ Mother's health during pregnancy: medications taken, gestational diabetes, unexplained fever, illicit drug use

⚘ Children

+ Tiring during play: amount of time before tiring, activities that are tiring, inability to keep up with other children
+ Naps: longer than expected
+ Knee-chest position or squatting after shortness of breath
+ Headaches
+ Nosebleeds
+ Unexplained joint pain
+ Expected height and weight gain (and any substantiating records)
+ Expected physical and cognitive development (and any substantiating records)

⚘ Pregnant Women

+ History of cardiac disease or surgery
+ Dizziness or syncope or near-syncope on standing
+ Indications of heart disease during pregnancy, including progressive or severe dyspnea, progressive orthopnea, paroxysmal nocturnal dyspnea, hemoptysis, syncope with exertion, and chest pain related to effort or emotion

⚘ Older Adults

+ Common symptoms of cardiovascular disorders: confusion, dizziness, blackouts, syncope, palpitations, coughs and wheezes, hemoptysis, shortness of breath, chest pains or chest tightness, impotence, fatigue, leg edema: pattern, frequency, time of day most pronounced
+ If heart disease has been diagnosed: drug reactions: potassium excess (weakness, bradycardia, hypotension, confusion); potassium depletion (weakness, fatigue, muscle cramps, dysrhythmias); digitalis toxicity (anorexia, nausea, vomiting, diarrhea, headache, confusion, dysrhythmias, halo, yellow vision); interference with activities of daily living; ability of the patient and family to cope with the condition, perceived and actual; orthostatic hypotension

EXAMINATION AND FINDINGS

Equipment

+ Stethoscope
+ Marking pencil
+ Centimeter ruler

The examination of the heart includes the following: inspection, palpation, and percussion of the chest and then auscultation of the heart. Performing a successful examination requires a competence of each procedure and an ability to integrate and interpret the findings in relation to the cardiac events they reflect.

Findings from examinations of other body systems have a significant impact on judgments made about the cardiovascular system. For example, crackles auscultated in the lungs, palpation of an enlarged liver, and observation of peripheral edema are signs of heart failure. Examples of other influencing factors may include the following:

> ### Staying Well
>
> *Importance of a Healthy Lifestyle*
>
> Elevated serum cholesterol is a potent risk factor for myocardial infarction. Hyperlipidemia is one of the most common metabolic diseases because of the increasing obesity epidemic.
> - Lower levels of total cholesterol and low-density lipoprotein (LDL) cholesterol further reduce the risk of myocardial infarction.
> - National Institutes of Health Adult Treatment Panel III guidelines (2004): desirable level of total cholesterol of <200 mg/dL, LDL cholesterol of <100 mg/dL, (LDL goal with previous myocardial infarction or diabetes mellitus is 70 mg/dL), HDL >40 mg/dL, and triglycerides <150 mg/dL
>
> Use some of the time during your cardiac examination to remind the patient of the importance of healthy lifestyle in maintaining good cardiac health:
> - Enjoy a diet low in cholesterol. If indicated, consider referral to a nutritionist. Consider medication if diet alone is not sufficient to reduce cholesterol to goal.
> - Exercise regularly. Even brisk walking increases and maintains cardiac health.
> - Cease smoking. Various behavioral programs and medications may assist.
> - Monitor blood pressure, blood glucose, inflammatory markers, and lipids annually.

+ Effect of a barrel chest or pectus deformity
+ Xanthelasma (yellowish deposit of fat underneath the skin)
+ Funduscopic changes of hypertension
+ Ascites or pitting edema
+ Abdominal aortic bruit

In assessing cardiac function, it is a common error to auscultate the heart first. It is important to follow the proper sequence, beginning with inspection and proceeding to palpation, percussion, and performing auscultation last. Use a tangential light source to inspect the chest, allowing shadows to accent the surface flicker of any underlying cardiac movement. The room should be quiet because subtle, low-pitched sounds are hard to hear. Stand to the patient's right, at least at the start. A thorough examination of the heart requires the patient to assume a variety of positions: sitting erect and leaning forward, lying supine, and left lateral recumbent position. These changes in position mandate a comfortable examining table on which movement is easy. Large breasts can make examination difficult. Either you or the patient can move the left breast up and to the left.

Inspection

In most adults the apical impulse is visible at about the midclavicular line in the fifth left intercostal space, but it is easily obscured by obesity, large breasts, or muscularity. In some patients it may be visible in the fourth left intercostal space. It should be seen in only one intercostal space if the heart is healthy. In some adults the apical impulse may become visible only when the patient sits up and the heart is brought closer to the anterior wall.

FIGURE 14-12 Sequence for palpation of the precordium. **A,** Apex. **B,** Left sternal border. **C,** Base.

Examination findings are affected by the shape and thickness of the chest wall and the amount of tissue, air, and fluid through which the impulses are transmitted. For example, a readily visible and palpable impulse when the patient is supine suggests an intensity that may be the result of a problem. The absence of an apical impulse in addition to faint heart sounds, particularly when the patient is in the left lateral recumbent position, suggests some intervening extracardiac problem, such as pleural or pericardial fluid.

Inspection of other organs may reflect important information about the cardiac status. For example, inspecting the skin for cyanosis or venous distention and inspecting the nail bed for cyanosis and capillary refill time provide valuable clues to the cardiac evaluation.

Palpation

Make sure that your hands are warm, and with the patient supine, palpate the precordium. Use the proximal halves of the four fingers held gently together or use the whole hand. Touch lightly and let the cardiac movements rise to your hand because sensation decreases as you increase pressure.

As always, be methodical. One suggested sequence is to begin at the apex, move to the inferior left sternal border, then move up the sternum to the base and down the right sternal border and into the epigastrium or axillae if the circumstance dictates (Fig. 14-12).

Feel for the apical impulse and identify its location by the intercostal space and the distance from the midsternal line. The point at which the apical impulse is most readily seen or felt should be described as the *point of maximal impulse* (PMI).

Angle of Louis

FIGURE 14-13 Palpation of the apical pulse.

The PMI is typically noted at the left 5th intercostal space, midclavicular line in adults and 4th intercostal space medial to the nipple in children. Determine the diameter of the area in which it is felt. Usually it is palpable within a small diameter—no more than 1 cm. The impulse is usually gentle and brief, not lasting as long as systole. In some adults, the apical impulse is not felt because of the thickness of the chest wall (Fig. 14-13).

If the apical impulse is more vigorous than expected, characterize it as a *heave* or *lift.* An apical impulse that is more forceful and widely distributed, fills systole, or is displaced laterally and downward may indicate increased cardiac output or left ventricular hypertrophy. A lift along the left sternal border may be caused by right ventricular hypertrophy. A loss of thrust

EXAMINATION AND FINDINGS

Box 14-4 The Thrill of Heart Examination

A murmur at the grade IV level or more can be felt (see Tables 14-4 and 14-5). This palpable sensation is called a *thrill*. It may be appreciated in systole or diastole. The following are common:

Timing	Location	Probable Cause
Systole	Suprasternal notch and/or second and third right intercostal space	Aortic stenosis
	Suprasternal notch and/or second and third left intercostal space	Pulmonic stenosis
	Fourth left intercostal space	Ventricular septal defect
	Apex	Mitral regurgitation
	Left lower sternal border	Tetralogy of Fallot
	Left upper sternal border, often with extensive radiation	Patent ductus arteriosus
Diastole	Right sternal border	Aortic regurgitation
		Aneurysm of ascending aorta
	Apex	Mitral stenosis

FIGURE 14-14 Palpation of the carotid artery to time events felt over the precordium.

may be related to overlying fluid or air or to displacement beneath the sternum. Displacement of the apical impulse to the right without a loss or gain in thrust suggests dextrocardia, diaphragmatic hernia, distended stomach, or a pulmonary abnormality.

Feel for a *thrill*—a fine, palpable, rushing vibration, a palpable murmur, often, but not always, over the base of the heart in the area of the right or left second intercostal space. It generally indicates turbulence or a disruption of the expected blood flow related to some defect in the closure of the aortic or pulmonic valve (generally aortic or pulmonic stenosis), pulmonary hypertension, or atrial septal defect (Box 14-4). Locate each sensation in terms of its intercostal space and relationship to the midsternal, midclavicular, or axillary lines. Chapter 13 describes the method for counting ribs and intercostal spaces.

While palpating the precordium, use your other hand to palpate the carotid artery so that you can describe the finding in relation to the cardiac cycle. The carotid pulse and S_1 are practically synchronous. The carotid pulse is located just medial to and below the angle of the jaw (Fig. 14-14).

Percussion

Percussion is of limited value in defining the borders of the heart or determining its size because the shape of the chest is relatively rigid and can make the more malleable heart conform. Left ventricular size is better judged by the location of the apical impulse. The right ventricle tends to enlarge in the anteroposterior diameter rather than laterally, thus diminishing the value of percussion of the right heart border. Obesity, unusual muscular development, and some pathologic conditions (e.g., presence of

air or fluids) can also easily distort the findings. A chest radiograph is far more useful in defining the heart borders.

If radiographic facilities are unavailable, percussion can be used to estimate the size of the heart. Begin tapping at the anterior axillary line, moving medially along the intercostal spaces toward the sternal border. The change from a resonant to a dull note marks the cardiac border. Note these points with a marking pen and the outline of the heart is visually defined. On the left, the loss of resonance will generally be close to the PMI at the apex of the heart. Measure this point from the midsternal line at each intercostal space and record that distance. When percussing the right cardiac border, a change in resonance is usually noted when the right sternal border is encountered. The right heart border is only found if it extends beyond the sternal border.

Auscultation

Because all heart sounds are of relatively low frequency, in a range somewhat difficult for the human ear to detect, you must ensure a quiet environment. Because shivering and movement increase adventitious sound, and because comfort is important, make certain the patient is warm and relaxed before beginning. Always place a comfortably warm stethoscope on the unclothed chest. You must also learn to appreciate the differences in findings when the chest is thin and nonmuscular (i.e., sounds are louder, closer) or muscular or obese (i.e., sounds are dimmer, more distant).

Because sound is transmitted in the direction of blood flow, specific heart sounds are best heard in areas where the blood flows after it passes through a valve (see Clinical Pearl, "Heart Sounds"). Approach each of the precordial areas systematically in a sequence that is comfortable for you, working your way from base to apex or apex to base (Box 14-5). Because the site of the apex of the heart may be changed by elevation of the diaphragm from pregnancy, ascites, or other intraabdominal condition, many health care providers prefer to begin their examination at the base of the heart.

Second right
interspace

PULMONIC
VALVE

AORTIC VALVE

Second left
interspace

MITRAL VALVE

Third left
interspace

TRICUSPID
VALVE

Fourth left
interspace

Fifth left
interspace
(mitral apical)

FIGURE 14-15 Areas for auscultation of the heart.

Clinical Pearl

Heart Sounds

It is a common error to try to hear all of the sounds in the cardiac cycle at once. Take the time to isolate each sound and each pause in the cardiac cycle, listening separately and selectively for as many beats as necessary to evaluate the sounds. It takes time to tune in; do not rush. Avoid jumping the stethoscope from one site to another; instead, inch the endpiece along the route. This maneuver helps prevent missing important sounds, such as more widely transmitted abnormal sounds. It also allows you to track a sound from its loudest point to its farthest reach (e.g., into the axilla or the back).

Auscultation should be performed in, but not be limited to, each of the five cardiac areas, using first the diaphragm and then the bell of the stethoscope. Use firm pressure with the diaphragm (best for higher frequency sounds) and light pressure with the bell (best with low-frequency sounds). The five traditional auscultatory areas are located as follows (Fig. 14-15):

+ Aortic valve area: second right intercostal space at the right sternal border
+ Pulmonic valve area: second left intercostal space at the left sternal border
+ Second pulmonic area: third left intercostal space at the left sternal border
+ Tricuspid area: fourth left intercostal space along the lower left sternal border
+ Mitral (or apical) area: at the apex of the heart in the fifth left intercostal space at the midclavicular line

Assess the rate and rhythm of the heart at one auscultatory site where the tones are easily heard. Note that site. If the cardiac rhythm is irregular, compare the beats per minute over the heart (apical heart rate) with the radial pulse rate. Note any deficit.

Instruct the patient to breathe normally and then hold the breath in expiration. Listen for S_1 while you palpate the carotid pulse. S_1 marks the beginning of systole. S_1 coincides with the

rise (upswing) of the carotid pulse. Note the intensity, any variations, the effect of respirations, and any splitting of S_1.

Concentrate on systole, listening for any extra sounds or murmurs.

S_2 marks the initiation of diastole and closure of the aortic and pulmonic valves. Concentrate on diastole, usually a longer interval than systole, listening for any extra sounds or murmurs. Keep in mind that systole and diastole are equal in duration when the heart rate is rapid.

Instruct the patient to inhale deeply, listening closely for S_2 to become two components (split S_2) during inspiration. Split S_2 is best heard in the pulmonic auscultatory area.

Areas for inspection, palpation, and auscultation change if the heart is not located in its expected place in the left mediastinum. In situs inversus and dextrocardia, the heart is rotated to the right. In such a circumstance, adjust to the anatomic alteration by thinking of the examination sites as they would be in a mirror image of the expected location.

Basic Heart Sounds

Heart sounds are characterized in much the same way as respiratory and other body sounds: by pitch, intensity, duration, and timing in the cardiac cycle. Heart sounds are relatively low in pitch, except in the presence of significant pathologic events. Table 14-2 summarizes their relative differences in intensity by auscultatory area (also see Fig. 14-19).

The four basic heart sounds are S_1, S_2, S_3, and S_4. Of these, S_1 and S_2 are the most distinct heart sounds and should be characterized separately because variations can offer important clues to cardiac function. S_3 and S_4 may or may not be present. Their absence is not an unusual finding, and their presence does not necessarily indicate a pathologic condition. Thus, evaluate S_3 and S_4 in relation to other sounds and events in the cardiac cycle.

S_1 and S_2. S_1, which results from closure of the mitral and tricuspid (AV) valves, indicates the beginning of systole. It is best

Box 14-5 | **Procedure for Auscultating the Heart**

Adopt a routine for the various positions the patient is asked to assume for auscultating the heart; however, be prepared to alter the sequence if the patient's condition requires it. Instruct the patient when to breathe comfortably and when to hold the breath in expiration and inspiration. Listen carefully for each heart sound, isolating each component of the cardiac cycle, especially while the respirations are momentarily suspended. The following sequence is suggested:

Patient sitting up and leaning slightly forward and, preferably, in expiration: listen in all five areas (Fig. 14-16, *A*). This is the best position

to hear relatively high-pitched murmurs with the stethoscope diaphragm.

Patient supine: listen in all five areas (see Fig. 14-16, *B*).

Patient left lateral recumbent: listen in all five areas. This is the best position to hear the low-pitched filling sounds in diastole with the stethoscope bell (see Fig. 14-16, *C*).

Other positions depend on your findings. Patient right lateral recumbent is the best position for evaluating a right rotated heart of dextrocardia. Listen in all five areas.

FIGURE 14-16 Auscultation positions.

heard toward the apex where it is usually louder than S_2 (Box 14-6). At the base, S_1 is louder on the left than on the right but softer than S_2 in both areas. It is lower in pitch and a bit longer than S_2, and it occurs immediately after diastole (Fig. 14-17).

Although there is some asynchrony between closure of the mitral and tricuspid valves, S_1 is usually heard as one sound. If the asynchrony is more marked than usual, the sound may be split and is best heard in the tricuspid area. Other variations in S_1 depend on the competence of the pulmonary and systemic circulations, the structure of the heart valves, their position when ventricular contraction begins, and the force of the contraction.

S_2, the result of closure of the aortic and pulmonic (semilunar) valves, indicates the end of systole and is best heard in the aortic and pulmonic areas. It is of higher pitch and shorter duration than S_1. S_2 is louder than S_1 at the base of the heart; still, it is usually softer than S_1 at the apex (Box 14-7).

Splitting. Splitting occurs when the mitral and tricuspid valves or the pulmonic and aortic valves do not close simultane-

Table 14-2 | **Intensity of Heart Sounds According to Auscultatory Area**

	Aortic	Pulmonic	Second Pulmonic	Mitral	Tricuspid
Pitch	$S_1 < S_2$	$S_1 < S_2$	$S_1 < S_2$	$S_1 > S_2$	$S_1 = S_2$
Loudness	$S_1 < S_2$	$S_1 < S_2$	$S_1 < S_2$*	$S_1 > S_2$†	$S_1 > S_2$
Duration	$S_1 > S_2$	$S_1 > S_2$	$S_1 > S_2$	$S_1 > S_2$	$S_1 > S_2$
S_2 split	> inhalation in all auscultatory areas, the S_2 split may not be audible in the mitral area if P_2 is inaudible < exhalation in all auscultatory areas				
A_2	Loudest	Loud	Decreased		
P_2	Decreased	Louder	Loudest		

*S_1 is relatively louder in second pulmonic area than in aortic area.
†S_1 may be louder in mitral area than in tricuspid area.

Box 14-6 S₁ Intensity: Diagnostic Clues

When systole begins with the mitral valve open, the valve snaps shut more vigorously, producing a louder S_1. This occurs in the following situations:

- Blood velocity is increased (e.g., with anemia, fever, hyperthyroidism, anxiety, and during exercise).
- The mitral valve is stenotic.

  If the mitral valve is not completely open, ventricular contraction forces it shut. The loudness produced by valve closure depends on the degree of opening:

- S_1 intensity is increased in the following situations:
  - Complete heart block is present.
  - Gross disruption of rhythm occurs, such as during fibrillation.
- The intensity of S_1 is decreased in the following situations:
  - Increased overlying tissue, fat, or fluid (e.g., as in emphysema, obesity, or pericardial fluid) obscures sounds.
  - Systemic or pulmonary hypertension is present, which contributes to more forceful atrial contraction. If the ventricle is noncompliant, the contraction may be delayed or diminished, especially if the valve is partially closed when contraction begins.
  - Fibrosis and calcification of a diseased mitral valve can result from rheumatic heart disease. Calcification diminishes valve flexibility so that it closes with less force.

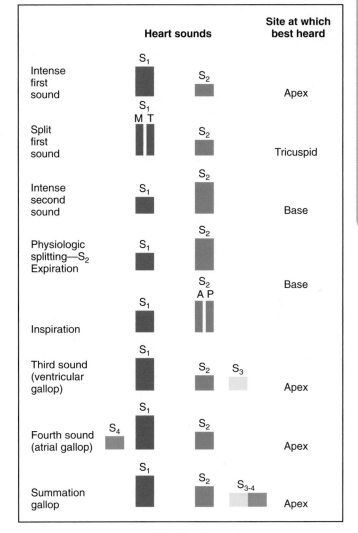

FIGURE 14-17 Heart sounds.

ously. Splitting of S_1 is not usually heard because the sound of the tricuspid valve closing is too faint to hear. Rarely, however, it may be audible in the tricuspid area, particularly on deep inspiration.

S_2 is actually two sounds that merge during expiration. The closure of the aortic valve (A_2) contributes most of the sound of S_2 when it is heard in the aortic or pulmonic areas. A_2 tends to mask the sound of pulmonic valve closure (P_2). During inspiration, P_2 occurs slightly later, giving S_2 two distinct components; this is a split S_2. Splitting is more often heard and easier to detect in the young; it is not well heard in older adults. This may be because of the tendency of the anteroposterior diameter of the chest to increase with age.

Splitting of S_2 is an expected event because pressures are higher and depolarization occurs earlier on the left side of the heart. During inspiration, the lungs fill with air as the chest wall expands. The intrathoracic pressure becomes more negative and this increases venous blood return from the body into the right atrium, and right ventricle. Simultaneously, the blood volume returning from the lungs into the left ventricle is reduced (the blood wants to stay in the lungs because of the negative intrathoracic pressure). The increased blood volume in the right ventricle during inspiration causes the pulmonary valve (P_2) to stay open longer during systole, whereas the aortic valve (A_2) closes slightly earlier due to reduced blood volume in the left ventricle (see Fig. 14-17). Ejection times tend to equalize when the breath is held in expiration, so this maneuver also tends to eliminate the split. The respiratory cycle is not always the dominant factor in splitting; the interval between the components may remain easily discernible throughout the respiratory cycle (Box 14-8).

Box 14-7 S₂ Intensity: Diagnostic Clues

The intensity of S_2 increases in the following conditions:
- Systemic hypertension (S_2 may ring or boom), syphilis of the aortic valve, exercise, or excitement accentuates S_2.
- Pulmonary hypertension, mitral stenosis, and congestive heart failure accentuate P_2.
- The valves are diseased but still fully mobile; the component of S_2 affected depends on which valve is compromised.

  The intensity of S_2 decreases in the following conditions:
- A shocklike state with arterial hypotension causes loss of valvular vigor.
- The valves are immobile, thickened, or calcified; the component of S_2 affected depends on which valve is compromised.
- Aortic stenosis affects A_2.
- Pulmonic stenosis affects P_2.
- Overlying tissue, fat, or fluid mutes S_2.

Box 14-8　Unexpected Splitting of Heart Sounds

Wide Splitting

The split becomes wider when delayed activation of contraction or right ventricle emptying slows pulmonic closure. This occurs, for example, in right bundle branch block, which splits both S_1 and S_2. Wide splitting of S_2 also occurs when stenosis delays closure of the pulmonic valve, when pulmonary hypertension delays ventricular emptying, or when mitral regurgitation induces early closure of the aortic valve. The split becomes narrower and is even eliminated or paradoxical when closure of the aortic valve is delayed, such as in left bundle branch block.

Fixed Splitting

Splitting is said to be fixed when it is unaffected by respiration. This occurs with delayed closure of the pulmonic valve when output of the right ventricle is greater than that of the left. This can occur with large atrial septal defects, a ventricular septal defect with left-to-right shunting, or right ventricular failure.

Paradoxical (Reversed) Splitting

Paradoxical splitting occurs when closure of the aortic valve is delayed (e.g., as in left bundle branch block) so that P_2 occurs first, followed by A_2. In this case, the interval between P_2 and A_1 is heard during expiration and disappears during inspiration.

　　See Figure 14-18 for a visual depiction of variations in splitting of S_2 heart sounds.

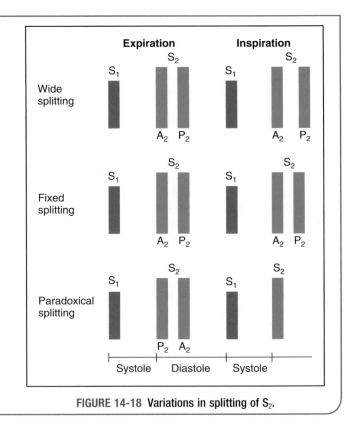

FIGURE 14-18　Variations in splitting of S_2.

S_3 and S_4. During diastole, the ventricles fill in two steps: the early, passive flow of blood from the atria is followed by a more vigorous atrial ejection. The passive phase occurs relatively early in diastole, distending the ventricular walls and causing vibration. The resulting S_3 sound is quiet, low-pitched, and often difficult to hear (see Fig. 14-17). In the second phase of ventricular filling, vibration in the valves, papillae, and ventricular walls produces S_4 (see Fig. 14-17). Because it occurs so late in diastole (presystole), S_4 may be confused with a split S_1.

S_3 and S_4 should be quiet and therefore somewhat difficult to hear. Increasing venous return (by asking the patient to raise a leg or inhale) or arterial pressure (by asking the patient to grip your hand vigorously and repeatedly) may make these sounds easier to hear (see Fig. 14-19). When S_3 becomes intense and easy to hear, the resulting sequence of sounds simulates a gallop; this is the early diastolic gallop rhythm. It may be best heard when the patient is in the left lateral decubitus (recumbent) position. S_4 may also become more intense, producing a readily discernible presystolic gallop rhythm. S_4 is most commonly heard in older patients, but it may be heard at any age when there is increased resistance to filling because the ventricular walls have lost compliance (e.g., in hypertensive disease and coronary artery disease) or with the increased stroke volume of high-output states (e.g., in profound anemia, pregnancy, and thyrotoxicosis). The rhythm of the heart sound when an S_3 is heard resembles the rhythm of pronouncing the word Ken-TUCK-y. When an S_4 is heard, it resembles the rhythm of pronouncing the word TEN-nes-see. A loud S_4 always suggests pathology and deserves additional evaluation.

The cardiac valves generally open noiselessly unless thickened, roughened, or otherwise altered as a result of disease. Valvular stenosis may produce an opening snap (mitral valve), ejection clicks (semilunar valves), or mid to late nonejection systolic clicks (mitral prolapse). The pulmonary ejection click is best heard on expiration in the second left intercostal space and is seldom heard on inspiration; aortic ejection clicks are less sharp, are less involved with S_1, and may be heard in the second right intercostal space. Extra heart sounds often accompany murmurs and should always be considered indicative of a pathologic process.

Extra Heart Sounds

A pericardial friction rub can be easily mistaken for cardiac-generated sounds. Inflammation of the pericardial sac causes a roughening of the parietal and visceral surfaces, which produces a rubbing machine-like sound audible on auscultation. It occupies both systole and diastole and overlies the intracardiac sounds. A pericardial friction rub may have three components that are associated in sequence with the atrial component of systole, ventricular systole, and ventricular diastole. It is usually heard widely but is more distinct toward the apex. A three-component friction rub may be intense enough to obscure the heart sounds. If there are only one or two components, the sound may not be intense or machine-like and may then be more

Heart sounds	First heart sound [$S_1(M_1T_1)$]	Second heart sound [$S_2(A_2P_2)$]	Third heart sound (S_3, ventricular gallop)	Fourth heart sound (S_4, atrial gallop)
Anatomic reference				
Preferable position of patient	Any position	Sitting or supine	Supine or left lateral	Supine or left semilateral
Area for auscultation	Entire precordium (apex)	A_2 at 2nd RICS P_2 at 2nd LICS	Apex	Apex
Endpiece	Diaphragm	Diaphragm	Bell	Bell
Pitch	High	High	Low	Low
Effects of respiration	Softer on inspiration	Fusion of A_2P_2 on expiration; physiologic split on inspiration	Increased on inspiration	Increased on inspiration
External influences	Increased with excitement, exercise, amyl nitrate, epinephrine, and atropine	Increased with thin chest walls and with exercise	Increased with exercise, fast heart rate, elevation of legs, and increased venous return	Increased with exercise, fast heart rate, elevation of legs, and increased venous return
Cause	Closure of tricuspid and mitral valves	Closure of pulmonic and aortic valves	Rapid ventricular filling	Forceful atrial ejection into distended ventricle

Continued

FIGURE 14-19 **Assessment of heart sounds.** *LICS*, Left intercostal space; *RICS*, right intercostal space. *(Modified from Guzzetta and Dossey, 1992.)*

difficult to distinguish from an intracardiac murmur. The detection of extra heart sounds is detailed in Table 14-3, along with associated causes (Fig. 14-19). See Clinical Pearl, "Heart Sounds after Surgical Procedures."

Clinical Pearl

Heart Sounds After Surgical Procedures
You should always know, based on history and chest inspection, if a patient has had a cardiac surgical procedure. If this involves placement of a prosthetic mitral valve, listen for a distinct click early in diastole, loudest at the apex and transmitted precordially. A prosthetic aortic valve causes a sound in early systole. The intensity of these sounds depends on the type of material used for the prosthesis. Animal tissue is the quietest and may even be silent. Pacemakers do not cause a sound.

Heart Murmurs

Heart murmurs are relatively prolonged extra sounds heard during systole or diastole. They often indicate a problem. Murmurs are caused by some disruption in the flow of blood into, through, or out of the heart. The characteristics of a murmur depend on the adequacy of valve function, the size of the opening, the rate of blood flow, the vigor of the myocardium, and the thickness and consistency of the overlying tissues through which the murmur must be heard.

Diseased valves, a common cause of murmurs, either do not open or close well. When the leaflets are thickened and the passage narrowed, forward blood flow is restricted (stenosis). When valve leaflets, which are intended to fit together snugly, lose competency and leak, blood flows backward (regurgitation). Table 14-4 summarizes the characteristics of the heart murmurs. Murmurs are described in many ways (e.g., harsh, blowing,

Audio: Friction Rubs

Audio: Various Types of Murmurs

EXAMINATION AND FINDINGS

Quadruple rhythm	Summation gallop (triple gallop)	Ejection sounds	Systolic click	Opening snap
S_4S_1 S_2 S_3 S_4S_1 S_2	S_{3-4} S_1 S_2 S_{3-4} S_1 S_2	S_1 S_2 S_1 S_2	S_1 S_2 S_1 S_2	S_1 S_2 S_1 S_2
Supine or left lateral	Supine or left lateral	Sitting or supine	Sitting or supine	Any position
Apex	Apex	2nd RICS, 2nd LICS, or apex	Apex	Apex
Bell	Bell	Diaphragm	Diaphragm	Diaphragm
Low	Low	High	High	High
Increased on inspiration	Increased on inspiration	Increased on expiration with pulmonary stenosis	Increased on inspiration	Uninfluenced by inspiration
Aortic ejection sound same as S_1 and S_2; pulmonary ejection sound increased on expiration	Aortic ejection sound same as S_1 and S_2; pulmonary ejection sound increased on expiration	Aortic ejection sound same as S_1 and S_2; pulmonary ejection sound increased on expiration	Occurs later in systole with increased venous return (e.g., with elevated legs or supine position)	May be confused with S_3
S_1, S_2, S_3, and S_4, all heard separately	S_3 and S_4 fuse with fast heart rates	Opening of deformed semi-lunar valves	Prolapse of mitral valve leaflet	Abrupt recoil of stenotic mitral or tricuspid valve

FIGURE 14-19, cont'd

musical). Such descriptions may or may not be consistent with the way you hear the sounds. Do not hesitate to use words that best suit your interpretation.

The most common source of significant murmurs is anatomic disorders of the heart valves (Fig. 14-20 and Table 14-5).

The discovery of a heart murmur requires careful assessment and diagnosis. Although some murmurs are benign (Box 14-9), others represent a pathologic process. Often additional testing is mandatory before a murmur is dismissed as functional.

Not all murmurs, however, are the result of valvular defects. Other causes include the following:

+ High output demands that increase speed of blood flow (e.g., fever, thyrotoxicosis, anemia, pregnancy)

+ Structural defects, either congenital or acquired, that allow blood to flow through inappropriate pathways (e.g., atrial or ventricular septal defects)
+ Diminished strength of myocardial contraction
+ Altered blood flow in the major vessels near the heart
+ Transmitted murmurs resulting from valvular aortic stenosis, ruptured chordae tendineae of the mitral valve, or severe aortic regurgitation
+ Vigorous left ventricular ejection (more common in children than in adults)
+ Persistence of fetal circulation (e.g., patent ductus arteriosus)

It is not always possible on physical examination to identify with consistency the cause of a systolic murmur.

Table 14-3 | Extra Heart Sounds

Sounds	Detection	Timing and Description
Increased S_3	Bell at apex; patient in left lateral recumbent position	Early diastole, low pitch
Increased S_4	Bell at apex, patient supine or in left lateral recumbent position	Late diastole or early systole, low pitch
Gallops	Bell at apex; patient supine or in left lateral recumbent position	Presystole, intense, easily heard
Mitral valve opening snap	Diaphragm medial to apex, may radiate to base; any position, second left intercostal space	Early diastole briefly, before S_3; high pitch, sharp snap or click; not affected by respiration; easily confused with S_2
Aortic valve ejection click	Apex, base in second right intercostal space; patient sitting or supine	Early systole, intense, high pitch; radiates; not affected by respirations
Pulmonary valve ejection click	Second left intercostal space at sternal border; patient sitting or supine	Early systole, less intense than aortic click; intensifies on expiration, decreased on inspiration
Pericardial friction rub	Widely heard, sound clearest toward apex	May occupy all of systole and diastole; intense, grating, machine-like; may have three components and obliterate heart sounds; if only one or two components, may sound like murmur

Table 14-4 | Characterization of Heart Murmurs

	Classification	Description
Timing and duration*	Early systolic	Begins with S_1, decrescendos, ends well before S_2
	Midsystolic (ejection)	Begins after S_1, ends before S_2; crescendo-decrescendo quality sometimes difficult to discern
	Late systolic	Begins mid to late systole, crescendos, ends at S_2; often introduced by mid to late systolic clicks
	Early diastolic	Begins with S_2
	Mid-diastolic	Begins at clear interval after S_2
	Late diastolic (presystolic)	Begins immediately before S_1
	Holosystolic (pansystolic)	Begins with S_1, occupies all of systole, ends at S_2
	Holodiastolic (pandiastolic)	Begins with S_2, occupies all of diastole, ends at S_1
	Continuous	Starts in systole, continues without interruption through S_2, into all or part of diastole; does not necessarily persist throughout entire cardiac cycle
Pitch	High, medium, low	Depends on pressure and rate of blood flow; low pitch is heard best with the bell
Intensity†	Grade I	Barely audible in quiet room
	Grade II	Quiet but clearly audible
	Grade III	Moderately loud
	Grade IV	Loud, associated with thrill
	Grade V	Very loud, thrill easily palpable
	Grade VI	Very loud, audible with stethoscope not in contact with chest, thrill palpable and visible
Pattern	Crescendo	Increasing intensity caused by increased blood velocity
	Decrescendo	Decreasing intensity caused by decreased blood velocity
	Square or plateau	Constant intensity
Quality	Harsh, raspy, machine-like, vibratory, musical, blowing	Quality depends on several factors, including degree of valve compromise, force of contractions, blood volume
Location	Anatomic landmarks (e.g., second left intercostal space on sternal border)	Area of greatest intensity, usually area to which valve sounds are normally transmitted
Radiation	Anatomic landmarks (e.g., to axilla or carotid arteries)	Site farthest from location of greatest intensity at which sound is still heard; sound usually transmitted in direction of blood flow
Respiratory phase	Intensity, quality, and timing may vary	Variations associated with venous return increase on inspiration or decrease on expiration

*Systolic murmurs are best described according to time of onset and termination; diastolic murmurs are best classified according to time of onset only.
†Discrimination among the six grades is more difficult for the diastolic murmur than for the systolic.

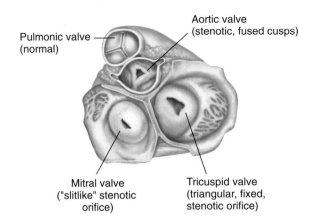

Pulmonic valve (normal)

Aortic valve (stenotic, fused cusps)

Mitral valve ("slitlike" stenotic orifice)

Tricuspid valve (triangular, fixed, stenotic orifice)

FIGURE 14-20 Valvular heart disease. *(Modified from Canobbio, 1990.)*

Table 14-5   Heart Murmurs

Type and Detection	Findings on Examination	Description	
Mitral Stenosis Heard with bell at apex, patient in left lateral decubitus position	Low-frequency diastolic rumble, more intense in early and late diastole, does not radiate; systole usually quiet; palpable thrill at apex in late diastole common; S₁ increased and often palpable at left sternal border; S₂ split often with accented P₂; opening snap follows P₂ closely Visible lift in right parasternal area if right ventricle hypertrophied Arterial pulse amplitude decreased	Narrowed valve restricts forward flow; forceful ejection into ventricle Often occurs with mitral regurgitation Caused by rheumatic fever or cardiac infection	Mitral valve Mitral valve stenosis
Aortic Stenosis Heard over aortic area; ejection sound at second right intercostal border	Midsystolic (ejection) murmur, medium pitch, coarse, diamond-shaped,* crescendo-decrescendo; radiates along left sternal border (sometimes to apex) and to carotid with palpable thrill; S₁ often heard best at apex, disappearing when stenosis is severe, often followed by ejection click; S₂ soft or absent and may not be split; S₄ palpable; ejection sound muted in calcified valves; the more severe the stenosis, the later the peak of the murmur in systole Apical thrust shifts down and left and is prolonged if left ventricular hypertrophy is also present	Calcification of valve cusps restricts forward flow; forceful ejection from ventricle into systemic circulation Caused by congenital bicuspid (rather than the usual tricuspid) valve, rheumatic heart disease, atherosclerosis May be the cause of sudden death, particularly in children and adolescents, either at rest or during exercise; risk apparently related to degree of stenosis	Aortic valve Aortic valve stenosis

In the image for Mitral Stenosis row: "Mitral valve" with label "Mitral valve stenosis"

In the image for Aortic Stenosis row: "Aortic valve" with label "Aortic valve stenosis"

Table 14-5   Heart Murmurs—cont'd

Type and Detection	Findings on Examination	Description	
Subaortic Stenosis Heard at apex and along left sternal border	Murmur fills systole, diamond-shaped, medium pitch, coarse; thrill often palpable during systole at apex and right sternal border; multiple waves in apical impulses; S_2 usually split; S_3 and S_4 often present Arterial pulse brisk, double wave in carotid common; jugular venous pulse prominent	Fibrous ring, usually 1 to 4 mm below aortic valve; most pronounced on ventricular septal side; may become progressively severe with time; difficult to distinguish from aortic stenosis on clinical grounds alone	Subaortic fibrous ring Subaortic stenosis
Pulmonic Stenosis Heard over pulmonic area radiating to left and into neck; thrill in second and third left intercostal spaces	Systolic (ejection) murmur, diamond-shaped, medium pitch, coarse; usually with thrill; S_1 often followed quickly by ejection click; S_2 often diminished, usually wide split; P_2 soft or absent; S_4 common in right ventricular hypertrophy; murmur may be prolonged and confused with that of a ventricular septal defect	Valve restricts forward flow; forceful ejection from ventricle into pulmonary circulation Cause is almost always congenital	Pulmonic valve Pulmonic valve stenosis
Tricuspid Stenosis Heard with bell over tricuspid area	Diastolic rumble accentuated early and late in diastole, resembling mitral stenosis but louder on inspiration; diastolic thrill palpable over right ventricle; S_2 may be split during inspiration Arterial pulse amplitude decreased; jugular venous pulse prominent, especially a wave; slow fall of v wave (see Chapter 15)	Calcification of valve cusps restricts forward flow; forceful ejection into ventricles Usually seen with mitral stenosis, rarely occurs alone Caused by rheumatic heart disease, congenital defect, endocardial fibroelastosis, right atrial myxoma	Tricuspid valve Tricuspid valve stenosis

Continued

EXAMINATION AND FINDINGS

Table 14-5   Heart Murmurs—cont'd

Type and Detection	Findings on Examination	Description	
Mitral Regurgitation Heard best at apex; loudest there, transmitted into left axilla	Holosystolic, plateau-shaped intensity, high pitch, harsh blowing quality, often quite loud and may obliterate S_2; radiates from apex to base or to left axilla; thrill may be palpable at apex during systole; S_1 intensity diminished; S_2 more intense with P_2 often accented; S_3 often present; S_3-S_4 gallop common in late disease If mild, late systolic murmur crescendos; if severe, early systolic intensity decrescendos; apical thrust more to left and down in ventricular hypertrophy	Valve incompetence allows backflow from ventricle to atrium Caused by rheumatic fever, myocardial infarction, myxoma, rupture of chordae	Mitral regurgitation (heart in systole)
Mitral Valve Prolapse Heard at apex and left lower sternal border; easily missed in supine position; also listen with patient upright	Typically late systolic murmur preceded by midsystolic clicks, but both murmur and clicks highly variable in intensity and timing	Valve is competent early in systole but prolapses into atrium later in systole; may become progressively severe, resulting in a holosystolic murmur; often concurrent with pectus excavatum	Mitral valve Mitral valve prolapse (heart in systole)
Aortic Regurgitation Heard with diaphragm, patient sitting and leaning forward; Austin-Flint murmur heard with bell; ejection click heard in second intercostal space	Early diastolic, high pitch, blowing, often with diamond-shaped midsystolic murmur, sounds often not prominent; duration varies with blood pressure; low-pitched, rumbling murmur at apex common (Austin-Flint); early ejection click sometimes present; S_1 soft; S_2 split may have drumlike quality; M_1 and A_2 often intensified, S_3-S_4 gallop common In left ventricular hypertrophy, prominent prolonged apical impulse down and to left Pulse pressure wide; water-hammer or Corrigan pulse common in carotid, brachial, and femoral arteries (see Chapter 15)	Valve incompetence allows backflow from aorta to ventricle Caused by rheumatic heart disease, endocarditis, aortic diseases (Marfan syndrome, medial necrosis), syphilis, ankylosing spondylitis, dissection, cardiac trauma	Aortic regurgitation (heart in diastole)

Table 14-5	Heart Murmurs—cont'd		
Type and Detection	**Findings on Examination**	**Description**	
Pulmonic Regurgitation	Difficult to distinguish from aortic regurgitation on physical examination	Valve incompetence allows backflow from pulmonary artery to ventricle Secondary to pulmonary hypertension or bacterial endocarditis	
Tricuspid Regurgitation Heard at left lower sternum, occasionally radiating a few centimeters to left	Holosystolic murmur over right ventricle, blowing, increased on inspiration; S_3 and thrill over tricuspid area common In pulmonary hypertension, pulmonary artery impulse palpable over second left intercostal space and P_2 accented; in right ventricular hypertrophy, visible lift to right of sternum Jugular venous pulse has large v waves (see Chapter 15)	Valve incompetence allows backflow from ventricle to atrium Caused by congenital defects, bacterial endocarditis (especially in IV drug abusers), pulmonary hypertension, cardiac trauma	

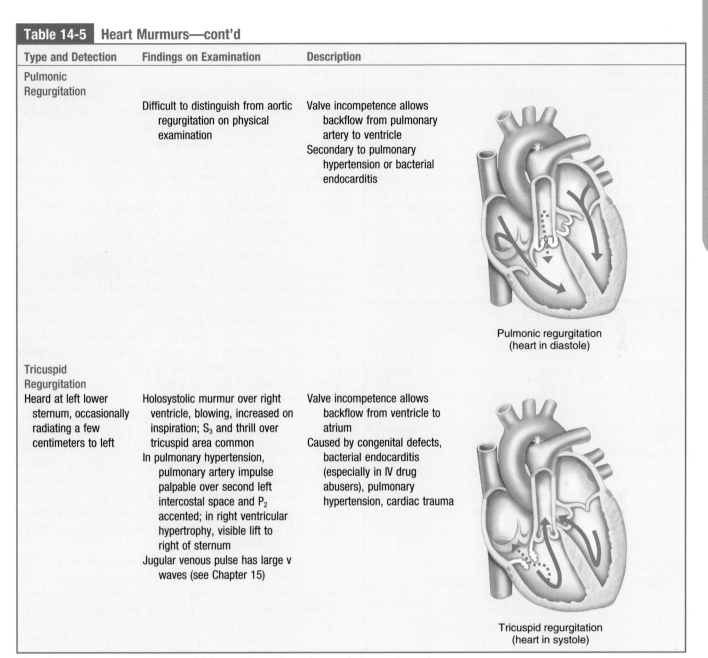

Pulmonic regurgitation
(heart in diastole)

Tricuspid regurgitation
(heart in systole)

*Diamond-shaped murmur is named for its recorded shape on phonocardiogram (a crescendo-decrescendo sound).

Box 14-9 Are Some Murmurs Innocent?

Many murmurs—particularly in children, adolescents, and especially in young athletes—have no apparent cause and are also called *Still murmurs* (named after the physician who first described them). They are presumably a result of vigorous myocardial contraction, the consequent stronger blood flow in early systole or midsystole, and the rush of blood from the larger chamber of the heart into the smaller bore of a blood vessel. The thinner chests of the young make these sounds easier to hear, particularly with a lightly held bell. They are usually grade I or II, usually midsystolic, without radiation, medium pitch, blowing, brief, and often accompanied by splitting of S_2. They are often located in the second left intercostal space near the left sternal border. Such murmurs heard in a recumbent position may disappear when the patient sits or stands because of the tendency of the blood to pool. Do not confuse an "innocent" murmur with one that is "benign," the result of a structural anomaly that is not severe enough to cause a clinical problem.

Evidence-Based Practice in Physical Examination

Cardiac Murmurs in Children

Structural heart disease is more likely when the murmur is:

- Holosystolic
- Diastolic
- Grade 3 or higher
- Associated with a systolic click
- Increased in intensity with standing
- Of a harsh quality

Chest radiography and electrocardiography rarely assist in the diagnosis of heart murmurs in children. Order echocardiography and consider referral to a pediatric cardiologist for newborns with a heart murmur, even if the child is asymptomatic, because of the higher prevalence of structural heart lesions in this population.

(Frommelt, 2004; Danford, 2000.)

DIFFERENTIAL DIAGNOSIS

Comparison of Systolic Murmurs

Origin	Maneuver	Effect of Intensity
Right-sided chambers	Inspiration	Increase
	Expiration	Decrease
Hypertrophic Cardiomyopathy	Valsalva	Increase
	Squatting to standing	Increase
	Standing to squatting	Decrease
	Passive leg elevation to 45 degrees, patient supine	Decrease
Mitral regurgitation*	Handgrip	Increase
Ventricular septal defect*	Transient arterial occlusion (sphygmomanometer placed on each of patient's upper arms and simultaneously inflated to 20 to 40 mm Hg above patient's previously recorded blood pressures; intensity noted after 20 seconds)	Increase
Aortic stenosis	No maneuver distinguishes this murmur; the diagnosis can be made by exclusion	

*The combination of handgrip, transient arterial occlusion, and inhalation of amyl nitrate will distinguish mitral regurgitation and ventricular septal defect from other causes of systolic murmurs; more than just auscultation is needed to make further distinction.

Rhythm Disturbance

Determine the regularity of the heart rhythm, which should be regular. If it is irregular, determine whether there is a consistent pattern. A heart rate that is irregular but occurs in a repeated pattern may indicate sinus arrhythmia, a cyclic variation of the heart rate characterized by an increasing rate on inspiration and decreasing rate on expiration. An unpredictable, irregular rhythm may indicate heart disease or conduction system impairment (e.g., atrial fibrillation). Please see Chapter 4, Vital Signs, pp. 53-55.

�֍ Infants

Cardiac examination of the newborn presents a challenge because of the immediate change from fetal to systemic and pulmonary circulation. Examine the heart within the first 24 hours of life and again at about 2 to 3 days of age.

Complete evaluation of heart function includes examination of the skin, lungs, and liver. Infants with right-sided congestive heart failure have large, firm livers with the inferior edge as much as 5 to 6 cm below the right costal margin. Unlike adults, this finding may precede that of pulmonary crackles.

Inspect the color of the skin and mucous membranes. The well newborn should be reassuringly pink. A purplish plethora is associated with polycythemia (increased red cell mass), an ashen white color indicates shock, and central cyanosis (i.e., cyanosis of the skin and mucous membranes of the face and upper body) suggests congenital heart disease. Note the distribution and intensity of discoloration, as well as the extent of change after vigorous exertion (e.g., crying). Acrocyanosis, cyanosis of the hands and feet without central cyanosis, does not signify pathology; it usually disappears within a few days, or even a few hours, after birth.

Cyanosis is a characteristic of congenital heart defects that allow mixture of arterial and venous blood or prevent blood flow to the lungs. Severe cyanosis evident at birth or shortly thereafter suggests transposition of the great vessels, tetralogy of Fallot, tricuspid atresia, a severe septal defect, or severe pulmonic stenosis. Cyanosis that does not appear until after the neonatal period suggests pulmonic stenosis, Eisenmenger complex (heart defect that can lead to a right-to-left shunt), tetralogy of Fallot, or large septal defects.

Expect to see and palpate the apical impulse in the newborn at the fourth to fifth left intercostal space just medial to the midclavicular line. The smaller the baby or the thinner the chest, the more obvious it will be. It may be somewhat farther to the right in the first few hours of life, sometimes even substernal.

Note any enlargement of the heart. It is especially important to note the position of the heart if a baby is having trouble breathing. A pneumothorax (lung collapse) shifts the apical impulse away from the area of the pneumothorax. A diaphragmatic hernia, more commonly found on the left, shifts the heart to the right. Dextrocardia results in an apical impulse on the right.

The right ventricle is relatively more vigorous than the left in a well, full-term newborn. If the baby is thin, you might even be able to feel the closure of the pulmonary valve in the second left intercostal space.

S_2 in infants is somewhat higher in pitch and more discrete than S_1. The vigor and quality of the heart sounds of the newborn (and throughout infancy and early childhood) are major indicators of heart function. Diminished vigor may be the only apparent change when an infant is already in heart failure. Splitting of the heart sounds is common. S_2 is usually heard without a split at birth, and then often splits within a few hours. See Clinical Pearl, "The Infant Heart and Liver."

> ### Clinical Pearl
>
> **The Infant Heart and Liver**
> If you push up on the liver, thereby increasing right atrial pressure, the murmur of a left-to-right shunt through a septal opening or patent ductus will disappear briefly, whereas the murmur of a right-to-left shunt will intensify.

S_3 and S_4 are commonly heard in pediatric patients. Increased intensity of either sound is suspect.

Murmurs are relatively common in the newborn until about 48 hours of age. Most are innocent, caused by the transition from fetal to pulmonic circulation rather than by a significant congenital abnormality. These murmurs are usually of grade I or II intensity, systolic, and unaccompanied by other signs and symptoms; they usually disappear within 2 to 3 days. Paradoxically, a significant congenital abnormality may be unaccompanied by a murmur.

If you cannot tell a murmur from respiration, listen while the baby is feeding, or time the sound with the carotid pulsation. Because of the rapid heart rate in infants, the heart sounds are more difficult to evaluate. A murmur heard immediately at birth is apt to be less significant than one continuously noted after the first few hours of life. If a murmur persists beyond the second or third day of life, is intense, fills systole, occupies diastole to any extent, or radiates widely, it must be investigated.

Murmurs that extend beyond S_2 and occupy diastole are said to have a machine-like quality; they may be associated with a patent ductus arteriosus. The murmur should disappear when the patent ductus closes in the first 2 or 3 days of life. Diastolic murmurs, almost always significant, may be transient and possibly related to early closure of the ductus arteriosus or a mild, brief, pulmonary insufficiency.

� Children

The precordium of a child tends to bulge over an enlarged heart if the enlargement is longstanding. A child's thoracic cage, being more cartilaginous and yielding than that of an adult, responds more to the thrust of cardiac enlargement.

Sinus arrhythmia is a physiologic event during childhood. The heart rate varies in a cyclic pattern, usually faster on inspiration and slower on expiration. Most often, other dysrhythmias in children are ectopic in origin (e.g., supraventricular and ventricular ectopic beats). These and a variety of other seeming irregularities require extensive investigation only occasionally. Heart rates in children are discussed in Chapter 4, p. 58.

Most murmurs in infants and children are the result of congenital heart disease; however, Kawasaki disease accounts for most acquired murmurs (see Chapter 15, p. 349).

Some murmurs are innocent. A Still murmur, so-named after the physician who first described it, occurs in active, healthy children between the ages of 3 to 7 years. Caused by the vigorous expulsion of blood from the left ventricle into the aorta, it increases in intensity with activity and diminishes when the child is quiet. It is often described as musical (see Box 14-9).

When examining a child with known heart disease, take careful note of weight gain (or loss), developmental delay, cyanosis, and clubbing of fingers and toes. Cyanosis is a major clue to congenital heart defects that impede oxygenation of blood.

✂ Pregnant Women

The heart position is shifted during pregnancy, but the position varies with the size and position of the uterus. The apical impulse is upward and more lateral by 1 to 1.5 cm. Expect some changes in auscultated heart sounds because of the increased blood volume and extra effort of the heart. More audible splitting of S_1 and S_2, and S_3 may be readily heard after 20 weeks of gestation. A fourth heart sound is abnormal. In addition, systolic ejection murmurs may be heard over the pulmonic area in 90% of pregnant women. The murmur is intensified during inspiration or expiration but should not be louder than grade II (see Table 14-4). There is no significant change in the ECG.

The presence of cyanosis, clubbing, or persistent neck vein distention or the development of a diastolic murmur suggests an abnormality.

✂ Older Adults

You may need to slow the pace of your examination when asking an older patient to assume positions that may be uncomfortable or perhaps too difficult. Some older patients may not be able to lie flat for an extended time, and some may not be able to control their breathing pattern at your request. The cardiac response to even minimal demand may be slowed or insufficient. An abrupt position change may cause a transient light-headedness because of a drop in arterial pressure.

The apical impulse may be harder to find in many persons because of the increased anteroposterior diameter of the chest. In obese older adults, the diaphragm is raised and the heart is more transverse.

Older adults who exercise regularly may reverse or avoid some of the age-associated changes.

S_4 is more common in older adults and may indicate decreased left ventricular compliance. Early, soft physiologic murmurs may be heard, caused by aortic lengthening, tortuosity, and sclerotic changes.

Common ECG changes in older patients include first-degree atrioventricular block, bundle branch blocks, ST-T wave abnormalities, premature systole (atrial and ventricular), left anterior hemiblock, left ventricular hypertrophy, and atrial fibrillation. Occasional ectopic beats are fairly common and may or may not be significant.

ABNORMALITIES

Sample Documentation

History and Physical Examination

Subjective

A 56-year-old man comes to the emergency department complaining of substernal chest pain radiating to the jaw and into the left shoulder for past hour. No relief with antacid tablets. Nauseated. Rates pain as 8 on a scale of 10. Known history of hyperlipidemia.

Objective

Diaphoretic, pale, and grimacing in pain. Heart rate of 124 beats per minute, S_1 and S_2 with a regular rhythm, no murmurs or rubs S_4 noted.

Blood pressure 100/66 mm Hg. Precordium with no visible pulsations and no palpable lifts, heaves, or thrills. There is cyanosis of the finger tips and around lips.

For additional sample documentation, see Chapter 26, pp. 628-631.

ABNORMALITIES

HEART

Angina

Pain caused by myocardial ischemia

Pathophysiology

- Occurs when myocardial oxygen demand exceeds supply
- Can be recurrent or present as initial incidence

Subjective Data

- Substernal pain or intense pressure radiating to the neck, jaws, and arms, particularly the left
- Often accompanied by shortness of breath, fatigue, diaphoresis, faintness, and syncope

Objective Data

- No definitive examination findings suggest angina.
- Tachycardia, tachypnea, hypertension, and/or diaphoresis
- Ischemia may lead to presence of crackles due to pulmonary edema or a reduction in the S_1 intensity or an S_4.
- Physical examination may suggest other comorbidities that place the patient at higher risk for angina symptoms, such as COPD, xanthelasma, hypertension, evidence of peripheral arterial disease, abnormal pulsations on palpation over precordium, murmurs, or arrhythmias.

Bacterial Endocarditis

Bacterial infection of the endothelial layer of the heart and valves

Pathophysiology

- Individuals with congenital or acquired valve defects and those with history of previous endocarditis or who use intravenous drugs are particularly susceptible (Fig. 14-21).

Subjective Data

- Fever, fatigue
- Sudden onset of congestive heart failure (e.g., shortness of breath, ankle edema)

Objective Data

- Murmur
- Signs of neurologic dysfunction
- Janeway lesion (small erythematous or hemorrhagic macules appearing on the palms and soles)
- Osler nodes (appear on the tips of fingers or toes and are caused by septic emboli)

FIGURE 14-21 Bacterial endocarditis. *(Modified from Canobbio, 1990.)*

Congestive Heart Failure (CHF)—Left-Sided

Heart fails to propel blood forward with its usual force, resulting in congestion in the pulmonary circulation

Pathophysiology

- Many causes
- Left ventricular hypertrophy (high blood pressure leading to thickening of the left heart muscle)
- Cardiomyopathy (weakened heart muscle)
- Damaged aortic or mitral heart valves
- Ischemic cardiomyopathy (from coronary artery disease)
- Nonischemic cardiomyopathy
- Toxic exposures, such as alcohol or cocaine
- Viruses, such as coxsackie B
- Left-sided CHF is characterized as systolic or diastolic.
- Diastolic CHF is result of advanced glycation cross-linking collagen and creating a stiff ventricle unable to dilate actively
- Diastolic CHF occurs in older adults with diabetes mellitus whose tissue is exposed to glucose for a longer period of time.

Subjective Data

- Fatigue
- Breathing difficulty, shortness of breath
- Orthopnea
- Exercise intolerance

Objective Data

- Sudden with acute pulmonary edema or gradual symptom onset
- Crackles on pulmonary exam
- Systolic CHF has a narrow pulse pressure.
- Diastolic CHF has a wide pulse pressure.

Evidence-Based Practice in Physical Examination

Can the Clinical Examination Diagnose Left-Sided Heart Failure in Adults?

The most helpful physical exam findings in the diagnosis of left-sided congestive heart failure is jugular venous distention (see Chapter 15, Fig. 15-7, p. 337). Somewhat helpful symptoms and exam findings were the following:

- Dyspnea
- Orthopnea
- Tachycardia
- Decreased systolic or pulse pressure
- Third heart sound
- Crackles on auscultation of the lungs

Edema was found to be helpful diagnostically only if present; the absence of edema is not helpful in ruling out the diagnosis.

(From Badgett et al, 1997.)

Congestive Heart Failure (CHF)—Right-Sided

Heart fails to propel blood forward with its usual force, resulting in congestion in the systemic circulation

Pathophysiology

- Decreased cardiac output causes decreased blood flow to the tissues
- Many causes (see above)

Subjective Data

- Peripheral edema, particularly at the end of the day or after prolonged sitting
- Weight gain

Objective Data

- Pitting edema in lower extremities
- Jugular venous distention

Pericarditis

Inflammation of the pericardium

Pathophysiology

- Often the result of a viral infection such as echovirus or coxsackie virus
- May be seen in:
  - Cancer (including leukemia)
  - HIV infection and AIDS
  - Hypothyroidism
  - Kidney failure
  - Rheumatic fever
  - Tuberculosis
  - Kawasaki disease
- Other causes include:
  - Heart attack
  - Heart surgery or trauma to the chest, esophagus, or heart
  - Certain medications, such as procainamide, hydralazine, phenytoin, isoniazid
  - Radiation therapy to the chest
  - May cause a pericardial effusion, and may increase and result in cardiac tamponade (Fig. 14-22)

Subjective Data

- Sharp and stabbing chest pain (caused by the heart rubbing against the pericardium)
- Pain worse with coughing, swallowing, deep breathing or lying flat, or movement
- Pain relieved by sitting up and leaning forward
- Pain may be most severe when supine, relieved when leaning forward
- Pain in the back, neck or left shoulder
- Difficulty breathing when lying down
- A dry cough
- Anxiety or fatigue

Objective Data

- Scratchy, grating, triphasic friction rub on auscultation, comprises ventricular systole, early diastolic ventricular filling, and late diastolic atrial systole
- Friction rub easily heard just left of the sternum in third and fourth intercostal spaces

FIGURE 14-22 Pericarditis. *(Modified from Canobbio, 1990.)*

Cardiac Tamponade

Excessive accumulation of effused fluids or blood between the pericardium and the heart (Fig. 14-23)

Pathophysiology

- Seriously constrains cardiac relaxation, impairing blood return to the right heart
- Common causes: pericarditis, malignancy, aortic dissection, and trauma

Subjective Data

- Anxiety, restlessness
- Chest pain
- Difficulty breathing
- Discomfort, sometimes relieved by sitting upright or leaning forward
- Syncope, light-headedness
- Pale, gray, or blue skin
- Palpitations
- Rapid breathing
- Swelling of the abdomen or arms or neck veins

Objective Data

- Beck triad (jugular venous distention, hypotension, and muffled heart sounds)
- Chronically and severely involved pericardium may also scar and constrict, limiting cardiac filling; heart sounds are muffled, blood pressure drops, the pulse becomes weakened and rapid, and paradoxic pulse (see Chapter 15) becomes exaggerated.

FIGURE 14-23 Hemopericardium and cardiac tamponade. *(Modified from Canobbio, 1990.)*

Cor Pulmonale

Enlargement of the right ventricle secondary to chronic lung disease (Fig. 14-24)

Pathophysiology

- Usually chronic, occasionally acute
- In acute phase, the right side of the heart is dilated and fails.
  - Acute causes: massive pulmonary embolism and acute respiratory distress syndrome (ARDS)
- In chronic cor pulmonale, gradual hypertrophy of the right ventricle progresses until ultimate heart failure.
  - Results from chronic obstructive pulmonary disease (COPD) and pulmonary arterial hypertension

Subjective Data

- Fatigue
- Tachypnea
- Exertional dyspnea
- Cough
- Hemoptysis
- Light-headedness
- Syncope

Objective Data

- Evidence of pulmonary disease
  - Wheezes and crackles on auscultation
  - Increase in chest diameter
  - Labored respiratory efforts with chest wall retractions
- Evidence of right heart failure and hypertrophy
  - Distended neck veins with prominent A or V waves (Chapter 15, p. 336)
- Cyanosis
- Left parasternal systolic heave
  - Loud S_2 exaggerated in the pulmonic region
  - Lower extremity edema

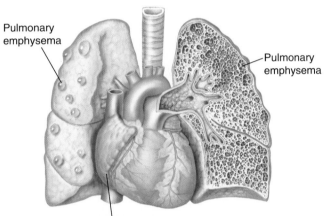

Pulmonary emphysema

Pulmonary emphysema

Right ventricular hypertrophy

FIGURE 14-24 Cor pulmonale. Notice extensive pulmonary emphysema and right ventricular hypertrophy. *(Modified from Wilson and Thompson, 1990.)*

Myocardial Infarction

Ischemic myocardial necrosis caused by abrupt decrease in coronary blood flow to a segment of the myocardium

Pathophysiology

- Most commonly affects left ventricle
- Results from atherosclerosis of the coronary blood vessels
- Atherosclerotic plaques rupture, and thrombosis (a clot) forms, rapidly causing a sudden obstruction of blood flow

Subjective Data

- Deep substernal or visceral pain that often radiates to the jaw, neck, and left arm (see Box 14-1, p. 302)
- Discomfort may be mild, especially in older adults or patients with diabetes mellitus
- Nausea
- Fatigue
- Shortness of breath

Objective Data

- Dysrhythmias are common.
- S_4 is usually present.
- Distant heart sounds
- Soft, systolic, blowing apical murmur
- Thready pulse
- Blood pressure varies, although hypertension is usual in the early phases.

Myocarditis

Focal or diffuse inflammation of the myocardium

Pathophysiology

- Inflammation can occur from direct cytotoxic effect of secondary immune response
- Causes:
  - Viral—enterovirus, coxsackie B, adenovirus, influenza, cytomegalovirus,
  - Bacterial—tuberculosis, streptococci
  - Spirochetal—syphilis, Lyme disease
  - Fungal—candidiasis, aspergillosis, cryptococcosis, histoplasmosis
  - Protozoal—Chagas disease, toxoplasmosis, malaria
  - Helminthic—trichinosis, schistosomiasis
  - Bites/stings—scorpion venom, snake venom, black widow spider venom
  - Chemotherapeutic medications
  - Amphetamines, cocaine, catecholamines
  - Physical agents
  - Systemic inflammatory disease—giant cell myocarditis, sarcoidosis, Kawasaki disease, Crohn disease, systemic lupus erythematosus
  - Peripartum cardiomyopathy

Subjective Data

- Initial symptoms vague
- Fatigue
- Dyspnea
- Fever
- Palpitations
- History of recent (within 1 to 2 weeks) flu-like syndrome of fevers, arthralgias, and malaise or pharyngitis, tonsillitis, or upper respiratory tract infection

Objective Data

- Cardiac enlargement
- Murmurs
- Gallop rhythms
- Tachycardia
- Dysrhythmias
- Pulsus alternans (alternation of strong and weak arterial pulse due to alternate strong and weak ventricular contractions)

ABNORMALITIES IN HEART RATE AND RHYTHM

Conduction Disturbances

Conduction disturbances either proximal to the bundle of His or diffusely throughout the conduction system

Pathophysiology

- May result from a variety of causes: ischemic, infiltrative or, rarely, neoplastic
- Antidepressant medications, digitalis, quinidine, and many other medications can be precipitating factors.

Subjective Data

- Transient weakness
- Syncope, may occur acutely without warning, sometimes as a "gray-out" instead of a "black-out," may precede the event
- Strokelike episodes
- Palpitations

Objective Data

- Rapid or irregular heartbeat
- Rhythm disturbances (Table 14-6)

Sick Sinus Syndrome

Arrhythmias caused by a malfunction of the sinus node

Pathophysiology

- Occurs secondary to hypertension, arteriosclerotic heart disease, or rheumatic heart, or without known cause (idiopathic)

Subjective Data

- Fainting, transient dizzy spells, light-headedness, seizures, palpitations, and angina

Objective Data

- Dysrhythmias
- Signs of congestive heart failure

Table 14-6	Abnormalities in Rates and Rhythms	
Type and Detection	Findings on Examination	Description
Atrial (Auricular) Flutter		
	Atrial rate far in excess of ventricular rate; heart sounds not necessarily weak	Regular uniform atrial contractions occur in excess of 200 beats/min, but the ventricular response is limited as a result of physiologic heart block. The conduction system cannot respond to the rapidity of the atrial rate, causing variance from the ventricular rate. The ECG may look like a saw-tooth cog.
Atrial flutter with a constant 4:1 conduction ratio		
Sinus Bradycardia		
	Slow rate below 50 or 60/min	No disruption in conduction is not necessarily suggestive of a problem.
Sinus bradycardia		
Atrial Fibrillation		
	Dysrhythmic contraction of the atria gives way to rapid series of irregular spasms of the muscle wall; no discernible regularity in rhythm or pattern	The conduction system is malfunctioning and is in an anarchic state. Any contraction of the atria that is best described as *irregularly* irregular.
Atrial fibrillation with rapid ventricular response		

Continued

ABNORMALITIES

Table 14-6	Abnormalities in Rates and Rhythms—cont'd	
Type and Detection	**Findings on Examination**	**Description**
Heart Block	Heart rate slower than expected; incomplete heart block rate is often 25 to 45/min at rest	Conduction from atria to ventricles partially or completely disrupted. Conduction either occurs: 1. All the time (but taking a little longer than usual): first-degree heart block 2. Some of the time: second-degree heart block i. Type 1: Wenckebach/Mobitz 1 ii. Type 2: Mobitz 2 3. None of the time: third-degree; complete heart block ECG is necessary to determine the nature of heart block in conduction. 1. First-degree heart block: PR interval longer than 0.20 second 2i. Second-degree heart block, type 1: Wenckebach/Mobitz 1: benign, PR interval increases each beat until a QRS is dropped 2ii. Second-degree heart block, type 2/Mobitz 2: may progress to compete heart block; PR interval stays the same then a QRS is dropped 3. Third-degree, complete heart block: none of the P waves are conducted to the AV node, AV node generates a rate by itself (nodal or junctional rhythm)

Table 14-6	Abnormalities in Rates and Rhythms—cont'd	
Type and Detection	**Findings on Examination**	**Description**
Supraventricular Tachycardia (SVT)	Rapid, regular heart rate and narrow QRS complex	Rapid heart rhythm originating at or above the atrioventricular node. The rate will occasionally decrease with vagal stimulation, holding a deep breath, or gentle massage of a carotid sinus. (Massage must always be done with care.) (See Chapter 15.)
Paroxysmal atrial tachycardia (PAT)		
Ventricular Tachycardia	Rapid, relatively regular heartbeat (often nearly 200/min) without loss in apparent strength	The electrical source of the beat is in an unusual focus somewhere in the ventricles. This usually arises in serious heart disease and is a grave prognostic sign.
Ventricular tachycardia		
Ventricular Fibrillation	Complete loss of regular heart rhythm with expected conduction pattern absent if weakened and rapid, ventricular contraction is irregular	The ventricle has lost the rhythm of its expected response, and all evidence of vigorous contraction is gone. It calls for immediate action and may immediately precede sudden death.
Ventricular fibrillation		

ABNORMALITIES

✿ Infants and Children

Tetralogy of Fallot

Congenital heart defect composed of four cardiac defects: ventricular septal defect, pulmonic stenosis, dextroposition of the aorta, and right ventricular hypertrophy

Pathophysiology

- Increased right ventricular outflow tract obstruction leads to increased right-to-left shunting of blood through the underdeveloped interventricular septum. Degree of right ventricular outflow tract obstruction varies among patients and determines clinical symptoms and disease progression.
- Results in cyanosis during hypercontractile episodes, associated with agitation/crying

Subjective Data

- Dyspnea with feeding, poor growth, exercise intolerance
- Paroxysmal dyspnea with loss of consciousness and central cyanosis (tetralogy spell)

Objective Data

- Parasternal heave and precordial prominence, systolic ejection murmur over the third intercostal space, sometimes radiating to the left side of the neck; a single S_2 is heard (Fig. 14-25).
- Older children develop clubbing of fingers and toes.
- May develop heart failure if not surgically corrected

The four abnormalities:
Stenotic pulmonary valve
Ventricular septal defect
Overriding aortic valve
Hypertrophy of right ventricle

FIGURE 14-25 Tetralogy of Fallot. *(Modified from Canobbio, 1990.)*

Ventricular Septal Defect (VSD)

Opening between the left and right ventricles

Pathophysiology

- During ventricular contraction, some blood from the left ventricle goes into the right ventricle, passes through the lungs, and reenters the left ventricle via the pulmonary veins and left atrium.
- Significant number (30% to 50%) of small defects close spontaneously during the first 2 years of life

Subjective Data

- Recurrent respiratory infections
- If large VSD, rapid breathing, poor growth, symptoms of congestive heart failure

Objective Data

- Arterial pulse is small, and jugular venous pulse is unaffected.
- Holosystolic murmur, often loud, coarse, high-pitched, and best heard along the left sternal border in the third to fifth intercostal spaces
- Left peristernal lift
- A smaller defect causes a louder murmur and a more easily felt thrill than a large one (Fig. 14-26; see Table 14-5).

FIGURE 14-26 **Ventricular septal defect.** *(Modified from Canobbio, 1990.)*

Patent Ductus Arteriosus

Failure of the ductus arteriosus to close after birth (Fig. 14-27)

Pathophysiology

- Blood flows through the ductus during systole and diastole, increasing pressure in the pulmonary circulation and consequently the workload of the right ventricle.

Subjective Data

- Small shunt can be asymptomatic; a larger one causes dyspnea on exertion.

Objective Data

- Dilated and pulsatile neck vessels
- Wide pulse pressure
- Harsh, loud, continuous murmur heard at the first to third intercostal spaces and the lower sternal border, with a machine-like quality
- Murmur usually unaltered by postural change, unlike murmur of a venous hum

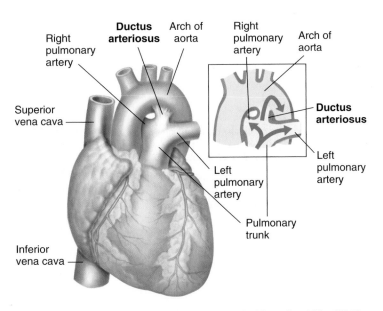

FIGURE 14-27 **Patent ductus arteriosus.** *(Modified from Canobbio, 1990.)*

ABNORMALITIES

Atrial Septal Defect (ASD)

Congenital defect in the septum dividing the left and right atria (Fig. 14-28)

Pathophysiology

- Large ASD (>9 mm), allows left-to-right shunting of blood
- Extra blood from the left atrium may cause a volume overload of the right atrium and the ventricle.
- Untreated ASD can result in enlargement of the right side of the heart and shunt reversal (right to left shunt) and heart failure.

Subjective Data

- Often asymptomatic
- Heart failure rarely occurs in children but can often occur in adults.

Objective Data

- Diamond-shaped systolic ejection murmur often loud, high-pitched, and harsh, heard over the pulmonic area
- May be accompanied by a brief, rumbling, early diastolic murmur
- Does not usually radiate beyond the precordium
- Systolic thrill may be felt over the area of the murmur, along with a palpable parasternal thrust.
- S_2 may be widely split.
- Sometimes murmur may not sound particularly impressive, especially in overweight children; if there is a palpable thrust and radiation to the back, it is more apt to be significant.

FIGURE 14-28 Atrial septal defect. *(From Canobbio, 1990.)*

Acute Rheumatic Fever

Systemic connective tissue disease occurring after streptococcal pharyngitis or skin infection

Pathophysiology

- Characterized by a variety of major and minor manifestations (Box 14-10)
- May result in serious cardiac valvular involvement of mitral or aortic valve; tricuspid and pulmonic are not often affected
- Affected valve becomes stenotic and regurgitant
- Children between 5 and 15 years of age are most commonly affected
- Prevention—adequate treatment for streptococcal pharyngitis or skin infections—is the best therapy.

Subjective Data

- Fever
- Inflamed swollen joints
- Flat or slightly raised, painless rash with pink margins with pale centers and a ragged edge (erythema marginatum)
- Aimless jerky movements (Sydenham chorea or St. Vitus dance)
- Small, painless nodules beneath the skin
- Chest pain
- Palpitations
- Fatigue
- Shortness of breath

Objective Data

- Characterized by a variety of major and minor manifestations (Box 14-10)
- Murmurs of mitral regurgitation and aortic insufficiency
- Cardiomegaly
- Friction rub of pericarditis
- Signs of congestive heart failure

Box 14-10 Jones Criteria for Diagnosis of Rheumatic Fever

Major Manifestations	Minor Manifestations
Carditis	Clinical
Polyarthritis	Previous rheumatic fever or rheumatic heart disease
Chorea	Arthralgia
Erythema marginatum	Fever
Subcutaneous nodules	Laboratory
	Acute phase reactions: erythrocyte sedimentation rate, C-reactive protein, leukocytosis
	Prolonged PR interval on ECG

Supporting Evidence of Streptococcal Infection
- Increased titer of antistreptolysin antibodies (antistreptolysin O in particular)
- Positive throat culture for group A streptococci
- Recent scarlet fever

The presence of two major or one major and two minor manifestations suggests a high probability of acute rheumatic fever if supported by evidence of a preceding group A streptococcal infection. Do not make the diagnosis on the basis of laboratory findings and two minor manifestations alone.

From Ferrieri P, for the Jones Criteria Working Group, 2002; Special Writing Group of the Committee on Rheumatic Fever, Endocarditis,

✂ Older Adults

Atherosclerotic Heart Disease (Atherosclerosis, Coronary Heart Disease)
Narrowing of the small blood vessels that supply blood and oxygen to the heart

Pathophysiology
- Caused by deposition of cholesterol, other lipids, by a complex inflammatory process
- Leads to vascular wall thickening and narrowing of the lumen

Subjective Data
- May be asymptomatic
- Angina pectoris, shortness of breath, palpitations
- Family history of close relatives with atherosclerotic disease, early death, or dyslipidemia

Objective Data
- Dyslipidemia
- Dysrhythmias and signs of congestive heart failure

Mitral Insufficiency, Regurgitation
Abnormal leaking of blood through the mitral valve, from left ventricle into left atrium

Pathophysiology
- Most common causes:
  - Rheumatic heart disease
  - Infective endocarditis
  - Annular calcification of the mitral valve
  - Cardiomyopathy
  - Ischemic heart disease
  - Mitral valve prolapse
  - Ruptured chordae tendineae
  - Myxomatous valvular degeneration

Subjective Data
- Acute mitral regurgitation has symptoms of decompensated congestive heart failure.
- Shortness of breath
- Pulmonary edema
- Orthopnea
- Paroxysmal nocturnal dyspnea
- Decreased exercise tolerance
- Chronic compensated mitral regurgitation may be asymptomatic.
- Patients may be sensitive to small shifts in intravascular volume and are prone to develop congestive heart failure.

Objective Data
- High-pitched pansystolic murmur radiating to axilla
- May also have a third heart sound

Senile Cardiac Amyloidosis
Amyloid, fibrillary protein produced by chronic inflammation or neoplastic disease, deposition in the heart

Pathophysiology
- Heart contractility may be reduced.
- Causes heart failure

Subjective Data
- Palpitations, lower extremity edema, fatigue, reduced activity tolerance

Objective Data
- Pleural effusion
- Arrhythmia
- Lower extremity edema
- Dilated neck veins
- Hepatomegaly or ascites
- Electrocardiography or echocardiography shows small, thickened left ventricle; right ventricle may also be thickened.

CHAPTER 15

Blood Vessels

The physical examination of the venous and arterial structures of the vascular system is a critical component of the patient's evaluation. You can gain great insight into his or her overall cardiovascular status, specifically the detection of peripheral artery disease (PAD) of the lower extremities, which is associated with an increased risk of stroke and cardiovascular events.

evolve *http://evolve.elsevier.com/Seidel*

- Physical Exam Key Points
- NCLEX Review Questions
- Interactive Activities
- Animations
- Videos
- Student Checklist

Physical Examination Preview

Here is a preview of the steps involved in conducting a physical examination of the blood vessels. ⓔ These procedures are explained in detail in this chapter and are available on Evolve in printable formats.

Blood Vessels

1. Palpate the arterial pulses in distal extremities, comparing characteristics bilaterally for the following (p. 338):
   - Rate
   - Rhythm
   - Contour
   - Amplitude
2. Auscultate the carotid, abdominal aorta, and renal, iliac, and femoral arteries for bruits (p. 340).
3. With the patient reclining at a 45-degree angle, inspect for jugular venous pulsations and distention; differentiate jugular and carotid pulse waves, and measure jugular venous pressure (p. 342).
4. Inspect the extremities for sufficiency of arteries and veins through the following (p. 343):
   - Color, skin texture, and nail changes
   - Presence of hair
   - Muscular atrophy
   - Edema or swelling
   - Varicose veins
5. Palpate the extremities for the following (p. 344):
   - Warmth
   - Pulse quality
   - Tenderness along any superficial vein
   - Pitting edema

ANATOMY AND PHYSIOLOGY

The great vessels, the arteries leading from and the veins leading to the heart, are located in close proximity at the base of the heart. They include the aorta, superior and inferior venae cavae, pulmonary arteries, and pulmonary veins (Fig. 15-1). The aorta carries oxygenated blood out of the left ventricle to the body. The pulmonary artery, which leaves the right ventricle and divides almost immediately into right and left branches, carries deoxygenated blood to the lungs. The superior and inferior venae cavae carry deoxygenated blood from the upper and lower body, respectively, to the right atrium. The pulmonary veins return oxygenated blood from the lungs to the left atrium.

Blood Circulation

Once it leaves the heart, blood flows through two circulatory systems, the pulmonary and the systemic (Fig. 15-2). The pulmonary circulation routes blood through the lungs, where it is oxygenated before returning to the left atrium and ventricle of the heart. Venous blood arrives at the right atrium via the superior and inferior vena cavae and moves through the tricuspid valve to the right ventricle. During systole, deoxygenated blood is ejected through the pulmonic valve into the pulmonary artery; it travels through the pulmonary arteries, arterioles, and capillaries until it reaches the alveoli, where gas exchange occurs.

Oxygenated blood of the systemic circulation returns to the heart and enters the systemic circulation through the pulmonary veins into the left atrium and then through the mitral valve into the left ventricle. The left ventricle contracts, forcing a volume of blood with each beat (stroke volume) through the aortic valve into the aorta where it is distributed systemically through the arteries and capillaries. In the capillary bed, oxygen is provided to the tissues of the body; the now deoxygenated blood is carbon dioxide-rich and passes into the venous system and returns to the heart via the superior and inferior vena cavae and into the right atrium (Fig. 15-3).

The structure of the arteries and veins reflects their function. The arteries are thicker with a greater smooth muscle layer and less ability to stretch and expand (distension) from internal pressure. They are subjected to much more pressure than are the

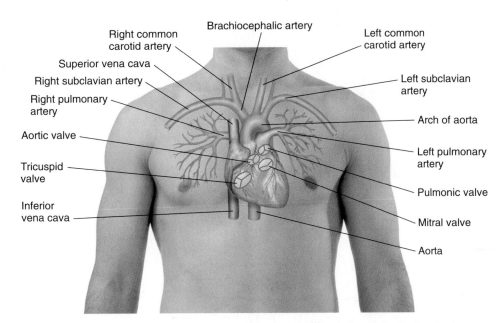

FIGURE 15-1 Anatomic location of the great vessels and their relationship to the heart valves.

FIGURE 15-2 Circulatory system.

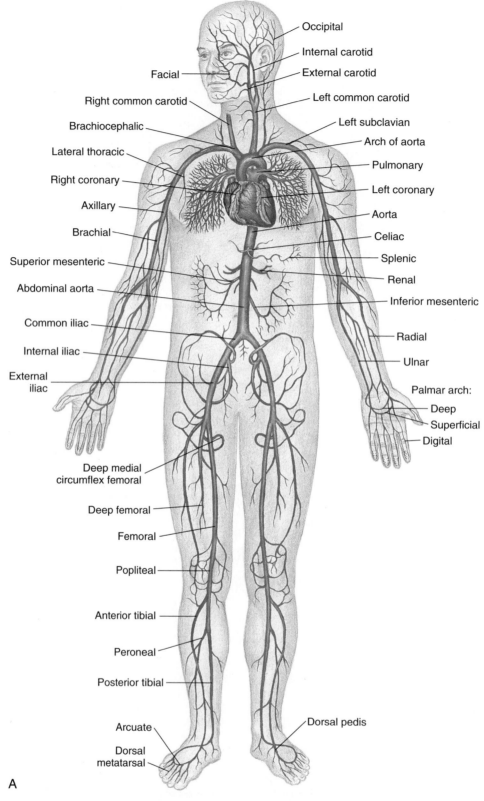

A

FIGURE 15-3 Systemic circulation. A, Arteries.

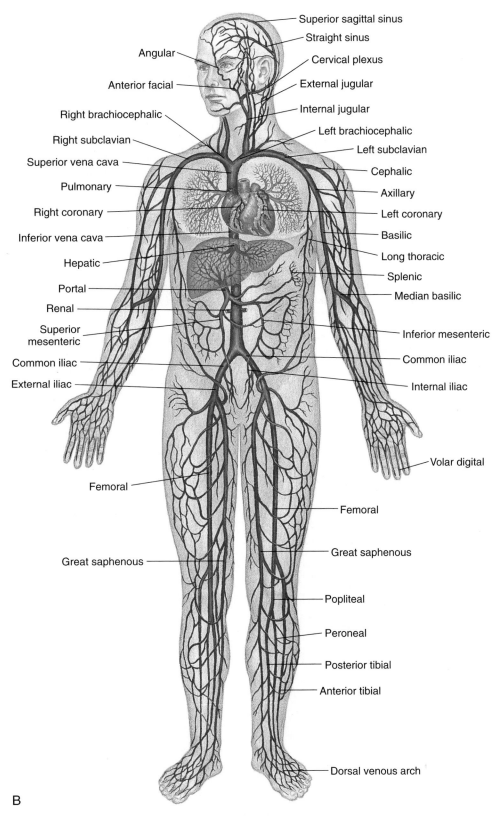

FIGURE 15-3, cont'd B, Veins.

veins. The veins are less sturdy and more distensible than the arteries (Fig. 15-4). Venous return is less forceful than blood flow through the arteries, and veins contain valves to keep blood flowing in one direction. If blood volume increases significantly, the veins can expand and act as a repository for extra blood. This compensatory mechanism helps diminish stress on the heart.

Arterial Pulse and Pressure

The palpable and sometimes visible arterial pulses are the result of ventricular systole, which produces a pressure wave throughout the arterial system (arterial pulse). It takes barely 0.2 second for the impact of this wave to be felt in the dorsalis pedis artery within the foot and considerably more than 2 seconds for a red blood cell to travel the same distance. The arterial blood pressure is the force exerted by the blood against the wall of an artery as a result of a bolus of blood exiting the left ventricle of the heart as it contracts.

The pulse usually is felt as a forceful wave that is smooth and more rapid on the ascending part of the wave; it becomes domed, less steep, and slower on the descending part (Fig. 15-5). Because the carotid arteries are the most accessible of the arteries closest to the heart, they have the most definitive pulse for evaluation of cardiac function.

The following variables contribute to the characteristics of the pulses:

- Volume of blood ejected (stroke volume)
- Distensibility of the aorta and large arteries
- Obstruction of blood flow (e.g., narrowing of aortic valve [stenosis] or aorta [coarctation], vasculitis—blood vessel inflammation with narrowing—or PAD)
- Peripheral artery resistance
- Viscosity of the blood

Jugular Venous Pulse and Pressure

The jugular veins, which empty directly into the superior vena cava, reflect the activity of the right side of the heart and offer clues to its competency. The level at which the jugular venous pulse is visible gives an indication of right atrial pressure.

The external jugular veins are more superficial and more visible bilaterally above the clavicle, close to the insertion of the sternocleidomastoid muscles. The larger internal jugular veins run deep to the sternocleidomastoids, near the carotid arteries, and are less accessible to inspection (Fig. 15-6).

The activity of the right side of the heart is transmitted back through the jugular veins as a pulse* that has five identifiable components—three peaks and two descending slopes (Fig. 15-7):

a wave	The a wave, the first and most prominent component, is the result of a brief backflow of blood to the vena cava during right atrial contraction.
c wave	The c wave is a transmitted impulse from the vigorous backward push produced by closure of the tricuspid valve during ventricular systole.
v wave	The v wave is caused by the increasing volume and concomitant increasing pressure in the right atrium. It occurs after the c wave, late in ventricular systole.
x slope	The downward x slope is caused by passive atrial filling.
y slope	The y slope following the v wave reflects the open tricuspid valve and the rapid filling of the ventricle.

✢ Infants and Children

At birth the cutting of the umbilical cord, through which oxygen has been provided in utero, requires the infant to begin breathing. The onset of respiration expands the lungs and carries air to the alveoli. Pulmonary vascular resistance drops, allowing blood to flow more freely to the lungs. Systemic vascular resistance

---

*Although often referred to as a pulse, this is not the same as an arterial pulse because it is reflected back from the right heart rather than pushed forward by the left heart. Unlike arterial pulses, it cannot be palpated, only visualized.

FIGURE 15-4 Structure of arteries and veins. Note the relative thickness of the arterial wall.

FIGURE 15-5 Diagram of usual pulse.

increases. The ductus arteriosus closes, usually within the first 12 to 14 hours of life. Once pulmonary vascular resistance is lower than systemic resistance, blood flows into the pulmonary arteries rather than across the interatrial foramen ovale. The interatrial foramen ovale is functionally closed by the shifting pressures between the right and left sides of the heart.

�֍ Pregnant Women

During pregnancy, the systemic vascular resistance decreases and peripheral vasodilation occurs, often resulting in palmar erythema and spider telangiectasias. The systolic blood pressure decreases slightly. There is a greater decrease in the diastolic pressure. The lowest levels occur in the second trimester and then rise but still remain below prepregnancy levels. Maternal position affects blood pressure. Lower blood pressure can be noted when the patient is supine during the third trimester. This lower pressure is secondary to venous compression of the vena cava and impaired venous return. Blood in the lower extremities tends to pool in later pregnancy—except when the woman is in the lateral recumbent position—as a result of compression of the pelvic veins and inferior vena cava from pressure created by the enlarged uterus. The compression may result in an increase in dependent edema, varicosities of the legs and vulva, and hemorrhoids.

�֍ Older Adults

Calcification and plaque buildup in the walls of the arteries can cause stiffness as well as dilation of the aorta, aortic branches, and carotid arteries. The arterial walls lose elasticity and vasomotor tone and are less distensible. The resulting increased

peripheral vascular resistance may lead to elevated blood pressure, especially systolic.

REVIEW OF RELATED HISTORY

For each of the symptoms or conditions discussed in this section, targeted topics to include in the history of the present illness are listed. Responses to questions about these topics provide clues for focusing the physical examination and the development of an appropriate diagnostic evaluation. Questions regarding medication use (prescription and over the counter preparations) as well as complementary or alternative therapies are relevant for each.

History of Present Illness

+ Leg pain or cramps
    + Onset and duration: with activity or rest, recent injury or immobilization
    + Character
    + Continuous burning in toes, pain in thighs or buttocks, pain over specific location, induced by activity
    + Skin changes: cold skin, pallor, sores, redness or warmth over vein, visible veins, darkened or ischemic skin
    + Swelling of the leg
    + Limping: pain in buttock or calf with walking (claudication)
    + Waking at night with leg pain
+ Swollen ankles
    + Onset and duration: present in the morning, appearing as the day progresses, sudden onset, insidious onset
    + Related circumstances: recent and long airplane travel, recent travel to high elevations
    + Associated symptoms: onset of nocturia, increased frequency of urination, increasing shortness of breath
    + Treatment attempted (including rest, massage, heat, elevation)
    + Medications: heparin, warfarin, diuretics, antihypertensive medications

Past Medical History

+ Cardiac surgery or hospitalization for cardiac evaluation or disorder, congenital heart defect, surgical or interventional vascular catheterization procedures

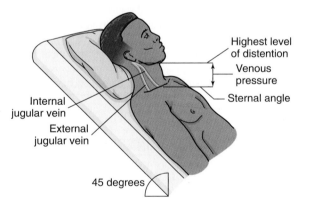

FIGURE 15-6 Inspection of jugular venous pressure. *(From Mohan et al, 2007.)*

FIGURE 15-7 Expected venous pulsations.

+ Chronic illness: hypertension and studies to define its cause, bleeding disorder, hyperlipidemia, diabetes, thyroid dysfunction, stroke, vasculitis, thrombosis, transient ischemic attacks, coronary artery disease, atrial fibrillation or other type of dysrhythmia,

Family History

Family members with risk factors, morbidity, and mortality related to cardiovascular system; hypertension, dyslipidemia, diabetes, heart disease, thrombosis, peripheral vascular disease, abdominal aortic aneurysms, ages at time of illness or death

Personal and Social History

+ Employment: physical demands; environmental hazards such as heat, chemicals, dust; sources of emotional stress
+ Tobacco: type (cigarettes, cigars, pipe, chewing tobacco, snuff); duration of use; amount; efforts to quit and methods used; age started and, perhaps, stopped; pack-years (Number of years smoking × Number of packs per day)
+ Nutritional status
+ Usual diet: proportion of fat, food preferences, history of dieting
+ Weight: loss or gain, amount and rate
+ Exercise: type, amount, frequency, intensity
+ Use of alcohol: amount consumed, frequency, duration of current intake
+ Use of recreational drugs: intravenous drug use, cocaine

Staying Well

Components of a Healthy Diet

Those who eat a diet common to the Mediterranean region have taught us that we should use olive oil consistently in our diets. This, in addition to a disciplined, *moderate* intake of wine (no more than 1 to 2 glasses per day), is helpful in the effort to decrease the risk of hypertension and associated cardiac problems. An undisciplined, immoderate habit of alcohol consumption negates any advantage. The message then: olive oil in abundance, wine in moderation.

❀ Infants and Children

+ Hemophilia
+ Sickle cell disease
+ Renal disease
+ Coarctation of the aorta
+ Leg pains during exercise

❀ Pregnant Women

+ Blood pressure: prepregnancy levels, elevation during pregnancy; evidence of preeclampsia with associated symptoms and signs such as headaches, visual changes, nausea and vomiting, epigastric pain, right upper quadrant pain, oliguria, rapid onset of edema (facial, abdominal, or peripheral), hyperreflexia, proteinuria, unusual bruising or bleeding
+ Legs: edema, varicosities, pain or discomfort

Risk Factors

Preeclampsia

- Older than 40 years of age
- First pregnancy
- Preexisting chronic hypertension
- Renal disease or diabetes mellitus
- Multifetal gestation
- Family history of preeclampsia or gestational hypertension
- Previous preeclampsia or gestational hypertension
- Obesity

❀ Older Adults

+ Leg edema: pattern, frequency, time of day most pronounced
+ Interference with activities of daily living
+ Ability of the patient and family to cope with the condition
+ Claudication: area involved, unilateral or bilateral, distance one can walk before its onset, sensation, length of time required for relief
+ Medications used for relief; efficacy of drugs

Risk Factors

Varicose Veins

- Gender; women four times more common than men (during pregnancy in particular, increased hormonal levels weaken the walls of the vein and result in failure of the valves)
- Genetic predisposition (children of women with varicosities)
- Tobacco use, sedentary lifestyle (habitual inactivity allows blood to pool in the veins, resulting in edema), increased body mass index
- Age (the veins of older adults are less elastic and more likely to be varicose)
- History of lower extremity trauma or venous thrombosis

EXAMINATION AND FINDINGS

Equipment

+ Marking pencil
+ Two separate centimeter rulers at least 15 cm long
+ Stethoscope with bell and diaphragm

Peripheral Arteries

Palpation

The pulses are best palpated over arteries that are close to the surface of the body and lie over bones. These include the carotid, brachial, radial, femoral, popliteal, dorsalis pedis, and posterior tibial arteries (Fig. 15-8).

An arterial pulsation is essentially a bounding wave of blood that diminishes with increasing distance from the heart. The carotid pulses are most easily accessible and closest to the cardiac

FIGURE 15-8 Palpation of arterial pulses. A, Carotid. **B,** Brachial. **C,** Radial. **D,** Femoral. **E,** Popliteal.
F, Dorsalis pedis. **G,** Posterior tibial.

source, making them most useful in evaluating heart function. Examine the arterial pulses in the extremities to determine the sufficiency of the entire arterial circulation. Palpate at least one pulse point in each extremity, usually at the most distal point (see Clinical Pearl, "Carotid Palpation").

Clinical Pearl

Carotid Palpation
When palpating the carotid arteries, never palpate both sides simultaneously. Excessive carotid sinus massage can cause slowing of the pulse and a drop in blood pressure and compromise blood flow to the brain, leading to syncope. If you have difficulty feeling the pulse, rotate the patient's head to the side being examined to relax the sternocleidomastoid muscle.

When examining the arterial pulses, the thumb may be used, especially if vessels have a tendency to move when probed by fingers. In this setting the thumb is particularly useful in "fixing" the brachial and even the femoral pulses. Palpate firmly but not so hard as to occlude the artery. The exception to this is when doing the Allen test to ensure ulnar artery patency prior to radial artery puncture (Box 15-1).

Palpate the arterial pulses (most often the radial) to assess the heart rate and rhythm, pulse contour (waveform), amplitude (force), symmetry, and sometimes obstructions to blood flow. Variations from the expected findings are described in Figure 15-9.

The contour of the pulse wave is pliable. Healthy arteries have a smooth, rounded, or dome shape. Pay attention to the ascending portion, the peak, and the descending portion. Compare each wave crest with the next to detect cyclic differences.

Video: Blood Vessels: Assessing Arterial Pulses

Box 15-1   The Allen Test

This test assesses the patency of the ulnar artery. Perform this test prior to radial artery puncture for arterial blood gas sampling or the insertion of a radial arterial catheter.
1. With the patient's palm facing upward, compress the radial and ulnar artery with your fingers *(A)*.
2. Have the patient close and open the fist five times and then leave the blanched palm open.
3. Release pressure on the ulnar artery alone and watch for palmar reperfusion within 4 to 5 seconds.
4. If palmar reperfusion does not occur, suspect ulnar artery insufficiency and do not puncture the radial artery *(B)*.

(From Skirven et al, 2011.)

The amplitude of the pulse is described on a scale of 0 to 4:

4	Bounding, aneurysmal
3	Full, increased
2	Expected
1	Diminished, barely palpable
0	Absent, not palpable

Determine the regularity of the heart rhythm. If it is irregular, determine whether there is a consistent pattern. An irregular heart rate that occurs in a repeated pattern may indicate sinus arrhythmia, a cyclic variation of the heart rate characterized by an increasing rate on inspiration and decreasing rate on expiration. A patternless, unpredictable, irregular rate may indicate heart disease or an impaired conduction system such as atrial fibrillation. If you note an irregular rate, record the beats per minute and compare it with the rate heard when auscultating the heart (see Chapter 14). Note the strength of the pulse.

Lack of symmetry (in pulse contour or strength) between the left and right extremities suggests impaired circulation. Compare the strength of the upper extremity pulses with those of the lower extremities and the left with the right. Ordinarily, the femoral is as strong as or stronger than the radial pulse. If the femoral pulsation is absent or diminished, proximal obstruction should be suspected, which may be due to such conditions as coarctation of the aorta, atherosclerotic peripheral arterial disease, or vasculitis.

Auscultation

Auscultate over an artery for a bruit (i.e., a murmur or unexpected sound) if you are following the radiation of murmurs first noted during the cardiac examination or looking for evidence of local obstruction. These sounds are usually low-pitched and relatively hard to hear. Place the bell of the stethoscope directly over the artery. Sites to auscultate for a bruit are over the carotid, subclavian, abdominal aorta, renal, iliac, and femoral arteries. See Chapter 17 for auscultation of abdominal bruits. When listening over the carotid vessels, ask the patient to suspend his or her breathing for a few heartbeats so that respiratory sounds will not interfere with auscultation (Fig. 15-10). Sounds heard over the neck include venous hums and carotid bruits (Box 15-2).

Assessment for Peripheral Arterial Disease

Arteries in any location can become narrowed, leading to decreased blood flow. The reduced circulation to the tissues will lead to signs and symptoms that are related to the following:
- Site
- Degree of narrowing
- Ability of collateral channels to compensate
- Rapidity with which the problem develops

The first symptom is pain that results from muscle ischemia, referred to as *claudication*. This pain can be characterized as a dull ache with accompanying muscle fatigue and cramps. It usually appears during sustained exercise, such as walking a distance or climbing several flights of stairs. Just a few minutes of rest will ordinarily relieve it. It recurs again with the same amount of activity. Continued activity causes worsening pain.

The site of pain is distal to the narrowing. After determining the distinguishing characteristics of the pain, note the following:
- Pulses (strong, weak or possibly absent)
- Possible systolic bruits over the arteries that may extend through diastole
- Loss of expected body warmth in the affected area
- Localized pallor and cyanosis
- Collapsed superficial veins, with delay in venous filling
- Thin, atrophied skin; muscle atrophy (particularly with long-term insufficiency)

To judge the degree of narrowing and the potential severity of the arterial insufficiency, perform the following steps:
- Have the patient lie supine.
- Elevate the extremity.
- Note the degree of blanching.
- Have the patient sit on the edge of the bed or examining table in order to lower the extremity.
- Note the time for maximal return of color after the extremity has been elevated. Slight pallor on elevation and a return to full color as soon as the leg becomes dependent are the expected findings. A delay of many seconds or even minutes before the extremity regains full color indicates arterial insufficiency. When return to full color takes as long as 2 minutes, the problem is severe.

A measurement of the *capillary refill time* provides another method of assessing severity (Box 15-3).

PULSE

POSSIBLE CAUSE

Alternating pulse (pulsus alternans)

Left ventricular failure (more significant if pulse slow)

Pulsus alternans is characterized by alternation of a pulsation of small amplitude with the pulsation of large amplitude while the rhythm is regular.

A

Pulsus bisferiens

Aortic stenosis combined with aortic insufficiency

Pulsus bisferiens is best detected by palpation of the carotid artery. This pulsation is characterized by two main peaks. The first is termed *percussion wave* and the second, *tidal wave*. Although the mechanism is not clear, the first peak is believed to be the pulse pressure and the second, reverberation from the periphery.

B

Bigeminal pulse

Disorder of rhythm

Bigeminal pulsations result from a normal pulsation followed by a premature contraction. The amplitude of the pulsation of the premature contraction is less than that of the normal pulsation.

C

Large, bounding pulse

Exercise
Anxiety
Fever
Hyperthyroidism
Aortic rigidity or atherosclerosis

The large bounding (also called hyperkinetic or strong) pulse is readily palpable. It does not "fade out" and is not easily obliterated by the examining fingers. This pulse is recorded as 3+.

D

Paradoxic pulse (pulsus paradoxus)

Inspiration   Expiration   Inspiration

Premature cardiac contraction
Tracheobronchial obstruction
Bronchial asthma
Emphysema
Pericardial effusion
Constrictive pericarditis

Pulsus paradoxus is characterized by an exaggerated decrease (>10 mm Hg) in the amplitude of pulsation during inspiration and increased amplitude during expiration. (See text for measurement with sphygmomanometer.)

E

Water-hammer pulse (Corrigan pulse)

Patent ductus arteriosus
Aortic regurgitation

The water-hammer pulse (also known as collapsing pulse) has a greater amplitude than expected, a rapid rise to a narrow summit, and a sudden descent.

F

FIGURE 15-9 Pulse abnormalities.

FIGURE 15-10 Auscultation for bruits in the carotid artery.

Box 15-2 | Listening to the Neck

Venous Hum
- Heard at medial end of clavicle and anterior border of sternocleidomastoid muscle
- Usually of no clinical significance
- Confused with carotid bruit, patent ductus arteriosus, and aortic regurgitation
- In adults, may occur with anemia, pregnancy, thyrotoxicosis, or intracranial arteriovenous malformation

Carotid Artery Bruits
- Heard at just above the medial end of clavicle and anterior margin of sternocleidomastoid muscle
- Mild obstruction produces a short, not particularly intense, localized bruit; greater stenosis lengthens the duration and increases the pitch.
- Complete stenosis may eliminate the bruit.
- Transmitted murmurs: valvular aortic stenosis, ruptured chordae tendineae of mitral valve, or severe aortic regurgitation.
- Can be heard with vigorous left ventricular ejection (more commonly in children than in adults)
- Occurs with arterial narrowing in cervical arteries (e.g., atherosclerotic carotid arteries, fibromuscular dysplasia, and arteritis)

The following list provides a general guideline for assessment of possible causes of pain:

Pain Location	Probable Obstructed Artery
Calf muscles	Superficial femoral artery
Thigh	Common femoral artery or external iliac artery
Buttock	Common iliac artery or distal aorta (erectile dysfunction may accompany stenosis of distal aorta)

If the pain is constant, the narrowing is critical and probably acute; if it is excruciating, a major artery has probably been severely compromised.

Box 15-3 | Capillary Refill Time

The capillary bed joins the arterial and venous systems. The capillary structure allows fluid exchange between the vascular and interstitial spaces, determined by the hydrostatic pressures of the blood and interstitial tissues and the colloid osmotic pressures of plasma and interstitial fluids. In the healthy person the dominance of hydrostatic pressure at the arterial end of the capillary bed (pushing fluid out) and of the colloid osmotic pressure at the venous end (pulling fluid in) maintains the balance of fluids in the intravascular and extravascular spaces.

The capillary refill time is the time it takes the capillary bed to fill after it is occluded by pressure, indicating the health of the vascular system. To gauge the *capillary refill time*, perform the following:
- Blanch the nail bed with a sustained pressure of several seconds on a fingernail or toenail.
- Release the pressure.
- Observe the time elapsed before the nail regains its full color.

If the vascular system is intact, the refill time is less than 2 seconds. If, however, the system is compromised (e.g., peripheral arterial disease, hypovolemic shock, or hypothermia), the refill time will be *more than 2 seconds*, and much longer if circulatory compromise is severe.

CAUTION: Environmental influences, such as a moderately cool room temperature, may prolong the capillary refill time, suggesting a problem that may not exist. Variability among examiners in calculating the time may also be a problem. One strategy is to say "capillary refill" as you release the pressure on the nail bed, which takes about 2 seconds, as a guide.

Peripheral Veins

Jugular Venous Pressure

Careful measurement of the jugular venous pressure (JVP) is an important and, in some cases, critical portion of the physical examination. Several techniques may be used. The simplest, most reproducible and reliable method requires two pocket rulers at least 15 cm long. Place the patient in the supine position using a bed or examining table with an adjustable back support. Use a light to supply tangential illumination across the right side of the patient's neck to accentuate the appearance of the jugular venous pulsations (Fig. 15-11).

When the supine patient is initially placed flat, note the engorgement of the jugular veins. Gradually raise the head of the bed until the jugular venous pulsations become evident between the angle of the jaw and the clavicle (see Fig. 15-6). Palpating the carotid pulse helps identify the venous pulsations and distinguish them from the carotid pulsations. Table 15-1 provides instructions on differentiating between jugular and carotid pulses. The jugular pulse can only be visualized; it cannot be palpated.

Several conditions may make the JVP examination more difficult: (1) severe right heart failure, tricuspid insufficiency, constrictive pericarditis, and cardiac tamponade may each cause extreme elevation of the JVP so that it is not apparent until the patient is sitting upright; (2) severe volume depletion makes the JVP difficult to detect even when the patient is flat; and (3) in

FIGURE 15-11 Measuring jugular venous pressure.

Table 15-1	Comparison of the Jugular and Carotid Pulse Waves	
	Jugular	**Carotid**
Quality and Character	Three positive waves in normal sinus rhythm	One wave
Palpate the carotid artery on one side of the neck and look at the jugular vein on the other to tell the difference.	More undulating	More brisk
Effect of Respiration	Level of pulse wave decreased on inspiration and increased on expiration	No effect
Venous Compression Apply gentle pressure over vein at base of neck above clavicle.	Easily eliminates pulse wave	No effect
Abdominal Pressure Place the palm with moderate firmness over the right upper quadrant of the abdomen for 30 seconds.	May cause some increased prominence even in well persons; with right-sided heart failure, jugular vein may be more visible.	No effect

extreme obesity, overlying adipose tissue obscures the jugular venous pulsations.

Place a ruler with its tip at the midaxillary line (the position of the heart within the chest) at the level of the nipple and extended vertically. Place the second ruler at the level of the meniscus of the JVP, extended horizontally to where it intersects the vertical ruler. The vertical distance above the level of the heart is noted as the mean JVP in centimeters of water (see Fig. 15-11). A value of less than 9 cm H_2O is the expected value.

Maneuvers useful for confirming the JVP measurement include hepatojugular reflux and evaluation of the venous engorgement of the hands at various levels of elevation above the heart.

Hepatojugular Reflux

The hepatojugular reflux is exaggerated when right heart failure is present, and its measurement is used to evaluate that condition. To assess the hepatojugular reflux maneuver, use your hand to apply firm and sustained pressure to the abdomen in the mid-epigastric region and instruct the patient to breathe regularly. Observe the neck for an elevation in JVP followed by an abrupt fall in JVP as the hand pressure is released. The JVP quickly equilibrates to its true level between the positions it achieved with and immediately after removal of the abdominal hand pressure.

If the JVP is not obvious with this maneuver, the pressure is either much higher or much lower. Repeat the maneuver with the patient more supine if you suspect the pressure to be lower. Position the patient more upright if you suspect the JVP to be higher.

Evaluation of Hand Veins

The veins of the hand can be used as an "auxiliary manometer" of the right heart pressure when the patient does not have thrombosis or arteriovenous fistula in that arm or superior vena cava syndrome. With the patient semirecumbent, place the hand on the examination table or mattress. Palpate the hand veins, which should be engorged, to make sure they are compressible. Slowly raise the hand until the hand veins collapse (Fig. 15-12). Use a ruler to note the vertical distance between the midaxillary line at the nipple level (level of the heart) and the level of collapse of the hand veins. Confirm this level by lowering the hand slowly until the veins distend again and raise it back until they once again collapse. This distance should be identical to the mean JVP.

The hand vein measurement is particularly helpful to evaluate severe right heart failure when the pressure may be 20 to 30 cm H_2O (i.e., JVP is not evident with the patient sitting upright) or with volume depletion (i.e., JVP not visible with the patient supine).

Assessment for Venous Obstruction and Insufficiency

Obstruction of the venous system and a consequent insufficiency results in signs and symptoms that vary depending on how rapidly the obstruction develops and on the degree of localization. An acute obstruction may result from injury, external compression, or thrombosis. In the affected area, constant pain occurs simultaneously with the following:

+ Swelling and tenderness over the muscles
+ Engorgement of superficial veins
+ Erythema and/or cyanosis

Inspect the extremities for signs of venous insufficiency (e.g., thrombosis, varicose veins, or edema). Examine the patient in both the standing and supine positions, particularly in the case of a suspected chronic venous occlusion. Ultrasound studies can confirm the presence of venous occlusion. See Clinical Pearl, "Calf Pain."

Thrombosis. Note any redness, thickening, and tenderness along a superficial vein, suggesting thrombophlebitis of a superficial vein. Suspect a deep vein thrombosis if swelling, pain, and tenderness occur over a vein. It cannot be confirmed on physical examination alone.

FIGURE 15-12 **Evaluation of hand veins. A,** Engorged veins in dependent hand. **B,** Collapsed veins in elevated hand.

FIGURE 15-13 Assessing for pitting edema.

> **Clinical Pearl**
>
> Calf Pain
> Do not confuse calf pain with Achilles tendon pain. This is a common finding in athletes who frequently stress the Achilles tendon and in women who wear high-heeled shoes. Directly palpate the Achilles for tenderness to identify the source of pain.

Homan Sign. Flex the patient's knee slightly with one hand and, with the other, dorsiflex the foot. The description of calf pain with this procedure is a positive sign and may indicate venous thrombosis. Absence of the Homan sign does not preclude venous thrombosis.

Edema. Inspect the extremities for edema, manifested as a change in the usual contour of the leg. Press your index finger over the bony prominence of the tibia or medial malleolus for several seconds. A depression that does not rapidly refill and resume its original contour indicates orthostatic (pitting) edema. This finding is not usually accompanied by thickening or pigmentation of the overlying skin. Right-sided heart failure leads to an increased fluid volume, which in turn elevates the hydrostatic pressure in the vascular space, causing edema in dependent parts of the body.

The severity of edema may be characterized by grading 1+ through 4+ (Fig. 15-13). Any concomitant pitting can be mild or severe, as evidenced by the following:

1+   Slight pitting, no visible distortion, disappears rapidly

2+   A somewhat deeper pit than in 1+, but again no readily detectable distortion; disappears in 10 to 15 seconds

3+   Noticeably deep pit that may last more than a minute; dependent extremity looks fuller and swollen

4+   Very deep pit that lasts as long as 2 to 5 minutes; dependent extremity is grossly distorted

> **Clinical Pearl**
>
> Edema
> If edema is unilateral, suspect the occlusion of a major vein. If edema is bilateral, consider congestive heart failure. If edema occurs without pitting, suspect arterial insufficiency or lymphedema.

Edema accompanied by some thickening and ulceration of the skin is frequently associated with deep venous obstruction or venous valvular incompetence (see Clinical Pearl, "Edema"). Edema related to valvular incompetence or an obstruction of a deep vein (usually in the legs) is caused by the mechanical pressure of increased blood volume in the area served by the affected vein. Circulatory disorders that cause edema so tense that it does not pit must be distinguished from lymphedema (see Chapter 9).

Varicose Veins. Varicose veins are dilated and swollen, with a diminished rate of blood flow and an increased intravenous pressure. These characteristics result from incompetence of the vessel wall or venous valves or an obstruction in a more proximal vein.

Inspect the legs for superficial varicosities when the patient is standing. With varicosities, the veins appear dilated and often tortuous. If varicose veins are suspected, have the patient stand on the toes 10 times in succession. Palpate the legs to feel the venous distention. When the venous system is competent, the distention of the veins disappears in a few seconds. If the distention of the veins is sustained for a longer time then venous insufficiency is suspected.

To evaluate the direction of blood flow and the competency of the valves in the venous system, distend visible veins by putting the limb in a dependent position. Compress the vein with the finger or thumb of one hand and strip the vein of blood by compressing the vein and moving the fingers of the second hand proximally. If the compressed vessel fills before either compressing finger is released, collateral circulation exists. If the compressing finger nearest the heart is released, the vessel should fill backward to the first valve only. If the entire venous column fills, the valves in that vessel are incompetent.

✤ Infants

The brachial, radial, and femoral pulses of the newborn are easily palpated. When the pulse is weaker than expected, cardiac output may be diminished or peripheral vasoconstriction may be present. A bounding pulse is associated with a large left-to-right shunt produced by a patent ductus arteriosus. In coarctation of the aorta, a difference is noted in pulse amplitude between the upper extremities or between the femoral and radial pulses, or the femoral pulses are absent.

Capillary refill times in infants and children younger than 2 years of age are rapid, less than 1 second. A prolonged capillary refill time, longer than 2 seconds, indicates dehydration or hypovolemic shock.

✤ Children

A venous hum, common in children, usually has no pathologic significance (see Box 15-2). It is caused by the turbulence of blood flow in the internal jugular veins. To detect a venous hum, ask the child to sit with the head turned away from you and tilted slightly upward. Auscultate over the supraclavicular space at the medial end of the clavicle and along the anterior border of the sternocleidomastoid muscle (Fig. 15-14). The intensity of the hum is increased when the patient is sitting with the head turned away from the area of auscultation, and it is diminished with a Valsalva maneuver. When present, the hum is a continuous, low-pitched sound that is louder during diastole. It may be interrupted by gentle pressure over the vein in the space between the

FIGURE 15-14 Auscultation for venous hum.

trachea and the sternocleidomastoid muscle at about the level of the thyroid cartilage. The venous hum can be confused with patent ductus arteriosus, aortic regurgitation, and the murmur of valvular aortic stenosis transmitted into the carotid arteries.

Venous thrombosis occurs less commonly in children than in adults and is most often associated with placement of venous access devices. They can occur in any peripheral vessel and cause swollen, painful extremities.

✤ Pregnant Women

With increasing cardiac output beginning in the first trimester, the pulse may be more easily palpated, with an abrupt rise and rapid fall. With increasing blood volume in the second trimester jugular a and v waves may be easier to see. JVP should remain normal. Peripheral edema is a common finding as the pregnancy progresses. Varicose veins can develop during pregnancy and in the postpartum period.

✤ Older Adults

The dorsalis pedis and posterior tibial pulses may be more difficult to find, and the superficial vessels are more apt to appear tortuous and distended.

Sample Documentation
History and Physical Examination

Subjective

A 67-year-old man with a history of carcinoma of the lung noted the onset of pain in his right leg 1 day ago, accompanied by erythema. Pain is severe when he tries to stand upright and is reduced when supine. On a scale of 0 to 10, the patient judges his pain to be a 6.

Objective

Circumference of the leg 7 cm above the medial malleolus is 23 cm on the left and 27 cm on the right. At 15 cm below the patellar tip, the circumference is 37 cm on the left and 40 cm on the right. The right lower extremity is diffusely erythematous. Homan sign is positive on the right.

For additional sample documentation, see Chapter 26, pp. 628-631.

ABNORMALITIES

ABNORMALITIES

BLOOD VESSELS

VESSEL DISORDERS

Temporal Arteritis (Giant Cell Arteritis)

An inflammatory disease of the branches of the aortic arch, including the temporal arteries

Pathophysiology
- Etiology is unknown
- Inflammatory infiltrates develop in the thoracic aorta and neighboring arteries of the head and neck.
- Arterial wall thickening and thrombosis can lead to reduced blood supply and ischemia of structures such as the masseter muscle, tongue, or optic nerve.

Subjective Data
- Usually affects persons older than 50 years of age
- Flu-like symptoms (e.g., low-grade fever, malaise, anorexia) may be accompanied by polymyalgia involving the hips and shoulders.
- Headache in the temporal region on one or both sides, although the headache can occur in other regions
- Ocular symptoms, including loss of vision, are common.
- Ischemia can also cause tongue pain and jaw claudication.

Objective Data
- Area over the temporal artery may be red, swollen, tender, and nodular
- Temporal pulse may be strong, weak, or absent

Arterial Aneurysm

An aneurysm is a localized dilation, generally defined as 1.5 times the diameter of the normal artery, caused by a weakness in the arterial wall (Fig. 15-15).

Pathophysiology
- Usually the result of atherosclerosis with family history, tobacco use, and hypertension playing important roles
- Abdominal aneurysms are four times more common in men than in women.
- Occurs most commonly in the aorta, although renal, femoral, and popliteal arteries are also common sites

Subjective Data
- Generally asymptomatic until they dissect or compress an adjacent structure
- With dissection, the patient may describe a severe ripping pain.

Objective Data
- Pulsatile swelling along the course of an artery
- A thrill or bruit may be evident over the aneurysm.

Normal　　　Aneurysm

Stretched intima
and media

FIGURE 15-15 Aortic aneurysm.

Arteriovenous Fistula

An arteriovenous fistula is a pathologic communication between an artery and a vein.

Pathophysiology
- May be congenital or acquired
- Damage to vessels caused by catheterization is the most common acquired etiology
- If the fistula is large, there may be significant arterial to-venous shunting of blood.
- May result in an aneurysmal dilation

Subjective Data
- Patients may present with lower extremity edema, varicose veins, or claudication due to ischemia.

Objective Data
- A continuous bruit or thrill over the area of the fistula suggests its presence.
- Edema or ischemia may develop in the involved extremity.

Peripheral Arterial Disease

Stenosis of the blood supply to the extremities by atherosclerotic plaques

Pathophysiology	Subjective Data	Objective Data
• Most common cause is peripheral atherosclerosis • Diabetes, hypertension, dyslipidemia, and tobacco use are all risk factors. • Can also be a result of vascular trauma, radiation therapy, or vasculitis	• Pain in muscle after exercise that disappears with rest • The amount of exercise needed to cause discomfort is predictable (e.g., occurring each time the same distance is walked).	• Limb appears healthy, but pulses are weak or absent • Progressive stenosis results in severe ischemia, in which the foot or leg is painful at rest, is cold and numb, and has skin changes (e.g., dry and scaling, with poor hair and nail growth). • Edema seldom accompanies this disorder, but ulceration is common in severe disease, and the muscles may atrophy.

Raynaud Phenomenon

An exaggerated spasm of the digital arterioles (occasionally in the nose and ears) usually in response to cold exposure (Fig. 15-16)

Pathophysiology	Subjective Data	Objective Data
• Primary Raynaud phenomenon occurs most commonly in young, otherwise healthy individuals, most commonly women, with no evidence of underlying cause. • Secondary Raynaud phenomenon is associated with an underlying connective tissue disease such as scleroderma or systemic lupus erythematosus.	• Involved areas feel cold and achy, improve on rewarming • In secondary Raynaud, there can be intense pain from digital ischemia.	• With primary Raynaud phenomenon, there is a triphasic demarcated skin pallor (white), cyanosis (blue), and reperfusion (red) in the extremities. • The vasospasm may last from minutes to less than an hour. • In secondary Raynaud, ulcers may appear on the tips of the digits, and eventually the skin over the digits can appear smooth, shiny, and tight from loss of subcutaneous tissue.

FIGURE 15-16 Raynaud phenomenon. *(From Hallett et al, 2009.)*

Arterial Embolic Disease

Atrial fibrillation can lead to clot formation within the atrium; if the clot is unstable, emboli may be dispersed throughout the arterial system (Fig. 15-17).

Pathophysiology	Subjective Data	Objective Data
• Emboli can also be caused by atherosclerotic plaques, infectious material from fungal and bacterial endocarditis, and atrial myxomas (a mass of connective tissue).	• Pain is the most common symptom. • Paresthesias may also develop.	• Occlusion of small arteries and necrosis of the tissue supplied by that vessel (e.g., blue toe syndrome) • With endocarditis, splinter hemorrhages are seen in the nail beds.

FIGURE 15-17 Embolic phenomenon. *(From Crawford et al, 2005.)*

ABNORMALITIES

Venous Thrombosis

Thrombosis can occur suddenly or gradually and with varying severity of symptoms; it can be the result of trauma or prolonged immobilization.

Pathophysiology	Subjective Data	Objective Data
• Risk factors for venous thrombosis include prolonged immobilization (e.g., bed rest, recent surgery, long airplane flight), malignancy, trauma, use of contraceptive medication, and family or personal history of previous thrombosis.	• Tenderness in area of thrombus, such as along the iliac vessels or the femoral canal, in the popliteal space, or over the deep calf veins • Deep vein thrombosis in the femoral and pelvic circulations may be asymptomatic. • Pulmonary embolism may occur without warning.	• Swelling may be distinguished only by measuring and comparing the circumference of the upper and lower legs bilaterally. • Minimal ankle edema, low-grade fever, and tachycardia • Homan sign can be helpful but is not absolutely reliable in suggesting deep vein thrombosis.

JUGULAR VENOUS PRESSURE DISORDER

Tricuspid Regurgitation

The backflow of blood into the right atrium during systole; a mild degree of tricuspid regurgitation can be seen in up to 75% of the normal adult population.

Pathophysiology	Subjective Data	Objective Data
• Most commonly due to conditions that lead to dilation of the right ventricle (e.g., hypertension, pulmonary thrombosis) • Less frequently it can also result from primary valvular disease.	• With mild to moderate tricuspid regurgitation, there are typically no symptoms. • With severe disease, you may see symptoms of right-sided heart failure such as ascites or peripheral edema.	• The v wave is much more prominent and occurs earlier, often merging with the c wave (Fig. 15-18; for expected normal venous pulsations, see Fig. 15-7). • A holosystolic murmur in the tricuspid region, a pulsatile liver, and peripheral edema

FIGURE 15-18 Diagram of pulsation in tricuspid regurgitation.

✤ Children

Coarctation of the Aorta

Coarctation of the aorta is a stenosis seen most commonly in the descending aortic arch near the origin of the left subclavian artery and ligamentum arteriosum (Fig. 15-19).

Pathophysiology	Subjective Data	Objective Data
• Frequently due to congenital defect of the underlying vascular wall • May also be acquired due to inflammatory aortic disease or severe atherosclerosis	• May be asymptomatic unless severe hypertension or vascular insufficiency develops • If symptomatic, may have symptoms of heart failure or vascular insufficiency of an involved upper extremity with activity	• Differences in systolic blood pressure readings between the arm and leg readings • Femoral pulses are weaker than radial pulses, or femoral pulses are absent.

FIGURE 15-19 Coarctation of the aorta. *(From Shiland, 2006.)*

Kawasaki Disease

An acute small vessel vasculitic illness of uncertain cause affecting young males more often than females; the critical concern is cardiac involvement in which coronary artery aneurysms may develop.

Pathophysiology	Subjective Data	Objective Data
• The cause of the vasculitis is unknown. • Immune-mediated blood vessel damage can result in both vascular stenosis and aneurysm formation.	• The symptoms are diffuse and typified by fever lasting 5 days or more. • The effects of a systemic vasculitis include weight loss, fatigue, and myalgias, as well as arthritis.	• Findings may include fever, conjunctival injection, strawberry tongue, and edema of the hands and feet. • Lymphadenopathy and polymorphous nonvesicular rashes (Fig. 15-20)

FIGURE 15-20 Strawberry tongue. *(From Crawford et al, 2009.)*

✂ Pregnant Women

Preeclampsia-Eclampsia

Preeclampsia-eclampsia defines a syndrome specific to pregnancy; it is determined by hypertension that occurs after the 20th week of pregnancy and the presence of proteinuria; eclampsia is preeclampsia with seizures when no other cause for the seizures can be found.

Pathophysiology	Subjective Data	Objective Data
• Theorized to result from a combination of vascular and immunologic abnormalities within the uteroplacental circulation	• May be diagnosed without proteinuria if other systemic symptoms are present (e.g., visual changes, headache, abdominal pain, pulmonary edema)	• Sustained elevation of the blood pressure (systolic >160 mm Hg, diastolic >110 mm Hg)

✂ Older Adults

Venous Ulcers

This results from chronic venous insufficiency in which lack of venous flow leads to lower extremity venous hypertension (Fig. 15-21).

Pathophysiology	Subjective Data	Objective Data
• Obstruction of venous flow may result from incompetent valves, obstruction of blood flow, or loss of the pumping effect of the leg muscles.	• Frequently asymptomatic in the early stages • Patients may describe a leg heaviness and discomfort progressing to edema and ulceration.	• Ulcers are generally found on the medial or lateral aspects of the lower limbs. • Induration, edema, and hyperpigmentation are common associated findings.

FIGURE 15-21 Venous stasis ulcer. *(From Lemmi and Lemmi, 2000.)*

CHAPTER 16

Breasts and Axillae

The breast examination is typically performed when a patient presents with a specific breast concern, as a follow-up to an abnormal examination or increased risk for breast cancer, or as part of an overall health visit for both women and men. Examination of the breasts includes examination of the axillae and relevant lymph node chains. A major focus of the examination in adults is identification of breast masses, skin, or vascular changes that could indicate malignancy. Breast examination is important in children for Tanner staging and as part of an evaluation regarding premature or delayed puberty.

evolve *http://evolve.elsevier.com/Seidel*
- Physical Exam Key Points
- NCLEX Review Questions
- Interactive Activities
- Videos
- Student Checklist

ANATOMY AND PHYSIOLOGY

The breasts are paired mammary glands located on the anterior chest wall, superficial to the pectoralis major and serratus anterior muscles (Fig. 16-1). In women, the breast extends from the

---

Physical Examination Preview

Here is a preview of the steps involved in conducting a physical examination of the breasts and axillae. ⓔ These procedures are explained in detail in this chapter and are available on Evolve in printable formats.

Breasts and Axillae

Females
1. Inspect with patient seated. Compare breasts for (p. 355):
   - Size
   - Symmetry
   - Contour
   - Retractions or dimpling
   - Skin color and texture
   - Venous patterns
   - Lesions
   - Supernumerary nipples
2. Inspect both areolae and nipples and compare for (p. 356):
   - Shape
   - Symmetry
   - Color
   - Smoothness
   - Size
   - Nipple inversion, eversion, or retraction
3. Reinspect breasts with the patient in the following positions (p. 357):
   - Arms extended over head or flexed behind the neck
   - Hands pressed on hips with shoulder rolled forward

   - Seated and leaning over
   - In recumbent position
4. Perform a chest wall sweep (p. 360).
5. Perform bimanual digital palpation (p. 360).
6. Palpate for lymph nodes in the axilla, down the arm to the elbow, and in the axillary, supraclavicular, and infraclavicular areas (p. 360).
7. Palpate breast tissue with patient supine, using light, medium, and deep pressure (p. 361).
8. Depress the nipple into the well behind the areola (p. 361).

Males
1. Inspect breasts for the following (p. 355):
   - Symmetry
   - Enlargement
   - Surface characteristics
2. Inspect both areolae and nipples and compare for (p. 356):
   - Shape
   - Symmetry
   - Color
   - Smoothness
   - Size
   - Nipple inversion, eversion, or retraction
3. Palpate breasts and over areolae for lumps or nodules (p. 363).
4. Palpate for lymph nodes in the axilla, down the arm to the elbow, and in the axillary, supraclavicular, and infraclavicular areas (p. 360).

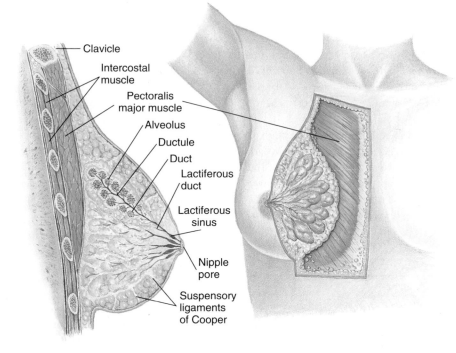

FIGURE 16-1 Anatomy of the breast showing position and major structures.

second or third rib to the sixth or seventh rib and from the sternal margin to the midaxillary line. The nipple is located centrally, surrounded by the areola. The male breast consists of a small nipple and areola overlying a thin layer of breast tissue.

The female breast is composed of glandular and fibrous tissue and subcutaneous and retromammary fat. The glandular tissue is arranged into 15 to 20 lobes per breast that radiate about the nipple. Each lobe is composed of 20 to 40 lobules; each lobule consists of milk-producing acini cells that empty into lactiferous ducts. These cells are small and inconspicuous in nonpregnant, nonlactating women. A lactiferous duct drains milk from each lobe onto the surface of the nipple.

The layer of subcutaneous fibrous tissue provides support for the breast. Suspensory ligaments (Cooper ligaments) extend from the connective tissue layer through the breast and attach to the underlying muscle fascia, providing further support. The muscles forming the floor of the breast are the pectoralis major, pectoralis minor, serratus anterior, latissimus dorsi, subscapularis, external oblique, and rectus abdominis.

Vascular supply to the breast is primarily through branches of the internal mammary artery and the lateral thoracic artery. This network provides most of the blood supply to the deeper tissues of the breast and to the nipple. The subcutaneous and retromammary fat that surrounds the glandular tissue constitutes most of the bulk of the breast and gives the breast its soft consistency. The proportions of each of the component tissues vary with age, nutritional status, pregnancy, lactation, and genetic predisposition.

For the purposes of examination the breast is divided into five segments, four quadrants and a tail (Fig. 16-2). The greatest amount of glandular tissue lies in the upper outer quadrant.

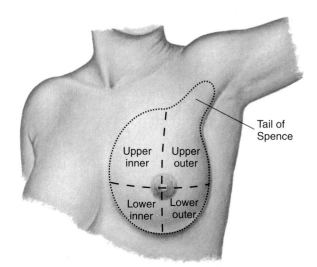

FIGURE 16-2 Quadrants of the left breast and axillary tail of Spence.

Breast tissue extends from this quadrant into the axilla, forming the tail of Spence. In the axillae the mammary tissue is in direct contact with the axillary lymph nodes.

The nipple is located centrally on the breast and is surrounded by the pigmented areola. The nipple is composed of epithelium that is infiltrated with circular and longitudinal smooth muscle fibers. Contraction of the smooth muscle, induced by tactile, sensory, or autonomic stimuli, produces erection of the nipple and causes the lactiferous ducts to empty. Tiny sebaceous glands may be apparent on the areola surface (Montgomery tubercles or follicles). Hair follicles may be found about the circumference of

ANATOMY AND PHYSIOLOGY

the areola. Supernumerary nipples or breast tissue is sometimes present along the mammary ridge that extends from the axilla to the groin (see Fig. 16-10).

Each breast contains a lymphatic network that drains the breast radially and deeply to underlying lymphatics. Superficial lymphatics drain the skin, and deep lymphatics drain the mammary lobules. Table 16-1 summarizes the patterns of lymph drainage.

The complex of lymph nodes, their locations, and direction of drainage are illustrated in Figure 16-3. The axillary nodes are more superficial and accessible to palpation when enlarged. The anterior axillary (pectoral) nodes are located along the lower border of the pectoralis major, inside the lateral axillary fold. The midaxillary (central) nodes are high in the axilla close to the ribs.

The posterior axillary (subscapular) nodes lie along the lateral border of the scapula and deep in the posterior axillary fold, whereas the lateral axillary (brachial) nodes can be felt along the upper humerus.

�֍ Children and Adolescents

The breast evolves in structure and function throughout life. Childhood and preadolescence represent a latent phase of breast development (see Physical Variations, "Breast Development"). Thelarche (breast development) represents the first sign of puberty in girls. The developmental process can be classified using the five Tanner stages of breast development and sexual maturation rating, as discussed in Chapter 6.

Table 16-1	Patterns of Lymph Drainage
Area of Breast	**Drainage**
Superficial	
Upper outer quadrant	Scapular, brachial, intermediate nodes toward axillary nodes
Medial portion	Internal mammary chain toward opposite breast and abdomen
Deep	
Posterior chest wall and portion	Posterior axillary nodes (subscapular) of the arm
Anterior chest wall	Anterior axillary nodes (pectoral)
Upper arm	Lateral axillary nodes (brachial)
Retroareolar area	Interpectoral (Rotter) nodes into the axillary chain
Areola and Nipple	Midaxillary, infraclavicular, and supraclavicular nodes

Physical Variations

Breast Development
As girls approach puberty they often worry about when their breasts will begin to develop. Thelarche occurs earlier in black girls than in white girls. For Hispanic girls the age is between that of the other two groups. Racial and ethnic differences reflect a combination of genetic, social, and environmental factors.

Euling et al, 2008.

In using the Tanner system to stage breast development, it is important to note temporal relationships. It is unusual for the onset of menses to occur before stage 3. About 25% of females begin menstruation at stage 3. Approximately 75% are menstruating at stage 4 and are beginning a regular menstrual cycle. Some 10% of young women do not begin to menstruate until stage 5. The average interval from the appearance of the breast bud (stage 2) to menarche is 2 years. Breasts develop at

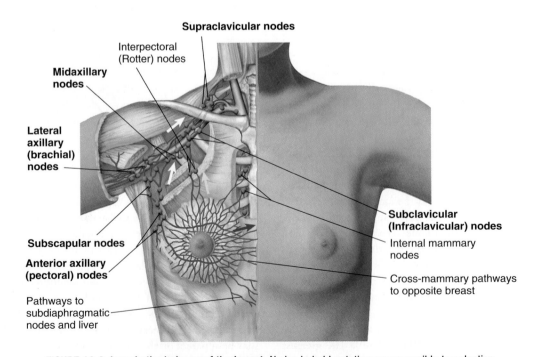

FIGURE 16-3 Lymphatic drainage of the breast. Nodes in bold notation are accessible to palpation.

different rates in the individual, which can result in temporary asymmetry.

✤ Pregnant Women

Striking changes occur in the breasts during pregnancy. In response to luteal and placental hormones, the lactiferous ducts proliferate and the alveoli increase extensively in size and number, which may cause the breasts to enlarge two to three times their prepregnancy size. The increase in glandular tissue displaces connective tissue and the breasts become softer and looser. Toward the end of pregnancy, as epithelial secretory activity increases, colostrum is produced and accumulates in the acinus cells (alveoli).

The areolae become more deeply pigmented and their diameter increases. The nipples become more prominent, darker, and more erectile. Montgomery tubercles often develop as sebaceous glands hypertrophy.

Mammary vascularization increases, causing veins to engorge and become visible as a blue network beneath the surface of the skin.

✤ Lactating Women

In the first few days after delivery, small amounts of colostrum are secreted from the breasts. Colostrum contains more protein and minerals than does mature milk. Colostrum also contains antibodies and other host resistance factors. Milk production replaces colostrum 2 to 4 days after delivery in response to surging prolactin levels, declining estrogen levels, and the stimulation of sucking. As the alveoli and lactiferous ducts fill, the breasts may become full and tense. This, combined with tissue edema and a delay in effective ejection reflexes, produces breast engorgement.

At the termination of lactation, involution occurs over a period of about 3 months. Breast size decreases without loss of lobular and alveolar components; the breasts rarely return to their prelactation size.

✤ Older Adults

After menopause, glandular tissue atrophies gradually and is replaced by fat. The inframammary ridge at the lower edge of the breast thickens. The breasts tend to hang more loosely from the chest wall as a result of the tissue changes and relaxation of the suspensory ligaments. The nipples become smaller and flatter and lose some erectile ability.

The skin may take on a relatively dry, thin texture. Loss of axillary hair may also occur.

REVIEW OF RELATED HISTORY

For each of the symptoms or conditions discussed in this section, targeted topics to include in the history of the present illness are listed. Responses to questions about these topics help fully assess the patient's condition and provide clues for focusing the physical examination and the development of an appropriate diagnostic evaluation. Questions regarding medication use (prescription and over the counter preparations) as well as complementary and alternative therapies are relevant for each.

History of Present Illness

*   Breast discomfort/pain
    *   Temporal sequence: onset gradual or sudden; length of time symptom has been present; does symptom come and go or is it always present
    *   Relationship to menses: timing, severity
    *   Character: stinging, pulling, burning, drawing, stabbing, aching, throbbing; unilateral or bilateral; localization; radiation
    *   Associated symptoms: lump or mass, discharge from nipple
    *   Contributory factors: skin irritation under breasts from tissue-to-tissue contact or from rubbing of undergarments; strenuous activity; recent injury to breast
    *   Medications: hormones or bioidentical hormones; oral contraceptives
*   Breast mass or lump
    *   Temporal sequence: length of time since lump first noted; does lump come and go or is it always present; relationship to menses
    *   Symptoms: tenderness or pain (characterize as described previously), dimpling or change in contour
    *   Changes in lump: size, character, relationship to menses (timing or severity)
    *   Associated symptoms: nipple discharge or retraction, tender lymph nodes
    *   Medications: hormones or bioidentical hormones
*   Nipple discharge
    *   Character: spontaneous or provoked; unilateral or bilateral, onset gradual or sudden, duration, color, consistency, odor, amount
    *   Associated symptoms: nipple retraction; breast lump or discomfort
    *   Associated factors: relationship to menses or other activity; recent injury to breast
    *   Medications: contraceptives; hormones, phenothiazines, digitalis, diuretics, steroids
*   Breast enlargement in men
    *   History of hyperthyroidism, testicular cancer, Klinefelter syndrome
    *   Medications: cimetidine, omeprazole, spironolactone, antiandrogens (finasteride), human immunodeficiency virus (HIV) medications (efavirenz), some chemotherapy agents, some antihypertensives, some antipsychotics
    *   Treatment for prostate cancer with antiandrogens or gonadotropin-releasing hormone analogs
    *   Illicit drugs: anabolic steroids, marijuana

Past Medical History

*   Previous breast disease: cancer, fibroadenomas, fibrocystic changes
*   Known *BRCA1*, *BRCA2*, or other genetic mutation; known hereditary cancer syndrome (hereditary nonpolyposis colorectal cancer [HNPCC], Li-Fraumeni syndrome, or Cowden syndrome)

Box 16-1 Screening Recommendations for Breast Cancer

Breast cancer is the most common cancer among women in the United States and is the second leading cause of cancer death in women. Early detection through screening is important for timely treatment and prevention of death. Authorities do not completely agree on the need for, frequency of, and timing of screening (see the Evidence-Based Practice box). CBE, mammography, MRI, and breast self-awareness are the currently available modalities for screening asymptomatic women.

Summary of Recommendations

CBE
- Younger than 40 years of age: every 3 years (ACS, 2012)
- Older than 40 years of age: annually (ACS, 2012)
- Insufficient evidence to assess the additional benefits and harms of CBE beyond screening mammography in women 40 years or older (USPSTF, 2009)

Mammogram
- Yearly starting at 40 years of age and continuing for as long as a woman is in good health (ACS 2012)
- Biennial screening mammography for women between the ages of 50 and 74 years (USPSTF, 2009)
- Insufficient evidence to assess the additional benefits and harms in women 75 years or older (USPSTF, 2009)

MRI
- Women at high risk:
  - Known *BRCA* mutation or untested but have a first-degree relative with a *BRCA* mutation
  - Greater than 20% lifetime risk based primarily on family history
  - Prior mantle radiation
- MRI in addition to mammogram every year (ACS, 2012)

Breast Self-Awareness
- Women should be familiar with their breasts and report any changes to their health care provider (ACS, 2012)
- Not addressed by USPSTF (USPSTF, 2009)

ACS, American Cancer Society; *USPSTF*, United States Preventive Services Task Force.

- Previous other related cancers: ovarian, colorectal, endometrial
- Surgeries: breast biopsies, aspirations, implants, reductions, reconstructions, oophorectomy
- Risk factors for breast cancer (see the Risk Factors box)
- Mammogram and other breast imaging history: frequency, date of last imaging, results (Box 16-1)
- Menstrual history: first day of last menstrual period; age at menarche and menopause; cycle length, duration, amount of flow, and regularity; associated breast symptoms (nipple discharge; pain or discomfort)
- Pregnancy: age at each pregnancy, length of each pregnancy, date of delivery or termination
- Lactation: number of children breast-fed; duration of time for breast-feeding; date of termination of last breast-feeding; medications used to suppress lactation
- Menopause: onset, course, associated problems, residual problems

- Use of hormonal medications: name and dosage, reason for use (contraception, menstrual control, menopausal symptom relief), length of time on hormones, date of termination
- Other medications: nonprescription or prescription; hormones (estrogen, progesterone), selective estrogen receptor modulators (SERMS) (tamoxifen, raloxifene), aromatase inhibitors (e.g., anastrozole, letrozole, exemestane)

Risk Factors
Breast Cancer

Nonmodifiable Factors

Age: Risk increases with aging.

Gender: Female. More women than men develop breast cancer.

Genetic risk factors: Women with an inherited *BRCA1* or *BRCA2* mutation have a 35% to 85% chance of developing breast cancer during their lifetime as compared to the average risk of about 12%.

Personal history of breast cancer: Cancer in one breast increases risk of developing a new cancer in the other breast.

Family history of breast cancer: Having one first-degree relative (mother, sister, or daughter) with breast cancer approximately doubles a woman's risk and having two first-degree relatives increases her risk fivefold.

Previous breast biopsies: Atypical hyperplasia or lobular cancer in situ (LCIS) substantially increases breast cancer risk. Fibrocystic changes without proliferative breast disease do not affect breast cancer risk.

Race: White women are higher risk than other racial/ethnic groups.

Previous breast radiation: Radiation therapy to the chest area as treatment for another cancer (such as Hodgkin disease or non-Hodgkin lymphoma) significantly increases risk for breast cancer.

Menstrual periods: Menarche before age 12 or menopause after age 55 slightly increases risk.

Breast density: Breast tissue may be dense or fatty. Older women whose mammograms show more dense tissue are at increased risk.

Diethylstilbestrol (DES) therapy: Women who received diethylstilbestrol in the 1940s through the 1960s during their pregnancies have a slightly increased risk. Women exposed to DES in utero—daughters whose mothers took DES while they were pregnant—may have a slightly increased risk of breast cancer after age 40.

Modifiable/Lifestyle Factors

Childbirth: Nulliparity or late age at birth of first child (after age 30) is associated with an increased risk.

Hormone therapy: Use of combined estrogen and progesterone hormone replacement therapy (HRT) after menopause (more than 4 years of use) increases risk.

Alcohol: Risk increases with amount of alcohol consumed.

Obesity and high-fat diets: Obesity is associated with an increased risk, especially for women after menopause. Having more fat tissue can increase estrogen levels and increase the likelihood of developing breast cancer.

Lack of physical activity: Women who are physically inactive throughout life may have an increased risk of breast cancer.

From American Cancer Society, 2011; National Cancer Institute, 2012.

Family History

+ Breast cancer: primary relatives, secondary relatives; type of cancer; age at time of occurrence; treatment and results; known *BRCA1*, *BRCA2*, or other mutation
+ Other cancers: ovarian, colorectal, known hereditary cancer syndromes (breast-ovarian cancer syndrome, HNPCC, Li-Fraumeni syndrome, or Cowden syndrome)
+ Other breast disease in female and male relatives: type of disease; age at time of occurrence; treatment and results

Personal and Social History

+ Age
+ Breast support used with strenuous exercise or sports activities
+ Amount of caffeine intake; impact on breast tissue
+ Breast self-awareness/self-examination: frequency; at what time in the menstrual cycle; see Staying Well, "Breast Self-Examination and Self-Awareness"
+ Use of alcohol; daily amounts
+ Use of anabolic steroids or marijuana

Staying Well

Breast Self-Examination and Self-Awareness

Breast self-awareness has largely replaced breast self-examination (BSE) as a tool in the detection of breast cancer. The American Cancer Society supports both options and recommends that women be informed about the potential benefits and limitations associated with BSE (ACS, 2014). The U.S. Preventive Services Task Force (USPSTF, 2009) recommends against teaching BSE. The lesson learned from a randomized clinical trial is that intensive teaching of BSE does not improve its effectiveness (Thomas et al, 2002) and that self-awareness may be more effective for detecting breast cancer than structured BSE. Every woman should be familiar with her own breasts and should report any breast change promptly to her health care provider. Women can notice changes in their breasts by being aware of how their breasts normally feel and feeling their breasts for changes. As you discuss self-awareness, it would be an appropriate time to review the accepted recommendations for early breast cancer detection (Box 16-1) and to discuss the issues related to breast cancer screening.

✼ Pregnant Women

+ Sensations: fullness, tingling, tenderness
+ Presence of colostrum and knowledge about how to care for breasts and nipples during pregnancy
+ Use of supportive bra
+ Knowledge and information about breast-feeding
+ Plans to breastfeed, experience, expectations, concerns

✼ Lactating Women

+ Cleaning procedures for breasts: use of soap products that can remove natural lubricants, frequency of use; nipple preparations

+ Use of breast-feeding bra
+ Nipples: tenderness, pain, cracking, bleeding; retracted; related problems with feeding; exposure to air
+ Associated problems: engorgement, leaking breasts, plugged duct (localized tenderness and lump), fever, infection; treatment and results; infant with oral candidal infection
+ Breast-feeding routine: length of feeding, frequency, rotation of breasts, positions used
+ Breast milk pumping devices used, frequency of use
+ Cultural beliefs about breast-feeding
+ Food and environmental agents that can affect breast milk (e.g., chocolate, alcohol, pesticides)
+ Medications that can cross the milk-blood barrier (e.g., cimetidine, clemastine, thiouracil); all medications—prescription and nonprescription—should be evaluated for potential side effects in the newborn.

✼ Older Adults

+ Skin irritation under pendulous breasts from tissue-to-tissue contact or from rubbing of undergarments; treatment
+ Hormone therapy during or since menopause: name and dosage of medication; duration of therapy

---

EXAMINATION AND FINDINGS

Equipment

+ Small pillow or folded towel
+ Ruler
+ Flashlight with transilluminator
+ Glass slide and cytologic fixative, if nipple discharge is present

Adequate lighting is essential for revealing shadows and subtle variations in skin color and texture. Adequate exposure is also essential, requiring that the patient be disrobed to the waist. Simultaneous observation of both breasts is necessary to detect minor differences between them that may be significant. Stay attentive for modesty concerns and convey the need for full exposure. The presence of a chaperone may ease discomfort and protect both the patient and the examining health care provider and is recommended with adolescent patients.

Inspection

Breasts

As the patient sits with arms hanging loosely at the sides, inspect each breast and compare it with the other for size, symmetry, contour, skin color and texture, venous patterns, and lesions. Perform this portion of the examination for both women and men. With female patients, lift the breasts with your fingertips, inspecting the lower and lateral aspects to determine changes in the color or texture of the skin.

Women's breasts vary in shape, from convex to pendulous or conical, and often one breast is somewhat smaller than the other (Fig. 16-4). Men's breasts are generally even with the chest wall, although some men, particularly those who are overweight, have breasts with a convex shape.

FIGURE 16-4 Variations in breast size and contour. A, Conical. B, Convex. C, Pendulous. D, Large pendulous. E, Right larger than left.

The skin texture should appear smooth and the contour should be uninterrupted. Alterations in contour are best seen on bilateral comparison of one breast with the other. Retractions and dimpling signify the contraction of fibrotic tissue that may occur with carcinoma. A peau d'orange (orange skin) appearance of the skin indicates edema of the breast caused by blocked lymph drainage in advanced or inflammatory breast cancer (Fig. 16-5). The skin appears thickened with enlarged pores and accentuated skin markings. Healthy skin may look similar if the pores of the skin are large.

Venous networks may be visible, although they are usually pronounced only in the breasts of pregnant or obese women. Venous patterns should be symmetric. Unilateral venous patterns can be produced by dilated superficial veins as a result of increased blood flow to a malignancy. This finding requires further investigation.

Other markings and nevi that are long-standing, unchanging, or nontender are usually of little concern. Changes in or the recent appearance of any lesions always signal the need for closer investigation.

Nipples and Areolae

Inspect the areolae and nipples of both men and women. The areola should be round or oval and bilaterally symmetrical or nearly so. The color ranges from pink to black. In light-skinned

FIGURE 16-5 Peau d'orange appearance from edema. *(From Gallager, 1978.)*

women the areola usually turns brown with the first pregnancy and remains dark. In women with dark skin, the areola is brown before pregnancy. A peppering of nontender, nonsuppurative Montgomery tubercles is a common expected finding (Fig. 16-6). The surface should be otherwise smooth. The peau d'orange skin associated with cancer is often seen first in the areola.

Most nipples are everted, but one or both nipples may be inverted (Fig. 16-7), with the nipple tucked inward. In these instances, ask whether there is a lifetime history of inversion.

FIGURE 16-6 **Montgomery tubercles. A,** Light-skinned woman. **B,** Dark-skinned woman. *(A, from Mansel and Bundred, 1995.)*

FIGURE 16-7 **A,** Left nipple inverted; right nipple everted. **B,** Close-up of nipple inversion. *(From Lemmi and Lemmi, 2000.)*

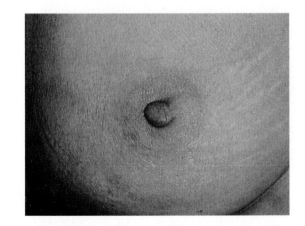

FIGURE 16-8 **Nipple retraction laterally and swelling behind right nipple in Asian woman with breast cancer.** *(From Mansel and Bundred, 1995.)*

Recent unilateral inversion of a previously everted nipple suggests malignancy.

Simultaneous bilateral inspection is necessary to detect nipple retraction or deviation. Retraction is seen as a flattening or pulling back of the nipple and areola, which indicates inward pulling by inflammatory or malignant tissue (Fig. 16-8; also see

Fig. 16-19). The fibrotic tissue of carcinoma can also change the axis of the nipple, causing it to point in a direction different from that of the other nipple.

The nipples should be a homogeneous color and match that of the areolae. Their surface may be either smooth or wrinkled but should be free of crusting, cracking, or discharge. Areola color varies from light pink to very dark brown or black (Fig. 16-9). Inflammation of the sebaceous glands in the areola can result in retention cysts that are tender and suppurative.

Supernumerary nipples, which are more common in black women than in white women, appear as one or more extra nipples located along the embryonic mammary ridge (the "milk line") (Fig. 16-10). These nipples and areolae may be pink or brown, are usually small, and are commonly mistaken for moles (Fig. 16-11). Infrequently, some glandular tissue may accompany these nipples. In some cases, supernumerary nipples may be associated with congenital renal or cardiac anomalies, particularly in whites.

Reinspection in Varied Positions

Reinspect the woman's breasts with the patient in the following positions:

+ Seated with arms over the head or flexed behind the neck. This adds tension to the suspensory ligaments, accentuates

EXAMINATION AND FINDINGS

Evidence-Based Practice in Physical Examination

Breast Cancer Screening

Are clinical breast examination (CBE), mammography, and magnetic resonance imaging (MRI) effective in screening for breast cancer? A clear distinction must be made between screening asymptomatic women and the clinical assessment of women who have breast symptoms. The evidence is controversial and mixed.

CBE

The sensitivity of CBE in detecting breast cancer ranges from 40% to 69% and the specificity from 88% to 99% (USPSTF, 2012). No trial has compared CBE alone with no screening. The sensitivity of the CBE combined with mammography is greater than that of mammography alone because CBE can detect cancer missed by mammography. Proportions of breast cancers found by CBE but missed by mammography range from 5.2% to 29%. The value of detecting breast cancers by CBE that are not detected by mammography is not known. The results of randomized trials using both modalities did not demonstrate improved results over those using only mammography. The mortality rate in women in whom breast cancer is missed by mammography and detected by CBE was higher in women whose cancers were detected by mammography alone (Barton and Harris, 2009).

Mammography

The sensitivity of mammography screening is 77% to 95%, whereas specificity is 94% to 97% (USPSTF, 2012). However, estimates of the sensitivity and specificity of mammography in detecting breast cancer vary and multiple factors, including age, time since last examination, breast tissue density, equipment, and the skill of the interpreting radiologist can affect sensitivity and specificity. Sensitivity is lower among women who are younger than 50 years of age, have denser breasts, or are taking hormone replacement therapy. Specificity is increased with a shorter screening interval and the availability of prior mammograms. A decision analysis performed for the USPSTF projected that biennial screening produced 70% to 99% of the benefit of annual screening and that screening between the ages of 50 and 69 years produced a projected 17% reduction in mortality compared with no screening (USPSTF, 2009). In comparison, using the same data, another analysis showed a 39.6% mortality reduction from annual screening in women 40 to 84 years old (Hendrick and Helvie, 2011).

MRI

MRI in high-risk women without cancer has a sensitivity of 71% to 100% and a specificity of 81% to 97%. Therefore MRI is used to supplement mammography and clinical breast examination for screening of women who are at high risk of developing breast cancer from genetic mutations (see Box 16-1). Data from a systematic review indicate that screening with both MRI and mammography might rule out cancerous lesions better than mammography alone in women who are known or likely to have an inherited predisposition to breast cancer (Warner et al, 2011). No studies have been done using MRI to screen women at average risk. Therefore, for average-risk women, MRI is reserved for diagnostic evaluation.

It is important to educate patients about the likelihood and significance of both false-positive and false-negative test results and address the associated issues of uncertainty, anxiety, and cost.

FIGURE 16-9 Variations in color of areola. **A**, Pink. **B**, Brown. **C**, Black.

dimpling, and may reveal variations in contour and symmetry (Fig. 16-12, *A*).

+ Seated with hands pressed against hips with shoulders rolled forward (or alternatively have the patient push her palms together): This contracts the pectoral muscles, which can reveal deviations in contour and symmetry (Fig. 16-12, *B* and *C*).

+ Seated and leaning forward from the waist: This also causes tension in the suspensory ligaments. The breasts should hang equally. This maneuver can be particularly helpful in assessing the contour and symmetry of large breasts because the breasts fall away from the chest wall and hang freely. As the patient leans forward, support her by the hands (Fig. 16-12, *D*).

For all patient positions, the breasts should appear bilaterally symmetrical, with an even contour and absence of dimpling, retraction, or deviation.

Palpation

After a thorough inspection, systematically palpate the breasts, axillae, and supraclavicular and infraclavicular regions. Palpation of male breasts can be brief but should not be omitted.

FIGURE 16-10 Supernumerary nipples and tissue may arise along the "milk line," an embryonic ridge. *(From Thompson et al, 1997.)*

FIGURE 16-11 **A,** Supernumerary nipple without glandular tissue. **B,** Supernumerary breast and nipple on left side and supernumerary nipple alone on right side. *(B, From Mansel and Bundred, 1995.)*

FIGURE 16-12 **Inspect the breasts in the following positions. A,** Arms extended overhead. **B,** Hands pressed against hips. **C,** Pressing hands together (an alternative way to flex the pectoral muscles). **D,** Leaning forward from the waist.

FIGURE 16-13 **Chest wall sweep.** With the palm of your hand, sweep from the clavicle to the nipple, covering the area from the sternum to the midaxillary line.

FIGURE 16-15 Palpation of the axilla for lymph nodes.

FIGURE 16-14 **Bimanual digital palpation.** Walk your fingers across the breast tissue, compressing it between your fingers and the palmar surface of your other hand.

Patient in Seated Position

Chest Wall Sweep. Have the patient sit with arms hanging freely at the sides. Place the palm of your right hand at the patient's right clavicle at the sternum. Sweep downward from the clavicle to the nipple, feeling for superficial lumps. Repeat the sweep until you have covered the entire right chest wall. Repeat the procedure using your left hand for the left chest wall (Fig. 16-13).

Bimanual Digital Palpation. Place one hand, palmar surface facing up, under the patient's right breast. Position your hand so that it acts as a flat surface against which to compress the breast tissue. With the fingers of the other hand, walk across the breast tissue, feeling for lumps as you compress the tissue between your fingers and your flat hand. Repeat the procedure for the other breast (Fig. 16-14).

Lymph Node Palpation. Palpate for lymph nodes in both male and female patients. To palpate the axillae, have the patient seated with arms flexed at the elbow. Support the patient's left lower arm with your left hand while examining the left axilla with your right hand, as shown in Figure 16-15. With the palmar surface of your fingers, reach deeply into the axillary hollow,

pushing firmly so that you are gently rolling the soft tissue against the chest wall and muscles of the axilla. From the apex, palpate downward to the bra line and also along the inner aspect of the upper arm down to the elbow. Reposition your fingers to palpate the medial aspect along the rib cage and into the anterior wall along the pectoral muscles. Reposition again to palpate the posterior wall along the border of the scapula. Repeat the mirror image of this maneuver for the right axilla.

Palpate the supraclavicular and infraclavicular areas for the presence of enlarged nodes. Hook your fingers over the clavicle and rotate them over the entire supraclavicular fossa. Have the patient turn his or her head toward the side being palpated and raise the same shoulder, allowing your fingers to reach more deeply into the fossa. Have the patient bend the head forward to relax the sternocleidomastoid muscle. These nodes are considered to be sentinel nodes (Virchow nodes), so any enlargement is highly significant. Sentinel nodes are indicators for invasion of the lymphatics by cancer. Move your fingers to the infraclavicular area and palpate along the clavicle using a rotary motion with your fingers.

Lymph nodes in these areas are not usually palpable in the healthy adult. Palpable nodes may be the result of an inflammatory or malignant process. Move your fingers to the infraclavicular area and palpate along the clavicle using a rotary motion with your fingers. Nodes that are detected should be described according to location, size, shape, consistency, tenderness, fixation, and delineation of borders (see Chapter 9).

Patient in Supine Position

Have the patient raise one arm behind her head; then place a small pillow or folded towel under that shoulder to spread the breast tissue more evenly over the chest wall (Fig. 16-16). The ideal position for examination is to have the nipple pointing toward the ceiling. Women with large breasts may need to roll slightly to achieve this position. Palpate each breast separately.

Palpate all areas of breast tissue, feeling for lumps or nodules (Box 16-2). Remember that the breast tissue extends from the second or third rib to the sixth or seventh rib, and from the sternal margin to the midaxillary line. It is essential to include

Box 16-2   Documenting Breast Masses

If a breast mass is felt, characterize it by its location, size, shape, consistency, tenderness, mobility, delineation of borders, and retraction (see Figs. 16-21 and 16-22). Ultrasound can be used to confirm the presence of fluid in certain masses. These characteristics are not diagnostic by themselves but in conjunction with a thorough history, they provide a great deal of clinical information for correlation with findings from diagnostic testing.

Describe any breast mass or lump that you encounter using the following characteristics:

- Location: clock positions and distance from nipple
- Size (in centimeters): length, width, thickness
- Shape: round, discoid, lobular, stellate, regular or irregular
- Consistency: firm, soft, hard
- Tenderness
- Mobility: movable (in what directions) or fixed to overlying skin or subadjacent fascia
- Borders: discrete or poorly defined
- Retraction: presence or absence of dimpling; altered contour

All new solitary or dominant masses must be investigated with further diagnostic testing.

FIGURE 16-16 Supine position for palpation.

the tail of Spence in palpation. Recall that the greatest amount of glandular tissue lies in the upper outer quadrant of the breast, with tissue extending from this quadrant into the axilla to form the tail of Spence.

Palpate using your finger pads as they are more sensitive than your fingertips. Palpate systematically, pushing gently but firmly, toward the chest wall, as you rotate your fingers in a clockwise or counterclockwise pattern. At each point, as you rotate your fingers, press inward, using three depths of palpation: light, then medium, and finally deep. The exact sequence you select for palpation is not critical, but a systematic approach will help ensure that all portions of the breast are examined. Figure 16-17 illustrates three methods that are commonly used. In the vertical strip technique, begin at the top of the breast and palpate, first downward, then upward, working your way down over the entire breast. In the concentric circle technique, begin at the outermost edge of the breast tissue and spiral your way inward toward the nipple. To use the wedge method, palpate from the center of the breast in radial fashion, returning to the areola to begin each spoke. Regardless of the method, glide your fingers from one point to the next. Avoid lifting your fingers off the breast tissue because doing so makes it easy to miss tissue.

Early lesions can be tiny and may be detected only through meticulous technique. If a breast mass is felt, note its characteristics and palpate its dimensions, consistency, and mobility (Fig. 16-18) and whether it causes dimpling or retraction (Fig. 16-19; see Box 16-2). Also see Staying Well, "Breast Health."

At the completion of the examination, return to the nipple and with two fingers, gently depress the tissue inward into the well behind the areola. Your fingers and tissue should move easily inward (Fig. 16-20).

Nipple compression should be performed only if the patient reports spontaneous nipple discharge (see Clinical Pearl, "Nipple Compression"). Determine whether the discharge is bilateral or unilateral. Use a magnifying glass to look closely at the nipple to determine whether the discharge is from a single duct or multiple

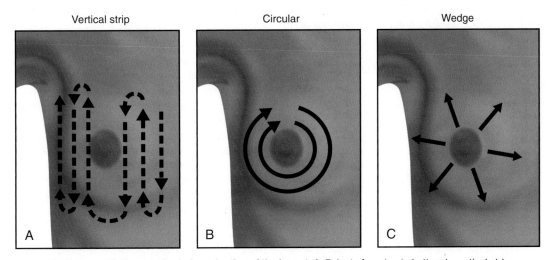

Vertical strip   Circular   Wedge

FIGURE 16-17 **Various methods for palpation of the breast. A,** Palpate from top to bottom in vertical strips.
B, Palpate in concentric circles. **C,** Palpate out from the center in wedge sections.

FIGURE 16-18 A, Palpating for consistency of a breast lesion. **B,** Palpating for delineation of borders of breast mass. **C,** Palpating for mobility of breast mass.

FIGURE 16-19 A, Clinical signs of cancer. **B,** Nipple retraction and dimpling of skin. *(B, From Lemmi and Lemmi, 2000.)*

FIGURE 16-20 Depressing nipple inward into well behind the areola.

Staying Well

Breast Health: Can Breast Cancer Be Prevented?

At this time there is no guaranteed way to prevent breast cancer. The best preventive health strategy is to reduce known risk factors whenever possible. Maintaining a healthy weight, engaging in regular physical activity, reducing alcohol intake to no more than one drink a day for women, and avoiding the use of postmenopausal combination hormone therapy are lifestyle changes that can decrease the risk of breast cancer.

Women who are at increased risk of breast cancer may consider chemoprevention. Tamoxifen has been shown to reduce the risk by almost 50% in women who are at high risk (Fisher et al, 1998). Raloxifene is equally effective in reducing the risk of invasive breast cancer (Vogel et al, 2006). Women at very high risk may elect prophylactic mastectomy, which has been shown to reduce the risk of developing breast cancer by about 90% (Hartmann et al, 2001).

FIGURE 16-21 **Types of nipple discharge. A,** Milky discharge. **B,** Multicolored sticky discharge. **C,** Purulent discharge. **D,** Watery discharge. **E,** Serous discharge. **F,** Serosanguineous discharge. *(From Gallager, 1978.)*

ducts. Characteristics of concern include spontaneous discharge that is unilateral and from a single duct. Figure 16-21 shows various types of nipple discharge.

Clinical Pearl

Nipple Compression

Nipple compression to provoke discharge is no longer performed as part of routine clinical breast examination. Many benign circumstances including prior breast-feeding and nipple stimulation as a part of sexual activity can result in nipple discharge when the nipple is compressed.

Females. The breast tissue of adult women will feel dense, firm, and elastic. Expected variations include the lobular feel of glandular tissue (soft nondiscrete bumps diffusely dispersed throughout the breast tissue) and the fine, granular feel of breast tissue in older women. A firm transverse ridge of compressed tissue (the inframammary ridge) may be felt along the lower edge of the breast. It is easy to mistake this for a breast mass. A cyclical pattern of breast enlargement, increased nodularity, and tenderness is a common response to hormonal changes during the menstrual cycle. Be aware of where the woman is in her cycle because these changes are most likely to occur premenstrually and during menses. They are least noticeable during the week after menses. The procedure for examining the patient who has had a mastectomy is described in Box 16-3.

Males. In most men, expect to feel a thin layer of fatty tissue overlying muscle. Obese men may have a somewhat thicker fatty layer, giving the appearance of breast enlargement. A firm disk of glandular tissue can be felt in some men.

✿ Infants

The breasts of many well newborns, male and female, are enlarged for a relatively brief time as a result of passively transferred maternal estrogen. If you squeeze the breast bud gently, a small amount of clear or milky white fluid, commonly called "witch's milk," is sometimes expressed. The enlargement is rarely more than 1 to 1.5 cm in diameter and can be easily palpated behind the nipple. It usually disappears within 2 weeks and rarely lasts beyond 3 months of age.

✿ Children and Adolescents

The right and left breasts of the adolescent female may not develop at the same rate. Reassure the girl that this asymmetry is common and that her breasts are developing appropriately. Chapter 6 describes the stages of breast development. Breast tissue of the adolescent female feels homogeneous, dense, firm, and elastic. Although malignancy in this age group is rare, routine examination provides an excellent opportunity for reassurance and education for the girl and the parent.

Many males at puberty have transient unilateral or bilateral subareolar masses. These are firm, sometimes tender, and are often a source of great concern to the patient and his parents. Reassure them that these breast buds will most likely disappear,

Box 16-3 Examining the Patient Who Has Had a Mastectomy

- The patient who has had a mastectomy has special examination needs. In addition to examining the unaffected breast in the usual manner, you must examine the mastectomy site, with particular attention to the scar. If malignancy recurs, it may be at the scar site. Be aware that a woman who has had a mastectomy may feel uncomfortable removing her bra and prosthesis if she wears one.
- Inspect the mastectomy site and axilla for any visible signs of swelling, lumps, thickening, redness, color change, rash, or irritation to the scar. Note muscle loss or lymphedema that may be present, depending on the type and extent of the surgical procedure.
- Palpate the surgical scar with two fingers, using small, circular motions to assess for swelling, lumps, thickening, or tenderness. Then palpate the chest wall using three or four fingers in a sweeping motion across the area, being sure not to miss any spots. Intercostal residual breast tissue may exist. Position your fingers on either side of each rib and run your fingers along the anterior ribs, using a stripping motion. Remember to use your finger pads and not your fingertips. Finally, palpate for lymph nodes in the axillary and supraclavicular and infraclavicular areas.
- If the patient has had breast reconstruction, augmentation, or a lumpectomy, perform breast examination in the usual manner, with particular attention to any scars and new tissue.

Have this patient demonstrate her breast self-examination procedures. Regular monthly breast self-examination is an essential component of continuing health care for these women.

usually within a year. They seldom enlarge to a point of cosmetic difficulty.

Occasionally, pubescent males experience gynecomastia, breast enlargement that is readily noticeable. Fortunately, it is usually temporary and benign and resolves spontaneously. If the enlargement is extreme, it can be corrected surgically for psychologic or cosmetic reasons. In rare instances, biopsy is required to rule out the presence of cancer. Gynecomastia can be associated with the use of either prescription or illicit drugs, particularly marijuana. Symptoms resolve after the drugs are discontinued.

FIGURE 16-22 Breast changes in pregnancy. A, Note venous network, darkened areolae and nipples, and vascular spider. **B,** Increased pigmentation and the development of raised sebaceous glands known as Montgomery tubercles. **C,** Marked pigmentation in woman with dark skin. *(B, C, From Symonds and Macpherson, 1994.)*

❧ Pregnant Women

Many changes in the breasts occur during pregnancy. Most become obvious during the first trimester. The woman may experience a sensation of fullness with tingling, tenderness, and a bilateral increase in size. It is important to ascertain that the woman is providing adequate support for her breasts with a properly fitting bra. As her breasts continue to enlarge, she may need to alter the size and style of the bra.

Generally, the nipples enlarge and are more erectile. As the pregnancy progresses, the nipples sometimes become flattened or inverted. A crust caused by dried colostrum can be evident on the nipple. Inspect the breasts and expect to see areolae that are broader and darker. Montgomery tubercles are common (Fig. 16-22).

Palpation reveals a generalized coarse nodularity, and the breasts feel lobular because of hypertrophy of the mammary alveoli. Dilated subcutaneous veins may create a network of blue tracing across the breasts.

During the second trimester, telangiectasias (called spider angiomas or vascular spiders) may develop on the upper chest, arms, neck, and face as a result of elevated levels of circulating estrogen. The spiders are bluish in color and do not blanch with pressure. Striae may be evident as a result of stretching as the breasts increase in size.

✤ Lactating Women

During lactation, it is important to assess whether the breasts are adequately supported with a properly fitting bra. Palpate the breasts to determine the degree of softness. Full breasts, which are firm, dense, and slightly enlarged, may become engorged. Engorged breasts feel hard and warm and are enlarged, shiny, and painful. Engorgement is not an unusual condition in the first 24 to 48 hours after the breasts fill with milk; however, its later development may signal the onset of mastitis.

Clogged milk ducts are a relatively common occurrence in lactating women. A clogged duct may result from either inadequate emptying of the breast or a bra that is too tight. The clogged duct will create a tender spot on the breast that may feel lumpy and hot. Frequent breast-feeding and/or expression of the milk, along with local application of heat, will help open the duct. A clogged duct left unattended may result in the development of mastitis.

Examine the nipples for signs of irritation (redness and tenderness) and for blisters or petechiae, which are precursors of overt cracking. Cracked nipples will be sore and may be bleeding. Lighter-colored nipples are no more prone to damage from breast-feeding than are darker nipples. Nipple damage from breast-feeding is associated with placement of the nipple in the infant's mouth.

After pregnancy and lactation, there is regression of most of these changes. The areolae and nipples tend to retain their darker color, and the breasts become less firm than in their pre-pregnant state.

✤ Older Adults

The breasts in postmenopausal women may appear flattened, elongated, and suspended more loosely from the chest wall as the result of glandular tissue atrophy and relaxation of the suspensory ligaments. A finer granular feel on palpation replaces the lobular feel of glandular tissue. The inframammary ridge thickens and can be felt more easily. The nipples become smaller and flatter.

Sample Documentation
History and Physical Examination

Subjective
A 42-year-old woman noticed a lump in her right lower breast last week. Denies nipple discharge or skin changes. Reports normal mammogram 2 years ago. Has never had a breast lump or breast biopsy. Currently on last day of menses. Has breast tenderness just before menses but denies breast pain today. No personal or family history of breast cancer or related cancers.

Objective
Breasts: moderate size, conical shape, breasts symmetric with left slightly larger than right. No skin lesions; contour smooth bilaterally without dimpling or retraction; venous patterns symmetric. Nipples symmetric without discharge; Montgomery tubercles bilaterally. Tissue diffusely nodular particularly in upper quadrants. In left lower quadrant of the right breast, a 3 cm × 3 cm × 2 cm soft mass, 5 cm from nipple. Mobile, nontender, borders smooth. Nipples depress into wells easily. No supraclavicular, infraclavicular, or axillary lymphadenopathy.

For additional sample documentation, see Chapter 26, pp. 628-631.

Audio Examination Summaries: Physical examination of the breasts and axillae

ABNORMALITIES

BREASTS

BREAST LUMPS

See the Differential Diagnosis table for characteristic differences between fibrocystic changes, fibroadenomas, and breast cancer. The differential signs and symptoms will help guide the next step(s) for diagnosis.

DIFFERENTIAL DIAGNOSIS
Signs and Symptoms of Breast Masses

Characteristic	Fibrocystic Changes	Fibroadenoma	Cancer
Age range (yr)	20 to 49	15 to 55	30 to 80
Occurrence	Usually bilateral	Usually bilateral	Usually unilateral
Number	Multiple or single	Single; may be multiple	Single
Shape	Round	Round or discoid	Irregular or stellate
Consistency	Soft to firm; tense	Firm, rubbery	Hard, stonelike
Mobility	Mobile	Mobile	Fixed
Retraction signs	Absent	Absent	Often present
Tenderness	Usually tender	Usually nontender	Usually nontender
Borders	Well delineated	Well delineated	Poorly delineated; irregular
Variation with menses	Yes	No	No

Fibrocystic Changes

Benign fluid-filled cyst formation caused by ductal enlargement

Pathophysiology

- Usually bilateral and multiple
- Most common in women 30 to 55 years of age
- Associated with a long follicular or luteal phase of the menstrual cycle

Subjective Data

- Tender and painful breasts and/or palpable lumps that fluctuate with menses
- Usually worse premenstrually

Objective Data

- Round, soft to firm, tense, mobile masses with well-delineated borders
- Usually tender
- Usually bilateral
- Multiple or single

Fibroadenoma

Benign tumors composed of stromal and epithelial elements that represent a hyperplastic or proliferative process in a single terminal ductal unit

Pathophysiology

- May occur in girls and women of any age during their reproductive years
- After menopause, the tumors often regress.

Subjective Data

- Painless lumps that do not fluctuate with the menstrual cycle
- May be asymptomatic with discovery on clinical breast examination or breast imaging

Objective Data

- Round or discoid, firm, rubbery, mobile masses with well-delineated borders
- Usually nontender
- Usually bilateral
- Single; may be multiple
- Biopsy often performed to rule out carcinoma

Malignant Breast Tumors

Ductal carcinoma arises from the epithelial lining of ducts; lobular carcinoma originates in the glandular tissue of the lobules.

Pathophysiology

- Mutations to normal cells result in uncontrolled cell division and tumor formation; as the tumor grows and invades surrounding tissue, metastases occur through the lymph and vascular systems.
- Peak incidence between ages 40 and 75 years, with the majority of malignant breast tumors occurring in women older than 50 years

Subjective Data

- Painless lump; change in size, shape, or contour of breast
- Axilla may be tender if lymph nodes involved
- May be asymptomatic with discovery on clinical breast examination or breast imaging

Objective Data

- May have palpable mass that is usually single; unilateral, irregular, or stellate in shape; poorly delineated borders; fixed; hard or stonelike; and nontender
- Breast may have dimpling, retraction, prominent vasculature
- Skin may have peau d'orange or thickened appearance.
- Nipple may be inverted or deviate in position (Fig. 16-23).

FIGURE 16-23 A, Patient with lump and nipple retraction in left breast. **B,** Patient with altered nipple height resulting from breast cancer in left breast. *(From Mansel and Bundred, 1995.)*

Fat Necrosis

Benign breast lump occurs as inflammatory response to local injury

Pathophysiology

- Necrotic fat and cellular debris become fibrotic and may contract into a scar.

Subjective Data

- History of trauma to the breast (including surgery)
- Painless lump

Objective Data

- Firm, irregular mass, often appearing as an area of discoloration (Fig. 16-24)
- May mimic breast malignancy on clinical examination or breast imaging, requiring biopsy for diagnosis

FIGURE 16-24 Fat necrosis presenting as a hard mass in the breast following an episode of trauma sufficient to cause bruising. *(From Mansel and Bundred, 1995.)*

NIPPLES AND AREOLAE

Intraductal Papillomas and Papillomatosis
Benign tumors of the subareolar ducts that produce nipple discharge

Pathophysiology
- Epithelial hyperplasia produces a wartlike tumor in a lactiferous duct.
- 2 to 3 cm in diameter
- May occur singly or in multiples

Subjective Data
- Spontaneous nipple discharge
- Usually unilateral
- Usually serous or bloody

Objective Data
- Single-duct unilateral nipple discharge provoked on physical examination
- Mass behind the nipple may or may not be present
- May need to be excised and examined to rule out malignancy

Duct Ectasia
Benign condition of the subareolar ducts that produces nipple discharge

Pathophysiology
- Subareolar ducts become dilated and blocked with desquamating secretory epithelium, necrotic debris, and chronic inflammatory cells.
- Occurs most commonly in menopausal women

Subjective Data
- Spontaneous unilateral or bilateral nipple discharge
- Discharge often green or brown in color
- Discharge may be sticky

Objective Data
- Single or multiductal, unilateral or bilateral nipple discharge provoked on physical examination
- Mass behind the nipple may or may not be present
- Breast may or may not be tender
- Nipple retraction may be present.

Galactorrhea
Lactation not associated with childbearing

Pathophysiology
- Elevated levels of prolactin, resulting in milk production, occur as a result of disruption of the communication between the pituitary and hypothalamus glands.
- Common causes include pituitary secreting tumors, hypothalamic-pituitary disorders, systemic diseases, numerous medications and herbs, physiologic conditions, or local factors.

Subjective Data
- Spontaneous nipple discharge, usually bilateral; usually serous or milky
- Possible related medical history: amenorrhea, pregnancy, post abortion, hypothyroidism, Cushing syndrome, chronic renal failure
- Possible medication history: phenothiazines, tricyclic antidepressants, some antihypertensive agents, estrogens, H2 receptor blockers, marijuana, amphetamines, opiates
- Possible physiologic history: suckling, stress, dehydration, exercise, nipple stimulation

Objective Data
- Multiductal nipple discharge may or may not be provoked on physical examination (Fig. 16-25).
- No mass

ABNORMALITIES

FIGURE 16-25 Galactorrhea produced by a prolactin-secreting pituitary tumor. *(From Mansel and Bundred, 1995.)*

Paget Disease

Surface manifestation of underlying ductal carcinoma

Pathophysiology

- Migration of malignant epithelial cells from the underlying intraductal carcinoma via the lactiferous sinuses into nipple skin
- Tumor cells disrupt the epithelial barrier, allowing extracellular fluid to seep out onto the nipple surface.

Subjective Data

- Crustiness of the nipple, areola, and surrounding skin
- Pruritus of the nipple common

Objective Data

- Red, scaling, crusty patch on the nipple, areola, and surrounding skin (Fig. 16-26)
- May be unilateral or bilateral
- Appears eczematous but, unlike eczema, does not respond to steroids

FIGURE 16-26 **Paget disease.** *(From Callen et al, 2000.)*

Mastitis

Inflammation and infection of the breast tissue

Pathophysiology

- Most infections are staphylococcal, often *Staphylococcus aureus*.
- Most common in lactating women after milk is established, usually the second to third week after delivery; however, it may occur at any time.
- Abscess formation can result.

Subjective Data

- Characterized by sudden onset of swelling, tenderness, redness, and heat in the breast
- Usually accompanied by chills, fever

Objective Data

- Tender, hard breast mass, with an area of fluctuation, erythema, and heat
- May have discharge of pus (suppuration)
- Underlying pus-filled abscess may impart a bluish tinge to the skin (Fig. 16-27).

FIGURE 16-27 Mastitis. *(From Lemmi and Lemmi, 2000)*

Gynecomastia

Breast enlargement in men

Pathophysiology

- Result of increased body fat; hormone imbalance from puberty or aging; by testicular, pituitary, or hormone-secreting tumors; by liver failure; or by a variety of medications including anabolic steroids, marijuana, some antihypertensives, some antipsychotics, or those containing estrogens or antiandrogens
- When testosterone levels are low relative to estrogen, breasts grow larger and are more noticeable.
- Increased body fat, which in turn produces more estrogen, can also cause breast enlargement.

Subjective Data

- Breast enlargement (Figs. 16-28 and 16-29)
- Relevant medication history

Objective Data

- Smooth, firm, mobile, tender disk of breast tissue located behind the areola
- Usually nontender
- May be unilateral or bilateral
- Amount of breast tissue varies; can be small overgrowth of breast tissue around the areola and nipple, to larger, more "female"-looking breasts

FIGURE 16-28 Adult gynecomastia. *(From Mansel and Bundred, 1995.)*

FIGURE 16-29 Prepubertal gynecomastia, small and subareolar. *(Courtesy Wellington Hung, MD; Children's National Medical Center; Washington, DC.)*

✤ Children

Premature Thelarche

Breast enlargement in girls before onset of puberty

Pathophysiology

- Cause unknown
- Breasts continue to enlarge slowly throughout childhood until full development is reached during adolescence.

Subjective Data

- Breast enlargement

Objective Data

- Degree of enlargement varies from very slight to fully developed breasts.
- Usually occurs bilaterally
- Other signs of sexual maturation may be absent.

CHAPTER 17

Abdomen

The abdominal examination is performed as part of the comprehensive physical examination or when a patient presents with signs or symptoms of an abdominal disease process. It involves the core examination skills in a particular sequence: inspection, auscultation, percussion, and palpation. Additional procedures are used to detect serious abdominal pathology. During the abdominal examination, pay careful attention to the patient's comfort level or degree of distress.

evolve *http://evolve.elsevier.com/Seidel*
- Physical Exam Key Points
- NCLEX Review Questions
- Interactive Activities
- Animations
- Videos
- Audio Clips
- Student Checklist

ANATOMY AND PHYSIOLOGY

The abdominal cavity contains several of the body's vital organs (Fig. 17-1). The peritoneum, a serous membrane, lines the cavity and forms a protective cover for many of the abdominal organs. Double folds of the peritoneum around the stomach constitute the greater and lesser omentum. The mesentery, a fan-shaped fold of the peritoneum, covers most of the small intestine and anchors it to the posterior abdominal wall.

Alimentary Tract

The alimentary tract, a tube approximately 27 feet long, runs from the mouth to the anus and includes the esophagus, stomach,

Physical Examination Preview

Here is a preview of the steps involved in conducting a physical examination of the abdomen. ⓔ These procedures are explained in detail in this chapter and are available on Evolve in printable formats.

Abdomen
1. Inspect the abdomen for the following (pp. 378-81):
   - Skin characteristics
   - Venous return patterns
   - Symmetry
   - Surface motion
2. Inspect abdominal muscles as patient raises head to detect presence of the following (p. 381):
   - Masses
   - Hernia
   - Separation of muscles
3. Auscultate with stethoscope diaphragm for the following (p. 381):
   - Bowel sounds
4. Auscultate with bell of stethoscope for the following (p. 381):
   - Bruits over aorta, renal, iliac, and femoral arteries
5. Percuss the abdomen for the following (pp. 381-83):
   - Tone in all four quadrants (or nine regions)
   - Liver borders to estimate span

- Splenic dullness in left midaxillary line
- Gastric air bubble
6. Lightly palpate in all quadrants or regions for the following (p. 383):
   - Muscular resistance
   - Tenderness
   - Masses
7. Deeply palpate for the following (pp. 384-88):
   - Bulges and masses around the umbilicus and umbilical ring
   - Liver border in right costal margin
   - Gallbladder below liver margin at lateral border of the rectus muscle
   - Spleen in left costal margin
   - Right and left kidneys
   - Aortic pulsation in midline
   - Other masses
8. With patient sitting, percuss the left and right costovertebral angles for kidney tenderness (p. 383).

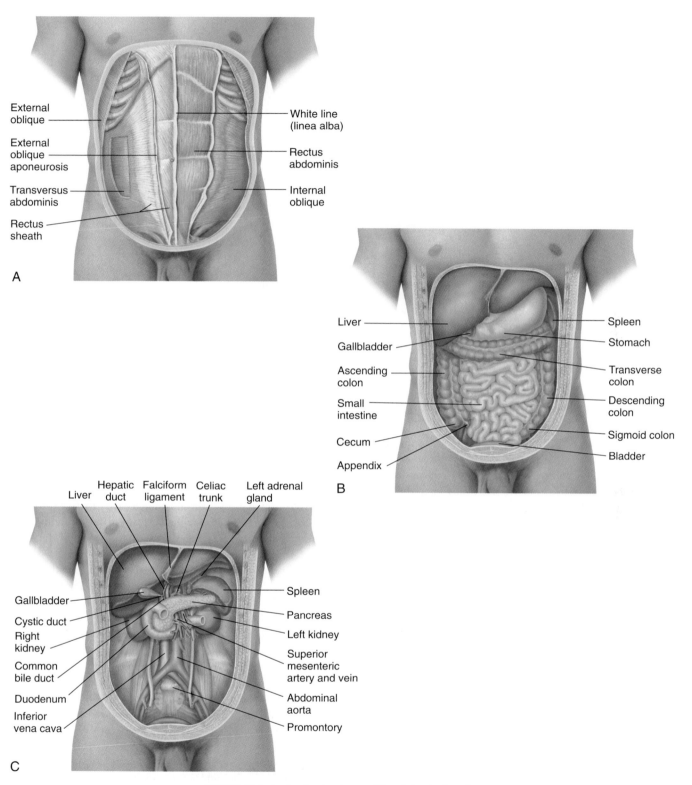

External
oblique

External
oblique
aponeurosis

Transversus
abdominis

Rectus
sheath

White line
(linea alba)

Rectus
abdominis

Internal
oblique

A

Liver

Gallbladder

Ascending
colon

Small
intestine

Cecum

Appendix

Spleen

Stomach

Transverse
colon

Descending
colon

Sigmoid colon

Bladder

B

Liver   Hepatic   Falciform   Celiac   Left adrenal
        duct   ligament   trunk   gland

Gallbladder

Cystic duct

Right
kidney

Common
bile duct

Duodenum

Inferior
vena cava

Spleen

Pancreas

Left kidney

Superior
mesenteric
artery and vein

Abdominal
aorta

Promontory

C

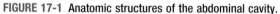

FIGURE 17-1 Anatomic structures of the abdominal cavity.

ANATOMY AND PHYSIOLOGY

Animation: Digestion

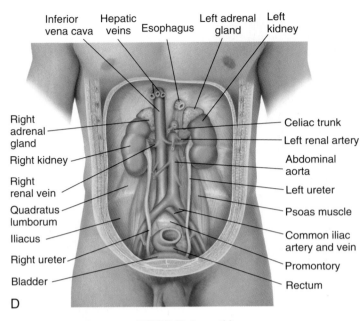

Inferior vena cava
Hepatic veins
Esophagus
Left adrenal gland
Left kidney

Right adrenal gland
Right kidney
Right renal vein
Quadratus lumborum
Iliacus
Right ureter
Bladder

Celiac trunk
Left renal artery
Abdominal aorta
Left ureter
Psoas muscle
Common iliac artery and vein
Promontory
Rectum

D

FIGURE 17-1, cont'd

small intestine, and large intestine. It functions to ingest and digest food; absorb nutrients, electrolytes, and water; and excrete waste products. Food and the products of digestion are moved along the length of the alimentary tract by peristalsis under autonomic nervous system control.

The esophagus, a collapsible tube about 10 inches long, connects the pharynx to the stomach. Just posterior to the trachea, the esophagus descends through the mediastinal cavity and diaphragm, entering the stomach at the cardiac orifice.

The stomach lies transversely in the upper abdominal cavity, just below the diaphragm. It consists of three sections: the fundus, lying above and to the left of the cardiac orifice; the middle two thirds, or body; and the pylorus, the most distal portion that narrows and terminates in the pyloric orifice. The stomach secretes hydrochloric acid and digestive enzymes that break down fats and proteins. Pepsin acts to digest proteins, whereas gastric lipase acts on emulsified fats. Little absorption takes place in the stomach.

The small intestine, about 21 feet long, begins at the pylorus. Coiled in the abdominal cavity, it joins the large intestine at the ileocecal valve. The first 12 inches of the small intestine, the duodenum, forms a C-shaped curve around the head of the pancreas. The common bile duct and pancreatic duct open into the duodenum at the duodenal papilla, about 3 inches below the pylorus of the stomach. The next 8 feet of intestine, the jejunum, gradually becomes larger and thicker. The ileum makes up the remaining 12 feet of the small intestine. The ileocecal valve between the ileum and large intestine prevents backward flow of fecal material.

The small intestine completes digestion through the action of pancreatic enzymes, bile, and several other enzymes. Nutrients are absorbed through the mucosa of the small intestine. The functional surface area of the small intestine is increased by its circular folds and villi.

The large intestine begins at the cecum, a blind pouch about 2 to 3 inches long. The ileal contents empty into the cecum through the ileocecal valve, and the vermiform appendix extends from the base of the cecum. The ascending colon rises from the cecum along the right posterior abdominal wall to the undersurface of the liver. The ascending colon turns toward the midline at the hepatic flexure and becomes the transverse colon. The transverse colon crosses the abdominal cavity toward the spleen and turns downward at the splenic flexure. The descending colon continues along the left abdominal wall to the rim of the pelvis, where it turns medially and inferiorly to form the S-shaped sigmoid colon. The rectum extends from the sigmoid colon to the muscles of the pelvic floor. It continues as the anal canal and terminates at the anus.

The large intestine is about 4½ to 5 feet long, with a diameter of 2½ inches. Its main functions are to absorb water and transport waste. Mucous glands secrete large quantities of alkaline mucus that lubricate the intestinal contents and neutralize acids formed by intestinal bacteria. Live bacteria decompose undigested food residue, unabsorbed amino acids, cell debris, and dead bacteria through a process of putrefaction.

Liver

The liver lies in the right upper quadrant of the abdomen, just below the diaphragm and above the gallbladder, right kidney, and hepatic flexure of the colon. The heaviest organ in the body, the liver weighs about 3 pounds in the adult. It is composed of four lobes containing lobules, the functional units. Each lobule is made up of liver cells radiating around a central vein. Branches of the portal vein, hepatic artery, and bile duct penetrate to the periphery of the lobules. Bile secreted by the liver cells drains from the bile ducts into the hepatic duct, which joins the cystic duct from the gallbladder to form the common bile duct.

The hepatic artery transports blood to the liver directly from the aorta, and the portal vein carries blood from the digestive tract and spleen to the liver. Repeated branching of both vessels makes the liver a highly vascular organ. Three hepatic veins carry blood from the liver and empty into the inferior vena cava.

The liver plays an important role in the metabolism of carbohydrates, fats, and proteins. Glucose is converted and stored as glycogen until, in response to varying levels of insulin and regulator hormones, it is reconverted and released again as glucose. The liver also can convert amino acids to glucose (gluconeogenesis). Fats, arriving at the liver in the form of fatty acids, are oxidized to two-carbon components in preparation for entry into the tricarboxylic acid cycle. Cholesterol is used by the liver to form bile salts. Synthesis of fats from carbohydrates and proteins also occurs in the liver. Proteins are broken down to amino acids through hydrolysis, and their waste products are converted to urea for excretion.

Other functions of the liver include storage of several vitamins and iron; detoxification of potentially harmful substances; production of antibodies; conjugation and excretion of steroid hormones; and the production of prothrombin, fibrinogen, and other substances for blood coagulation. The liver is responsible for the production of the majority of proteins circulating in the plasma. It serves as an excretory organ through the synthesis of bile, the secretion of organic wastes into bile, and the conversion of fat-soluble wastes to water-soluble material for renal excretion.

Gallbladder

The gallbladder is a saclike, pear-shaped organ about 4 inches long, lying recessed in the inferior surface of the liver. It concentrates and stores bile from the liver. In response to cholecystokinin, a hormone produced in the duodenum, the gallbladder releases bile into the cystic duct. The cystic duct and hepatic duct form the common bile duct. Contraction of the gallbladder propels bile along the common duct and into the duodenum at the duodenal papilla. Composed of cholesterol, bile salts, and pigments, bile serves to maintain the alkaline pH of the small intestine, permitting emulsification of fats so that absorption of lipids can be accomplished.

Pancreas

The pancreas lies behind and beneath the stomach, with its head resting in the curve of the duodenum and tip extending across the abdominal cavity to almost touch the spleen. As an exocrine gland, the acinar cells of the pancreas produce digestive juices containing inactive enzymes for the breakdown of proteins, fats, and carbohydrates. Collecting ducts empty the juice into the pancreatic duct (duct of Wirsung), which runs the length of the organ. The pancreatic duct empties into the duodenum at the duodenal papilla, alongside the common bile duct. Once introduced into the duodenum, the digestive enzymes are activated. As an endocrine gland, islet cells scattered throughout the pancreas produce the hormones insulin and glucagon.

Spleen

The spleen is in the left upper quadrant, lying above the left kidney and just below the diaphragm. White pulp (lymphoid tissue) constitutes most of the organ and functions as part of the reticuloendothelial system to filter blood and manufacture lymphocytes and monocytes. The red pulp of the spleen contains a capillary network and venous sinus system that allow for storage and release of blood, permitting the spleen to accommodate up to several hundred milliliters at once.

Kidneys, Ureters, and Bladder

The two kidneys are located in the retroperitoneal space of the upper abdomen. Each extends from about the vertebral level of T12 to L3. The right kidney is usually slightly lower than the left, presumably because of the large, heavy liver just above it. Both kidneys are embedded in fat and fascia, which anchor and protect these organs. Each contains more than 1 million nephrons, the structural and functional units of the kidneys. The nephrons are composed of a tuft of capillaries, the glomerulus, a proximal convoluted tubule, the loop of Henle, and a distal convoluted tubule. The distal tube empties into a collecting tubule.

Each kidney receives about one eighth of the cardiac output through the renal artery. The glomeruli filter blood at a rate of about 125 mL/min in the adult male and about 110 mL/min in the adult female. Most of the filtered material, including electrolytes, glucose, water, and small proteins, is actively resorbed in the proximal tubule. Some organic acids are also actively secreted in the distal tubule. Urinary volume is carefully controlled by antidiuretic hormone (ADH) to maintain a constant total body fluid volume. Urine passes into the renal pelvis via the collecting tubules and then into the ureter. Peristaltic waves move urine to the urinary bladder, which has a capacity of about 400 to 500 mL in the adult.

The kidney also serves as an endocrine gland responsible for the production of renin, which controls aldosterone secretion. It is the primary source of erythropoietin production in adults, thus influencing the body's red cell mass. In addition to synthesizing several prostaglandins, the kidney produces the biologically active form of vitamin D.

Musculature and Connective Tissues

The rectus abdominis muscles anteriorly and the internal and external oblique muscles laterally form and protect the abdominal cavity. The linea alba, a tendinous band, is located in the midline of the abdomen between the rectus abdominis muscles. It extends from the xiphoid process to the symphysis pubis and contains the umbilicus. The inguinal ligament (Poupart ligament) extends from the anterior superior spine of the ilium on each side to the pubis.

Vasculature

The abdominal portion of the descending aorta travels from the diaphragm through the abdominal cavity, just to the left of

ANATOMY AND PHYSIOLOGY

midline. At about the level of the umbilicus, the aorta branches into the two common iliac arteries. The splenic and renal arteries, which supply their respective organs, also branch off within the abdomen.

✤ Infants

The pancreatic buds, liver, and gallbladder all begin to form during week 4 of gestation, by which time the intestine already exists as a single tube. The motility of the gastrointestinal tract develops in a cephalocaudal direction, permitting amniotic fluid to be swallowed by 17 weeks of gestation. Production of meconium, an end product of fetal metabolism, begins shortly thereafter. By 36 to 38 weeks of gestation, the gastrointestinal tract is capable of adapting to extrauterine life. However the elasticity, musculature, and control mechanisms of the gastrointestinal tract continue to develop, reaching adult function at 2 to 3 years of age.

During gestation, the liver begins to form blood cells at about week 6, synthesize glycogen by week 9, and produce bile by week 12. The liver's role as a metabolic and glycogen storage organ accounts for the large size at birth. The liver remains the heaviest organ in the body.

Pancreatic islet cells are developed by 12 weeks of gestation and begin producing insulin. The spleen is active in blood formation during fetal development and the first year of life. Afterward, the spleen aids in the destruction of blood cells and functions as a lymphatic organ for immunologic response.

Nephrogenesis begins during the second embryologic month. By 12 weeks, the kidney is able to produce urine, and the bladder expands as a sac. Development of new nephrons ceases by 36 weeks of gestation. After birth, the kidney increases in size because of enlargement of the existing nephrons and adjoining tubules. The glomerular filtration rate is approximately 0.5 mL/min before 34 weeks of gestation and gradually increases in a linear fashion to the adulthood rate.

✤ Pregnant Women

As the uterus enlarges, the muscles of the abdominal wall stretch and lose tone. During the third trimester the rectus abdominis muscles may separate, allowing abdominal contents to protrude at the midline.

The umbilicus flattens or protrudes. The abdominal contour changes when lightening occurs (about 2 weeks before term in a nullipara), and the fetal presenting part descends into the true pelvis. Striae may form as the skin is stretched. A line of pigmentation at the midline (linea nigra) often develops (Fig. 17-2). Abdominal muscles have less tone and are less active. After pregnancy, the muscles gradually regain tone, although separation of the rectus abdominis muscles (diastasis recti) may persist.

During the second trimester lower esophageal sphincter pressure decreases. Peristaltic wave velocity in the distal esophagus also decreases. Gastric emptying appears to be normal; however, gastrointestinal transit time is prolonged in the second and third trimesters, leading to constipation. Incompetence of the pyloric sphincter may result in alkaline reflux of duodenal

FIGURE 17-2 Linea nigra in the third trimester of pregnancy.

contents into the stomach. Heartburn (gastroesophageal reflux) is a common concern.

The gallbladder may become distended, accompanied by decreased emptying time and change in tone. The combination of gallbladder stasis and secretion of lithogenic bile increases formation of cholesterol crystals and the development of gallstones. Gallstones are more common in the second and third trimesters.

The kidneys enlarge slightly (by about 1 cm in length) during pregnancy. The renal pelvis and ureters dilate from the effects of hormones and pressure from the enlarging uterus. Dilation of the ureter is greater on the right side than on the left, probably because it is affected by displacement of the uterus to the right by an enlarged right ovarian vein. The ureters also elongate and form single and double curves of varying sizes and angulation. These changes can lead to urinary stasis and pyelonephritis in gravid women with asymptomatic bacteriuria. Renal function is most efficient if the woman lies in the lateral recumbent position, which helps prevent compression of the vena cava and aorta. These changes can last up to 3 or 4 months after delivery.

The bladder has increased sensitivity and compression during pregnancy, leading to frequency and urgency of urination during the first and third trimesters. After the fourth month, the increase in uterine size, hyperemia of all pelvic organs, and hyperplasia of muscle and connective tissue elevate the bladder trigone and cause thickening of the posterior margin. This process produces a marked deepening and widening of the trigone by the end of the pregnancy and may result in microhematuria. During the third trimester, compression may also result from the descent of the fetus into the pelvis; this, in turn, causes a sense of urgency and/or incontinence, even with a small amount of urine in the bladder.

The colon is displaced laterally upward and posteriorly, peristaltic activity may decrease, and water absorption is increased. As a result, bowel sounds are diminished, and constipation and flatus are more common. The appendix is displaced upward and laterally, away from McBurney's point, an anatomic landmark one-third of the distance from the anterior superior iliac spine to the umbilicus.

In the postpartum period, the uterus involutes rapidly. Immediately after delivery, the uterus is approximately the size of a 20-week pregnancy (palpable at the level of the umbilicus). By the end of the first week, it is about the size of a 12-week pregnancy, palpable at the symphysis pubis. The muscles of the pelvic floor and the pelvic supports gradually regain tone during the postpartum period and may require 6 to 7 weeks to recover. Stretching of the abdominal wall during pregnancy may result in persistent striae and diastasis of the rectus muscles.

⚘ Older Adults

The process of aging results in changes in the functional abilities of the gastrointestinal tract. Motility of the intestine is the most severely affected; secretion and absorption are affected to a lesser degree. Altered motility may be caused by age-related changes in neurons of the central nervous system and by changes in collagen properties that increase the resistance of the intestinal wall to stretching. Reduced circulation to the intestine often follows other system changes associated with hypoxia and hypovolemia. Thus, functional abilities of the intestine can decrease secondary to systemic changes in the older adult.

As a result of epithelial atrophy, the secretion of both digestive enzymes and protective mucus decreases in the intestinal tract. Particular elements of the mucosal cells show a lesser degree of differentiation and are associated with reduction in secretory ability. These cells are also more susceptible to both physical and chemical agents, including ingested carcinogens. Bacterial flora of the intestine can undergo both qualitative and quantitative changes and become less biologically active. These changes may impair digestive ability and thereby cause food intolerances in the older adult.

Liver size decreases after 50 years of age, which parallels the decrease in lean body mass. Hepatic blood flow decreases as a result of a decline in cardiac output associated with aging. The liver loses some ability to metabolize certain drugs. Increasing obesity and the development of type 2 diabetes mellitus also put the liver at risk for the development of nonalcoholic steatohepatitis.

The size of the pancreas is unaffected by aging, although the main pancreatic duct and branches widen. With aging there is an increase in fibrous tissue and fatty deposition with acinar cell atrophy; however, the large reserve of the organ results in no significant physiologic changes.

There may be an increase of biliary lipids, specifically the phospholipids and cholesterol, resulting in the formation of gallstones.

REVIEW OF RELATED HISTORY

For each of the symptoms or conditions discussed in this section, targeted topics to include in the history of the present illness are listed. Questions regarding these topics will help focus the physical examination and develop an appropriate diagnostic evaluation. Questions regarding medication use (prescription and over the counter preparations) as well as complementary and alternative therapies are relevant for each area.

History of Present Illness

- Abdominal pain
  - Onset and duration: when it began; sudden or gradual; persistent, recurrent, intermittent
  - Character: dull, sharp, burning, gnawing, stabbing, cramping, aching, colicky
  - Location: of onset, change in location over time, radiating to another area, superficial or deep
  - Associated symptoms: vomiting, diarrhea, constipation, passage of flatus, belching, jaundice, change in abdominal girth, weight loss or weight gain
  - Relationship to: menstrual cycle, abnormal menses, intercourse, urination, defecation, inspiration, change in body position, food or alcohol intake, stress, time of day, trauma
  - Recent stool characteristics: color, consistency, odor, frequency
  - Urinary characteristics: frequency, color, volume congruent with fluid intake, force of stream, ease of starting stream, ability to empty bladder
  - Medications: high doses of aspirin, steroids, nonsteroidal antiinflammatory drugs (NSAIDs)
- Indigestion
  - Character: feeling of fullness, heartburn, discomfort, excessive belching, flatulence, loss of appetite, severe pain
  - Location: localized or general, radiating to arms or shoulders
  - Relationship to: amount, type, and timing of food intake; date of last menstrual period
  - Onset of symptoms: time of day or night, sudden or gradual
  - Symptom relieved by antacids, rest, activity
  - Medications: antacids
- Nausea: associated with vomiting, particular stimuli (odors, activities, time of day, food intake), date of last menstrual period
  - Medications: antiemetics
- Vomiting
  - Character: nature (color, bright red blood or coffee grounds, bilious, undigested food particles), quantity, duration, frequency, ability to keep any liquids or food in stomach
  - Relationship to: previous meal, change in appetite, diarrhea or constipation, fever, weight loss, abdominal pain, medications, headache, nausea, date of last menstrual period
  - Medications: antiemetics
- Diarrhea
  - Character: watery, copious, explosive; color; presence of blood, mucus, undigested food, oil, or fat; odor; number of times per day, duration; change in pattern
  - Associated symptoms: fever, chills, thirst, weight loss, abdominal pain or cramping, fecal incontinence
  - Relationship to: amount, type and timing of food intake, stressful life events or daily stressors
  - Travel history and/or ill contacts
  - Medications: laxatives or stool softeners; antidiarrheals

+ Constipation
  + Character: presence of bright red blood, black or tarry appearance of stool; diarrhea alternating with constipation; accompanied by abdominal pain or discomfort
  + Pattern: last bowel movement, pain with defecation, change in pattern or size of stool
  + Diet: recent change in diet, inclusion of high-fiber foods
  + Medications: laxatives, stool softeners, iron, diuretics
+ Fecal incontinence
  + Character: stool characteristics, timing in relation to meals, number of episodes per day; occurring with or without warning sensation
  + Associated with: use of laxatives, presence of underlying disease (cancer, inflammatory bowel disease, diverticulitis, colitis, proctitis, diabetic neuropathy)
  + Relationship to: fluid and dietary intake, immobilization
  + Medications: laxatives, stool softeners, iron, diuretics
+ Jaundice
  + Onset and duration
  + Color of stools or urine
  + Associated with abdominal pain, chills, fever
  + Exposure to hepatitis, use of illicit drugs, high-risk sexual activity
  + Medications: high doses of acetaminophen; antiepileptics
+ Dysuria
  + Character: location (suprapubic, distal urethra), pain or burning, frequency or volume changes

+ Associated fever or other systemic signs of illness: bacterial infection, tuberculosis, fungal or viral infection, parasitic infection
+ Increased frequency of sexual intercourse
+ Amount of daily fluid intake
+ Urinary frequency
  + Change in usual pattern and/or volume
  + Associated with dysuria or other urinary characteristics: urgency, hematuria, incontinence, nocturia
  + Change in urinary stream; dribbling
  + Medications: diuretics
+ Urinary incontinence
  + Character: amount and frequency, constant or intermittent, dribbling versus frank incontinence
  + Associated with: urgency, previous surgery, coughing, sneezing, walking up stairs, nocturia, menopause
  + Medications: diuretics
+ Hematuria
  + Character: color (bright red, rusty brown, cola-colored); present at beginning, end, or throughout voiding
  + Associated symptoms: flank or costovertebral pain, passage of wormlike clots, pain on voiding
  + Alternate possibilities: ingestion of foods containing red vegetable dyes (may cause red urinary pigment); ingestion of laxatives containing phenolphthalein
  + Medications: aspirin, NSAIDs, anticoagulants, diuretics, antibiotics

Risk Factors

Persons at Risk for Viral Hepatitis

Risk Factor	Hepatitis A	Hepatitis B	Hepatitis C
People who have sex with an infected individual		√	√
Men who have sex with men	√	√	√
People who have multiple sex partners (e.g., >1 sex partner in the previous 6 months)		√	√
People who live with chronically infected individuals		√	
Travelers to countries with intermediate or high prevalence	√	√	
Household family members and close contacts of children adopted from countries with high rates of infection	√		
Children in day care, employees, and household contacts	√		
Infants born to infected mothers		√	√
People with human immunodeficiency virus infection			√
People with clotting factor disorders	√		
People who received clotting factor concentrates made before 1987			√
People who received blood transfusions or solid organ transplants before July 1992			√
Hemodialysis patients		√	√
Injection and noninjection drug users	√		
Injection drug users		√	√
Health care and public safety workers at risk for occupational exposure to blood or blood-contaminated products		√	√
Residents and staff of facilities for developmentally disabled persons		√	

Modified from Centers for Disease Control and Prevention, 2012.

Past Medical History

+ Gastrointestinal disorder: peptic ulcer, polyps, inflammatory bowel disease, irritable bowel syndrome, intestinal obstruction, pancreatitis, hyperlipidemia
+ Hepatitis or cirrhosis of the liver
+ Abdominal or urinary tract surgery or injury
+ Urinary tract infection: number of episodes, treatment
+ Major illness: cancer, arthritis (steroids, NSAIDs or aspirin use), kidney disease, cardiac disease
+ Blood transfusions
+ Immunization status (hepatitis A and hepatitis B)
+ Colorectal cancer or related cancers—breast, ovarian, endometrial

Family History

+ Colorectal cancer and familial colorectal cancer syndromes—familial adenomatous polyposis, hereditary nonpolyposis colorectal cancer (Lynch syndrome)
+ Gallbladder disease
+ Kidney disease: renal stone, polycystic disease, renal tubular acidosis, renal or bladder carcinoma
+ Malabsorption syndrome: cystic fibrosis, celiac disease
+ Hirschsprung disease (aganglionic megacolon)
+ Familial Mediterranean fever (periodic peritonitis)

Personal and Social History

+ Nutrition: 24-hour dietary recall; food preferences and dislikes; ethnic foods, religious food restrictions, food intolerances, lifestyle effects on food intake, use of probiotics or dietary supplements; voluntary and involuntary weight gain or loss
+ First day of last menstrual period
+ Alcohol intake: frequency, type, and usual amounts
+ Recent major stressful life events or chronic daily stressors: physical, social, and psychologic changes
+ Exposure to infectious diseases: hepatitis, influenza; travel history; occupational or environmental exposures
+ Trauma: through type of work, physical activity, physical or emotional abuse, intimate partner violence
+ Use of recreational or intravenous drugs
+ Tobacco use—smoking: frequency, amount, duration, pack-years

❀ Infants

+ Gestational age and birth weight (preterm and less than 1500 g at higher risk for necrotizing enterocolitis)
+ Passage of first meconium stool within 24 hours, constipation
+ Jaundice: in newborn period; exchange transfusions, prolonged use of total parenteral nutrition, phototherapy; breast-fed infant; appearance later in first month of life
+ Vomiting: increasing in amount or frequency, forceful or projectile, failure to gain weight, insatiable appetite, blood in emesis (pyloric stenosis or gastroesophageal reflux); associated with intermittent abdominal pain or drawing up of the legs (intussusception)
+ Diarrhea, colic, failure to gain weight, weight loss, steatorrhea (malabsorption)
+ Apparent enlargement of abdomen (with or without pain)

❀ Children

+ Constipation: toilet training methods; soiling; diarrhea; abdominal distention; size, shape, consistency, and time of last stool; rectal bleeding; painful passage of stool
+ Dietary habits: lack of fiber in diet, change in appetite, daily fluid intake; pica
+ Abdominal pain: splinting of abdominal movement, resists movement, keeps knees flexed
+ Psychosocial stressors: home, school and peers

❀ Pregnant Women

+ Urinary symptoms: frequency, urgency, nocturia (common in early and late pregnancy); burning, dysuria, odor (signs of infection)
+ Abdominal pain: weeks of gestation (pregnancy can alter usual location of pain)
+ Fetal movement
+ Contractions: onset, frequency, duration, intensity; accompanying symptoms; lower back pain; leakage of fluid, vaginal bleeding

❀ Older Adults

+ Urinary symptoms: nocturia, change in stream, dribbling, incontinence
+ Change in bowel patterns, constipation, diarrhea, fecal incontinence
+ Dietary habits: inclusion of fiber in diet, change in ability to tolerate certain foods, change in appetite, daily fluid intake

EXAMINATION AND FINDINGS

Equipment

+ Stethoscope
+ Centimeter ruler and measuring tape
+ Marking pen

Preparation

To perform the abdominal examination, you will need a good light source; full exposure of the abdomen; warm hands with short fingernails; and, ideally, a comfortable, relaxed patient. Have the patient empty his or her bladder before the examination begins; a full bladder interferes with accurate examination of nearby organs and makes the examination uncomfortable. Place the patient in a supine position with arms at the sides. Approach the patient from the right side. The patient's abdominal musculature should be relaxed to allow access to the underlying structures. It may be helpful to place a small pillow under the patient's head and another under slightly flexed knees. Drape a towel or sheet over the patient's chest for warmth and privacy.

FIGURE 17-3 Four quadrants of the abdomen. *(From Wilson and Giddens, 2009.)*

FIGURE 17-4 Nine regions of the abdomen. 1, Epigastric; 2, umbilical; 3, hypogastric; 4 and 5, right and left hypochondriac; 6 and 7, right and left lumbar; 8 and 9, right and left inguinal. *(Modified from Wilson and Giddens, 2009.)*

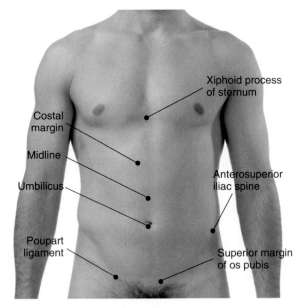

FIGURE 17-5 Landmarks of the abdomen. *(From Wilson and Giddens, 2009.)*

Make your approach slow and gentle, avoiding sudden movements. Ask the patient to point to any tender areas, and examine those last.

For the purposes of examination, the abdomen is commonly divided into four. To divide the abdomen into quadrants, draw an imaginary line from the sternum to the pubis through the umbilicus. Draw a second imaginary line perpendicular to the first, horizontally across the abdomen through the umbilicus (Fig. 17-3). Alternatively the abdomen is divided into nine regions using following imaginary lines: two horizontal lines,

one across the lowest edge of the costal margin and the other across the edge of the iliac crest, and two vertical lines running bilaterally from the midclavicular line to the middle of the Poupart ligament, approximating the lateral borders of the rectus abdominis muscles (Fig. 17-4). Choose one of these mapping methods and use it consistently. Box 17-1 lists the contents of the abdomen in each of the quadrants and regions. Mentally visualize the underlying organs and structures in each of the zones as you proceed with the examination. Certain other anatomic landmarks are useful in describing the location of pain, tenderness, and other findings. These landmarks are illustrated in Figure 17-5.

Inspection

Surface Characteristics

Begin by inspecting the abdomen from a seated position at the patient's right side. This position allows a tangential view that enhances shadows and contouring. Observe the skin color and surface characteristics. The skin of the abdomen will have the same expected variations in color and surface characteristics as the rest of the body. The skin may be somewhat paler if not exposed to the sun. A fine venous network is often visible. Above the umbilicus, venous return should be toward the head; below the umbilicus, it should be toward the feet (Fig. 17-6, *A*). To determine the direction of venous return, use the following procedure. Place the index fingers of both hands side by side perpendicularly over a vein. Press and separate the fingers, milking empty a section of vein. Release one finger and time the refill. Release the other finger and time the refill. The flow of venous blood is in the direction of the faster filling. Flow patterns are altered in some disease states (see Fig. 17-6, *B* and *C*).

Box 17-1 Landmarks for Abdominal Examination

Anatomic Correlates of the Four Quadrants of the Abdomen

Right Upper Quadrant (RUQ)	Left Upper Quadrant (LUQ)
Liver and gallbladder	Left lobe of liver
Pylorus	Spleen
Duodenum	Stomach
Head of pancreas	Body of pancreas
Right adrenal gland	Left adrenal gland
Portion of right kidney	Portion of left kidney
Hepatic flexure of colon	Splenic flexure of colon
Portions of ascending and transverse colon	Portions of transverse and descending colon

Right Lower Quadrant (RLQ)	Left Lower Quadrant (LLQ)
Lower pole of right kidney	Lower pole of left kidney
Cecum and appendix	Sigmoid colon
Portion of ascending colon	Portion of descending colon
Bladder (if distended)	Bladder (if distended)
Ovary and salpinx	Ovary and salpinx
Uterus (if enlarged)	Uterus (if enlarged)
Right spermatic cord	Left spermatic cord
Right ureter	Left ureter

Anatomic Correlates of the Nine Regions of the Abdomen

Right Hypochondriac	*Epigastric*	*Left Hypochondriac*
Right lobe of liver	Pylorus	Stomach
Gallbladder	Duodenum	Spleen
Portion of duodenum	Pancreas	Tail of pancreas
Hepatic flexure of colon	Portion of liver	Splenic flexure of colon
Portion of right kidney	*Umbilical*	Upper pole of left kidney
Right adrenal gland	Omentum	Left adrenal gland
Right Lumbar	Mesentery	*Left Lumbar*
Ascending colon	Lower part of duodenum	Descending colon
Lower half of right kidney	Jejunum and ileum	Lower half of left kidney
Portion of duodenum and jejunum		Portions of jejunum and ileum
Right Inguinal	*Hypogastric (Pubic)*	*Left Inguinal*
Cecum	Ileum	Sigmoid colon
Appendix	Bladder	Left ureter
Lower end of ileum	Uterus (if enlarged)	Left spermatic cord
Right ureter		Left ovary
Right spermatic cord		
Right ovary		

Unexpected findings include generalized color changes such as jaundice or cyanosis. A glistening, taut appearance suggests ascites. Inspect for bruises and localized discoloration. Areas of redness may indicate inflammation. A bluish periumbilical discoloration (Cullen sign) suggests intraabdominal bleeding. Striae often result from pregnancy or weight gain. Striae of recent origin are pink or blue in color but turn silvery white over time. Abdominal tumors or ascites can produce striae. The striae of Cushing disease remain purplish.

Inspect for any lesions, particularly nodules. Lesions are of particular importance because gastrointestinal diseases often produce secondary skin changes. A pearl-like, enlarged and sometimes painful umbilical nodule, known as Sister Mary Joseph's nodule, may be the first sign of an intraabdominal malignancy (Iavazzo et al, 2012). Skin and gastrointestinal lesions may arise from the same cause or may occur without relationship to one another. See Clinical Pearl, "Scars."

Clinical Pearl

Scars

Note any scars and draw their location, configuration, and relative size on an illustration of the abdomen. If the cause of a scar was not explained during the history, now is a good time to pursue that information. The presence of scarring should alert you to the possibility of intraabdominal adhesions.

Contour

Inspect the abdomen for contour, symmetry, and surface motion, using tangential lighting to illuminate contour and visible peristalsis. Contour is the abdominal profile from the rib margin to the pubis, viewed on the horizontal plane. The expected contours can be described as flat, rounded, or scaphoid. A flat contour is common in well-muscled, athletic adults. The rounded or convex contour is characteristic of young children, but in adults it is the result of subcutaneous fat or poor muscle tone. The abdomen should be evenly rounded with the maximum height of convexity at the umbilicus. The scaphoid or concave contour is seen in thin adults.

Note the location and contour of the umbilicus. It should be centrally located without displacement upward, downward, or laterally. The umbilicus may be inverted or protrude slightly, but it should be free of inflammation, swelling, or bulge that may indicate a hernia.

Inspect for symmetry from a seated position at the patient's side, then move to a standing position behind the patient's head, if possible. Contralateral areas of the abdomen should be symmetric in appearance and contour. Look for any distention or bulges.

Generalized symmetric distention may occur as a result of obesity, enlarged organs, and fluid or gas. Distention from the umbilicus to the symphysis can be caused by an ovarian tumor, pregnancy, uterine fibroids, or a distended bladder. Distention of the upper half, above the umbilicus, can be due to tumor, pancreatic cyst, or gastric dilation. Asymmetric distention or protrusion may indicate hernia, tumor, cysts, bowel obstruction, muscle or soft tissue hematoma, or enlargement of abdominal organs. See Clinical Pearl, "Abdominal Distention."

Risk Factors

Colon Cancer

- Age older than 50 years
- Family history of colorectal cancer or adenomatous polyps in one or more first-degree relatives and family history of syndromic colon cancer, including familial adenomatous polyposis (FAP), hereditary nonpolyposis colorectal cancer (HNPCC), Turcot syndrome (also associated with brain tumors), Peutz-Jeghers syndrome, and MUYTH-associated polyposis (MAP; mutation in the gene *MUYTH*)
- Personal history of colon cancer, intestinal polyps, inflammatory bowel disease (Crohn disease, ulcerative colitis), FAP, HNPCC
- Personal history of ovarian or endometrial cancer
- Race: African American
- Ethnic background: Jewish, Eastern European descent (Ashkenazi)
- Diet: low-fiber, high in red meat and processed meats, low fruit and vegetable intake
- Obesity
- Smoking cigarettes
- Lack of regular physical activity
- Heavy alcohol use
- Type 2 diabetes

American Cancer Society, 2012.

Clinical Pearl

Abdominal Distention

You are with a patient whose abdomen is significantly distended and whose bowel sounds are hypoactive or even absent. There is no particular pain and you feel no masses. The deep tendon reflexes are diminished. You know that the patient is on diuretics for treatment of hypertension. Think of hypokalemia as a cause of a paralytic ileus (intestinal pseudo-obstruction).

Diuretics/distention/deficiency of potassium. Narcotics and hypothyroidism can do the same thing.

Ask the patient to take a deep breath and hold it. The contour should remain smooth and symmetric. This maneuver lowers the diaphragm and compresses the organs of the abdominal cavity, which may cause previously unseen bulges or masses to appear. Next, ask the patient to raise his or her head from the table. This contracts the rectus abdominis muscles, which produces muscle prominence in thin or athletic adults. Superficial abdominal wall masses may become visible. If a hernia is present, the increased abdominal pressure may cause it to protrude.

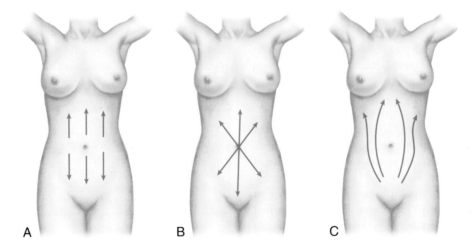

FIGURE 17-6 **Abdominal venous patterns.** **A,** Expected. **B,** Portal hypertension. **C,** Inferior vena cava obstruction.

An incisional hernia is caused by a defect in the abdominal musculature that develops after a surgical incision, resulting in a protrusion in the area of the surgical scar. Protrusion of the navel indicates an umbilical hernia. The adult type develops during pregnancy, in longstanding ascites, or when intrathoracic pressure is repeatedly increased, as occurs in chronic respiratory disease. Hernias may also occur in the midline of the epigastrium (i.e., hernia of the linea alba). This type of hernia contains a bit of fat and is felt as a small, tender nodule. Most hernias are reducible, meaning that the contents of the hernia can be pushed back into place. If not, the hernia is nonreducible or incarcerated (blood supply to the protruded contents may become obstructed and require immediate surgery).

In addition to hernias, separation of the rectus abdominis muscles may become apparent when the patient raises his or her head from the table. Diastasis recti occurs more often in pregnancy and the postpartum period. The condition is of little clinical significance.

Movement

With the patient's head again resting on the table, inspect the abdomen for movement. Smooth, even movement should occur with respiration. Males exhibit primarily abdominal movement with respiration, whereas females show mostly costal movement. Limited abdominal motion associated with respiration may indicate peritonitis in an ill-appearing adult male. Surface motion from peristalsis, seen as a rippling movement across the abdomen, may be seen in thin individuals but can also be a sign of intestinal obstruction. Abdominal aortic pulsations seen in the upper midline are often visible in thin adults. Marked pulsations may occur as the result of increased pulse pressure or abdominal aortic aneurysm.

Auscultation

Unlike the usual sequence, always perform auscultation of the abdomen prior to percussion and palpation because these maneuvers may alter the frequency and intensity of bowel sounds.

Bowel Sounds

Lightly place the diaphragm of a warmed stethoscope on the abdomen. Some health care providers say they prefer to use the bell; in reality, they tend to pull the skin tight with the bell and, in effect, make a diaphragm. A cold stethoscope, like cold hands, may initiate contraction of the abdominal muscles. Listen for bowel sounds and note frequency and character. They are usually heard as clicks and gurgles that occur irregularly and range from 5 to 35 per minute. Bowel sounds are generalized so most often they can be assessed adequately by listening in one place. Loud prolonged gurgles are called borborygmi (stomach growling). Increased bowel sounds may occur with gastroenteritis, early intestinal obstruction, or hunger. High-pitched tinkling sounds suggest intestinal fluid and air under pressure, as in early obstruction. Decreased bowel sounds occur with peritonitis and paralytic ileus. Auscultate in all four quadrants if you have a concern. Absent bowel sounds, referring to an inability to hear

any bowel sounds after 5 minutes of continuous listening, is typically associated with abdominal pain and rigidity and is a surgical emergency.

Additional Sounds and Bruits

Listen with the diaphragm for friction rubs over the liver and spleen. Friction rubs are high pitched and are heard in association with respiration. Although friction rubs in the abdomen are rare, they indicate inflammation of the peritoneal surface of the organ from tumor, infection, or infarct. A bruit is a harsh or musical intermittent auscultatory sound, which may reflect blood flow turbulence and indicate vascular disease. Listen with the bell of the stethoscope in the epigastric region and for bruits in the aortic, renal, iliac, and femoral arteries. Vascular sounds are usually well localized. Keep their specific locations in mind as you listen at those sites (Fig. 17-7). Auscultate with the bell of the stethoscope in the epigastric region and around the umbilicus for a venous hum, which is soft, low pitched, and continuous. A venous hum occurs with increased collateral circulation between the portal and systemic venous systems.

Percussion

Percussion (generally indirect) is used to assess the size and density of the organs in the abdomen and to detect the presence of fluid (as with ascites), air (as with gastric distention), and fluid-filled or solid masses. Percussion is used either independently or concurrently with palpation of specific organs and can validate palpatory findings. For simplicity, percussion and palpation are discussed separately.

First percuss all quadrants or regions of the abdomen for a sense of overall tympany and dullness (Table 17-1). Tympany is the predominant sound because air is present in the stomach and intestines. Dullness is heard over organs and solid masses. A distended bladder produces dullness in the suprapubic area. Develop a systematic route for percussion.

Liver Span

Now go back and percuss individually the liver, spleen, and stomach. Begin liver percussion at the right midclavicular line over an area of tympany. Always begin with an area of tympany and proceed to an area of dullness because that sound change is easiest to detect. Percuss upward along the midclavicular line, as shown in Figure 17-8, to determine the lower border of the liver. The area of liver dullness is usually heard at the costal margin or slightly below it. Mark the border with a marking pen. A lower liver border that is more than 2 to 3 cm ($\frac{3}{4}$ to 1 inch) below the costal margin may indicate organ enlargement or downward displacement of the diaphragm because of emphysema or other pulmonary disease.

To determine the upper border of the liver, begin percussion on the right midclavicular line at an area of lung resonance around the third intercostal space. Continue downward until the percussion tone changes to one of dullness; this marks the upper border of the liver. Mark the location with the pen. The upper border is usually in the fifth intercostal space. An upper border below this may indicate downward displacement or liver atrophy.

Animation: Abdominal Aortic Aneurysm

Video: Abdomen: Auscultating the Abdomen

Video: Abdomen: Assessing the Liver Span

FIGURE 17-7 Sites to auscultate for bruits: renal arteries, iliac arteries, aorta, and femoral arteries. *(Modified from Wilson and Giddens, 2009.)*

Table 17-1	Percussion Notes of the Abdomen	
Note	**Description**	**Location**
Tympany	Musical note of higher pitch than resonance	Over air-filled viscera
Hyperresonance	Pitch lies between tympany and resonance	Base of left lung
Resonance	Sustained note of moderate pitch	Over lung tissue and sometimes over the abdomen
Dullness	Short, high-pitched note with little resonance	Over solid organs adjacent to air-filled structures

Dullness extending above the fifth intercostal space suggests upward displacement from abdominal fluid or masses.

Measure the distance between the marks to estimate the vertical span of the liver. The usual span is approximately 6 to 12 cm (2½ to 4½ inches). A span greater than this may indicate liver enlargement, whereas a lesser span suggests atrophy. Age and gender influence liver size. Liver span is usually greater in males and in tall individuals.

Percussion provides a gross estimate of liver size. Errors in estimating liver span can occur when the dullness of a pleural effusion or lung consolidation obscures the upper liver border. Similarly, gas in the colon may produce tympany in the right upper quadrant and obscure the dullness of the lower liver border.

If liver enlargement is suspected, additional percussion maneuvers can provide further information. Percuss upward and then downward over the right midaxillary line. Liver dullness is

FIGURE 17-8 Liver percussion routes along midclavicular and midsternal lines. *(Modified from Wilson and Giddens, 2009.)*

usually detected around the seventh intercostal space. You can also percuss along the midsternal line to estimate the midsternal liver span (see Fig 17-8). The usual span at the midsternal line is 4 to 8 cm (1½ to 3 inches). Spans exceeding 8 cm suggest liver enlargement.

To assess the descent of the liver, ask the patient to take a deep breath and hold it while you percuss upward again from the abdomen at the right midclavicular line. The area of lower border dullness should move downward 2 to 3 cm. This maneuver will guide subsequent palpation of the organ. See Clinical Pearl, "Assessing Liver Size."

FIGURE 17-9 Percussion of the spleen. *(From Wilson and Giddens, 2009.)*

Spleen

Percuss the spleen just posterior to the midaxillary line on the left side as shown in Figure 17-9. Percuss in several directions beginning at areas of lung resonance. You may hear a small area of splenic dullness from the sixth to the ninth rib. Traube's space is a semilunar region defined by the sixth rib superiorly, the midaxillary line laterally, and the left costal margin inferiorly. This area is typically tympanitic because it overlies the fundus of the stomach. With splenic enlargement, tympany changes to dullness as the spleen is brought forward and downward with inspiration (splenic percussion sign). However, a full stomach, feces-filled intestine, or left-sided pleural effusion may also produce dullness.

Gastric Bubble

Percuss for the gastric air bubble in the area of the left lower anterior rib cage and left epigastric region. The tympany produced by the gastric bubble is lower in pitch than the tympany of the intestine.

Kidneys

To assess each kidney for tenderness, ask the patient to assume a sitting position. Place the palm of your hand over the right costovertebral angle and strike your hand with the ulnar surface of the fist of your other hand (Fig. 17-10, *A*). Repeat the maneuver over the left costovertebral angle. Direct percussion with the fist over each costovertebral angle may also be used (see Fig. 17-10, *B*). The patient should perceive the blow as a thud, but it should not cause pain. For efficiency of time and motion, this maneuver is performed while examining the back rather than the abdomen.

Palpation

Use palpation to assess the organs of the abdominal cavity and to detect muscle spasm, masses, fluid, and areas of tenderness. Evaluate the abdominal organs for size, shape, mobility, and consistency. Stand at the patient's right side with the patient in the supine position. Attempt to make the patient as comfortable and relaxed as possible. Use warm hands and bend the patient's knees to help relax the abdominal muscles. Ticklishness may be a challenge (Box 17-2).

Light Palpation

Begin with a light, systematic palpation of all four quadrants, or nine regions, initially avoiding any areas that have been identified as problem spots. Lay the palm of your hand lightly on the abdomen, with the fingers extended and held together (Fig. 17-11). With the palmar surface of your fingers, depress the abdominal wall no more than 1 cm, using a light and even pressing circular motion. Avoid short, quick jabs. The abdomen should feel smooth, with a consistent softness. The patient's abdomen may tense if you press too deeply, your hands are cold, the patient is ticklish, or inflammation is present. Guarding, tensing of the abdominal musculature to protect inflamed viscera, should alert you to move cautiously through the remainder of the examination.

Light palpation is useful in identifying muscular resistance and areas of tenderness. A large mass or distended structure may be appreciated on light palpation as a sense of resistance. If resistance is present, determine whether it is voluntary or involuntary in the following way: Place a pillow under the patient's knees and ask the patient to breathe slowly through the mouth as you feel for relaxation of the rectus abdominis muscles on expiration. If the tenseness remains, it is probably an involuntary response to localized or generalized rigidity. Rigidity is a boardlike hardness of the abdominal wall overlying areas of peritoneal irritation.

Moderate Palpation

Continue palpation with the same hand position and technique used for light palpation, exerting moderate pressure as

FIGURE 17-10 Fist percussion of the costovertebral angle for kidney tenderness. **A,** Indirect percussion. **B,** Direct percussion.

Box 17-2	Examining the Abdomen in a Ticklish Patient

The ticklishness of a patient can sometimes make it difficult to palpate the abdomen satisfactorily; however, there are ways to overcome this problem. Ask the patient to perform self-palpation, and place your hands over the patient's fingers, not quite touching the abdomen itself. After a time, let your fingers drift slowly onto the abdomen while still resting primarily on the patient's fingers. You can still learn a good deal, and ticklishness might be less of a problem. You might also use the diaphragm of the stethoscope (making sure it is warm enough) as a palpating instrument. This serves as a starting point, and again your fingers can drift over the edge of the diaphragm and palpate without eliciting an excessively ticklish response. Applying a stimulus to another, less sensitive part of the body with your non-palpating hand can also decrease a ticklish response. In some instances, a patient's ticklishness cannot be overcome and you just have to palpate as best you can.

FIGURE 17-12 Moderate palpation using the side of the hand.

FIGURE 17-11 Light palpation of the abdomen. With fingers extended and approximated, press in no more than 1 cm.

an intermediate step to gradually approach deep palpation. Tenderness not elicited on light palpation may become evident with deeper pressure. An additional maneuver of moderate palpation is performed with the side of your hand (Fig. 17-12). This maneuver is useful in assessing organs that move with

respiration, specifically the liver and spleen. Palpate during the entire respiratory cycle. As the patient inspires, the organ is displaced downward, and you may be able to feel it as it bumps gently against your hand.

Deep Palpation

Deep palpation is necessary to thoroughly delineate abdominal organs and to detect less obvious masses. Use the palmar surface of your extended fingers, pressing deeply and evenly into the abdominal wall (Fig. 17-13). Palpate all four quadrants or nine regions, moving the fingers back and forth over the abdominal contents. Often you are able to feel the borders of the rectus abdominis muscles, the aorta, and portions of the colon. Tenderness not elicited with light or moderate palpation may become evident. Deep pressure may also evoke tenderness in the healthy person over the cecum, sigmoid colon, aorta, and in the midline near the xiphoid process. If deep palpation is difficult because of obesity or muscular resistance, you can use a bimanual technique with one hand atop the other, as shown in Figure 17-14. Exert pressure with the top hand while concentrating on sensation with the other hand. Some examiners prefer to use the bimanual technique for all patients.

Masses

Identify any masses and note the following characteristics: location, size, shape, consistency, tenderness, pulsation, mobility, and movement with respiration. To determine whether a mass is superficial (i.e., located in the abdominal wall) or intraabdominal, have the patient lift his or her head from the examining table, thus contracting the abdominal muscles. Masses in the abdominal wall will continue to be palpable, but those located in the

abdominal cavity will be more difficult to feel because they are obscured by abdominal musculature. The presence of feces in the colon, often mistaken for an abdominal mass, can be felt as a soft, rounded, boggy mass in the cecum and in the ascending, descending, or sigmoid colons. Other structures that are sometimes mistaken for masses are the lateral borders of the rectus abdominis muscles, uterus, aorta, sacral promontory, and common iliac artery (Fig. 17-15). By mentally visualizing the placement of the abdominal structures, you can distinguish between what ought to be there and an unexpected finding.

Umbilical Ring

Palpate the umbilical ring and around the umbilicus. The area should be free of bulges, nodules, and granulation. The umbilical ring should be round and free of irregularities. Note whether it is incomplete or soft in the center, which suggests the potential for herniation. The umbilicus may be either slightly inverted or everted, but it should not protrude.

Palpation of Specific Organs and Structures

Liver. Place your left hand under the patient at the 11th and 12th ribs, pressing upward to elevate the liver toward the abdominal wall. Place your right hand on the abdomen, fingers pointing toward the head and extended so the tips rest on the right midclavicular line below the level of liver dullness, as shown in Figure 17-16, *A.* Alternatively, you can place your right hand parallel to the right costal margin, as shown in Figure 17-16, *B.* In either case, press your right hand gently but deeply, in and up. Have the patient breathe regularly a few times and then take a deep breath. Try to feel the liver edge as the diaphragm pushes it down to meet your fingertips. Ordinarily, the liver is not palpable, although it may be felt in some thin persons without pathologic conditions. If the liver edge is felt, it should be firm, smooth, even, and nontender. Feel for nodules, tenderness, and irregularity. If the liver is palpable, repeat the maneuver medially and laterally to the costal margin to assess the liver contour and surface.

FIGURE 17-13 Deep palpation of the abdomen. Press deeply and evenly with the palmar surface of extended fingers.

FIGURE 17-14 Deep bimanual palpation.

FIGURE 17-15 Abdominal structures commonly felt as masses.

FIGURE 17-16 **Palpating the liver. A,** Fingers are extended, with tips on right midclavicular line below the level of liver dullness and pointing toward the head. **B,** Alternative method for liver palpation with the fingers parallel to the costal margin.

FIGURE 17-17 **Palpating the liver with fingers hooked over the costal margin.**

FIGURE 17-18 **Scratch technique for auscultating the liver.** With the stethoscope over the liver, lightly scratch the abdominal surface, moving toward the liver. The sound will be intensified over the liver.

Liver: Alternative Techniques. An alternative technique is to hook your fingers over the right costal margin below the border of liver dullness, as shown in Figure 17-17. Stand on the patient's right side facing his or her feet. Press in and up toward the costal margin with your fingers, and ask the patient to take a deep breath. Try to feel the liver edge as it descends to meet your fingers.

If the abdomen is distended or the abdominal muscles tense, the usual techniques for determining the lower liver border may be unproductive, and the scratch test may be useful (Fig. 17-18). This technique uses auscultation to detect the differences in sound transmission over solid and hollow organs. Place the diaphragm of the stethoscope over the liver and with the finger of your other hand scratch the abdominal surface lightly, moving toward the liver border. When you encounter the liver, the sound you hear intensifies.

To check for liver tenderness when the liver is not palpable, use indirect fist percussion. Place the palmar surface of one hand over the lower right rib cage, and then strike your hand with the ulnar surface of the fist of your other hand. The healthy liver is not tender to percussion.

Gallbladder. Palpate below the liver margin at the lateral border of the rectus abdominis muscle for the gallbladder. A

healthy gallbladder will not be palpable. A palpable, tender gallbladder indicates cholecystitis, whereas nontender enlargement suggests common bile duct obstruction. If you suspect cholecystitis, have the patient take a deep breath during deep palpation. As the inflamed gallbladder comes in contact with the examining fingers, the patient will experience pain and abruptly halt inspiration (Murphy sign).

Spleen. While still standing on the patient's right side, reach across with your left hand and place it beneath the patient over the left costovertebral angle. Press upward with that hand to lift the spleen anteriorly toward the abdominal wall. Place the palmar surface of your right hand with fingers extended on the patient's abdomen below the left costal margin (Fig. 17-19, *A*). Use findings from percussion as a guide. Press your fingertips inward toward the spleen as you ask the patient to take a deep breath. Try to feel the edge of the spleen moving downward toward your fingers. The spleen is not usually palpable in an adult; if you can feel it, it is probably enlarged (Box 17-3). Be sure to palpate with your fingers below the costal margin so that you will not miss the lower edge of an enlarged spleen. Be gentle

FIGURE 17-19 Palpating the spleen. A, Press upward with the left hand at the patient's left costovertebral angle. Feel for the spleen with the right hand below the left costal margin. **B,** Palpating the spleen with the patient lying on the side. Press inward with the left hand and tips of the right fingers.

Box 17-3	An Enlarged Spleen or an Enlarged Left Kidney?

When an organ is palpable below the left costal margin, it may be difficult to differentiate an enlarged spleen from an enlarged left kidney. Percussion should help distinguish between the organs. The percussion note over an enlarged spleen is dull because the spleen displaces the bowel. The usual area of splenic dullness will be increased downward and toward the midline. The percussion note over an enlarged kidney is resonant because the kidney is deeply situated behind the bowel. In addition, the edge of the spleen is sharper than that of the kidney. A palpable notch along the medial border suggests an enlarged spleen rather than an enlarged kidney.

FIGURE 17-20 Palpating the left kidney. Elevate the left flank with the left hand. Palpate deeply with the right hand.

in palpation. Patients with splenomegaly from infectious mononucleosis have a small risk for spontaneous splenic rupture (Won and Ethell, 2012).

Repeat the palpation while the patient is lying on the right side with hips and knees flexed (see Fig. 17-19, *B*). Still standing on the right side, press inward with your left hand to assist gravity in bringing the spleen forward. Press inward with the fingertips of your right hand and feel for the edge of the spleen. Again, you will not usually feel it; if you can, it is probably enlarged.

Left Kidney. Standing on the patient's right side, reach across with your left hand as you did in spleen palpation and place your hand over the left flank. Place your right hand at the patient's left costal margin. Have the patient take a deep breath and then elevate the left flank with your left hand and palpate deeply (because of the retroperitoneal position of the kidney) with your right hand (Fig. 17-20). Try to feel the lower pole of the kidney with your fingertips as the patient inhales. The left kidney is ordinarily not palpable.

Another approach is to capture the kidney. Move to the patient's left side and position your hands as before, with the left hand over the patient's left flank and the right hand at the left costal margin. Ask the patient to take a deep breath. At the height of inspiration, press the fingers of your two hands together to capture the kidney between the fingers. Ask the patient to

FIGURE 17-21 Capture technique for palpating the kidney (left kidney palpation shown). As the patient takes a deep breath, press the fingers of both hands together. As the patient exhales, slowly release the pressure and feel for the kidney to slip between the fingers.

breathe out and hold the exhalation while you slowly release your fingers (Fig. 17-21). If you have captured the kidney you may feel it slip beneath your fingers as it moves back into place. Although the patient may feel the capture and release, the maneuver should not be painful. Again, a left kidney is seldom palpable.

EXAMINATION AND FINDINGS

FIGURE 17-22 Palpating the aorta. Place the thumb on one side of the aorta and the fingers on the other side.

Right Kidney. Stand on the patient's right side, placing one hand under the patient's right flank and the other hand at the right costal margin. Perform the same maneuvers as you did for the left kidney. Because of the anatomic position of the right kidney, it is more commonly palpable than the left kidney. If it is palpable, it should be smooth, firm, and nontender. It may be difficult to distinguish the kidney from the liver edge. The liver edge tends to be sharp, whereas the kidney is more rounded. The liver also extends more medially and laterally and cannot be captured.

Aorta. Palpate deeply slightly to the left of the midline, and feel for the aortic pulsation. If the pulsation is prominent, try to determine the direction of pulsation. A prominent lateral pulsation suggests an aortic aneurysm. If you are unable to feel the pulse on deep palpation, an alternate technique may help. Place the palmar surface of your hands with fingers extended on the midline. Press the fingers deeply inward on each side of the aorta, and feel for the pulsation. In thin individuals, you can use one hand, placing the thumb on one side of the aorta and the fingers on the other side (Fig. 17-22).

Evidence-Based Practice in Physical Examination

Detecting Abdominal Aortic Aneurysms

Although health care providers can detect asymptomatic abdominal aortic aneurysms (AAAs) by palpation, the overall sensitivity is somewhat low. A negative examination does not rule out the diagnosis, especially in obese patients and in those who are unable to relax their abdominal musculature during the exam. In general palpation has a moderate sensitivity for detecting aneurysms large enough to be referred for surgery. The United States Preventive Services Task Force (USPSTF) currently recommends a one-time screening ultrasound for AAA in men 65-75 years of age who have ever smoked.

From Lederle, 2009; USPSTF, 2005.

Urinary Bladder. The urinary bladder is not palpable in a healthy patient unless the bladder is distended with urine, at which time you will feel it as a smooth, round, tense mass. You can determine the distended bladder outline with percussion; a distended bladder will elicit a lower percussion note than the surrounding air-filled intestines.

Advanced Skills

Ascites Assessment

Ascites, a pathologic increase in fluid in the peritoneal cavity, may be suspected in the patient with risk factors who has a protuberant abdomen or bulging flank when lying supine. Percuss for areas of dullness and resonance with the patient supine. Because ascites fluid settles with gravity, expect to hear dullness in the dependent parts of the abdomen and tympany in the upper parts where the relatively lighter bowel has risen. Mark the borders between tympany and dullness. There are several physical examination maneuvers used to detect the presence of ascites.

Shifting Dullness. After identifying the borders between tympany and dullness, have the patient lie on one side and again percuss for tympany and dullness and mark the borders. In the patient without ascites, the borders will remain relatively constant. With ascites, the border of dullness shifts to the dependent side (approaches the midline) as the fluid resettles with gravity (Fig. 17-23).

Fluid Wave. This procedure requires three hands, so you will need assistance from the patient or another examiner (Fig. 17-24). With the patient supine, ask him or her or another person to press the edge of the hand and forearm firmly along the vertical midline of the abdomen. This positioning helps stop the transmission of a wave through adipose tissue. Place your hands on each side of the abdomen and strike one side sharply with your fingertips. Feel for the impulse of a fluid wave with the fingertips of your other hand. An easily detected fluid wave suggests ascites. However, a fluid wave can sometimes be felt in people without ascites and, conversely, may not occur in people with early ascites.

Evidence-Based Practice in Physical Examination

Detecting Ascites

The most sensitive maneuvers for detecting ascites are flank dullness (84%) and the presence of bulging flanks (81%), both of which have a specificity of 59%. The most specific test is the presence of a fluid wave (90%), although its sensitivity is fair (62%). Because these maneuvers may miss smaller amounts of peritoneal fluid, radiologic studies may be necessary.

From McGibbon, 2007; Simel, 2009.

Pain Assessment

Abdominal pain is a common symptom but often difficult to evaluate. How bad is the pain? Has there been recent trauma? Pain that is severe enough to make the patient unwilling to move, accompanied by nausea and vomiting, and marked by areas of localized tenderness generally suggests underlying pathology. While examining the abdomen, keep your eyes on the patient's

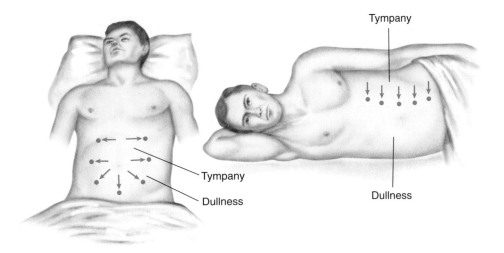

FIGURE 17-23 Testing for shifting dullness. Dullness shifts to the dependent side.

FIGURE 17-24 Testing for fluid wave. Strike one side of the abdomen sharply with the fingertips. Feel for the impulse of a fluid wave with the other hand. *(From Wilson and Giddens, 2009.)*

---

face. The facial response is as important in your evaluation as the patient's verbal response to questions about the quality and degree of pain. Ask the patient to cough or take a deep breath. Assess the patient's willingness to jump or to walk. Is the pain exacerbated by movement? (See Box 17-4.)

Common causes of abdominal pain are described in Tables 17-2 and 17-3. Careful assessment of the quality (Table 17-4) and location of pain (Box 17-5) can usually narrow the possible causes, allowing you to select additional diagnostic studies with greater efficiency.

Findings associated with peritoneal irritation are summarized in Box 17-6. The Evidence-Based Practice box describes the use of history and physical examination in diagnosing appendicitis.

Several tools have been developed based on history, physical examination, and laboratory values. The Alvarado score (also known as the MANTRELS [Migration of pain, Anorexia, Nausea/vomiting, Tenderness in the right lower quadrant, Rebound pain, Elevation of temperature, Leukocytosis, Shift to the left] score) has been validated in children and adults and remains the most widely accepted and simplest decision tool (Wagner, 2009). The Pediatric Appendicitis Score, which uses pain with cough, hopping, or rebound tenderness with

---

Box 17-4 Clues in Diagnosing Abdominal Pain

There are all types of rules for identifying whether pain in the abdomen has significance. The following are a few of them:

Patients may give a "touch-me-not" warning—that is, not to touch in a particular area; however, these patients may not actually have pain if their faces seem relaxed and unconcerned, even smiling. When you touch they might recoil, but the unconcerned face persists. (This sign is helpful in other areas of the body, as well as the abdomen.)

Patients with an organic cause for abdominal pain are generally not hungry. A negative response to the "Do you want something to eat?" question is probable, particularly with appendicitis or intraabdominal infection.

Ask the patient to point a finger to the location of the pain. If it is not directed to the umbilicus but goes immediately to a fixed point, there is a greater likelihood that this has significant pathologic importance. The farther from the umbilicus the pain, the more likely it will be organic in origin (Apley rule). If the finger goes to the umbilicus and the patient seems otherwise well to you, you should include psychosomatic causes in the differential diagnosis.

Patients with nonspecific abdominal pain may keep their eyes closed during abdominal palpation, whereas patients with organic disease usually keep their eyes open.

Patients with nonsignificant pain will have abdominal pain when you manually palpate the abdomen. However, if you then tell the patient you want to listen to the painful area and push just as hard with the stethoscope and elicit no pain response, the pain is likely not significant.

---

percussion in place of right lower quadrant pain, has also been used. The Ohmann score, which uses patient age, history, physical examination and laboratory findings, is another tool to help identify patients at low, moderate, and high risk of having appendicitis. Experts recommend observation for patients at low risk, diagnostic testing and imaging studies (computed tomography or ultrasound) for moderate-risk patients and urgent surgical evaluation for high-risk patients (Ebell, 2008).

EXAMINATION AND FINDINGS

Evidence-Based Practice in Physical Examination

Diagnosing Appendicitis

Appendicitis is the most common indication for emergency abdominal surgery. Although it is most common in the second decade of life, each year in the United States, more than 70,000 pediatric hospital discharges are for appendicitis and related conditions (Bundy et al, 2007). An accurate diagnosis based on history and physical examination can facilitate immediate surgical evaluation and definitive treatment and prevent unnecessary use of radiologic imaging. In adults, historical symptoms that increase the likelihood of appendicitis are right lower quadrant (RLQ) pain, initial periumbilical pain with migration to the RLQ, and the presence of pain before vomiting. The presence of rigidity, a positive psoas sign (see p. 393), fever, and/or rebound tenderness are

physical examination findings that increase the likelihood of appendicitis. Conversely, the absence of RLQ pain, the absence of the migration of the pain, and the presence of similar pain previously are historical findings that make appendicitis less likely. On physical examination, the lack of RLQ pain, rigidity, or guarding makes appendicitis less likely. Health care providers rarely rely on a single symptom or sign to make a diagnosis; however, the precision and accuracy of combinations of these findings have not been reported. No finding effectively rules out appendicitis. In children, vomiting, rebound tenderness, rectal tenderness, and fever are more helpful, whereas right lower quadrant tenderness is less helpful (Bundy et al, 2007).

Table 17-2   Conditions Producing Acute Abdominal Pain

Condition	Usual Pain Characteristics	Possible Associated Signs and Symptoms
Appendicitis	Initially periumbilical or epigastric; colicky; later becomes localized to RLQ, often at McBurney's point	Guarding, tenderness; + iliopsoas and + obturator signs, RLQ skin hyperesthesia; anorexia, nausea, or vomiting after onset of pain; low-grade fever; + Aaron, Rovsing, Markle, and McBurney signs*
Peritonitis	Onset sudden or gradual; pain generalized or localized, dull or severe and unrelenting; guarding; pain on deep inspiration	Shallow respiration; + Blumberg, Markle, and Ballance signs; reduced or absent bowel sounds, nausea and vomiting; + obturator + iliopsoas signs
Cholecystitis	Severe, unrelenting RUQ or epigastric pain; may be referred to right subscapular area	RUQ tenderness and rigidity, + Murphy sign, palpable gallbladder, anorexia, vomiting, fever, possible jaundice
Pancreatitis	Dramatic, sudden, excruciating LUQ, epigastric, or umbilical pain; may be present in one or both flanks; may be referred to left shoulder and penetrates to back	Epigastric tenderness, vomiting, fever, shock; + Grey Turner sign; + Cullen sign: both signs occur 2 to 3 days after onset
Salpingitis	Lower quadrant, worse on left	Nausea, vomiting, fever, suprapubic tenderness, rigid abdomen, pain on pelvic examination
Pelvic inflammatory disease	Lower quadrant, increases with activity	Tender adnexa and cervix, cervical discharge, dyspareunia
Diverticulitis	Epigastric, radiating down left side of abdomen especially after eating; may be referred to back	Flatulence, borborygmus, diarrhea, dysuria, tenderness on palpation
Perforated gastric or duodenal ulcer	Abrupt RUQ; may be referred to shoulders	Abdominal free air and distention with increased resonance over liver; tenderness in epigastrium or RUQ; rigid abdominal wall, rebound tenderness
Intestinal obstruction	Abrupt, severe, colicky, spasmodic; referred to epigastrium, umbilicus	Distention, minimal rebound tenderness, vomiting, localized tenderness, visible peristalsis; bowel sounds absent (with paralytic obstruction) or hyperactive high pitched (with mechanical obstruction)
Volvulus	Referred to hypogastrium and umbilicus	Distention, nausea, vomiting, guarding; sigmoid loop volvulus may be palpable
Leaking abdominal aneurysm	Steady throbbing midline over aneurysm; may penetrate to back, flank	Nausea, vomiting, abdominal mass, bruit
Biliary stones, colic	Episodic, severe, RUQ, or epigastrium lasting 15 minutes to several hours; may be lower	RUQ tenderness, soft abdominal wall, anorexia, vomiting, jaundice, subnormal temperature

Table 17-2	Conditions Producing Acute Abdominal Pain—cont'd	
Condition	**Usual Pain Characteristics**	**Possible Associated Signs and Symptoms**
Renal calculi	Intense; flank, extending to groin and genitals; may be episodic	Fever, hematuria; + Kehr sign
Ectopic pregnancy	Lower quadrant; referred to shoulder; with rupture is agonizing	Hypogastric tenderness, symptoms of pregnancy, spotting, irregular menses, soft abdominal wall, mass on bimanual pelvic examination; ruptured: shock, rigid abdominal wall, distention; + Kehr and Cullen signs
Ruptured ovarian cyst	Lower quadrant, steady, increases with cough or motion	Vomiting, low-grade fever, anorexia, tenderness on pelvic examination
Splenic rupture	Intense; LUQ, radiating to left shoulder; may worsen with foot of bed elevated	Shock, pallor, lowered temperature

LUQ, Left upper quadrant; *RLQ*, right lower quadrant; *RUQ*, right upper quadrant.
*See Table 17-5 for explanation of signs.

Table 17-3	Conditions Producing Chronic Abdominal Pain	
Condition	**Usual Pain Characteristics**	**Possible Associated Signs and Symptoms**
Irritable bowel syndrome	Hypogastric pain; crampy, variable, infrequent; associated with bowel function	Unremarkable physical examination Pain associated with gas, bloating, distention; relief with passage of flatus, feces
Lactose intolerance	Crampy pain after drinking milk or eating milk products	Associated diarrhea; unremarkable physical examination
Diverticular disease	Localized pain	Abdominal tenderness, fever
Constipation	Colicky or dull and steady pain that does not progress and worsen	Fecal mass palpable, stool in rectum
Uterine fibroids	Pain related to menses, intercourse	Palpable myoma(s)
Hernia	Localized pain that increases with exertion or lifting	Hernia on physical examination
Esophagitis/gastroesophageal reflux disease	Burning or gnawing pain in midepigastrium, worsens with recumbency and certain foods	Unremarkable physical examination
Peptic ulcer	Burning or gnawing pain	May have epigastric tenderness on palpation
Gastritis	Constant burning pain in epigastrium	May be accompanied by nausea, vomiting, diarrhea, or fever Unremarkable physical examination

Modified from Dains et al, 2007.

Table 17-4	Quality and Onset of Abdominal Pain
Characteristic	**Possible Related Conditions**
Burning	Peptic ulcer
Cramping	Biliary colic, gastroenteritis
Colicky	Appendicitis with impacted feces; renal stone
Aching	Appendiceal irritation
Knifelike	Pancreatitis
Ripping, tearing	Aortic dissection
Gradual onset	Infection
Sudden onset	Duodenal ulcer, acute pancreatitis, obstruction, perforation

Abdominal Signs

"Classic" abdominal pain signs have often been given the name of the person who first described them. Some of the most common and historic signs are included in Table 17-5.

Rebound Tenderness

There are several maneuvers that can be used to assess for peritoneal inflammation (Box 17-6). Rebound tenderness is identified in the following manner. Holding your hand at a 90-degree angle to the abdomen with the fingers extended, press gently and deeply into a region remote from the area of abdominal discomfort. Rapidly withdraw your hand and fingers (Fig. 17-25). The return to position—or "rebound" of the structures that were compressed by your fingers—causes a sharp stabbing pain at the

Box 17-5	Some Causes of Pain Perceived in Anatomic Regions

Right Upper Quadrant

Duodenal ulcer
Hepatitis
Hepatomegaly
Lower lobe pneumonia
Cholecystitis

Left Upper Quadrant

Ruptured spleen
Gastric ulcer
Aortic aneurysm
Perforated colon
Lower lobe pneumonia

Right Lower Quadrant

Appendicitis
Salpingitis
Ovarian cyst
Ruptured ectopic
  pregnancy
Tubo-ovarian abscess
Renal/ureteral stone
Strangulated hernia
Meckel diverticulitis
Regional ileitis
Perforated cecum

Periumbilical

Intestinal
  obstruction
Acute pancreatitis
Early appendicitis
Mesenteric
  thrombosis
Aortic aneurysm
Diverticulitis

Left Lower Quadrant

Sigmoid diverticulitis
Salpingitis
Ovarian cyst
Ruptured ectopic
  pregnancy
Tubo-ovarian abscess
Renal/ureteral stone
Strangulated hernia
Perforated colon
Regional ileitis
Ulcerative colitis

Box 17-6	Findings in Peritoneal Irritation

- Involuntary rigidity of abdominal muscles
- Tenderness and guarding
- Absent bowel sounds
- Positive obturator test (p. 393)
- Positive iliopsoas test (p. 393)
- Rebound tenderness (Blumberg sign and McBurney sign; see Table 17-5)
- Abdominal pain on walking
- Positive heel jar test (Markle sign; see Table 17-5)
- Right lower quadrant pain intensified by left lower quadrant abdominal palpation (Rovsing sign; see Table 17-5)

Table 17-5	Abdominal Signs Associated with Common Abdominal Conditions

Sign	Description	Associated Conditions
Aaron	Pain or distress occurs in area of patient's heart or stomach on palpation of McBurney's point	Appendicitis
Ballance	Fixed dullness to percussion in left flank and dullness in right flank that disappears on change of position	Peritoneal irritation
Blumberg	Rebound tenderness	Peritoneal irritation; appendicitis
Cullen	Ecchymosis around umbilicus	Hemoperitoneum; pancreatitis; ectopic pregnancy
Dance	Absence of bowel sounds in right lower quadrant	Intussusception
Grey Turner	Ecchymosis of flanks	Hemoperitoneum; pancreatitis
Kehr	Abdominal pain radiating to left shoulder	Spleen rupture; renal calculi; ectopic pregnancy
Markle (heel jar)	Patient stands with straightened knees, then raises up on toes, relaxes, and allows heels to hit floor, thus jarring body. Action will cause abdominal pain if positive.	Peritoneal irritation; appendicitis
McBurney	Rebound tenderness and sharp pain when McBurney's point is palpated	Appendicitis
Murphy	Abrupt cessation of inspiration on palpation of gallbladder	Cholecystitis
Romberg-Howship	Pain down the medial aspect of the thigh to the knees	Strangulated obturator hernia
Rovsing	Right lower quadrant pain intensified by left lower quadrant abdominal palpation	Peritoneal irritation; appendicitis

FIGURE 17-25 **Testing for rebound tenderness. A,** Press deeply and gently into the abdomen. **B,** Then rapidly withdraw the hands and fingers.

> **Clinical Pearl**
>
> *Ectopic Pregnancy*
>
> Unfortunately, ectopic pregnancy is often not diagnosed before rupture because symptoms are mild. Big clue: a sudden, dramatic change from mild, even vague abdominal pain that is not particularly distressing to a sudden onset of severe abdominal tenderness in the hypogastric area, particularly on the involved side. Rigidity and rebound may come on early or late. The main point: If a woman presents with vague abdominal symptoms, be sure to inquire about her sexual activity and menstrual history, conduct a pelvic examination, and strongly consider performing a urine pregnancy test. Do not disregard the mild tenderness that might be evoked. Try, at least, to anticipate the emergency of a rupture.

site of peritoneal inflammation (positive Blumberg sign). Rebound tenderness over McBurney's point in the lower right quadrant suggests appendicitis (positive McBurney sign). The maneuver for rebound tenderness should be performed at the end of the examination because a positive response produces pain and muscle spasm that can interfere with any subsequent examination. Because light percussion produces a mild localized response in the presence of peritoneal inflammation, assessing for rebound tenderness is considered unnecessary by many examiners. See Clinical Pearl, "Ectopic Pregnancy."

Iliopsoas Muscle Test

This test is performed when you suspect appendicitis because an inflamed appendix may cause irritation of the lateral iliopsoas muscle. Ask the patient to lie supine and then place your hand over the lower right thigh. Ask the patient to raise the right leg, flexing at the hip, while you push downward (Fig. 17-26). An alternative technique is to position the patient on the left side and ask that the right leg be raised from the hip while you press downward against it. A third technique is to hyperextend the right leg by drawing it backward while the patient is lying on the left side. Pain with any of these techniques is considered a positive psoas sign, indicating irritation of the iliopsoas muscle.

FIGURE 17-26 **Iliopsoas muscle test. A,** The patient raises the leg from the hip while the examiner pushes downward against it. **B,** Alternate technique. The examiner hyperextends the right leg by drawing it backward while the patient lies on the left side. *(B, From Swartz, 2006.)*

Obturator Muscle Test

This test can be performed when you suspect a ruptured appendix or a pelvic abscess due to irritation of the obturator muscle. While in the supine position, ask the patient to flex the right leg at the hip and knee to 90 degrees. Hold the leg just above the knee, grasp the ankle, and rotate the leg laterally and medially (Fig. 17-27). Pain in the right hypogastric region is a positive sign, indicating irritation of the obturator muscle.

Ballottement

Ballottement is a palpation technique used to assess an organ or a mass. To perform abdominal ballottement with one hand, place

EXAMINATION AND FINDINGS

your extended fingers, hand, and forearm at a 90-degree angle to the abdomen. Push in toward the organ or mass with the fingertips (Fig. 17-28, *A*). If the mass is freely movable, it will float upward and touch the fingertips as fluid and other structures are displaced by the maneuver. To perform bimanual ballottement, place one hand on the anterior abdominal wall and one hand against the flank. Push inward on the abdominal wall while palpating with the flank hand to determine the presence and size of the mass (Fig. 17-28, *B*).

FIGURE 17-27 Obturator muscle test. With the right leg flexed at the hip and knee, rotate the leg laterally and medially. *(From Swartz, 2006.)*

✿ Infants and Children

If possible, the infant's abdomen should be examined during a time of relaxation and quiet. It is often best to do this at the start of the overall examination, especially before initiating any procedure that might cause distress (Fig. 17-29). Sucking on a pacifier may help relax the infant. The parent's lap often makes the best examining surface as the infant or toddler will feel most secure. Sit facing the parent and conduct the abdominal examination entirely on the parent's lap. This works well during the first several months—and often the first 2 to 3 years—of life (Fig. 17-30).

Inspection

Inspect the abdomen, noting its shape, contour, and movement with respiration. It should be rounded and dome-shaped because the abdominal musculature has not fully developed. Note any localized fullness. Abdominal and chest movements should be synchronous, with a slight bulge of the abdomen at the beginning of respiration. Note whether the abdomen protrudes above the level of the chest or is scaphoid. A distended or protruding abdomen can result from feces, a mass, or organ enlargement. A scaphoid abdomen in a newborn suggests that the abdominal contents are displaced into the thorax.

Note any pulsations over the abdomen. Pulsations in the epigastric area are common in newborns and infants. Superficial veins are usually visible in the thin infant; however, distended veins across the abdomen are an unexpected finding suggestive of vascular obstruction or abdominal distention or obstruction. Spider nevi may indicate liver disease.

Inspect the umbilical cord of the newborn, counting the number of vessels. Two arteries and one vein should be present. A single umbilical artery should alert you to the possibility of congenital anomalies. Any intestinal structure present in the umbilical cord or protruding into the umbilical area and visible through a thick transparent membrane suggests an omphalocele (see Clinical Pearl, "Umbilical Cord").

The umbilical stump area should be dry and odorless. Inspect it for discharge, redness, induration, and skin warmth. Once the stump has separated, typically by 2 weeks of age, serous or serosanguineous discharge may indicate a granuloma when no other signs of infection are present. Inspect all folds of skin in the umbilicus for a nodule of granulomatous tissue. If drainage

FIGURE 17-28 Ballottement technique. A, Single-handed ballottement. Push inward at a 90-degree angle. If the object is freely movable, it will float upward to touch the fingertips. **B,** Bimanual ballottement: *P,* pushing; *R,* receiving hand.

FIGURE 17-29 Positioning for examination of the infant's abdomen.

FIGURE 17-31 Umbilical hernia in an infant. *(From Zitelli and Davis, 2012.)*

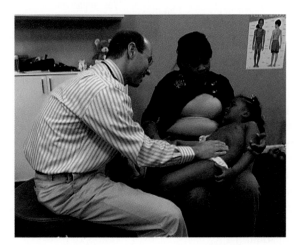

FIGURE 17-30 Positioning for examination of a toddler in a parent's lap.

persists after cord separation, consider the possibility of a patent urachal cyst or remnant.

Note any protrusion through the umbilicus or rectus abdominis muscles when the infant strains. The umbilicus is usually inverted. A small umbilical hernia (i.e., the protrusion of omentum and intestine through the umbilical opening, forming a visible and palpable bulge) is a common finding in infants. Umbilical hernias can be very large and impressive (Fig. 17-31). It is ordinarily easy to reduce them temporarily by pushing the contents back into the intraabdominal position. Measure the diameter of the umbilical opening rather than the protruding contents to determine the size. The maximum size is generally reached by 1 month of age, and most hernias will close spontaneously by 1 to 2 years of age.

Diastasis rectus abdominis, a separation 1 to 4 cm wide in the midline, usually between the xiphoid and the umbilicus, is a common finding when the rectus abdominis muscles do not approximate each other. Ordinarily, there is no need to repair this. Although rare, herniation through the rectus abdominis muscles can be a problem.

If the infant is vomiting frequently, use tangential lighting and observe the abdomen at eye level for peristaltic waves. Peristalsis is not usually visible. Peristaltic waves may sometimes be seen in thin, malnourished infants, but their presence usually suggests an intestinal obstruction such as pyloric stenosis.

Clinical Pearl

Umbilical Cord

A thick umbilical cord suggests a well-nourished fetus; a thin cord suggests otherwise.

Auscultation and Percussion

The procedures of auscultation and percussion of the abdomen do not differ from those used for adults. Peristalsis is detected when metallic tinkling is heard every 10 to 30 seconds, and bowel sounds should be present within 1 to 2 hours after birth. A scaphoid abdomen in a newborn with respiratory distress suggests a diaphragmatic hernia. In this instance, bowel sounds may be appreciated in the chest. Bruits and venous hums should not be heard on abdominal auscultation.

Renal bruits are associated with renal artery stenosis and rarely with a renal arteriovenous fistula. The bruit of stenosis has a high frequency and is soft; the bruit of an arteriovenous fistula is continuous. Both are difficult to hear. When suspicious, try first with the patient held upright or sitting, listening at the posterior flank; then try with the patient supine, listening over the abdomen.

The abdomen may produce more tympany on percussion than is found in adults because infants swallow air when feeding or crying. As with adults, tympany in a distended abdomen is usually the result of gas, whereas dullness may indicate fluid or a solid mass.

Palpation

Palpate the abdomen with the infant's feet slightly elevated and knees flexed to promote relaxation of the abdominal musculature (see Clinical Pearl, "Palpating an Infant's Abdomen"). Begin with superficial palpation to detect the spleen, liver, and masses close to the surface. The spleen is usually palpable 1 to 2 cm below the left costal margin during the first few weeks after birth. A detectable spleen tip at the left costal margin is a common finding in well infants and young children. An enlarged spleen may indicate congenital hemolytic disease or sepsis.

EXAMINATION AND FINDINGS

Clinical Pearl

Palpating an Infant's Abdomen

The abdomen of an infant can seem very tiny in relation to the size of your hand. One technique for palpating a very small abdomen is as follows. Place your right hand gently on the abdomen with the thumb at the right upper quadrant and the index finger at the left upper quadrant. Press very gently at first, only gradually increasing pressure (never too vigorously) as you palpate over the entire abdomen.

Clinical Pearl

Enlarged Liver

An infant of a mother with poorly controlled insulin-dependent diabetes mellitus (IDDM) or gestational diabetes may have an enlarged liver. This history and/or finding should alert the health care provider to check for hypoglycemia in the infant.

DIFFERENTIAL DIAGNOSIS

Abdominal Masses in Infants and Children

Neonates	Infants and Children
Hydronephrosis	Feces (constipation)
Multicystic dysplastic kidney	Pyloric stenosis
Polycystic kidney disease	Gastrointestinal duplication
Renal vein thrombosis	Meckel diverticulum
Wilms tumor	Neuroblastoma
Ovarian cyst	Wilms tumor
Hydrocolpos	Lymphoma
Hydrometrocolpos	Hepatoblastoma
Gastrointestinal duplication	Embryonal sarcoma
	Ovarian cyst
	Teratoma

Modified from Rahhal et al, 2006.

Liver Palpation

To assess the liver, superficially palpate at the right midclavicular line 3 to 4 cm below the costal margin. As the infant inspires, wait to feel a narrow mass tap your finger. Gradually move your fingers up the midclavicular line until the sensation is felt. The liver edge is usually palpable just below the right costal margin in the newborn. The liver edge may be palpable at 1 to 3 cm below the right costal margin in infants and toddlers. Estimation of true liver size can be accomplished only by percussing the upper border, as well as palpating the lower edge. The upper edge of the liver should be detected by percussion at the sixth intercostal space. Together, the techniques provide an estimate of liver span, rather than just a projection of size below the costal margin (see Clinical Pearl, "Enlarged Liver").

Hepatomegaly is present when the liver is more than 3 cm below the right costal margin, suggesting infection, cardiac failure, or liver disease. Before 2 years of age, females have a slightly larger liver span than males. The mean range of liver spans in infants and children is as follows:

Age	Liver Span (cm)	Age	Liver Span (cm)
6 months	2.4 to 2.8	5 years	4.5 to 4.8
12 months	2.8 to 3.1	6 years	4.8 to 5.1
24 months	3.5 to 3.6	8 years	5.1 to 5.6
3 years	4.0	10 years	5.5 to 6.1
4 years	4.3 to 4.4		

Deep Palpation

Following light palpation, perform deep palpation in all quadrants or regions. Note the location, size, shape, tenderness, and consistency of any masses. More than half of all masses detected in newborns are genitourinary in origin; hydronephrosis and multicystic dysplastic kidney are the most common. Abdominal masses should be investigated with radiologic studies.

The olive-shaped mass of pyloric stenosis may be detected with deep palpation in the right upper quadrant immediately after the infant vomits. It can be helpful to sit the infant in your lap, folding the upper body gently against your palpating hand and bringing the pyloric mass into opposition with your hand. Almost all other palpable masses in the abdomen of the newborn are typically renal in origin. A sausage-shaped mass in the left or right upper quadrant may indicate intussusception in an ill-appearing or lethargic infant or toddler. A midline suprapubic mass suggests Hirschsprung disease, in which feces fills the rectosigmoid colon. A soft mass in the left lower quadrant of child of any age may indicate feces in the sigmoid colon associated with constipation.

In the infant and toddler, the bladder can usually be palpated and percussed in the suprapubic area. A distended bladder, felt as a firm, central, dome-shaped structure in the lower abdomen, may indicate urethral obstruction or central nervous system defects. Compared to newborns, abdominal tumors are more commonly palpated in infants and toddlers, the most common being neuroblastoma, Wilms tumor, and lymphoma. Palpation of the femoral arteries is performed during the abdominal examination as described in Chapter 15.

Tenderness or pain on palpation may be difficult to detect in the infant; however, pain and tenderness are assessed by such behaviors as change in the pitch of crying, facial grimacing, rejection of the opportunity to suck, and drawing the knees to the abdomen with palpation. Examine the infant on the parent's lap. If the infant continues to cry throughout the examination, seize the quiet moment in the respiratory cycle to palpate to distinguish between a firm and soft abdomen. The abdomen should be soft during inspiration. If the abdomen remains hard, with a noticeable rigidity or resistance to pressure during both respiratory phases, peritoneal irritation may be present. It is often necessary to delay examination of a distressed infant, waiting for a quieter moment, unless there is reason for urgency. Causes of abdominal pain in pediatric patients vary by age.

The abdomen of the young child protrudes slightly, giving a potbellied appearance when the child is standing, sitting, and supine (Fig. 17-32). After age 5 years, the contour of the child's abdomen, when supine, may become convex and will not extend

EXAMINATION AND FINDINGS

DIFFERENTIAL DIAGNOSIS
Causes of Acute Abdominal Pain in Infants, Children, and Adolescents

Diagnosis	Infancy (<2 Years)	Preschool Age (2 to 5 Years)	School Age (>5 Years)	Adolescent
Appendicitis		✓	✓	✓
Cholecystitis				✓
Constipation	✓	✓	✓	✓
Functional			✓	✓
Gastritis				✓
Gastroenteritis	✓	✓	✓	✓
Gastroesophageal reflux disease	✓			✓
Hepatitis				✓
Incarcerated hernia	✓			
Inflammatory bowel disease			✓	✓
Henoch-Schönlein purpura		✓		
Intussusception	✓	✓		
Milk protein allergy	✓			
Pancreatitis				✓
Volvulus	✓			
Extraabdominal				
Dysmenorrhea				✓
Ectopic pregnancy				✓
Epididymitis				✓
Group A streptococcal pharyngitis			✓	✓
Nephrolithiasis				✓
Ovarian torsion				✓
Pelvic inflammatory disease				✓
Pneumonia		✓	✓	✓
Pregnancy				✓
Testicular torsion			✓	✓
Urinary tract infection	✓		✓	✓

Modified from Marin and Alpern, 2011.
Diagnoses are included for age groups in which they are most commonly seen.

above an imaginary line drawn from the xiphoid process to the symphysis pubis. Respirations will continue to be abdominal until the child is 6 to 7 years old. Restricted abdominal respiration in young children can be caused by peritoneal irritation or an acute abdomen.

Palpate the abdomen of a child who is ticklish with a firm rather than soft touch. If this is unsuccessful, place the child's hand under the palm of your examining hand, leaving your fingers free to palpate. Localization of abdominal tenderness or pain may be difficult in the young child who cannot verbally describe the site or character of pain. Distract the child with a toy, or question the child about a favorite activity as you begin palpating in the abdominal region believed most distant from the area of pain. Observe for changes in facial expression during palpation to identify the location of greatest pain. Check for rebound tenderness and make the same observations of the child's facial expression. As with adults, check for rebound tenderness cautiously. Once a child has experienced palpation that is too intense, a subsequent examiner has little chance for a successful abdominal examination.

❧ Adolescents

The techniques of abdominal examination of the adolescent are the same as those used for adults. Do not overlook the possibility

FIGURE 17-32 Potbellied stance of a toddler.

Evidence-Based Practice in Physical Examination

In a study of 82 young girls and adolescent women found to have ovarian torsion, most reported severe intermittent pain for 24 hours duration. More often patients reported pain in the right lower quadrant compared to the left lower quadrant (61% vs. 34%). Most (91%) had abdominal tenderness, 27% had guarding, and 18% had rebound tenderness on exam.

Rossi et al, 2012.

of pregnancy or ovarian torsion as a cause of abdominal pain or lower abdominal mass, even in young adolescent females.

✤ Pregnant Women

Uterine changes that can be detected on pelvic examination are discussed in Chapter 18. Nausea and vomiting are common in the first trimester. Constipation is a common occurrence, and hemorrhoids often develop later in pregnancy. Bowel sounds will be diminished as a result of decreased peristaltic activity. Striae and a midline band of pigmentation (linea nigra) may be present (see Fig. 17-2). Assessment of the abdomen of pregnant women includes uterine size estimation for gestational age, fetal growth, position of the fetus, monitoring of fetal well-being, and presence of uterine contractions (see Chapter 18).

✤ Older Adults

The techniques of examination are the same as those used for younger adults. The abdominal wall of the older adult becomes thinner and less firm as a result of the loss of connective tissue and muscle mass that accompanies aging. Palpation, therefore, may be relatively easier and yield more accurate findings. A pulsating abdominal aortic aneurysm may be more readily palpable than in younger patients. Deposition of fat over the abdominal

area is common despite concurrent loss of fatty tissue over the extremities. The abdominal contour is often rounded as a result of loss of muscle tone.

The only modifications in examination techniques require some common sense. Use judgment in determining whether a patient is able to assume a particular position. Rotation of joints, such as with the obturator muscle test, may cause discomfort in patients who have decreased muscle flexibility or increased joint tenderness.

Be aware that respiratory changes can produce corresponding findings in the abdominal examination. The liver in patients with hyperexpanded lungs from chronic obstructive pulmonary disease may be displaced downward, but not necessarily enlarged. In this case, both the upper and lower borders of the liver may be detected 1 to 2 cm below the usual markers, but the liver span should still be between 6 and 12 cm. On the other hand, with the decrease in liver size after 50 years of age, you may find a smaller midclavicular liver span.

With decreased intestinal motility associated with aging, intestinal disorders are common in older adults, so be particularly sensitive to patient concerns and related findings in this regard. Constipation is a common symptom, and you are more likely to feel stool in the sigmoid colon. The sensation of bloating or increased gas may be reflected by increased tympany on percussion. Fecal impaction is a common finding in older adults with severe or chronic constipation. See Clinical Pearl, "Constipation with Diarrhea."

Obstruction may be a problem with older adults, occurring as a result of hypokalemia, myocardial infarction, and infections such as pneumonia, sepsis, peritonitis, and pancreatitis. Vomiting, distention, diarrhea, and constipation can signal obstruction.

The incidence of gastrointestinal cancer increases with age. Symptoms depend on the site of the tumor and include dysphagia, nausea, vomiting, anorexia, and hematemesis. Patients may also report changes in stool frequency, size, consistency, or color. See Chapter 20 for a discussion of the rectal digital examination, an important step in the detection of colon cancer.

Pain perception may be altered as part of the aging process, and older patients may exhibit atypical pain symptoms. These can include less severe or totally absent pain with disease states that characteristically produce pain in younger adults. Therefore, evaluation of pain in the older adult must take into account concurrent symptoms and accompanying findings.

Clinical Pearl

Constipation with Diarrhea

Be aware that people with apparent diarrhea may still be seriously constipated. Some may have loose stools around a major fecal impaction and develop overflow incontinence.

Sample Documentation

History and Physical Examination

Subjective

A 44-year-old woman describes a burning sensation in epigastric area and chest. Occurs after eating, especially spicy foods. Lasts 1 to 2 hours. Is worse when lying down. Sometimes causes bitter taste in mouth. Also feels bloated. Antacids do not relieve the symptoms. Denies nausea, vomiting, diarrhea. No cough or shortness of breath.

Objective

Abdomen rounded and symmetric with white striae adjacent to umbilicus in all quadrants. A well-healed, 5-cm white surgical scar evident in right lower quadrant. No areas of visible pulsations or peristalsis. Active bowel sounds audible in all four quadrants. Percussion tones tympanic over epigastrium and resonant over remainder of abdomen. Liver span 8 cm at right midclavicular line. On inspiration, liver edge firm, smooth, and nontender. No splenomegaly. Musculature soft and relaxed to light palpation. No masses or areas of tenderness to deep palpation. No costovertebral angle tenderness.

For additional sample documentation, see Chapter 26, pp. 628-631.

ABNORMALITIES

ABDOMEN

ALIMENTARY TRACT

Acute Diarrhea

Frequent liquid or loose stools lasting less than 4 weeks' duration

Pathophysiology

- Most commonly, viral and self-limited in those without signs or symptoms or other organ involvement
- International travelers may acquire foodborne infection (e.g., enterotoxigenic *Escherichia coli, Salmonella, Shigella,* or *Entamoeba histolytica*).
- Camping or well water exposes individuals to *Giardia* and *Campylobacter* through untreated water.
- *Cryptosporidium* is a potential cause from contaminated water in urban areas of the United States.
- *Salmonella* or *Campylobacter jejuni* from undercooked poultry
- Undercooked beef or unpasteurized milk may contain *E. coli* 0157:H7.
- Raw shellfish is a potential source of Norwalk virus.
- Consider food poisoning if diarrhea develops in two or more persons following ingestion of the same food.

Subjective Data

- Usually abrupt onset and lasts less than 2 weeks
- Abdominal pain
- Nausea
- Vomiting
- Fever
- Tenesmus (feeling of incomplete defecation)
- Vomiting within several hours of ingesting a particular food suggests food poisoning
- Bloody diarrhea may occur with organisms such as *Campylobacter* and *Shigella.*

Objective Data

- Diffuse abdominal tenderness
- Examination can mimic peritoneal inflammation with right lower quadrant pain or guarding
- If severe, may have findings consistent with moderate to severe dehydration, particularly in infants, children, and older adults (e.g., tachycardia, hypotension, and altered mental status)

ABNORMALITIES

Gastroesophageal Reflux Disease

Backward flow of gastric contents, which are typically acidic, into the esophagus

Pathophysiology

- Caused by relaxation or incompetence of the lower esophageal sphincter
- Delayed gastric emptying is a predisposing factor
- More common among older adults and in pregnant women

Subjective Data

- Heartburn or acid indigestion (burning chest pain, localized behind the breastbone that moves up toward the neck and throat)
- Bitter or sour taste of acid in the back of the throat
- Hoarseness
- Infants and toddlers exhibit back arching, fussiness with feeding, or regurgitation and vomiting; can be severe enough to cause weight loss and failure to thrive
- Can precipitate an acute asthma exacerbation or cause chronic respiratory problems from aspiration, and esophageal bleeding

Objective Data

- Generally unremarkable examination
- With severe disease may have erythema of the posterior pharynx and edematous vocal cords

Irritable Bowel Syndrome

Disorder of intestinal motility

Pathophysiology

- Common; occurs in about one in five Americans, more often in women
- Usually begins in late adolescence or early adult life and rarely appears for the first time after 50 years of age

Subjective Data

- Commonly report a cluster of symptoms, consisting of abdominal pain, bloating, constipation, and diarrhea (see Table 17-3)
- Some experience alternating diarrhea and constipation.
- Mucus may be present around or in the stool.
- Bouts may occur at times of emotional stress.

Objective Data

- Generally unremarkable examination
- Diagnosis is typically made after excluding other potential causes.
- Rome III diagnostic criteria (2006) requires recurrent abdominal pain or discomfort at least 3 days per month during the previous 3 months associated with two or more of the following:
  - Relieved by defecation
  - Onset associated with change in stool frequency
  - Onset associated with change in stool form or appearance
- Supporting symptoms include:
  - Altered stool passage (straining and/or urgency)
  - Mucorrhea

Staying Well

Avoiding Foodborne Infection

Adults and children are susceptible to foodborne infection, both at home and while traveling. Prevention measures that you can recommend:

- Cook all ground beef and poultry thoroughly. Send restaurant food back if it is not cooked well. Eat only food that has been cooked thoroughly and is still hot.
- Do not drink unpasteurized juices or milk.
- Refrigerate ground beef and perishable food right away after shopping.
- Wash hands and food utensils with hot, soapy water after handling meat and poultry.
- Avoid cooked food that has been kept at room temperature for several hours.

Travelers can minimize their risk for "traveler's diarrhea" by practicing the following effective preventive measures:

- Avoid eating foods or drinking beverages purchased from street vendors or other establishments where unhygienic conditions are present.
- Avoid eating raw or undercooked meat and seafood.
- Avoid eating raw fruits (e.g., oranges, bananas, avocados) and vegetables unless the traveler peels them.
- Avoid ice unless it has been made from safe water.
- Avoid dishes containing raw or undercooked eggs.
- NOTE: Boiling kills most bacteria; hot tea and coffee can generally be considered safe to drink.

Hiatal Hernia with Esophagitis

Part of the stomach passes through the esophageal hiatus in the diaphragm into the chest cavity

Pathophysiology	Subjective Data	Objective Data
• Very common; occurs most often in women and older adults • Associated with obesity, pregnancy, ascites, and the use of tight-fitting belts and clothes; muscle weakness is a predisposing factor.	• Epigastric pain and/or heartburn that worsens with lying down and is relieved by sitting up or antacids • Water brash (mouth fills with fluid from the esophagus) • Dysphagia • Most are asymptomatic and discovered incidentally • Symptoms of incarcerated hernia include sudden onset of vomiting, pain, and complete dysphagia.	• Generally unremarkable examination • With severe disease may have erythema of the posterior pharynx and edematous vocal cords

Duodenal Ulcer (Duodenal Peptic Ulcer Disease)

Chronic circumscribed break in the duodenal mucosa that scars with healing

Pathophysiology	Subjective Data	Objective Data
• May develop from infection with *Helicobacter pylori* and increased gastric acid secretion (e.g., Zollinger-Ellison syndrome [or gastrinoma]) • Occurs approximately twice as often in men as in women	• Localized epigastric pain that occurs when the stomach is empty and is relieved by food or antacids • With upper gastrointestinal bleeding, symptoms include hematemesis and melena; significant blood loss may result in dizziness and syncope.	• Anterior wall ulcers may produce tenderness on palpation of the abdomen. • Ulcers occur on both the anterior and posterior walls of the duodenal bulb; anterior ulcers are more likely to perforate, whereas posterior ulcers are more likely to bleed. • Perforation of the duodenum presents with signs of an acute abdomen (abdominal distention, rebound, and guarding). • With significant bleeding, may show hypotension and tachycardia

Crohn Disease

Chronic inflammatory disorder that can affect any part of the gastrointestinal tract that produces ulceration, fibrosis, and malabsorption; terminal ileum and colon are the most common sites

Pathophysiology	Subjective Data	Objective Data
• Cause is unknown but is thought to occur from an imbalance between proinflammatory and antiinflammatory mediators	• Chronic diarrhea with compromised nutritional status • Other systemic manifestations may include arthritis, iritis, and erythema nodosum. • Disease course characterized by unpredictable flares and remissions	• May have right lower quadrant tenderness • Abdominal mass may be palpated secondary to thickened or inflamed bowel • Perianal skin tags, fistulae, and abscesses may be seen. • Extraintestinal examination findings include erythema nodosum and pyoderma gangrenosum, as well as arthritis involving the large joints. • Colonoscopy and pathology show characteristic cobblestone appearance of the mucosa. • Fistula and abscess formation, sometimes extending to the skin, is common (Fig. 17-33), as well as perianal skin tags (Fig. 17-34).

ABNORMALITIES

FIGURE 17-33 Crohn disease showing a perianal abscess, raised and erythematous lesion, above a small scar from a prior incision and drainage procedure. *(From Zitelli and Davis, 2012.)*

FIGURE 17-34 **Crohn disease.** Note a scar from a previous incision and drainage. Perianal skin tags are common in Crohn disease and a good clue to diagnosis. *(From Zitelli and Davis, 2012.)*

Ulcerative Colitis

Chronic inflammatory disorder of the colon and rectum that produces mucosal friability and areas of ulceration

Pathophysiology

- Cause unknown, but immunologic and genetic factors have been implicated
- Active chronic ulcerative colitis predisposes an individual to developing colon cancer.

Subjective Data

- Bloody, frequent, watery diarrhea, with as many as 20 to 30 diarrheal stools per day
- May exhibit weight loss, fatigue, and general debilitation
- May range from mild to severe, depending on the degree of colon involvement
- May remain in remission for years after an acute phase of the illness
- Sclerosing cholangitis (inflammation, scarring and destruction of bile ducts) may present with fatigue and jaundice

Objective Data

- Generally do not have fistulae or perianal disease
- Contrast radiographs typically show loss of the normal mucosal pattern.
- Sclerosing cholangitis may occur with a cholestatic pattern of elevated transaminase levels.
- Endoscopic findings show mucosal edema with ulcerations and bleeding (Fig. 17-35).

FIGURE 17-35 Ulcerative colitis showing severe mucosal edema and inflammation with ulcerations and bleeding. *(From Doughty and Jackson, 1993.)*

Stomach Cancer

Arises from epithelial cells of the mucous membrane

Pathophysiology	Subjective Data	Objective Data
• Most commonly found in lower half of the stomach • In early stages, the growth is confined to the mucosa and submucosa; as disease progresses, the muscular layer of the stomach becomes involved; metastases, local and distant, are common.	• May have vague and nonspecific symptoms, including loss of appetite, feeling of fullness, weight loss, dysphagia, and persistent epigastric pain	• May have midepigastric tenderness, hepatomegaly, enlarged supraclavicular nodes, and ascites • An epigastric mass may be palpable in the late stages of disease.

Diverticular Disease

Pathophysiology	Subjective Data	Objective Data
• Diverticula are saclike mucosal outpouchings through colonic muscle (Fig. 17-36) • May involve any part of the gastrointestinal tract; the sigmoid is the most commonly affected location. • Cause unknown, but may be caused by colonic dysmotility, defective muscular structure, and defects in collagen and aging	• Most patients are asymptomatic. • With diverticulitis (when diverticula become inflamed), may experience left lower quadrant pain, anorexia, nausea, vomiting, and altered bowel habits (usually constipation) • Pain usually localizes to the site of inflammation.	• May have abdominal distention and be tympanic to percussion with decreased bowel sounds and localized tenderness (see Table 17-2) • Lower gastrointestinal bleeding may occur.

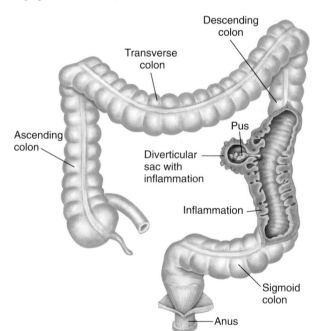

FIGURE 17-36 Diverticulosis (diverticulitis). *(From Doughty and Jackson, 1993.)*

Colon Cancer (Colorectal Cancer)

Pathophysiology	Subjective Data	Objective Data
• May involve the rectum, sigmoid, proximal and descending colon • Second most common cancer in the United States; see Risk Factors box on p. 378	• Symptoms depend on cancer location, size, and presence of metastases. • May describe abdominal pain, blood in the stool, or a recent change in the frequency or character of stools • Earliest sign may be occult blood in the stool, which can be detected by fecal occult blood testing (FOBT)	• Few early examination findings • If disease has progressed, may have palpable abdominal mass in right or left lower quadrants or show signs of anemia from occult blood loss (e.g., pallor and tachycardia) • Rectal cancer may be palpable by digital rectal examination (see Chapter 20). • Evidence-Based Practice box on p. 404 highlights some colon cancer screening test concerns and recommendations.

Evidence-Based Practice in Physical Examination

Screening for Colorectal Cancer

Of cancers affecting women and men, colorectal cancer is the second leading cause of cancer-related deaths in the United States, accounting for about 53,000 deaths each year (U.S. Cancer Statistics Working Group, 2010.) Many of these deaths are preventable through appropriate screening. Colorectal cancer can be prevented by the detection and removal of adenomatous polyps. Five-year survival is 90% when the cancer is diagnosed in the localized stage. In 2006-2007, the American Cancer Society, the U.S. Multi-Society Task Force on Colorectal Cancer, and the American College of Radiology developed consensus guidelines for the detection of adenomatous polyps and colorectal cancer in asymptomatic, average-risk adults. Persons are defined as being at average risk for colorectal cancer if they are 50 years or older and have no risk factors for colorectal cancer other than age. Colorectal screening tests fall into two categories: (1) fecal tests to primarily identify colorectal cancer; and (2) partial or full structural examinations to detect both cancer and premalignant adenomatous polyps.

Options for screening asymptomatic adults 50 years or older include the following:

- Tests that primarily detect cancer
  - Annual guaiac-based fecal occult blood test (gFOBT) with high test sensitivity

- Annual fecal immunochemical test (FIT) with high test sensitivity
- Stool DNA test with high sensitivity (testing interval uncertain)
- Tests that detect adenomatous polyps and cancer
  - Flexible sigmoidoscopy (FSIG) every 5 years
  - Colonoscopy every 10 years
  - Double-contrast barium enema every 5 years
  - Computed tomography colography every 5 years

Which to Recommend?

Several large randomized controlled trials have shown that patients screened with gFOBT have cancers detected at earlier stages than unscreened patients, with a reduction in mortality between 15% and 33% over time. To date, no clear difference has been demonstrated in test performance comparing the two types of fecal blood tests (gFOBT and FIT). Screening for molecular markers using stool-based DNA testing is considered an acceptable option and may evolve over time with technologic advances. Evidence for screening using FSIG was demonstrated in two case-control studies, with a 60% to 80% reduction in colorectal cancer mortality. Experts recommend that patients with positive screening tests undergo colonoscopy.

Levin et al, 2008.

HEPATOBILIARY SYSTEM

Hepatitis

Inflammatory process characterized by diffuse or patchy hepatocellular necrosis

Pathophysiology	Subjective Data	Objective Data
- Most commonly caused by viral infection, alcohol, drugs, or toxins - Acute viral hepatitis is caused by at least five distinct agents; see Risk Factors box on p. 376 regarding hepatitis A, B, and C. - Hepatitis D occurs only in those infected with hepatitis B, either as a coinfection in acute hepatitis B or as a superinfection in chronic hepatitis B. - Hepatitis E is a self-limited type that may occur after a natural disaster because of fecal-contaminated water or food.	- Some are asymptomatic; others report jaundice, anorexia, abdominal pain, clay-colored stools, tea-colored urine, and fatigue.	- Liver function tests are abnormal - Examination findings may include jaundice and hepatomegaly. - With severe or progressive disease, may develop cirrhosis with its associated examination findings (see p. 405)

Cirrhosis

Diffuse hepatic process characterized by fibrosis and alteration of normal liver architecture into structurally abnormal nodules

Pathophysiology	Subjective Data	Objective Data
- Progression of liver disease to cirrhosis can happen over weeks to years - Signs and symptoms occur as a result of decreased liver synthetic function, decreased detoxification capabilities, or portal hypertension. - Most common causes in the United States are hepatitis C and alcoholic liver disease - Less common causes include autoimmune hepatitis, primary biliary cirrhosis, Wilson disease, hemochromatosis, α_1-antitrypsin deficiency, and sarcoidosis.	- Some are asymptomatic; others report jaundice, anorexia, abdominal pain, clay-colored stools, tea-colored urine, and fatigue. - May describe prominent abdominal vasculature, cutaneous spider angiomas, hematemesis, and abdominal fullness	- On examination, the liver is initially enlarged with a firm, nontender border on palpation; as scarring progresses, the liver size is reduced, and it generally cannot be palpated. - Neurologic examination abnormalities may be seen (e.g., hepatic encephalopathy). - With progressive disease, portal hypertension and ascites may occur (Fig. 17-37). - Muscle wasting and nutritional deficiencies may be evident in late-stage disease. - May have abnormal laboratory values (e.g., liver function tests and coagulopathy)

FIGURE 17-37 Marked ascites and an umbilical hernia, which had ruptured a few days before the photograph, in a patient with cirrhosis and portal hypertension secondary to hepatitis C.

Primary Hepatocellular Carcinoma

Pathophysiology

- Frequently arises in the setting of cirrhosis, approximately 20 to 30 years after liver injury or disease onset; however, about 25% have no prior risk factors for cirrhosis.
- Most patients die from tumor progression with the median survival time from diagnosis around 6 months.
- Can metastasize to the lungs, portal vein, periportal nodes, bone, and brain
- Widespread vaccination for hepatitis A and B and routine screening for hepatitis B and C may reduce the incidence.

Subjective Data

- Symptoms may include jaundice, anorexia, fatigue, abdominal fullness, clay-colored stools, and tea-colored urine.

Objective Data

- On examination, hepatomegaly with a hard, irregular liver border may be palpated.
- Liver nodules may be present and palpable, and the liver may be tender or nontender.
- Examination findings related to cirrhosis may be seen (see earlier).

Cholelithiasis

Stone formation in the gallbladder occurs when certain substances reach a high concentration in bile and produce crystals.

Pathophysiology

- Crystals mix with mucus and form gallbladder sludge; over time, the crystals enlarge, mix, and form stones.
- Main substances involved in gallstone formation are cholesterol (>80%) and calcium bilirubinate
- Chronic disease can result in fibrosis and gallbladder dysfunction and predispose to gallbladder cancer.

Subjective Data

- Many patients are asymptomatic.
- Symptoms may include indigestion, colic, and mild transient jaundice.

Objective Data

- Condition commonly produces episodes of acute cholecystitis (see p. 406)

ABNORMALITIES

Cholecystitis

Inflammatory process of the gallbladder most commonly due to obstruction of the cystic duct from cholelithiasis, which may be acute or chronic

Pathophysiology	Subjective Data	Objective Data
• With cystic duct obstruction, the gallbladder becomes distended, and blood flow is compromised, leading to ischemia and inflammation. • Acute cholecystitis has associated stone formation (cholelithiasis) in 90% of cases, causing obstruction and inflammation. • Acute cholecystitis without stones (acalculous) results from any condition that affects the regular emptying and filling of the gallbladder, such as immobilization with major surgery, trauma, sepsis, or long-term total parenteral nutrition. • Chronic cholecystitis refers to repeated attacks of acute cholecystitis in a gallbladder that is scarred and contracted.	• Primary symptom is right upper quadrant pain with radiation around the midtorso to the right scapular region; pain is abrupt and severe and lasts for 2 to 4 hours. • May have associated symptoms including fever, jaundice, and anorexia • With chronic cholecystitis may exhibit fat intolerance, flatulence, nausea, anorexia, and nonspecific abdominal pain	• In acute cholecystitis, classic examination finding is marked tenderness in the right upper quadrant (RUQ) or epigastrium (see Table 17-2). • Involuntary guarding or rebound tenderness may be present. • Some may have a full palpable gallbladder in the RUQ. • Some may have subtle examination findings, including diffuse abdominal pain, whereas others may have an unremarkable examination. • In chronic cholecystitis, a palpable gallbladder is typically not appreciated due to gallbladder fibrosis.

Nonalcoholic Fatty Liver Disease (NAFLD)

Spectrum of hepatic disorders not associated with excessive alcohol intake, ranging from steatosis to cirrhosis and hepatocellular carcinoma

Pathophysiology	Subjective Data	Objective Data
• Hepatic cell inflammation and injury thought to result from accumulation of triglycerides in the liver • Genetic and environmental factors are likely to contribute to disease development. • Insulin resistance is an important factor; as such, NAFLD is associated with the metabolic syndrome (obesity, hypertriglyceridemia, and diabetes). • Currently the most common cause of chronic liver disease in the United States • Occurs fairly equally in males and females, but ethnic differences include a higher prevalence in Hispanic individuals	• Most patients are asymptomatic but some describe right upper quadrant pain, fatigue, malaise, and jaundice.	• Usually identified after discovering abnormal liver function tests; most will have elevated transaminases with aspartate aminotransferase (AST) and alanine aminotransferase (ALT) being two to three times the upper limits of normal. • Other than an elevated body mass index (BMI) (overweight or obese by criteria), the physical examination is typically unremarkable. • About half of patients have hepatomegaly. • In more severe disease, patients may have jaundice and ascites. • Magnetic resonance spectroscopy (MRS) and liver biopsy are most sensitive diagnostic techniques

PANCREAS

Acute Pancreatitis

Acute inflammatory process in which release of pancreatic enzymes results in glandular autodigestion

Pathophysiology	Subjective Data	Objective Data
• Although unclear what pathophysiologic mechanism initiates acute pancreatitis, there are a number of known causes, including biliary disease (cholelithiasis) and chronic alcohol use, accounting for approximately 80% of cases.	• Symptoms range from mild to severe sudden onset of persistent epigastric pain that may radiate to the back; pain is typically described as constant and dull. • Often associated with nausea, vomiting, abdominal distention, fever, and anorexia	• Most patients have diffuse abdominal tenderness to palpation; involuntary guarding and abdominal distention can occur (see Table 17-2). • Decreased bowel sounds may be appreciated as a result of an ileus. • In severe necrotizing pancreatitis, Cullen and Grey Turner signs may be appreciated on examination (see Table 17-5). • Some may present with fever and tachycardia. • Others may have dyspnea due to diaphragm irritation. • Pancreatic enzymes (amylase and lipase) are elevated.

Chronic Pancreatitis

Chronic inflammatory process of the pancreas, characterized by irreversible morphologic changes resulting in atrophy, fibrosis, and pancreatic calcifications

Pathophysiology	Subjective Data	Objective Data
• Most common cause is chronic alcohol use; other causes include congenital structural abnormalities of the pancreas, hereditary pancreatitis, cystic fibrosis, medication-induced disease, and autoimmune pancreatitis.	• Symptoms may include constant, unremitting abdominal pain, weight loss, and steatorrhea.	• Examination findings are similar to those in acute pancreatitis; however, with chronic disease, there is a greater likelihood of pseudocyst formation. • With advanced disease, some may exhibit signs of malnutrition with decreased subcutaneous fat and temporal wasting. • Pancreatic enzyme levels (amylase and lipase) are elevated, and glucose intolerance may be seen.

SPLEEN

Spleen Laceration/Rupture

Pathophysiology	Subjective Data	Objective Data
• Most commonly injured organ in abdominal trauma because of its anatomic location • Mechanism of injury can be either blunt or penetrating, but is more often blunt (e.g., from motor vehicle accidents)	• Symptoms include pain in the left upper quadrant with radiation to the left shoulder (positive Kehr sign); see Table 17-5. • Depending on degree of blood loss, may have symptoms of hypovolemia (e.g., lightheadedness, syncope)	• Examination is remarkable for left upper quadrant pain with palpation; signs of peritoneal irritation may be seen (involuntary guarding or rebound tenderness) (see Table 17-2). • Diagnosis is made by paracentesis or computed tomography. • Depending on the degree of blood loss, patients may present with hypotension and a decreasing hematocrit.

KIDNEY

Acute Glomerulonephritis

Inflammation of the capillary loops of the renal glomeruli

Pathophysiology	Subjective Data	Objective Data
• Results from immune complex deposition or formation • Many causes; most common include infection (poststreptococcal) and immune-mediated (IgA nephropathy)	• Symptoms usually nonspecific and include nausea and malaise; flank pain may be reported as well as headache secondary to hypertension. • Some patients report tea-colored urine or gross hematuria. • About 85% of affected children develop peripheral and periorbital edema.	• May have an unremarkable examination and normal blood pressure • Examination findings may include edema, hypertension, and oliguria. • Microscopic hematuria occurs in all affected patients (red blood cell casts are seen on urine microscopy).

Hydronephrosis

Dilation of the renal pelvis and calyces due to an obstruction of urine flow anywhere from the urethral meatus to the kidneys

Pathophysiology	Subjective Data	Objective Data
• Increasing ureteral pressure results in changes in glomerular filtration, tubular function, and renal blood flow.	• With an acute obstruction, may have intermittent, severe pain (renal colic) with nausea and vomiting • With secondary infection, may report abdominal pain, flank pain hematuria, and fever	• Most will have an unremarkable physical examination. • In severe cases, the kidneys may be palpable during the abdominal examination; costovertebral angle tenderness may be present. • With lower urinary tract obstruction, a distended bladder may be palpable (e.g., posterior urethral valves in a newborn). • Most are asymptomatic; hydronephrosis is found during radiologic screening (e.g., fetal ultrasound) or diagnostic imaging.

Pyelonephritis

Infection of the kidney and renal pelvis

Pathophysiology	Subjective Data	Objective Data
• Gram-negative bacilli (*Escherichia coli* and *Klebsiella*) and *Enterococcus faecalis* are the most common pathogens. • Less common organisms occur in hospitalized patients and/or those with indwelling catheters. • Risk factors include indwelling catheters, diabetes mellitus, sexual activity, prior history of urinary tract infections (UTIs), vesicoureteral reflux (infants and children), and urinary incontinence (older adults).	• Typically present with fever, dysuria, and flank pain • Other symptoms include rigors, polyuria, urinary frequency, urgency, and hematuria.	• Most are generally ill-appearing with significant pain or discomfort. • Fever and costovertebral angle (CVA) tenderness distinguish pyelonephritis from uncomplicated urinary tract infections (UTIs). • On laboratory evaluation, pyuria and bacteriuria are present and confirm the diagnosis.

Renal Abscess

Localized infection in the medulla or cortex of the kidney

Pathophysiology	Subjective Data	Objective Data
• Abscesses in the renal cortex are often caused by gram-positive organisms (*Staphylococcus aureus* and *Enterococcus faecalis*) • Medullary abscesses are commonly caused by gram-negative bacilli (*E. coli* and *Klebsiella*)	• Symptoms of pyelonephritis (chills, fever, dysuria, and flank pain) persist beyond 72 hours of appropriate antibiotic therapy.	• Similar to pyelonephritis, most are generally ill appearing, with fever and significant pain or discomfort. • CVA tenderness is typically present on examination. • Urinalysis may show pyuria and bacteriuria if the abscess is in the renal medulla; pyuria may be the only lab finding if the abscess is located in the cortex. • Renal imaging: ultrasound, computed tomography (CT), or magnetic resonance imaging (MRI) are common diagnostic tools.

Renal Calculi

Stones formed in the pelvis of the kidney from a physiochemical process associated with obstruction and infections in the urinary tract

Pathophysiology

- Stones are composed of calcium salts, uric acid, cystine, and struvite.
- Situations leading to alkaline urine are conducive to stone formation because uric acid, calcium, and phosphate are all more soluble in a low pH; urine temperature, ionic strength, and concentration also affect stone formation.
- Much more prevalent in men than in women

Subjective Data

- Symptoms include fever, dysuria, hematuria, and flank pain.
- Renal colic is marked by severe cramping flank pain with nausea and vomiting; as the stone passes through the ureter, the pain typically moves from the flank to the groin and then to the scrotal or labial area (see Table 17-2).

Objective Data

- Most present to an emergency or urgent care facility with severe cramping pain
- Examination findings may include CVA tenderness and/or abdominal tenderness with palpation.
- Urinalysis may show microscopic hematuria; an elevated urinary calcium-to-creatinine ratio is suggestive.

Acute Renal Failure

Sudden impairment of renal function over hours to days, resulting in an acute uremic episode

Pathophysiology

- No universally accepted definition of acute renal failure (ARF); a common clinical laboratory definition is an absolute rise in serum creatinine concentration of 0.5 to 1.0 mg/dL.
- Retention of nitrogenous and metabolic waste products and extracellular fluid results from a decrease in glomerular filtration rate (GFR)
- Intrinsic ARF most commonly results from renal parenchymal injury: acute tubular necrosis from nephrotoxic medications, sepsis or ischemia; interstitial nephritis from medications, infections or autoimmune disease, or glomerulonephritis

Subjective Data

- Urine output may be normal, decreased, or absent (anuria).
- In prerenal ARF, may have had symptoms resulting in dehydration and decreased kidney perfusion (e.g., vomiting, diarrhea, decreased intake, or diuretic use); patients may also have had symptoms resulting in intravascular volume depletion (e.g., shortness of breath and peripheral edema with congestive heart failure).
- In postrenal ARF, patients may have had symptoms from urinary tract obstruction depending on the level of obstruction (i.e., anuria with complete obstruction).
- Patients with intrinsic ARF may present with symptoms related to the underlying cause of their renal failure (tea- or cola-colored urine in glomerulonephritis or malar rash with systemic lupus erythematosus).

Objective Data

- Examination findings are nonspecific.
- Some may display signs of either fluid overload (increased jugular venous distention and peripheral edema) or deficit (hypotension, orthostatic pulse and blood pressure changes, dry mucous membranes).
- In postrenal ARF, with complete obstruction, may have abdominal distention (bladder distention) and suprapubic tenderness to palpation

ABNORMALITIES

❧ Infants

Intussusception

Prolapse, or telescoping, of one segment of intestine into another causes intestinal obstruction

Pathophysiology

- Commonly occurs in infants between 3 and 12 months old and is the most common cause of bowel obstruction in infants and children 3 months to 6 years of age; four times as likely to occur in females as in males
- Some episodes may resolve spontaneously, but if untreated most cases result in bowel infarction, perforation, and peritonitis.
- Although the cause of most cases is unknown, lymph tissue hyperplasia is thought to lead to mucosal prolapse with the most common site being the terminal ileum into the colon; in a small percentage of children, lead points are identified (Meckel diverticulum, polyp, lymphoma); lead points are more common in children older than 2 years.
- In adults, about 1% to 5% of bowel obstruction is from intussusception; usually there is a pathologic lead point (malignancy in over half of cases) (Marinis et al, 2009) (Fig. 17-38).

Subjective Data

- Symptoms include acute intermittent abdominal pain, abdominal distention, and vomiting.
- Symptoms can be dramatic in onset; previously well child may start with paroxysms of crying and severe abdominal pain, sometimes awakening from sleep; intermittent bouts of lethargy may also occur.
- Child is often inconsolable, sometimes with legs and knees flexed (doubled up) with pain
- Stool appears normal in the early stages; as ischemia progresses, subsequent stools may be mixed with blood and mucus with a red currant jelly appearance

Objective Data

- Sausage-shaped mass may be palpated in the right or left upper quadrant, whereas the right lower quadrant feels empty (positive Dance sign)
- As disease progresses, may display findings of bowel perforation (abdominal distention and guarding)
- Diagnosis and treatment most often carried out with the use of an air-contrast enema

FIGURE 17-38 Jejunojejunal intussusception in an adult patient.

Pyloric Stenosis

Hypertrophy of the circular muscle of the pylorus leading to obstruction of the pyloric sphincter

Pathophysiology

- Occurs in 1 to 3/1000 infants in the United States and is more common in whites; males are affected about four times as often as females, and there is a strong familial tendency.
- Cause is unknown; an association has been found with use of erythromycin

Subjective Data

- Symptoms typically develop after several weeks of age and include regurgitation progressing to projectile vomiting (i.e., vigorous, shoots out of the mouth, and carries a short distance); feeding eagerly (even after a vomiting episode); and failure to gain weight.

Objective Data

- Epigastric distention from an obstructed stomach may be seen as well as a visible wave of peristalsis (left to right) (Fig. 17-39).
- Small, rounded olive-shaped mass sometimes palpable in the right upper quadrant, particularly after the infant vomits
- Ultrasound and/or surgical consult should be obtained with suspected cases.

FIGURE 17-39 Epigastric distention and a visible wave of peristalsis in an infant with pyloric stenosis. *(From Zitelli and Davis, 2012.)*

Meconium Ileus

Distal intestinal obstruction caused by thick inspissated impacted meconium in the lower intestine

Pathophysiology	Subjective Data	Objective Data
• May be the first manifestation of cystic fibrosis (CF); about 10% to 20% of newborns with CF have meconium ileus.	• Most affected newborns present with failure to pass meconium in the first 24 hours after birth in the nursery	• Newborns will present with abdominal distention.
• Pancreatic insufficiency or congenital pancreatic anomalies (pancreatic duct stenosis) are thought to be contributing factors; however, many affected infants have normal pancreatic function and structure.	• Symptoms related to distal intestinal obstruction develop (vomiting and abdominal distention).	• In complicated cases (volvulus), infants can present with signs of shock (e.g., tachycardia and hypotension).
• In uncomplicated cases, the distal ileum narrows with proximal intestinal distention; up to one half of cases are complicated (volvulus, atresia, or meconium peritonitis).		• Uncomplicated cases are treated with hyperosmolar enemas (e.g., Gastrografin) under fluoroscopic guidance; resolution occurs in more than half of affected infants.
• If condition occurs in utero, fetal volvulus may cause intestinal atresia		

ABNORMALITIES

Biliary Atresia

Congenital obstruction or absence of some or all of the bile duct system resulting in bile flow obstruction; most have complete absence of entire extrahepatic biliary tree

Pathophysiology

- Now classified as postnatal onset (85% to 90% of cases) or embryonic onset
- In postnatal onset, disease inflammation and necrosis of extrahepatic bile ducts are thought to result from a perinatal insult (e.g., viral infection).
- Embryonic onset is thought to result from gene mutations controlling bile duct formation and differentiation early in gestation; intrahepatic cholestasis and biliary tract fibrosis develop; this type is associated with other congenital anomalies (polysplenia syndrome).

Subjective Data

- Symptoms of neonatal cholestasis develop in the first several weeks of life and include jaundice, light clay-colored stools, and dark urine.
- Newborns may show failure to gain weight or have normal weight gain.

Objective Data

- Most infants are full term and develop jaundice in the first 2 months of life; hepatomegaly may be firm to palpation.
- Splenomegaly may occur and indicates progressive disease with portal hypertension (Fig. 17-40).
- In the embryonic type, infants may have heart murmurs indicating associated congenital heart disease.
- Abdominal ultrasound is diagnostic; without prompt surgical correction, secondary biliary cirrhosis occurs.

FIGURE 17-40 Child with biliary atresia and cirrhosis with prominent abdominal veins. *(From Zitelli and Davis, 2012.)*

Meckel Diverticulum

Outpouching of the ileum that varies in size from a small appendiceal process to a segment of bowel several inches long, often in the proximity of the ileocecal valve (Fig. 17-41)

Pathophysiology

- Develops from incomplete obliteration of the vitelline duct resulting in a blind-ending pouch that contains all the mucosal layers in the ileum (see Fig. 17-41)
- Most common congenital anomaly of the gastrointestinal tract, occurring in about 2% of the general population

Subjective Data

- Most are asymptomatic.
- Often found as an incidental finding during a radiologic study or intraabdominal surgery for other reasons
- In children, bright or dark red rectal bleeding with little, if any, abdominal pain is a common presenting concern.
- Some present with abdominal pain that can be severe in character; others may present with signs of intestinal obstruction or diverticulitis, similar to acute appendicitis with bilious emesis.

Objective Data

- Painless rectal bleeding is the most common presenting finding on examination.
- Some patients present with intestinal obstruction (abdominal tenderness, involuntary guarding) and rebound tenderness); in severe cases, perforation can occur with peritoneal signs and hypovolemic shock (tachycardia and hypotension).

FIGURE 17-41 Meckel diverticulum.

Necrotizing Enterocolitis

Inflammatory disease of the gastrointestinal mucosa associated with prematurity and gut immaturity

Pathophysiology	Subjective Data	Objective Data
• Most common gastrointestinal emergency in neonates • Varying degrees of mucosal or transmural intestinal necrosis occur, most commonly in the distal ileum and proximal colon. • Cause is unknown but likely multifactorial; an infectious cause is thought to have a primary role in the development; coagulation necrosis is found on intestinal specimens at surgery. • Incidence is 1% to 5% of infants in neonatal intensive care units; incidence and mortality are inversely related to gestational age.	• Symptoms may be subtle, including inability to tolerate feedings (oral or nasogastric); may also present suddenly and progress quickly • Abdominal distention, vomiting, and bloody stools often prompt an evaluation in at-risk neonates.	• May display temperature instability and subtle signs of distress • Examination signs may include lethargy, abdominal distention, apnea, and respiratory distress. • Plain abdominal radiograph may show pneumatosis intestinalis (air in the bowel wall) • Often fatal due to complications of intestinal perforation and sepsis

�֎ Children

Neuroblastoma

Solid malignancy of embryonal origin in the peripheral sympathetic nervous system

Pathophysiology	Subjective Data	Objective Data
• Considered a spectrum of tumors of varying degrees of neural differentiation • Although commonly arising from the adrenal medulla, may occur anywhere along the craniospinal axis • Cause is unknown, but genetic and environmental factors are proposed causes associations have been found with parental occupational chemical exposures, and familial cases have been reported.	• Typically presents as an asymptomatic abdominal mass in a young child • Symptoms may include malaise, loss of appetite, weight loss, and protrusion of one or both eyes. • Other symptoms arise from compression of the mass or metastasis to adjacent organs.	• Examination findings include a firm, fixed, nontender, irregular, and nodular abdominal mass that crosses the midline. • Metastases to the periorbital region result in proptosis and infraorbital ecchymoses. • Horner syndrome, ataxia, and opsomyoclonus ("dancing eyes and dancing feet") may be seen on physical examination. • Radiologic studies may show a calcified mass with hemorrhage into surrounding structures.

Wilms Tumor (Nephroblastoma)

Most common intraabdominal tumor of childhood; usually appears at 2 to 3 years of age

Pathophysiology	Subjective Data	Objective Data
• Most cases are sporadic; a small percentage have a family history. • Wilms tumor gene, *WT1,* is located on chromosome 11 and regulates normal kidney development; about 20% of affected children have mutations of this gene. • Associated with several syndromes; WAGR includes Wilms tumor, aniridia, genitourinary abnormalities, and mental retardation.	• Most present with painless enlargement of the abdomen or an abdominal mass (often found while parents are bathing their young child). • Some present with abdominal pain, vomiting, and hematuria. • Some are identified during screening due to associated congenital abnormalities.	• May be felt on abdominal examination as a firm, nontender mass deep within the flank, only slightly movable and not usually crossing the midline (Fig. 17-42); sometimes bilateral • Hypertension may be present.

FIGURE 17-42 **Wilms tumor.** Large left-sided flank mass seen on visual inspection.

Hirschsprung Disease (Congenital Aganglionic Megacolon)

Primary absence of parasympathetic ganglion cells in a segment of the colon, which interrupts intestinal motility

Pathophysiology	Subjective Data	Objective Data
• Abnormal intestinal innervation results in the absence of peristalsis, which leads to the accumulation of stool proximal to the defect and intestinal obstruction. • Most common cause of lower intestinal obstruction in newborns • Four times as common in males as in females • Genetic mutations have been identified in some patients.	• Symptoms typically begin at birth with failure to pass meconium in the first 24 to 48 hours after birth. • Other symptoms include failure to thrive, constipation, abdominal distention, and episodes of bilious vomiting and diarrhea. • Older infants and young children may present with severe constipation.	• Examination findings consistent with severe constipation include abdominal distention and stool palpated in the left lower abdomen.

Hemolytic Uremic Syndrome (HUS)

Triad of microangiopathic hemolytic anemia, thrombocytopenia, and uremia

Pathophysiology	Subjective Data	Objective Data
• One of the most common causes of acute renal failure in children, generally occurring in those younger than 4 years • Most common cause of HUS in the United States is the Shiga-like toxin produced by E. coli O157:H7; other bacterial pathogens such as *Shigella* can cause HUS, as well as some viruses • Risk factors include ingestion of undercooked meat or unpasteurized milk.	• Most have a preceding upper respiratory infection or gastroenteritis with fever, abdominal pain, and vomiting; diarrhea often becomes bloody. • Gastrointestinal involvement may lead to symptoms of an acute abdomen, with occasional perforation. • Some present with a sudden onset of pallor, weakness, lethargy, and decreased urine output.	• Typically present with dehydration, edema, petechiae, and hepatosplenomegaly • With severe gastrointestinal disease, may display peritoneal signs (abdominal distention, involuntary guarding, rebound tenderness)

⚘ Older Adults

Fecal Incontinence

Inability to control bowel movements leading to leakage of stool; associated with three major causes—fecal impaction, underlying disease, and neurogenic disorders

Pathophysiology

- Fecal impaction (most common cause) is associated with immobilization and poor fluid and dietary intake; laxative overuse may also be a cause.
- Local neurogenic disorders refers to any process that causes degeneration of the mesenteric plexus and lower bowel, resulting in a lax sphincter muscle, diminished sacral reflex, and decreased puborectal muscle tone.
- Cognitive neurogenic disorders usually result from stroke or dementia.

Subjective Data

- Most have "overflow incontinence" (a soft stool that oozes around the impaction).
- Unable to recognize rectal fullness and with an inability to inhibit intrinsic rectal contractions; stools normally formed and occur in a set pattern, usually after a meal

Objective Data

- Diagnosed through digital rectal examination when assessing rectal tone or other abnormalities
- Radiologic and manometry studies are often helpful in determining the underlying cause such as cancer, inflammatory bowel disease, diverticulitis, colitis, proctitis, or diabetic neuropathy.

DIFFERENTIAL DIAGNOSIS

Urinary Incontinence

Condition	History	Physical Findings
Stress incontinence	Small-volume incontinence with coughing, sneezing, laughing, running; history of prior pelvic surgery	Pelvic floor relaxation; cystocele, rectocele; lax urethral sphincter; loss of urine with provocative testing; atrophic vaginitis; postvoid residual less than 100 mL
Urge incontinence	Uncontrolled urge to void; large volume incontinence; history of central nervous system disorders such as stroke, multiple sclerosis, parkinsonism	Unexpected findings only as related to central nervous system disorder; postvoid residual less than 100 mL
Overflow incontinence	Small-volume incontinence, dribbling, hesitancy; in men, symptoms of enlarged prostate; nocturia, dribbling, hesitance, deceased force and caliber of stream	Distended bladder; prostate hypertrophy; stool in rectum, fecal impaction; postvoid residual greater than 100 mL
	In neurogenic bladder: history of bowel problems, spinal cord injury, or multiple sclerosis	Evidence of spinal cord disease or diabetic neuropathy; lax sphincter; gait disturbance
Functional incontinence	Change in mental status; impaired mobility; new environment	Impaired mental status; impaired mobility
	Medications: hypnotics, diuretics, anticholinergic agents, alpha-adrenergic agents, calcium channel blockers	Impaired mental status or unexpected findings only as related to other physical conditions

CHAPTER 18

Female Genitalia

Examination of the female genitalia is typically performed when a patient presents with a specific concern, as part of the newborn examination, for the sexually active adolescent, or as part of an overall health visit. Examination of the anus and rectum (Chapter 20) is often performed at the same time.

evolve http://evolve.elsevier.com/Seidel
- Physical Exam Key Points
- NCLEX Review Questions
- Activities
- Animations
- Videos
- Student Checklist

ANATOMY AND PHYSIOLOGY

External Genitalia

The vulva, or external female genital organs, include the mons pubis, labia majora, labia minora, clitoris, vestibular glands, vaginal vestibule, vaginal orifice, and urethral opening (Fig. 18-1). The symphysis pubis is covered by a pad of adipose tissue called the mons pubis or mons veneris, which in the postpubertal female is covered with coarse terminal hair. Extending downward

Physical Examination Preview

Here is a preview of the steps involved in conducting physical examination of the female genitalia. ⓔ These procedures are explained in detail in this chapter and are available on Evolve in printable formats.

The following steps are performed with the patient in the lithotomy position unless alternate positions are necessary: (see p. 428)

External Genitalia

1. Inspect the pubic hair characteristics and distribution (p. 428).
2. Inspect and palpate the labia for the following (pp. 428, 429):
   - Symmetry of color
   - Caking of discharge
   - Inflammation
   - Irritation or excoriation
   - Swelling
3. Inspect the urethral meatus and vaginal opening for the following (p. 429):
   - Discharge
   - Lesions or caruncles
   - Polyps
   - Fistulas
4. Milk the Skene glands (p. 428).
5. Palpate the Bartholin glands (p. 429).
6. Inspect and palpate the perineum for the following (p. 429):
   - Smoothness
   - Tenderness, inflammation
   - Fistulas
   - Lesions or growths
7. Inspect for prolapse and urinary incontinence as the patient bears down (p. 430).

8. Inspect the perineal area and anus for the following (p. 430):
   - Skin characteristics
   - Lesions
   - Fissures or excoriation
   - Inflammation

Internal Genitalia Speculum Examination

1. Insert the speculum along the path of least resistance (p. 430).
2. Inspect the cervix for the following (p. 431):
   - Color
   - Position
   - Size
   - Surface characteristics
   - Discharge
   - Size and shape of os
3. Collect necessary specimens (p. 433).
4. Inspect vaginal walls for the following (p. 435):
   - Color
   - Surface characteristics
   - Secretions

Bimanual Examination

1. Insert the index and middle fingers of one hand into the vagina and place the other hand on the abdominal midline (p. 435).
2. Palpate the vaginal walls for the following (p. 436):
   - Smoothness
   - Tenderness
   - Lesions (cysts, nodules, or masses)

Physical Examination Preview—cont'd

3. Palpate the cervix for the following (p. 436):
   * Size, shape, and length
   * Position
   * Mobility
4. Palpate the uterus for the following (p. 437):
   * Location
   * Position
   * Size, shape, and contour
   * Mobility
   * Tenderness
5. Palpate the ovaries for the following (p. 437):
   * Size
   * Shape
   * Consistency
   * Tenderness
6. Palpate adnexal areas for masses and tenderness (p. 437).

Rectovaginal Examination
1. Insert the index finger into the vagina and the middle finger into the anus (p. 438).
2. Assess sphincter tone (p. 438).
3. Palpate the rectovaginal septum for the following (p. 439):
   * Thickness
   * Tone
   * Nodules
4. Palpate the posterior aspect of the uterus (p. 439).
5. Palpate the anterior and posterior rectal wall for the following (p. 439):
   * Masses, polyps, or nodules
   * Strictures, other irregularities, tenderness
6. Note characteristics of feces when the gloved finger is removed (p. 439).

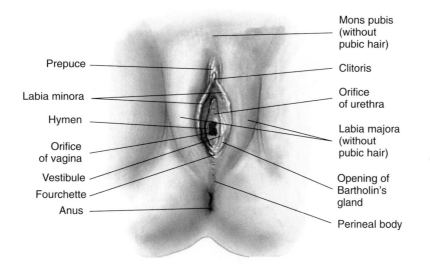

FIGURE 18-1 External female genitalia. *(From Lowdermilk and Perry, 2007.)*

and backward from the mons pubis are the labia majora, two folds of adipose tissue covered by skin. The labia majora vary in appearance depending on the amount of adipose tissue present. The outer surfaces of the labia majora are also covered with hair in the postpubertal female.

Lying inside and usually hidden by the labia majora are the labia minora, two hairless, flat, reddish folds. The labia minora meet at the anterior of the vulva, where each labium divides into two lamellae, the lower pair fusing to form the frenulum of the clitoris and the upper pair forming the prepuce. Tucked between the frenulum and the prepuce is the clitoris, a small bud of erectile tissue, the homolog of the penis and a primary center of sexual excitement. Posteriorly, the labia minora meet as two ridges that fuse to form the fourchette.

The labia minora enclose the area designated as the vestibule, which contains six openings: the urethra, the vagina, two ducts of Bartholin glands, and two ducts of Skene glands. The lower two thirds of the urethra lie immediately above the anterior

vaginal wall and terminate in the urethral meatus at the midline of the vestibule just above the vaginal opening and below the clitoris. Skene ducts drain a group of urethral glands and open onto the vestibule on each side of the urethra. The ductal openings may be visible.

The vaginal opening occupies the posterior portion of the vestibule and varies in size and shape. Surrounding the vaginal opening is the hymen, a connective tissue membrane that may be circular, crescentic, or fimbriated. After the hymen tears and becomes permanently divided, the edges either disappear or form hymenal tags. Bartholin glands, located posteriorly on each side of the vaginal orifice, open onto the sides of the vestibule in the groove between the labia minora and the hymen. The ductal openings are not usually visible. During sexual excitement, Bartholin glands secrete mucus into the introitus for lubrication.

The pelvic floor consists of a group of muscles that form a supportive sling for the pelvic contents. The muscle fibers insert

ANATOMY AND PHYSIOLOGY

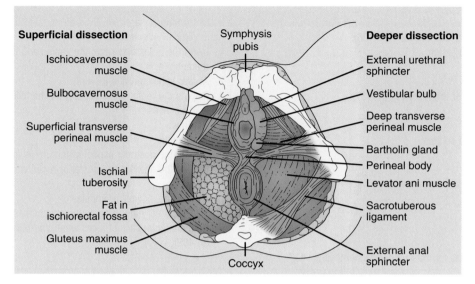

FIGURE 18-2 Musculature of the perineum. *(From Black et al, 2008.)*

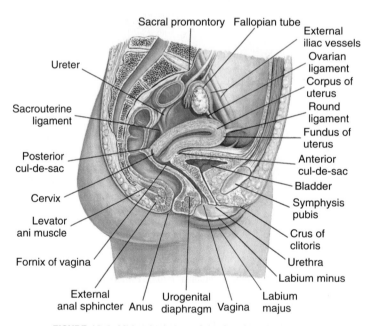

FIGURE 18-3 Midsagittal view of the female pelvic organs.

at various points on the bony pelvis and form functional sphincters for the vagina, rectum, and urethra (Fig. 18-2).

Internal Genitalia

The vagina is a musculomembranous tube that has transverse rugae (anatomic folds) during the reproductive phase of life. It inclines posteriorly at an angle of approximately 45 degrees with the vertical plane of the body (Fig. 18-3). The anterior wall of the vagina is separated from the bladder and urethra by connective tissue called the vesicovaginal septum. The posterior vaginal wall is separated from the rectum by the rectovaginal septum. Usually, the anterior and posterior walls of the vagina lie in close proximity, with only a small space between them. The upper end of the vagina is a blind vault into which the uterine cervix

projects. The pocket formed around the cervix is divided into the anterior, posterior, and lateral fornices. These are of clinical importance because the internal pelvic organs can be palpated through their thin walls. The vagina carries menstrual flow from the uterus, serves as the terminal portion of the birth canal, and is the receptive organ for the penis during sexual intercourse.

The uterus sits in the pelvic cavity between the bladder and the rectum. It is an inverted pear-shaped, muscular organ that is relatively mobile (Fig. 18-4). The uterus is covered by the peritoneum and lined by the endometrium, which is shed during menstruation. The rectouterine cul-de-sac (pouch of Douglas) is a deep recess formed by the peritoneum as it covers the lower posterior wall of the uterus and upper portion of the vagina, separating it from the rectum. The uterus is flattened anteroposteriorly and usually inclines forward at a 45-degree angle,

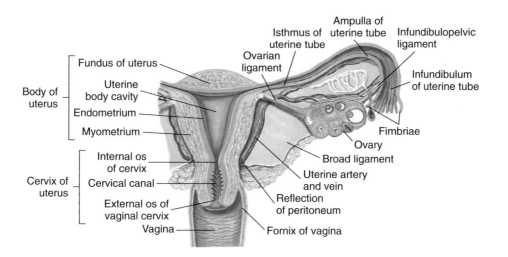

FIGURE 18-4 Cross-sectional view of internal female genitalia and pelvic contents.

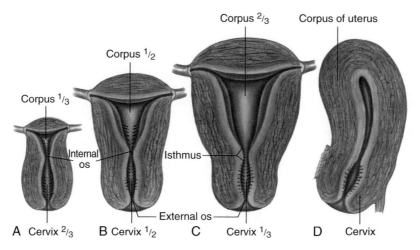

FIGURE 18-5 Comparative sizes of uteri at various stages of development. **A,** Prepubertal. **B,** Adult nulliparous. **C,** Adult multiparous. **D,** Lateral view, adult multiparous. The fractions give the relative proportion of the size of the corpus and the cervix.

although it may be anteverted, anteflexed, retroverted, or retroflexed. In nulliparous women the size is approximately 5.5 to 8 cm long, 3.5 to 4 cm wide, and 2 to 2.5 cm thick. The uterus of a parous woman may be larger by 2 to 3 cm in any of the dimensions. The uterus of a nulliparous woman weighs approximately 40 to 50 g (Fig. 18-5), and that of a multiparous woman is 20 to 30 g heavier.

The uterus is divided anatomically into the corpus and cervix. The corpus consists of the fundus, which is the convex upper portion between the points of insertion of the fallopian tubes; the main portion or body; and the isthmus, which is the constricted lower portion adjacent to the cervix. The cervix extends from the isthmus into the vagina. The uterus opens into the vagina via the external cervical os.

The adnexa of the uterus comprise the fallopian tubes and ovaries. The fallopian tubes insert into the upper portion of the uterus and extend laterally to the ovaries. Each tube ranges from 8 to 14 cm long and is supported by a fold of the broad ligament called the mesosalpinx. The isthmus end of the fallopian tube

opens into the uterine cavity. The fimbriated end opens into the pelvic cavity, with a projection that extends to the ovary and captures the ovum. Rhythmic contractions of the tubal musculature transport the ovum to the uterus.

The ovaries are a pair of oval organs resting in a slight depression on the lateral pelvic wall at the level of the anterosuperior iliac spine. The ovaries are approximately 3 cm long, 2 cm wide, and 1 cm thick in the adult woman during the reproductive years. Ovaries secrete estrogen and progesterone, hormones that have several functions, including controlling the menstrual cycle (Fig. 18-6 and Table 18-1) and supporting pregnancy.

The internal genitalia are supported by four pairs of ligaments: the cardinal, uterosacral, round, and broad ligaments.

Bony Pelvis

The pelvis is formed from four bones: two innominate (each consisting of ilium, ischium, and pubis), the sacrum, and the coccyx (Fig. 18-7). The bony pelvis is important in

ANATOMY AND PHYSIOLOGY

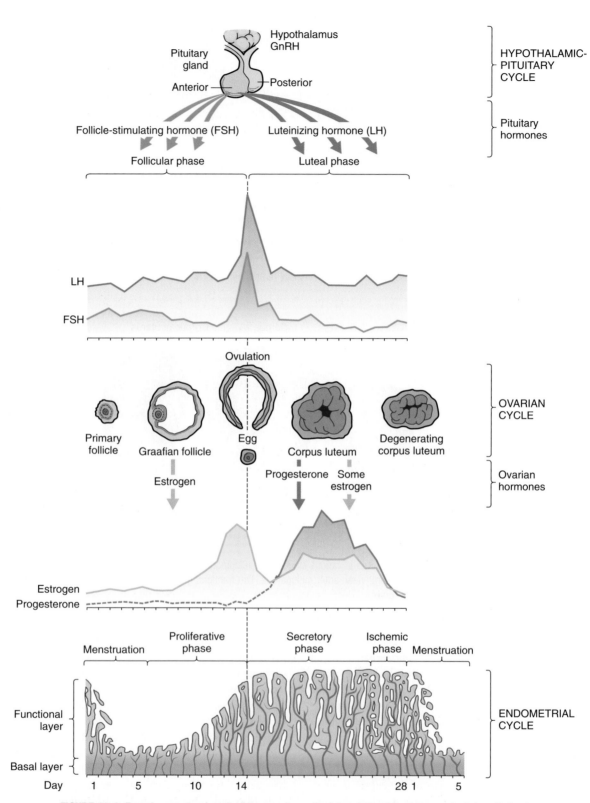

FIGURE 18-6 Female menstrual cycle. Diagram shows the interrelationship of the cerebral, hypothalamic, pituitary, and uterine functions throughout a standard 28-day menstrual cycle. *(From Lowdermilk and Perry, 2007.)*

Table 18-1 The Menstrual Cycle

Phase		Process Description
Menstrual Phase: Days 1 to 4	Ovary	Estrogen levels begin to rise, preparing follicle and egg for next cycle
	Uterus	Progesterone stimulates endometrial prostaglandins that cause vasoconstriction; upper layers of endometrium shed
	Breast	Cellular activity in the alveoli decreases; breast ducts shrink.
	Central nervous system (CNS) hormones	Follicle-stimulating hormone (FSH) and luteinizing hormone (LH) levels decrease.
	Symptoms	Menstrual bleeding may vary, depending on hormones and prostaglandins.
Postmenstrual, Preovulatory Phase: Days 5 to 12	Ovary	Ovary and maturing follicle produce estrogen; *follicular phase*—egg develops within follicle
	Uterus	*Proliferative phase*—uterine lining thickens
	Breast	Parenchymal and proliferation (increased cellular activity) of breast ducts occurs
	CNS hormones	FSH stimulates ovarian follicular growth.
Ovulation: Day 13 or 14	Ovary	Egg is expelled from follicle into abdominal cavity and drawn into the uterine (fallopian) tube by fimbriae and cilia; follicle closes and begins to form corpus luteum; fertilization of egg may occur in outer third of tube if sperm are unimpeded
	Uterus	End of proliferative phase; progesterone causes further thickening of the uterine wall.
	CNS hormones	LH and estrogen levels increase rapidly; LH surge stimulates release of egg
	Symptoms	Mittelschmerz may occur with ovulation; cervical mucus is increased and is stringy and elastic (spinnbarkeit).
Secretory Phase: Days 15 to 20	Ovary	Egg (ovum) is moved by cilia into the uterus
	Uterus	After the egg is released, the follicle becomes a corpus luteum; secretion of progesterone increases and predominates.
	CNS hormones	LH and FSH levels decrease.
Premenstrual, Luteal Phase: Days 21 to 28	Ovary	If implantation does not occur, the corpus luteum degenerates; progesterone production decreases, and estrogen production drops and then begins to rise as a new follicle develops.
	Uterus	Menstruation starts around day 28, which begins day 1 of the menstrual cycle.
	Breast	Alveolar breast cells differentiate into secretory cells.
	CNS hormones	Increased levels of gonadotropin-releasing hormone (GnRH) cause increased secretion of FSH.
	Symptoms	Vascular engorgement and water retention may occur.

Modified from Edge and Miller, 1994.

ANATOMY AND PHYSIOLOGY

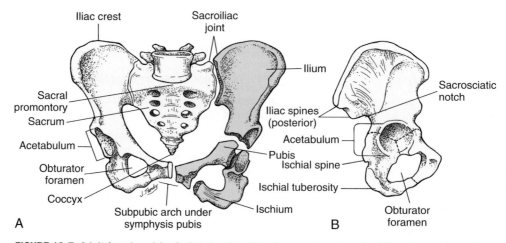

FIGURE 18-7 **Adult female pelvis. A,** Anterior view. The three embryonic parts of the left innominate bone are lightly shaded. **B,** External view of right innominate bone (fused). *(From Lowdermilk and Perry, 2007.)*

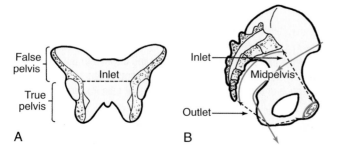

FIGURE 18-8 **Female pelvis. A,** Cavity of the false pelvis is a shallow basin above the inlet; the true pelvis is a deeper cavity below the inlet. **B,** Cavity of the true pelvis is an irregularly curved canal *(arrows)*. *(From Lowdermilk and Perry, 2007.)*

accommodating a growing fetus during pregnancy and in the birth process. The four pelvic joints—the symphysis pubis, the sacrococcygeal, and the two sacroiliac joints—usually have little movement.

The pelvis is divided into two parts. The shallow upper section is considered the false pelvis, which consists mainly of the flared-out iliac bones. The true pelvis is the lower curved bony canal, including the inlet, cavity, and outlet; the fetus must pass through these during birth. The upper border of the outlet is at the level of the ischial spines, which project into the pelvic cavity and serve as important landmarks during labor. The lower border of the outlet is bounded by the pubic arch and the ischial tuberosities (Fig. 18-8).

❧ Infants and Children

The vagina of the female infant is a small narrow tube with fewer epithelial layers than those of the adult. The uterus is approximately 35 mm long, with the cervix constituting about two thirds of the entire length of the organ. The ovaries are tiny and functionally immature. The labia minora are relatively avascular, thin, and pale. The labia majora are hairless and nonprominent. The hymen is a thin diaphragm just inside the introitus, usually with

a crescent-shaped opening in the midline. The clitoris is small. External genitalia may be swollen at birth due to estrogen from the mother. The swelling will decrease after several days.

During childhood, the genitalia, except for the clitoris, grow incrementally at varying rates. Anatomic and functional development accelerate with the onset of puberty and the accompanying hormonal changes.

❧ Adolescents

During puberty, the external genitalia increase in size and begin to assume adult proportions. The clitoris becomes more erectile and the labia minora more vascular. The labia majora and mons pubis become more prominent and begin to develop hair, often occurring simultaneously with breast development. Growth changes and secondary sex characteristic developments that occur during puberty are discussed in Chapter 6.

If the hymen is intact, the vaginal opening is about 1 cm. The vagina lengthens, and the epithelial layers thicken. The vaginal secretions become acidic.

The uterus, ovaries, and fallopian tubes increase in size and weight. The uterine musculature and vascular supply increase. The endometrial lining thickens in preparation for the onset of menstruation (menarche). The average age at menarche in the United States is between 12 and 13 years (Walvoord, 2010). Just before menarche, vaginal secretions increase. Functional maturation of the reproductive organs is reached during puberty. Irregular menstrual cycles are not unusual during adolescence as a result of anovulatory cycles

❧ Pregnant Women

The high levels of estrogen and progesterone that are necessary to support pregnancy are responsible for uterine enlargement during the first trimester. After the third month, uterine enlargement is primarily the result of mechanical pressure of the growing fetus. As the uterus enlarges, the muscular walls strengthen and become more elastic. As the uterus becomes larger and more ovoid, it rises out of the pelvis; by 12 weeks of gestation it reaches into the abdominal cavity. During the first months the walls become thicker, but then gradually thin to about 1.5 cm or less at term. Uterine weight at term, excluding the fetus and placenta, will usually have increased more than 10-fold and the capacity increases 500 to 1000 times that of the nonpregnant uterus. In the postpartum period the uterus involutes rapidly. Immediately after delivery the uterus is approximately the size of a 20-week pregnancy (at the level of the umbilicus). By the end of the first week, it is about the size of a 12-week pregnancy, palpable at the symphysis pubis.

Hormonal activity (relaxin and progesterone) is responsible for the softening of the pelvic cartilage and strengthening of the pelvic ligaments. As a consequence, the pelvic joints separate slightly, allowing some mobility; this results in the characteristic "waddle" gait. The symphysis pubis relaxes and increases in width, and there is marked mobility of the pelvis at term with resolution of changes occurring within 3 to 5 months postpartum. Protrusion of the abdomen as the uterus grows causes the pelvis to tilt forward, placing additional strain on the back and sacroiliac joints.

During pregnancy, an increase in uterine blood flow and lymph causes pelvic congestion and edema. As a result the uterus, cervix, and isthmus soften, and the cervix takes on a bluish color (Chadwick sign). Softening of the cervix from this increase in vascularity is called the Goodell sign. The cervical canal is obstructed by thick mucus soon after conception, protecting the infant from infection. When this plug dislodges at the beginning of labor it produces a sign of labor called "bloody show." The glands near the external os proliferate with eversion of the columnar endocervical glands, which tend to be friable. The softness and compressibility of the isthmus result in exaggerated uterine anteflexion during the first 3 months of pregnancy, causing the fundus to press on the urinary bladder.

The vaginal changes are similar to the cervical changes and result in the characteristic bluish color.

Both the mucosa of the vaginal walls and the connective tissue thicken, and smooth muscle cells hypertrophy. These changes result in an increased length of the vaginal walls, so that at times they can be seen protruding from the vulvar opening. The papillae of the mucosa have a hobnailed appearance. The vaginal secretions increase and have an acidic pH due to an increase in lactic acid production by the vaginal epithelium. The increase in pH helps keep bacteria from multiplying in the vagina but also can cause *Candida* infection. Figure 18-9 compares the changes that occur in a woman experiencing her first pregnancy with those in a woman who has experienced more than one pregnancy.

⚘ Older Adults

Concurrent with endocrine changes, ovarian function diminishes during a woman's 40s, and menstrual periods begin to cease although fertility may continue. The median age of menopause of women in the United States is 51 years (range 41 to 59 years). Menopause is defined as 1 year with no menses (amenorrhea). Just as menarche in the adolescent is one aspect of puberty, similarly cessation of menses is one aspect of this transitional phase of the life cycle. During this time, estrogen levels decrease, causing the labia and clitoris to become smaller. The labia majora also become flatter as body fat is lost. Pubic hair turns gray and is

FIGURE 18-9 Comparison of vulva and cervix in a nullipara **(A)** and a multipara **(B)** woman at the same stage of pregnancy. *(From Lowdermilk and Perry, 2007.)*

usually sparser. Both adrenal androgens and ovarian testosterone levels markedly decrease after menopause, which may account in part for decreases in libido and in muscle mass and strength.

The vaginal introitus gradually constricts. The vagina narrows, shortens, and loses its rugae, and the mucosa becomes thin, pale, and dry, which may result in pain with sexual intercourse (dyspareunia). The cervix becomes smaller and paler. The uterus decreases in size, and the endometrium thins.

The ovaries also decrease to approximately 1 to 2 cm. Follicles gradually disappear, and the surface of the ovary convolutes. Ovulation usually ceases about 1 to 2 years before menopause.

The ligaments and connective tissue of the pelvis sometimes lose their elasticity and tone, thus weakening the supportive sling for the pelvic contents. The vaginal walls may lose some of their structural integrity.

Menopause has systemic effects, which include an increase in body fat and intraabdominal deposition of body fat (tendency toward male pattern of body fat distribution). Levels of total and low-density lipoprotein cholesterol increase. Thermoregulation is altered, which produces the hot flashes associated with menopause.

REVIEW OF RELATED HISTORY

For each of the symptoms or conditions discussed in this section, targeted topics to include in the history of the present illness are listed. Responses to questions about these topics provide clues for focusing the physical examination and the development of an appropriate diagnostic evaluation. Questions regarding medication use (prescription and over the counter preparations) as well as complementary and alternative therapies are relevant for each.

History of Present Illness

- Abnormal bleeding: postmenopausal bleeding, menstrual abnormalities (see Box 18-1)
  - Character: interval between periods, amount of flow and duration during menses, bleeding between periods; postmenopausal bleeding

Box 18-1   Abnormal Uterine Bleeding: Terminology

- Amenorrhea: absence of menstruation
- Polymenorrhea: shortened interval between periods—less than 19 to 21 days
- Oligomenorrhea: lengthened interval between periods—more than 35 days
- Hypermenorrhea: excessive flow during normal duration of regular periods
- Hypomenorrhea: decreased flow during normal duration of regular periods
- Menorrhagia: regular and normal interval between periods, excessive flow and duration
- Metrorrhagia: irregular interval between periods, excessive flow and duration
- Menometrorrhagia: irregular or excessive bleeding during periods and between periods

- Change in flow: nature of change, number of pads or tampons used in 24 hours (tampons/pads soaked?), presence of clots
- Temporal sequence: onset, duration, precipitating factors, course since onset
- Associated symptoms: pain, cramping, abdominal distention, pelvic fullness, change in bowel habits, weight loss or gain
- Medications; oral contraceptives; hormones; tamoxifen
- Pain
  - Temporal sequence: date and time of onset, sudden versus gradual onset, course since onset, duration, recurrence
  - Character: specific location, type, and intensity of pain
  - Associated symptoms: vaginal discharge or bleeding, gastrointestinal symptoms, abdominal distention or tenderness, pelvic fullness
  - Association with menstrual cycle: timing, location, duration, changes
  - Relationship to body functions and activities: voiding, eating, defecation, flatus, exercise, walking up stairs, bending, stretching, sexual activity
  - Aggravating or relieving factors
  - Previous medical care for this problem
  - Efforts to treat
  - Medications: analgesics
- Vaginal discharge
  - Character: amount, color, odor, consistency, changes in characteristics
  - Occurrence: acute or chronic
  - Douching habits
  - Clothing habits: use of underwear or pantyhose with crotch that is not cotton or ventilated, tight pants or jeans
  - Sexual history—see in personal and social history
  - Presence of discharge or symptoms in sexual partner
  - Use of spermicide or latex condoms
  - Associated symptoms: itching; tender, inflamed, or bleeding external tissues; dyspareunia; dysuria or burning on urination; abdominal pain or cramping; pelvic fullness

- Efforts to treat: vaginal cream
- Medications: oral contraceptives, antibiotics
- Premenstrual symptoms
  - Symptoms: headaches, weight gain, edema, breast tenderness, irritability or mood changes
  - Frequency: every period?
  - Interference with activities of daily living
  - Relief measures
  - Aggravating factors
  - Medications: analgesics, diuretics
- Menopausal symptoms
  - Age at menopause or currently experiencing
  - Symptoms: menstrual changes, mood changes, tension, hot flashes, sleep disruption
  - Postmenopausal uterine bleeding
  - General feelings about menopause: self-image, effect on intimate relationships
  - Mother's experience with menopause
  - Birth control measures during menopause
  - Medications: hormones—dose and duration; serum estrogen receptor modulators
  - Use of complementary or alternative therapy: soy, other natural estrogen products; black cohosh (used as an alternative to hormonal treatment for menopause)
- Infertility
  - Length of time attempting pregnancy, sexual activity practices, knowledge of fertile period in menstrual cycle, length of cycle
  - Abnormalities of vagina, cervix, uterus, fallopian tubes, ovaries
  - Contributing factors: stress, nutrition, chemical substances
  - Partner factors (see Chapter 19)
  - Diagnostic evaluation to date
- Urinary symptoms: dysuria, burning on urination, frequency, urgency
  - Character: acute or chronic; frequency of occurrence; last episode; onset; course since onset; feel like bladder is empty or not after voiding; pain at start, throughout, or at cessation of urination
  - Description of urine: color, presence of blood or particles, clear or cloudy
  - Associated symptoms: vaginal discharge or bleeding, abdominal pain or cramping, abdominal distention, pelvic fullness or pressure, flank pain
  - Medications: urinary tract analgesics, antispasmodics

Past Medical History

- Menstrual history
  - Age at menarche and/or menopause
  - Date of last normal menstrual period: first day of last cycle
  - Number of days in cycle and regularity of cycle
  - Character of flow: amount (number of pads or tampons used in 24 hours on heaviest days), duration, presence and size of clots

- Dysmenorrhea: characteristics, duration, frequency (occurs with each cycle?), relief measures
- Intermenstrual bleeding or spotting: amount, duration, frequency, timing in relation to phase of cycle
- Intermenstrual pain: severity, duration, timing; association with ovulation
- Premenstrual symptoms: see History of Present Illness (HPI)
- Obstetric history
  - **G:** Gravidity (total number of pregnancies)
  - **T:** number of Term pregnancies
  - **P:** number of Preterm pregnancies
  - **A:** number of Abortions, spontaneous or induced
  - **L:** number of Living children
  - Complications of pregnancy, delivery, abortion, or with fetus or neonate
- Menopausal history: see HPI
- Gynecologic history
  - Prior Papanicolaou (Pap) smears, human papillomavirus (HPV) testing and results
  - Prior abnormal Pap smears or HPV test—when, how treated, follow-up
  - Recent and past gynecologic procedures or surgery—tubal ligation, hysterectomy, oophorectomy, laparoscopy, cryo-surgery, conization, colposcopy
  - Sexually transmitted infections (STIs)
  - Pelvic inflammatory disease
  - Vaginal infections
  - Diabetes
  - Cancer of reproductive organs or related cancers (breast, colorectal)

Family History

- Diabetes
- Cancer of reproductive organs
- Pregnancies with multiple births (e.g., twins, triplets)
- Congenital anomalies

Personal and Social History

- Cleansing routines: use of sprays, powders, perfume, antiseptic soap, deodorants, or ointments
- Contraceptive history
  - Current method: length of time used, effectiveness, consistency of use, side effects, satisfaction with method
  - Previous methods: duration of use for each, side effects, and reasons for discontinuing each
- Douching history: Frequency: length of time since last douche; number of years douching, method, solution used, reason for douching
- Sexual history
  - Current sexual activity: number of current and previous partners; number of their partners; gender of partner(s), sexual preference
  - Use of barrier protection for STIs

Risk Factors
Cervical Cancer

HPV infection: Human papillomavirus (HPV) infection is common and only a small percentage of women infected with untreated HPV will develop cervical cancer. The "high-risk" types include HPV 16, HPV 18, HPV 31, HPV 33, and HPV 45, as well as some others.

HPV vaccination: protective factor; decreases risk of cervical cancer

Pap smear history: lack of regular screening for cervical cancer

High parity: Women who have had three or more full-term pregnancies have an increased risk of developing cervical cancer.

Young age at parity: Women who were younger than 17 years when they had their first full-term pregnancy are almost twice as likely to develop cervical cancer later in life than women who were not pregnant until they were 25 years or older.

Cigarette smoking: doubles the risk; tobacco byproducts have been found in the cervical mucus of women who smoke.

HIV infection: increased susceptibility to HPV infections

Diet: Diets low in fruits and vegetables may increase risk for cervical cancer; overweight women are more likely to develop this cancer.

DES exposure: women whose mothers took diethylstilbestrol (DES) during pregnancy (prescribed to women at high risk of miscarriages between 1940 and 1971)

Oral contraceptives: Some evidence indicates that long-term use (more than 5 years) may slightly increase the risk of cervical cancer.

Low socioeconomic status: likely related to access to health care services, including cervical cancer screening and treatment of precancerous cervical disease

From American Cancer Society, 2012; National Cancer Institute, 2012.

Risk Factors
Ovarian Cancer

Age: Risk increases with age. Most ovarian cancers develop after menopause; half are found in women older than 63 years.

Inherited genetic mutation: known inherited mutation of the *BRCA1* or *BRCA2* gene

Family history: one or more first-degree relatives (mother, sister, daughter) with ovarian and/or breast cancer; strong family history of colon cancers; Ashkenazi Jewish descent; and a family history of breast and/or ovarian cancer

Obesity: Women with a body mass index of at least 30 have a higher risk of developing ovarian cancer.

Reproductive history: Nulliparity increases the risk.

Use of fertility drugs: increased risk in some studies, especially if pregnancy is not achieved

Personal history: breast, endometrial, and/or colon cancers

Hormone replacement therapy: In postmenopausal women, this increases the risk. The risk seems to be higher in women taking estrogen alone (without progesterone) for at least 5 or 10 years.

Diet: high-fat diet associated with higher rates of ovarian cancer in industrialized nations, but the link remains unproved

Use of oral contraceptives: Protective use for 4 or more years is associated with an approximately 50% reduction in ovarian cancer risk in the general population.

From American Cancer Society, 2012; National Cancer Institute, 2012.

Risk Factors

Endometrial Cancer

Early menarche: before 12 years of age; increases the number of years during which the endometrium is exposed to estrogen

Late menopause: after 50 years of age; increases the number of years during which the endometrium is exposed to estrogen. Women with increased bleeding during perimenopause have an increased risk of endometrial cancer.

Total years of menstruation (length of time from menarche to menopause): may be a more important factor than age at menarche or menopause. For example, early menarche is less a risk factor for women who also have early menopause. Likewise, early menarche *and* late menopause would be higher risk.

Infertility or nulliparity: During pregnancy, the hormonal balance shifts toward more progesterone. Therefore, having many pregnancies reduces endometrial cancer risk, and women who have not been pregnant have a higher risk.

Obesity: Having more fat tissue can increase a woman's estrogen levels and therefore increase her endometrial cancer risk.

Tamoxifen: an antiestrogen drug that acts like an estrogen in the uterus

Estrogen replacement therapy (ERT): estrogen alone (without progestins) in women with a uterus

Ovarian diseases: Polycystic ovaries and some ovarian tumors such as granulosa–theca cell tumors cause an increase in estrogen relative to progestin. Some of these conditions lead to hysterectomy and oophorectomy, ending the risk for endometrial cancer.

Diet: diet high in animal fat

Diabetes: endometrial cancer more common in women with both type 1 and type 2 diabetes

Age: Risk increases with age; 95% of endometrial cancers occur in women 40 years of age or older. The average age at diagnosis is 60.

Family history: history of endometrial, breast, ovarian, or colorectal cancers

Personal history: breast or ovarian cancer, or hereditary nonpolyposis colorectal cancer syndrome; known genetic mutation in *BRCA1* or *BRCA2*

Prior pelvic radiation therapy: Radiation used to treat some other cancers can damage the DNA of cells, sometimes increasing the risk of developing a second type of cancer such as endometrial cancer.

From American Cancer Society, 2012; National Cancer Institute, 2012.

Staying Well

Genital Self-Examination for Women

Genital self-examination (GSE) is recommended for anyone who is at risk for contracting a sexually transmitted infection (STI). This includes sexually active persons who have had more than one sexual partner or whose partner has had other partners. The purpose of GSE is to detect any signs or symptoms that might indicate the presence of an STI. Many people who have an STI do not know that they have one, and some STIs can remain undetected for years. GSE should become a regular part of routine self–health care practices.

You should explain and demonstrate the following procedure to your patient and give her the opportunity to perform a GSE under your guidance. Emphasize hand washing before and afterward.

Instruct the patient to start by examining the area that the pubic hair covers. Patients may want to use a mirror and position it so that they can see their entire genital area. The pubic hair should then be spread apart with the fingers, and the woman should carefully look for any bumps, sores, or blisters on the skin. Bumps and blisters may be red or light-colored or resemble pimples. Also instruct the patient to look for warts, which may look similar to warts on other parts of the body. At first they may be small, bumpy spots; left untreated, however, they could develop a fleshy, cauliflower-like appearance (see Fig. 18-47).

Next, instruct the patient to spread the outer vaginal lips and look closely at the hood of the clitoris. She should gently pull the hood up to see the clitoris and again look for any bumps, blisters, sores, or warts. Then both sides of the inner vaginal lips should be examined for the same signs.

Have the patient move on to examine the area around the urinary and vaginal openings, looking for any bumps, blisters, sores, or warts (see Figs. 18-48 through 18-51). Some signs of STIs may be out of view—in the vagina or near the cervix. Therefore, if patients believe that they have come in contact with an STI, they should see their health care provider even if no signs or symptoms are discovered during self-examination.

Also educate patients about other symptoms associated with STIs—specifically, pain or burning on urination, pain in the pelvic area, bleeding between menstrual periods, or an itchy rash around the vagina. Some STIs may cause a vaginal discharge. Because most women have a vaginal discharge from time to time, they should try to be aware of what their normal discharge looks like. Discharge caused by an STI will be different from the usual; it may be yellow and thicker and have an odor.

Instruct patients to see a health care provider if they have any of the above signs or symptoms.

- Prior STIs
- Partner testing for STIs
- Satisfaction with relationship(s), sexual pleasure achieved, frequency
- Problems: pain on penetration (entry or deep); decreased lubrication, lack of orgasm
- Sexual assault or abuse
  - Screening for intimate partner violence (IPV) and domestic violence: see Chapter 1.
- Performance of genital self-examination (see Staying Well, "Genital Self-Examination for Women")
- Date of last pelvic examination
- Use of illicit drugs

�֍ Infants and Children

Usually no special questions are required unless there is a specific concern from the parent or child.

- Bleeding
  - Character: onset, duration, precipitating factor if known, course since onset
  - Age of mother at menarche
  - Signs of breast development
  - Associated symptoms: pain, change in crying of infant, child fearful of parent or other adults
  - Parental suspicion about insertion of foreign objects by child
  - Parental suspicion about possible sexual abuse

| Box 18-2 | Evaluation of Masturbation in Children |

Masturbation is a common, healthy, self-discovery activity in children. Parents sometimes express concern about their child's masturbation activity. The following guidelines can help you determine when such activity might be a cause for concern.

Healthy Activity	Needs Further Assessment
Occasional	Frequent, compulsive excessive/obsessive
Discreet, private	No regard for privacy Age-inappropriate public masturbation
Not preferred over other activity or play	Often preferred over other activity or play Combined with other emotional and/or behavioral problems
No physical signs or symptoms	Produces genital discomfort, irritation, or physical signs
External stimulation of genitalia only	Involves penetration of the genital orifices; aggressive; includes bizarre practices or rituals

From Haka-Ikse and Mian, 1993; Mallants and Casteels, 2008.

+ Pain
  + Character: type of pain, onset, course since onset, duration
  + Specific location
  + Associated symptoms: vaginal discharge or bleeding, urinary symptoms, gastrointestinal symptoms, child fearful of parent or other adults
  + Contributory problems: use of bubble bath, irritating soaps, or detergents; parental suspicion about insertion of foreign objects by child or about possible sexual abuse
+ Vaginal discharge
  + Relationship to diapers: use of powder or lotions, how frequently diapers are changed
  + Associated symptoms: pain, bleeding
  + Contributory problems: parental suspicion about insertion of foreign objects by child or about possible sexual abuse
+ Masturbation (Box 18-2)

�֍ Adolescents

As the older child matures, you should ask her the same questions that you ask adult women. You should not assume that youthful age precludes sexual activity or any of the related concerns. While taking the history, it is necessary at some point to talk with the adolescent alone while the parent is out of the room in order to provide a confidential safe space for discussion of sensitive topics. Your questions should be posed in a gentle, matter-of-fact, and nonjudgmental manner.

✖ Pregnant Women

+ Expected date of delivery (EDD) or weeks of gestation
+ Previous obstetric history: GPTAL, prenatal complications, infertility treatment
+ Previous birth history: length of gestation at birth, birth weight, fetal outcome, length of labor, fetal presentation, type of delivery, use of forceps, lacerations and/or episiotomy, complications (natal and postnatal)
+ Previous menstrual history (see menstrual history under Past Medical History)
+ Surgical history: prior uterine surgery and type of scar
+ Family history: diabetes mellitus, multiple births, preeclampsia, genetic disorder
+ Involuntary passage of fluid, which may result from rupture of membranes (ROM); determine onset, duration, color, odor, amount, and if still leaking
+ Bleeding
  + Character: onset, duration, precipitating factor if known (e.g., intercourse, trauma), course since onset, amount
  + Associated symptoms
+ Pain: type (e.g., sharp or dull, intermittent or continuous), onset, location, duration
+ Gastrointestinal symptoms: nausea, vomiting, heartburn

✖ Older Adults

+ Menopausal history: See HPI
+ Symptoms associated with age-related physiologic changes: itching, urinary symptoms, dyspareunia
+ Changes in sexual desire or behavior in self or partner(s)

EXAMINATION AND FINDINGS

Equipment

+ Lamp or light source
+ Drapes
+ Speculum
+ Gloves
+ Water-soluble lubricant
+ Pap smear/HPV collection equipment
  + Collection device: (wooden or plastic spatula, cervical brush or broom)
  + Glass slides and cytologic fixative or fluid collection media
+ Other specimen collection equipment as needed:
  + Cotton swabs
  + Culture plates or media
  + DNA tests for organisms

Preparation

Although most women express lack of enthusiasm in anticipation of a pelvic examination, most do not experience anxiety (see Clinical Pearl, "Anxiety"). Explain in general terms what you are going to do. Maintain eye contact with the patient, both before and, as much as possible, during the examination. Women from some cultural or ethnic groups may not return eye contact as a show of respect. Be sensitive to cultural variations in behavior. If the patient has not seen the equipment before, show it to her, and explain its use.

EXAMINATION AND FINDINGS

Assure the patient that you will explain to her what you are doing as the examination proceeds. Let her know that you will be as gentle as possible, and tell her to let you know if she feels any discomfort.

Have the patient empty her bladder before the examination. Bimanual examination is uncomfortable for the woman if her bladder is full. A full bladder also makes it difficult to palpate the pelvic organs.

Make sure that the room temperature is comfortable. Do what you can to ensure privacy. The door should be securely closed and should be opened only with permission of both the patient and examiner. The examination table should be positioned so that the patient faces away from it during the examination. A drawn curtain can ensure that any door opening will not expose the patient. Ideally, examiners of either gender will be accompanied by a female chaperone. A chaperone is often required by practice or institution policy and protects both the examiner and patient. Some patients may be reluctant to reveal confidential and sensitive information in the presence of an observer chaperone.

Positioning

Assist the patient into the lithotomy position on the examining table. (If a table with stirrups is not available or if the woman is unable to assume the lithotomy position, the examination can be performed in other positions, see p. 448). Help the woman stabilize her feet in the stirrups and slide her buttocks down to the edge of the examining table. If the patient is not positioned correctly, you will have difficulty with the speculum examination.

Draping and Gloving

The patient can be draped in such a way that allows minimal exposure. A good method is to cover her knees and symphysis, depressing the drape between her knees. This allows you to see the woman's face (and she, yours) throughout the examination (Fig. 18-10).

Once the patient is positioned and draped, make sure that any equipment is nearby and in easy reach. Arrange the examining lamp so that the external genitalia are clearly visible. Wash or sanitize your hands and put gloves on both hands (see Clinical Pearl, "Gloving").

FIGURE 18-10 Draped patient in dorsal lithotomy position.

Ask the woman to drop open her knees. Never try to separate her legs forcibly or even gently. The pelvic examination is an intrusive procedure, and you may need to wait a moment until the woman is ready. Tell her that you are going to begin, then start with a neutral touch on her lower thigh, moving your examining hand along the thigh without breaking contact to the external genitalia.

External Examination

Inspection and Palpation

Sit at the end of the examining table and inspect and palpate the external genitalia. Look at the hair distribution and notice the surface characteristics of the mons pubis and labia majora. The skin should be smooth and clean, and the hair should be free of nits or lice.

Labia Majora

The labia majora may be gaping or closed and may appear dry or moist. They are usually symmetric and may be either shriveled or full. The tissue should feel soft and homogeneous. Labial swelling, redness, or tenderness, particularly if unilateral, may be indicative of a Bartholin gland infection. Look for excoriation, rashes, or lesions, which suggest an infectious or inflammatory process. If any of these signs are present, ask the woman if she has been scratching. Observe for discoloration, varicosities, obvious stretching, or signs of trauma or scarring.

FIGURE 18-11 Separation of the labia.

FIGURE 18-13 Urethral caruncle, a red fleshy lesion at the urethral meatus. *(From Lemmi and Lemmi, 2009.)*

FIGURE 18-12 Normal vulva with finely textured papular sebaceous glands on the inner labia majora and labia minora. *(From Morse et al, 2003.)*

Labia Minora

Separate the labia majora with the fingers of one hand and inspect the labia minora. Use your other hand to palpate the labia minora between your thumb and second finger; then separate the labia minora and inspect and palpate the inside of the labia minora, clitoris, urethral orifice, vaginal introitus, and perineum (Fig. 18-11).

The labia minora may appear symmetric or asymmetric, and the inner surface should be moist and dark pink. The tissue should feel soft, homogeneous, and without tenderness (Fig. 18-12). Look for inflammation, irritation, excoriation, or caking of discharge in the tissue folds, which suggests vaginal infection or poor hygiene. Discoloration or tenderness may be the result of traumatic bruising. Ulcers or vesicles may be signs of an STI. Palpate for irregularities or nodules.

Clitoris

Inspect the clitoris for size. Generally, the clitoris is about 2 cm or less in length and 0.5 cm in diameter. Enlargement may be a sign of a masculinizing condition. Observe also for atrophy, inflammation, or adhesions.

Urethral Orifice

The urethral orifice appears as an irregular opening or slit. It may be close to or slightly within the vaginal introitus and is usually in the midline. Inspect for discharge, polyps, caruncles, and fistulas. A caruncle is a bright red polypoid growth that protrudes from the urethral meatus; most urethral caruncles cause no symptoms (Fig. 18-13).

Signs of irritation, inflammation, or dilation suggest repeated urinary tract infections or insertion of foreign objects. Ask questions about any findings at a later time—not during the pelvic examination when the woman feels most vulnerable.

Vaginal Introitus

The vaginal introitus can be a thin vertical slit or a large orifice with irregular edges from hymenal remnants (myrtiform caruncles). The tissue should be moist. Look for swelling, discoloration, discharge, lesions, fistulas, or fissures.

Skene and Bartholin Glands

With the labia still separated, examine the Skene and Bartholin glands. Tell the woman you are going to insert one finger in her vagina and that she will feel you pressing forward with it. With your palm facing upward, insert the index finger of the examining hand into the vagina as far as the second joint of the finger. Exerting upward pressure, milk the Skene glands by moving the finger outward. Do this on both sides of the urethra, and then directly on the urethra (Fig. 18-14). Look for discharge and note any tenderness. If a discharge occurs, note its color, consistency, and odor, and obtain a culture. Discharge from the Skene glands or urethra usually indicates an infection—most commonly, but not necessarily, gonococcal.

With your finger still in place, you can then locate the cervix and note the direction in which it points. This may help you locate the cervix when you insert the speculum.

Maintaining labial separation and with your finger still in the vaginal opening, tell the patient that she will feel you pressing around the entrance to the vagina. Palpate the lateral tissue between your index finger and thumb. Palpate the entire area,

FIGURE 18-14 **Palpation of Skene glands.**

FIGURE 18-16 **Palpating the perineum.**

FIGURE 18-15 **Palpation of Bartholin glands.**

paying particular attention to the posterolateral portion of the labia majora where the Bartholin glands are located. Note any swelling, tenderness, masses, heat, or fluctuation. Observe for discharge from the opening of the Bartholin gland duct. Palpate and observe bilaterally, because each gland is separate (Fig. 18-15). Note the color, consistency, and odor of any discharge, and obtain a specimen for laboratory evaluation. Swelling that is painful, hot to the touch, and fluctuant is indicative of infection of the Bartholin gland. The infection is usually gonococcal or staphylococcal in origin and is filled with pus. A nontender mass is indicative of a Bartholin cyst, which is the result of chronic inflammation of the gland.

Muscle Tone

Test muscle tone if the woman has borne children or has told you about signs of weak muscle tone (e.g., urinary incontinence or the sensation of something "falling out"). To test, ask the patient to squeeze the vaginal opening around your finger, explaining that you are testing muscle tone. Then ask the patient to bear down as you watch for urinary incontinence and uterine prolapse. Uterine prolapse is marked by protrusion of the cervix or uterus on straining.

Perineum

Inspect and palpate the perineum (Fig. 18-16). The perineal surface should be smooth; episiotomy scarring may be evident in

women who have borne children. The tissue will feel thick and smooth in the nulliparous woman. It will be thinner and rigid in multiparous women. In either case, it should not be tender. Look for inflammation, fistulas, lesions, or growths.

Anus

The anal surface is more darkly pigmented, and the skin may appear coarse. It should be free of scarring, lesions, inflammation, fissures, lumps, skin tags, or excoriation. If you touch the anus or perianal skin, be sure to change your gloves so that you do not introduce bacteria into the vagina during the internal examination.

Internal Examination

Preparation

It is essential that you become familiar with how the speculum operates before you begin the examination so that you do not inadvertently hurt the woman through mishandling of the instrument. Chapter 3 describes the proper use of the speculum. Become familiar with both the reusable stainless steel and the disposable plastic specula because their mechanisms of action are somewhat different.

Lubricate the speculum (and the gloved fingers) with water or a water-soluble lubricant. Most health care providers routinely lubricate with water only. An added advantage of using water as a lubricant is that a cold speculum can be warmed by rinsing in warm (but not hot) water. A speculum can also be warmed by holding it in your hand (if it is warm) or under the lamp for a few minutes.

Select the appropriate size speculum (see Chapter 3) and hold it in your hand with the index finger over the top of the proximal end of the anterior blade and the other fingers around the handle. This position controls the blades as the speculum is inserted into the vagina.

Insertion of Speculum

Tell the patient that she is going to feel you touching her again, and gently insert a finger of your other hand just inside the vaginal introitus and apply pressure downward. Ask the woman to breathe slowly and try to consciously relax her muscles or the

Evidence-Based Practice in Physical Examination

Lubricating the Speculum

The conventional wisdom has been that gel lubricants should not be used when collecting a Pap smear specimen because the gel could obscure cellular elements and interfere with specimen analysis and interpretation. Recent studies (Gilson et al, 2006; Griffith et al, 2005; Harer et al, 2003) question this premise and show evidence that using a water-soluble gel lubricant does not adversely affect cellular analysis with either conventional or liquid-based Pap smears. However, another report (Zardawi et al, 2003) documents contamination by excess gel in some instances with both conventional and liquid-based Pap smears, and two other studies (Charoenkwan et al, 2008; Köşüş et al, 2012) document a higher proportion of unsatisfactory smears that were contaminated with gel. Charoenkwan et al (2008) also reported discordance in cytologic diagnosis between the gel-contaminated and uncontaminated smears from the same patient. Our advice: Until further studies conclusively determine that gel lubricant does not adversely interfere with specimen analysis, we continue to recommend lubrication with water. However, if gel lubricant is used, a thin layer on the external surface of the blades only will help avoid contamination of the specimen.

muscles of her buttocks. Wait until you feel the relaxation (Fig. 18-17, *A*). Use the fingers of that hand to separate the labia minora so that the vaginal opening becomes clearly visible. Then slowly insert the speculum along the path of least resistance, often slightly downward, avoiding trauma to the urethra and vaginal walls. Some health care providers insert the speculum blades at an oblique angle; others prefer to keep the blades horizontal. In either case, avoid touching the clitoris, catching pubic hair, or pinching labial skin (Fig. 18-17, *B* and *C*). Insert the speculum the length of the vaginal canal. While maintaining gentle downward pressure with the speculum, open it by pressing on the thumb piece. Sweep the speculum slowly upward until the cervix comes into view. Gently reposition the speculum, if necessary, to locate the cervix. Adjust the light source.

Once you visualize the cervix, manipulate the speculum to fully expose the cervix between the anterior and posterior blades. Lock the speculum blades into place to stabilize the distal spread of the blades, and adjust the proximal spread as needed (Fig. 18-17, *D*).

Cervix

Inspect the cervix for color, position, size, surface characteristics, discharge, and size and shape of the os.

Color. Expect the cervix to be pink, with the color evenly distributed. A bluish color indicates increased vascularity, which may be a sign of pregnancy. Symmetric circumscribed redness around the os is an expected finding that indicates exposed columnar epithelium from the cervical canal. However, beginning health care providers should consider any reddened areas as an unexpected finding, especially if patchy or if the borders are irregular. A pale cervix is associated with anemia.

Position. The anterior-posterior position of the cervix correlates with the position of the uterus. A cervix that is pointing anteriorly indicates a retroverted uterus; one pointing posteriorly indicates an anteverted uterus. A cervix in the horizontal position indicates a uterus in midposition. The cervix should be located in the midline. Deviation to the right or left may indicate a pelvic mass, uterine adhesions, or pregnancy. The cervix may protrude 1 to 3 cm into the vagina. Projection greater than 3 cm may indicate a pelvic or uterine mass. The cervix of a woman of childbearing age is usually 2 to 3 cm in diameter.

Surface Characteristics. The surface of the cervix should be smooth. Usually the transformation zone (the junction of squamous and columnar epithelium) is just barely visible inside the external os. Some squamocolumnar epithelium of the cervical canal may be visible as a symmetric reddened circle around the os (Fig. 18-18). Cervical ectropion occurs when eversion of the endocervix exposes columnar epithelium. The everted epithelium has a red, shiny appearance around the os and may bleed easily. Ectropion is common in adolescents, pregnant women, or those taking estrogen-containing contraceptives. Ectropion is not an abnormality, but because it is indistinguishable from early cervical carcinoma, further diagnostic studies (e.g., Pap smear, biopsy) must be performed for differential diagnosis.

Nabothian cysts may be observed as small, white or yellow, raised, round areas on the cervix. These are mucinous retention cysts of the endocervical glands and are considered an expected finding. They occur during the process of metaplasia at the transformation zone when endocervical columnar cells continue to secrete but are covered by squamous epithelium. An infected nabothian cyst becomes swollen with fluid and may distort the shape of the cervix, giving it an irregular appearance. Infected nabothian cysts vary in size and may occur singly or in multiples.

Look for friable tissue, red patchy areas, granular areas, and white patches that could indicate cervicitis, infection, or carcinoma.

Note the presence of any cervical polyps, which are bright red, soft, and fragile. They usually arise from the endocervical canal (Fig. 18-19).

Discharge. Note any discharge. Determine whether the discharge comes from the cervix itself, or whether it is vaginal in origin and has only been deposited on the cervix. Usual discharge is odorless; may be creamy or clear; may be thick, thin, or stringy; and is often heavier at midcycle or immediately before menstruation. The discharge of a bacterial or fungal infection will more likely have an odor and will vary in color from white to yellow, green, or gray.

Size and Shape. The os of the nulliparous woman is small and round or oval. The os of a multiparous woman is usually a horizontal slit or may be irregular and stellate. Cervical lacerations caused by trauma from childbirth can produce lateral transverse, bilateral transverse, or stellate scarring. Trauma from induced abortion or difficult removal of an intrauterine device may also change the shape of the os to a slit (Fig. 18-20).

Obtain specimens for Pap smear, HPV testing, culture, DNA testing, or other laboratory analysis as indicated in Box 18-3.

FIGURE 18-17 **Examination of the internal genitalia with a speculum.** Begin by inserting a finger and applying downward pressure to relax the vaginal muscles. **A,** Gently insert the closed speculum blades into the vagina. **B,** Direct the speculum along the path of least resistance. **C,** Insert the speculum the length of the vaginal canal. **D,** Speculum is in place, locked, and stabilized. Note cervix in full view. *(D, Photograph from Edge and Miller, 1994.)*

FIGURE 18-18 **Normal cervix.** The squamocolumnar junction and lower part of the endocervical canal are seen. *(From Morse et al, 2003.)*

FIGURE 18-19 Polyp protruding through the cervical os. *(From Baggish, 2003.)*

FIGURE 18-20 Common appearances of the cervix. A, Normal nulliparous cervix. The surface is covered with pink squamous epithelium that is uniform in consistency. The os is small and round. A small area of ectropion is visible inferior to the os. **B,** Parous cervix. Note slit appearance of os. **C,** Multiparous, lacerated. **D,** Everted. Columnar mucosal cells usually found in the endocervical canal have extended out into the surface of the cervix, creating a circular raised erythematous appearance. Note the normal nonpurulent cervical mucus. This normal variant is not to be confused with cervicitis. **E,** Eroded. **F,** Nabothian cysts. *(Photographs from Zitelli and Davis, 1997; **A,** courtesy C. Stevens; **D,** courtesy E. Jerome, MD.)*

| **Box 18-3** | **Obtaining Vaginal Smears and Specimens** |

Vaginal specimens for smears and cultures are often obtained during the speculum examination. Vaginal specimens are obtained while the speculum is in place but after the cervix and its surrounding tissue have been inspected. Collect specimens as indicated for Pap smear, HPV testing, sexually transmitted infection screening, and wet mount. Label the specimen with the patient's name and a description of the specimen (e.g., cervical smear, vaginal smear, and culture). Be sure to follow Standard Precautions for the safe collection of human secretions.

Conventional Papanicolaou Smear

Brushes and brooms are now being used in conjunction with, or instead of, the conventional spatula to improve the quality of cells obtained. The cylindric-type brush collects endocervical cells only. First, collect a sample from the ectocervix with a spatula (Figs. 18-21 and 18-22, *A*). Insert the longer projection of the spatula into the cervical os; rotate it 360 degrees, keeping it flush against the cervical tissue. Withdraw the spatula, and spread the specimen on a glass slide. A single light stroke with each side of the spatula is sufficient to thin the specimen out over the slide. Immediately spray with cytologic fixative and label the slide as the ectocervical specimen. Then introduce the brush device into the vagina and insert it into the cervical os until only the bristles closest to the handle are exposed (Fig. 18-22, *B* and *C*). Slowly rotate one-half turn. Remove and prepare the endocervical smear by rolling and twisting the brush with moderate pressure across a glass slide. Fix the specimen with spray and label as the endocervical specimen.

FIGURE 18-21 Scrape the cervix with the bifid end of the spatula for obtaining pap smear. *(From Symonds and Macpherson, 1994.)*

The broom-type device is used for collecting both ectocervical and endocervical cells at the same time (see Fig. 18-22, *D*). This broom uses flexible plastic bristles, which are reported to cause less blood spotting after the examination. Introduce the brush into the vagina and

Continued

Box 18-3	**Obtaining Vaginal Smears and Specimens—cont'd**

FIGURE 18-22 Implements used to obtain a Pap smear. **A,** Close-up of spatula. **B,** Brush device. **C,** Close-up of brush. **D,** Broom device. *(Courtesy Therapak Corporation, Irwindale, CA.)*

insert the central long bristles into the cervical os until the lateral bristles bend fully against the ectocervix. Maintain gentle pressure and rotate the brush by rolling the handle between the thumb and forefinger three to five times to the left and right. Withdraw the brush, and transfer the sample to a glass slide with two single paint strokes: Apply first one side of the bristle, turn the brush over, and paint the slide again in exactly the same area. Apply fixative and label as the ectocervical and endocervical specimen.

Liquid-Based Pap Testing
The liquid-based cytology requires use of the broom-type device. Insert the central bristles of the broom into the endocervical canal deep enough to allow the shorter bristles to fully contact the ectocervix. Push gently, and rotate the broom in a clockwise direction five times. Rinse the broom into the solution vial by pushing the broom into the bottom of the vial 10 times, forcing the bristles apart. As a final step, swirl the broom vigorously to further release material. Discard the collection device. Alternatively, deposit the broom end of the device directly into the collection vial. With any collection device, be sure to follow the manufacturer's and laboratory instructions to collect and preserve the specimen appropriately. Close the vial tightly to prevent leakage and loss of the sample during transport. The liquid sample is also used to test for HPV.

Gonococcal Culture Specimen
Immediately after the Pap smear is obtained, introduce a sterile cotton swab into the vagina and insert it into the cervical os (Fig. 18-23); hold it in place for 10 to 30 seconds. Withdraw the swab and spread the

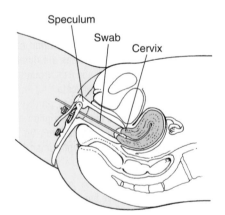

FIGURE 18-23 Obtaining a cervical specimen by inserting a swab into the cervical os. *(From Grimes, 1991.)*

specimen in a large Z pattern over the culture medium, rotating the swab at the same time. Label the tube or plate, and follow agency routine for transporting and maintaining appropriate temperature of the specimen of the specimen. If indicated, an anal culture can be obtained after the vaginal speculum has been removed. Insert a fresh, sterile cotton swab about 2.5 cm into the rectum and rotate it full circle; hold it in place for 10 to 30 seconds. Withdraw the swab and prepare the specimen as described for the vaginal culture. Gonococcal cultures are now used less commonly than the combined DNA probe for chlamydia and gonorrhea.

Box 18-3   Obtaining Vaginal Smears and Specimens—cont'd

DNA Testing for Organisms

These tests involve the construction of a nucleic acid sequence that will match to a sequence in the DNA or RNA of the target tissue. The results are rapid and sensitive. Use a Dacron swab (with plastic or wire shaft) when collecting your specimen, because wooden cotton-tipped applicators may interfere with the test results. Also be sure to check the expiration date so as not to use out-of-date materials. Insert the swab into the cervical os and rotate the swab in the endocervical canal for 30 seconds to ensure adequate sampling and absorption by the swab. Avoid contact with the vaginal mucous membranes, which would contaminate the specimen. Remove the swab and place it in the tube containing the specimen reagent. Single or dual organism tests are available for *Chlamydia trachomatis* and *N. gonorrhea*. Multiorganism tests are available for *Trichomonas vaginalis*, *Gardnerella vaginalis*, and *Candida* species

Wet Mount and Potassium Hydroxide (KOH) Procedures

In a woman with vaginal discharge, these microscope examinations can demonstrate the presence of *Trichomonas vaginalis*, bacterial vaginosis, or candidiasis. For the wet mount, obtain a specimen of vaginal discharge using a swab. Smear the sample on a glass slide and add a drop of normal saline. Place a coverslip on the slide, and view under the microscope. The presence of trichomonads indicates *T. vaginalis*. The presence of bacteria-filled epithelial cells (clue cells) indicates bacterial vaginosis. On a separate glass slide, place a specimen of vaginal discharge, apply a drop of aqueous 10% KOH, and put a coverslip in place. The presence of a fishy odor (the "whiff test") suggests bacterial vaginosis. The KOH dissolves epithelial cells and debris and facilitates visualization of the mycelia of a fungus. View under the microscope for the presence of mycelial fragments, hyphae, and budding yeast cells, which indicate candidiasis.

Withdrawal of Speculum

Unlock the speculum and remove it slowly and carefully so that you can inspect the vaginal walls. Note color, surface characteristics, and secretions. The color should be about the same color pink as the cervix, or a little lighter. Reddened patches, lesions, or pallor indicates a local or systemic pathologic condition. The surface should be moist and homogeneous. The walls will have rugae in premenopausal women and be smooth in postmenopausal women. Look for cracks, lesions, bleeding, nodules, and swelling. Secretions that may be expected are usually thin, clear or cloudy, and odorless. Secretions indicative of infection are often profuse; may be thick, curdy, or frothy; appear gray, green, or yellow; and may have a foul odor.

Look for the presence of a cystocele or rectocele. A cystocele is a hernial protrusion of the urinary bladder through the anterior wall of the vagina, sometimes even exiting the introitus (Fig. 18-24). The bulging can be seen and felt as the woman bears down. More severe degrees of cystocele are accompanied by urinary stress incontinence. Seen as a bulge on the posterior wall of the vagina, a rectocele (or proctocele) is a hernial protrusion of part of the rectum through the posterior vaginal wall (Fig. 18-25).

As you withdraw the speculum, the blades will tend to close themselves. Avoid pinching the cervix and vaginal walls. Maintain downward pressure of the speculum to avoid trauma to the urethra. Hook your index finger over the anterior blade as it is removed. Keep one thumb on the handle lever and control closing of the speculum. Make sure that the speculum is fully closed when the blades pass through the hymenal ring. Note the odor of any vaginal discharge that has pooled in the posterior blade and obtain a specimen, if you have not already done so. Deposit the speculum in the proper container.

Bimanual Examination

Inform the woman that you are going to examine her internally with your fingers. Change your gloves or remove the outer glove

FIGURE 18-24 Cystocele. *(From Lemmi and Lemmi, 2000.)*

FIGURE 18-25 Rectocele. *(From Lemmi and Lemmi, 2000.)*

FIGURE 18-26 Bimanual palpation of the uterus.

and lubricate the index and middle fingers of your examining hand. Insert the tips of the gloved index and middle fingers into the vaginal opening and press downward, again waiting for the muscles to relax. Gradually and gently insert your fingers their full length into the vagina. Palpate the vaginal wall as you insert your fingers. It should be smooth, homogeneous, and nontender. Feel for cysts, nodules, masses, or growths.

Be careful where you place your thumb during the bimanual examination. You can tuck it into the palm of your hand, but that will cut down on the distance you can insert your fingers. Be aware of where the thumb is and keep it from touching the clitoris, which can produce discomfort (Fig. 18-26).

Box 18-4 describes the examination of a woman who has had a hysterectomy.

Evidence-Based Practice in Physical Examination

Cervical Cancer Screening After Hysterectomy?

Experts agree that women who have had a hysterectomy for noncancer reasons, with the cervix removed, no evidence of malignancy, and no history of abnormal cancerous cell growth, can discontinue screening for cervical cancer. The yield of cytologic screening is very low in women after hysterectomy, and there is no evidence that continuing screening improves health outcomes.

American Cancer Society, 2012; National Cancer Institute, 2012; Moyer for the U.S. Preventive Services Task Force, 2012.

Cervix

Locate the cervix with the palmar surface of your fingers, feel its end, and run your fingers around its circumference to feel the fornices. Feel the size, length, and shape, which should correspond with your observations from the speculum examination. The consistency of the cervix in a nonpregnant woman will be firm, like the tip of the nose; during pregnancy the cervix is softer. Feel for nodules, hardness, and roughness. Note the position of the cervix as discussed in the speculum examination. The cervix should be in the midline and may be pointing anteriorly or posteriorly.

Grasp the cervix gently between your fingers and move it from side to side. Observe the patient for any expression of pain or

---

Box 18-4   **Examining the Woman Who Has Had a Hysterectomy**

Examination of a woman who has had a hysterectomy is essentially no different from the usual procedure. The same examination steps and sequence are followed, with minor variation in what you are assessing. Getting an accurate history before the examination will assist you in knowing what to look for. Determine whether the surgical approach was vaginal or abdominal, whether the woman had a total hysterectomy, a supracervical hysterectomy (cervix left intact) or a partial hysterectomy (fallopian tubes and ovaries left intact), the reason for the hysterectomy, if there have been bladder or bowel changes since the surgery, and the presence of menopausal symptoms.

Examine the external genitalia for atrophy, skin changes, decreased resilience, and discharge. In these patients, specimens for gonococci or chlamydia are often taken at the vestibule rather than internally. On speculum examination, the cervix will be absent except when a supracervical hysterectomy was performed. The surgical scar (vaginal cuff) will be visible at the end of the vaginal canal and will be an identifiable white or pink suture line in the posterior fornix. If indicated, a Pap smear should be taken from this suture line with the blunt end of the spatula or blunt broom. Be sure to label the specimen as vaginal cells; otherwise, the report may be sent back as incomplete or unsatisfactory because of a lack of endocervical cell sample. Assess the walls, mucosa, and secretions as you ordinarily would. The vaginal canal of a woman who has had a total hysterectomy might show the same changes as those that occur with menopause (e.g., a decrease in rugae and secretions), especially if the woman is not receiving hormone therapy. Examine for a cystocele or rectocele. Stress incontinence may be a problem, so observe for this when having the patient bear down.

On bimanual examination, the uterus will obviously not be present; further findings will depend on whether the hysterectomy was total or partial. If partial, proceed with the examination as usual, assessing the ovaries and surrounding area. If the hysterectomy was total, assess the adnexal area for masses, adhesions, or tenderness. The bladder and bowel may feel more prominent than usual.

---

discomfort with movement (cervical motion tenderness). The cervix should move 1 to 2 cm in each direction with minimal or no discomfort. Painful cervical movement suggests a pelvic inflammatory process such as pelvic inflammatory disease or a ruptured tubal pregnancy.

Uterus

Position. Palpate the uterus. Place the palmar surface of your other hand on the abdominal midline, midway between the umbilicus and the symphysis pubis. Place the intravaginal fingers in the anterior fornix. Slowly slide the abdominal hand toward the pubis, pressing downward and forward with the flat surface of your fingers. At the same time, push inward and upward with the fingertips of the intravaginal hand while you push downward on the cervix with the backs of your fingers. Think of it as trying to bring your two hands together as you press down on the cervix. If the uterus is anteverted or anteflexed (the position of most uteri), you will feel the fundus between the fingers of your two hands at the level of the pubis (Fig. 18-27, *A* and *B*).

If you do not feel the uterus with the previous maneuver, place the intravaginal fingers together in the posterior fornix, with the abdominal hand immediately above the symphysis pubis. Press firmly downward with the abdominal hand while you press against the cervix inward with the other hand. A retroverted or retroflexed uterus should be felt with this maneuver (Fig. 18-27, *C* and *D*).

If you still cannot feel the uterus, move the intravaginal fingers to each side of the cervix. Keeping contact with the cervix, press inward and feel as far as you can. Then slide your fingers so that one is on top of the cervix and one is underneath. Continue pressing inward while moving your fingers to feel as much of the uterus as you can. When the uterus is in the midposition, you will not be able to feel the fundus with the abdominal hand (Fig. 18-27, *E*).

Confirm the location and position of the uterus by comparing your inspection findings with your palpation findings. The uterus should be located in the midline regardless of its position.

Deviation to the right or left is indicative of possible adhesions, pelvic masses, or pregnancy. Knowing the position of the uterus is essential before performing any intrauterine procedure, including insertion of an intrauterine contraceptive device.

Size, Shape, and Contour. Palpate the uterus for size, shape, and contour. It should be pear-shaped and 5.5 to 8 cm long, although it is larger in all dimensions in multiparous women. A uterus larger than expected in a woman of childbearing age is indicative of pregnancy, fibroid, or tumor. The contour should be rounded, and the walls should feel firm and smooth in the nonpregnant woman. The contour smoothness will be interrupted by pregnancy or tumor.

Mobility. Gently move the uterus between the intravaginal hand and abdominal hand to assess for mobility and tenderness. The uterus should be mobile in the anteroposterior plane. A fixed uterus indicates adhesions. Tenderness on movement suggests a pelvic inflammatory process or ruptured tubal pregnancy.

Adnexa and Ovaries

Palpate the adnexal areas and ovaries. Place the fingers of your abdominal hand on the right lower quadrant. With the intravaginal hand facing upward, place both fingers in the right lateral fornix. Press the intravaginal fingers deeply inward and upward toward the abdominal hand while sweeping the flat surface of the fingers of the abdominal hand deeply inward and obliquely downward toward the symphysis pubis. Palpate the entire area by firmly pressing the abdominal hand and intravaginal fingers together. Repeat the maneuver on the left side (Fig. 18-28).

The ovaries, if palpable, should feel firm, smooth, ovoid, and approximately 3 by 2 by 1 cm in size. The healthy ovary is slightly to moderately tender on palpation. Marked tenderness, enlargement, and nodularity are unexpected. Usually no other structures are palpable except for round ligaments. Fallopian tubes are usually not palpable, so a problem may exist if they are felt. You are also palpating for adnexal masses, and if any are found they should be characterized by size, shape, location, consistency, and tenderness.

The adnexa are often difficult to palpate because of their location and position and the presence of excess adipose tissue in some women. If you are unable to feel anything in the adnexal areas with thorough palpation, you can assume that no abnormality is present, provided no clinical symptoms exist (see Clinical Pearl, "Mittelschmerz and Adnexal Tenderness").

Clinical Pearl

Mittelschmerz and Adnexal Tenderness

Mittelschmerz, lower abdominal pain associated with ovulation, may be accompanied by tenderness on the side in which ovulation took place that month. The timing is, of course, essential in the history. The onset of pain is usually sudden, and remission is spontaneous. On a pelvic examination you may discover a bit of adnexal tenderness but the examination will otherwise be reassuringly negative.

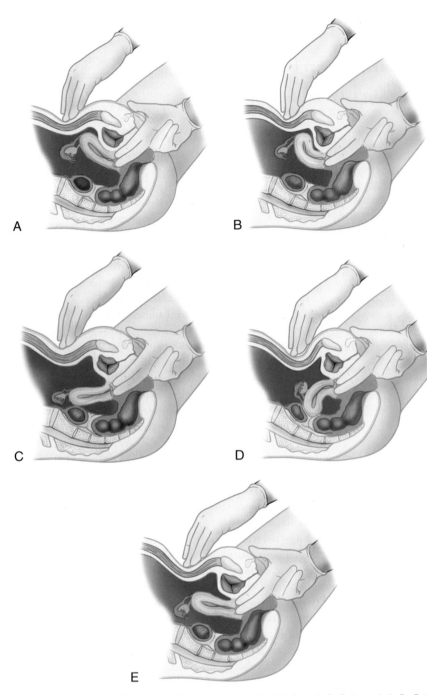

FIGURE 18-27 Varying positions of uteri. A, Anteverted. **B,** Anteflexed. **C,** Retroverted. **D,** Retroflexed.
E, Midposition.

Rectovaginal Examination

Preparation

The rectovaginal examination is an important part of the total pelvic examination. It allows you to reach almost 2.5 cm (1 inch) higher into the pelvis, which enables you to better evaluate the pelvic organs and structures. It is an uncomfortable examination for the patient, however, and she may ask you to omit it. Nevertheless, it is important to perform, and you should explain to the woman why it is necessary.

As you complete the bimanual examination, withdraw your examining fingers, change gloves, and lubricate fingers. Tell the patient that she may feel the urgency of a bowel movement. Assure her that she will not have one, and ask her to breathe slowly and consciously try to relax her sphincter, rectum, and buttocks because tightening the muscles makes the examination more uncomfortable for her.

Anal Sphincter

Place your index finger in the vagina, and then press your middle finger against the anus and ask the patient to bear down. As she

FIGURE 18-28 Bimanual palpation of adnexa. Sweep abdominal fingers downward to capture ovary.

FIGURE 18-29 Rectovaginal palpation. *(From Lowdermilk and Perry, 2007.)*

does, slip the tip of the finger into the rectum just past the sphincter. Palpate the area of the anorectal junction and just above it. Ask the woman to tighten and relax her anal sphincter. Observe sphincter tone. An extremely tight sphincter may be the result of anxiety about the examination; may be caused by scarring; or may indicate spasticity caused by fissures, lesions, or inflammation. A lax sphincter suggests neurologic deficit, whereas an absent sphincter may result from improper repair of a third-degree perineal laceration after childbirth or trauma.

Rectal Walls and Rectovaginal Septum

Slide both your vaginal and rectal fingers in as far as they will go, and then ask the woman to bear down. This will bring an additional centimeter within reach of your fingers. Rotate the rectal finger to explore the anterior rectal wall for masses, polyps, nodules, strictures, irregularities, and tenderness. The wall should feel smooth and uninterrupted. Palpate the rectovaginal septum along the anterior wall for thickness, tone, and nodules. You may feel the uterine body and occasionally the uterine fundus in a retroflexed uterus.

Uterus

Press firmly and deeply downward with the abdominal hand just above the symphysis pubis while you position the vaginal finger in the posterior vaginal fornix, and press strongly upward against the posterior side of the cervix. Palpate as much of the posterior side of the uterus as possible, confirming your findings from the vaginal examination regarding location, position, size, shape, contour, consistency, and tenderness of the uterus. This maneuver is particularly useful in evaluating a retroverted uterus (Fig. 18-29).

Adnexa

If you were unable to palpate the adnexal areas on bimanual examination or if the findings were questionable, repeat the adnexal examination using the same maneuvers described in the bimanual examination.

Stool

As you withdraw your fingers, rotate the rectal finger to evaluate the posterior rectal wall just as you did earlier for the anterior

wall. Gently remove your examining fingers and observe for secretions and stool. Note the color and presence of any blood. Prepare a specimen for occult blood testing, if indicated. Unless the woman is unable to, let her wipe off the lubricating gel herself. She can do a more thorough and comfortable job. Be sure to provide tissues and an appropriate disposal receptacle.

Completion

Assist the woman into a sitting position and give her the opportunity to regain her equilibrium and composure. Provide a sanitary pad if she is menstruating. Share with her the findings and ask her to voice her feelings about the examination. This conversation may be brief, but it should never be avoided. Some health care providers prefer to leave the room and give the woman the opportunity to dress before discussing findings.

❀ Infants

The appearance of the external genitalia can help in the assessment of gestational age in the newborn. Examination is conducted with the infant's legs held in a frog position. The labia majora appear widely separated, and the clitoris is prominent up to 36 weeks of gestation, but by full term the labia majora completely cover the labia minora and clitoris.

The newborn's genitalia reflect the influence of maternal hormones. The labia majora and minora may be swollen, with the labia minora often more prominent. The hymen is often protruding, thick, and vascular, and it may simulate an extruding mass. These are all transient phenomena and will disappear in a few weeks (Fig. 18-30).

The clitoris may appear relatively large; this usually has no significance. True hypertrophy is not common; however, in newborns, an enlarged clitoris must alert the health care provider to the possibility of congenital adrenal hyperplasia.

The central opening of the hymen is usually about 0.5 cm in diameter. It is important to determine the presence of an opening; however, make no effort to stretch the hymen. An imperforate hymen is rare but can cause difficulty later, including hydrocolpos in the child and hematocolpos in the adolescent.

Malformations in the external genitalia are often difficult to discern. If the baby was a breech delivery, her genitalia may be swollen and bruised for many days after delivery. Any

FIGURE 18-30 Normal appearance of the female genitalia. A, Genitalia of a newborn girl. The labia majora are full, and the thickened labia minora protrude between them. **B,** Genitalia of a 2-year-old girl. The labia majora are flattened, and the labia minora and hymen are thin and flat. *(From Zitelli and Davis, 2007; A, courtesy Ian Holzman, MD, NY.)*

ambiguous appearance or unusual orifice in the vulvar vault or perineum must be expeditiously explored before gender assignment occurs.

A mucoid, whitish vaginal discharge is commonly seen during the newborn period and sometimes as late as 4 weeks after birth. The discharge is occasionally mixed with blood. This is the result of passive hormonal transfer from the mother and is an expected finding. Parental reassurance is often necessary.

Thin but difficult-to-separate adhesions between the labia minora are often seen during the first few months or even years of life. Sometimes they completely cover the vulvar vestibule. There may be just the smallest of openings through which urine can escape. These may require separation, using the gentlest of teasing or the application of estrogen creams.

Vaginal discharge in infants and young children may occur as the result of irritation from the diaper or powder. The discharge is usually mucoid.

⚘ Children

Indications for Examination

The extent of the gynecologic examination depends on the child's age and concerns or parental concerns. For the well child, the examination includes only inspection and palpation of the external genitalia. The internal vaginal examination is performed on a young child only when there is a specific problem such as bleeding, discharge, trauma, or suspected sexual abuse. Bubble bath vaginitis is common in young girls and does not require an internal examination. Speculum examination on a young child requires special equipment and an experienced and knowledgeable gynecologist or pediatrician.

The young child usually cooperates with examination of the external genitalia if your approach is very matter of fact. The very young child might prefer to lie in the parent's lap, with legs held in a frog position by the parent. The preschool child can be placed on the examining table, lying back against the head of the table, which should be raised about 30 degrees. The parent can help the child hold her legs up in a frog position.

A school-age child may not like the examination but is likely to cooperate if you take the time to reassure her that you will only look at and touch the outside. However, you must realize that a child in this circumstance, lying down, underpants off, will most often feel quite vulnerable. You might have the child help by taking her hand and first having her touch herself and even retracting the labia majora herself to help you. She should be positioned on the table on her back with her knees flexed and drawn up. The examination should be approached with the same degree of respect, explanation, and caution as with the adult woman.

It is always necessary to have a chaperone during examination of the genitalia.

Inspection and Palpation

Inspect the perineum, all the structures of the vulvar vestibule, and the urethral and vaginal orifices by separating the labia with the thumb and forefinger of one hand.

Adequate visualization of the interior of the vagina and the hymenal opening can be difficult in prepubertal girls. A technique that can be helpful is that of anterior labial traction. Firmly grasp both labia majora (not the minora) with the thumb and index finger of each hand, then gently but firmly pull the labia forward and slightly to the side. Gentle but firm traction will not cause discomfort. A previously obscured hymenal opening almost always becomes visible with this technique, as does the interior of the vagina, nearly to the cervix. Most foreign bodies are visible with this method. With the help of an assistant, a swab is easily inserted through the hymenal opening to obtain cultures if needed.

EXAMINATION AND FINDINGS

Bartholin and Skene glands are usually not palpable; if they are, enlargement exists. This indicates infection, which is most often (but not always) gonococcal. If there is concern about an imperforate hymen, ask the girl to cough, and as she does so, observe the hymen. An imperforate hymen will bulge, whereas one with an opening will not.

Discharge

Vaginal discharge often irritates the perineal tissues, causing redness and perhaps excoriation. Other sources of perineal irritation include bubble baths, soaps, detergents, and urinary tract infections. Carefully question the parent for a history of hematuria, dysuria, or other symptoms that would indicate urinary tract infection. A foul odor is more likely indicative of a foreign body (particularly in preschool children), especially if a secondary infection is present. Vaginal discharge may also result from trichomonal, gonococcal, or monilial infection.

Injuries

Swelling of vulvar tissues, particularly if accompanied by bruising or foul-smelling discharge, should alert you to the possibility of sexual abuse (Box 18-5). It must always be suspected if a young child has an STI or if there is injury to the external genitalia. Injuries to the softer structure of the external genitalia are not caused by bicycle seats. A straddle injury from a bicycle seat is generally evident over the symphysis pubis where the structures are more fixed. The injuries resulting from sexual abuse are generally more posterior and may involve the perineum grossly. The knee-chest position may be necessary for sexual abuse evaluation because it provides a clearer view of anatomic features.

Such findings cannot be ignored. Careful questioning of the parent or guardian is mandatory, as well as a report to the appropriate social service agencies for further investigation. In most cases of sexual abuse, the physical examination is normal. A normal examination does not rule out sexual abuse if there is suspicion.

Bleeding

Vaginal bleeding in children is often the result of unintentional injury, experimentation with a foreign body (e.g., toy), or sexual abuse. Rarely there may be an ovarian tumor or carcinoma of the cervix. Remember, too, that some girls may have precocious puberty and begin menstruation well before the expected time (Box 18-6). If this occurs, further evaluation is necessary.

Rectal Examination

On occasion, a rectal examination may be indicated to determine the presence or absence of the uterus or the presence of a foreign body in the vagina. The parent or guardian can assist and offer reassurance to the child during the examination. The rectal examination may be performed with the patient lying on her back, feet held together and knees bent up on the abdomen. Place one hand on the child's knees to steady her, slipping the gloved examining finger into the rectum. Most examiners prefer the index finger, but this is not mandatory. Once your finger is introduced, you may release the legs and use your free hand to simultaneously palpate the abdomen. If the child is old enough to

---

Box 18-5 Red Flags for Sexual Abuse

The following signs and symptoms in children or adolescents should raise your suspicion for sexual abuse. Remember, however, that any sign or symptom by itself is of limited significance; it may be related to sexual abuse, or it may be from another cause altogether. Also, the physical examination is often normal. This is an area in which good clinical judgment is imperative. Each sign or symptom must be considered in context with the particular child's health status, stage of growth and development, and entire history.

Medical Concerns and Findings
- Evidence of general physical abuse or neglect
- Evidence of trauma and/or scarring in genital, anal, and perianal areas
- Unusual changes in skin color or pigmentation in genital or anal area
- Presence of sexually transmitted infection (oral, anal, genital)
- Anorectal problems such as itching, bleeding, pain, fecal incontinence, poor anal sphincter tone, bowel habit dysfunction
- Genitourinary problems such as rash or sores in genital area, vaginal odor or discharge, pain (including abdominal pain), itching, bleeding, discharge, dysuria, hematuria, urinary tract infections, enuresis

Examples of Nonspecific Behavioral Manifestations
- Problems with school
- Dramatic weight changes or eating disturbances
- Depression
- Anxiety
- Sleep problems or nightmares
- Sudden change in personality or behavior
- Increased aggression and impulsivity, sudden avoidance of certain people or places

Examples of Sexual Behaviors That Are Concerning
- Use of sexually provocative mannerisms
- Excessive masturbation or sexual behavior that cannot be redirected
- Age-inappropriate sexual knowledge or experience
- Repeated object insertion into vagina and/or anus
- Child asking to be touched or kissed in genital area
- Sex play between children with 4 years or more age difference
- Sex play that involves the use of force, threats, or bribes

Modified from Hornor, 2004; Kellog, 2005; Koop, 1988; McClain et al, 2000.

Box 18-6 Causes of Genital Bleeding in Children

Vaginal bleeding during childhood is always clinically important and requires further evaluation. Common causes in children include the following:
- Genital lesions
- Vaginitis
- Foreign body
- Trauma
- Tumors
- Endocrine changes
- Estrogen ingestion
- Precocious puberty
- Hormone-producing ovarian tumor

cooperate, have her pant like a puppy to relax the muscles. A foreign body may be palpable, as well as the cervix. The ovaries are not usually felt. There may be bleeding and even a transient mild rectal prolapse after the examination, so be sure to warn the parent of this.

❧ Adolescents

The adolescent requires the same examination and positioning as the adult. Ask whether this is the young woman's first gynecologic examination. The first examination is perhaps the most important because it will set the stage for how she views future examinations. Take time to explain to her what you will be doing. Use models or illustrations to show her what will happen and what you will look for. Techniques such as deep breathing throughout the procedure, alternating tightening and relaxation of the perineal muscles, or progressive muscle relaxation may help the adolescent stay relaxed during the examination. An adolescent should be allowed the privacy of having the examination without her parent or guardian present, but a chaperone is always necessary. An interview without the parent is always necessary to obtain an accurate sexual history, including sexual abuse and intimate partner violence, and to discuss sexual play (see Chapter 1). This is typically conducted prior to the pelvic examination.

Choose the appropriate size speculum. A pediatric speculum with blades that are 1 to 1.5 cm wide can be used and should cause minimal discomfort. If the adolescent is sexually active, a small adult speculum may be used.

As the girl goes through puberty, you will see the maturational changes of sexual development (see Fig. 6-10, Chapter 6). Just before menarche there is a physiologic increase in vaginal secretions. The hymen may or may not be stretched across the vaginal opening. By menarche, the opening should be at least 1 cm wide. As the adolescent matures, the findings are the same as those for the adult.

❧ Pregnant Women

The gynecologic examination for the pregnant woman follows the same procedure as that for the nonpregnant adult woman. Assessment of pregnant women includes gestational age estimation, uterine size and contour, pelvic size estimates, and cervical dilation and length. Examination also includes fetal assessment: growth, position, and well-being. During labor, fetal station and head position are also assessed.

Gestational Age

Calculation is performed to determine the EDD. The Naegele rule is often used to calculate EDD: Add 1 year to the first day of the last normal menstrual period, subtract 3 months, and add 7 days.

The average duration of pregnancy is considered to be 280 days, or 40 weeks. The pregnancy is then divided into trimesters, each of which is slightly more than 13 weeks, or 3 calendar months. The clinically appropriate unit of measure, however, is weeks of gestation completed. Weeks of gestation completed can be easily calculated by using an obstetric wheel or an electronic pregnancy calculator.

Uterus Size and Contour

Estimate uterine size by manual measurement of fundal height. This technique provides an estimate for the length of the pregnancy, fetal growth, and gestational age. Have the patient empty her bladder before the procedure. Ask the patient to lie supine. Early uterine enlargement may not be symmetric, and you may feel deviation of the uterus to one side and an irregularity in its contour at the site of implantation. This uterine irregularity occurs around weeks 8 to 10 (Piskacek sign).

There is a lack of consensus about the accuracy of estimates of the size of the uterus at the various weeks; however, some estimate should be made. The size of various fruits is a common, although not reliable, means for describing the size of the uterus in early pregnancy. Centimeters are more accurate units of measurement and should be used as soon as possible. Table 18-2 provides estimates of uterine size.

With a nonstretchable tape measure, measure from the upper part of the pubic symphysis to the superior of the uterine fundus (Fig. 18-31). Record the measurement in centimeters. The same person should perform the measurement each time to decrease chances of individual variations.

This measurement is most accurate between 20 and 32 weeks of gestation when the fundal height in centimeters correlates well with the gestational age in weeks, ±2 cm. A 1-cm increase per week in fundal height is an expected pattern. Suspect twin pregnancy or other conditions that enlarge the uterus if during the second trimester the uterine size is larger than expected based on the EDD. A variation of more than 2 cm may indicate the need for further evaluation with an ultrasound. If the uterine size

Table 18-2	Estimates of Uterine Size in Early Pregnancy	
Weeks of Gestation	**Uterine Length (cm)**	**Uterine Width (cm)**
6	7.3 to 9.1	3.9
8	8.8 to 10.8	5.0
10	10.2 to 12.5	6.1
12	11.7 to 14.2	7.1
14	13.2 to 15.9	8.2

From Fox, 1985.

FIGURE 18-31 Measurement of fundal height from the symphysis pubis to the superior fundus uterus.

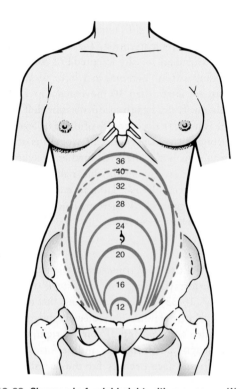

FIGURE 18-32 Changes in fundal height with pregnancy. Weeks 10 to 12: Uterus within pelvis; fetal heartbeat can be detected with Doppler. Week 12: Uterus palpable just above symphysis pubis. Week 16: Uterus palpable halfway between symphysis and umbilicus; ballottement of fetus is possible by abdominal and vaginal examination. Week 20: Uterine fundus at lower border of umbilicus; fetal heartbeat can be auscultated with a fetoscope. Weeks 24 to 26: Uterus changes from globular to ovoid shape; fetus palpable. Week 28: Uterus approximately halfway between umbilicus and xiphoid; fetus easily palpable. Week 34: Uterine fundus just below xiphoid. Week 40: Fundal height drops as fetus begins to engage in pelvis.

| Box 18-7 | Early Signs of Pregnancy |

The following are physical signs that occur early in pregnancy. These signs—along with internal ballottement, palpation of fetal parts, and positive test results for urine or serum human chorionic gonadotropin—are probable indicators of pregnancy. They are considered probable because clinical conditions other than pregnancy can cause any one of them. Their occurrence together, however, creates a strong case for the presence of a pregnancy.

Sign	Finding	Approximate Weeks of Gestation
Goodell	Softening of the cervix	4 to 6
Hegar	Softening of the uterine isthmus	6 to 8
McDonald	Fundus flexes easily on the cervix	7 to 8
Braun von Fernwald	Fullness and softening of the fundus near the site of implantation	7 to 8
Piskacek	Palpable lateral bulge or soft prominence of one uterine cornu	7 to 8
Chadwick	Bluish color of the cervix, vagina, and vulva	8 to 12

is smaller than expected, consider the possibility of intrauterine growth restriction. The accuracy of fundal height as a screening tool for intrauterine growth restriction is poor but can provide clinical suspicion indicating a need for sonography. Customized charts based on maternal height, weight, parity, and ethnicity are more accurate. Factors that can affect the accuracy of fundal height measurement are obesity, amount of amniotic fluid, myomata, multiple gestation, fetal size, and position of the uterus.

Changes in fundal height at the various weeks of gestation are shown in Figure 18-32, along with some changes that are detectable on examination.

Pelvic Examination

In early pregnancy you can feel a softening of the isthmus, whereas the cervix is still firm. In the second month of pregnancy, the cervix, vagina, and vulva acquire their bluish color from increased vascularity. The cervix itself softens and will feel more like lips than like the firmness of the nose tip. The fundus flexes easily on the cervix. There is slight fullness and softening of the fundus near the site of implantation. These findings are summarized in Box 18-7. You will notice increased vaginal secretions

as a result of increased vascularity. None of these findings is perfectly sensitive or specific for detecting pregnancy and should not replace human chorionic gonadotropin testing.

Cervical Effacement and Dilation

Other pregnancy conditions that are assessed during the pelvic examination include cervical effacement and dilation and effacement. Effacement refers to the thinning of the cervix that results when myometrial activity pulls the cervix upward, allowing the cervix to become part of the lower uterine segment during prelabor or early labor. The cervix is reduced in length. Ultrasonographic methods estimate its length at 3 to 4 cm at the end of the third trimester. Shortening of the cervix (less than 29 mm) noted on vaginal ultrasound in midpregnancy indicates risk for preterm delivery. Digital examinations are not as accurate as ultrasound and may miss the problem. The cervix gradually thins to only a few millimeters (paper thin). Record effacement in centimeters. Effacement usually precedes cervical dilation in the primipara and often occurs with dilation in the multipara.

Dilation involves the opening of the cervical canal to allow for the passage of the fetus. The process is measured in centimeters and progresses from a closed os (internal) to 10 cm, which is full or complete dilation. During labor, the time may vary among women for progression of cervical dilation related to parity, weeks of gestation (some dilation may be present late in pregnancy), and progress of labor.

Fetal Well-Being

Assessment of fetal well-being includes, but is not limited to, measurement of fetal heart rate (FHR) and fetal movement (FM). FHR is detected by Doppler by 11 to 12 weeks' gestation and heard by fetoscope at 19 to 20 weeks' gestation. Count the FHR or impulse for 1 minute, and compare it with the mother's pulse during that time. Note the quality and rhythm of the heart tones. Charting the results is sometimes done using a two-line figure in which the point of intersection is the umbilicus and the four quadrants are the maternal abdomen. Use an X or FHR to record the location of the maximal impulse on the maternal abdomen (see example below).

FM typically is appreciated by mothers between 16 and 20 weeks' gestation. Maternal assessment of FM can be used as an indicator of fetal well-being. Instruct the woman to note the pattern of movement over a given time. If the pattern shows a decrease, or if movement ceases, the woman should notify her health care provider immediately. One of the most commonly used techniques is the Cardiff count-to-10 method, where the woman counts 10 movements, noting the length of time for them to occur. There are no universally accepted FM count criteria, but the standard ranges from 10 times in 1 hour to 10 times in 12 hours. If there are fewer than 10 movements in 12 hours, the woman should notify her health care professional. If no monitoring technique is used, the occurrence of three or fewer FMs in 2 hours for 2 consecutive days while the woman is at rest in left lateral position signals the need for further evaluation of fetal well-being. If there are no identifiable risks of uteroplacental insufficiency, women may be asked to start recording FM between 34 and 36 weeks of gestation. If there are risk factors, monitoring should start as early as 28 weeks.

Fetal Position

In the latter half of the third trimester, assessment of fetal position can be performed using the four steps of the Leopold maneuvers (Fig. 18-33). After positioning the woman supine with her head slightly elevated and knees slightly flexed, place a small towel under her right hip. If you are right-handed, stand at the woman's right side facing her and perform the first three steps, then turn and face her feet for the last step; if you are

FIGURE 18-33 Leopold maneuvers. A, First maneuver. Place hand(s) over fundus and identify the fetal part. **B,** Second maneuver. Use the palmar surface of one hand to locate the back of the fetus. Use the other hand to feel the irregularities, such as hands and feet. **C,** Third maneuver. Use thumb and third finger to grasp presenting part over the symphysis pubis. **D,** Fourth maneuver. Use both hands to outline the fetal head. With a head presenting deep in the pelvis, only a small portion may be felt.

FIGURE 18-34 Abdominal palpation of twin pregnancy.

left-handed, stand on the woman's left for the first three steps, then turn and face her feet for the last step. The maneuvers are performed as follows:

1. Place hands over the fundus and identify the fetal part (Fig. 18-33, *A*). The head feels round, firm, and freely movable and is detectable by ballottement. The buttocks feel softer and less mobile and regular.
2. With the palmar surface of your hand, locate the back of the fetus by applying gentle but deep pressure (Fig. 18-33, *B*). The back feels smooth and convex, whereas the small parts (the feet, hands, knees, and elbows) will feel more irregular.
3. With the right hand (if you are right-handed) or with the left (if you are left-handed), using the thumb and third finger, gently grasp the presenting part over the symphysis pubis (Fig. 18-33, *C*). The head will feel firm and, if not engaged, will be movable from side to side and easily displaced upward. If the buttocks are presenting, they will feel softer. If the presenting part is not engaged, the fourth step is used.
4. Turn and face the woman's feet and use two hands to outline the fetal head (Fig. 18-33, *D*). If the head is presenting and is deep into the pelvis, only a small portion may be felt. Palpation of the cephalic prominence (the part of the fetus that prevents descent of the examiner's hand) on the same side as the small parts suggests that the head is flexed and the vertex

is presenting. This is the optimal position. Palpation of the cephalic prominence on the same side as the back suggests that the presenting part is extended.

When recording the information obtained from abdominal palpation, include the presenting part (i.e., vertex if the head, or breech if the buttocks), the lie (the relationship of the long axis of the fetus to the long axis of the mother) as longitudinal, transverse (perpendicular), or oblique, and the attitude of the fetal head if it is the presenting part (flexed or extended). With experience, you will also be able to estimate the weight of the fetus. A bedside ultrasound can confirm the position.

Twins are a variation, often suspected when there is the presence of two fetal heart tones or on abdominal palpation when a second set of fetal parts is detected. Diagnosis is made by ultrasound. The technique for abdominal palpation in twin pregnancy is depicted in Figure 18-34.

The FHR can also be used to estimate the position of the fetus. The areas of maximal intensity of the FHR and the position of the fetus are depicted in Figure 18-35.

Station

Station is the relationship of the presenting part to the ischial spines of the mother's pelvis. Vaginal examination and palpation are performed during labor to estimate the descent of the

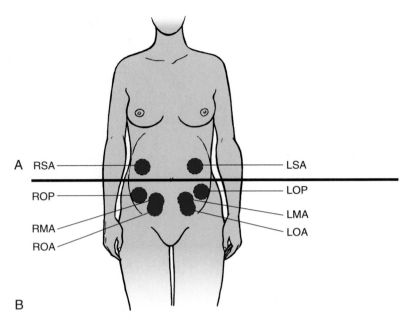

FIGURE 18-35 Areas of maximal intensity of fetal heart rate (FHR) for differing positions: *RSA*, right sacrum anterior; *ROP*, right occipitoposterior; *RMA*, right mentum anterior; *ROA*, right occipitoanterior; *LSA*, left sacrum anterior; *LOP*, left occipitoposterior; *LMA*, left mentum anterior; and *LOA*, left occipitoanterior. **A,** Presentation is breech if FHR is heard above umbilicus. **B,** Presentation is vertex if FHR is heard below umbilicus. *(From Lowdermilk et al, 1997.)*

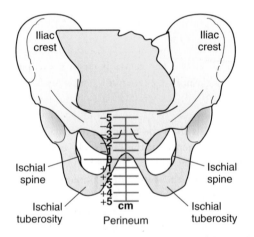

FIGURE 18-36 Stations of presenting part (degree of descent). Silhouette shows head of infant at station 0. *(Courtesy Ross Products Division, Abbott Laboratories Inc., Columbus, OH. From Lowdermilk and Perry, 2007.)*

presenting part. The measurement is determined by centimeters above and below the ischial spines and is recorded by plus and minus signs (Fig. 18-36). For example, the station at 1 cm below the spines is recorded as a +1, at the spines as a 0, and at 1 cm above the spines as a −1. Record (in centimeters) the routine cervical examination findings for dilation, cervical length, and station, in that order.

Contractions

Uterine contractions may begin as early as the third month of gestation and are called Braxton Hicks contractions. They may go unnoticed by the woman but may become painful at times, especially as the pregnancy progresses and with increased gravidity. The regular occurrence of more than 4 to 6 uterine contractions per hour before 37 weeks of gestation requires evaluation.

You can assess uterine contractions with abdominal palpation, but more accuracy is obtained through the use of electronic monitoring equipment, either indirectly through the abdominal wall or directly with the placement of an intrauterine pressure catheter. Assessment through abdominal palpation is helpful when equipment is not available to determine the onset or course of labor, either preterm or term. Practice is needed to determine the difference between mild, moderate, and strong contractions. Place the fingertips on the abdomen so that you are able to detect the contraction and relaxation of the uterus, and keep them there throughout the entire contraction, including the period of relaxation.

The strength of the contraction is classified as follows:

Mild: slightly tense fundus that is easy to indent with the fingertips

Moderate: firm fundus that is difficult to indent with the fingertips

Strong: rigid or hard, boardlike fundus or one that does not indent with fingertips

The duration of the contraction is measured in seconds from the beginning until relaxation occurs. The frequency of contractions is measured from the beginning of one contraction to the beginning of the next. The frequency of contractions is assessed for regularity (at regular intervals, such as every 5 minutes, or at irregular or sporadic intervals). Each woman's experience of the discomfort created by the contracting uterus varies because of physiologic makeup, past experiences, cultural

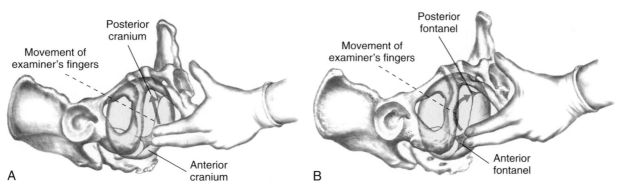

FIGURE 18-37 A, Locating the sagittal suture on vaginal examination. **B,** Differentiating the fontanels on vaginal examination.

influences, expectations, prenatal education, support, and other factors. Her sense of the event should not be discounted based on physiologic and subjective measures.

Fetal Head Position

The position of the fetal head can be determined by vaginal examination once dilation has begun. Insert your fingers anteriorly into the posterior aspect of the vagina and then move your fingers upward over the fetal head as you turn them, locating the sagittal suture with the posterior and anterior fontanels at either end (Fig. 18-37, *A*). The position of the fontanels is determined by examining the anterior aspect of the sagittal suture and then using a circular motion to pass alongside the head until the other fontanel is felt and differentiated (Fig. 18-37, *B*). The position of the face and breech are easier to determine because the various parts are more distinguishable.

Other Pregnancy-Associated Changes

The uterus may become more anteflexed during the first 3 months from softening of the isthmus. As a result, the fundus may press on the urinary bladder, causing the woman to experience urinary frequency.

Vulvar varicosities occur commonly during pregnancy. The varicosities may involve both the vulva and the rectal area. Pressure from the pregnant uterus and possibly hereditary factors contribute to the formation of the varicosities.

Breast and skin changes that occur with pregnancy are discussed in Chapters 8 and 16.

♣ Older Adults

The temptation with older women is to defer the examination because of their age. This is often not appropriate. The examination procedure for the older woman is the same as that for the woman of childbearing age, with a few modifications for comfort. The older woman may require more time and assistance to assume the lithotomy position. She may need assistance from another individual to help hold her legs, because they may tire easily when the hip joints remain in abduction for an extended period. Patients with orthopnea will need to have their head and chest elevated during examination. You may need to use a smaller speculum, depending on the degree of introital constriction that occurs with aging.

Note that the labia appear flatter and smaller, corresponding with the degree of loss of subcutaneous fat elsewhere on the body. The skin is drier and shinier than that of a younger adult, and the pubic hair is gray and may be sparse. The clitoris is smaller than that of a younger adult.

The urinary meatus may appear as an irregular opening or slit. It may be located more posteriorly than in younger women, very near or within the vaginal introitus, as a result of relaxed perineal musculature.

The vaginal introitus may be constricted and may admit only one finger. In some multiparous older women, the introitus may gape, with the vaginal walls rolling toward the opening.

The vagina is narrower and shorter, and you will see and feel the absence of rugae. The cervix is smaller and paler than in younger women, and the surrounding fornices may be smaller or absent. The cervix may seem less mobile if it protrudes less far into the vaginal canal. The os may be smaller but should still be palpable.

The uterus diminishes in size and may not be palpable, and the ovaries are rarely palpable because of atrophy. Ovaries that are palpable should be considered suspicious for tumor, and additional workup to exclude cancer is required.

The rectovaginal septum will feel thin, smooth, and pliable. Anal sphincter tone may be somewhat diminished. As the pelvic musculature relaxes, look particularly for stress incontinence and prolapse of the vaginal walls or uterus.

As with younger women, as you inspect and palpate you are evaluating for signs of inflammation (older women are particularly susceptible to atrophic vaginitis), infection, trauma, tenderness, masses, nodules, enlargement, irregularity, and changes in consistency.

♣ Women with Disabilities

Preparation

The health care provider and/or woman with disabilities can do a number of things to promote a comfortable pelvic examination experience. See Chapter 3 for a discussion of common approaches to patients with mobility or sensory impairments and patients with spinal cord injury or lesions.

FIGURE 18-38 The knee-chest position.

FIGURE 18-39 The diamond-shaped position.

FIGURE 18-40 The obstetric stirrups position.

Alternative Positions for the Pelvic Examination

A number of alternatives in positioning for the pelvic examination are possible. The woman is the best judge of which position will work for her and how to use assistants most effectively. These decisions should be made by the patient and the health care provider together.

An assistant will help the woman and the health care provider facilitate a comfortable, thorough pelvic examination. For example, the assistant may help the woman position herself on the examination table. At least one assistant should be available throughout the examination in addition to the health care provider. The assistant might be a staff member or an attendant or friend of the patient.

Many women cannot comfortably assume the traditional (lithotomy) pelvic examination position. A woman who experiences one or more conditions such as joint stiffness, pain, paralysis, or lack of muscle control may require the use of an alternative position.

Knee-Chest Position. In the knee-chest position, the woman lies on her side with both knees bent, with her top leg brought closer to her chest (Fig. 18-38). A variation of this position would allow the woman to lie with her bottom leg straightened while the top leg is still bent close to her chest. Insert the speculum with the handle pointed in the direction of the woman's abdomen or back. Because the woman is lying on her side, be sure to angle the speculum toward the small of the patient's back and not straight up toward her head. Once the speculum has been removed, the woman will need to roll onto her back.

The assistant may provide support for the patient while she is on the examination table, help the woman straighten her bottom leg if she prefers the variation of this position, or support the patient in rolling onto her back for the bimanual examination. If the patient cannot separate her legs, the assistant may help her elevate one leg.

The knee-chest position does not require the use of stirrups. It is particularly good for a woman who feels most comfortable and balanced lying on her side.

Diamond-Shaped Position. In the diamond-shaped position, the woman lies on her back with her knees bent so that both legs are spread flat and her heels meet at the foot of the table (Fig. 18-39). Insert the speculum with the handle up and perform the bimanual examination from the side or foot of the table.

The assistant may help the patient support herself on the table and hold her feet together in alignment with her spine to maintain this position. A woman may be more comfortable using pillows or an assistant to elevate her thighs and/or using a pillow under the small of the back.

The diamond-shaped position does not require the use of stirrups. A woman must be able to lie flat on her back to use this position. You can also use the diamond-shaped position with children.

Obstetric Stirrups Position. In the obstetric stirrups position, the woman lies on her back near the foot of the table with her legs supported under the knee by obstetric stirrups (Fig. 18-40). Insert the speculum with the handle down and perform the bimanual examination from the foot of the table.

The patient may require assistance in putting her legs into the stirrups. The stirrups can be padded to increase comfort and reduce irritation. A strap can be attached to each stirrup to hold a woman's legs securely in place if the woman prefers this increased support.

Obstetric stirrups provide much more support than the traditionally used foot stirrups. This position allows a woman who has difficulty using the foot stirrups to assume the traditional pelvic examination position.

M-Shaped Position. In the M-shaped position, the woman lies on her back, knees bent and apart, and feet resting on the examination table close to her buttocks (Fig. 18-41). Insert the

FIGURE 18-41 The M-shaped position.

FIGURE 18-43 Positioning the visually impaired woman.

FIGURE 18-42 The V-shaped position.

FIGURE 18-44 Positioning the hearing-impaired woman.

speculum with the handle up and perform the bimanual examination from the foot of the table.

If the woman feels her legs are not completely stable on the examination table, an assistant may support her feet or knees. If a woman has had bilateral leg amputations, assistants may elevate her residual limbs to simulate this position.

The M-shaped position does not require the use of stirrups. This position allows the patient to lie with her entire body supported by the table.

V-Shaped Position. In the V-shaped position, the woman lies on her back with her straightened legs separated widely to either side of the table (Fig. 18-42). If a woman is able to put one foot in the stirrup, a variation of this position would allow the woman to hold one leg out straight and keep one foot in a stirrup. Insert the speculum with the handle up, and perform the bimanual examination from the side or foot of the table.

At least one and possibly two assistants are needed to enable the woman to maintain this position. The assistants should

support each straightened leg at the knee and ankle. The patient may be more comfortable if her legs are slightly elevated or if a pillow is used under the small of her back or tailbone.

The V-shaped position may or may not require stirrups. The patient must be able to lie comfortably on her back to use this position.

Women with Sensory Impairment

A woman with visual or hearing impairment will probably want to utilize the usual foot-stirrup position for the pelvic examination (Figs. 18-43 and 18-44). Before the examination, you can ask the patient if she would like to examine the speculum, swab, or other instruments that will be used during the examination. If three-dimensional genital models are available, they can be used to familiarize the woman with the examination process. You may elevate the head of the table for a woman with a hearing impairment so that she can see the health care provider and/or interpreter. The drape that is used to cover the woman's body below her waist should be kept low between her legs.

Sample Documentation

History and Physical Examination

Subjective

A 45-year-old female with vaginal discharge and itching for the past week. Has had several yeast infections before. No history of sexually transmitted infections. Completed course of antibiotics for sinusitis 2 days ago. LMP 2 weeks ago. Sexually active, one partner, mutually monogamous. No unusual vaginal bleeding. Does not douche.

Objective

External: Hair in female hair pattern distribution; no masses, lesions, or swelling. Urethral meatus intact without erythema or discharge. Perineum intact with a healed episiotomy scar present. No lesions.

Internal: Vaginal mucosa pink and moist with rugae present. No unusual odors. Profuse thick, white, curdy discharge present in vaginal vault. Cervix pink with horizontal slit, midline; no lesions or discharge.

Bimanual: Cervix smooth, firm, mobile. No cervical motion tenderness. Uterus midline, anteverted, firm, smooth, and nontender; not enlarged. Ovaries not palpable. No adnexal tenderness.

Rectovaginal: Septum intact. Sphincter tone intact; anal ring smooth and intact. No masses or tenderness. Rectal exam confirms bimanual findings.

For additional sample documentation, see Chapter 26, pp. 628-631.

ABNORMALITIES

FEMALE GENITALIA

Premenstrual Syndrome (PMS)

A collection of physical, psychologic, and mood symptoms related to a woman's menstrual cycle

Pathophysiology

- Etiology unclear; likely causes include hormonal factors and responses to hormonal factors.
- Usually begins in a woman's late 20s and increases in incidence and severity as menopause approaches

Subjective Data

- Symptoms may include breast swelling and tenderness, acne, bloating and weight gain, headache or joint pain, food cravings, irritability, difficulty concentrating, mood swings, crying spells, and depression.
- Symptoms occur 5 to 7 days before menses (luteal phase) and subside with onset of menses.

Objective Data

- None
- Diagnosis based on symptoms and temporal relationship to menstrual cycle

Infertility

The inability to conceive over a period of 1 year of unprotected sexual intercourse

Pathophysiology

- Many causes, including both male and female conditions
- Contributing factors in the woman include abnormalities of the vagina, cervix, uterus, fallopian tubes, and ovaries.
- Male infertility can be caused by insufficient, nonmotile, or immature sperm; ductal obstruction of sperm; and transport-related factors.
- Factors influencing fertility in both women and men include stress, nutrition, chemical substances, chromosomal abnormalities, certain disease processes, sexual and relationship problems, and hematologic and immunologic disorders.

Subjective Data

- Unsuccessful attempts to become pregnant

Objective Data

- Varies with underlying cause
- Often no findings on physical examination

Endometriosis

The presence and growth of endometrial tissue outside the uterus (Figs. 18-45 and 18-46)

Pathophysiology

- Pathogenesis not definitive
- Thought to be due to retrograde reflux of menstrual tissue from the fallopian tubes during menstruation

Subjective Data

- Pelvic pain, dysmenorrhea, and heavy or prolonged menstrual flow

Objective Data

- No findings
- On bimanual examination, tender nodules may be palpable along the uterosacral ligaments.
- Diagnosis confirmed by laparoscopy

FIGURE 18-45 Endometriosis. *(From Fedele et al, 2005.)*

FIGURE 18-46 **Common sites of endometriosis.** *(From Stenchever et al, 2001.)*

LESIONS FROM SEXUALLY TRANSMITTED INFECTIONS

Condyloma Acuminatum (Genital Warts)

Warty lesions due to sexually transmitted infection with HPV

Pathophysiology

- HPV invades the basal layer of the epidermis; virus penetrates through skin and causes mucosal microabrasions
- Latent viral phase begins with no signs or symptoms and can last from a month to several years
- Following latency, viral DNA, capsids, and particles are produced; host cells become infected and develop the characteristic skin lesions.
- Considered a sexually transmitted infection

Subjective Data

- Soft, painless, wartlike lesions
- History of sexual contact

Objective Data

- Flesh-colored, whitish pink to reddish brown, discrete, soft growths on labia, vestibule or perianal area (Fig. 18-47)
- Lesions may occur singly or in clusters and may enlarge to form cauliflower-like masses.

FIGURE 18-47 **Condyloma acumi-natum.** *(From Morse et al, 2003.)*

Molluscum Contagiosum

Viral infection of the skin and mucous membranes; considered a sexually transmitted infection in adults, in contrast to the common non–sexually transmitted infection occurring in young children (Fig. 18-48)

Pathophysiology

- Caused by a poxvirus, the virus enters the skin through small breaks of hair follicles.
- Spreads through direct person-to-person contact and through contact with contaminated object
- After incubation period, growths appear.
- Genital lesions are sexually transmitted.

Subjective Data

- Painless lesions in genital area
- Sexually active

Objective Data

- White or flesh-colored, dome-shaped papules that are round or oval
- Surface has a characteristic central umbilication from which a thick creamy core can be expressed
- Lesions may last from several months to several years.
- Diagnosis usually based on the clinical appearance of the lesions
- Direct microscopic examination of stained material from the core will reveal typical molluscum bodies within the epithelial cell.

FIGURE 18-48 **Molluscum contagiosum.** Note that these have occurred around the eyes. *(Courtesy Walter Tunnesen, MD, Chapel Hill, NC.)*

Syphilitic Chancre

Skin lesion associated with primary syphilis

Pathophysiology

- Sexually transmitted infection caused by the bacterium *Treponema pallidum*
- Transmitted through direct contact with a syphilis sore
- Lesions of primary syphilis generally occur 2 weeks after exposure.
- Chancre lasts 3 to 6 weeks, heals without treatment

Subjective Data

- Often no lesion noted, as may be internal (Fig. 18-49)
- Painless genital ulcer
- Sexually active

Objective Data

- Solitary lesion; firm, round, small, painless ulcer
- Lesion has indurated borders with a clear base
- Scrapings from the ulcer, examined microscopically, show spirochetes.

FIGURE 18-49 Primary syphilitic chancre in vagina.

Condyloma Latum

Lesions of secondary syphilis

Pathophysiology

- Sexually transmitted infection caused by the bacterium *T. pallidum*
- Appear about 6 to 12 weeks after infection

Subjective Data

- Healed solitary genital lesion
- Sexually active

Objective Data

- Flat, round, or oval papules covered by a gray exudate (Fig. 18-50)

FIGURE 18-50 Condyloma latum.
(From Lemmi and Lemmi, 2000.)

ABNORMALITIES

Genital Herpes

Genital herpes is a sexually transmitted viral infection of the skin and mucosa.

Pathophysiology

- Caused by the herpes simplex virus (HSV)
- Most transmission of HSV occurs when individuals shed virus in the absence of symptoms.

Subjective Data

- Painful lesions in genital area
- History of sexual contact
- May report burning or pain with urination

Objective Data

- Superficial vesicles in the genital area; internal or external (Figs. 18-51 and 18-52); may be eroded
- Initial infection is often extensive, whereas recurrent infection is usually confined to a small localized patch on the vulva, perineum, vagina, or cervix

FIGURE 18-51 Herpes lesions. Scattered erosions covered with exudate. *(From Habif, 2004.)*

FIGURE 18-52 Herpetic cervicitis. Erythema, purulent exudate, and erosions are present on the cervix. *(From Morse et al, 2003.)*

VULVA AND VAGINA

Inflammation of Bartholin Gland

Pathophysiology

- Commonly, but not always, caused by *Neisseria gonorrhea*
- May be acute or chronic

Subjective Data

- Pain and swelling in the groin

Objective Data

- Hot, red, tender, fluctuant swelling of the Bartholin gland that may drain pus (Fig. 18-53)
- Chronic inflammation results in a nontender cyst on the labium.

FIGURE 18-53 Inflammation of Bartholin gland. *(A, From Elsevier; B, from Swartz, 2006.)*

Vaginal Carcinoma

Classified according to the type of tissue from which the cancer arises: squamous cell, adenocarcinoma, melanoma, and sarcoma

Pathophysiology

- Squamous cell carcinoma begins in the epithelial lining of the vagina; may be caused by HPV; develops over a period of many years from precancerous changes called vaginal intraepithelial neoplasia (VAIN)
- Adenocarcinoma begins in the glandular tissue.
- Malignant melanoma develops from pigment-producing cells called melanocytes.
- Sarcomas form deep in the wall of the vagina, not on its surface epithelium.

Subjective Data

- Abnormal vaginal bleeding
- Difficult or painful urination
- Pain during sexual intercourse
- Pain in the pelvic area, back, or legs
- Edema in the legs
- Risk factor includes patient's mother having taken DES during pregnancy

Objective Data

- Vaginal discharge, lesions, and masses
- Melanoma tends to affect the lower or outer portion of the vagina.
- Tumors vary greatly in size, color, and growth pattern.
- Diagnosis is based on tissue biopsy.

ABNORMALITIES

Vulvar Carcinoma

Classified according to the type of tissue from which the cancer arises: squamous cell, adenocarcinoma, melanoma, and basal cell

Pathophysiology

- Squamous cell carcinoma arises from epithelial cells; most common form of vulvar cancer
- Adenocarcinoma starts in the Bartholin glands or vulvar sweat glands and accounts for a small percentage of vulvar cancer cases.
- Melanoma accounts for about 2% to 4% of vulvar cancer; women with melanoma on other parts of their body have an increased risk of developing vulvar melanoma.
- Basal cell carcinoma, common on sun-exposed areas, is a rare form of vulvar cancer.

Subjective Data

- Lump or growth in or on the vulvar area or a patch of skin that is differently textured or colored
- Ulcer that persists for longer than 1 month
- Bleeding from vulvar area
- Change in the appearance of an existing mole (specific to vulvar melanoma)
- Persistent itching, pain, soreness, or burning in the vulvar area
- Painful urination

Objective Data

- Squamous cell carcinoma: ulcerated or raised lesion on the vulva; usually found on the labia (Fig. 18-54, *A*)
- Adenocarcinoma: ulcerated or raised lesion usually found on the sides of the vaginal opening
- Melanoma: dark-colored lesion most often on the clitoris or the labia minora
- Basal cell: ulcerated lesion (Fig. 18-54, *B*)
- Diagnosis is based on tissue biopsy

FIGURE 18-54 A, Ulcerative squamous cell carcinoma of the vulva. **B,** Basal cell carcinoma of the vulva. *(From Symonds and Macpherson, 1994.)*

Vaginal Infections

Vaginal infections often produce a discharge (Figs. 18-55 and 18-56); see Differential Diagnosis table.

FIGURE   18-55 Trichomoniasis.   The vaginal mucosa is inflamed and often speckled with petechial lesions. In adolescents, petechial hemorrhages may also be found on the cervix, resulting in the so-called strawberry cervix. *(From Zitelli and Davis, 2007.)*

FIGURE 18-56 Microscopic differentiation of vaginal infections. A, Bacterial vaginosis: "clue cells." **B,** Candida vulvovaginitis: "budding, branching hyphae." **C,** Trichomoniasis: motile trichomonads. *(From Zitelli and Davis, 2007.)*

ABNORMALITIES

DIFFERENTIAL DIAGNOSIS
Vaginal Discharges and Infections

Condition	History	Physical Findings	Diagnostic Tests
Physiologic vaginitis	Increase in discharge	Clear or mucoid discharge	Wet mount: up to 3 to 5 WBCs; epithelial cells
Bacterial vaginosis (*Gardnerella vaginalis*)	No foul odor, itching or edema Foul-smelling discharge; complains of "fishy odor"	Homogenous thin, white or gray discharge; pH >4.5	+ KOH "whiff" test; wet mount: + clue cells (see Fig. 18-56, *A*)
Candida vulvovaginitis (*Candida albicans*)	Pruritic discharge; itching of labia; itching may extend to thighs	White, curdy discharge; pH 4.0 to 5.0; cervix may be red; may have erythema of perineum and thighs	KOH prep: mycelia, budding, branching yeast, pseudohyphae (see Fig. 18-56, *B*)
Trichomoniasis (*Trichomonas vaginalis*)	Watery discharge; foul odor; dysuria and dyspareunia with severe infection	Profuse, frothy, greenish discharge; pH 5.0 to 6.6; red friable cervix with petechiae ("strawberry" cervix) (see Fig. 18-55)	Wet mount: round or pear-shaped protozoa; motile "gyrating" flagella (see Fig. 18-56, *C*)
Gonorrhea (*Neisseria gonorrhoeae*)	Partner with STI; often asymptomatic or may have symptoms of PID	Purulent discharge from cervix; Skene/Bartholin gland inflammation; cervix and vulva may be inflamed	Gram stain Culture DNA probe
Chlamydia (*Chlamydia trachomatis*)	Partner with nongonococcal urethritis; often asymptomatic; may complain of spotting after intercourse or urethritis	± Purulent discharge; cervix may or may not be red or friable	DNA probe
Atrophic vaginitis	Dyspareunia; vaginal dryness; perimenopausal or postmenopausal	Pale, thin vaginal mucosa; pH >4.5	Wet mount: folded, clumped epithelial cells
Allergic vaginitis	New bubble bath, soap, douche, or other hygiene products	Foul smell; erythema; pH may be altered	Wet mount: WBCs
Foreign body	Red and swollen vulva; vaginal discharge; history of use of tampon, condom, or diaphragm	Bloody or foul-smelling discharge	Wet mount: WBCs

KOH, Potassium hydroxide; *PID,* pelvic inflammatory disease; *STI,* sexually transmitted infection; *WBC,* white blood cell.

CERVIX

Cervical Cancer

Classified according to the type of tissue from which the cancer arises: squamous cell carcinoma and adenocarcinoma. There are a few other rare types of cervical cancer.

Pathophysiology
- Typically originates from a dysplastic or premalignant lesion present at the active squamocolumnar junction
- Lesions gradually progress through recognizable stages before developing into invasive disease.
- The transformation from mild dysplastic to invasive carcinoma generally occurs slowly over several years.
- HPV is now recognized as the most important causative agent in cervical carcinogenesis at the molecular level.
- HPV vaccine is available.

Subjective Data
- Usually asymptomatic
- May report unexpected vaginal bleeding or spotting

Objective Data
- Often no findings on physical examination
- A hard granular surface at or near the cervical os
- Lesion can evolve to form an extensive irregular cauliflower growth that bleeds easily (Fig. 18-57)
- Early lesions are indistinguishable from ectropion.
- Ulcerated area
- Precancerous and early cancer changes are detected by Pap smear, not by physical examination.

ABNORMALITIES

FIGURE 18-57   The cervical cancer lesion is predominantly around the external os. *(From Symonds and Macpherson, 1994.)*

UTERUS

Uterine Prolapse

Descent or herniation of the uterus into or beyond the vagina

Pathophysiology

- Result of weakening of the supporting structures of the pelvic floor, often occurring concurrently with a cystocele and rectocele
- Uterus becomes progressively retroverted and descends into the vaginal canal (Fig. 18-58)

Subjective Data

- Sensation of pelvic heaviness and/or uterus falling out
- Tissue protruding from vagina
- May report urine leakage or urge incontinence, difficulty having a bowel, movement, or low back pain

Objective Data

- First-degree prolapse: The cervix remains within the vagina.
- Second-degree prolapse: The cervix is at the introitus.
- Third-degree prolapse: The cervix and vagina drop outside the introitus (Fig. 18-59).

FIGURE 18-58 Uterine prolapse. A, Expected uterine position. **B,** First-degree prolapse of the uterus. **C,** Second-degree prolapse of the uterus. **D,** Complete prolapse of the uterus.

FIGURE 18-59 A third-degree prolapse of the uterus and vaginal walls. *(From Symonds and Macpherson, 1994.)*

Uterine Bleeding

Abnormality in menstrual bleeding and inappropriate uterine bleeding are common gynecologic problems (Table 18-3)

Pathophysiology	Subjective Data	Objective data
Dysfunctional uterine bleeding: • Abnormal uterine bleeding in the absence of disease in the pelvis, pregnancy, or medical illness. 90% caused by anovulation; 10% ovulatory in origin—can be caused by dysfunction of corpus luteum or midcycle bleeding • Endocrinopathies such as polycystic ovary syndrome, thyroid dysfunction, and hyperprolactinemia produce bleeding as a result of imbalance of the hypothalamic-pituitary-ovarian (HPO) axis. • Coagulopathies can produce uterine bleeding.	Dysfunctional uterine bleeding: • Shortened or lengthened interval between periods • Absence of menstruation • Normal intervals between periods with excessive flow and/or duration or decreased flow • Irregular intervals between periods with excessive flow and duration • Bleeding between periods; see Box 18-1.	Dysfunctional uterine bleeding: • None Endocrinopathies: • Pelvic examination normal; other physical findings consistent with the endocrine disorder Coagulopathies: • Findings consistent with the specific coagulopathy
Pregnancy-related: • Pregnancy implantation, placental abnormalities, threatened abortion and ectopic pregnancy	Pregnancy-related: • Vaginal bleeding • Pain may or may not be present.	Pregnancy-related: • Findings consistent with stage of pregnancy
Reproductive tract disorders: • Leiomyomas, reproductive tract infection, and malignancy can produce bleeding (see specific abnormalities).	Reproductive tract disorders: • See specific abnormalities.	Reproductive tract disorders: • See specific abnormalities

Table 18-3	Types of Uterine Bleeding and Associated Causes	
Type	**Common Causes**	
Mid-cycle spotting	Mid-cycle estradiol fluctuation associated with ovulation	
Delayed menstruation	Anovulation or threatened abortion with excessive bleeding	
Frequent bleeding	Chronic PID, endometriosis, DUB, anovulation	
Profuse menstrual bleeding	Endometrial polyps, DUB, adenomyosis, submucous bleeding leiomyomas, IUD	
Intermenstrual or irregular bleeding	Endometrial polyps, DUB, uterine or cervical cancer, oral contraceptives	
Postmenopausal bleeding	Endometrial hyperplasia, estrogen therapy, endometrial cancer	

Modified from Thompson et al, 1997.
DUB, Dysfunctional uterine bleeding; *IUD*, intrauterine device; *PID*, pelvic inflammatory disease.

Myomas (Leiomyomas, Fibroids)

Common, benign, uterine tumors (Fig. 18-60)

Pathophysiology	Subjective Data	Objective Data

• Arise from the overgrowth of smooth muscle and connective tissue in the uterus
• May occur singly or in multiples and vary greatly in size
	• Fibroid symptoms are related to the number of tumors, as well as to their size and location. Symptoms may include the following:
	  • Heavy menses
	  • Abdominal cramping usually felt during menstruation
	  • Urinary frequency, urgency, and/or incontinence from pressure on the bladder
	  • Constipation, difficult defecation, or rectal pain from pressure on the colon
	  • Abdominal cramping from pressure on the small bowel
	  • Generalized pelvic and/or lower abdominal discomfort
		• Firm, irregular nodules in the contour of the uterus on bimanual examination
		• Uterus may be enlarged

ABNORMALITIES

FIGURE 18-60 **Myomas of the uterus (fibroids). A,** Common location of myomas. **B,** Multiple uterine fibroids. **C,** Multiple uterine fibroids with enlarged ovaries resulting from multiple small cysts. *(B, C from Symonds and Macpherson, 1994.)*

Endometrial Cancer

Pathophysiology

- Occurs most often in postmenopausal women
- Nearly all endometrial cancers are cancers of the glandular cells found in the lining of the uterus; most known risk factors for endometrial cancer are linked to the imbalance between estrogen and progesterone in the body.
- Women taking tamoxifen are at increased risk.

Subjective Data

- Postmenopausal vaginal bleeding—red flag for endometrial cancer

Objective Data

- None; diagnosed by endometrial biopsy

ADNEXA

Ovarian Cysts

Fluid-filled sac in an ovary (Fig. 18-61)

Pathophysiology

- Follicle undergoes varying rates of maturation and cysts can occur as the result of hypothalamic-pituitary dysfunction or because of native anatomic defects in the reproductive system.
- Can occur unilaterally or bilaterally
- Can be present from the neonatal period to postmenopause
- Most ovarian cysts occur during infancy and adolescence, which are hormonally active periods of development.
- Most are functional in nature and resolve with minimal treatment.

Subjective Data

- Usually asymptomatic
- May report lower abdominal pain: sharp, intermittent, sudden, and severe
- Sudden onset of abdominal pain may suggest cyst rupture

Objective Data

- Pelvic mass may be palpated
- Cervical motion tenderness may be elicited.
- Often an incidental finding during ultrasonography performed for other reasons

One or both sides, usually nontender

FIGURE 18-61 **Ovarian cyst.** *(Photograph from Symonds and Macpherson, 1994.)*

Ovarian Cancer

Classified by the cells from which the cancer arises: epithelial, stromal, or germ cell

Pathophysiology	Subjective Data	Objective Data
• Epithelial tumors: arise from a layer of germinal epithelium on the outside of the ovary; most common form of ovarian cancer • Stromal tumors develop from connective tissue cells that help form the structure of the ovary and produce hormones. • Germ cell tumors arise from germ cells (cells that produce the egg); develop most often in young women (including teenage girls)	• Often asymptomatic at first • Suspect ovarian cancer in a woman older than 40 years with persistent and unexplained vague gastrointestinal symptoms such as generalized abdominal discomfort and/or pain, gas, indigestion, pressure, swelling, bloating, cramps, or feeling of fullness even after a light meal.	• May have no physical findings • On bimanual examination, an ovary that is enlarged in premenopausal woman or a palpable ovary in a postmenopausal woman should be considered suspicious for cancer. • Further diagnostic tests are required.

Tubal (Ectopic) Pregnancy

Ectopic pregnancy occurring outside the uterus

Pathophysiology	Subjective Data	Objective Data
• Most common site is in one of the fallopian tubes but can occur in other areas. • Ectopic pregnancy usually caused by a condition that blocks or slows the movement of a fertilized egg through the fallopian tube to the uterus • May be caused by a physical blockage in the tube; most cases from scarring caused by past ectopic pregnancy, past infection in the fallopian tubes, pelvic inflammatory disease, or surgery of the fallopian tubes	• Abnormal vaginal bleeding • Low back pain • Mild cramping on one side of the pelvis • Pain in the lower abdomen or pelvic area • If the area of the abnormal pregnancy ruptures and bleeds, symptoms may worsen. • Feeling lightheaded or syncope • Pain that is felt in the shoulder area • Severe, sharp, and sudden pain in the lower abdomen	• Marked pelvic tenderness, with tenderness and rigidity of the lower abdomen • Cervical motion tenderness; a tender, unilateral adnexal mass may indicate the site of the pregnancy (Fig. 18-62) • Tachycardia and hypotension reflect hemorrhage of a ruptured tubal pregnancy into the peritoneal cavity and impending cardiovascular collapse. • A ruptured tubal pregnancy is a surgical emergency.

Unilateral, tender

Movement of cervix painful

FIGURE 18-62 **Ruptured tubal pregnancy.**

Pelvic Inflammatory Disease (PID)

Infection of the uterus, fallopian tubes, and other reproductive organs; a common and serious complication of some sexually transmitted infections (Fig. 18-63)

Pathophysiology

- Often caused by *Neisseria gonorrhoeae* and *Chlamydia trachomatis*
- May be acute or chronic

Subjective Data

- Symptoms may be mild or absent.
- Unusual vaginal discharge that may have a foul odor
- Symptoms include painful intercourse, painful urination, irregular menstrual bleeding, and pain in the right upper abdomen.

Objective Data

- Acute PID produces very tender, bilateral adnexal areas; the patient guards and usually cannot tolerate bimanual examination.
- Symptoms of chronic PID are bilateral, tender, irregular, and fairly fixed adnexal areas.

FIGURE 18-63 Pelvic inflammatory disease. Photograph shows sheet of fine adhesions covering the fallopian tubes and ovary, which is buried beneath the fallopian tubes. *(Photograph from Symonds and Macpherson, 1994.)*

Salpingitis

Inflammation or infection of the fallopian tubes, often associated with PID; can be acute or chronic (Fig. 18-64)

Pathophysiology

- Most cases of acute salpingitis occur in two stages: the first involves acquisition of a vaginal or cervical infection; the second involves ascent of the infection to the upper genital tract.
- Organisms most commonly associated with acute salpingitis are *Neisseria gonorrhoeae* and *C. trachomatis*

Subjective Data

- Lower quadrant pain; constant and dull or cramping; pain may be accentuated by motion or sexual activity; coexisting purulent vaginal discharge; abnormal vaginal bleeding, nausea, vomiting, fever

Objective Data

- Cervical motion tenderness and/or adnexal tenderness on bimanual examination
- Mucopurulent cervical discharge

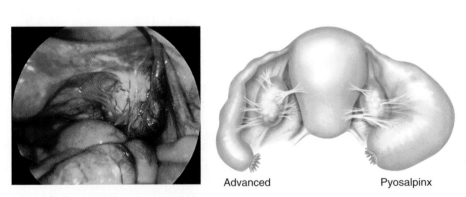

FIGURE 18-64 Salpingitis. Photograph shows acute salpingitis with adhesions. Dye has been instilled into the grossly swollen fallopian tube on the right. Dense adhesions obscure the ovary. *(Photograph from Morse et al, 2003.)*

⚗ Infants and Children

Ambiguous Genitalia

The newborn's genitalia are not clearly either male or female (Fig. 18-65).

Pathophysiology

- Presence or absence of male hormones controls the development of the sex organs during fetal development; male genitalia develop because of male hormones from the fetal testicles; in the female fetus, without the effects of male hormones, the genitalia develop as female.
- A deficiency of male hormones in a genetic male fetus results in ambiguous genitalia; in a female fetus, the presence of male hormones during development results in ambiguous genitalia.
- Most causes of ambiguous genitalia are due to genetic abnormalities.

Subjective Data

- Family history of:
  - Genital abnormalities
  - Known congenital adrenal hyperplasia
  - Unexplained deaths in early infancy
  - Infertility in close relatives
  - Abnormal development during puberty

Objective Data

- Ambiguous genitalia in a genetic female:
  - An enlarged clitoris that has the appearance of a small penis
  - The urethral opening anywhere along, above, or below the surface of clitoris
  - Fused labia resembling a scrotum
  - A lump of tissue is felt within the fused labia, making it look like a scrotum with testicles.
- Ambiguous genitalia in a genetic male:
  - A small penis that resembles an enlarged clitoris
  - Urethral opening anywhere along, above, or below the penis; or as low as on the peritoneum, further making the infant appear to be female
  - Small scrotum with any degree of separation, resembling labia
  - Undescended testicles commonly accompany ambiguous genitalia
- Infant should have chromosomal studies performed

FIGURE 18-65 Ambiguous genitalia. *(Courtesy Patrick C. Walsh, MD, The Johns Hopkins School of Medicine, Baltimore.)*

Clinical Pearl

Looks Can Be Deceiving

Looks can be deceiving. Don't always jump to conclusions. The pictures below prove the point. The patient is not a male. The clitoris is enlarged; the labia are fused. Inspection must be very careful.

(Photograph from Biomedical Photography, Johns Hopkins University School of Medicine, Baltimore, MD.)

Normal infant female external genitalia. *(Lowdermilk and Perry, 2007.)*

Normal infant male external genitalia. *(Lowdermilk and Perry, 2007.)*

ABNORMALITIES

Hydrocolpos

Distention of the vagina caused by accumulation of fluid due to congenital vaginal obstruction

Pathophysiology

- Obstruction usually caused by an imperforate hymen or, less commonly, a transverse vaginal septum

Subjective Data

- None

Objective Data

- Small midline lower abdominal mass or a small cystic mass between the labia
- Condition may resolve spontaneously or may require surgical intervention
- Abdominal sonography is helpful in making the correct diagnosis, showing a large midline translucent mass displacing the bladder forward.

Vulvovaginitis

Inflammation of the vulvar and vaginal tissues

Pathophysiology

- Possible causes include sexual abuse; trichomonal, monilial, or gonococcal infection; secondary infection from a foreign body; nonspecific infection from bubble baths; diaper irritation; urethritis; injury; or pinworm infection.
- Recent pharyngitis can lead to group A beta-hemolytic streptococcal (GABHS) vaginitis
- Asymptomatic vaginal discharge often occurs in the months prior to menarche and represents a physiologic response to increasing estrogen levels.

Subjective Data

- Vaginal discharge
- Discomfort, pain, or pruritus
- Vulvar irritation
- Burning on urination
- With infants and young children, the parent may report a discharge on the diaper or panties, an abnormal vaginal odor, or redness of the vulva.
- Wiping the anus from posterior to anterior, wearing tight-fitting synthetic undergarments, and using vaginal irritants such as bubble baths
- Recent upper respiratory infection or pharyngitis

Objective Data

- Warm, erythematous, and swollen vulvar tissues (Fig. 18-66)
- Vaginal pruritus, especially at night, suggests pinworm infection.
- Itching, soreness, bleeding, and vaginal discharge; bloody and foul-smelling discharge may suggest a vaginal foreign body.

FIGURE 18-66 Nonspecific inflammation characteristic of chemical irritant vulvovaginitis. *(From Zitelli and Davis, 2007.)*

⚘ Pregnant Women

Premature Rupture of Membranes

The spontaneous premature rupture of the membranes (PROM) in a preterm pregnancy carries a high risk of perinatal morbidity and mortality, as well as maternal morbidity and mortality.

Pathophysiology	Subjective Data	Physical Findings
• Cause of PROM is not known; however, certain conditions such as infection and hydramnios have been implicated; some health care professionals also consider the rupture of membranes before the onset of labor in a term pregnancy to be premature rupture if labor does not begin within 12 hours.	• During pregnancy prior to term, premature passage of fluid from the vagina	• PROM should be verified with a sterile speculum examination to collect fluid for testing with Nitrazine paper and microscopic examination. • Amniotic fluid has a pH of 7.15 and will turn Nitrazine paper blue-green. • Amniotic fluid placed on a slide and air-dried will have a "fern" pattern. • Ultrasound evaluation of fluid will reveal decreased or absent amniotic fluid.

Vaginal Bleeding during Pregnancy

Vaginal bleeding that can occur early or late in pregnancy.

Pathophysiology	Subjective Data	Objective Data
• In early pregnancy, may be due to unknown causes of little consequence or due to a potentially life-threatening condition such as an ectopic pregnancy. • Late in pregnancy, causes of bleeding may range from benign conditions such as cervical changes to a potentially life-threatening abruptio placentae.	• Vaginal bleeding • May or may not be accompanied by pain	• Diagnosis based on the gestational age and the character of her bleeding (light or heavy, associated with pain or painless, intermittent or constant) • Women who are bleeding in labor or who have a suspected placenta previa (prepare for emergency cesarean section prior to examination) • Laboratory and imaging tests are used to confirm or revise the initial diagnosis.

⚘ Older Adults

Atrophic Vaginitis

Inflammation of the vagina due to the thinning and shrinking of the tissues, as well as decreased lubrication

Pathophysiology	Subjective Data	Objective Data
• Caused by lack of estrogen during perimenopause and menopause	• Vaginal soreness or itching • Discomfort or bleeding with sexual intercourse	• Vaginal mucosa is dry and pale, although it may become reddened and develop petechiae and superficial erosions • Accompanying vaginal discharge may be white, gray, yellow, green, or blood-tinged • Can be thick or watery and, although it varies in amount, rarely profuse

Urinary Incontinence

See Chapter 17.

CHAPTER 19

Male Genitalia

Examination of the male genitalia is typically performed when a patient presents with a specific concern, as part of the newborn examination, or as part of an overall child or adult health visit. In adults, examination of the anus, rectum, and prostate (see Chapter 20) is often performed at the same time.

evolve *http://evolve.elsevier.com/Seidel*
- Physical Exam Key Points
- NCLEX Review Questions
- Activities
- Animations
- Videos
- Student Checklist

ANATOMY AND PHYSIOLOGY

The penis, testicles, epididymides, scrotum, prostate gland, and seminal vesicles constitute the male genitalia (Fig. 19-1).

The penis serves as the final excretory organ for urine and, when erect, as the means of introducing semen into the vagina. The penis consists of the corpora cavernosa, which form the dorsum and sides, and the corpus spongiosum, which contains the urethra. The corpus spongiosum expands at its distal end to form the glans penis. The urethral orifice is a slitlike opening located approximately 2 mm ventral to the tip of the glans (Figs. 19-2 and 19-3). The skin of the penis is thin, redundant to permit erection, and free of subcutaneous fat. It is generally more darkly pigmented than body skin. Unless the patient has been circumcised, the prepuce (foreskin) covers the glans. In the uncircumcised male, smegma is formed by the secretion of sebaceous material by the glans and the desquamation of epithelial cells from the prepuce. It appears as a cheesy white material on the glans and in the fornix of the foreskin.

The scrotum, like the penis, is generally more darkly pigmented than body skin. A septum divides the scrotum into two pendulous sacs, each containing a testis, epididymis, spermatic cord, and a muscle layer termed the *cremasteric muscle* that allows the scrotum to relax or contract (Fig. 19-4). Testicular temperature is controlled by altering the distance of the testes from the body through muscular action. Spermatogenesis requires maintenance of temperatures lower than 37°C.

The testicles are responsible for the production of both spermatozoa and testosterone. The adult testis is ovoid and measures

Physical Examination Preview

Here is a preview of the steps involved in conducting physical examination of the male genitalia. ⓔ These procedures are explained in detail in this chapter and are available on Evolve as printable PDFs or downloadable formats for electronic device use.

Male Genitalia

The following steps are performed with the adult patient lying or standing:
1. Inspect the pubic hair characteristics and distribution (p. 471).
2. Retract the foreskin if the patient is uncircumcised (p. 471).
3. Inspect the glans of the penis with foreskin retracted, noting the following (p. 471):
   - Color
   - Smegma
   - External meatus of urethra
   - Urethral discharge
4. Palpate the penis, noting the following (p. 472):
   - Tenderness
   - Induration
5. Strip the urethra for discharge (p. 472).
6. Inspect the scrotum and ventral surface of the penis for the following (p. 472):
   - Color
   - Texture
   - Asymmetry
   - Lesions
   - Unusual thickening
   - Presence of hernia
7. Palpate the inguinal canal for a direct or indirect hernia (p. 472).
8. Palpate the testes, epididymides, and vasa deferentia for the following (p. 473):
   - Consistency
   - Size
   - Tenderness
   - Bleeding, masses, lumpiness, or nodules
9. Transilluminate any masses in the scrotum (p. 475).
10. Palpate for inguinal lymph nodes (p. 176).
11. Elicit the cremasteric reflex bilaterally (p. 474).

Rectum
Seminal vesicle
Levator ani muscle
Ejaculatory duct
Anus
Bulbocavernosus muscle
Epididymis
Testis

Urinary bladder
Symphysis pubis
Prostate gland
Corpus cavernosum
Corpus spongiosum
Urethra
Glans
Penis

FIGURE 19-1 Male pelvic organs.

Corpus cavernosum
Corpus spongiosum
Glans penis
Crus penis
Corpus cavernosum
Corpus spongiosum
Urethra
Glans penis

FIGURE 19-2 Anatomy of the penis.

Prostate
Cowper gland
Crus penis
Bulb
Corpus cavernosum
Corpus spongiosum
Lacunae of Morgagni with glands of Littre
Urethra
Glans penis
Fossa navicularis

Orifices of ejaculatory duct
Opening of Cowper glands

ROOF
FLOOR

FIGURE 19-3 Anatomy of urethra and penis. *(From Lowdermilk et al, 1997.)*

Spermatic cord
Vas deferens
Pampiniform plexis
Epididymis
Testis
Vas deferens
Vasa efferentia
Testis
Cremasteric muscle
Ductus epididymis
Scrotum

FIGURE 19-4 Scrotum and its contents.

approximately 4 × 3 × 2 cm. The epididymis is a soft, comma-shaped structure located on the posterolateral and upper aspect of the testis. It provides for storage, maturation, and transit of sperm. The vas deferens begins at the tail of the epididymis, ascends the spermatic cord, travels through the inguinal canal, and unites with the seminal vesicle to form the ejaculatory duct.

The prostate gland, which resembles a large chestnut and is approximately the size of a testis, surrounds the urethra at the bladder neck. It produces the major volume of ejaculatory fluid, which contains fibrinolysin. This enzyme liquefies the coagulated semen, a process that may be important for satisfactory sperm motility. The seminal vesicles extend from the prostate onto the posterior surface of the bladder.

Erection of the penis occurs when the two corpora cavernosa become engorged with blood, generally 20 to 50 mL. Arterial dilation and decreased venous outflow produce the increased blood supply; both processes are under the control of the autonomic nervous system and occur because of the local synthesis of nitric oxide. Ejaculation during orgasm consists of the emission of secretions from the vas deferens, epididymides, prostate, and seminal vesicles. Orgasm is followed by constriction of the vessels supplying blood to the corpora cavernosa and gradual detumescence (subsidence of the erection).

⚘ Infants and Children

The external genitalia are identical for males and females at 8 weeks of gestation, but by 12 weeks of gestation sexual differentiation has occurred. Any fetal insult during 8 or 9 weeks of gestation may lead to major anomalies of the external genitalia. Minor morphologic abnormalities arise during later stages of gestation.

During the third trimester, the testes descend from the retroperitoneal space through the inguinal canal to the scrotum. At full term, one or both testes may still lie within the inguinal canal, with the final descent into the scrotum occurring in the early postnatal period. Descent of the testicles may be arrested at any point, however, or they may follow an abnormal path.

Small separations between the glans and the inner preputial epithelium begin during the third trimester. Separation of the prepuce from the glans is usually incomplete at birth and often remains so until the age of 3 to 4 years in uncircumcised males.

⚘ Adolescents

With the onset of puberty, testicular growth begins and the scrotal skin reddens, thins, and becomes increasingly pendulous. Sparse, downy, straight hair appears at the base of the penis. The penis enlarges in length and breadth. As maturation continues, the pubic hair darkens and extends over the entire pubic area, and the prostate gland enlarges. By the completion of puberty, the pubic hair is curly, dense, and coarse and forms a diamond-shaped pattern from the umbilicus to the anus. The growth and development of the testes and scrotum are complete (see Chapter 6 for stages of genital developmental and sexual maturation).

⚘ Older Adults

Pubic hair becomes finer and less abundant with aging, and pubic alopecia may occur. The scrotum becomes more pendulous.

Frequency of sexual activity may decline with aging. An erection may develop more slowly, and orgasm may be less intense.

REVIEW OF RELATED HISTORY

For each of the symptoms or conditions discussed in this section, targeted topics to include in the history of the present illness are listed. Responses to questions about these topics provide clues for focusing the physical examination and the development of an appropriate diagnostic evaluation. Questions regarding medication use (prescription and over the counter preparations) as well as complementary and alternative therapies are relevant for each.

History of Present Illness

- Discharge or lesion on the penis
  - Character of lumps, sores, rash
  - Discharge: color, consistency, odor, tendency to stain underwear
  - Symptoms: itching, burning, stinging
  - Exposure to sexually transmitted infection (STI): multiple partners, infection in partners, failure to use or incorrect condom use, history of prior STI
- Swelling in inguinal area
  - Intermittent or constant, association with straining or lifting, duration, presence of pain
  - Change in size or character of swelling
  - Pain in the groin: character (tearing, sudden, searing, or cutting pain), associated activity (lifting heavy object, coughing, or straining at stool)
  - Use of truss or other treatment
  - Frequent heavy lifting
  - Medications: analgesics
- Testicular pain or mass
  - Change in testicular size
  - Events surrounding onset: noted casually while bathing, after trauma, during a sporting event; sudden onset
  - Irregular lumps, soreness, or heaviness of testes
  - Medications: analgesics, antibiotics
- Curvature of penis in any direction with erection
  - Associated pain
  - Injury to penis
  - Personal history diabetes, contracture of fourth and fifth fingers of the hand (Dupuytren contracture)
  - Family history of condition
  - Medications: propranolol
- Persistent erections unrelated to sexual stimulation
  - Current history of sickle cell anemia, leukemia, multiple sclerosis, diabetes, spinal cord injury
  - Trauma to genitals or groin
  - Associated with alcohol ingestion or medication
  - Medications: erectile dysfunction agents, antidepressants, antipsychotics, anticoagulants, anxiolytics, recreational drugs

*   Difficulty with ejaculation
    *   Painful or premature, efforts to treat the problem
    *   Ejaculate color, consistency, odor, and amount
    *   Medications: alpha blockers, antidepressants, antipsychotics, clonidine, methyldopa
*   Difficulty achieving or maintaining erection
    *   Pain with erection, prolonged painful erection
    *   Constant or intermittent, with one or more sexual partners
    *   Associated with alcohol ingestion or medication
    *   Medications: diuretics, sedatives, antihypertensive agents, anxiolytics, estrogens, inhibitors of androgen synthesis, antidepressants, carbamazepine, erectile dysfunction agents
*   Infertility
    *   Lifestyle factors that may increase temperature of scrotum: tight clothing, briefs, hot baths, employment in high-temperature environment (e.g., a steel mill) or requiring prolonged sitting (e.g., truck driving)
    *   Length of time attempting pregnancy, sexual activity pattern, knowledge of fertile period of woman's reproductive cycle
    *   History of varicocele, hydrocele, or undescended testes
    *   Diagnostic evaluation to date: semen analysis, physical examination, sperm antibody titers
    *   Medications: testosterone, glucocorticoids, hypothalamic releasing hormone, marijuana

Past Medical History

*   Congenital anomaly and/or surgery of genitourinary tract: undescended testes, hypospadias, epispadias, hydrocele, varicocele, hernia, prostate; vasectomy
*   STIs: single or multiple infections, specific organism (gonorrhea, syphilis, herpes, human papillomavirus [HPV]), chlamydia), treatment, effectiveness, residual problems; vaccination for HPV
*   Chronic illness: testicular or prostatic cancer, neurologic or vascular impairment, diabetes mellitus, arthritis, cardiac or respiratory disease

Staying Well

HPV Immunization in Males

The Centers for Disease Control and Prevention (CDC) recommend routine use of quadrivalent human papillomavirus (HPV) vaccine in males aged 11 or 12 years. The CDC also recommends vaccination with HPV4 for males aged 13 through 21 years who have not been vaccinated previously or who have not completed the three-dose series. All men may receive the vaccine through age 26, and should speak with their health care provider to determine if getting vaccinated is right for them.

The vaccine is also recommended for any man who has sex with men and men with compromised immune systems (including human immunodeficiency virus [HIV]) through age 26 if they did not get fully vaccinated when they were younger.

Centers for Disease Control, 2012.

Family History

*   Infertility in siblings
*   History of prostate, testicular, or penile cancer
*   Hernias
*   Peyronie disease (contracture of penis)

Personal and Social History

*   Occupational risk of trauma to suprapubic region or genitalia, exposure to radiation or toxins
*   Exercise: use of a protective device with contact sports or bicycle riding
*   Concerns about genitalia: size, shape, surface characteristics, texture
*   Testicular/genital self-examination practices (see Staying Well box)
*   Concerns about sexual practices: sexual partners (single or multiple), sexual lifestyle (heterosexual, homosexual, bisexual)
*   Reproductive function: number of children, form of contraception used, frequency of ejaculation
*   Alcohol, marijuana use: quantity and frequency
*   Use of drugs

✤ Infants and Children

*   Maternal use of sex hormones or birth control pills during pregnancy
*   Circumcised: complications from procedure
*   Uncircumcised: hygiene measures, retractability of foreskin, interference with urinary stream
*   Scrotal swelling with crying or bowel movement
*   Congenital anomalies: hypospadias, epispadias, undescended testes, ambiguous genitalia
*   Parental concerns with masturbation, sexual exploration
*   Swelling, discoloration, or sores on the penis or scrotum, pain in the genitalia
*   Concern for sexual abuse

✤ Adolescents

*   Knowledge of reproductive function, source of information about sexual activity and function
*   Presence of nocturnal emissions, pubic hair, enlargement of genitalia, age at time of each occurrence
*   Concern of sexual abuse
*   Sexual activity, protection used for contraception and STI prevention

✤ Older Adults

*   Change in frequency of sexual activity or desire: related to loss of spouse or other sexual partner; no sexual partner; sexually restrictive environment; depression; physical illness resulting in fatigue, weakness, or pain
*   Change in sexual response: longer time required or inability to achieve full erection, less forceful ejaculation, more rapid detumescence, longer interval between erections, prostate surgery

REVIEW OF RELATED HISTORY

Staying Well

Genital Self-Examination for Men

Genital self-examination (GSE) is recommended for anyone who is at risk for contracting a sexually transmitted infection (STI). This includes sexually active persons who have had more than one sexual partner or whose partner has had other partners. The purpose of GSE is to detect any signs or symptoms that might indicate the presence of an STI. Many people who have an STI do not know they have one, and some STIs can remain undetected for years. GSE should become a part of routine self-examination health care practices. Explain and demonstrate the following procedure to your patients and give them the opportunity to perform a GSE with your guidance.

Instruct the patient to hold the penis in his hand and examine the head. If not circumcised, he should gently pull back the foreskin to expose the glans. Inspection and palpation of the entire head of the penis should be performed in a clockwise motion while the patient carefully looks for any bumps, sores, or blisters on the skin. Bumps and blisters may be red or light-colored, or may resemble pimples. Have the patient also look for genital warts, which may look similar to warts on other parts of the body. The urethral meatus should also be examined for any discharge.

Next the patient will examine the entire shaft and look for the same signs. Instruct him to separate the pubic hair at the base of the penis and carefully examine the skin underneath. Make sure he includes the underside of the shaft in the examination; a mirror may be helpful.

Instruct the patient to examine the scrotal skin and contents. He should hold each testicle gently and inspect and palpate the skin, including the underneath of the scrotum, looking for any lump, swelling, or soreness. He should also gently feel each testicle for lumps or irregularities. (Suggest to the patient that self-examination of the scrotum at home be performed while bathing, because the warmth is likely to make the scrotal skin less thick.) Although there is no evidence to support routine screening for testicular cancer through either clinical examination or self-examination (U.S. Preventive Services Task Force, 2011; American Academy of Family Physicians, 2012), testicular examination can be easily and quickly included as part of a genital self-examination.

Educate the patient about other symptoms associated with STIs, specifically pain or burning on urination or discharge from the penis. The discharge may vary in color, consistency, and amount.

If the patient has any of the above signs or symptoms, he should see a health care provider.

Left, Self-examination of penis. **Right,** Self-examination of scrotum and testicle.

Risk Factors

Cancer of the Male Genitalia

Penile
- Lack of circumcision with failure to maintain good hygiene
- Phimosis
- Infection with high-risk types of HPV (human papillomavirus)
- Age: risk increases with age
- Smoking (smoking alone increases risk; smokers with HPV infection at even higher risk)
- HIV infection
- UV light treatment of psoriasis if genitalia exposed

Testicular
- Undescended testicle (cryptorchidism): risk elevated for both testicles
- Personal history of testicular cancer (the opposite testicle is at increased risk)
- Family history of testicular cancer
- Abnormal testicle development: Klinefelter syndrome
- Age: 20 to 54 years
- Race: white; 5 times that of black men and more than 3 times that of Asian American and Native American men

American Cancer Society, 2012; National Cancer Institute, 2012; Pow-Sang et al, 2010.

FIGURE 19-5 Appearance of male genitalia. A, Circumcised. B, Uncircumcised.

EXAMINATION AND FINDINGS

Equipment

+ Gloves
+ Drapes
+ Penlight for transillumination

Examination of the genitalia involves inspection, palpation, and transillumination of any mass found. The patient may be anxious about examination of his genitalia, so it is important to examine the genitalia carefully and completely but also expeditiously (Box 19-1). The patient may be lying or standing for this part of the examination. A chaperone protects both the examiner and patient and one is often required by policy. Some patients may be reluctant to reveal confidential and sensitive information in the presence of a chaperone.

Inspection and Palpation

Genital Hair Distribution

First inspect the genital hair distribution. Genital hair is coarser than scalp hair. It should be abundant in the pubic region and may continue in a narrowing midline pattern to the umbilicus (the male escutcheon pattern). Depending on how the patient is positioned, it may be possible to note that the distribution continues around the scrotum to the anal orifice. The penis itself is not covered with hair, and the scrotum generally has a scant amount.

Penis

Examine the penis. The dorsal vein should be apparent on inspection. Note whether the patient is circumcised or uncircumcised (Fig. 19-5). If the patient is uncircumcised, retract the foreskin or ask the patient to do so. It should retract easily, and a bit of smegma (white cheesy sebaceous matter that collects between the glans penis and the foreskin) may be seen over the glans. Occasionally the foreskin is tight and cannot be retracted. This condition is called phimosis (Fig. 19-6) and may occur during the first 6 years of life or as a result of recurrent balanitis (inflammation of the glans) (Fig. 19-7), or balanoposthitis (inflammation of the glans penis and prepuce), which occur in

| Box 19-1 | Minimizing the Patient's Anxiety |

The physical examination is laden with anxiety-provoking elements for most people, but no part of the body is likely to arouse as much psychic discomfort for the male patient as examination of his genitals. Adolescents and men are often fearful of having an erection during the examination. Boys and adolescents may worry about whether their genitals are "normal," and misinformation on sexual matters (such as "the evils of masturbation") can add to their concerns. Your attitude and ability to communicate can reassure the apprehensive patient. Some important elements to remember:

• Know the language. It is inappropriate to talk down to anyone, but you and the patient must understand each other. You may not be entirely comfortable with some of the common words and phrases you hear from the patients, but the common language may be appropriate in certain circumstances. You will not lose your dignity if you maintain your composure and succeed in communicating effectively. Know the language and use it effectively, without apology, and in a nondemeaning fashion.

• Never make jokes. Light, casual talk or jokes about the genitalia or sexual function are always inappropriate, no matter how well you know the patient. Feelings about one's own sexuality run deep and are often well masked. Do not pull at the edges of a mask you may not suspect is there.

• Remember that your face is easily seen by the patient when you are examining the genitalia. An unexpected finding may cause a sudden change in your expression. You must guard against what you communicate by the unspoken.

• You need not be defensive if you are a woman examining a man, any more than if you are a man examining a woman—an ordinary event, historically. Here again, you communicate much by demeanor and hesitancy in speech. Do not be apologetic in any obvious or subtle way. Remember that you are a professional, fulfilling the responsibility of a professional.

Video: Male Genitalia: Examining the Penis

uncircumcised individuals, and may be caused by either bacterial or fungal infections. It is most commonly seen in men with poorly controlled diabetes mellitus. Phimosis may also be caused by previous unsuccessful efforts to retract the foreskin that have caused radial tearing of the preputial ring, resulting in adhesions of the foreskin to the glans.

If the patient is circumcised, the glans is exposed and appears erythematous and dry. No smegma will be present.

FIGURE 19-6 Phimosis. *(From Wolfe, 1984.)*

FIGURE 19-8 Examination of urethral orifice.

FIGURE 19-7 Balanitis. *(From Lloyd-Davies et al, 1994.)*

FIGURE 19-9 Priapism. *(From Lloyd-Davies et al, 1994.)*

Urethral Meatus

Examine the external meatus of the urethra. The orifice should appear slitlike and be located on the ventral surface just millimeters from the tip of the glans. Press the glans between your thumb and forefinger to open the urethral orifice (Fig. 19-8). You can ask the patient to perform this procedure. The opening should be glistening and pink. Bright erythema or a discharge indicates inflammatory disease, whereas a pinpoint or round opening may result from meatal stenosis.

Penile Shaft

Palpate the shaft of the penis for tenderness and induration. Strip the urethra for any discharge by firmly compressing the base of the penis with your thumb and forefinger and moving them toward the glans. The presence of a discharge may indicate an STI. The texture of the flaccid penis should be soft and free of nodularity. Reposition the foreskin after performing these maneuvers.

Rarely, you may see a patient with a prolonged penile erection, called priapism (Fig. 19-9). It is often painful. Although in the majority of cases the condition is idiopathic, it can occur in patients with leukemia or hemoglobinopathies such as sickle cell disease, or as a result of medications for impotence.

Scrotum

Inspect the scrotum (Fig. 19-10). It may appear more deeply pigmented than the body skin, and the surface may be coarse.

The scrotal skin is often reddened in red-haired individuals; however, reddened skin in other individuals may indicate an inflammatory process. The scrotum usually appears asymmetric because the left testicle has a longer spermatic cord and therefore is often lower. The thickness of the scrotum definitely varies with temperature and age. Lumps in the scrotal skin are commonly caused by sebaceous cysts, also called epidermoid cysts. They appear as small lumps on the scrotum, but they may enlarge and discharge oily material (Fig. 19-11).

Occasionally you may observe unusual thickening of the scrotum caused by edema, often with pitting. This does not generally imply disease related to the genitalia, but is more likely a consequence of general fluid retention associated with cardiac, renal, or hepatic disease.

Hernia

Examine for evidence of a hernia. Figure 19-16 shows the anatomy of the region and the three common types of hernias. With the patient standing, ask him to bear down as if having a bowel movement. While he is straining, inspect the area of the inguinal canal and the region of the fossa ovalis. After asking the patient to relax again, insert your examining finger into the lower

FIGURE 19-10 Inspection of scrotum and ventral surface of penis as the patient positions his penis.

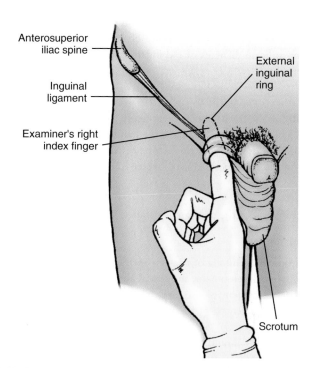

FIGURE 19-12 Checking for inguinal hernia; gloved finger inserted through inguinal canal. *(From Phipps et al, 2007.)*

FIGURE 19-11 Sebaceous glands on the scrotum. *(From Morse et al, 2003.)*

FIGURE 19-13 Palpating contents of the scrotal sac.

part of the scrotum and carry it upward along the vas deferens into the inguinal canal (Fig. 19-12). You can auscultate for bowel sounds, which will be present in uncomplicated reducible hernias.

Which finger you use depends on the size of the patient. In the young child, the little finger is appropriate; in the adult, the index or middle finger is generally used. You should be able to feel the oval external ring. Ask the patient to cough. If an inguinal hernia is present, you should feel the sudden presence of a viscus against your finger. The hernia is described as indirect if it lies within the inguinal canal. It may also come through the external canal and even pass into the scrotum. Because an indirect hernia on one side strongly suggests the possibility of bilateral herniation, be sure to examine both sides thoroughly. If the viscus is felt medial to the external canal, it probably represents a direct inguinal hernia.

Testes

Palpate the testes using the thumb and first two fingers. The testes should be sensitive to gentle compression but not tender, and they should feel smooth and rubbery and be free of nodules (Fig. 19-13). In some diseases (e.g., syphilis and diabetic

neuropathy), a testis may be totally insensitive to painful stimuli. Irregularities in texture or size may indicate an infection, a cyst, or a tumor.

The epididymis, located on the posterolateral surface of the testis, should be smooth, discrete, larger cephalad, and nontender. You may be able to feel the appendix epididymidis as an irregularity on the cephalad surface.

Next palpate the vas deferens. It has accompanying arteries and veins, but they cannot be precisely identified by palpation. The vas deferens itself feels smooth and discrete; it should not be beaded or lumpy in its course as you palpate from the testicle to the inguinal ring. The presence of such unexpected findings might indicate diabetes or old inflammatory changes, especially tuberculosis.

Cremasteric Reflex

Finally, evaluate the cremasteric reflex. Stroke the inner thigh with a blunt instrument such as the handle of the reflex hammer, or for a child, with your finger. The testicle and scrotum should rise on the stroked side (see Chapter 22).

Prostate

Examination of the prostate is detailed in Chapter 20.

❀ Infants

Examine the genitalia of the newborn for congenital anomalies, incomplete development, and sexual ambiguity. Inspect the penis for size, placement of the urethral meatus, and any anomalies. The nonerect length of the penis at birth is usually 2 to 3 cm. Transitory erection of the penis during infancy is common, and the penis should have a straight projection. An unusually small penis (microphallus) may be associated with conditions of abnormal testicular development (e.g., Klinefelter syndrome) and may not be appropriate for circumcision if the mother desires one. The small penis must also be differentiated from the unusually large clitoris (clitoromegaly) that may be seen at birth in congenital adrenal hyperplasia. A hooked, downward bowing of the penis suggests a chordee.

Inspection and Palpation

Inspect the glans penis of the neonate. The foreskin in the uncircumcised infant is commonly tight, but it should retract enough to permit a good urinary stream. Do not retract the foreskin more than necessary to see the urethra, especially if the neonate will not be circumcised. Mobility of the foreskin increases with time, and for most boys it is fully retractable by 3 or 4 years of age (Kliegman et al, 2011). The slitlike urethral meatus should be located near the tip. Inspect the glans of the circumcised infant for ulcerations, bleeding, and inflammation (Box 19-2). The urinary stream should be strong, with good caliber. Dribbling or a reduced force or caliber of the urinary stream may indicate stenosis of the urethral meatus.

Clinical Pearl

Retraction of the Foreskin

It is important not to force the retraction of the foreskin because forced retraction may contribute to the formation of binding adhesions. Some adherence of the prepuce to the glans may continue until 6 years of age.

Inspect the scrotum for size, symmetry, shape, rugae, presence of testicles, and any anomalies (Fig. 19-14). The scrotum of the premature infant may appear underdeveloped, without rugae and without testes, whereas the full-term neonate should have a loose, pendulous scrotum with rugae and a midline raphe. The

Box 19-2 Male Circumcision

There has been much discussion about the appropriateness of routine circumcision in neonates. In 2007, the American Academy of Pediatrics (AAP) convened a multidisciplinary workgroup to evaluate the evidence regarding male circumcision. In 2012, the AAP released the following policy statement: "Evaluation of current evidence indicates that the health benefits of newborn male circumcision outweigh the risks; furthermore, the benefits of newborn male circumcision justify access to this procedure for families who choose it" (AAP, 2012).

Specific benefits from male circumcision were identified for the prevention of urinary tract infections, acquisition of HIV, transmission of some sexually transmitted infections, and penile cancer. Male circumcision did not appear to adversely affect penile sexual function/sensitivity or sexual satisfaction. Adequate training for both sterile techniques and effective pain management was imperative.

The AAP recognizes the sociocultural and ethical issues embedded in the circumcision decision and advises that parents should weigh the health benefits and risks in light of their own religious, cultural, and personal preferences, as the medical benefits alone may not outweigh these other considerations for individual families. Your role as a health care provider is to provide factually correct, nonbiased information about circumcision and assist parents by explaining, in a nonbiased manner, the potential benefits and risks and by ensuring that they understand the elective nature of the procedure.

FIGURE 19-14 Palpating the scrotum of an infant.

proximal end of the scrotum should be the widest area. The scrotum in infants usually appears large compared with the rest of the genitalia. Edema of the external genitalia is common, especially after a breech delivery. A deep cleft in the scrotum (bifid scrotum) is usually associated with other genitourinary anomalies or ambiguous genitalia.

The cremasteric reflex, in which the scrotal contents retract, can occur in response to cold hands and abrupt handling. Before you palpate the scrotum, place the thumb and index finger of one hand over the inguinal canals at the upper part of the scrotal sac. This maneuver helps prevent retraction of the testes into the inguinal canal or abdomen. Palpate each side of the scrotum to detect the presence of the testes or other masses. The testicle of the newborn is approximately 1 cm in diameter.

If either of the testicles is not palpable, place a finger over the upper inguinal ring and gently push toward the scrotum. You may feel a soft mass in the inguinal canal. Try to push it toward the scrotum and palpate it with your thumb and index finger. If the testicle can be pushed into the scrotum, it is considered a descended testicle, even though it retracts to the inguinal canal. A retractile testis has a significant risk of becoming an ascending or an acquired undescended testis and so requires regular long-term follow-up examinations. A testicle that is either palpable in the inguinal canal but cannot be pushed into the scrotum or not palpable at all is considered an undescended testicle.

Palpate over the internal inguinal canal with the flat part of your fingers. Roll the spermatic cord beneath the fingers to feel the solid structure going through the ring. If the feeling of smoothness disappears as you palpate, the peritoneum is passing through the ring, indicating an invisible hernia. An apparent bulge in the inguinal area suggests a visible hernia. Palpation may elicit a sensation of crepitus.

Transillumination

When any mass other than the testicle or spermatic cord is palpated in the scrotum, determine whether it is filled with fluid, gas, or solid material. It will most likely be a hernia or hydrocele. Attempt to reduce the size of the mass by pushing it back through the external inguinal canal. If a bright penlight transilluminates the mass, and there is no change in size when reduction is attempted, it most likely contains fluid (hydrocele with a closed tunica vaginalis). A mass that does not transilluminate but does change in size when reduction is attempted is probably a hernia. A mass that neither changes in size nor transilluminates may represent an incarcerated hernia (a surgical emergency) or testicular cancer.

✤ Children

The external genitalia of the toddler and preschooler are examined as described for infants. Preschoolers may have developed a sense of modesty, so you should explain what you are doing throughout the examination and involve the parent or caregiver to help position the child (e.g., child lying on parent's lap). Reassure the child that he is developing appropriately whenever such reassurance is possible.

Inspection and Palpation

Inspect the penis for size, lesions, swelling, inflammation, and malformation. Retract the foreskin in the uncircumcised boy without forcing it, and inspect the glans for lesions, discharge, and the location and appearance of the urethral meatus. The penis may appear relatively small if obscured by fatty tissue. If the penis appears swollen or tender or if bruises are present, be concerned about the possibility of sexual abuse.

The scrotum is inspected for size, shape, color, and presence of testicles or other masses. Well-formed rugae indicate that the testes have descended during infancy, even if the testes are not apparent in the scrotum. Palpate the scrotum to identify the testes and epididymides. Again, bruises on the scrotum or in the groin area raise the suspicion of sexual abuse.

Some testes are very retractile and therefore hard to find. Warm hands, a warm room, and a gentle approach will help. If the patient is old enough to cooperate, ask him to sit in tailor position with legs crossed, or have the child sit on a chair with

FIGURE 19-15 Position of child to push testicles into the scrotum. An alternative maneuver is to seat the child in tailor position.

the heels of his feet on the chair seat and his hands on his knees. Either position places pressure on the abdominal wall that will help push the testicles into the scrotum. If an inguinal hernia exists, this maneuver is also useful in eliciting that finding (Fig. 19-15). A scrotum that remains small, flat, and undeveloped indicates cryptorchidism (undescended testes).

A hard, enlarged, painless testicle may indicate a tumor. Acute swelling in the scrotum with discoloration can result from torsion of the spermatic cord or orchitis. Acute painful swelling without discoloration and a thickened or nodular epididymis suggests epididymitis. An enlarged penis without enlargement of the testes occurs with precocious puberty, adrenal hyperplasia, and some central nervous system lesions.

✤ Adolescents

The examination of older children and adolescents is the same as for adults. Because of their modesty and great sensitivity to development, this portion of the physical examination is usually performed last. The changes of puberty follow a predictable sequence, but their timing is variable. Sexual maturation is rated from 1 to 5 according to the stages (see Chapter 6; sexual maturation for the male is based on changes in pubic hair, development of the testes and scrotum, and penis). Each of these areas is evaluated separately. It is possible for a male to have a different sexual maturation rating (SMR) for each area, but SMRs for pubic hair and genitalia usually are closely correlated. SMR correlates highly with physical maturity as measured by bone age compared with chronologic age (Kliegman et al, 2011).

> **Clinical Pearl**
>
> *Concerns of Adolescence*
>
> The adolescent male may need to be reassured that his genital development is proceeding as expected. If he has an erection during the examination, consider explaining that this is a common response to touch and that it is not a problem.

✤ Older Adults

The examination procedure for older adults is that same as that for younger men. Age-related changes that you may note include graying and less abundant pubic hair, and as well as a pendulous scrotal sac and contents.

ABNORMALITIES

Sample Documentation

History and Physical Examination

Subjective

Two days ago, this 19-year-old male noted swelling in his left groin after lifting weights. Reports mild pain on straining. No fever, chills, recent illness. No history of sexually transmitted infections.

Objective

No discharge from urinary meatus. No external genital lesions. Penile shaft smooth. Testes descended bilaterally; smooth without nodularity, induration, or masses. No tenderness along the course of the spermatic cords, no inguinal lymphadenopathy. Soft swelling in left inguinal area. Palpable hernia to fingertip on examination. Reduces easily. No bulging on right.

For additional sample documentation, see Chapter 26, pp. 628-631.

ABNORMALITIES

INFERTILITY

See Chapter 18.

Hernia

Protrusion of a peritoneal-lined sac through some defect in the abdominal wall. Figure 19-16 shows the anatomy of the region and the three common types of pelvic hernias.

Pathophysiology

- Hernias arise along the course that the testicle traveled as it exited the abdomen and entered the scrotum during intrauterine life.
- Occur because there is a potential space for protrusion of some abdominal organ, commonly the bowel but occasionally the omentum
- Femoral hernias occur at the fossa ovalis, where the femoral artery exits the abdomen.
- Strangulated hernias occur when the blood supply to the protruded tissue is compromised.

Subjective Data

- Soft swelling or bulge in inguinal area
- May have pain on straining (indirect, femoral)

Objective Data

- Indirect: soft swelling in area of internal ring; hernia comes down canal and touches fingertip on examination
- Large hernia may be present in scrotum (Fig. 19-17)
- Direct: bulge in area of Hesselbach triangle; easily reduced; hernia bulges anteriorly, pushes against side of finger on examination
- Femoral: inguinal canal empty on examination
- Strangulated: hernia is nonreducible; this condition requires prompt surgical intervention.

FIGURE 19-16 Anatomy of region of common pelvic hernias. A, Indirect inguinal hernia. **B,** Direct inguinal hernia. **C,** Femoral hernia.

FIGURE 19-17 Large indirect inguinal hernia. *(From Lemmi and Lemmi, 2009.)*

DIFFERENTIAL DIAGNOSIS
Distinguishing Characteristics of Hernias

	Indirect Inguinal	Direct Inguinal	Femoral
Incidence	Most common type of hernia; both genders are affected; often patients are children and young males.	Less common than indirect inguinal; occurs more often in males than females; more common in those older than 40 years of age	Least common type of hernia; occurs more often in females than in males; rare in children
Pathway	Through internal inguinal ring; can remain in canal, exit the external ring, and pass into scrotum; may be bilateral	Through external inguinal ring; located in region of the Hesselbach triangle; rarely enters scrotum	Through femoral ring, femoral canal, and fossa ovalis
Presentation	Soft swelling in area of internal ring; pain on straining; hernia comes down canal and touches fingertip on examination	Bulge in area of Hesselbach triangle; usually painless; easily reduced; hernia bulges anteriorly, pushes against side of finger on examination	Right-sided presentation more common than left; pain may be severe; inguinal canal empty on examination

PENIS

Paraphimosis

The inability to replace the foreskin to its usual position after it has been retracted behind the glans

Pathophysiology

- Almost always an iatrogenically or inadvertently induced condition caused by retracting the prepuce and then inadvertently leaving it in its retracted position
- In most cases, the foreskin reduces on its own, but if reduction does not occur, swelling and paraphimosis can occur.
- When the foreskin becomes trapped behind the corona for a prolonged period, a constricting band of tissue forms around the penis and impairs blood and lymphatic flow to the glans penis and prepuce.

Subjective Data

- Retraction of the foreskin during penile examination, cleaning, urethral catheterization, or cystoscopy
- Penile pain and swelling
- Children may report obstructive voiding symptoms.

Objective Data

- Glans penis is congested and enlarged (Fig. 19-18)
- Foreskin edematous
- Constricting band of tissue directly behind the head of the penis
- If untreated, necrosis and gangrene of the glans penis may be present (discolored, blackened, ulcerated).

FIGURE 19-18 Paraphimosis. *(Courtesy Patrick C. Walsh, MD, The Johns Hopkins University School of Medicine, Baltimore.)*

Syphilitic Chancre

Skin lesion associated with primary syphilis

Pathophysiology

- Sexually transmitted infection caused by the bacterium *Treponema pallidum*
- Contracted through direct contact with a syphilis sore
- Lesion of primary syphilis generally occurs 2 weeks after exposure

Subjective Data

- Painless lesion on penis
- History of sexual contact

Objective Data

- Solitary lesion; firm, round, small, commonly located on the glans but can be located on the foreskin (Fig. 19-19)
- Lesion has indurated borders with a clear base
- Scrapings from the ulcer, when examined microscopically, show spirochetes.

FIGURE 19-19 Syphilitic chancre. *(From Lemmi and Lemmi, 2009.)*

Genital Herpes

Genital herpes is a sexually transmitted infection caused by the herpes simplex virus (HSV).

Pathophysiology

- Genital herpes most commonly caused by the HSV-2 virus
- Most transmission of HSV occurs when individuals shed virus in the absence of symptoms.

Subjective Data

- Painful lesions on penis, genital area, perineum
- History of sexual contact
- May report burning or pain with urination

Objective Data

- Superficial vesicles on the glans, penile shaft, or at the base of the penis (Fig. 19-20)
- Often associated with inguinal lymphadenopathy and systemic symptoms, including fever
- Men who have sex with men may also get blisters in or around the anus.

FIGURE 19-20 Genital herpes. *(From Lemmi and Lemmi, 2009.)*

Condyloma Acuminata

"Genital warts" caused by human papillomavirus (HPV)

Pathophysiology

- HPV invades the basal layer of the epidermis; virus penetrates through skin and causes mucosal microabrasions
- Latent viral phase begins with no signs or symptoms and can last from a month to several years
- Following latency, viral DNA, capsids and particles are produced; host cells become infected and develop the characteristic skin lesions.
- Considered a sexually transmitted infection

Subjective Data

- Soft painless wartlike lesions on penis
- History of sexual contact

Objective Data

- Single or multiple papular lesions
- May be pearly, filiform, fungating (ulcerating and necrotic) cauliflower, or plaquelike (Figs. 19-21 and 19-22)
- Can be smooth, verrucous, or lobulated
- May be the same color as the skin, or may be reddish or hyperpigmented
- Lesions are commonly present on the prepuce, glans penis, and penile shaft, but they may be present within the urethra as well.

FIGURE 19-21 Condyloma acuminatum (genital warts). *(From Wolfe, 1984.)*

FIGURE 19-22 Condyloma acuminatum (genital warts). *(From Lemmi and Lemmi, 2009.)*

Lymphogranuloma Venereum

Sexually transmitted infection of the lymphatics

Pathophysiology

- Caused by *Chlamydia trachomatis*
- Organism enters through skin breaks and abrasions, or it crosses the epithelial cells of mucous membranes
- Initial lesion occurs at the site of entry
- Travels via lymphatics to regional lymph nodes, where organism replicates within macrophages
- Subsequently, local lymph nodes become involved; draining sinus tracts may form.

Subjective Data

- Painless lesion on penis
- Symptoms may be systemic (fever, malaise)
- History of sexual contact

Objective Data

- Initial lesion is a painless erosion at or near the coronal sulcus (Fig. 19-23)
- Enlarged regional lymph nodes
- If lymphatic drainage is blocked, penile and scrotal lymphedema may ensue.
- Draining sinus tract in untreated infection

FIGURE 19-23 Lymphogranuloma venereum. *(From Meheus, 1982.)*

Molluscum Contagiosum

Viral infection of the skin and mucous membranes; considered a sexually transmitted infection in adults

Pathophysiology	Subjective Data	Objective Data
• Caused by a poxvirus that infects only the skin • Spread by skin-to-skin contact or by contact with an object that has touched infected skin • Virus enters the skin through small breaks in the skin barrier. • After an incubation period, growths appear	• Painless lesions on penis • Contact with an infected person	• Lesions are pearly gray, often umbilicated, smooth, dome-shaped, and with discrete margins (Fig. 19-24) • Lesions most common on the glans penis

FIGURE 19-24 Molluscum contagiosum. Close-up showing central umbilication. *(From Lemmi and Lemmi, 2009.)*

Peyronie Disease

Peyronie disease is characterized by a fibrous band in the corpus cavernosum.

Pathophysiology	Subjective Data	Objective Data
• Dense, fibrous scar tissue (plaque) forms in the tunica albuginea (wall of the corpus cavernosum). • Plaque focally interferes with expansion of the corpus cavernosum during erection • Etiology unclear; may occur as the result of trauma, inflammation, or inherited disorder • It is generally unilateral. • The mid-top of the penis is the area most commonly involved.	• Bending and/or indentation of the erection (Fig. 19-25) • Loss of penile length • May have pain with erection • Family history of the condition • History of Dupuytren contracture (finger joint flexion contractures; most commonly fourth and fifth fingers of the hand)	• One or more palpable hardened areas • Reduced elasticity of the flaccid penis • Radiography or ultrasound can show plaque calcification.

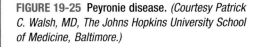

FIGURE 19-25 Peyronie disease. *(Courtesy Patrick C. Walsh, MD, The Johns Hopkins University School of Medicine, Baltimore.)*

Penile Cancer

Almost all cases are squamous cell carcinoma usually originating in the glans or foreskin.

Pathophysiology	Subjective Data	Objective Data
• Associated with HPV types 16 and 18 (Pow-Sang et al, 2010; Chaux and Cubilla, 2012) • Men who have been circumcised rarely develop penile cancer. • Lesions start as superficial neoplasms of the prepuce or glans penis and then progress to invade the corpora cavernosa and urethra, with subsequent development of metastases to the inguinal lymph nodes.	• Painless ulceration that fails to heal • Uncircumcised • Poor penile hygiene	• Lesion, usually on glans, may present as a reddened area • Papule or pustule • Warty growth, shallow erosion, or a deep ulceration with rolled edges (Fig. 19-26) • May have a phimosis that obscures the lesion

ABNORMALITIES

FIGURE 19-26 **Cancer of the penis.** *(Courtesy Patrick C. Walsh, MD, The Johns Hopkins University School of Medicine, Baltimore.)*

SCROTUM

Hydrocele

Fluid accumulation in the scrotum

Pathophysiology

- Fluid accumulates in the scrotum as a result of a defect in the tunica vaginalis; this condition is common in infancy; if the tunica vaginalis is not patent, the hydrocele will generally disappear spontaneously in the first 6 months of life.

Subjective Data

- Painless enlargement or swelling of the scrotum

Objective Data

- Nontender, smooth, firm mass superior and anterior to the testes (Fig. 19-27)
- Transilluminates
- Confined to the scrotum and does not enter the inguinal canal, unless it has been present for a long time and is very large and taut

FIGURE 19-27 **Hydrocele.** *(From Lloyd-Davies et al, 1994.)*

Spermatocele

Benign cystic accumulation of sperm occurring on the epididymis

Pathophysiology

- Etiology and pathophysiology unknown

Subjective Data

- Asymptomatic; incidental finding on physical examination or self-examination

Objective Data

- Smooth, spherical, nontender mass at epididymis (superior and posterior to the testis) (Fig. 19-28)
- Usually smaller than 1 cm

FIGURE 19-28 **Spermatocele.** *(From Lloyd-Davies et al, 1994.)*

Varicocele

Abnormal tortuosity and dilation of veins of the pampiniform plexus within the spermatic cord (Fig. 19-29)

Pathophysiology

- More common in the left testicle than in the right because of several anatomic factors, including the angle at which the left testicular vein enters the left renal vein, the lack of effective antireflux valves at the juncture of the testicular vein and renal vein, and the increased renal vein pressure due to its compression between the superior mesenteric artery and the aorta
- May be associated with reduced fertility, probably from increased venous pressure and elevated testicular temperature

Subjective Data

- Usually asymptomatic (and found in course of evaluation for infertility)
- May report scrotal pain or heaviness

Objective Data

- Often visible only when the patient is standing; is classically described as a "bag of worms"
- Graded as:
  - Small: palpated only during Valsalva maneuver
  - Moderate: easily palpated without Valsalva maneuver
  - Large: causing visible bulging of the scrotum

FIGURE 19-29 Varicocele.

Orchitis

Acute inflammation of the testis secondary to infection

Pathophysiology

- Uncommon except as a complication of mumps in the adolescent or adult
- Is generally unilateral and results in testicular atrophy in 50% of the cases
- In older adults may result from bacterial migration from a prostatic infection

Subjective Data

- Acute onset testicular pain and swelling
- Pain ranges from mild discomfort to severe pain
- Associated systemic symptoms: fatigue, malaise, myalgias, fever
- Mumps orchitis follows the development of parotitis by 4 to 7 days.

Objective Data

- Enlarged, tender testis (Fig. 19-30)
- Erythematous and edematous scrotal skin
- Enlarged epididymis associated with epididymo-orchitis

FIGURE 19-30 Orchitis.

ABNORMALITIES

Epididymitis

Inflammation of the epididymis (a major consideration in the differential diagnosis is testicular torsion, a surgical emergency; see the Differential Diagnosis table, Acute Testicular Swelling)

Pathophysiology
- Often seen in association with a urinary tract infection
- May also occur as a result of an STI
- Occasionally, chronic epididymitis may occur as a consequence of tuberculosis.

Subjective Data
- Painful scrotum
- Urethral discharge
- Fever
- Pyuria
- Recent sexual activity

Objective Data
- Epididymis feels firm and lumpy; is tender (Fig. 19-31)
- Vasa deferentia may be beaded
- Overlying scrotum may be markedly erythematous

FIGURE 19-31 **Epididymitis.** *(From Lloyd-Davies et al, 1994.)*

Testicular Torsion

Twisting of testis on spermatic cord; testicular torsion is a surgical emergency (see the Differential Diagnosis table, Acute Testicular Swelling).

Pathophysiology
- Twisting of the spermatic cord cuts off the blood supply to the testicle.
- Occurs in newborns to adolescents; most common in adolescents

Subjective Data
- Acute onset of scrotal pain, often accompanied by nausea and vomiting
- Absence of systemic symptoms such as fever and myalgia
- Risk factors: trauma and strenuous physical activity

Objective Data
- The testicle is exquisitely tender.
- Scrotal discoloration is often present.
- Absence of cremasteric reflex on side of acute swelling

DIFFERENTIAL DIAGNOSIS

Acute Testicular Swelling

	Torsion	Epididymitis
Cause	Twisting of testis on spermatic cord	Bacterial infection (STI or UTI)
Age	Newborn to adolescence	Adolescence to adulthood
Onset of pain	Acute	Gradual
Vomiting	Common	Uncommon
Anorexia	Common	Uncommon
Fever	Uncommon	Possible
Dysuria	Uncommon	Possible
Supporting findings	Absence of cremasteric reflex on side of acute swelling Scrotal discoloration	Urethral discharge History of recent sexual activity Fever Pyuria Thickened or nodular epididymis

STI, Sexually transmitted infection; *UTI,* urinary tract infection.

Testicular Cancer

Classified by the cells from which the cancer arises

Pathophysiology

- Seminomas and nonseminomas arise from germ cells (sperm-producing cells).
- Non–germ cell tumors arise from supportive and hormone-producing tissue.
- Most testicular cancers are germ cell cancers.
- Germ cell tumors tend to occur in young men and are the most common tumor in males 15 to 30 years of age.

Subjective Data

- Presence of painless mass in testicle
- May report scrotal enlargement or swelling
- Sensation of heaviness in the scrotum
- Dull ache in the lower abdomen, back, or groin
- Sudden collection of fluid in the scrotum

Objective Data

- Irregular, nontender mass fixed on the testis (Fig. 19-32)
- Does not transilluminate
- May also have hydrocele (does transilluminate)
- May have associated inguinal lymphadenopathy

FIGURE 19-32 Testicular tumor. *(From 400 Self-assessment picture tests in clinical medicine, 1984. By permission of Mosby International.)*

Klinefelter Syndrome

Congenital anomaly associated with XXY chromosomal inheritance

Pathophysiology

- Caused by an extra X chromosome
- Infant with Klinefelter syndrome appears normal at birth; condition becomes apparent in puberty when secondary sexual characteristics fail to develop
- Symptoms depend on how many XXY cells a man has, how much testosterone is in his body, and his age when the condition is diagnosed.

Subjective Data

- Differences in physical, language, and social development compared with other males of the same age

Objective Data

- Hypogonadism, including a small scrotum
- Diminished pubic, axillary, and facial hair
- Enlarged breast tissue
- Tall stature, long legs, short trunk (Fig. 19-33)
- In mild cases, no abnormalities will be present; however, the individual will be infertile.

FIGURE 19-33 Klinefelter syndrome. *(From Thibodeau and Patton, 2010.)*

ABNORMALITIES

✤ Infants

AMBIGUOUS GENITALIA

See Chapter 18.

Hypospadias

Congenital defect in which the urethral meatus is located on the ventral surface of the glans penile shaft or the base of the penis

Pathophysiology	Subjective Data	Objective Data
• Congenital defect that is thought to occur embryologically during urethral development, from 8 to 20 weeks of gestation • Several etiologies suggested, including genetic, endocrine, and environmental factors • Presence of hypospadias puts the infant at greater risk of having undescended testicles.	• Parent may note penile defect or may be discovered by a nurse or other health care provider in the nursery	• Diagnosis generally made on examination of the newborn infant • Urethral meatus located on the ventral surface of the glans penile shaft or the base of the penis (Fig. 19-34) • Dorsal hood of foreskin and glanular groove are evident, but prepuce is incomplete ventrally • Penis may have ventral shortening and curvature, called chordee, with more proximal urethral defects

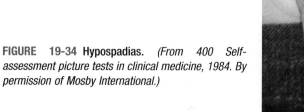

FIGURE 19-34 **Hypospadias.** *(From 400 Self-assessment picture tests in clinical medicine, 1984. By permission of Mosby International.)*

CHAPTER 20

Anus, Rectum, and Prostate

xamination of the anus and rectum may be performed as part of a routine health visit for both men and women. In men, it includes examination of the prostate. The examination is also performed when the patient has a specific concern.

evolve *http://evolve.elsevier.com/Seidel*
- Physical Exam Key Points
- NCLEX Review Questions
- Activities
- Animations
- Videos
- Student Checklist

ANATOMY AND PHYSIOLOGY

The rectum and anus form the terminal portions of the gastro-intestinal (GI) tract (Fig. 20-1). The anal canal is approximately 2.5 to 4 cm long and opens onto the perineum. The tissue visible at the external margin of the anus is moist, hairless mucosa. Juncture with the perianal skin is characterized by increased pigmentation and, in the adult, the presence of hair.

The anal canal is normally kept securely closed by concentric rings of muscle, the internal and external sphincters. The internal

Physical Examination Preview

Here is a preview of the steps involved in conducting physical examination of the anus, rectum, and prostate. ⓔ These procedures are explained in detail in this chapter and are available on Evolve in printable formats.

Anus, Rectum, and Prostate

1. Inspect the sacrococcygeal and perianal area for the following (p. 489):
   - Skin characteristics
   - Lesions
   - Pilonidal dimpling and/or tufts of hair
   - Inflammation
   - Excoriation
2. Inspect the anus for the following (p. 489):
   - Skin characteristics and tags
   - Lesions, fissures, hemorrhoids, or polyps
   - Fistulae
   - Prolapse
3. Insert finger and assess sphincter tone (p. 489).
4. Palpate the muscular ring for the following (pp. 489-490):
   - Smoothness
   - Evenness of pressure against examining finger
5. Palpate the lateral, posterior, and anterior rectal walls for the following (p. 490):
   - Nodules, masses, or polyps
   - Tenderness
   - Irregularities

6. In males, palpate the posterior surface of the prostate gland through the anterior rectal wall for the following (p. 491):
   - Size
   - Contour
   - Consistency
   - Mobility
7. In females, palpate the cervix and uterus through the anterior rectal wall for the following (p. 491):
   - Size
   - Shape
   - Position
   - Smoothness
   - Mobility
8. Have the patient bear down and palpate deeper for the following (p. 490):
   - Tenderness
   - Nodules
9. Withdraw the finger and examine fecal material for the following (p. 491):
   - Color
   - Consistency
   - Blood or pus
   - Occult blood by chemical test if indicated

ANATOMY AND PHYSIOLOGY

FIGURE 20-1 **Anatomy of the anus and rectum.**

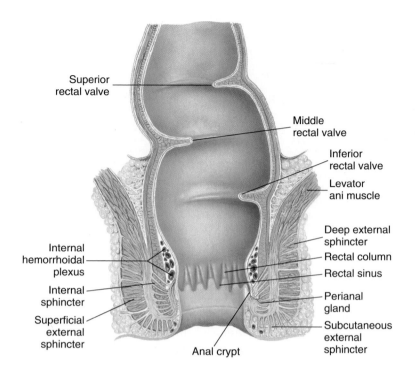

Superior rectal valve

Middle rectal valve

Inferior rectal valve

Levator ani muscle

Deep external sphincter

Rectal column

Rectal sinus

Internal hemorrhoidal plexus

Internal sphincter

Superficial external sphincter

Perianal gland

Subcutaneous external sphincter

Anal crypt

ring of smooth muscle is under involuntary autonomic control. The urge to defecate occurs when the rectum fills with feces, which causes reflexive stimulation that relaxes the internal sphincter. Defecation is controlled by the striated external sphincter, which is under voluntary control. The lower half of the canal is supplied with somatic sensory nerves, making it sensitive to painful stimuli, whereas the upper half is under autonomic control and is relatively insensitive. Therefore conditions of the lower anus cause pain, whereas those of the upper anus may not.

Internally the anal canal is lined by columns of mucosal tissue (columns of Morgagni) that fuse to form the anorectal junction. The spaces between the columns are called crypts, into which anal glands empty. Inflammation of the crypts can result in fistula or fissure formation. Anastomosing veins cross the columns, forming a ring called the zona hemorrhoidalis. Internal hemorrhoids result from dilation of these veins. The lower segment of the anal canal contains a venous plexus that drains into the inferior rectal veins. Dilation of this plexus results in external hemorrhoids.

The rectum lies superior to the anus and is approximately 12 cm long. Its proximal end is continuous with the sigmoid colon. The distal end, the anorectal junction, is visible on proctoscopic examination as a sawtooth-like edge but is not palpable. Above the anorectal junction, the rectum dilates and turns posteriorly into the hollow of the coccyx and sacrum, forming the rectal ampulla, which stores flatus and feces. The rectal wall contains three semilunar transverse folds (Houston valves). The lowest of these folds can be palpated by the examiner.

In males, the prostate gland is located at the base of the bladder and surrounds the urethra. It is composed of muscular and glandular tissue and is approximately 4 × 3 × 2 cm. The posterior surface of the prostate gland is in close contact with the anterior rectal wall and is accessible by digital examination. It is convex and is divided by a shallow median sulcus into right and

left lateral lobes. A third or median lobe, not palpable on examination, is composed of glandular tissue and lies between the ejaculatory duct and the urethra. It contains active secretory alveoli that contribute to ejaculatory fluid. The seminal vesicles extend outward from the prostate (Fig. 20-2).

In females, the anterior rectal wall lies in contact with the vagina and is separated from it by the rectovaginal septum. See Chapter 18 for a more detailed discussion.

✀ Infants and Children

At 7 weeks of gestation, a portion of the caudal hindgut is divided by an anorectal septum into a urogenital sinus and a rectum. The urogenital sinus is covered by a membrane that develops into the anal opening by 8 weeks of gestation. Most anorectal malformations result from abnormalities in this partitioning process.

The first meconium stool is ordinarily passed within the first 24 to 48 hours after birth and indicates anal patency. Thereafter, it is common for newborns, especially those who are breastfed, to have a stool after each feeding (the gastrocolic reflex). Both the internal and external sphincters are under involuntary reflexive control because myelination of the spinal cord is incomplete.

By the end of the first year, the infant may have one or two bowel movements daily. Children are developmentally ready to begin toilet training at age 2 to 4 years. Girls typically acquire bladder control before boys; bowel control typically is achieved before bladder control (Katz and DeMaso, 2011).

In males, the prostate is small, inactive, and not palpable on rectal examination. The prostate remains undeveloped until puberty, at which time androgenic influences prompt its growth and maturation. The initially minimal glandular component develops active secretory alveoli, and the prostate becomes functional.

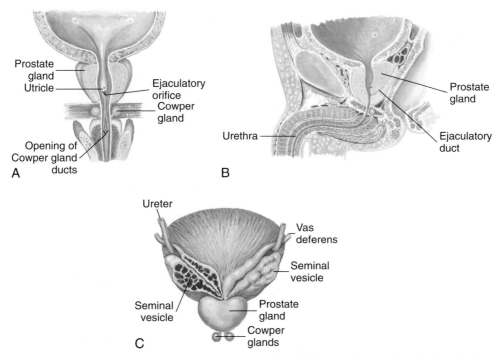

FIGURE 20-2 **Anatomy of the prostate gland and seminal vesicles. A,** Cross section. **B,** Lateral view. **C,** Posterior view.

❧ Pregnant Women

During pregnancy pressure increases in the veins below the enlarged uterus. Dietary habits and hormonal changes that decrease gastrointestinal tract tone and motility produce constipation. These factors predispose pregnant women to the development of hemorrhoids. Labor, which results in pressure on the pelvic floor by the presenting part of the fetus and expulsive efforts of the woman, may also aggravate the condition, causing protrusion and inflammation of hemorrhoids.

❧ Older Adults

Degeneration of afferent neurons in the rectal wall interferes with the process of relaxation of the internal sphincter in response to distention of the rectum. This can result in an elevated pressure threshold for the sensation of rectal distention in the older adult, with consequent retention of stool. Conversely, as the autonomically controlled internal sphincter loses tone, the external sphincter cannot by itself control the bowels, and the older adult may experience fecal incontinence.

In men, the fibromuscular structures of the prostate gland atrophy, with loss of function of the secretory alveoli; however, the atrophy of aging is often obscured by benign hyperplasia of the glandular tissue. The muscular component of the prostate is progressively replaced by collagen.

REVIEW OF RELATED HISTORY

For each of the symptoms or conditions discussed in this section, targeted topics to include in the history of the present illness are listed. Responses to questions about these topics provide clues for focusing the physical examination and the development of an

appropriate diagnostic evaluation. Questions regarding medication use (prescription and over the counter preparations) as well as complementary and alternative therapies are relevant for each.

History of Present Illness

- ◆ Changes in bowel function
    - ◆ Character: number, frequency, consistency of stools; presence of mucus or blood; color (dark, bright red, black, light, or clay-colored); odor
    - ◆ Onset and duration: sudden or gradual, relation to dietary change, relation to stressful events
    - ◆ Accompanying symptoms: incontinence, flatus, pain, fever, nausea, vomiting, cramping, abdominal distention
    - ◆ Medications: iron, laxatives, stool softeners
- ◆ Anal discomfort: itching, pain, stinging, burning
    - ◆ Relation to body position and defecation
    - ◆ Straining at stool
    - ◆ Presence of mucus or blood
    - ◆ Interference with activities of daily living or sleep
    - ◆ Medications: hemorrhoid preparations
- ◆ Rectal bleeding
    - ◆ Color: bright or dark red, black
    - ◆ Relation to defecation
    - ◆ Amount: spotting on toilet paper versus active bleeding
    - ◆ Accompanying changes in stool: color, frequency, consistency, shape, odor, presence of mucus
    - ◆ Associated symptoms: incontinence, flatus, rectal pain, abdominal pain or cramping, abdominal distention, weight loss
    - ◆ Medications: iron, fiber additives

+ Males: changes in urinary function
  + History of enlarged prostate or prostatitis
  + Symptoms: hesitancy, urgency, nocturia, dysuria, change in force or caliber of stream, dribbling, urethral discharge
  + Medications: antihistamines, anticholinergics, tricyclic antidepressants, 5-alpha-reductase inhibitors

Past Medical History

+ Hemorrhoids
+ Spinal cord injury
+ Bowel habits and characteristics: timing, frequency, number, consistency, shape, color, odor
+ Males: prostatic hypertrophy or carcinoma
+ Females: episiotomy or fourth-degree laceration during delivery
+ Colorectal cancer or related cancers: breast, ovarian, endometrial

Family History

+ Rectal polyps
+ Colon cancer or familial cancer syndromes (see Risk Factors box, Chapter 17)
+ Prostate cancer (see Risk Factors box)

Personal and Social History

+ Travel history: areas with high incidence of parasitic infestation, including zones in the United States
+ Diet: inclusion of fiber foods (cereals, breads, nuts, fruits, vegetables) and concentrated high-fiber foods; amount of animal fat
+ Risk factors for colorectal, prostate, or anal cancer (see Risk Factors Box in Chapter 17)
+ Males: having sex with males (see Box 20-1)
+ Vaccination status for the human papilloma virus (HPV)
+ Use of alcohol

Risk Factors

Prostate Cancer

- Older than 50 years
- Race: twice the risk in black men compared to white men
- Nationality: common in North America and northwestern Europe; less common in Asia, Africa, Central America, and South America
- Family history of prostate cancer: twice the risk with one first-degree relative; risk increases with more than one first-degree relative
- Inherited cancer syndromes: *BRCA1*, *BRCA2* mutations
- Diet high in animal fat, dairy products, or calcium
- Hormones: cumulative exposure of the prostate to high levels of androgens
- Physical inactivity (regular physical activity reduces risk)

American Cancer Society, 2012; National Cancer Institute, 2012.

Box 20-1   Screening for Sexually Transmitted Infections in Men Who Have Sex with Men (MSM)

The Centers for Disease Control and Prevention (CDC) recommend routine laboratory screening for common sexually transmitted infections (STIs) in all sexually active MSM. The tests should be performed at least annually.

- Human immunodeficiency virus (HIV) serology, if HIV-negative or not tested within the previous year
- Syphilis serology
- HBsAg to detect hepatitis B virus HBV infection
- Test for the following infections in men who have had receptive oral intercourse during the preceding year regardless of history of condom use during exposure:
  - Urethral infection and rectal infection with *N. gonorrhoeae* and *C. trachomatis*
  - Pharyngeal infection with *N. gonorrhoeae*
- Consider evaluation for herpes simplex virus (HSV)-2 infection with type-specific serologic tests if infection status is unknown. Routine testing for anal cytologic abnormalities or anal HPV infection can be considered but evidence is limited concerning the natural history of anal intraepithelial neoplasias, the reliability of screening methods, the safety and response to treatments, and the programmatic support needed for such a screening activity.
- More frequent STI screening (e.g., at 3- to 6-month intervals) is indicated for MSM who have multiple or anonymous partners, have sex in conjunction with illicit drug use, who use methamphetamine, or whose sex partners participate in these activities.

From CDC, 2010.

Risk Factors

Anal Cancer

- Infection with high-risk type HPV
- Multiple sexual partners
- Receptive anal intercourse
- Cigarette smoking
- Immunosuppression
- Race: black

American Cancer Society, 2012.

✽ Infants and Children

+ Newborns: characteristics of stool
+ Bowel movements accompanied by crying, straining, bleeding
+ Feeding habits: types of foods, milk (formula or breast for infants), appetite
+ Age at which bowel control and toilet training were achieved
+ Encopresis (involuntary "fecal soiling" in children who have usually already been toilet-trained)
+ Associated symptoms: episodes of diarrhea or constipation; tenderness when cleaning after a stool; perianal irritations; weight loss; nausea, vomiting
+ Congenital anomaly: imperforate anus, myelomeningocele, aganglionic megacolon

❈ Pregnant Women

+ Weeks of gestation and estimated date of delivery
+ Exercise
+ Fluid intake and dietary habits
+ Medications: prenatal vitamins, iron, fiber supplements
+ Use of complementary or alternative therapies

❈ Older Adults

+ Changes in bowel habits or character: frequency, number, color, consistency, shape, odor
+ Associated symptoms: weight loss, rectal or abdominal pain, incontinence, flatus, episodes of constipation or diarrhea, abdominal distention, rectal bleeding
+ Dietary changes: intolerance for certain foods, inclusion of high-fiber foods, regularity of eating habits, appetite
+ Males: history of enlarged prostate, urinary symptoms (hesitancy, urgency, nocturia, dysuria, force and caliber of urinary stream, dribbling)

EXAMINATION AND FINDINGS

Equipment

+ Gloves
+ Water-soluble lubricant
+ Drapes
+ Penlight or other light source
+ Fecal occult blood testing materials if indicated

Preparation

Although the rectal examination is generally uncomfortable and sometimes embarrassing for the patient, it provides important information that is a necessary part of a comprehensive examination. Be calm, slowly paced, and gentle in your touch. Explain what will happen step by step and let the patient know what to expect. A hurried or rough examination can cause unnecessary pain and sphincter spasm, and you can easily lose the trust and cooperation of the patient.

Clinical Pearl

In Pain?

The patient with a really acute rectal problem will often shift uncomfortably from side to side when sitting.

Positioning

The rectal examination can be performed with the patient in any of these positions: knee-chest; lithotomy; left lateral with hips and knees flexed; or standing with the hips flexed and the upper body supported by the examining table. In adult males, the latter two positions are satisfactory for most purposes and allow adequate visualization of the perineal and sacrococcygeal areas. In women, the rectal examination is most often performed as part of the rectovaginal examination while the woman is in the lithotomy position (see Chapter 18).

Ask the patient to assume one of the examining positions, guiding gently with your hands when necessary. Use drapes but retain good visualization of the area. Glove one or both hands.

Sacrococcygeal and Perianal Areas

Inspect the sacrococcygeal (pilonidal) and perianal areas. The skin should be smooth and uninterrupted. Inspect for lumps, rashes, inflammation, excoriation, scars, pilonidal dimpling, and tufts of hair at the pilonidal area. Fungal infection and pinworm infestation can cause perianal irritation. Fungal infection is more common in adults with diabetes, and pinworms are more common in children. The best time to visualize pinworms in children is after they fall asleep. Inspection of the anus often reveals them. Palpate the area. The discovery of tenderness and inflammation should alert you to the possibility of a perianal abscess, anorectal fistula or fissure, pilonidal cyst, or pruritus ani.

Anus

Spread the patient's buttocks apart and inspect the anus. Use a penlight or lamp to assist in visualization. The skin around the anus will appear coarser and more darkly pigmented. Look for skin lesions, skin tags or warts, external hemorrhoids, fissures, and fistulae. Ask the patient to bear down. This will make fistulae, fissures, rectal prolapse, polyps, and internal hemorrhoids more readily apparent.

Sphincter

Lubricate your index finger of your gloved hand and press the pad of it against the anal opening (Fig. 20-3, *A*). Ask the patient to bear down to relax the external sphincter. As relaxation occurs, slip the tip of the finger into the anal canal (see Fig. 20-3, *B*). Warn the patient that there may be a feeling of urgency for a bowel movement, and assure him or her that this will not happen. Ask the patient to tighten the external sphincter around your finger (Fig. 20-4, *A*), noting its tone; it should tighten evenly with no discomfort to the patient. A lax sphincter may indicate neurologic deficit or sexual abuse. An extremely tight sphincter can result from scarring, spasticity caused by a fissure or other lesion, inflammation, or anxiety about the examination.

An anal fistula or fissure may produce such extreme tenderness that you are not able to complete the examination without local anesthesia. Rectal pain is almost always indicative of a local disease. Look for irritation, rock-hard constipation, rectal fissures, fluctuance from a perirectal abscess, or thrombosed hemorrhoids. Always inquire about previous episodes of pain.

Anal Ring

Rotate your finger to examine the muscular anal ring (Fig. 20-4, *B*). It should feel smooth and exert even pressure on the finger. Note any nodules or irregularities.

EXAMINATION AND FINDINGS

Video: Anus, Rectum, and Prostate: Examining the Anus and Anal Sphincter

Video: Anus, Rectum, and Prostate: Palpating the Posterior and Lateral Rectal Walls

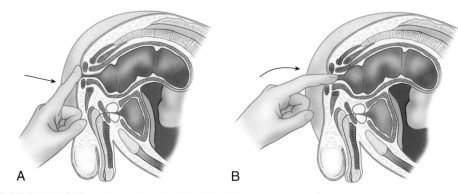

FIGURE 20-3 A, Correct procedure for introducing finger into rectum. Press pad of finger against the anal opening. **B,** As external sphincter relaxes, slip the fingertip into the anal canal. Note that patient is in the hips-flexed position.

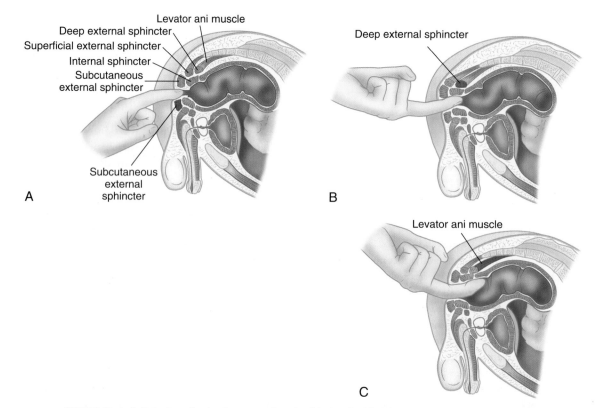

FIGURE 20-4 A, Palpation of subcutaneous external sphincter. Feel it tighten around the examining finger. **B,** Palpation of deep external sphincter. **C,** Palpation of the posterior rectal wall.

Lateral and Posterior Rectal Walls

Insert your finger farther and palpate in sequence the lateral and posterior rectal walls, noting any nodules, masses, irregularities, polyps, or tenderness (Fig. 20-4, C). The walls should feel smooth, even, and uninterrupted. Internal hemorrhoids are not ordinarily felt unless they are thrombosed. The examining finger can palpate a distance of about 6 to 10 cm into the rectum.

Bidigital Palpation

Bidigital palpation with the thumb and index finger can sometimes reveal more information than palpating with the index finger alone. To perform bidigital palpation, gently press your thumb against the perianal tissue and bring your index finger toward the thumb. This technique is particularly useful for detecting a perianal abscess.

Anterior Rectal Wall

Rotate the index finger to palpate the anterior rectal wall as above. Ask the patient to bear down. This allows you to reach a few centimeters farther into the rectum. Because the anterior rectal wall is in contact with the peritoneum, you may be able to detect the tenderness of peritoneal inflammation and the nodularity of peritoneal metastases. The nodules, called shelf lesions,

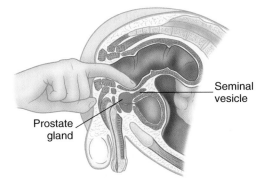

FIGURE 20-5 Palpation of the posterior surface of the prostate gland. Feel for the lateral lobes and median sulcus.

Prostate gland

Seminal vesicle

Box 20-2	Prostate Enlargement

Prostate enlargement is classified by the amount of protrusion into the rectum:

  Grade I: 1 to 2 cm
  Grade II: 2 to 3 cm
  Grade III: 3 to 4 cm
  Grade IV: more than 4 cm

are palpable just above the prostate in males and in the cul-de-sac of females. These can be felt as a hard, nodular shelf at the tip of the examining finger.

Prostate

In males, you can palpate the posterior surface of the prostate gland (Fig. 20-5) on the anterior wall. Tell the patient that he may feel the urge to urinate but that he will not. Note the size, contour, consistency, and mobility of the prostate. The gland should feel like a pencil eraser—firm, smooth, and slightly movable—and it should be nontender. A healthy prostate has a diameter of about 4 cm, with less than 1 cm protrusion into the rectum. Greater protrusion denotes prostatic enlargement, which should be noted with the amount of protrusion recorded (Box 20-2). The median sulcus may be obliterated when the lobes are hypertrophied or neoplastic. A rubbery or boggy consistency is indicative of benign hypertrophy, whereas stony hard nodularity may indicate carcinoma, prostatic calculi, or chronic fibrosis. A tender fluctuant softness suggests prostatic abscess. Identify the lateral lobes and the median sulcus. The prostatic lobes should feel symmetric. The seminal vesicles are not palpable unless they are inflamed. The Evidence-Based Practice box discusses screening for prostate cancer.

Palpation of the prostate can force secretions through the urethral orifice. Any secretions that appear at the meatus should be cultured and examined microscopically. Specimen preparation techniques are described in Chapter 18.

Uterus and Cervix

In females, a retroflexed or retroverted uterus is usually palpable through rectal examination. The cervix may be palpable through

the anterior rectal wall (see Chapter 18). Do not mistake these structures for a tampon or a tumor.

Stool

Slowly withdraw your finger and examine it for any fecal material, which should be soft and brown (Box 20-3). Note any blood or pus. Very light tan or gray stool could indicate obstructive jaundice, whereas tarry black stool should make you suspect upper intestinal tract bleeding. A more subtle blood loss can result in a virtually unchanged color of the stool, but even a small amount will yield a positive test for occult blood. If indicated, fecal material can be tested for blood using a chemical guaiac procedure. Common causes of rectal bleeding are identified in Box 20-4.

Further evaluation is indicated if there is persistent anal or rectal bleeding; any interruption in the smooth contour of the rectal wall on palpation; persistent pain with negative findings on rectal examination; or unexplained, persistent stool changes.

⚘ Infants and Children

Rectal examination is not always performed on infants and children unless there is a particular problem. An examination is

Box 20-3   Stool Characteristics in Disease

Changes in the shape, content, or consistency of stool suggest that some disease process is present. Stool characteristics can sometimes point to the type of disorder present; therefore, you should be familiar with the following characteristics and associated disorders:

- Intermittent, pencil-like stools suggest a spasmodic contraction in the rectal area.
- Persistent, pencil-like stools indicate permanent stenosis from scarring or from pressure of a malignancy.
- Decreased caliber (pencil-thin stools) indicate lower rectal stricture.
- A large amount of mucus in the fecal matter is characteristic of intestinal inflammation and mucous colitis.
- Small flecks of bloodstained mucus in liquid feces are indicative of amebiasis.
- Fatty stools are seen in patients with pancreatic disorders and malabsorption syndromes, such as cystic fibrosis.
- Stools the color of aluminum (caused by a mixture of melena and fat) occur in tropical sprue, carcinoma of the hepatopancreatic ampulla, and children treated with sulfonamides for diarrhea.

Box 20-4   Common Causes of Rectal Bleeding

There are numerous reasons that blood can appear in the feces, ranging from benign, self-limiting events to serious, life-threatening disease. Following are some common causes:

- Anal fissures
- Anaphylactoid purpura
- Aspirin-containing medications
- Bleeding disorders
- Coagulation disorders
- Colitis
- Dysentery, acute and amebic
- Esophageal varices
- Familial telangiectasia
- Foreign body trauma
- Hemorrhoids
- Hiatal hernia
- Hookworm
- Intussusception
- Iron poisoning
- Meckel diverticulum
- Neoplasms of any type
- Oral steroids
- Peptic ulcers, acute and chronic
- Polyps, single or multiple
- Regional enteritis
- Strangulated hernia
- Swallowed blood
- Thrombocytopenia
- Volvulus

Table 20-1   Sequence and Description of Stools in Infants

Infants	Type of Stool
Newborn meconium	Greenish black, viscous, contains occult blood; first stool is sterile
3 to 6 days old	Transitional: thin, slimy, brown to green
Breast-fed	Mushy, loose, seedy, golden (mustard) yellow; frequency varies from after each feeding to every few days; nonirritating to skin
Formula-fed	Light yellow, characteristic odor, irritating to skin

Data from Lowdermilk and Perry, 2004.

Candida, or other irritants of the diaper area. Rectal prolapse results from constipation, diarrhea, or sometimes severe coughing or straining. Hemorrhoids are rare in children, and their presence suggests a serious underlying problem such as portal hypertension. Small flat flaps of skin around the rectum (condylomas) are commonly from HPV infection. Sinuses, tufts of hair, and dimpling in the pilonidal area may indicate lower occult spinal deformities; the presence of these should alert the examiner for the need of an ultrasound to evaluate for potential spinal deformities.

Lightly touch the anal opening, which should produce anal contraction (the "anal wink"). Lack of contraction may indicate a lower spinal cord lesion or chronic abuse.

Examine the patency of the anus and its position in all newborn infants. Patency is usually confirmed by passage of meconium or initial rectal temperature. To determine patency when there is concern, insert a lubricated catheter no more than 1 cm into the rectum. Occasionally a perianal fistula may be confused with an anal orifice. Be careful in making this judgment. Sometimes the anal orifice can seem appropriate, yet there may be atresia just inside or a few centimeters within the rectum. Rectal examination or insertion of a catheter does not always provide definitive assessment, and radiologic studies may be necessary. If there is no passage of stool in 24 hours in a newborn, suspect rectal atresia, Hirschsprung disease (congenital megacolon), or cystic fibrosis.

Perform the rectal examination in infants and young children with the child lying on his or her back. You may hold the child's feet together and flex the knees and hips on the abdomen with one hand, using the gloved index finger of your other hand for the examination (Fig. 20-6). Some health care providers are reluctant to use the index finger because of its size, choosing instead the fifth finger; however, even with the smallest of adult fingers, some bleeding and transient prolapse of the rectum often occur right after examination. Always warn the parents of this possibility.

Assess the tone of the rectal sphincter. It should feel snug but neither too tight nor too loose. A very tight sphincter can cause enough tension to produce a stenosis, which leads to stool retention and pain during a bowel movement. A lax sphincter is associated with lesions of the peripheral spinal nerves or spinal cord, *Shigella* infection, and previous fecal impactions. The presence of bruises around the anus, scars, anal tears (especially those that

required whenever there is any symptom that suggests an intraabdominal or pelvic problem, a mass or tenderness, bladder distention, bleeding, or rectal or bowel abnormalities. Deviation from the expected stool pattern in infants demands investigation (Table 20-1).

It is imperative that you respect the child's modesty and apprehension. Careful explanation of each step in the process is necessary for the child who is old enough to understand.

Routinely inspect the anal region and perineum, examining the surrounding buttocks for redness, bruising, masses, or swelling. Inspect for swollen, tender perirectal protrusion, abscesses, and possibly rectal fistulae. A variety of problems can be discovered by this inspection. Shrunken buttocks suggest a chronic debilitating disease. They are also common in premature infants. Asymmetric creases occur with congenital dislocation of the hips. Perirectal redness and irritation are suggestive of pinworms,

FIGURE 20-6 Positioning the infant or child for rectal examination.

extend into the surrounding perianal skin), and anal dilation may be evidence of sexual abuse.

Feel for feces in the rectum. Chronic constipation in children with cognitive deficiency or emotional problems is often associated with a rectum distended with feces. A consistently empty rectum in the presence of constipation is a clue to the diagnosis of Hirschsprung disease. A fecal mass in the rectum accompanying diarrhea suggests overflow diarrhea. Stool recovered on the examining finger should be tested for occult blood.

A rectal examination in the young female gives good access to information about the cervix and uterus (see Chapter 18). The ovaries are not usually palpable on rectal examination.

In boys, the prostate is usually not felt. A palpable prostate in preadolescent boys suggests precocious puberty or a virilizing disease process, which should be apparent from examination of the genitalia.

The rectum can be further evaluated for suspected fissures, fistulae, or polyps by using a small proctoscope or even a wide-mouth speculum on the otoscope.

Rectal examination should be part of the physical examination for adolescents who have symptoms related to the lower intestinal tract. The same procedures and guidelines that are used for adults apply to adolescents. Be especially sensitive to a first examination, and spend additional time explaining what to expect. Illustrations and models can be helpful.

✤ Pregnant Women

The examination of the rectum provides information about rectovaginal musculature and more specific information about the cervix and uterus (see Chapter 18). Assessment for hemorrhoids should include both external and internal evaluation. Hemorrhoids are usually not found early in pregnancy; however, they may be an expected variation late in pregnancy. Evaluate hemorrhoids for size, extent, location (internal or external), discomfort to the patient, and signs of infection or bleeding.

Clinical Pearl

Stool Changes in Pregnant Women

During pregnancy, the stool color may be dark green or black if the woman is taking iron supplements. Iron may also cause diarrhea or constipation.

✤ Older Adults

The examination procedure and findings for the older adult are much the same as those for the younger adult. The older patient may be more limited in ability to assume a position other than the left lateral. Sphincter tone may be somewhat decreased. Older adults commonly experience fecal impaction resulting from constipation. Older men are far more likely to have an enlarged prostate, which will be felt as smooth, rubbery, and symmetric. The median sulcus may or may not be obliterated. Older adults are more likely to have polyps and are at higher risk for carcinoma, making the rectal examination particularly important in this age group.

Sample Documentation

History and Physical Examination

Subjective

A 57-year-old man reports nighttime urination for the past several months, at least twice per night. Restricts fluid intake after 8 PM. Notices difficulty in starting stream. No pain or bleeding on urination. No change in caliber of stream. Denies change in bowel habits or stool characteristics. No history of prostatitis or enlarged prostate.

Objective

Perianal area intact without lesions or visible hemorrhoids. An external skin tag is visible at the 6 o'clock position. No fissures or fistulae. Sphincter tightens evenly. Prostate is symmetric, smooth, boggy, with 1-cm protrusion into rectum. Median sulcus present. Nontender, no nodules. Rectal walls free of masses. Moderate amount of soft stool present.

For additional sample documentation, see Chapter 26, pp. 628-631.

Staying Well

Sexually Transmitted Infections

Infected persons may spread sexually transmitted infections (STIs) through anal sex practices in which blood, semen, or other fluid is shared. Practicing safer sex can prevent STIs in men and women. STIs that affect the anus include the following:
- HSV infection of the skin and mucosa causing recurring sores and pain
- Gonorrheal infection of the mucosa, producing an infectious discharge
- HPV, causing anal warts
- Parasites that affect the entire gastrointestinal tract
- Syphilis, early infection causing a painless lesion

Hepatitis and HIV are two STIs whose symptoms do not appear on the anus but can be transmitted through anal sex practices.

It is possible to acquire an STI without penetration. Oral–anal contact, whether from kissing or from oral contact with fingers that have been touching the anus, can spread bacteria and cause infection. The use of sex toys may transmit certain infections.

Box 20-1 discusses screening recommendations for STIs in a high-risk group.

ABNORMALITIES

ANUS, RECTUM, AND SURROUNDING SKIN

Pilonidal Cyst

Cyst or sinus near the cleft of the buttocks

Pathophysiology

- Loose hairs penetrate the skin in the sacrococcygeal area.
- Local inflammatory reaction causes a cyst to form around the ingrown hair
- Excessive pressure or repetitive trauma to the sacrococcygeal predisposes to development of the cyst.
- Most first diagnosed in young adults, although they are usually a congenital anomaly

Subjective Data

- Usually asymptomatic
- May have pain with sitting and inflammation from secondary infection

Objective Data

- Cyst or sinus seen as a dimple with a sinus tract opening
- Located in the midline, superficial to the coccyx and lower sacrum (Fig. 20-7)
- Opening may contain a tuft of hair and be surrounded by erythema
- A cyst may be palpable.

FIGURE 20-7 Pilonidal cyst. *(From Zitelli and Davis, 2007.)*

Anal Warts (Condyloma Acuminata)

Growths in or around the anus and genital area

Pathophysiology

- Result of infection with HPV
- Virus transmitted from person to person, almost always by direct sexual contact; considered an STI

Subjective Data

- Patients may be unaware that the warts are present.

Objective Data

- Single or multiple papular lesions in or around the anus and genital area
- May be pearly, filiform, fungating (ulcerating and necrotic) cauliflower, or plaquelike (Fig. 20-8)

FIGURE 20-8 Anal warts (condyloma acuminata). *(From Morse et al, 2003.)*

Perianal and Perirectal Abscesses

Infection of the anal tissue or glands

Pathophysiology

- Perianal abscess: infection of the soft tissues surrounding the anal canal, with formation of a discrete abscess cavity
- Perirectal abscesses; infection of the mucus-secreting anal glands, which drain into the anal crypts; abscess formation occurs in the deeper tissues (Fig. 20-9).
- Infections caused by anaerobic organisms, usually polymicrobial

Subjective Data

- Painful and tender
- Fever
- Pain on defecation or with sitting or walking
- Risk factors:
  - Crohn disease
  - Immunosuppression

Objective Data

- Perianal abscess: tender swollen fluctuant mass in the superficial subcutaneous tissue just adjacent to the anus
- Perirectal abscess: tender mass that may be indurated, fluctuant, or draining

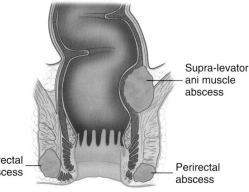

FIGURE 20-9 Perianal and perirectal abscesses. Common sites of abscess formation.

Anorectal Fissure

Tear in the anal mucosa (Fig. 20-10)

FIGURE 20-10 Lateral anal fissure in adult. *(Courtesy Gershon Efron, MD, Sinai Hospital of Baltimore.)*

ABNORMALITIES

Pathophysiology
- Tear usually caused by traumatic passage of large, hard stools

Subjective Data
- History of hard stools
- Bleeding seen in toilet or on toilet paper
- Pain, itching, or bleeding

Objective Data
- Examination is painful and may require local anesthesia.
- Fissure most often in the posterior midline, although it can also occur in the anterior midline
- Sentinel skin tag may be seen at the lower edge of the fissure
- May be ulceration through which muscles of the internal sphincter are seen
- Internal sphincter is spastic

Anal Fistula

Inflammatory tract that runs from the anus or rectum and opens onto the surface of the perianal skin or other tissue

Pathophysiology
- Caused by inflammation from a perianal or perirectal abscess; the abscess degrades the tissue until a tract and an opening in the skin is created.

Subjective Data
- May report chills, fever, nausea, vomiting, and malaise

Objective Data
- External opening of a fistula appears as a pink or red, elevated, elevated red granular tissue on the skin near the anus
- Palpable indurated tract may be present on digital rectal examination
- Serosanguineous or purulent drainage may appear with compression of the area.

Pruritus Ani

Itching of the anal area

Pathophysiology
- Commonly caused by fungal infection in adults and by parasites in children

Subjective Data
- Anal burning or itching that may interfere with sleep

Objective Data
- Excoriation, thickening, and pigmentation of anal and perianal tissue

Hemorrhoids

Swollen veins in the lower portion of the rectum or anus

Pathophysiology
- External hemorrhoids: varicose veins that originate below the anorectal line and are covered by anal skin (Fig. 20-11, *A*)
- Internal hemorrhoids: varicose veins that originate above the anorectal junction and are covered by rectal mucosa (Fig. 20-11, *B*)
- Caused by pressure on the veins in the pelvic and rectal area from straining, diarrhea, constipation, prolonged sitting, or pregnancy

Subjective Data
- May cause itching and bleeding and discomfort
- Internal: no discomfort unless they are thrombosed, prolapsed, or infected
- Bleeding may occur with or without defecation.

Objective Data
- Usually not visible at rest, they can protrude on standing and on straining at stool.
- If not reduced, they can become edematous and thrombosed and may require surgical removal.
- Thrombosed hemorrhoids appear as blue, shiny masses at the anus.
- Internal: soft swellings that are not palpable on rectal examination and are not visible unless they prolapse through the anus; proctoscopy usually required for diagnosis
- Hemorrhoidal skin tags, which can appear at the site of resolved hemorrhoids, are fibrotic or flaccid and painless.

FIGURE 20-11 A, Prolapsed hemorrhoids. **B,** Primary internal hemorrhoids. *(Courtesy Gershon Efron, MD, Sinai Hospital of Baltimore.)*

Polyps

Abnormal growth of tissue projecting from the mucous membrane

Pathophysiology	Subjective Data	Objective Data
• Occur anywhere in the intestinal tract • May be malignant or benign or have malignant potential • Can occur singly or in profusion	• Asymptomatic • Rectal bleeding	• Rectal polyp may protrude through rectum (Fig. 20-12) • Rectal polyps sometimes palpable on rectal examination as soft nodules and can be either pedunculated (on a stalk) or sessile (closely adhering to the mucosal wall) • Colonoscopy or proctoscopy is usually required for diagnosis, and biopsy is necessary to distinguish benign from malignant

FIGURE 20-12 A, Fibroepithelial polyp of the rectum. **B,** Infant with prolapsed rectal polyp. *(Courtesy Gershon Efron, MD, Sinai Hospital of Baltimore.)*

Anal Cancer

Cancer of the anal skin, mucosa, or glands

Pathophysiology	Subjective Data	Objective Data
• Most are squamous cell carcinomas, which are associated with HPV infection. • About 15% are adenocarcinomas, which originate in the glands near the anus. • Remaining anal cancers are basal cell carcinoma and malignant melanoma. • Melanoma in the anus is difficult to see and is often discovered at a late stage, after the cancer has spread through layers of tissue.	• May be asymptomatic • May report • Bleeding from the anus or rectum • Pain or pressure in the area around the anus • Itching or discharge from the anus • A lump near the anus • A change in bowel habits such as constipation, diarrhea, and the thinning of the stools	• Raised erythematous mucosa • White scaling mucosa • Pigmented mucosa • Mucosal ulceration • Verrucous lesion

ABNORMALITIES

Colorectal Cancer

Cancer of the large intestine or rectum

Pathophysiology

- Adenocarcinomas comprise the large majority of colorectal cancers.
- Accumulation of genetic and epigenetic alterations that affect essential cellular and tissue-level functions
- Begins with cell proliferation with progression to adenoma and invasive carcinoma
- The APC tumor suppressor gene is defective in more than 80% of adenomatous polyps and colon cancers.

Subjective Data

- Bleeding most common symptom
- Often asymptomatic
- May report change in bowel habits or stool characteristics
- May report abdominal pain or tenderness
- May report personal or family history of colon polyps
- May report family history of colon cancer

Objective Data

- Rectal cancer may be felt as a sessile polypoid mass with nodular raised edges and areas of ulceration; the consistency is often stony, and the contour is irregular.
- Carcinoma higher in the colon not palpable
- Polyps or lesions visualized on colonoscopy or flexible sigmoidoscopy

PROSTATE

Prostatitis

Inflammation and infection of the prostate gland (Fig. 20-13)

Pathophysiology

- Acute: bacterial infection including *Escherichia coli, Klebsiella,* and *Proteus*
- May be acquired as a sexually transmitted disease or from infection of an adjacent organ, or as a complication of prostate biopsy
- Chronic: may be bacterial or nonbacterial (chronic pelvic pain syndrome)

Subjective Data

- Acute
  - Pain
  - Urination problems
  - Sexual dysfunction
  - Fever, chills, shakes
- Chronic
  - Asymptomatic
  - Frequent bladder infections
  - Frequent urination
  - Persistent pain in the lower abdomen or back

Objective Data

- Acute
  - Gentle exam imperative; massage of the prostate can cause bacteremia.
  - Prostate enlarged, acutely tender, and often asymmetric
  - Abscess may develop, felt as a fluctuant mass in the prostate.
  - Seminal vesicles are often involved and may be dilated and tender on palpation; however, the prostate may feel boggy, enlarged, and tender or have palpable areas of fibrosis that simulate neoplasm
  - Bacteria in the urine
- Chronic
  - Prostate may be normal in size and consistency
  - May be enlarged and boggy

FIGURE 20-13 Prostatitis.

> **Clinical Pearl**
>
> *Unexplained Fever*
>
> The search for an unexplained fever should always include the rectal examination—a rectal condition or prostatitis may be the cause.

Benign Prostatic Hypertrophy (BPH)

Nonmalignant enlargement of the prostate

Pathophysiology

- Common in men older than 50 years
- Gland begins to grow at adolescence, continuing to enlarge with advancing age (Fig. 20-14)
- Growth of the prostate parallels the increased incidence of BPH

Subjective Data

- Symptoms of urinary obstruction: hesitancy, decreased force and caliber of stream, dribbling, incomplete emptying of the bladder, frequency, urgency, nocturia, and dysuria

Objective Data

- Prostate feels smooth, rubbery, symmetric, and enlarged
- Median sulcus may or may not be obliterated

FIGURE 20-14 Benign pros-tatic hypertrophy.

Prostate Cancer

Cancer of the prostate

Pathophysiology

- Over 99% of prostate cancers are adenocarcinomas, developing from the gland cells in the prostate (Fig. 20-15).
- In most cases, prostate cancer is a relatively slow-growing cancer; a small percentage is a rapidly growing, aggressive form.
- Incidence increases with age and is less frequent in men younger than 50 years of age.
- Pathogenesis poorly understood. Following the initial transformation event, further mutations of a multitude of genes lead to tumor progression and metastasis.

Subjective Data

- Early carcinoma asymptomatic
- As the malignancy advances, symptoms of urinary obstruction occur (see symptoms listed in BPH).

Objective Data

- A hard, irregular nodule may be palpable on prostate examination
- Prostate feels asymmetric, and the median sulcus may be obliterated
- Biopsy required for diagnosis

FIGURE 20-15 Cancer of prostate.

✿ Infants and Children

Imperforate Anus

Congenital defect in which the opening to the anus is missing or blocked

Pathophysiology

- A variety of anorectal malformations can occur during fetal development.
- Rectum may end blindly, be stenosed, or have a fistulous connection to the perineum, urinary tract or, in females, the vagina (Fig. 20-16)

Subjective Data

- None

Objective Data

- Condition is usually diagnosed during newborn examination on rectal examination and confirmed by lack of passage of stool within the first 48 hours of life (Figs. 20-17 and 20-18); radiographic confirmation may be necessary
- Be aware that the imperforation may be just out of the reach of the examining finger on infrequent occasions.

FIGURE 20-16 Imperforate anus: various anorectal malformations. **A,** Congenital anal stenosis. **B,** Anal membrane atresia. **C,** Anal agenesis. **D,** Rectal atresia. **E,** Rectoperineal fistula. **F,** Rectovaginal fistula.

FIGURE 20-17 Imperforate anus. *(From 400 self-assessment picture tests in clinical medicine, 1984. By permission of Mosby International.)*

FIGURE 20-18 Rectal atresia. *(Courtesy Gershon Efron, MD, Sinai Hospital of Baltimore.)*

Enterobiasis (Roundworm, Pinworm)

Infection caused by a small, thin, white roundworm, *Enterobius vermicularis*

Pathophysiology

- Adult nematode (parasite) lives in the rectum or colon and emerges onto perianal skin to lay eggs while the child sleeps

Subjective Data

- Intense itching of the perianal area
- Parents often describe unexplained irritability in the infant or child, especially at night.

Objective Data

- Perianal irritation often results from scratching.
- Can be diagnosed using Scotch tape test: press the sticky side of cellulose tape against the perianal folds and then press the tape on a glass slide; nematodes can be seen on microscopic examination.

CHAPTER 21

Musculoskeletal System

The musculoskeletal system provides the stability and mobility necessary for physical activity. Physical performance requires bones, muscles, and joints that function smoothly and effortlessly. Because the musculoskeletal system serves as the body's main line of defense against external forces, injuries are common. Moreover, numerous disease processes affect the musculoskeletal system and can ultimately cause disability. The purpose of this chapter is to review a systematic approach to the evaluation of the musculoskeletal system.

ANATOMY AND PHYSIOLOGY

The musculoskeletal system is a bony structure that provides stability to the soft tissues of the body. Its joints are held together by ligaments, attached to muscles by tendons, and cushioned by cartilage, which facilitates movement (Figs. 21-1 and 21-2). The musculoskeletal system protects vital organs, provides storage space for minerals, and produces blood cells (hematopoiesis).

Most joints are synovial—freely moving articulations containing ligaments and cartilage covering the ends of the opposing bones, which are enclosed by a fibrous capsule. A synovial membrane lines the joint and secretes the serous lubricating synovial fluid. Bursae develop in the spaces of connective tissue between

Physical Examination Preview

Here is a preview of the steps involved in conducting a physical examination of the musculoskeletal system. ⓔ These procedures are explained in detail in this chapter and are available on Evolve in printable formats.

The following steps are performed with the patient standing, sitting, and walking:
1. Inspect the skeleton and extremities and compare sides for the following (p. 510):
   • Alignment
   • Contour and symmetry
   • Size
   • Gross deformity
2. Inspect the skin and subcutaneous tissues over muscles and joints for the following (p. 510):
   • Color
   • Number of skinfolds
   • Swelling
   • Masses
3. Inspect muscles and compare sides for the following (p. 510):
   • Size
   • Symmetry
   • Fasciculations or spasms
4. Palpate all bones, joints, and surrounding muscles for the following (p. 510):
   • Muscle tone
   • Heat
   • Tenderness
   • Swelling
   • Crepitus
5. Test each major joint for active and passive range of motion and compare sides (p. 511).
6. Test major muscle groups for strength and compare sides (p. 511).

Joints that deserve particular attention include the following:

Hands and Wrists
1. Inspect the dorsum and palm of hands for the following (p. 512):
   • Contour
   • Position
   • Shape
   • Number and completeness of digits
2. Palpate each joint in the hand and wrist (p. 513).
3. Test range of motion by the following maneuvers (p. 513):
   • Metacarpophalangeal flexion (90 degrees) and hyperextension (30 degrees)
   • Thumb opposition
   • Forming a fist
   • Finger adduction and abduction
   • Wrist extension, hyperextension (70 degrees), and flexion (90 degrees)
   • Radial (20 degrees) and ulnar motion (55 degrees)
4. Test muscle strength by the following maneuvers (p. 513):
   • Wrist extension and hyperextension
   • Hand grip

Continued

Elbows

1. Inspect the elbows in flexed and extended positions for the following (p. 513):
   - Contour
   - Carrying angle (5 to 15 degrees)
2. Palpate the extensor surface of the ulna, olecranon process, and medial and lateral epicondyles of the humerus (p. 514).
3. Test range of motion by the following maneuvers (p. 514):
   - Flexion (160 degrees)
   - Extension (180 degrees)
   - Pronation and supination (90 degrees)

Shoulders

1. Inspect shoulders and shoulder girdle for contour (p. 514).
2. Palpate the joint spaces and bones of the shoulders (p. 514).
3. Test range of motion by the following maneuvers (p. 514):
   - Shrugging the shoulders
   - Forward flexion (180 degrees) and hyperextension (up to 50 degrees)
   - Abduction (180 degrees) and adduction (50 degrees)
   - Internal and external rotation (90 degrees)
4. Test muscle strength by the following maneuvers (p. 514):
   - Shrugged shoulders
   - Abduction with forward flexion
   - Medial rotation
   - Lateral rotation

Temporomandibular Joint

1. Palpate the joint space for clicking, popping, and pain (p. 516).
2. Test range of motion by having the patient perform the following (p. 516):
   - Opening and closing mouth
   - Moving jaw laterally to each side
   - Protruding and retracting jaw
3. Test strength of temporalis muscles with the patient's teeth clenched (p. 516).

Cervical Spine

1. Inspect the neck for the following (p. 516):
   - Alignment
   - Symmetry of skinfolds and muscles
2. Test range of motion by the following maneuvers (p. 518):
   - Forward flexion (45 degrees)
   - Hyperextension (55 degrees)
   - Lateral bending (40 degrees)
   - Rotation (70 degrees)
3. Test strength of sternocleidomastoid and trapezius muscles (cranial nerve XI, spinal accessory) (p. 518).

Thoracic and Lumbar Spine

1. Inspect the spine for alignment (p. 518).
2. Palpate the spinal processes and paravertebral muscles (p. 519).
3. Percuss for spinal tenderness (p. 519).
4. Test range of motion by the following maneuvers (p. 519):
   - Forward flexion (75 degrees)
   - Hyperextension (30 degrees)
   - Lateral bending (35 degrees)
   - Rotation

Hips

1. Inspect the hips for symmetry and level of gluteal folds (p. 519).
2. Palpate hips and pelvis for the following (p. 520):
   - Instability
   - Tenderness
   - Crepitus

3. Test range of motion by the following maneuvers (p. 520):
   - Flexion (120 degrees), extension (90 degrees), and hyperextension (30 degrees)
   - Adduction (30 degrees) and abduction (45 degrees)
   - Internal rotation (40 degrees)
   - External rotation (45 degrees)
4. Test muscle strength of hips with the following maneuvers (p. 520):
   - Knee in flexion and extension
   - Abduction and adduction

Legs and Knees

1. Inspect the knees for natural concavities (p. 520).
2. Palpate the popliteal space and joint space (p. 522).
3. Test range of motion by flexion (130 degrees) and extension (0 to 15 degrees) (p. 522).
4. Test the strength of muscles in flexion and extension (p. 522).

Feet and Ankles

1. Inspect the feet and ankles during weight bearing and non–weight bearing for the following (p. 522):
   - Contour
   - Alignment with tibias
   - Size
   - Number of toes
2. Palpate the Achilles tendon and each metatarsal joint (p. 522).
3. Test range of motion by the following maneuvers (p. 522):
   - Dorsiflexion (20 degrees) and plantar flexion (45 degrees)
   - Inversion (30 degrees) and eversion (20 degrees)
   - Flexion and extension of the toes
4. Test strength of muscles in plantar flexion and dorsiflexion (p. 522).

Additional procedures include the following:

Hand and Wrist Assessment (p. 524)

- Katz hand diagram
- Thumb abduction test
- Tinel sign
- Phalen test

Shoulder Assessment (p. 524)

- Neer test
- Hawkins test

Lower Spine Assessment (p. 526)

- Straight leg raising test
- Femoral stretch test

Hip Assessment (p. 526)

- Thomas test
- Trendelenburg test

Knee Assessment (p. 527)

- Ballottement
- Bulge sign
- McMurray test
- Anterior and posterior drawer tests
- Lachman test
- Varus and valgus stress tests

Limb Measurement (p. 529)

ANATOMY AND PHYSIOLOGY

FIGURE 21-1 A, Bones of the upper and lower extremities. **B,** Muscles of the upper extremities.

Anterior

- Iliopsoas
- Pectineus
- Tensor of fascia lata
- Adductor longus
- Sartorius
- Adductor magnus
- Rectus femoris
- Gracilis
- Vastus lateralis
- Vastus medialis
- Tendon of rectus femoris
- Patella
- Patellar ligament
- Peroneus longus
- Tibialis anterior
- Extensor digitorum longus

Posterior

- Fascia over gluteus medius
- Gluteus maximus
- Semitendinosus
- Biceps femoris long head
- Semimembranosus
- Iliotibial tract
- Biceps femoris short head
- Semimembranosus
- Plantaris
- Gastrocnemius
- Peroneus longus
- Soleus
- Peroneus brevis
- Flexor hallucis longus
- Calcaneal tendon (Achilles tendon)

C

FIGURE 21-1—cont'd C, Muscles of the lower extremities.

Anterior

- Clavicle
- Manubrium of sternum
- Coracoid process
- Glenoid cavity
- Body of sternum
- Scapula
- Xyphoid of sternum
- Ilium
- Pubis
- Acetabulum
- Ischium
- Symphysis pubis

A

Posterior

- Acromion process
- Thoracic vertebrae
- Lumbar vertebrae
- Sacrum
- Coccyx

B

FIGURE 21-2 A, Bones of the trunk, anterior view. **B,** Bones of the trunk, posterior view. **C,** Superficial muscles of the trunk, anterior view. **D,** Superficial muscles of the trunk, posterior view.

Anterior

- Sternocleidomastoid
- Trapezius
- Clavicle
- Deltoid
- Pectoralis major
- Serratus anterior
- Latissimus dorsi
- External oblique
- Transversus abdominis
- Internal oblique
- Pyramidalis
- Rectus sheath (cut edges)
- Rectus abdominis

C

Posterior

- Splenius capitis
- Levator scapulae
- Rhomboideus minor
- Supraspinatus
- Trapezius
- Deltoid
- Infraspinatus
- Infraspinatus fascia
- Rhomboideus major
- Teres minor
- Teres major
- Teres minor
- Teres major
- Serratus anterior
- Latissimus dorsi
- External oblique
- Lumbodorsal fascia
- Serratus posterior inferior
- External oblique
- Gluteus maximus
- Gluteus medius

D

tendons, ligaments, and bones to promote ease of motion at points where friction would occur.

Upper Extremities

The radiocarpal joint (wrist) consists of the articulation of the radius and the carpal bones. Additional articulations occur between the proximal and distal rows of carpal bones. An articular disk separates the ulna and carpal bones, and the joint is protected by ligaments and a fibrous capsule. The wrist moves in two planes (flexion and extension movement; radial and ulnar [or rotational] movement). The hand has articulations between the carpals and metacarpals, metacarpals and proximal phalanges, and middle and distal phalanges (Fig. 21-3). The forearm joints consist of the articulations between the radius and ulna at both the proximal and distal locations. They are important for pronation and supination.

The elbow consists of the articulation of the humerus, radius, and ulna. Its three contiguous surfaces are enclosed in a single synovial cavity, with the ligaments of the radius and ulna protecting the joint. A bursa lies between the olecranon and the skin (Fig. 21-4). The elbow is a hinge joint, permitting movement of the humerus and ulna in one plane (flexion and extension).

The glenohumeral joint (shoulder) consists of the articulation between the humerus and the glenoid fossa of the scapula. The acromion and coracoid processes and the ligament between them form the arch surrounding and protecting the joint (Fig. 21-5, *A*). Four muscles (supraspinatus, infraspinatus, teres minor, and subscapularis) and their tendons comprise the rotator cuff, reinforcing the glenohumeral joint to stabilize the shoulder and the position of the humeral head within the joint (Fig. 21-5, *B*). The shoulder is a ball-and-socket joint that permits movement of the humerus in many axes.

Two additional joints adjacent to the glenohumeral joint complete the articulation of the shoulder girdle. The acromioclavicular joint consists of the articulation between the acromion process and the clavicle, and the sternoclavicular joint consists of the articulation between the manubrium of the sternum and the clavicle.

Head and Spine

The temporomandibular joint consists of the articulation between the mandible and the temporal bone in the cranium. Each is located in the depression just anterior to the tragus of the ear. The hinge action of the joint opens and closes the mouth. The gliding action permits lateral movement, protrusion, and retraction of the mandible (Figs. 21-6 and 21-7). See Chapter 10 for a description of the fused bones of the cranium.

The spine is composed of cervical, thoracic, lumbar, and sacral vertebrae. All but the sacral vertebrae are separated from each other by fibrocartilaginous disks. Each disk has a nucleus of fibrogelatinous material that cushions the vertebral bodies (Fig. 21-8). The vertebrae form a series of joints that glide slightly

FIGURE 21-4 Structures of the left elbow joint, posterior view.

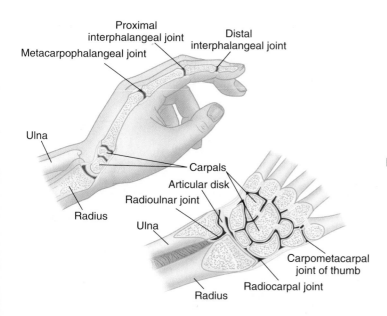

FIGURE 21-3 Structures of the wrist and hand joints.

ANATOMY AND PHYSIOLOGY

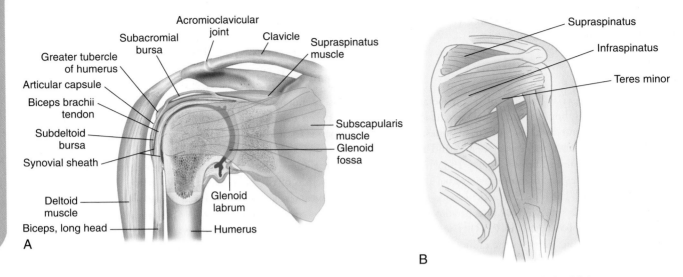

FIGURE 21-5 **Structures of the shoulder. A,** Structures of glenohumeral and acromioclavicular joints, anterior view. **B,** Rotator cuff muscles of shoulder, posterior view.

FIGURE 21-6 **Muscles of the face and head, left lateral view.**

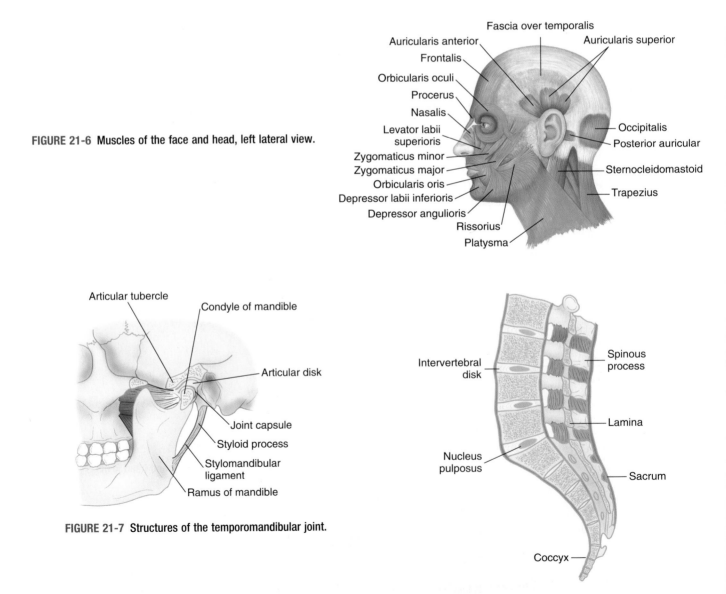

FIGURE 21-7 **Structures of the temporomandibular joint.**

FIGURE 21-8 **Structures of vertebral joints.**

over each other's surfaces, permitting movement on several axes. The cervical vertebrae are the most mobile. Flexion and extension occur between the skull and C1, whereas rotation occurs between C1 and C2. The sacral vertebrae are fused, and with the coccyx form the posterior portion of the pelvis.

Lower Extremities

The hip joint consists of the articulation between the acetabulum and the femur. The depth of the acetabulum in the pelvic bone—as well as the joint, which is supported by three strong ligaments—helps stabilize and protect the head of the femur in the joint capsule. Three bursae reduce friction in the hip. The hip is a ball-and-socket joint, permitting movement of the femur on many axes (Fig. 21-9).

The knee consists of the articulation of the femur, tibia, and patella. Fibrocartilaginous disks (medial and lateral menisci), which cushion the tibia and femur, are attached to the tibia and the joint capsule. Collateral ligaments give medial and lateral stability to the knee. Two cruciate ligaments cross obliquely within the knee, adding anterior and posterior stability. The anterior cruciate ligament protects the knee from hyperextension. The suprapatellar bursa separates the patella, quadriceps tendon, and muscle from the femur. The knee is a hinge joint, permitting movement (flexion and extension) between the femur and tibia on one plane (Fig. 21-10).

The tibiotalar joint (ankle) consists of the articulation of the tibia, fibula, and talus. It is protected by ligaments on the medial and lateral surfaces. The tibiotalar joint is a hinge joint that permits flexion and extension (dorsiflexion and plantar flexion)

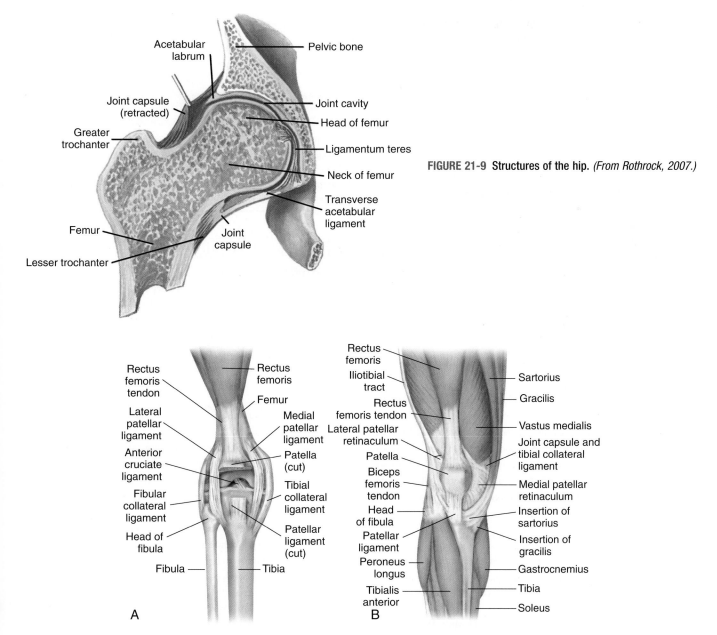

FIGURE 21-9 Structures of the hip. *(From Rothrock, 2007.)*

FIGURE 21-10 Structures of the knee, anterior view. A, Bones and ligaments of the joint. **B,** Muscles attaching at the knee.

FIGURE 21-11 Bones and joints of the ankle and foot.

in one plane. Additional joints in the ankle—the talocalcaneal joint (subtalar) and transverse tarsal joint—permit it to pivot or rotate (pronation and supination). Articulations of the foot between the tarsals and metatarsals, the metatarsals and proximal phalanges, and the middle and distal phalanges allow flexion and extension (Fig. 21-11) to occur.

✤ Infants and Children

During fetal development, the skeletal system emerges from embryologic connective tissues to form cartilage that calcifies and eventually becomes bone. Throughout infancy and childhood, long bones increase in diameter by the growth of new bone tissue around the bone shaft. Increased length of long bones results from the proliferation of cartilage at the growth plates (epiphyses). In the smaller bones, such as the carpals, ossification centers form in calcified cartilage. There is a specific sequence and timing of bone growth and ossification during childhood. Ligaments are stronger than bone until adolescence; therefore, injuries to long bones and joints are more likely to result in fractures than in sprains.

✤ Adolescents

Rapid growth during Tanner stage 3 (see Chapter 6, pp. 88-90) results in decreased strength in the epiphyses, as well as overall decreased strength and flexibility, leading to greater potential for injury. Bone growth is completed at about age 20 years, when the last epiphysis closes and becomes firmly fused to the shaft. Once bone growth stops, bone density and strength continue to increase. Peak bone mass is not achieved in either gender until about 35 years of age.

✤ Pregnant Women

Increased hormone levels contribute to the elasticity of ligaments and softening of the cartilage in the pelvis at about 12 to 20 weeks of gestation. Increased mobility of the sacroiliac, sacrococcygeal, and symphysis pubis joints results.

As the fetus grows, lordosis (inward curvature of the lower spine) occurs in an effort to shift the center of gravity back over the lower extremities. The ligaments and muscles of the lower spine may become stressed, leading to lower back pain in many pregnant women.

✤ Older Adults

With aging, the equilibrium between bone deposition and bone resorption changes, so that resorption dominates. For menopausal women, decreased estrogen increases bone resorption and decreases calcium deposition, resulting in bone loss and decreased bone density. By 80 years of age, a woman can lose up to 30% of her bone mass. The loss of bone density affects the entire skeleton, but the long bones and the vertebrae are particularly vulnerable. Weight-bearing bones may become predisposed to fractures. Bony prominences become more apparent with the loss of subcutaneous fat. Cartilage around joints deteriorates.

The muscle mass also undergoes alteration as increased amounts of collagen collect in the tissues initially, followed by fibrosis of connective tissue. Tendons become less elastic. This results in a reduction of total muscle mass, tone, and strength. A progressive decrease in reaction time, speed of movement, agility, and endurance also occurs.

Staying Well

Slowing Musculoskeletal Changes with Aging

A sedentary lifestyle and health problems that contribute to reduced physical activity promote and hasten the musculoskeletal changes associated with aging. Routine exercise and a well-balanced diet at all ages, including adequate intake of calcium and vitamin D, help slow the progression of the musculoskeletal changes.

REVIEW OF RELATED HISTORY

For each of the symptoms or conditions discussed in this section, targeted topics to include in the history of the present illness are listed. Responses to questions about these topics provide clues for focusing the physical examination and the development of an appropriate diagnostic evaluation. Questions regarding medication use (prescription and over the counter preparations) as well as complementary and alternative therapies are relevant for each.

History of Present Illness

- Joint symptoms
    - Character: stiffness or limitation of movement, change in size or contour, swelling or redness, constant pain or pain with particular motion, unilateral or bilateral involvement, interference with daily activities, joint locking or giving way
    - Associated events: time of day, activity, specific movements, injury, strenuous activity, weather
    - Temporal factors: change in frequency or character of episodes, better or worse as day progresses, nature of onset (slow versus rapid)
    - Efforts to treat: exercise, rest, weight reduction, physical therapy, heat, ice, braces or splints
    - Medications: nonsteroidal antiinflammatory drugs (NSAIDs), acetaminophen, biologic modifiers and other

immunosuppressants, corticosteroids, topical analgesics; glucosamine, chondroitin, hyaluronic acid

- Muscular symptoms
  - Character: limitation of movement, weakness or fatigue, paralysis, tremor, tic, spasms, clumsiness, wasting, aching or pain
  - Precipitating factors: injury, strenuous activity, sudden movement, stress
  - Efforts to treat: heat, ice, splints, rest, massage
  - Medications: muscle relaxants, statins, salicylates, NSAIDs
- Skeletal symptoms
  - Character: difficulty with gait or limping; numbness, tingling, or pressure sensation; pain with movement, crepitus; deformity or change in skeletal contour
  - Associated event: injury, recent fractures, strenuous activity, sudden movement, stress; postmenopause
  - Efforts to treat: rest, splints, chiropractic, acupuncture
  - Medications: hormone therapy, calcium; calcitonin, bisphosphonates
- Injury
  - Sensation at time of injury: click, pop, tearing, numbness, tingling, catching, locking, grating, snapping, warmth or coldness, ability to bear weight
  - Mechanism of injury: direct trauma, overuse, sudden change of direction, forceful contraction, overstretch
  - Pain: location, type, onset (sudden or gradual), aggravating or alleviating factors, position of comfort
  - Swelling: location, timing (with activity or injury)
  - Efforts to treat: rest, ice, heat, splints
  - Medications: analgesics, antiinflammatory drugs
- Back pain
  - Abrupt or gradual onset
  - Character of pain and sensation: tearing, burning, or steady ache; tingling or numbness; location and distribution (unilateral or bilateral), radiation to buttocks, groin, or legs; triggered by coughing or sneezing and sudden movements
  - Associated event: trauma, lifting of heavy weights, long distance driving, sports activities, change in posture or deformity
  - Efforts to treat: rest, avoid standing or sudden movements, chiropractic, acupuncture
  - Medications: muscle relaxants, analgesics, antiinflammatory drugs

Past Medical History

- Trauma: nerves, soft tissue, bones, joints; residual problems; bone infection
- Surgery on joint or bone; amputation, arthroscopy
- Chronic illness: cancer, arthritis, sickle cell disease, hemophilia, osteoporosis, renal or neurologic disorder
- Skeletal deformities or congenital anomalies

Family History

- Congenital abnormalities of hip or foot
- Scoliosis or back problems

- Arthritis: rheumatoid, osteoarthritis, ankylosing spondylitis, gout
- Genetic disorders: osteogenesis imperfecta, skeletal dysplasia, rickets, hypophosphatemia, hypercalciuria

---

Risk Factors

Osteoarthritis

- Obesity
- Family history of osteoarthritis
- Hypermobility syndromes
- Aging (older than 40 years)
- Injury, high level of sports activities
- Occupation requiring overuse of joints

Personal and Social History

- Employment: past and current, lifting and potential for unintentional injury, repetitive motions, typing/computer use, safety precautions, use of spinal support, chronic stress on joints
- Exercise: extent, type, and frequency; weight bearing; stress on specific joints; overall conditioning; sport (level of competition, type of shoes and athletic gear); warm-up and cool-down routines with exercise
- Functional abilities: personal care (eating, bathing, dressing, grooming, elimination); other activities (housework, walking, climbing stairs, caring for pet); use of prosthesis
- Weight: recent gain, overweight or underweight for body frame
- Height: maximum height achieved, any changes
- Nutrition: amount of calcium, vitamin D, calories, and protein
- Tobacco or alcohol use

⚗ Infants and Children

- Birth history
  - Presentation, large for gestational age, birth injuries (may result in fractures or nerve damage), type of delivery (vaginal versus cesarean section), use of forceps
  - Low birth weight, premature, resuscitation efforts, intrauterine insult or perinatal asphyxia, fetal stroke, maternal infections leading to muscle tone disorders, required ventilator support (may result in anoxia leading to muscle tone disorders)
- Fine and gross motor developmental milestones, appropriate for chronologic age
- Overweight or obese
- Quality of movement: spasticity, flaccidity, cog wheel rigidity
- Arm or leg pain
  - Character: localized or generalized; in muscle or joint; limitation of movement; associated with movement, trauma, or growth spurt
  - Onset: age, sudden or gradual, at night with rest, after activity
  - Participation in organized or competitive sports, weightlifting

❧ Pregnant Women

- Muscle cramps: nature of onset, frequency and time of occurrence, muscles involved, efforts to treat
- Back pain
  - Weeks of gestation, associated with multiple pregnancies, efforts to treat
  - Associated symptoms: uterine tightening, nausea, vomiting, fever, malaise (could signify musculoskeletal discomfort if not from another condition)
  - Type of shoes (heels may increase lordosis)

❧ Older Adults

- Weakness
  - Onset: sudden or gradual, localized or generalized, with activity or after sustained activity
  - Associated symptoms: stiffness of joints, muscle spasms or tension, any particular activity, dyspnea
- Increase in minor injuries: stumbling, falls, limited agility; association with poor vision
- Change in ease of movement: loss of ability to perform sudden movements, change in exercise endurance, pain, stiffness, localized to particular joints or generalized
- Nocturnal muscle spasm: frequency, associated back pain, numbness or coldness of extremities
- History of injuries or excessive use of a joint or group of joints, known joint abnormalities
- Previous fractures, bone mineral density screening
- Medications: steroids, calcium, bisphosphonates, NSAIDs

Risk Factors

Osteoporosis

- Race (white, Asian, Native American/American Indian); northwestern European descent
- Light body frame, thin
- Family history of osteoporosis, previous fractures
- Nulliparous
- Amenorrhea or menopause before 45 years of age, postmenopausal
- Sedentary lifestyle, lack of aerobic or weight-bearing exercise
- Constant dieting, inadequate calcium and vitamin D intake, excessive carbonated soft drinks per day
- Scoliosis, rheumatoid arthritis, cancer, multiple sclerosis, chronic illness, previous fractures
- Metabolic disorders (e.g., diabetes, hypercortisolism, hypogonadism, hyperthyroidism)
- Drugs that decrease bone density (e.g., thyroxine, corticosteroids, heparin, lithium, anticonvulsants, antacids with aluminum)
- Cigarette smoking or heavy alcohol use

EXAMINATION AND FINDINGS

Equipment

- Skin-marking pencil
- Goniometer
- Tape measure
- Reflex hammer

Begin your examination of the musculoskeletal system by observing the gait and posture when the patient enters the exam room. Note how the patient walks, sits, rises from sitting position, takes off a coat, and responds to other directions given during the examination.

As you give specific attention to bones, joints, and muscles, expose the body surface and view under good lighting. Position the patient to provide the greatest stability to the joints. Examine each region of the body for limb and trunk stability, muscular strength and function, and joint function. Position the extremities uniformly as you examine and look for asymmetry.

Inspection

Inspect the anterior, posterior, and lateral aspects of the patient's posture (Fig. 21-12). Observe the patient's ability to stand erect, symmetry of body parts, and alignment of the extremities. Note any lordosis, kyphosis (over-curvature of the thoracic vertebrae), or scoliosis (curved from side to side) of the spine.

Inspect the skin and subcutaneous tissues overlying the muscles, cartilage, bones, and joints for discoloration, swelling, and masses.

Observe the extremities for overall size, gross deformity, bony enlargement, alignment, contour, and symmetry of length and position. Expect to find bilateral symmetry in length, circumference, alignment, and the position and number of skinfolds (see Clinical Pearl, "Bilateral Symmetry").

Inspect the muscles for gross hypertrophy or atrophy, fasciculations, and spasms. Muscle size should approximate symmetry bilaterally, without atrophy or hypertrophy. Fasciculation occurs after injury to a muscle's motor neuron. Muscle wasting occurs after injury as a result of pain, disease of the muscle, or damage to the motor neuron.

Clinical Pearl

Bilateral Symmetry

Bilateral symmetry should not be defined as absolute because there is no perfect symmetry. For example, the dominant forearm is expected to be larger in athletes who play racquet sports and in manual laborers.

Palpation

Palpate any bones, joints, and surrounding muscles if symptomatic. Palpate inflamed joints last. Note any heat, tenderness, swelling, crepitus, pain, and resistance to pressure. No discomfort should occur when you apply pressure to bones or joints. Muscle tone should be firm, not hard or doughy. Synovial thickening can sometimes be felt in joints that are close to the skin surface when the synovium is edematous or hypertrophied because of inflammation. Crepitus can be felt when two irregular bony surfaces rub together as a joint moves, when two rough edges of a broken bone rub together, or with the movement of a tendon inside the tendon sheath when tenosynovitis is present.

FIGURE 21-12 Inspection of overall body posture. Note the even contour of the shoulders, level scapulae and iliac crests, alignment of the head over the gluteal folds, and symmetry and alignment of extremities. **A,** Anterior view. **B,** Posterior view. **C,** Lateral view. The occiput, shoulders, buttocks, and heels should be able to touch the wall the patient stands against.

Range of Motion and Muscle Tone

Examine both the active and passive range of motion for each major joint and its related muscle groups. Muscle tone is often evaluated simultaneously. Allow adequate space for the patient to move each muscle group and joint through its full range. Instruct the patient to move each joint through its range of motion as detailed in specific joint and muscle sections. Pain, limitation of motion, spastic movement, joint instability, deformity, and contracture suggest a problem with the joint, related muscle group, or nerve supply.

Ask the patient to relax and allow you to passively move the same joints until the end of the range of motion is felt. Do not force the joint if there is pain or muscle spasm. Muscle tone may be assessed by feeling the resistance to passive stretch. During passive range of motion, the muscles should have slight tension. Passive range of motion often exceeds active range of motion by 5 degrees. Range of motion with active and passive maneuvers should be equal between contralateral joints. Discrepancies between active and passive range of motion may indicate true muscle weakness or a joint disorder. No crepitation or tenderness with movement should be apparent. Note the specific location of tenderness when present. Spastic muscles are harder to put through the range of motion. Measurements may vary if the muscle tested relaxes with gentle persistence.

When a joint appears to have an increase or limitation in its range of motion, a goniometer is used to precisely measure the angle. Begin with the joint in the fully extended or neutral position, and then flex the joint as far as possible. Measure the angles of greatest flexion and extension, comparing these with the expected joint flexion and extension values (Fig. 21-13).

Muscle Strength

Evaluating the strength of each muscle group is considered part of the neurologic examination. However, it is usually integrated

FIGURE 21-13 Use of goniometer to measure joint range of motion.

FIGURE 21-14 Evaluation of muscle strength: flexion of the elbow against opposing force.

with examination of the associated joint for range of motion. Ask the patient first to contract the muscle you indicate by extending or flexing the joint and then to resist as you apply force against that muscle contraction (Fig. 21-14). Alternatively, tell the patient to push against your hand to feel the resistance. Compare the muscle strength bilaterally. Expect muscle strength to be bilaterally symmetric with full resistance to opposition. Full muscle strength requires complete active range of motion.

Variations in muscle strength are graded from no voluntary contraction to full muscle strength, using the scale in Table 21-1.

Table 21-1	Assessing Muscle Strength	
Muscle Function Level		**Grade**
No evidence of movement		0
Trace of movement		1
Full range of motion, but not against gravity*		2
Full range of motion against gravity but not against resistance		3
Full range of motion against gravity and some resistance, but weak		4
Full range of motion against gravity, full resistance		5

*Passive movement.

When muscle strength is grade 3 or less, disability is present; activity cannot be accomplished in a gravity field, and external support is necessary to perform movements. Weakness may result from disuse atrophy, pain, fatigue, or overstretching.

Specific Joints and Muscles

Hands and Wrists

Inspect the dorsal and palmar aspects of the hands, noting the contour, position, shape, number, and completeness of digits. Note the presence of palmar and phalangeal creases. The palmar surface of each hand should have a central depression with a prominent, rounded mound (thenar eminence) on the thumb side of the hand and a less prominent hypothenar eminence on the little finger side of the hand. Expect the fingers to fully extend when in close approximation to each other and to be aligned with the forearm. The lateral finger surfaces should gradually taper from the proximal to the distal aspects (Fig. 21-15).

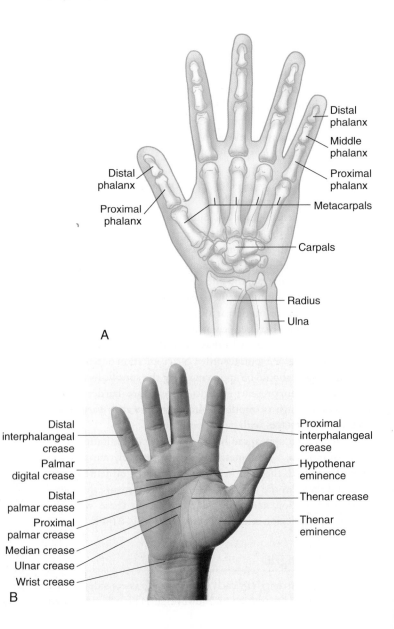

FIGURE 21-15 A, Bony structure of the right hand and wrist; note the alignment of the fingers with the radius. **B,** Features of the palmar aspect of the hand; note creases, thenar eminence and hypothenar eminence, and gradual tapering of the fingers.

Deviation of the fingers to the ulnar side and swan neck or boutonnière deformities of the fingers usually indicates rheumatoid arthritis (Fig. 21-16).

Palpate each joint in the hand and wrist. Palpate the interphalangeal joints with your thumb and index finger. The metacarpophalangeal joints are palpated with both thumbs. Palpate the wrist and radiocarpal groove with your thumbs on the dorsal surface and your fingers on the palmar aspect of the wrist (Fig. 21-17). Joint surfaces should be smooth and without nodules, swelling, bogginess, or tenderness. A firm mass over the dorsum of the wrist may be a ganglion.

Bony overgrowths in the distal interphalangeal joints, which are felt as hard, nontender nodules usually 2 to 3 mm in diameter but sometimes encompassing the entire joint, are associated with osteoarthritis. When located along the distal interphalangeal joints, they are called *Heberden nodes*; those along the proximal interphalangeal joints are called *Bouchard nodes*. Painful swelling of the proximal interphalangeal joints causes spindle-shaped fingers, which are associated with the acute stage of rheumatoid arthritis (Fig. 21-18). Cystic, round, nontender swellings along tendon sheaths or joint capsules that are more prominent with flexion may indicate ganglia.

Examine the range of motion of the hand and wrist by asking the patient to perform these movements:

+ Bend the fingers forward at the metacarpophalangeal joint; then stretch the fingers up and back at the knuckle. Expect metacarpophalangeal flexion of 90 degrees and hyperextension up to 30 degrees (Fig. 21-19, *A*).
+ Touch the thumb to each fingertip and to the base of the little finger; make a fist. All movements should be possible (Fig. 21-19, *B* and *C*).
+ Spread the fingers apart and then touch them together. Both movements should be possible (Fig. 21-19, *D*).
+ Bend the hand at the wrist up and down. Expect flexion of 90 degrees and hyperextension of 70 degrees (Fig. 21-19, *E*).
+ With the palm side down, turn each hand to the right and left. Expect radial motion of 20 degrees and ulnar motion of 55 degrees (Fig. 21-19, *F*).

Have the patient maintain wrist flexion and hyperextension while you apply opposing force to evaluate the strength of the wrist muscles. To evaluate hand strength, have the patient tightly grip two of your fingers. To avoid painful compression from an overzealous squeeze, offer your two fingers of one hand side by side in the handshake position. Finger extension, abduction, adduction, and thumb opposition may also be used to evaluate hand strength.

Elbows

Inspect the contour of the patient's elbows in both flexed and extended positions. Subcutaneous nodules along pressure points of the ulnar surface may indicate rheumatoid arthritis (Fig. 21-20) or gouty tophi.

Note any deviations in the carrying angle between the humerus and radius while the arm is passively extended, palm

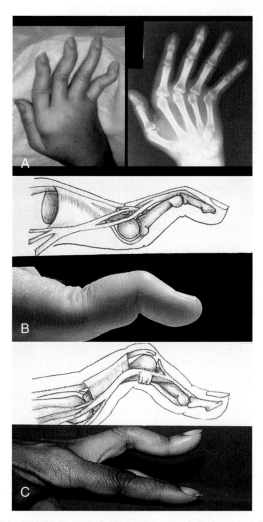

FIGURE 21-16 **Unexpected findings of the hand. A,** Ulnar deviation and subluxation of metacarpophalangeal joints. **B,** Swan neck deformities. **C,** Boutonnière deformity. *(Reprinted from the Clinical slide collection of the rheumatic diseases, 1991. Used by permission of the American College of Rheumatology.)*

FIGURE 21-17 **Palpation of joints of the hand and wrist. A,** Proximal interphalangeal joints. **B,** Metacarpophalangeal joints. **C,** Radiocarpal groove and wrist.

FIGURE 21-18 Unexpected findings of the fingers. A, Fusiform swelling or spindle-shaped enlargement of the proximal interphalangeal joints. **B,** Degenerative joint disease; Heberden nodes at the distal interphalangeal joints and Bouchard nodes at the proximal interphalangeal joints. **C,** Telescoping digits with hypermobile joints. *(Reprinted from the Clinical slide collection of the rheumatic diseases, 1991. Used by permission of the American College of Rheumatology.)*

forward. The carrying angle is usually 5 to 15 degrees laterally. Variations in carrying angle are cubitus valgus, a lateral angle exceeding 15 degrees, and cubitus varus, a medial carrying angle (Fig. 21-21).

Flex the patient's elbow 70 degrees and palpate the extensor surface of the ulna, the olecranon process, and the medial and lateral epicondyles of the humerus. Then palpate the groove on each side of the olecranon process for tenderness, swelling, and thickening of the synovial membrane (Fig. 21-22). Suspect epicondylitis or tendonitis when a boggy, soft, or fluctuant swelling; point tenderness at the lateral epicondyle or along the grooves of the olecranon process and epicondyles; and increased pain with pronation and supination of the elbow are found.

Examine the elbow's range of motion by asking the patient to perform the following movements:

+ With the elbow fully extended at 0 degrees, bend and straighten the elbow. Expect flexion of 160 degrees and extension returning to 0 degrees or 180 degrees of full extension (Fig. 21-23, *A*).
+ With the elbow flexed at a right angle, rotate the hand from palm side down to palm side up. Expect pronation of 90 degrees and supination of 90 degrees (Fig. 21-23, *B*).

Have the patient maintain flexion and extension while you apply opposing force to evaluate the strength of the elbow muscles.

Shoulders

Inspect the contour of the shoulders, the shoulder girdle, the clavicles and scapulae, and the surrounding musculature. Expect symmetry of size and contour of all shoulder structures. When the shoulder contour is asymmetric and one shoulder has hollows in the rounding contour, suspect a shoulder dislocation

(Fig. 21-24, *A*). Observe for a winged scapula, an outward prominence of the scapula, indicating injury to the nerve of the anterior serratus muscle (Fig. 21-24, *B*).

Palpate the sternoclavicular joint, clavicle, acromioclavicular joint, scapula, coracoid process, greater tubercle of the humerus, biceps groove, and area muscles. To palpate the biceps groove, rotate the arm and forearm externally. Locate the biceps muscle near the elbow and follow the muscle and its tendon into the biceps groove along the anterior aspect of the humerus. Palpate the muscle insertions of the supraspinatus, infraspinatus, and teres minor near the greater tuberosity of the humerus by lifting the elbow posteriorly to extend the shoulder. No tenderness should be noted over the muscle insertions.

Examine the range of motion of the shoulders by asking the patient to perform the following movements:

+ Shrug the shoulders. Expect the shoulders to rise symmetrically.
+ Raise both arms forward and straight up over the head. Expect forward flexion of 180 degrees.
+ Extend and stretch both arms behind the back. Expect hyperextension of 50 degrees (Fig. 21-25, *A*).
+ Lift both arms laterally and straight up over the head. Expect shoulder abduction of 180 degrees.
+ Swing each arm across the front of the body. Expect adduction of 50 degrees (Fig. 21-25, *B*).
+ Place both arms behind the hips, elbows out. Expect internal rotation of 90 degrees (Fig. 21-25, *C*).
+ Place both arms behind the head, elbows out. Expect external rotation of 90 degrees (Fig. 21-25, *D*).

Have the patient maintain shrugged shoulders while you apply opposing force to evaluate the strength of the shoulder

FIGURE 21-19 Range of motion of the hand and wrist. **A,** Metacarpophalangeal flexion and hyperextension. **B,** Finger flexion: thumb to each fingertip and to the base of the little finger. **C,** Finger flexion: fist formation. **D,** Finger abduction. **E,** Wrist flexion and hyperextension. **F,** Wrist radial and ulnar movement.

FIGURE 21-20 Subcutaneous nodules on the extensor surface of the forearm near the elbow. *(From Talley and O'Conner, 2010.)*

FIGURE 21-21 Expected carrying angle of the arm, at 5 to 15 degrees.

girdle muscles. Cranial nerve XI is simultaneously evaluated with this maneuver (Fig. 21-25, *E*).

Temporomandibular Joint

Locate the temporomandibular joints by placing your fingertips just anterior to the tragus of each ear. Allow your fingertips to slip into the joint space as the patient's mouth opens, and gently palpate the joint space (Fig. 21-26). An audible or palpable snapping or clicking in the temporomandibular joints is not unusual, but pain, crepitus, locking, or popping may indicate temporomandibular joint dysfunction.

Examine range of motion by asking the patient to perform the following movements:

+ Open and close the mouth. Expect a space of 3 to 6 cm between the upper and lower teeth when the jaw is open.
+ Laterally move the lower jaw to each side. The mandible should move 1 to 2 cm in each direction (Fig. 21-27).
+ Protrude and retract the chin. Both movements should be possible.

Strength of the temporalis and masseter muscles may be evaluated by asking the patient to clench the teeth while you palpate the contracted muscles and apply opposing force. This maneuver simultaneously tests cranial nerve V.

Cervical Spine

Inspect the patient's neck from both an anterior and a posterior position, observing for alignment of the head with the shoulders and symmetry of the skinfolds and muscles. Expect the cervical spine curve to be concave with the head erect and in appropriate alignment. No asymmetric skinfolds should be apparent.

Palpate the posterior neck, cervical spine, and paravertebral, trapezius, and sternocleidomastoid muscles. The muscles should have good tone and be symmetric in size, with no palpable tenderness or muscle spasm.

FIGURE 21-24 Contour changes of the shoulder. **A,** With dislocation. **B,** Winging of the scapula with abduction of the arm. *(European Journal of Paediatric Neurology, 2006.)*

FIGURE 21-22 Palpation of the olecranon process grooves.

FIGURE 21-23 Range of motion of the elbow. **A,** Flexion and extension. **B,** Pronation and supination.

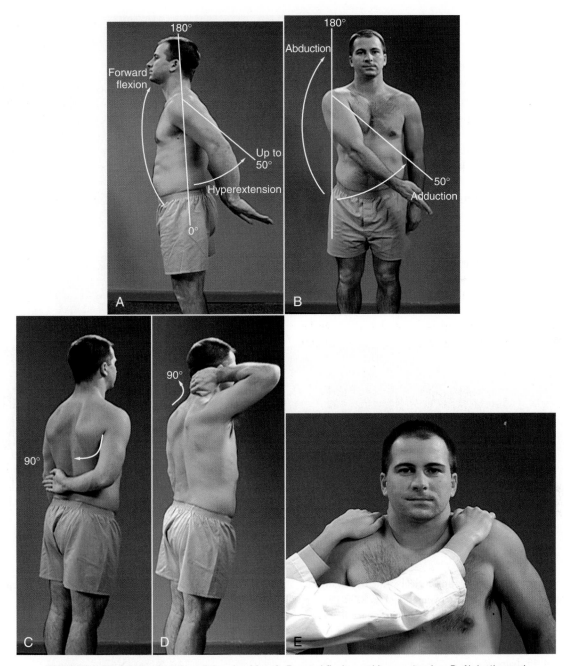

FIGURE 21-25 Range of motion of the shoulder. A, Forward flexion and hyperextension. **B,** Abduction and adduction. **C,** Internal rotation. **D,** External rotation. **E,** Shrugged shoulders.

FIGURE 21-26 Palpation of the temporomandibular joint.

FIGURE 21-27 Lateral range of motion in the temporomandibular joint.

FIGURE 21-28 Range of motion of the cervical spine. **A,** Flexion and hyperextension. **B,** Lateral bending. **C,** Rotation.

FIGURE 21-29 Examining the strength of the sternocleidomastoid and trapezius muscles. **A,** Flexion with palpation of the sternocleidomastoid muscle. **B,** Extension against resistance. **C,** Rotation against resistance.

Evaluate range of motion in the cervical spine by asking the patient to perform the following movements (Fig. 21-28):

+ Bend the head forward, chin to the chest. Expect flexion of 45 degrees.
+ Bend the head backward, chin toward the ceiling. Expect extension of 45 degrees.
+ Bend the head to each side, ear to each shoulder. Expect lateral bending of 40 degrees.
+ Turn the head to each side, chin to shoulder. Expect rotation of 70 degrees.

The strength of the sternocleidomastoid and trapezius muscles is evaluated with the patient maintaining each of the above positions while you apply opposing force. With rotation, cranial nerve XI is simultaneously tested (Fig. 21-29).

Thoracic and Lumbar Spine

Major landmarks of the back include each spinal process of the vertebrae (C7 and T1 are usually most prominent), the scapulae, iliac crests, and paravertebral muscles (Fig. 21-30). Expect the head to be positioned directly over the gluteal cleft and the vertebrae to be straight as indicated by symmetric shoulder, scapular, and iliac crest heights. The curve of the thoracic spine should

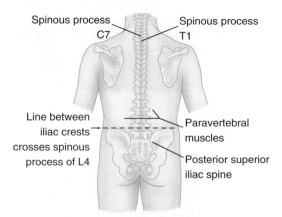

FIGURE 21-30 Landmarks of the back.

be convex. The curve of the lumbar spine should be concave (Fig. 21-31, *A*). The knees and feet should be in alignment with the trunk, pointing directly forward.

Kyphosis may be observed in aging adults (Fig. 21-31, *B*). Lordosis is common in patients who are obese or pregnant (Fig. 21-31, *C*). A sharp angular deformity, a gibbus, is associated with a collapsed vertebra from osteoporosis (Fig. 21-31, *D*).

A   B   C   D

FIGURE 21-31 Deviations in spinal column curvatures. **A,** Expected spine curvatures. **B,** Kyphosis. **C,** Lordosis. **D,** Gibbus.

FIGURE 21-32 Palpation of the spinal processes of the vertebrae.

With the patient standing erect, palpate along the spinal processes and paravertebral muscles (Fig. 21-32). No muscle spasms or spinal tenderness should be noted. Percuss for spinal tenderness, first by tapping each spinal process with one finger and then by percussing each side of the spine along the paravertebral muscles with the ulnar aspect of your fist. No muscle spasm or spinal tenderness with palpation or percussion should be elicited.

Ask the patient to bend forward slowly and touch the toes while you observe from behind. Inspect the spine for unexpected curvature. The patient's back should remain symmetrically flat as the concave curve of the lumbar spine becomes convex with forward flexion. A lateral curvature or rib hump should make you suspect scoliosis (Fig. 21-33). Then have the patient rise but remain bent at the waist to fully extend the back. Reversal of the lumbar curve should be apparent.

Evaluate range of motion by asking the patient to perform the following movements:

+ Bend forward at the waist and, without bending the knees, try to touch the toes. Expect flexion of 75 to 90 degrees (Fig. 21-34, *A*).
+ Bend back at the waist as far as possible. Expect hyperextension of 30 degrees (Fig. 21-34, *B*).
+ Bend to each side as far as possible. Expect lateral bending of 35 degrees bilaterally (Fig. 21-34, *C*).

FIGURE 21-33 Inspection of the spine for lateral curvature and lumbar convexity.

+ Swing the upper trunk from the waist in a circular motion front to side to back to side, while you stabilize the pelvis. Expect rotation of the upper trunk 30 degrees forward and backward (Fig. 21-34, *D*).

Hips

Inspect the hips anteriorly and posteriorly while the patient stands. Using the major landmarks of the iliac crest and the

---

Staying Well

Reducing the Risk for Lower Back Pain

Use appropriate techniques to lift heavy objects to reduce the risk for lower back injury. Rather than bend over to pick up a heavy object, keep the back straight and flex the knees to get closer to the object. Keep the object close to the body and lift with the knees. Avoid twisting the back during the lift.

FIGURE 21-34 Range of motion of the thoracic and lumbar spine. A, Flexion. **B,** Hyperextension. **C,** Lateral bending. **D,** Rotation of the upper trunk.

greater trochanter of the femur, note any asymmetry in the iliac crest height, the size of the buttocks, or the number and level of gluteal folds.

Examine the range of motion of the hips by asking the patient to perform the following movements:

+ While supine, raise the leg with the knee extended above the body. Expect up to 90 degrees of hip flexion (Fig. 21-35, *A*).
+ While either standing or prone, swing the straightened leg behind the body without arching the back. Expect hip hyperextension of 30 degrees or less (Fig. 21-35, *B*).
+ While supine, raise one knee to the chest while keeping the other leg straight. Expect hip flexion of 120 degrees (Fig. 21-35, *C*).
+ While supine, swing the leg laterally and medially with knee straight. With the adduction movement, passively lift the opposite leg to permit the examined leg full movement. Expect up to 45 degrees of abduction and up to 30 degrees of adduction (Fig. 21-35, *D*).

+ While supine, flex the knee keeping the foot on the table and then rotate the leg with the flexed knee toward the other leg. Expect internal rotation of 40 degrees (Fig. 21-35, *E*).
+ While supine, place the lateral aspect of the foot on the knee of the other leg; move the flexed knee toward the table (Patrick or FABER test—*F*lex, *AB*duct, and *E*xternally *R*otate). Expect 45 degrees of external rotation (Fig. 21-35, *F*).

To test hip flexion strength, apply resistance while the patient maintains flexion of the hip when the knee is flexed and then extended. Muscle strength can also be evaluated during abduction and adduction, as well as by resistance to uncrossing the legs while seated.

Legs and Knees

Inspect the knees and their popliteal spaces in both flexed and extended positions, noting the major landmarks: tibial tuberosity, medial and lateral tibial condyles, medial and lateral epicondyles of the femur, adductor tubercle of the femur, and patella (see Fig. 21-10). Inspect the extended knee for its natural

FIGURE 21-35 Range of motion of the hip. A, Hip flexion, knee extended. **B,** Hip extension, knee extended. **C,** Hip flexion, knee flexed. **D,** Abduction. **E,** Internal rotation. **F,** External rotation.

concavities on the anterior aspect, on each side, and above the patella. Loss of these concavities may suggest a knee effusion.

Observe the lower leg alignment. The angle between the femur and tibia is expected to be less than 15 degrees. Variations in lower leg alignment are genu valgum (knock-knees) and genu varum (bowlegs). Excessive hyperextension of the knee with

weight bearing (genu recurvatum) may indicate weakness of the quadriceps muscles.

An effusion of the knee fills the suprapatellar pouch and the concavity below the patella medially. When this occurs, the usual indentation above and on the medial side of the patella is filled out to be convex rather than concave.

FIGURE 21-36 Range of motion of the knee: flexion and extension.

FIGURE 21-37 **Pronation of heel.** Note that weight bearing is not through the midline of the foot. *(Courtesy Charles W. Bradley, DPM, MPA, and Caroline Harvey, DPM, California College of Podiatric Medicine.)*

Palpate the popliteal space, noting any swelling or tenderness. Fullness in the popliteal space may indicate a popliteal (Baker) cyst. Then palpate the tibiofemoral joint space, identifying the patella, the suprapatellar pouch, and the infrapatellar fat pad. The joint should feel smooth and firm, without tenderness, swelling, bogginess, nodules, or crepitus (see p. 527 for additional assessment procedures).

Examine the knees' range of motion by asking the patient to perform the following movements (Fig. 21-36):
+ Bend each knee. Expect 130 degrees of flexion.
+ Straighten the leg and stretch it. Expect full extension and up to 15 degrees of hyperextension.

The strength of the knee muscles is evaluated with the patient maintaining flexion and extension while you apply opposing force. The patient may be sitting or standing for this assessment.

Feet and Ankles

Inspect the feet and ankles while the patient is bearing weight (i.e., standing and walking) and while sitting. Landmarks of the ankle include the medial malleolus, the lateral malleolus, and the Achilles tendon. Expect smooth and rounded malleolar prominences, prominent heels, and prominent metatarsophalangeal joints. Calluses and corns indicate chronic pressure or irritation.

Observe the contour of the feet and the position, size, and number of toes. The feet should be in alignment with the tibias. Pes varus (in-toeing) and pes valgus (out-toeing) are common alignment variations. Weight bearing should be on the midline of the foot, on an imaginary line from the heel midline to between the second and third toes. Deviations in forefoot alignment (metatarsus varus or metatarsus valgus), heel pronation, and pain or injury often cause a shift in weight-bearing position (Fig. 21-37).

Expect the foot to have a longitudinal arch, although the foot may flatten with weight bearing (Fig. 21-38, *A*). Common variations include pes planus (Fig. 21-38, *B*), a foot that remains flat

even when not bearing weight, and pes cavus, a high instep (Fig. 21-38, *C*). Pes cavus may be associated with claw toes.

The toes should be straight forward, flat, and in alignment with each other. Several unexpected deviations of the toes can occur (Fig. 21-39). Hyperextension of the metatarsophalangeal joint with flexion of the toe's proximal joint is called hammertoe. A flexion deformity at the distal interphalangeal joint is called a mallet toe. Claw toe is hyperextension of the metatarsophalangeal joint with flexion of the toe's proximal and distal joints. Hallux valgus is lateral deviation of the great toe, which may cause overlapping with the second toe. A bursa often forms at the pressure point and, if it becomes inflamed, forms a painful bunion.

Heat, redness, swelling, and tenderness are signs of an inflamed joint, possibly caused by rheumatoid arthritis, gout, septic joint, fracture, or tendonitis. In particular, an inflamed metatarsophalangeal joint of the great toe should make you suspect gouty arthritis.

Palpate the Achilles tendon, the anterior surface of the ankle, and the medial and lateral malleoli. A persistently thickened Achilles tendon may indicate the tendonitis that can develop with spondyloarthritis or from xanthelasma of hyperlipidemia. Use the thumb and fingers of both hands to compress the forefoot and to palpate each metatarsophalangeal joint, looking for discomfort or swelling.

Assess range of motion of the foot and ankle by asking the patient to perform the following movements while sitting:
+ Point the foot toward the ceiling. Expect dorsiflexion of 20 degrees (Fig. 21-40, *A*).
+ Point the foot toward the floor. Expect plantar flexion of 45 degrees.
+ Bending the foot at the ankle, turn the sole of the foot toward and then away from the other foot. Expect inversion of 30 degrees and eversion of 20 degrees (Fig. 21-40, *B*).
+ Rotating the ankle, turn the foot away from and then toward the other foot while the examiner stabilizes the leg. Expect abduction of 10 degrees and adduction of 20 degrees (Fig. 21-40, *C*).
+ Bend and straighten the toes. Expect flexion and extension, especially of the great toes.

Have the patient maintain dorsiflexion and plantar flexion while you apply opposing force to evaluate strength of the ankle

FIGURE 21-38 Variations in the longitudinal arch of the foot. **A,** Commonly expected arch. **B1 and B2,** Pes planus (flatfoot). **C1 and C2,** Pes cavus (high instep). *(B2, Courtesy Charles W. Bradley, DPM, MPA, and Caroline Harvey, DPM, California College of Podiatric Medicine. C2, from Coughlin et al, 2007.)*

FIGURE 21-39 **Unexpected findings of the feet. A,** Hallux valgus with bunion. **B,** Protruding metatarsal heads with callosities. **C,** Hammertoes. **D,** Mallet toe. **E,** Claw toes. *(Courtesy Charles W. Bradley, DPM, MPA, and Caroline Harvey, DPM, California College of Podiatric Medicine.)*

FIGURE 21-40 **Range of motion of the foot and ankle. A,** Dorsiflexion and plantar flexion. **B,** Inversion and eversion. **C,** Abduction and adduction.

muscles. Abduction and adduction of the ankle and flexion and extension of the great toe may also be used to evaluate muscle strength.

For the assessment of gait, see Chapter 22.

Evidence-Based Practice in Physical Examination

Acute Ankle Injury in Adults

In cases of acute ankle injury, the Ottawa Ankle Rules help identify the characteristics of patients needing an ankle radiograph series. There must be pain in the malleolar zone and one of the following:
- Bone tenderness along the distal 6 cm of the posterior edge of the fibula or tip of the lateral malleolus
- Bone tenderness along the distal 6 cm of the posterior edge of the tibia or tip of the medial malleolus
- Inability to bear weight for 4 steps both immediately after the injury and in the emergency department

Absolute exclusion criteria for an ankle radiograph series include the following: age younger than 18, intoxication, multiple painful (distracting) injuries, pregnancy, head injury, and neurologic deficit.

The Ottawa Ankle Rules have 98.5% sensitivity for detecting an ankle fracture that is present on radiography.

Data from Dowling et al, 2009.

Advanced Skills

Various other procedures are performed for further evaluation of specific joints of the musculoskeletal system when problems are detected with routine procedures (Table 21-2).

Hand and Wrist Assessment

Several procedures are used to evaluate the integrity of the median nerve, which innervates the palm of the hand and the palmar surface of the thumb, index and middle fingers, and half of the ring finger. Ask the patient to mark the specific locations of pain, numbness, and tingling on the Katz hand diagram (Fig. 21-41). Certain patterns of pain, numbness, and tingling are associated with carpal tunnel syndrome.

The *thumb abduction test* isolates the strength of the abductor pollicis brevis muscle, innervated only by the median nerve. Have the patient place the hand palm up and raise the thumb perpendicular to it. Apply downward pressure on the thumb to test muscle strength (Fig. 21-42, *A*). Full resistance to pressure is expected. Weakness is associated with carpal tunnel syndrome.

To perform the *Phalen test*, ask the patient to hold both wrists in a fully palmar-flexed position with the dorsal surfaces pressed together for 1 minute (Fig. 21-42, *B*). Numbness and paresthesia in the distribution of the median nerve are suggestive of carpal tunnel syndrome. The reverse Phalen test is performed by placing the palms and fingers together with full wrist extension. The *Tinel sign* is tested by striking the patient's wrist with your index or middle finger where the median nerve passes under the flexor retinaculum and volar carpal ligament (Fig. 21-42, *C*). A tingling sensation radiating from the wrist to the hand in the distribution of the median nerve is a positive Tinel sign and is suggestive of carpal tunnel syndrome.

Table 21-2 Special Procedures for Assessment of the Musculoskeletal System

Procedure	Condition Detected
Limb measurement	Asymmetry in limb size
Neer test	Shoulder rotator cuff impingement or tear
Hawkins test	Shoulder rotator cuff impingement or tear
Katz hand diagram	Median nerve integrity
Thumb abduction test	Median nerve integrity
Tinel sign	Median nerve integrity
Phalen test	Median nerve integrity
Straight leg raising	L4, L5, S1 nerve root irritation
Femoral stretch test	L1, L2, L3, L4 nerve root irritation
Ballottement	Effusion in the knee
Bulge sign	Effusion in the knee
McMurray test	Torn meniscus in knee
Anterior and posterior drawer test	Anterior and posterior cruciate ligament integrity
Varus-valgus stress test	Medial or lateral collateral ligament instability in knee
Lachman test	Anterior cruciate ligament integrity
Thomas test	Flexion contracture of hip
Trendelenburg sign	Weak hip abductor muscles

Evidence-Based Practice in Physical Examination

Carpal Tunnel Syndrome

The likelihood that a patient will have a positive electrodiagnostic study for carpal tunnel syndrome is increased by the following: weakened thumb abduction; a classic or probable distribution of symptoms on the Katz hand diagram (see next page); and hypalgesia (decreased pain sensation along the thumb and median nerve distribution when compared to the little finger on the same hand). The Tinel and Phalen tests are less accurate.

Data from Watson et al, 2010.

Shoulder Assessment

Several procedures are used to evaluate the rotator cuff for impingement (tendonitis or overuse injury from repetitive overhead activities) or a tear.

To perform the *Neer test*, forward flex the patient's arm up to 150 degrees while depressing the scapula. This presses the greater tuberosity and supraspinatus muscle against the anteroinferior acromion. Increased shoulder pain is associated with rotator cuff inflammation or a tear (Fig. 21-43, *A*).

The *Hawkins test* is performed by abducting the shoulder to 90 degrees, flexing the elbow to 90 degrees, and then internally rotating the arm to its limit. Increased shoulder pain is associated with rotator cuff inflammation or a tear (Fig. 21-43, *B*).

To test the strength of the rotator cuff muscles, perform the following maneuvers. A normal result is indicated by the absence of pain or weakness with the following maneuvers:

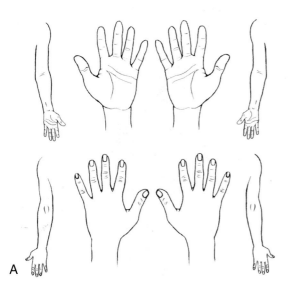

A

Classic pattern
Symptoms affect at least two of digits 1, 2, or 3. The classic pattern permits symptoms in the fourth and fifth digits, wrist pain, and radiation of pain proximal to the wrist, but it does not allow symptoms on the palm or dorsum of the hand.

FIGURE 21-41 Assessment for carpal tunnel syndrome. A, Katz hand diagram. B, Classic and probable patterns of pain, tingling, and numbness using the Katz hand diagram.

Probable pattern
Same symptom pattern as classic, except palmar symptoms are allowed unless confined solely to the ulnar aspect. In the **possible pattern,** *not shown,* symptoms involve only one of digits 1, 2, or 3.

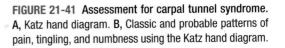

B   ▦ Numbness   ▨ Pain   ▧ Tingling   ▦ Decreased sensation

FIGURE 21-42 **Additional procedures for assessment of carpal tunnel syndrome. A,** Thumb abduction test. **B,** Phalen maneuver. **C,** Elicitation of Tinel sign.

FIGURE 21-43 **Assessment for rotator cuff inflammation or tear. A,** Neer test. **B,** Hawkins test.

To assess the supraspinatus muscle of the rotator cuff, have the patient place the arm in 90 degrees of abduction, 30 degrees of forward flexion, and internally rotated (thumbs pointing down). Apply downward pressure on the arm against patient resistance.

To assess the subscapularis muscle, have the patient hold the arm at the side, elbow flexed 90 degrees, and rotate the forearm medially against resistance.

To evaluate the infraspinatus and teres minor muscles have the patient hold the arm at the side, elbow flexed 90 degrees, and rotate the arm laterally against resistance.

Pain and weakness with opposing force is an unexpected finding and may be associated with inflammation or a tear.

Lower Spine Assessment

The *straight leg raising test* is used to test for nerve root irritation or lumbar disk herniation at the L4, L5, and S1 levels. Have the patient lie supine with the neck slightly flexed. Ask the patient to raise the leg, keeping the knee extended (see Fig. 21-35, *A*). No pain should be felt below the knee with leg raising. Radicular pain below the knee may be associated with disk herniation. Flexion of the knee often eliminates the pain with leg raising. Repeat the procedure on the unaffected leg. Crossover pain in the affected leg with this maneuver is more indicative of sciatic nerve impingements.

The *femoral stretch test* or hip extension test is used to detect inflammation of the nerve root at the L1, L2, L3, and sometimes L4 level. Have the patient lie prone and extend the hip. No pain is expected. The presence of pain on extension is a positive sign of nerve root irritation (Fig. 21-44).

Hip Assessment

The *Thomas test* is used to detect flexion contractures of the hip that may be masked by excessive lumbar lordosis. Have the

FIGURE 21-44 Femoral stretch test for high lumbar nerve root irritation.

FIGURE 21-45 Procedures for examination of the hip with the thomas test. Note the elevation of the extended leg off the examining table.

FIGURE 21-46 Test for the Trendelenburg sign. Note any asymmetry in the level of the iliac crests with weight bearing. *(From Van Tuijl, 2006).*

FIGURE 21-47 Procedure for ballottement examination of the knee.

patient lie supine; fully extend one leg flat on the examining table and flex the other leg with the knee to the chest. Observe the patient's ability to keep the extended leg flat on the examining table (Fig. 21-45). Lifting the extended leg off the examining table indicates a hip flexion contracture in the extended leg.

The *Trendelenburg test* is a maneuver to detect weak hip abductor muscles. Ask the patient to stand and balance first on one foot and then the other. Observing from behind, note any asymmetry or change in the level of the iliac crests. When the iliac crest drops on the side of the lifted leg, the hip abductor muscles on the weight-bearing side are weak (Fig. 21-46).

Knee Assessment

Ballottement is used to determine the presence of excess fluid or an effusion in the knee. With the knee extended, apply downward pressure on the suprapatellar pouch with the web or the thumb and forefinger of one hand, and then push the patella sharply downward against the femur with a finger of your other hand. If an effusion is present, a tapping or clicking will be sensed when the patella is pushed against the femur. Release the pressure against the patella, but keep your finger lightly touching it. If an effusion is present, the patella will float out as if a fluid wave were pushing it (Fig. 21-47).

Examination for the *bulge sign* is also used to determine the presence of excess fluid in the knee. With the patient's knee

extended, milk the medial aspect of the knee upward two or three times, and then milk the lateral side of the patella. Observe for a bulge of returning fluid to the hollow area medial to the patella (Fig. 21-48).

The *McMurray test* is used to detect a torn medial or lateral meniscus. Have the patient lie supine and flex one knee. Position your thumb and fingers on either side of the joint space. Hold the heel with your other hand, fully flexing the knee, and rotate the foot and knee outward (valgus stress) to a lateral position. Extend and then flex the patient's knee. Any palpable or audible click, grinding, pain, or limited extension of the knee is a positive sign of a torn medial meniscus. Repeat the procedure, rotating the foot and knee inward (varus stress) (Fig. 21-49). A palpable or audible click, pain, grinding, or lack of extension is a positive sign of a torn lateral meniscus.

The anterior and posterior *drawer test* is used to identify instability of the anterior and posterior cruciate ligaments. Have the patient lie supine and flex the knee 45 to 90 degrees, placing the foot flat on the table. Place both hands on the lower leg with

FIGURE 21-48 Testing for the Bulge sign in examination of the knee. **A,** Milk the medial aspect of the knee two or three times. **B,** Tap the lateral side of the patella.

FIGURE 21-49 Procedure for examination of the knee with the McMurray test. Knee is flexed after lower leg was rotated to medial position.

FIGURE 21-51 Valgus stress test of the knee with knee extended.

FIGURE 21-50 Examination of the knee with the drawer test for anterior and posterior stability.

Evidence-Based Practice in Physical Examination

Acute Knee Injury

In cases of acute knee injury, the Ottawa Knee Rules identify the characteristics of patients who should have a radiograph of the knee. The rules include any of the following findings:

- Age older than 55 years
- Tenderness at head of fibula
- Isolated tenderness of the patella
- Inability to flex the knee to 90 degrees

Data from Jalili et al, 2010.

the thumbs on the ridge of the anterior tibia just distal to the tibial tuberosity. Draw the tibia forward, forcing the tibia to slide forward of the femur. Then push the tibia backward (Fig. 21-50). Anterior or posterior movement of the knee greater than 5 mm in either direction is an unexpected finding.

The *Lachman test* is used to evaluate anterior cruciate ligament integrity. With the patient supine, flex the knee 10 to 15 degrees with the heel on the table. Place one hand above the knee to stabilize the femur and place the other hand around the proximal tibia. While stabilizing the femur, pull the tibia anteriorly. Attempt to have the patient relax the hamstring muscles for an optimal test. Increased laxity, greater than 5 mm compared to the uninjured side, indicates injury to the ligament.

The *varus (abduction)* and *valgus (adduction) stress tests* are used to identify instability of the lateral and medial collateral ligaments. Have the patient lie supine and extend the knee. Stabilize the femur with one hand and hold the ankle with your other hand. Apply varus force against the ankle (toward the midline) and internal rotation. Excessive laxity is felt as joint opening. Laxity in this position indicates injury to the lateral collateral ligament. Then apply valgus force against the ankle (away from the midline) and external rotation. Laxity in this position indicates injury to the medial collateral ligament (Fig. 21-51). Repeat the movements with the patient's knee flexed to 30 degrees. No excessive medial or lateral movement of the knee is expected.

FIGURE 21-52 Measuring limb length (A) and leg circumference (B).

Limb Measurement

When a difference in length or circumference of matching extremities is suspected, measure and compare the size of both extremities. Leg length is measured from the anterior superior iliac spine to the medial malleolus of the ankle, crossing the knee on the medial side (Fig. 21-52, *A*). Arm length is measured from the acromion process through the olecranon process to the distal ulnar prominence. The circumference of the extremities is measured in centimeters at the same distance on each limb from a major landmark (Fig. 21-52, *B*). Athletes who use the dominant arm almost exclusively in their activities (e.g., pitchers and tennis players) may have some discrepancy in circumference. For most people, no more than a 1-cm discrepancy in length and circumference between matching extremities should be found.

✿ Infants

Genetic and fetal conditions can produce musculoskeletal anomalies. The fetus may experience various postural pressures leading to reduced extension of the extremities and torsions of various bones.

Fully undress the infant and observe the posture and spontaneous generalized movements. Use a warming table when examining a newborn. No localized or generalized muscular twitching is expected. Inspect the back for tufts of hair, dimples, discolorations, cysts, or masses near the spine. A mass near the spine that transilluminates should cause you to suspect a meningocele or myelomeningocele.

From about age 2 months, the infant should be able to lift the head and trunk from the prone position, giving you an indication of forearm strength. Assess the curvature of the spine and the strength of the paravertebral muscles with the infant in a sitting position. Kyphosis of the thoracic and lumbar spine will be apparent in the sitting position until the infant can sit without support (Fig. 21-53).

Inspect the extremities, noting symmetric flexion of arms and legs. The axillary, gluteal, femoral, and popliteal creases should be symmetric, and the limbs should be freely movable. No unusual proportions or asymmetry of limb length or circumference, constricted annular bands, or other deformities should be noted.

Place the newborn in a fetal position to observe how that may have contributed to any asymmetry of flexion, position, or shape of the extremities. Newborns have some resistance to full

FIGURE 21-53 Kyphosis, expected convex curvature of the newborn's thoracic and lumbar spine.

extension of the elbows, hips, and knees. Movements should be symmetric.

All infants are flat-footed, and many newborns have a slight varus curvature of the tibias (tibial torsion) or forefoot adduction (metatarsus adductus) from fetal positioning. The midline of the foot may bisect the third and fourth toes, rather than the second and third toes. The forefoot should be flexible, straightening with abduction. It is necessary to follow tibial torsion and metatarsus adductus variations carefully, but it is seldom necessary to intervene. As growth and development take place, the expected body habitus is usually achieved.

The hands should open periodically with the fingers fully extended. Observe the palmar and phalangeal creases on each hand. A single crease extending across the entire palm may be associated with Down syndrome. Count the fingers and toes, noting polydactyly (six or more digits on an extremity) or syndactyly (two or more digits fused together) (Fig. 21-54).

Palpate the clavicles and long bones for fractures, dislocations, crepitus, masses, and tenderness. One of the most easily missed findings in the newborn is a fractured clavicle. This may be evident by a lump on the collarbone caused by the callus that forms on the healing clavicle noted in the first weeks after birth.

Position the baby with the trunk flexed, and palpate each spinal process. Feel the shape of each, noting whether it is thin and well formed, as expected, or whether it is split, possibly indicating a bifid defect (Fig. 21-55).

FIGURE 21-54 Anomalies of the newborn's hand. A, Simian crease. **B,** Syndactyly. **C,** Polydactyly. *(A, from Davidson, 2008; B, courtesy Dr. Joseph Imbriglia, Allegheny General Hospital; C, from Chung, 2009.)*

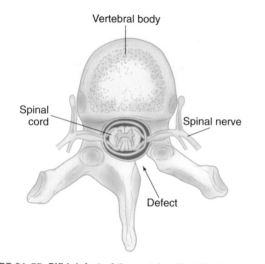

FIGURE 21-55 Bifid defect of the vertebra identified by palpation.

Palpate the muscles to evaluate muscle tone, grasping the muscle to estimate its firmness. Observe for spasticity or flaccidity and, when detected, determine whether it is localized or generalized. Use passive range of motion to examine joint mobility.

The *Barlow-Ortolani maneuver* to detect hip dislocation or subluxation should be performed each time you examine the infant during the first year of life. Using little force, test one hip at a time, stabilizing the pelvis with the other hand. With the infant supine, position yourself at the infant's feet, and flex the hip and knee to 90 degrees. For the Barlow maneuver, grasp the leg with your thumb on the inside of the thigh, the base of the thumb on the knee, and your fingers gripping the outer thigh with fingertips resting on the greater trochanter (Fig. 21-56). Adduct the thigh and gently apply downward pressure on the femur in an attempt to disengage the femoral head from the acetabulum. A positive sign is when a clunk or sensation is felt as the femoral head exits the acetabulum posteriorly. For the Ortolani maneuver, slowly abduct the thigh while maintaining axial pressure. With the fingertips on the greater trochanter, exert a lever movement in the opposite direction so that your fingertips press the head of the femur back toward the acetabulum center. If the head of the femur slips back into the acetabulum with a

palpable clunk when pressure is exerted, suspect hip subluxation or dislocation. High-pitched clicks are common and expected. By 3 months of age, muscles and ligaments tighten, and limited abduction of the hips becomes the most reliable sign of hip subluxation or dislocation (Fig. 21-57).

The test for the *Allis sign* is also used to detect hip dislocation or a shortened femur. With the infant supine on the examining table, flex both knees, keeping the feet flat on the table and the femurs aligned with each other. Position yourself at the child's feet, and observe the height of the knees (Fig. 21-58). When one knee appears lower than the other, the Allis sign is positive.

General muscle strength is evaluated by holding the infant in vertical suspension with your hands under the axillae (Fig. 21-59). Adequate shoulder muscle strength is present if the infant maintains the upright position. If the infant begins to slip through your fingers, proximal muscle weakness is present.

✣ Children

Watching young children play during the history can provide a great deal of information about the child's musculoskeletal system. Observe the child pick up and play with toys and move around the room. Observe the toddler's ability to sit, creep, and grasp and release objects during play. Knowledge of the expected sequence of motor development will facilitate your examination. If the child shows no limitation, the musculoskeletal examination may not reveal any additional information.

Position the young child to observe motor development and musculoskeletal function. Inspect the child's spine while he or she is standing. Young children will have a lumbar curvature of the spine and a protuberant abdomen (Fig. 21-60).

As you inspect the bones, joints, and muscles, pay particular attention to the alignment of the legs and feet because developmental stresses are placed on the musculoskeletal system. Remember to observe the wear of the child's shoes and ask about his or her favorite sitting posture. The W or reverse tailor position places stress on the joints of the hips, knees, and ankles. It is commonly seen in children with in-toeing associated with femoral anteversion (Fig. 21-61).

Inspect the longitudinal arch of the foot and the position of the feet with weight bearing. A fat pad obscures the longitudinal

FIGURE 21-56 Barlow-Ortolani maneuver to detect hip dislocation. A, Phase I, adduction. B, Phase II, abduction.

FIGURE 21-57 Signs of hip dislocation: limitation of abduction and asymmetric gluteal folds.

FIGURE 21-58 **Examination for the Allis sign.** Unequal upper leg length would indicate a positive sign.

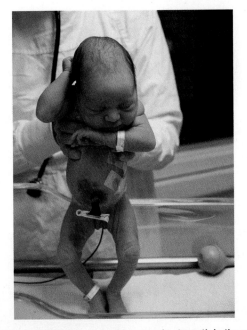

FIGURE 21-59 Evaluation of shoulder muscle strength in the newborn.

arch of the foot until about 3 years of age; after that time the arch should be apparent when the foot is not bearing weight. Metatarsus adductus should be resolved. The feet of the toddler will often pronate slightly inward until about 30 months of age. After that time, weight bearing should shift to the midline of the feet.

Assess for tibial torsion with the child prone on the examining table. Flex one knee 90 degrees and align the midline of the foot parallel to the femur. Using the thumb and index finger of one hand, grasp the medial and lateral malleoli of the ankle; grasp the knee, placing your thumb and index finger on the same side of the leg (Fig. 21-62). If your thumbs are not parallel to each

other, tibial torsion is present. Tibial torsion, a residual effect of fetal positioning, is expected to resolve within several years after weight bearing.

Assess for bowleg (genu varum) with the child standing, facing you, knees at your eye level. Measure the distance between the knees when the medial malleoli of the ankles are together. Genu varum is present if a space of 2.5 cm (1 inch) exists between

FIGURE 21-60 Lumbar curvature of the toddler's spine.

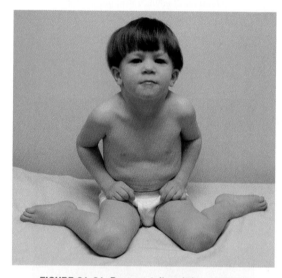

FIGURE 21-61 Reverse tailor sitting position.

FIGURE 21-62 Examination for tibial torsion.

FIGURE 21-63 Genu valgum (knock-knee) in the young child.

the knees. The expected 10- to 15-degree angle at the tibiofemoral articulation increases with genu varum but remains bilaterally symmetric. On future examinations, note any increase in the angle or increased space between the knees. Genu varum is a common finding in toddlers until 18 months of age. Asymmetry of the tibiofemoral articulation angle or space between the knees should not exceed 4 cm (1½ inches).

Evaluate knock-knee (genu valgum) with the child standing, facing you, knees at your eye level. With the knees together, measure the distance between the medial malleoli of the ankles. Genu valgum is present if a space of 2.5 cm (1 inch) exists between the medial malleoli. As with genu varum, the tibiofemoral articulation angle will increase with genu valgum. On future examinations, note any increase in the angle or increased space between the ankles. Genu valgum is a common finding of children between 2 and 4 years of age (Fig. 21-63). Asymmetry of the tibiofemoral articulation angle or a space between the medial malleoli should not exceed 5 cm (2 inches).

Palpate the bones, muscles, and joints, paying particular attention to asymmetric body parts. Use passive range of motion to examine a joint and muscle group if some limitation of movement is noted while the child is playing.

Ask the child to stand, rising from a supine position. The child with good muscle strength will rise to a standing position without using the arms for leverage. Proximal muscle weakness is indicated by the *Gower sign* in which the child rises from a sitting position by placing hands on the legs and pushing the trunk up (Fig. 21-64).

✿ Adolescents

Examine older children and adolescents with the same procedures used for adults. Specific procedures for the musculoskeletal examination for sports participation are found in Chapter 23.

The spine should be smooth, with balanced concave and convex curves. No lateral curvature or rib hump with forward flexion should be apparent. The shoulders and scapulae should

FIGURE 21-64 Gower sign of generalized muscle weakness. A, B, The child maneuvers to a position supported by both the arms and legs. **C, D,** The child pushes off the floor, rests the hand on the knee, and pushes self up with the hands and arms on the legs. **E,** The child stands upright. *(From Ball and Bindler, 2008.)*

be level with each other within ½ inch, and a distance between the scapulae of 3 to 5 inches is usual (see Fig. 21-12, B). Adolescents may have slight kyphosis and rounded shoulders with an interscapular space of 5 or 6 inches.

✤ Pregnant Women

Postural changes with pregnancy are common. The growing fetus shifts the woman's center of gravity forward, leading to increased lordosis and a compensatory forward cervical flexion (Fig. 21-65). Stooped shoulders and large breasts exaggerate the spinal curvature. Increased mobility and instability of the sacroiliac joints and symphysis pubis as the ligaments become less tense contribute to the "waddling" gait of late pregnancy. The pregnant woman can experience pain from the pubic symphysis down into the inner thigh when standing and may have a feeling that the bones are moving or snapping when walking.

During pregnancy, increases in the lumbosacral curve and anterior flexion of the head in the cervicodorsal region become apparent. To assess for lumbosacral hyperextension, ask the woman to bend forward at the waist toward her toes. Palpate the distance between the L4 and S1 spinal processes. As the woman rises to standing, from full flexion to full extension, note when the distance between L4 and S1 becomes fixed. If it becomes fixed before the spine is fully extended, the woman will be hyperextended when walking, possibly resulting

FIGURE 21-65 Postural changes with pregnancy.

in lower back pain. Most back pain resolves within 6 months after delivery.

Carpal tunnel syndrome (see p. 536) is experienced by some women during the last trimester because of the associated fluid retention during pregnancy. The symptoms should abate several weeks after delivery.

EXAMINATION AND FINDINGS

❀ Older Adults

The older adult should be able to participate in the physical examination as described for the adult, but the response to your requests may be more slow and deliberate. Fine and gross motor skills required to perform activities of daily living such as dressing, grooming, climbing steps, and writing will provide an evaluation of the patient's joint muscle agility (see the Functional Assessment box below). Joint and muscle agility have tremendous extremes among older adults.

The patient's posture may display increased dorsal kyphosis, accompanied by flexion of the hips and knees. The head may tilt backward to compensate for the increased thoracic curvature (see Fig. 21-31, *B*). The extremities may appear to be relatively long if the trunk has diminished in length due to vertebral collapse. The base of support may be broader with the feet more widely spaced, and the patient may hold the arms away from the body to aid balancing. The reduction in total muscle mass is often related to atrophy, either from disuse, as in patients with arthritis, or from loss of nerve innervation, as in patients with diabetic neuropathy.

Sample Documentation
History and Physical Examination

Subjective
A 13-year-old girl referred by school nurse because of uneven shoulder and hip heights. Active in sports, good strength, no back pain or stiffness.

Objective
Spine straight without obvious deformities when erect, but mild right curvature of thoracic spine with forward flexion. No rib hump. Right shoulder and iliac crest slightly higher than left. Muscles and extremities symmetric; muscle strength appropriate and equal bilaterally; active range of motion without pain, locking, clicking, or limitation in all joints.

For additional sample documentation, see Chapter 26, pp. 628-631.

FUNCTIONAL ASSESSMENT
Musculoskeletal Assessment

Activity to Observe	Indicators of Weakened Muscle Groups
Rising from lying to sitting position	Rolling to one side and pushing with arms to raise to elbows; grabbing a side rail or table to pull to sitting
Rising from chair to standing	Pushing with arms to supplement weak leg muscles; upper torso thrusts forward before body rises
Walking	Lifting leg farther off floor with each step; shortened swing phase; foot may fall or slide forward; arms held out for balance or move in rowing motion
Climbing steps	Holding handrail for balance; pulling body up and forward with arms; uses stronger leg
Descending steps	Lowering weakened leg first; often descends sideways holding rail with both hands; may watch feet
Picking up item from floor	Leaning on furniture for support; bending over at waist to avoid bending knees; uses one hand on thigh to assist with lowering and raising torso
Tying shoes	Using footstool to decrease spinal flexion
Putting on and pulling up trousers or stockings	Difficulty may indicate decreased shoulder and upper arm strength; these activities often performed in sitting position until clothing is pulled up
Putting on sweater	Putting sleeve on weaker arm or shoulder first; uses internal or external shoulder rotation to get remaining arm in sleeve
Zipping dress in back	Difficulty with this indicates weakened shoulder rotation
Combing hair	Difficulty indicates problems with grasp, wrist flexion, pronation and supination of forearm, and elbow rotation
Pushing chair away from table while seated	Standing and easing chair back with torso; difficulty indicates problems with upper arm, shoulder, lower arm strength, and wrist motion
Buttoning button or writing name	Difficulty indicates problem with manual dexterity and finger-thumb opposition

Modified from Wilson and Giddens, 2005.

ABNORMALITIES

MUSCULOSKELETAL

Ankylosing Spondylitis

A hereditary, chronic inflammatory disease, ankylosing spondylitis may affect the cervical, thoracic, and lumbar spine and will also involve the sacroiliac joints (Fig. 21-66).

Pathophysiology	Subjective Data	Objective Data
• Inflamed intervertebral disks and longitudinal ligaments ossify. • Leads to eventual fusion and severe deformity of the vertebral column	• Develops predominantly in men between 20 and 40 years of age • Begins insidiously with low back and buttock pain, also involving hips and shoulders • Buttock pain can fluctuate from one side to the other.	• Restriction in the lumbar flexion of the patient • Limited range of motion of the shoulders, chest wall, hips, and knees may develop. • Uveitis may be present.

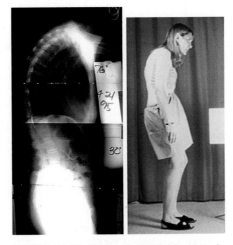

FIGURE 21-66 Gross postural changes in woman affected by ankylosing spondylitis. *(From Miller, 2010.)*

Lumbosacral Radiculopathy (Herniated Lumbar Disk)

Lumbosacral radiculopathy is herniation of a lumbar disk that irritates the corresponding spinal nerve root.

Pathophysiology	Subjective Data	Objective Data
• Generally caused by degenerative changes of the disk • Most commonly occurring at the L4, L5, and S1 nerve roots • Greatest incidence occurs between 31 and 50 years of age	• Can be associated with lifting heavy objects • Common symptoms include low back pain with radiation to the buttocks and posterior thigh or down the leg in the distribution of the dermatome of the nerve root. • Pain relief is often achieved by lying down.	• Spasm and tenderness over the paraspinal musculature may be present. • Potential difficulty with heel walking (L4 and L5) or toe walking (S1) • Numbness, tingling, or weakness in the involved extremity (Fig. 21-67)

ABNORMALITIES

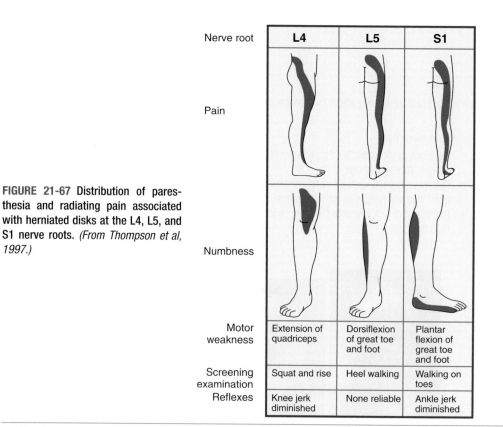

Nerve root	L4	L5	S1
Pain			
Numbness			
Motor weakness	Extension of quadriceps	Dorsiflexion of great toe and foot	Plantar flexion of great toe and foot
Screening examination	Squat and rise	Heel walking	Walking on toes
Reflexes	Knee jerk diminished	None reliable	Ankle jerk diminished

FIGURE 21-67 Distribution of paresthesia and radiating pain associated with herniated disks at the L4, L5, and S1 nerve roots. *(From Thompson et al, 1997.)*

Lumbar Stenosis

Spinal stenosis is narrowing of the spinal canal.

Pathophysiology

- Canal narrowing from bone and ligament hypertrophy may lead to entrapment of the spinal cord as it traverses the spinal canal.

Subjective Data

- Pain with walking or standing upright that often seems to originate in the buttocks and may then radiate down the legs
- Pain relief may occur with sitting or bending forward.
- Pain may be worsened by prolonged standing, walking, or hyperextending the back.

Objective Data

- In the early stages, the neurologic examination is frequently normal.
- With progression, the examination may show lower extremity weakness and sensory loss.

Carpal Tunnel Syndrome

Compression on the median nerve (see Fig. 21-41)

Pathophysiology

- Compression of the nerve within its flexor tendon sheath due to microtrauma, local edema, repetitive motion, or vibration of the hands
- Associated with rheumatoid arthritis, gout, acromegaly, hypothyroidism, and the hormonal changes of pregnancy

Subjective Data

- Numbness, burning, and tingling in the hands often occur at night.
- Can also be elicited by rotational movements of the wrist
- Pain may radiate to the arms.

Objective Data

- Weakness of the thumb and flattening of the thenar eminence of the palm
- Reproduction of symptoms with provocation of the Tinel and Phalen maneuvers

Gout

Gout, a form of arthritis, is a disorder of purine metabolism that results from an elevated serum uric acid level.

Pathophysiology

- Monosodium urate crystal deposition in joints and surrounding tissues results in acute inflammatory attacks.

Subjective Data

- Sudden onset of a hot, swollen joint; exquisite pain; limited range of motion
- Primarily affects men older than 40 years and women of postmenopausal age
- Usually affects the proximal phalanx of the great toe, although the wrists, hands, ankles, and knees may be involved

Objective Data

- The skin over the swollen joint may be shiny and red or purple.
- Uric acid crystals may form as tophi under the skin with chronic gout (Fig. 21-68).

FIGURE 21-68 Gouty tophus on right foot. *(From Thompson et al, 1997.)*

Temporomandibular Joint Syndrome

Painful jaw movement

Pathophysiology	Subjective Data	Objective Data
• Caused by congenital anomalies, malocclusion, trauma, arthritis, and other joint diseases	• Unilateral facial pain that usually worsens with joint movement • May be referred to any point on the face or neck	• Most patients have a muscle spasm, and many have clicking, popping, or crepitus in the affected joint.

Osteomyelitis

An infection in the bone

Pathophysiology	Subjective Data	Objective Data
• Usually results from an open wound or systemic infection • Purulent matter spreads through the cortex of the bone and into the soft tissue. • Decreased blood flow to the affected bone may lead to necrosis.	• Dull pain develops insidiously at the involved site and progresses over days to weeks. • Limp or decreased movement in infants and children	• Signs of infection include edema, erythema, and warmth at the site • Tenderness to palpation, pain with movement, and signs of inflammation such as fevers

Bursitis

Inflammation of the bursa

Pathophysiology	Subjective Data	Objective Data
• Due to repetitive movement and excessive pressure on the bursa • Can also be due to infection or gout	• Common sites include the shoulder, elbow, hip, and knee, with pain and stiffness surrounding the joint around the inflamed bursa. • The pain usually is worse during activity.	• Limitation of motion caused by swelling; pain on movement; point tenderness; and an erythematous, warm site (Fig. 21-69) • Soreness may radiate to tendons at the site.

FIGURE 21-69 Olecranon bursitis. *(Reprinted from the Clinical slide collection of the rheumatic diseases, 1991. Used by permission of the American College of Rheumatology.)*

Paget Disease of the Bone (Osteitis Deformans)

A focal metabolic disorder of the bone

Pathophysiology	Subjective Data	Objective Data
• Appears in persons older than 45 years • Excessive bone resorption and bone formation produce a mosaic pattern of lamellar bone.	• The bones of the skull are often affected, which can produce symptoms of vertigo and headache. • Progressive deafness from involvement of the ossicles or neural elements may develop.	• Bowed tibias, misshapen pelvis, or prominent skull forehead may be evident. • Frequent fractures may occur.

ABNORMALITIES

Osteoarthritis

The deterioration of the articular cartilage covering the ends of bone in synovial joints

Pathophysiology

- As a result of cartilage abrasion, pitting, and thinning, the bone surfaces are eventually exposed with bone rubbing against bone.
- Separately there can be remodeling of the bone surface and formation of bone spurs.

Subjective Data

- Pain in hands, feet, hips, knees, and cervical or lumbar spine (most commonly)
- Onset usually begins after 40 years of age and develops slowly over many years with nearly 100% of people older than 75 years being affected.

Objective Data

- The joints may be enlarged due to bone growths (osteophytes) (see Fig. 21-18, B).
- May have crepitus and limited, painful range of motion

Rheumatoid Arthritis

A chronic systemic inflammatory disorder of the synovial tissue surrounding the joints

Pathophysiology

- Cause is unknown
- Within the inflamed synovial tissue and fluid, polymorphonuclear leukocytes aggregate.
- Multiple inflammatory cytokines and enzymes are released that can result in subsequent damage to bone, cartilage, and other tissues.

Subjective Data

- Joint pain and stiffness, especially in the morning or after periods of inactivity
- Constitutional symptoms of fatigue, myalgias, weight loss, and low-grade fever are common.

Objective Data

- Involved joints include the hands, wrists, feet, and ankles as well as the hips, knees, and cervical spine.
- Synovitis, with soft tissue swelling and effusions, is present on examination.
- Nodules and characteristic deformities can develop (see Fig. 21-16).

The Differential Diagnosis table below contrasts rheumatoid arthritis and osteoarthritis.

DIFFERENTIAL DIAGNOSIS

Comparison of Osteoarthritis with Rheumatoid Arthritis

Signs and Symptoms	Osteoarthritis	Rheumatoid Arthritis
Onset	Insidious, over many years	Gradual although sometimes sudden (24 to 48 hours), typically weeks to months
Duration of stiffness	Few minutes, localized, but short "gelling" after prolonged rest	At least 1 hour, often longer, most pronounced after rest
Pain	On motion, with prolonged activity, relieved by rest	Even at rest, may disturb sleep
Weakness	Usually localized and not severe	Often pronounced, out of proportion with muscle atrophy
Fatigue	Unusual	Often severe, with onset 4 to 5 hours after rising
Emotional depression and lability	Unusual	Common, coinciding with fatigue and disease activity, often relieved if in remission
Tenderness localized over afflicted joint	Common	Almost always, most sensitive indicator of inflammation
Swelling	Noninflammatory effusion common, little synovial reaction	Fusiform soft tissue enlargement, inflammatory effusion common, synovial proliferation and thickening, often symmetric, rheumatoid nodules
Heat, erythema	Unusual, minimal if present	Sometimes present
Crepitus, crackling	Coarse to medium on motion	Medium to fine
Joint enlargement	Mild with bony consistency due to osteophytes	Moderate to severe if an inflammatory effusion is present

---

SPORTS INJURIES

Trauma to the musculoskeletal system results in a variety of injuries to muscles, bones, and supportive joint structures. The injury may be the result of an acute incident or overuse and repetitive trauma. Often a neurovascular assessment is necessary to detect any nerve damage or circulatory impairment (Box 21-1).

Box 21-1 Neurovascular Assessment

Assessment of circulation and nerve sensation is important when an extremity is injured. Perform the following steps to complete a neurovascular assessment distal to the injury. Use the contralateral extremity for comparison.

Assessment	Unexpected Findings
Color	Pallor or cyanosis
Temperature	Cool or cold
Capillary refill time	Greater than 4 seconds
Swelling	Significantly swollen
Pain	Presence of moderate to severe pain
Sensation	Numbness, tingling, pins and needles sensation
Movement	Decreased or no movement

Consider all the findings simultaneously to complete the neurovascular assessment. Presence of most or all of these unexpected findings indicates significantly impaired circulation and pressure or injury to the nerve, which needs emergency intervention.

Risk Factors

Sports Injury

- Poor physical conditioning
- Failure to warm up muscles adequately
- Intensity of competition
- Collision and contact sports participation
- Rapid growth
- Overuse of joints

Muscle Strain

Pathophysiology
- Can be due to excessive stretching or forceful contraction beyond the muscle's functional capacity
- Often associated with improper exercise warm-up, fatigue, or previous injury

Subjective Data
- Muscle pain
- Severity ranges from a mild intrafibrous tear to a total rupture of a single muscle

Objective Data
- Temporary muscle weakness, spasm, pain, and contusion

Dislocation

Complete separation of the contact between two bones in a joint

Pathophysiology
- Often caused by pressure or force pushing the bone out of the joint; usually occurs in the setting of acute trauma

Subjective Data
- Can occur more easily in patients with hyperextensibility conditions (e.g., Marfan, Ehlers-Danlös)

Objective Data
- Deformity and inability to use the extremity or joint as usual

---

Fracture

Partial or complete break in the continuity of a bone

Pathophysiology
- From trauma (direct, indirect, twisting, or crushing)

Subjective Data
- Pain, limited movement, cannot bear weight, swelling
- Felt a pop or snap with injury
- Can occur more easily in patients with bone disorders (e.g., osteogenesis imperfecta, osteoporosis, bone metastasis)

Objective Data
- Deformity, edema, pain, loss of function, color changes, and paresthesia

---

Tenosynovitis (Tendonitis)

Inflammation of the synovium-lined sheath around a tendon

Pathophysiology
- Seen with repetitive actions associated with occupational or sports activities
- Can occur in inflammatory conditions like rheumatoid arthritis

Subjective Data
- Pain with movement of such common sites as the shoulder, knee, heel, and wrist

Objective Data
- Point tenderness over the involved tendon
- Pain with active movement, and some limitation of movement in the affected joint

ABNORMALITIES

Rotator Cuff Tear

Microtrauma and tearing of the rotator cuff muscles, most often the supraspinatus

Pathophysiology

- Usually due to degeneration of the muscle and tendon from repeated overhead lifting and compression under the acromion
- An acute tear may also result from a fall on an outstretched arm

Subjective Data

- Pain in the shoulder and deltoid area is common. This can awaken the patient at night.

Objective Data

- Inability to maintain a lateral raised arm against resistance may develop
- Tenderness over the acromioclavicular joint
- Grating sound on movement, crepitus, and weakness in external shoulder rotation

✿ Infants and Children

Clubfoot (Talipes Equinovarus)

Fixed congenital defect of the ankle and foot

Pathophysiology

- Causes of clubfoot include genetic factors and external influences in the final trimester such as intrauterine compression.

Subjective Data

- Diagnosis is usually obvious at birth with the characteristic deformity.

Objective Data

- Most common combination of position deformities includes inversion of the foot at the ankle and plantar flexion, with the toes lower than the heel (Fig. 21-70)

FIGURE 21-70 Clubfoot deformity, talipes equinovarus (bilateral deviation). *(From Zitelli and Davis, 2007.)*

Metatarsus Adductus (Metatarsus Varus)

The most common congenital foot deformity, metatarsus adductus can be either fixed or flexible.

Pathophysiology

- Defect is caused by intrauterine positioning
- Medial adduction of the toes and forefoot results from angulation at the tarsometatarsal joint.

Subjective Data

- Diagnosis is usually obvious at birth with the characteristic deformity.
- The heel and ankle are uninvolved (Fig. 21-71).

Objective Data

- The lateral border of the foot is convex.
- A crease is sometimes apparent on the medial border of the foot.

FIGURE 21-71 Metatarsus adductus. *(From Beaty, 2003.)*

Legg-Calvé-Perthes Disease

Avascular necrosis of the femoral head

Pathophysiology	Subjective Data	Objective Data
• Results from a decreased blood supply to the femoral head	• Most commonly seen in boys between 3 and 11 years of age • Pain is often referred to the medial thigh, knee, or groin. • Bilateral involvement may occur in 10% of cases.	• Child may have a limp that is painless or antalgic (painful limp with shortened time on extremity) • Loss of internal rotation; abduction and decreased range of motion on the affected side are seen. • Muscle weakness of the upper leg may be present if symptoms have been present for a prolonged period.

Osgood-Schlatter Disease

A traction apophysitis (inflammation of a bony outgrowth) of the anterior aspect of the tibial tubercle

Pathophysiology	Subjective Data	Objective Data
• Inflammation of a bony outgrowth of the anterior aspect of the tibial tubercle • Develops in association with inflammation of the anterior patellar tendon • This self-limiting disorder is most common in boys between 9 and 15 years of age.	• The child is walking with a limp. • Often describes knee pain (especially with activity)	• Knee swelling that is aggravated by strenuous activity • Pain especially prominent with activity involving the quadriceps muscle • Pain with palpation over the tibial tuberosity

Slipped Capital Femoral Epiphysis

Disorder in which the capital femoral epiphysis slips over the neck of the femur

Pathophysiology	Subjective Data	Objective Data
• Most common between 8 and 16 years of age, although affected girls are often younger than affected boys • Majority of cases (75%) are unilateral; left side is involved more often than the right	• The child or adolescent presents with knee pain and a limp.	• The affected child has leg weakness and reduced internal hip rotation. • Characteristic plain radiograph shows slippage of femoral head

Muscular Dystrophy

This is a group of genetic disorders involving gradual degeneration of the muscle fibers.

Pathophysiology	Subjective Data	Objective Data
• Progressive symmetric weakness and muscle atrophy or pseudohypertrophy from fatty muscle infiltrates • Skeletal muscles and the heart may be involved • Some forms result in only mild disability, and these patients can expect a normal life span. • Other types produce severe disability, deformity, and death.	• Early signs may include clumsiness, difficulty climbing stairs, and frequent falls.	• Muscle atrophy and weakness with a waddling gait • A positive Gower sign (see Fig. 21-64) • Progressive loss of function, including ability to walk

Scoliosis

Physical deformity of the spine

Pathophysiology	Subjective Data	Objective Data
• A curvature of the vertebral bodies such that when viewed from the rear, the spine may look more like an "S" or a "C" than a straight line • Structural scoliosis most commonly affects girls and progresses during early adolescence. • There is no known cause.	• May lead to back discomfort and is often associated with a leg length discrepancy	• Lateral curvature of the spine, rib hump as the child flexes forward to touch the toes • In severe deformities, the patient has uneven shoulder and hip levels; may have crease on one side at the waist • Physiologic alterations occur in the spine, chest, and pelvis (Fig. 21-72).

FIGURE 21-72 Scoliosis, lateral curvature of the spine. Scapular asymmetry is easily discernible in the upright position. *(From Lemmi and Lemmi, 2000.)*

Radial Head Subluxation (Nursemaid's Elbow)

Known as nursemaid's elbow, this is a dislocation injury.

Pathophysiology

- Caused by jerking the arm upward while the elbow is extended
- The jerking pulls apart the elbow joint and tears the margin of the annular ligament around the radial head into the joint.

Subjective Data

- This injury is common in children 1 to 4 years of age.
- The child complains of pain in the elbow and wrist and refuses to move the arm.

Objective Data

- The child holds the arm slightly flexed and pronated.
- Supination motion is resisted.

❀ Older Adults

Osteoporosis

Disease in which a decrease in bone mass occurs because bone resorption is more rapid than bone deposition

Pathophysiology

- The bones become fragile and susceptible to spontaneous fractures.
- Most commonly seen in postmenopausal women, with a female-to-male ratio of 4:1
- Glucocorticoid excess and hypogonadism are also risk factors.

Subjective Data

- Presenting symptom is usually loss of height or an acute, painful fracture
- The most common fracture sites are the hip, vertebrae, and wrist.

Objective Data

- Affected persons lose height and have decreased abdominothoracic space (Fig. 21-73).
- In the spine, vertebral compression fractures lead to kyphosis or scoliosis.

FIGURE 21-73 Hallmark of osteoporosis: Dowager hump. *(From Hochberg et al, 2008.)*

Dupuytren Contracture

Contractures involving the flexor hand tendons

Pathophysiology

- Cause is unknown, although there may be a hereditary component

Subjective Data

- Flexion contractures develop insidiously.
- The incidence increases after the age of 40, occurring more frequently in men (Fig. 21-74).

Objective Data

- Flexor tendons generally of the fourth and fifth digits contract, causing the fingers to curl, with impaired extension.
- These tendons are easily palpable.

FIGURE 21-74 Dupuytren contracture.

ABNORMALITIES

CHAPTER 22

Neurologic System

The nervous system, with its central and peripheral divisions, maintains and controls all body functions by its voluntary and autonomic responses. The evaluation of motor, sensory, autonomic, cognitive, and behavioral elements makes neurologic assessment one of the most complex portions of the physical examination. This chapter focuses on assessment of the cranial nerves, cerebellar function and proprioception, sensory function, and the superficial and deep tendon reflexes. Assessment of mental status (cognitive function, communication, and behavior) is addressed in Chapter 5. Muscle strength assessment is addressed in Chapter 21.

evolve *http://evolve.elsevier.com/Seidel*
- Physical Exam Key Points
- NCLEX Review Questions
- Activities
- Animations
- Videos
- Student Checklist

ANATOMY AND PHYSIOLOGY

The central nervous system (brain and spinal cord) is the main network of coordination and control for the body. The peripheral nervous system, comprising the cranial and spinal nerves and the ascending and descending pathways, carries information to and from the central nervous system. The autonomic nervous system coordinates and regulates the internal organs of the body, such as cardiac muscle and smooth muscle. It has two divisions, each tending to balance the impulses of the other. The sympathetic division prods the body into action during times of physiologic and psychologic stress; the parasympathetic division functions in a complementary and a counterbalancing manner to conserve body resources and maintain day-to-day body functions such as digestion and elimination.

The intricate interrelationship of the nervous system permits the body to perform the following:

Physical Examination Preview

Here is a preview of the steps involved in conducting the portions of the physical examination of the neurologic system addressed in this chapter. ⓔ These procedures are explained in detail in this chapter and are available on Evolve in printable formats.

1. Test cranial nerves I through XII (pp. 553-557).

Cerebellar Function and Proprioception

2. Evaluate coordination and fine motor skills by the following (pp. 556-559):
   - Rapid rhythmic alternating movements
   - Accuracy of upper and lower extremity movements
3. Evaluate balance using the Romberg test (p. 559).
4. Observe the patient's gait (pp. 559-560).
   - Posture
   - Rhythm and sequence of stride and arm movements

Sensory Function

5. Test primary sensory responses to the following (pp. 559-561):
   - Superficial touch
   - Superficial pain

6. Test vibratory response to tuning fork over joints or bony prominences on upper and lower extremities (p. 561).
7. Evaluate perception of position sense with movement of the great toes or a finger on each hand (p. 561).
8. Assess ability to identify familiar object by touch and manipulation (p. 562).
9. Assess two-point discrimination (p. 562).
10. Assess ability to identify letter or number "drawn" on palm of hand (p. 562).
11. Assess ability to identify body area when touched (p. 562).

Superficial and Deep Tendon Reflexes

12. Test the plantar reflex (pp. 562-563).
13. Test abdominal reflexes (p. 563).
14. Test the cremasteric reflex in male patients (p. 564).
15. Test the following deep tendon reflexes: biceps, brachioradialis, triceps, patellar, and Achilles (pp. 564-565).
16. Test for ankle clonus (p. 565).

- Receive sensory stimuli from the environment
- Identify and integrate the adaptive processes needed to maintain body functions
- Orchestrate body function changes required for adaptation and survival
- Integrate the rapid responsiveness of the central nervous system with the more gradual responsiveness of the endocrine system
- Control cognitive and voluntary behavioral processes (see Chapter 5)
- Control subconscious and involuntary body functions

The brain and spinal cord are protected by the skull and vertebrae, the meninges, and the cerebrospinal fluid. Three layers of meninges surround the brain and spinal cord, assisting in the production and drainage of cerebrospinal fluid (Fig. 22-1). Cerebrospinal fluid circulates between an interconnecting system of ventricles in the brain and around the brain and spinal cord, serving as a shock absorber.

Brain

The brain receives its blood supply (approximately 20% of the total cardiac output) from the two internal carotid arteries and two vertebral arteries (Fig. 22-2). Blood drains from the brain through venous plexuses and dural sinuses that empty into the internal jugular veins. The three major units of the brain are the cerebrum, the cerebellum, and the brainstem.

Cerebrum

Two cerebral hemispheres, each divided into lobes, form the cerebrum. The gray outer layer, the cerebral cortex, houses the higher mental functions and is responsible for general movement, visceral functions, perception, behavior, and the integration of these functions. Commissural fibers (corpus callosum) interconnect the counterpart areas in each hemisphere, permitting the coordination of activities between the hemispheres (Fig. 22-3; see also Fig. 5-1).

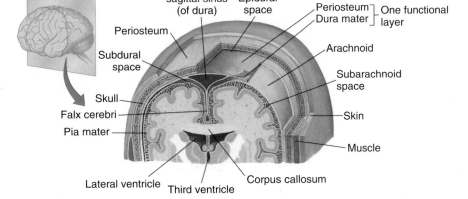

FIGURE 22-1 Frontal section of the superior portion of the head, as viewed from the front. Both bony and membranous coverings of the brain can be seen. *(From Thibodeau and Patton, 2003.)*

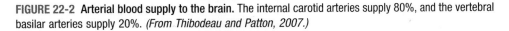

FIGURE 22-2 Arterial blood supply to the brain. The internal carotid arteries supply 80%, and the vertebral basilar arteries supply 20%. *(From Thibodeau and Patton, 2007.)*

ANATOMY AND PHYSIOLOGY

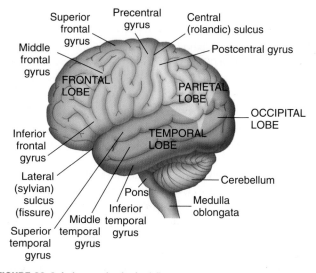

FIGURE 22-3 Lobes and principal fissures of the cerebral cortex, cerebellum, and brainstem (left hemisphere, lateral view). *(From McCance and Huether, 2006.)*

The *frontal lobe* contains the motor cortex associated with voluntary skeletal movement and fine repetitive motor movements, as well as the control of eye movements. Specific areas in the primary motor area are associated with the movement of specific parts of the body. The corticospinal tracts extend from the primary motor area into the spinal cord.

The *parietal lobe* is primarily responsible for processing sensory data as it is received. It assists with the interpretation of tactile sensations (i.e., temperature, pressure, pain, size, shape, texture, and two-point discrimination), as well as visual, taste, smell, and hearing sensations. Recognition of body parts and awareness of body position (proprioception) are dependent on the parietal lobe. Association fibers provide communication between the sensory and motor areas of the brain.

The *occipital lobe* contains the primary vision center and provides interpretation of visual data.

The *temporal lobe* is responsible for the perception and interpretation of sounds and determination of their source. It is also involved in the integration of taste, smell, and balance. The reception and interpretation of speech is located in the Wernicke area.

The *basal ganglia system* functions as the extrapyramidal pathway and processing station between the cerebral motor cortex and the upper brainstem. Through its interconnections with the thalamus, motor cortex, reticular formation, and spinal cord, the basal ganglia refine motor movements.

Cerebellum

The cerebellum aids the motor cortex of the cerebrum in the integration of voluntary movement. It processes sensory information from the eyes, ears, touch receptors, and musculoskeleton. In concert with the vestibular system, the cerebellum uses the sensory data for reflexive control of muscle tone, balance, and posture to produce steady and precise movements.

Brainstem

The brainstem is the pathway between the cerebral cortex and the spinal cord, and it controls many involuntary functions (Table 22-1). Its structures include the medulla oblongata, pons, midbrain, and diencephalon. The nuclei of the 12 cranial nerves arise from these structures. The thalamus is the major integrating center for perception of various sensations such as pain and temperature (along with the cortical processing for interpretation). The thalamus also relays sensory aspects of motor information between the basal ganglia and cerebellum. The pons transmits information between the brainstem and the cerebellum, relaying motor information from the cerebral cortex to the contralateral cerebellar hemisphere. The medulla oblongata is the site where the descending corticospinal tracts decussate (cross to the contralateral side).

Table 22-1	Structures of the Brainstem and Their Functions
Structure	**Function**
Medulla oblongata CN IX to XII	Respiratory, circulatory, and vasomotor activities; houses respiratory center Reflexes of swallowing, coughing, vomiting, sneezing, and hiccupping Relay center for major ascending and descending spinal tracts that decussate at the pyramid
Pons CN V to VIII	Reflexes of pupillary action and eye movement Regulates respiration; houses a portion of the respiratory center Controls voluntary muscle action with corticospinal tract pathway
Midbrain CN III and IV	Reflex center for eye and head movement Auditory relay pathway Corticospinal tract pathway
Diencephalon CN I and II Thalamus	Relays impulses between cerebrum, cerebellum, pons, and medulla (see Fig. 22-4) Conveys all sensory impulses (except olfaction) to and from cerebrum before their distribution to appropriate associative sensory areas Integrates impulses between motor cortex and cerebrum, influencing voluntary movements and motor response Controls state of consciousness, conscious perceptions of sensations, and abstract feelings
Epithalamus	Houses the pineal body Sexual development and behavior
Hypothalamus	Major processing center of internal stimuli for autonomic nervous system Maintains temperature control, water metabolism, body fluid osmolarity, feeding behavior, and neuroendocrine activity
Pituitary gland	Hormonal control of growth, lactation, vasoconstriction, and metabolism

Cranial Nerves

Cranial nerves are peripheral nerves that arise from the brain rather than the spinal cord. Each nerve has motor or sensory functions, and four cranial nerves have parasympathetic functions (Table 22-2).

Spinal Cord and Spinal Tracts

The spinal cord, 40 to 50 cm long, begins at the foramen magnum as a continuation of the medulla oblongata and terminates at L1

Table 22-2	The Cranial Nerves and Their Functions
Cranial Nerves	**Function**
Olfactory (I)	Sensory: smell reception and interpretation
Optic (II)	Sensory: visual acuity and visual fields
Oculomotor (III)	Motor: raise eyelids, most extraocular movements Parasympathetic: pupillary constriction, change lens shape
Trochlear (IV)	Motor: downward, inward eye movement
Trigeminal (V)	Motor: jaw opening and clenching, chewing, and mastication Sensory: sensation to cornea, iris, lacrimal glands, conjunctiva, eyelids, forehead, nose, nasal and mouth mucosa, teeth, tongue, ear, facial skin
Abducens (VI)	Motor: lateral eye movement
Facial (VII)	Motor: movement of facial expression muscles except jaw, close eyelids, labial speech sounds (b, m, w, and rounded vowels) Sensory: taste—anterior two thirds of tongue, sensation to pharynx Parasympathetic: secretion of saliva and tears
Acoustic (VIII)	Sensory: hearing and equilibrium
Glossopharyngeal (IX)	Motor: voluntary muscles for swallowing and phonation Sensory: sensation of nasopharynx, gag reflex, taste—posterior one third of tongue Parasympathetic: secretion of salivary glands, carotid reflex Motor: voluntary muscles of phonation (guttural speech sounds) and swallowing
Vagus (X)	Sensory: sensation behind ear and part of external ear canal Parasympathetic: secretion of digestive enzymes; peristalsis; carotid reflex; involuntary action of heart, lungs, and digestive tract
Spinal accessory (XI)	Motor: turn head, shrug shoulders, some actions for phonation
Hypoglossal (XII)	Motor: tongue movement for speech sound articulation (I, t, d, n) and swallowing

or L2 of the vertebral column. Fibers, grouped into tracts, run through the spinal cord carrying sensory, motor, and autonomic impulses between higher centers in the brain and the body. The gray matter, arranged in a butterfly shape with anterior and posterior horns, contains the nerve cell bodies associated with sensory pathways and the autonomic nervous system. The white matter of the spinal cord contains the ascending and descending spinal tracts (Fig. 22-4).

The *ascending spinal tracts* (e.g., spinothalamic, spinocerebellar) mediate various sensations. These spinal tracts manage the sensory signals necessary to perform complex discrimination tasks. They are capable of transmitting precise information about the type of stimulus and its location. The posterior (dorsal) column spinal tract (fasciculus gracilis and fasciculus cuneatus) carries the fibers for the sensations of fine touch, two-point discrimination, and proprioception. The spinothalamic tracts carry the fibers for the sensations of light and crude touch, pressure, temperature, and pain.

The *descending spinal tracts* (corticospinal, reticulospinal, vestibulospinal) convey impulses from the brain to various muscle groups by inhibiting or exciting spinal activity. They also have a role in the control of muscle tone, posture, and precise motor movements. The corticospinal (pyramidal) tract permits skilled, delicate, and purposeful movements. The vestibulospinal tract causes the extensor muscles of the body to suddenly contract when an individual starts to fall. The corticobulbar tract arising from the brainstem innervates the motor functions of the cranial nerves.

Upper motor neurons are nerve cell bodies for the motor pathways that all begin and end within the central nervous system. They comprise the descending pathways from the brain to the spinal cord. Their primary role is influencing, directing, and modifying spinal reflex arcs and circuits. The upper motor neurons can affect movement only through the lower motor neurons. The *lower motor neurons*, cranial and spinal motor neurons, originate in the anterior horn of the spinal cord and extend into the peripheral nervous system. They transmit neural signals directly to the muscles to permit movement. Injury to the upper motor neurons results in initial paralysis followed by partial recovery over an extended period. Injury to the lower motor neurons often results in permanent paralysis.

Spinal Nerves

Thirty-one pairs of spinal nerves arise from the spinal cord and exit at each intervertebral foramen (Fig. 22-5). The sensory and motor fibers of each spinal nerve supply and receive information in a specific body distribution called a *dermatome* (Fig. 22-6). The anterior branches of several spinal nerves combine to form a nerve plexus, so that a spinal nerve may lose its individuality to some extent. The spinal nerve may also complement the effort of an anatomically related nerve or even help compensate for some loss of function. A multitude of peripheral nerves originates from each nerve plexus.

Within the spinal cord, each spinal nerve separates into anterior and posterior roots. The motor or efferent fibers of the anterior root carry impulses from the spinal cord to the muscles

Animation: Cranial Nerves

Animation: Spine

ANATOMY AND PHYSIOLOGY

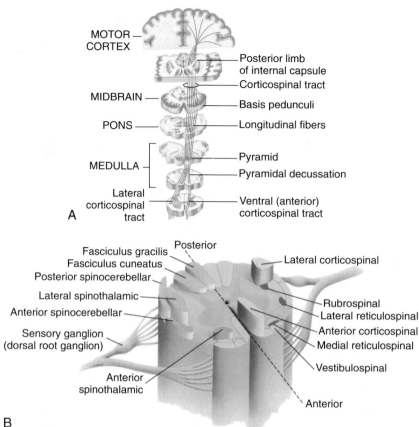

FIGURE 22-4 **Tracts of the spinal cord. A,** Pathway of spinal tracts from spinal cord to motor cortex. Note decussation of the pyramids at the level of the medulla. **B,** Major ascending (sensory) tracts, shown here only on the *left*, are highlighted in *blue*. Major descending (motor) tracts, shown here only on the *right*, are highlighted in *red*. (**A** *modified from Rudy, 1984;* **B** *from Thibodeau and Patton, 2003.*)

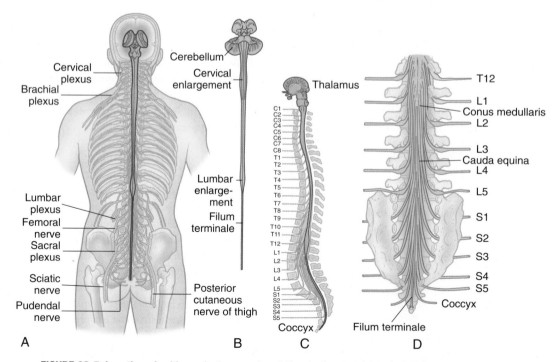

FIGURE 22-5 **Location of exiting spinal nerves in relation to the vertebrae. A,** Posterior view. **B,** Anterior view of brainstem and spinal cord. **C,** Lateral view showing relationship of spinal cord to vertebrae. **D,** Enlargement of caudal area with group of nerve fibers composing the cauda equina. *(Modified from Rudy, 1984.)*

FIGURE 22-6 Dermatomes of the body, the area of body surface innervated by particular spinal nerves; C1 usually has no cutaneous distribution. **A,** Anterior view. **B,** Posterior view. It appears that there is a distinct separation of surface area controlled by each dermatome, but there is almost always overlap between spinal nerves. C = cervical, T = thoracic, S = sacral, L = lumbar.

and glands of the body. The sensory or afferent fibers of the posterior root carry impulses from sensory receptors of the body to the spinal cord, and then on to the brain for interpretation by the cerebral sensory cortex.

A spinal afferent (sensory) neuron may initiate a reflex arc response when it receives an impulse stimulus such as a tap on a stretched muscle tendon. In this case, the response is transmitted outward by the efferent (motor) neuron in the anterior horn of the spinal cord via the spinal nerve and peripheral nerve of the skeletal muscle, stimulating a brisk contraction (Fig. 22-7). Such a reflex is dependent on intact afferent neurons, functional synapses in the spinal cord, intact efferent neurons, functional neuromuscular junctions, and competent muscle fibers.

�֍ Infants and Children

The major portion of brain growth occurs in the first year of life, along with myelinization of the brain and nervous system. Any event that disrupts brain development and growth during this period (e.g., infection, biochemical imbalance, or trauma) can have profound effects on eventual brain function. At birth, the neurologic impulses are primarily handled by the brainstem and spinal cord, such as the following reflexes: sucking, rooting, yawn, sneeze, hiccup, blink at bright light, and withdrawal from painful stimuli. Some primitive reflexes are present at birth (e.g., Moro, stepping, palmar and plantar grasp), and as the brain develops,

these reflexes are inhibited as more advanced cortical functions and voluntary control take over.

Motor maturation proceeds in a cephalocaudal direction. Motor control of the head and neck develops first, followed by the trunk and extremities. Motor development progresses, enabling more complex and independent functioning (see the table on Expected Motor Development Sequence in Children on ⓔ). Development occurs in an orderly sequence, but the timing varies considerably among children. Many capabilities may develop simultaneously in a child.

✖ Pregnant Women

Hypothalamic-pituitary neurohormonal changes occur with pregnancy; however, specific alterations in the neurologic system are not well identified. During the first trimester, women have increased sleep needs, but they may not feel rested, even with increased sleep. Late in pregnancy sleep can be affected due to multiple discomforts, such as back pain, frequent urination, leg cramps, and restless leg syndrome.

✖ Older Adults

The number of cerebral neurons decreases with aging, but this is not necessarily associated with deteriorating mental function (see Chapter 5). The vast number of reserve neurons inhibits the appearance of clinical signs. The velocity of nerve impulse conduction declines, so responses to various stimuli take longer.

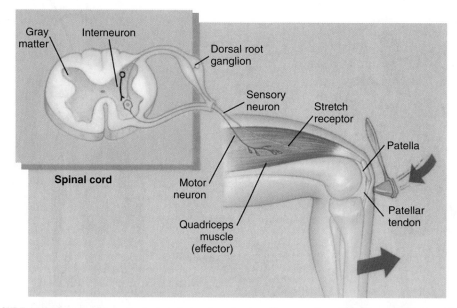

FIGURE 22-7 Cross section of spinal cord showing simple reflex arc. *(From Thibodeau and Patton, 1996.)*

REVIEW OF RELATED HISTORY

For each of the symptoms or conditions discussed in this section, particular topics to include in the history of the present illness are listed. Responses to questions about these topics provide clues for individualizing the physical examination and the development of a diagnostic evaluation appropriate for the particular patient. Questions regarding medication use (prescription and over the counter preparations) as well as complementary and alternative therapies are relevant for each area.

History of Present Illness

+ Seizures or convulsions
  + Sequence of events (independent observer's report): fall to ground, shrill cry, motor activity, transition phase, change in color of face or lips, pupil changes or eye deviations, loss of consciousness, loss of bowel or bladder control
  + Aura (perceptual sensation that may signal a seizure): irritability, tension, confusion, blurred vision, mood changes, initial focal motor seizure activity, gastrointestinal distress
  + Level of consciousness: loss, impairment, duration
  + Automatism: eyelid fluttering, chewing, lip smacking, swallowing
  + Muscle tone: flaccid, stiff, tense, twitching; where spasm began and moved through the body; change in character of motor activity during seizure
  + Postictal phase: weakness, transient paralysis, confusion, drowsiness, headaches, muscle aching, sleeping after seizure; any lateralization of signs
  + Relationship of seizure to time of day, meals, fatigue, emotional stress, excitement, menses, and discontinuing medications or poor compliance with medications; activity before episode

  + Frequency of seizures; total length of seizure activity; age at first seizure
  + Medications: anti-epileptic; initiation of medication or complementary or alternative therapy that interacts with prescribed anti-epileptic medication
+ Pain: see Chapter 4 for general topics, but consider "neurologic-specific" pain such as headaches associated with meningitis or encephalitis, space-occupying lesions, neck pain, sciatica, or trigeminal neuralgia.
  + Onset: sudden or progressive, associated with fever or injury
  + Quality and intensity: deep or superficial; aching, boring, throbbing, sharp or stabbing, burning, pressing, stinging, cramping, gnawing, prickling, shooting; duration and constancy
  + Location or path: along distribution of one or more peripheral nerves or a more general distribution; radiating from one part to another
  + Associated manifestations: crying, change in activity or energy level, sweating, muscle rigidity, tremor, impaired mental processes or concentration, weakness
  + Efforts to treat and impact on life
  + Medications: opioids and nonsteroidal antiinflammatory drugs; prescription, nonprescription
+ Gait coordination
  + Balance: sensation of leaning when walking to doorway; unsteadiness when walking
  + Falling: fall one way, backward, forward, consistent direction; associated with looking up; legs simply give way; stiffness of limbs
  + Associated problems: arthritis of cervical spine or in knees, ataxia, stroke, seizure, arrhythmias, sensory changes
  + Medications: phenytoin, pyrimethamine, etoposide, vinblastine; prescription, nonprescription

- Weakness or paresthesia
  - Onset: sudden, or with activity initiation or following sustained activity, time before symptoms begin; rapid or slow
  - Character: generalized or specific body area affected (face, extremity); progressively ascending or transient; proximal or distal extremities, unilateral, bilateral, or asymmetrical; difficulty walking; loss of balance or coordination; hypersensitivity to touch or burning sensation
  - Associated symptoms: tingling or numbness; confusion, trouble speaking or understanding speech; severe headache; impaired vision in one or both eyes; limb feels encased in tight bandage, pain, shortness of breath, stiffness of joints, spasms, muscle tension, sensory deficits; loss of urinary or bowel control
  - Concurrent chronic illness such as human immunodeficiency virus (HIV) infection, diabetes, nutritional or vitamin deficiency, or recent acute illness
  - Medications: zidovudine, chemotherapy, HIV medications, amphotericin B

Risk Factors

Stroke (Brain Attack or Cerebrovascular Accident)

- Hypertension
- Obesity
- Sedentary lifestyle
- Smoking tobacco products
- Stress
- Increased levels of serum cholesterol, lipoproteins, and triglycerides
- Use of oral contraceptives, sickle cell disease
- Family history of diabetes mellitus, cardiovascular disease, hypertension, and increased serum cholesterol levels
- Congenital cerebrovascular anomalies

- Tremor
  - Onset: sudden or gradual
  - Character: worse with rest, intentional movement, or anxiety; unilateral or bilateral; body location (distal extremities, head); interference with daily activities and impact on life
  - Associated problems: hyperthyroidism, familial tremor, liver or kidney disorder, consumption of alcohol, multiple sclerosis
  - Relieved by: rest, activity, alcohol
  - Medications: neuroleptics, valproate, phenytoin, albuterol, pseudoephedrine, antiarrhythmics, corticosteroids, caffeine (all may cause essential tremor)

Past Medical History

- Trauma: concussion or brain injury, spinal cord injury, or localized injury; central nervous system insult; birth trauma; stroke
- Meningitis, encephalitis, lead poisoning, poliomyelitis
- Deformities, congenital anomalies, genetic syndromes
- Cardiovascular, circulatory problems: hypertension, aneurysm, peripheral vascular disease

- Neurologic disorder, brain surgery, residual effects
- Headaches (e.g., migraines)

Family History

- Hereditary disorders: neurofibromatosis, Huntington chorea, muscular dystrophy, diabetes, pernicious anemia
- Alcoholism
- Intellectual disability
- Epilepsy or seizure disorder, headaches
- Alzheimer disease or other dementia, Parkinson disease
- Learning disorders
- Weakness or gait disorders, cerebral palsy
- Medical or metabolic disorder: thyroid disease, hypertension, diabetes mellitus

Personal and Social History

- Environmental or occupational hazards: exposure to lead, arsenic, insecticides, organic solvents, other chemicals; operate farm or other dangerous equipment or work at heights or in water (neurologic disorder may impact employment or personal safety)
- Hand, eye, and foot dominance; family patterns of dexterity and dominance
- Ability to care for self: hygiene, activities of daily living, finances, communication, shopping; ability to fulfill work expectations
- Sleeping or eating patterns; weight loss or gain; anxiety
- Use of alcohol or illicit drugs, especially mood-altering drugs

�֍ Infants

- Prenatal and maternal history: mother's health, medications taken, intrauterine infections such as toxoplasmosis, syphilis, tuberculosis, rubella, cytomegalovirus, herpes, fetal movement, prior history of hypertension, preeclampsia, bleeding, history of trauma or stress, persistent vomiting, hypertension, drug or alcohol use
- Birth history: Apgar score, gestational age, prematurity, birth weight, presentation, use of instruments to assist in delivery, prolonged or precipitate labor, fetal distress
- Respiratory status at birth: resuscitation needed, apnea, cyanosis, need for oxygen or mechanical ventilation
- Neonatal health: jaundice (from ABO blood type incompatibility, breast-feeding, or other causes), perinatal infections, seizures, irritability, poorly coordinated sucking and swallowing, need for intensive care, ototoxic medication exposure
- Congenital anomalies, congenital heart disease, or other physical disabilities
- Hypotonia or hypertonia in infancy, developmental delay

�֍ Children

- Developmental milestones
  - Age attained: smiling, head control in prone position, grasping, transferring objects between hands, rolling over,

sitting, crawling, independent walking, toilet-trained, says words other than "mama" and "dada"

+ Pattern of development: similar to other children; always slower than others; loss of previously achieved function; change in the child's rate of development; (progress occurred as expected until a certain age with slow progress afterward)

+ Performance of self-care activities: dressing, toileting, feeding

+ Hyperactive or impulsive behavior; problems with schedule changes, sitting for entire meal; poor organizational skills, unable to handle more than one instruction at a time, uncontrolled anger, poor social skills; school problems

+ Health problems:
  + Headaches, unexplained vomiting, lethargy, personality changes
  + Seizure activity: association with fever, frequency, duration, character of movement
  + Any clumsiness, unsteady gait, progressive muscular weakness, unexplained falling, problems going up and down stairs, problems getting up after lying down on floor

❀ Pregnant Women

+ Weeks of gestation or estimated date of delivery
+ Seizure activity: past history of seizures or pregnancy-induced hypertension; frequency, duration, character of movement
+ Headache: onset, character, frequency, association with hypertension; visual changes
+ Nutritional status: dietary supplements such as prenatal vitamins, calcium; salt depletion

❀ Older Adults

+ Pattern of increased stumbling, falls, unsteadiness, or decreased agility; worse in the dark; safety modifications used in home
+ Interference with performance of daily living tasks, social withdrawal, feelings about symptoms
+ Hearing loss, vision deficit, anosmia—transient or persistent
+ Urinary or fecal incontinence
+ Transient neurologic deficits (may indicate transient ischemic attacks)

Risk Factors

Falls in Older Adults

- One or more falls in the past year
- Past history of a stroke
- Neurologic condition such as Parkinson disease, dementia, or peripheral neuropathy
- Disorder of gait or balance
- Lower extremity weakness or sensory loss
- Impaired vision
- Use of an assistive device (e.g., walker or cane)

EXAMINATION AND FINDINGS

Equipment

+ Penlight
+ Tongue blades
+ Sterile needles
+ Tuning forks, 200 to 400 Hz and 500 to 1000 Hz
+ Familiar objects: coins, keys, paper clip
+ Cotton wisp
+ 5.07 monofilament
+ Reflex hammer
+ Vials of aromatic substances: coffee, orange, peppermint extract, oil of cloves
+ Vials of solutions: glucose, salt, lemon or vinegar, and quinine—with applicators for taste testing
+ Test tubes of hot and cold water for temperature sensation testing

Because the neurologic examination is complex, the discussion is divided into four sections for an organized approach. These sections include cranial nerves, proprioception and cerebellar function, sensory function, and reflex function. Assessment of mental status is detailed in Chapter 5. Evaluation of muscle tone and strength, an integral part of the neurologic examination, is detailed in Chapter 21.

The neurologic system is assessed during the entire patient visit. When the patient enters the room, his or her response to your suggestion about where to sit provides information about the functioning of the neurologic system. For example, you can observe balance, coordination and smoothness of gait, and ability to follow directions, all providing clues about the neurologic system. The musculoskeletal examination, particularly muscle tone and strength, provides important information about the neurologic examination because the systems are interdependent. When the history and examination findings have not yet revealed a potential neurologic problem, a neurologic screening examination may be performed (Box 22-1).

Box 22-1 | Procedure for the Neurologic Screening Examination

The shorter screening examination is commonly used for health visits when no known neurologic problem is apparent.

Cranial Nerves
Cranial nerves II through XII are routinely tested; however, taste is not tested unless some aberration is found (pp. 553-556).

Proprioception and Cerebellar Function
One test is administered for each of the following: rapid rhythmic alternating movements, accuracy of movements, balance (Romberg test is given), and gait and heel-toe walking (pp. 556-560).

Sensory Function
Superficial pain and touch at a distal point in each extremity are tested; vibration and position senses are assessed by testing the great toe (pp. 559-561).

Deep Tendon Reflexes
All deep tendon reflexes are tested, excluding the plantar reflex and the test for clonus (pp. 564-565).

Cranial Nerves

Evaluating the cranial nerves is an integral part of the neurologic examination. Ordinarily, taste and smell are not evaluated unless a problem is suspected. A patient may not recognize that some hearing, certain taste sensations, or some vision has been lost. When a sensory loss is suspected, be compulsive about determining the extent of loss when testing the relevant cranial nerve.

Examination of some cranial nerves is described in detail in other chapters, associated with the body system in which they are most commonly evaluated. Testing of the optic (II), oculomotor (III), trochlear (IV), and abducens (VI) nerves are described in Chapter 11; the acoustic (VIII) and hypoglossal (XII) nerves in Chapter 12; and the spinal accessory nerve (XI) in Chapter 21. Table 22-3 describes a review of all cranial nerve examination procedures. Unexpected findings (focal deficits) indicate trauma or a lesion in the cerebral hemisphere or local injury to the nerve. See Clinical Pearl, "Mnemonic for Cranial Nerve Names."

Olfactory (I)

The olfactory nerve is tested when a concern exists with the patient's ability to discriminate odors. Have available two or

---

Clinical Pearl

Mnemonic for Cranial Nerve Names

One way to remember the cranial nerves is the mnemonic for the first letter of each nerve: On Old Olympus Towering Tops A Finn and German Viewed Some Hops. Classification of each cranial nerves by function—Sensory (S), Motor (M), or Both (B) can be remembered by the mnemonic: Some Say Marry Money But My Brother Says Bad Business Marry Money.

---

three vials of familiar aromatic odors. Use the least irritating aromatic substance (e.g., orange or peppermint extract) first so that the patient's perception of weaker odors is not impaired. Before starting the assessment make sure the patient's nasal passages are patent. Occlude one naris at a time and ask the patient to breathe in and out.

Ask the patient to close his or her eyes and to occlude one naris. Hold an opened vial under the nose. Ask the patient to inspire deeply (so the odor reaches the upper nose and swirls around the olfactory mucosa) and to identify the odor (Fig. 22-8). Use a different odor to test the other side. Continue the assessment, alternating between sides with two or three odors,

---

Table 22-3   Procedure for Cranial Nerve Examination

Cranial Nerve (CN)	Procedure
CN I (olfactory)	Test ability to identify familiar aromatic odors, one naris at a time with eyes closed
CN II (optic)	Test distant and near vision Perform ophthalmoscopic examination of fundi
CN III (oculomotor), IV (trochlear), and VI (abducens)	Test visual fields by confrontation and extinction of vision Inspect eyelids for drooping Inspect pupils' size for equality and their direct and consensual response to light and accommodation. Test extraocular eye movements
CN V (trigeminal)	Inspect face for muscle atrophy and tremors Palpate jaw muscles for tone and strength when patient clenches teeth Test superficial pain and touch sensation in each branch (test temperature sensation if there are unexpected findings to pain or touch) Test corneal reflex
CN VII (facial)	Inspect symmetry of facial features with various expressions (e.g., smile, frown, puffed cheeks, wrinkled forehead) Test ability to identify sweet and salty tastes on each side of tongue
CN VIII (acoustic)	Test sense of hearing with whisper screening tests or by audiometry Compare bone and air conduction of sound Test for lateralization of sound
CN IX (glossopharyngeal), and X (vagus)	Test ability to identify sour and bitter tastes on each side of tongue Test gag reflex and ability to swallow Inspect palate and uvula for symmetry with speech sounds and gag reflex Observe for swallowing difficulty Evaluate quality of guttural speech sounds (presence of nasal or hoarse quality to voice)
CN XI (spinal accessory)	Test trapezius muscle strength (shrug shoulders against resistance) Test sternocleidomastoid muscle strength (turn head to each side against resistance)
CN XII (hypoglossal)	Inspect tongue in mouth and while protruded for symmetry, tremors, and atrophy Inspect tongue movement toward nose and chin Test tongue strength with index finger when tongue is pressed against cheek Evaluate quality of lingual speech sounds (l, t, d, n)

comparing the patient's ability to identify and discriminate between odors. Avoid offering multiple odors too quickly as this may confuse the olfactory sense.

Patients are expected to perceive an odor on each side, and usually to identify it. Inflammation of the mucous membranes, allergic rhinitis, and excessive tobacco smoking may all interfere with the ability to distinguish odors. The sense of smell may diminish with age. Anosmia, the loss of sense of smell or an inability to discriminate odors, can be caused by trauma to the cribriform plate or by an olfactory tract lesion.

Optic (II)

Visual acuity and visual fields are evaluated as in Chapter 11.

Oculomotor, Trochlear, and Abducens (III, IV, and VI)

Movement of the eyes through the six cardinal points of gaze, pupil size, shape, response to light and accommodation, and opening of the upper eyelids are described in Chapter 11.

When assessing patients with severe, unremitting headaches, the experienced examiner evaluates movement of the eyes for the presence or absence of lateral (temporal) gaze. The sixth cranial nerve is commonly one of the first to lose function in the presence of increased intracranial pressure.

Trigeminal (V)

Evaluate motor function by observing the face for muscle atrophy, deviation of the jaw to one side, and fasciculations (muscle twitches). Have the patient tightly clench the teeth as you palpate the muscles over the jaw, evaluating tone (Fig. 22-9). Muscle tone over the face should be symmetric, without fasciculations.

The three divisions of the trigeminal nerve are evaluated for sharp, dull, and light touch sensation (Fig. 22-10). With the patient's eyes closed, touch each side of the face at the scalp, cheek, and chin areas, alternately using the sharp and smooth edges of a broken tongue blade or a paper clip. Avoid using a predictable pattern. Ask the patient to report whether each sensation is sharp or dull. Then stroke the face in the same six areas

FIGURE 22-8 Examination of the olfactory cranial nerve. Occlude one naris, hold the vial with aromatic substance under the nose, and ask the patient to deeply inspire. If the patient's eyes are open, make sure there are no visual cues to odors. The patient should discriminate between odors.

FIGURE 22-9 Examination of the trigeminal cranial nerve for motor function. Have the patient tightly clench the teeth, and then palpate the muscles over the jaw for tone.

FIGURE 22-10 Examination of the trigeminal cranial nerve for sensory function. Touch each side of the face at the scalp, cheek, and chin areas alternately using no predictable pattern **(A)** with the point and rounded edge of a paper clip or broken tongue blade and **(B)** with a brush or cotton wisp. Ask the patient to discriminate between sensations.

with a cotton wisp, brush, or lightly with a fingerpad, asking the patient to tell when the stimulus is felt. A wooden applicator is used to test sensation over the buccal mucosa. Discrimination of all stimuli is expected over all areas of the face.

If sensation is impaired, use test tubes filled with hot and cold water to evaluate temperature sensation. Ask the patient to tell you if hot or cold is felt as you touch the same six areas of the face. Contrast the discrimination of temperature with the other sensations.

When the corneal reflex is clinically indicated, have the patient look up and away from you as you approach from the side (contact lenses, if used, should be removed). Avoiding the eyelashes and the conjunctiva, lightly touch the cornea of one eye with a cotton wisp. Repeat the procedure on the other cornea. A symmetric blink reflex to corneal stimulation is expected. Patients who wear contact lenses may have a diminished or absent reflex.

Facial (VII)

Evaluate motor function by observing a series of expressions you ask the patient to make: Raise the eyebrows, squeeze the eyes shut, wrinkle the forehead, frown, smile, show the teeth, purse the lips to whistle, and puff out the cheeks (Fig. 22-11). Observe for tics, unusual facial movements, and asymmetry of expression. Listen as the patient speaks and note any difficulties with labial speech sounds (b, m, and p). Drooping of one side of the mouth,

a flattened nasolabial fold, and a sagging lower eyelid are signs of muscle weakness. See the discussion of Bell palsy on p. 577 and Clinical Pearl, "Upper and Lower Neuron Disease."

> ### Clinical Pearl
> *Upper and Lower Neuron Disease*
>
> To distinguish between upper and lower neuron disease affecting the face, observe the patient's face when laughing or crying. When the upper motor neurons are affected, as in a stroke or brain attack, voluntary movements are paralyzed, but emotional movements are spared. In a lower motor neuron disorder, such as Bell palsy, all facial movements on the affected side are paralyzed.

To evaluate taste, a sensory function of cranial nerves VII and IX, have available the four solutions, applicators, and a card listing the tastes (bitter, sour, salty, sweet). Make sure the patient cannot see the labels on the vials. Ask the patient to keep the tongue protruded and to point out the taste perceived on the card. Apply one solution at a time to the lateral side of the tongue in the appropriate taste bud region (Fig. 22-12). Alternate the solutions, using a different applicator for each. Offer a sip of water after each stimulus. Each solution is used on both sides of

FIGURE 22-11 Examination of the facial cranial nerve for motor function. Ask the patient to **(A)** wrinkle the forehead by raising the eyebrows; **(B)** smile; **(C)** puff out the cheeks; **(D)** purse the lips and blow out; **(E)** show the teeth; and **(F)** squeeze the eyes shut.

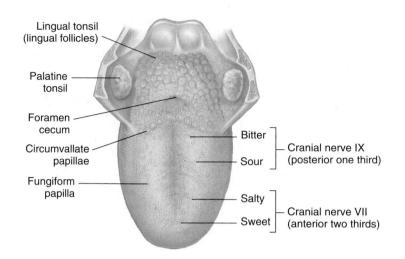

Lingual tonsil
(lingual follicles)

Palatine
tonsil

Foramen
cecum

Circumvallate
papillae

Fungiform
papilla

Bitter
Sour — Cranial nerve IX
(posterior one third)

Salty
Sweet — Cranial nerve VII
(anterior two thirds)

FIGURE 22-12 Location of the taste bud regions tested for the sensory function of the facial and glosso-pharyngeal cranial nerves.

the tongue to identify taste discrimination. The patient should identify each taste bilaterally when placed correctly on the tongue surface (see Clinical Pearl, "Evaluating Taste Sensation").

> ### Clinical Pearl
>
> *Evaluating Taste Sensation*
>
> Taste is rarely evaluated in the routine neurologic examination. Taste acuity decreases with advanced aging, but the extent of decline varies for the four different tastes—salty, sweet, sour, bitter that are tested. Most individuals who describe a loss of taste sensation actually have a dysfunction of olfactory sensation (Doty, 2012).

Acoustic (VIII)

Hearing is evaluated with the screening tests described in Chapter 12 or with an audiometer. Vestibular function is tested by the Romberg test (see p. 559). Other vestibular function tests are not routinely performed.

Glossopharyngeal (IX)

The sensory function of taste over the posterior third of the tongue may be tested during cranial nerve VII evaluation. The glossopharyngeal nerve is simultaneously tested during evaluation of the vagus nerve for nasopharyngeal sensation (gag reflex) and the motor function of swallowing.

Vagus (X)

To evaluate nasopharyngeal sensation, tell the patient you will be testing the gag reflex. Touch the posterior wall of the patient's pharynx with an applicator as you observe for upward movement of the palate and contraction of the pharyngeal muscles. Expect the uvula to remain in the midline. Drooping or absence of an arch on either side of the soft palate is unexpected.

Evaluate motor function by inspection of the soft palate for symmetry. Have the patient say "ah," and observe the movement of the soft palate and uvula for asymmetry. If the vagus or

glossopharyngeal nerve is damaged and the palate fails to rise, the uvula will deviate from the midline.

Have the patient sip and swallow water. You can do this while examining the thyroid gland (see Chapter 10). The patient should swallow easily. No retrograde passage of water through the nose after the nasopharynx has closed off or aspiration should occur.

Listen to the patient's speech, noting any hoarseness, nasal quality, or difficulty with guttural sounds.

Spinal Accessory (XI)

Evaluation of the size, shape, and strength of the trapezius and sternocleidomastoid muscles is described in Chapter 21.

Hypoglossal (XII)

Inspect the patient's tongue while at rest on the floor of the mouth and while protruded from the mouth (Fig. 22-13). Ask the patient to move the tongue in and out of the mouth, from side to side, curled upward as if to touch the nose, and curled downward as if to lick the chin. Test the tongue's muscle strength by asking the patient to push the tongue against the cheek as you apply resistance with an index finger. When listening to the patient's speech, expect no problems with lingual speech sounds (l, t, d, n). Any tongue fasciculations, asymmetry, atrophy, or deviation from the midline is unexpected.

Proprioception and Cerebellar Function

Coordination and Fine Motor Skills

When performing the following assessments, observe for any involuntary movements such as tremors (rhythmic oscillatory movements), tics, or fasciculations. Note the parts of the body affected, quality, rate and rhythm (see Differential Diagnosis: Tremors).

Rapid Rhythmic Alternating Movements. Ask the seated patient to pat his or her knees with both hands, alternately

FIGURE 22-13 Examination of the hypoglossal cranial nerve. **A,** Inspect the protruded tongue for size, shape, symmetry, and fasciculation. **B,** Observe movement of the tongue from side to side.

DIFFERENTIAL DIAGNOSIS

Tremors

Type of Tremor	Characteristics	Potential Cause
Enhanced physiologic tremor	Seen with arms held extended, disappears when limb is at rest; small amplitude	Drug or alcohol withdrawal Hyperthyroidism, hypoglycemia Toxicity associated with some medications (e.g., lithium, methylxanthines, valproate, tricyclic antidepressants)
Essential tremor	Bilateral, symmetric; primarily seen in hands or outstretched arms, intention tremor May be seen in head, trunk, voice, tongue May worsen with stress or fatigue; may improve temporarily with alcohol Progressive Usually absence of other neurologic signs Lower limbs rarely affected	No consistent cerebral pathology Autosomal dominant inheritance pattern
Intention tremor	Seen during intentional movements, such as writing, pouring water in a cup, finger to nose testing Does not occur at rest	May be associated with a cerebellar disorder such as multiple sclerosis or alcohol abuse
Resting tremor	Seen when limb is at rest Slow supination-pronation (pill-rolling) movements	Parkinson disease

turning up and down the palms of the hands and increasing the speed gradually (Fig. 22-14, *A* and *B*). As an alternate procedure, have the patient touch the thumb to each finger on the same hand, in sequence from the index finger to the little finger and back. Test one hand at a time, increasing speed gradually (Fig. 22-14, *C*). Expect the patient to smoothly execute these movements, maintaining rhythm with increasing speed. Stiff, slowed, nonrhythmic, or jerky clonic movements are unexpected.

Accuracy of Movements. The finger-to-nose test is performed with the patient's eyes open. Ask the patient to use an index finger and alternately touch his or her nose and your index finger (Fig. 22-15, *A* and *B*). Position your index finger about 18 inches from the patient, allowing the patient to reach full arm extension. Move your finger several times during the test. Repeat the procedure with the other hand. Expect the patient's movements to be rapid, smooth, and accurate. Consistent past pointing (i.e., missing the examiner's index finger) may indicate cerebellar disease.

An alternate finger-to-nose test involves asking the patient to close both eyes and touch his or her nose with the index finger of each hand. Alternate the hands used and increase speed gradually (Fig. 22-15, *C*). Expect the movement to be smooth, rapid, and accurate, even with increasing speed.

The heel-to-shin test is another alternate method, performed with the patient standing, sitting, or supine. Ask the patient to run the heel of one foot up and down the shin (from knee to ankle) of the opposite leg (Fig. 22-15, *D*). Repeat the procedure

FIGURE 22-14 Examination of coordination with rapid alternating movements. A, B, Pat the knees with both hands, alternately using the palm and back of the hand. **C,** Touch the thumb to each finger of the hand in sequence from index finger to small finger and back.

FIGURE 22-15 Examination of fine motor function. A and B, The patient alternately touches own nose and the examiner's index finger with the index finger of one hand; **C,** Alternately touches own nose with the index finger of each hand; and **D,** runs the heel of one foot down the shin or tibia of the other leg.

FIGURE 22-16 Evaluation of balance with the Romberg test.

FIGURE 22-17 Evaluation of gait and balance with heel-toe walking on a straight line.

with the other heel. Expect the patient to move the heel up and down the shin in a straight line, without irregular deviations to the side.

Balance

Equilibrium. Balance is initially evaluated with the Romberg test. Ask the patient (with eyes open and then closed) to stand, feet together and arms at the sides (Fig. 22-16). Stand close, prepared to catch the patient if he or she starts to fall. Slight swaying movement of the body is expected, but not to the extent that there is danger of falling. Loss of balance, a positive Romberg sign, indicates cerebellar ataxia, vestibular dysfunction, or sensory loss. If the patient staggers or loses balance with the Romberg test, postpone other tests of cerebellar function requiring balance.

To further evaluate balance, have the patient stand with feet slightly apart. Push the shoulders with enough effort to throw him or her off balance. Be ready to catch the patient if necessary. Recovery of balance should occur quickly.

Ask the patient to close his or her eyes and hold the arms straight at the side of the body and stand on one foot. Repeat the test on the opposite foot. Expect slight swaying along with the ability to maintain balance on each foot for 5 seconds.

Have the patient (eyes open) hop in place first on one foot and then on the other. Expect the patient to hop on each foot for 5 seconds without loss of balance. Note any instability, a need to continually touch the floor with the opposite foot, or a tendency to fall.

Gait. Observe the patient walk without shoes around the examining room or down a hallway, first with the eyes open. Observe the expected gait sequence, noting simultaneous arm movements and upright posture:

1. The first heel strikes the floor and then moves to full contact with the floor.
2. The second heel pushes off, leaving the ground.
3. Body weight is transferred from the first heel to the ball of its foot.
4. The leg swing is accelerated as weight is removed from the second foot.
5. The second foot is lifted and travels ahead of the weight-bearing first foot, swinging through.
6. The second foot slows in preparation for heel strike.

Expect the patient to continuously sequence stance and swing, step after step. The gait should have a smooth, regular rhythm and symmetric stride length. The trunk posture should sway with the gait phase, and arm swing should be smooth and symmetric.

Heel-toe walking (tandem gait) will exaggerate any unexpected finding in gait evaluation. Direct the patient to touch the toe of one foot with the heel of the other foot (Fig. 22-17). Have the patient walk a straight line, first forward and then backward, with eyes open and arms at the sides. Consistent contact between the heel and toe should occur, although slight swaying is expected. Note any extension of the arms for balance, instability, a tendency to fall, or lateral staggering and reeling. Note any shuffling, widely placed feet, toe walking, foot flop, leg lag, scissoring, loss of arm swing, staggering, or reeling. Figure 22-18 and Table 22-4 describe unexpected gait patterns.

Sensory Function

Evaluate both primary and cortical discriminatory sensation by having the patient identify various sensory stimuli at the following sites: hands, lower arms, abdomen, feet, and lower

FIGURE 22-18 Unexpected gait patterns. **A,** Spastic hemiparesis. **B,** Spastic diplegia (scissoring). **C,** Step-page gait. **D,** Cerebellar ataxia. **E,** Sensory ataxia.

Table 22-4 — Characteristics of Unexpected Gait Patterns

Gait Pattern	Characteristics
Spastic hemiparesis	The affected leg is stiff and extended with plantar flexion of the foot; movement of the foot results from pelvic tilting upward on the involved side; the foot is dragged, often scraping the toe, or it is circled stiffly outward and forward (circumduction); the affected arm remains flexed and adducted and does not swing (see Fig. 22-18, *A*).
Spastic diplegia (scissoring)	The patient uses short steps, dragging the ball of the foot across the floor; the legs are extended and the thighs tend to cross forward on each other at each step due to injury to the pyramidal system (see Fig. 22-18, *B*).
Steppage	The hip and knee are elevated excessively high to lift the plantar flexed foot off the ground; the foot is brought down to the floor with a slap; the patient is unable to walk on the heels (see Fig. 22-18, *C*).
Dystrophic (waddling)	The legs are kept apart, and weight is shifted from side to side in a waddling motion due to weak hip abductor muscles; the abdomen often protrudes, and lordosis is common.
Tabetic	The legs are positioned far apart, lifted high, and forcibly brought down with each step; the heel stamps on the ground.
Cerebellar gait (cerebellar ataxia)	The patient's feet are wide-based; staggering and lurching from side to side is often accompanied by swaying of the trunk (see Fig. 22-18, *D*).
Sensory ataxia	The patient's gait is wide-based; the feet are thrown forward and outward, bringing them down first on heels, then on toes; the patient watches the ground to guide his or her steps; a positive Romberg sign is present (see Fig. 22-18, *E*).
Parkinsonian gait	The patient's posture is stooped and the body is held rigid; steps are short and shuffling, with hesitation on starting and difficulty stopping (see Fig. 22-31, *C* on p. 580).
Dystonia	Jerky, dancing movements appear nondirectional.
Ataxia	Uncontrolled falling occurs.
Antalgic limp	The patient limits the time of weight bearing on the affected leg to limit pain.

legs. For the complete neurologic examination, assess each major peripheral nerve. Sensory discrimination of the face is performed by evaluating cranial nerve V.

Each sensory discrimination procedure is tested with the patient's eyes closed. Use minimal stimulation initially, increasing it gradually until the patient becomes aware of it. A stronger stimulus is needed over the back, buttocks, and heavily callused areas, where there are lower levels of sensitivity. Test contralateral areas of the body, and ask the patient to compare perceived sensations, side to side. With each type of sensory stimulus, expected findings include:

- Minimal differences side to side
- Correct description of sensations (e.g., hot/cold, sharp/dull)
- Recognition of the side of the body tested
- Location of sensation and whether proximal or distal to the previous stimuli

If evidence of sensory impairment is found, map the boundaries of the sensory deficit by the distribution of major peripheral nerves or dermatomes (see Fig. 22-6). Loss of sensation can indicate spinal tract, brainstem, or cerebral lesions.

Primary Sensory Functions

Superficial Touch. Touch the skin with a cotton wisp or with your fingertip, using light strokes. Do not depress the skin, and avoid stroking areas with hair (Fig. 22-19, *A*). Have the patient point to the area touched or tell you when the sensation is felt.

Superficial Pain. Alternating the sharp and smooth edges of a broken tongue blade or paper clip, touch the skin in an unpredictable pattern. Allow 2 seconds between each stimulus to avoid a summative effect (see Fig. 22-19, *B*). Ask the patient to identify each sensation as sharp or dull and where it is felt.

Evaluation of superficial pain and touch can be evaluated together. Alternate the use of the sharp and dull tongue blade edges with fingertip strokes to determine whether the patient can identify the change in sensation.

Temperature and Deep Pressure. Temperature and deep pressure sensation tests are performed only if superficial pain sensation is not intact. To evaluate temperature sensation, roll test tubes of hot and cold water against the skin, alternating in an unpredictable pattern between the various sites. Ask the patient to indicate which temperature is perceived and where it is felt. Deep pressure sensation is tested by squeezing the trapezius, calf, or biceps muscle. The patient should experience discomfort.

Vibration. Place the stem of a vibrating tuning fork (the tuning fork with lower Hz has slower reduction of vibration) against several bony prominences, beginning at toe and finger joints. The sternum, shoulder, elbow, wrist, shin, and ankle may also be tested (see Fig. 22-19, *C*). Ask the patient to tell you when and where the buzzing or tingling sensation is felt. Dampen the tines on occasion before application to determine if the patient distinguishes a difference.

Position of Joints. Assess the great toe of each foot and a finger on each hand. Hold the joint to be tested (e.g., great toe or finger) by the lateral aspects to avoid giving a clue about the direction moved. Beginning with the joint in neutral position, raise or lower the digit, and ask the patient which way the joint was moved (see Fig. 22-19, *D*). Expect patients to identify the joint position.

Loss of sensory modalities may indicate peripheral neuropathy. Symmetric sensory loss indicates a polyneuropathy. See Box 22-2 for patterns of sensory loss.

Cortical Sensory Functions

Cortical or discriminatory sensory functions test cognitive ability to interpret sensations. Inability to perform these tests may indicate a lesion in the sensory cortex or the posterior columns of

FIGURE 22-19 Evaluation of primary sensory function. A, Superficial tactile sensation; use a light stroke to touch the skin with a cotton wisp or brush. **B,** Superficial pain sensation; use the sharp and rounded edge of a broken tongue blade in an unpredictable alternate pattern. **C,** Vibratory sensation; place the stem of a vibrating tuning fork against several bony prominences. **D,** Position sense of joints; hold the toe or finger by the lateral aspects while raising and lowering the toe.

FIGURE 22-20 Evaluation of cortical sensory function. A, Stereognosis; patient identifies a familiar object by touch. **B,** Two-point discrimination; using two sterile needles or two points of a paper clip, alternately place one or two points simultaneously on the skin, and ask the patient to determine whether one or two sensations are felt. **C,** Graphesthesia; draw a letter or number on the body (without actually marking skin) and ask the patient to identify it.

| Box 22-2 | Patterns of Sensory Loss Injury or Defect and Description of Findings |

Single Peripheral Nerve
The area of sensory loss is generally less than the anatomic distribution of nerve. The lost sensation is greatest in the central portion of the nerve's anatomic distribution with a surrounding zone of partial loss due to overlap by adjacent nerves. All or selected forms of sensory discrimination may be lost.

Multiple Peripheral Nerves (Polyneuropathy)
The sensory loss is most severe over legs and feet or over hands (i.e., glove and stocking distribution). The change from expected to impaired sensation is often gradual. All forms of sensory discrimination are usually lost.

Multiple Spinal Nerve Roots
Incomplete loss of sensation in any area of the skin usually occurs when one nerve root is affected. When two or more nerve roots are completely divided, a zone of sensory loss is surrounded by partial loss. Tendon reflexes may also be lost.

Complete Transverse Lesion of the Spinal Cord
All forms of sensation are lost below the level of the lesion. Pain, temperature, and touch sensations are lost one to two dermatomes below the lesion.

Partial Spinal Sensory Syndrome (Brown-Séquard Syndrome)
Pain and temperature sensation are lost one to two dermatomes below the lesion on the opposite side of the body from the lesion. Proprioceptive loss and motor paralysis occur on the lesion side of the body.

Two-Point Discrimination. Use two sterile needles or ends of a paper clip, and alternate touching the patient's skin with one point or both points at various locations over the body (see Fig. 22-20, *B*). Ask the patient how many points are felt. On the fingertips and toes, two points are commonly felt when 2 to 8 mm apart. A greater distance is expected for discrimination of two points on other body parts, such as the back (40 to 70 mm) or chest and forearms (40 mm).

Extinction Phenomenon. Simultaneously touch two areas on each side of the body (e.g., cheek, hand, or other area) with the sharp edge of a broken tongue blade. Ask the patient to tell you how many stimuli there are and where they are. Expect similar sensations to be felt bilaterally.

Graphesthesia. With a blunt pen or an applicator stick, draw a letter, number, or shape on the palm of the patient's hand (see Fig. 22-20, *C*). Other body locations may also be used. Ask the patient to identify the figure. Repeat using a different figure on the other hand. Expect the figure to be readily recognized.

Point Location. Touch an area on the patient's skin and withdraw the stimulus. Ask the patient to point to the area touched. No difficulty localizing the stimulus should be noted. This procedure is often performed with superficial tactile sensation.

Table 22-5 provides a summary of procedures used to test the integrity of spinal tracts.

the spinal cord. The patient's eyes should be closed for these procedures.

Stereognosis. Hand the patient a familiar object (e.g., key, coin) to identify by touch and manipulation (Fig. 22-20, *A*). Tactile agnosia, an inability to recognize objects by touch, suggests a parietal lobe lesion.

Reflexes

Both superficial and deep tendon reflexes are used to evaluate the function of specific spine segmental levels (Table 22-6).

Superficial Reflexes

The plantar reflex is routinely performed. The abdominal and cremasteric reflexes are less commonly tested, but they are important when thoracic spinal nerves need to be evaluated.

Plantar Reflex. Use the end of a reflex hammer to stroke the lateral side of the foot from the heel to the ball and then across the ball of the foot to the medial side (Fig. 22-21, *A*). Expect plantar flexion of all toes. The Babinski sign is present when there is dorsiflexion of the great toe with or without fanning of the other toes. The Babinski sign indicates pyramidal tract disease in patients. It is, however, an expected finding in children younger than 2 years of age. The ticklish patient may respond with some degree of Babinski sign, but this can be avoided with a firm touch.

Abdominal Reflex. With the patient supine, stroke each quadrant of the abdomen with the end of a reflex hammer or edge of a tongue blade. Elicit the upper abdominal reflexes by stroking upward and away from the umbilicus. Elicit the lower abdominal reflexes by stroking downward and away from the umbilicus (Fig. 22-21, *B*). Expect a slight movement of the umbilicus toward each area of stimulation to be bilaterally equal. A diminished reflex may be present in patients who are obese or whose abdominal muscles have been stretched during pregnancy. Abdominal reflexes may be absent on the side of a corticospinal tract lesion, but their presence or absence may have little clinical significance.

Table 22-5	Procedures for Testing the Integrity of Individual Spinal Tracts for Upper and Lower Motor Neuron Disorders
Spinal Tracts	**Neurologic Tests**
Ascending Tracts—for Lower Motor Neuron Disorders	
Lateral spinothalamic	Superficial pain
	Temperature
Anterior spinothalamic	Superficial touch
	Deep pressure
Posterior column	Vibration
	Deep pressure
	Position sense
	Stereognosis
	Point location
	Two-point discrimination
Anterior and dorsal spinocerebellar	Proprioception
Descending Tracts—for Upper Motor Neuron Disorders	
Lateral and anterior corticospinal	Rapid rhythmic alternating movements
	Voluntary movement
	Deep tendon reflexes
	Plantar reflex
Medial and lateral reticulospinal	Posture and Romberg
	Gait
	Instinctual motor reactions

Table 22-6	Spinal Nerve Level Evaluated by Superficial and Deep Tendon Reflexes
Reflex	**Spinal Nerve Level Evaluated**
Superficial	
Upper abdominal	T8, T9, and T10
Lower abdominal	T10, T11, and T12
Cremasteric	T12, L1, and L2
Plantar	L5, S1, and S2
Deep Tendon	
Biceps	C5 and C6
Brachioradial	C5 and C6
Triceps	C6, C7, and C8
Patellar	L2, L3, and L4
Achilles	S1 and S2

FIGURE 22-21 Superficial reflexes. A, Plantar reflex indicating the direction of the stroke and the Babinski sign—dorsiflexion of the great toe with or without fanning of the toes. **B,** One of several approaches for the abdominal reflexes. Stroke the lower abdominal area downward, away from the umbilicus. Stroke the upper abdominal area upward, away from the umbilicus.

Cremasteric Reflex. Stroke the inner thigh of the male patient (proximal to distal) to elicit the cremasteric reflex. Expect the testicle and scrotum to rise on the stroked side.

Deep Tendon Reflexes

Evaluate deep tendon reflexes with the patient either sitting or lying down. Focus the patient's attention on an alternate muscle contraction (e.g., pulling clenched hands apart) to help prevent an exaggerated or diminished response. Position the limb with slight tension on the tendon to be tapped and palpate the tendon to locate the correct point for stimulation. Hold the reflex hammer loosely between your thumb and index finger and without striking too forcefully, briskly tap the tendon with a flick of the wrist.

Test each reflex, comparing responses between sides. Expect symmetric visible or palpable responses. Deep tendon reflex responses are scored as shown in Table 22-7. A method to document findings on a stick figure is illustrated in Chapter 26. Absent reflexes may indicate neuropathy or lower motor neuron disorder. Hyperactive reflexes suggest an upper motor neuron disorder. The characteristics of upper and lower motor neuron disorders are listed in the Differential Diagnosis: Characteristics of Upper and Lower Motor Neuron Disorders table.

Table 22-7   Scoring Deep Tendon Reflexes

Grade	Deep Tendon Reflex Response
0	No response
1+	Sluggish or diminished
2+	Active or expected response
3+	More brisk than expected, slightly hyperactive
4+	Brisk, hyperactive, with intermittent or transient clonus

Biceps Reflex. Flex the patient's arm to 45 degrees at the elbow. Palpate the biceps tendon in the antecubital fossa (Fig. 22-22, *A*). Place your thumb over the tendon and your fingers under the elbow. Strike your thumb, rather than the tendon directly, with the reflex hammer. Contraction of the biceps muscle causes visible or palpable flexion of the elbow.

Brachioradial Reflex. Flex the patient's arm up to 45 degrees and rest his or her forearm on your arm with the hand slightly pronated (see Fig. 22-22, *B*). Strike the brachioradial tendon (about 1 to 2 inches above the wrist) directly with the reflex hammer. Pronation of the forearm and flexion of the elbow should occur.

Triceps Reflex. Flex the patient's arm at the elbow up to 90 degrees, supporting the arm proximal to the antecubital fossa. Palpate the triceps tendon and strike it directly with the reflex hammer, just above the elbow (see Fig. 22-22, *C*). Contraction of the triceps muscle causes visible or palpable extension of the elbow.

Patellar Reflex. Flex the patient's knee to 90 degrees. Support the upper leg with your hand and allow the lower leg to hang loosely. Strike the patellar tendon just below the patella (see Fig. 22-22, *D*). Contraction of the quadriceps muscle causes extension of the lower leg.

Achilles Reflex. With the patient sitting, flex the knee to 90 degrees and keep the ankle in neutral position, holding the foot in your hand. (Alternatively, the patient may kneel on a chair with the toes pointing toward the floor.) Strike the Achilles tendon at the level of the ankle malleoli (see Fig. 22-22, *E*). Contraction of the gastrocnemius muscle causes plantar flexion of the foot.

DIFFERENTIAL DIAGNOSIS

Characteristics of Upper and Lower Motor Neuron Disorders

Assessment Parameters	Upper Motor Neuron	Lower Motor Neuron
Muscle tone	Increased tone, muscle spasticity, risk for contractures	Decreased tone, muscle flaccidity
Muscle atrophy	Little or no muscle atrophy, but decreased strength	Loss of muscle strength; muscle atrophy or wasting
Sensation	Sensation loss may affect entire limb	Sensory loss follows the distribution of dermatomes or peripheral nerves
Reflexes	Hyperactive deep tendon and abdominal reflexes; positive Babinski sign	Weak or absent deep tendon, plantar, and abdominal reflexes, negative plantar reflex, no pathologic reflexes
Fasciculation	No fasciculations	Fasciculations
Motor effect	Paralysis of voluntary movements	Paralysis of muscles
Location of insult	Damage above level of brainstem affects opposite side of body, damage below the brainstem affects the same side of the body	Damage affects muscle on same side of body

FIGURE 22-22 Location of tendons for evaluation of deep tendon reflexes. **A,** Biceps. **B,** Brachioradial. **C,** Triceps. **D,** Patellar. **E,** Achilles. **F,** Evaluation of ankle clonus.

Clonus. Test for ankle clonus, especially if the reflexes are hyperactive. Support the patient's knee in partially flexed position and briskly dorsiflex the foot with your other hand, maintaining the foot in flexion (see Fig. 22-22, *F*). No rhythmic oscillating movements between dorsiflexion and plantar flexion should be palpated. Sustained clonus is associated with upper motor neuron disease.

Advanced Skills

Other procedures for further evaluation of the neurologic system may be performed when problems are detected with routine examination.

Protective Sensation

Use the 5.07 monofilament to test for sensation on several sites of the foot in all patients with diabetes mellitus and peripheral neuropathy (Fig. 22-23). While the patient's eyes are closed, apply the monofilament in a random pattern to several sites on the plantar surface of the foot and on one site of the dorsal surface. Do not test over calluses or broken skin. Do not repeat a test site. The monofilament should be applied to each site for 1.5 seconds. When the filament bends, adequate pressure is applied. Patients should feel the sensation in all sites. Loss of sensation to the touch of the monofilament is an indication of peripheral neuropathy. It also indicates the loss of protective pain sensation that alerts patients to skin breakdown and injury on the foot.

Meningeal Signs

A stiff neck, or *nuchal rigidity, is* a sign that may be associated with meningitis and intracranial hemorrhage. With the patient supine, slip your hand under the head and raise it, flexing the neck. Try to make the patient's chin touch the sternum, but do

FIGURE 22-23 A, Sites for application of the 5.07 monofilament to test for protective sensation. Indicate presence (+) or absence (−) of sensory perception on a drawing of the foot. **B,** Apply the monofilament to the patient's foot with just enough pressure to bend the monofilament.

not force it. Placing your hand under the shoulders when the patient is supine and raising the shoulders slightly will help relax the neck, making the determination of true stiffness more accurate. Patients generally do not resist or complain of pain. Pain and a resistance to neck motion are associated with nuchal rigidity. Occasionally, painful swollen lymph nodes in the neck and superficial trauma may also cause pain and resistance to neck motion.

FIGURE 22-24 A, Brudzinski sign, flex the neck and observe for involuntary flexion of the hips and knees. **B,** Kernig sign, flex the leg at the knee and hip when the patient is supine, and then attempt to straighten the leg. Observe for pain in the lower back and resistance to straightening the leg.

The *Brudzinski sign* may also be present when neck stiffness is assessed. Involuntary flexion of the hips and knees when flexing the neck is a positive Brudzinski sign and may indicate meningeal irritation (Fig. 22-24, *A*).

The *Kernig sign* is evaluated by flexing the leg at the knee and hip when the patient is supine, then attempting to straighten the leg. A positive Kernig sign is present when the patient has pain in the lower back and resistance to straightening the leg at the knee. The presence of this sign may indicate meningeal irritation (see Fig. 22-24, *B*).

Staying Well

Vaccines to Reduce Risk for Meningitis

Vaccines are available to reduce the risk of developing meningitis caused by various organisms. Infants and young children are protected by the *Haemophilus influenzae* type b (Hib) and the pneumococcal vaccine (PCV13) administered as routine immunizations. Older children and adolescents are protected against four strains of *Neisseria meningitidis* by routine immunization with the conjugated meningococcal vaccine (MCV4). For those with continued high risk (e.g., an individual with functional asplenia), revaccination should occur every 5 years. Individuals up to age 55 years should receive the conjugated vaccine (MCV4). Adults over 55 years should receive the polysaccharide vaccine (MPSV4). Individuals with chronic medical conditions and older adults can be protected against many strains of pneumococci with the pneumococcal polysaccharide vaccine (PPSV) (Centers for Disease Control and Prevention, 2012).

Jolt Accentuation of Headache

For the patient presenting with fever and headache that leads to a suspected diagnosis of meningitis, jolt accentuation of headache may be performed. Ask the patient to move his or her head horizontally at a rate of 2 to 3 rotations per second. A positive sign is indicated by an increased headache over the baseline. This sign has potential as a diagnostic sign for meningitis, but this has not been confirmed by research (Hatala et al, 2009; Aminzadeh and Roudgari, 2010).

Posturing

Postures that may be found in unresponsive patients are associated with a severe brain injury. Decorticate or flexor posturing is

Evidence-Based Practice

Signs of Meningitis

The classic signs of acute meningitis are fever, a stiff neck, and altered mental status, but most patients do not have all three signs. Other potential presenting symptoms include headache, nausea, vomiting, chills, myalgia, and rash. Nuchal rigidity, Brudzinski sign, and Kernig sign have historically been considered important diagnostic signs for meningitis.

Prospective studies investigating physical signs associated with meningitis have not identified a single sign or information from the history that increases the likelihood of meningitis. Absence of the three classic signs of acute meningitis does not rule out meningitis as a diagnosis (Hatala et al, 2009; Waghdhare, 2010). A lumbar puncture is needed to confirm the presence of meningitis.

associated with injury to the corticospinal tracts above the brainstem (Fig. 22-25, *A*). Decerebrate or extensor posturing is associated with injury to the brainstem (Fig. 22-25, *B*).

❀ Infants

Neurologic problems are suspected in infants and young children when parents report they are not doing something expected of them or they have lost a skill they previously attained. The major clues are discovered with an accurate and thorough history. Observe for dysmorphic facial features that may be suggestive of congenital conditions that include neurologic problems (e.g., low-set ears or port-wine stain).

The cranial nerves are not routinely tested, but observations made during the physical examination provide an indirect evaluation (Table 22-8).

Observe the infant's spontaneous activity for symmetry and smoothness of movement (Fig. 22-26). Coordinated sucking and swallowing is also a function of the cerebellum. Hands are usually held in fists for the first 3 months of life, but not constantly. After 3 months the hands begin to open for longer periods. Purposeful movement (e.g., reaching and grasping for objects) begins at about 2 months of age. The infant progresses to taking objects with one hand at 6 months, transferring objects hand to hand at 7 months, and purposefully releasing objects by 10 months of age. No tremors or constant overshooting of movements is expected. See Clinical Pearl, "Infant Development—Rolling Over."

FIGURE 22-25 A, Decorticate or flexor posture. The upper arms are held tightly to the sides of the body. The elbows, wrists, and fingers are flexed, and the feet are plantar flexed. The legs are extended and internally rotated. Fine tremors or intense stiffness may be present. **B,** Decerebrate or extensor posture. The arms are fully extended with forearms pronated. The wrists and fingers are flexed, the jaw is clenched. The neck is extended and the back may be arched. The feet are plantar flexed.

Table 22-8 Indirect Cranial Nerve Evaluation in Newborns and Infants*

Cranial Nerves (CN)	Procedures and Observations
CN II, III, IV, and VI	Optical blink reflex: shine a light at the infant's open eyes; *observe the quick closure of the eyes and dorsal flexion of the infant's head;* no response may indicate poor light perception *Gazes intensely at close object or face* *Focuses on and tracks an object with both eyes* Doll's eye maneuver: (see CN VIII)
CN V	Rooting reflex: touch one corner of the infant's mouth; the infant should open its mouth and turn its head in the direction of stimulation; if the infant has been fed *recently*, minimal or no response is expected (see Table 22-9) Sucking reflex: place your finger in the infant's mouth, feeling the sucking action; *the tongue should push up against your finger with good strength;* note the pressure, strength, and pattern of sucking
CN VII	Observe the infant's facial expression when crying; *note the infant's ability to wrinkle the forehead and the symmetry of the smile*
CN VIII	Acoustic blink reflex: loudly clap your hands about 30 cm from the infant's head; avoid producing an air current; *note the blink in response to the sound;* no response after 2 to 3 days of age may indicate hearing problems; infant will habituate to repeated testing *Moves eyes in direction of sound; freezes position with high-pitched sound* Doll's eye maneuver: hold the infant under the axilla in an upright position, head held steady, facing you; rotate the infant first in one direction and then in the other; *the infant's eyes should turn in the direction of rotation and then the opposite direction when rotation stops;* if the eyes do not move in the expected direction, suspect a vestibular problem or eye muscle paralysis
CN IX and X	*Swallowing and gag reflex*
CN XII	*Coordinated sucking and swallowing ability* Pinch infant's nose; *mouth will open and tip of tongue will rise in a midline position*

*Italics indicate expected findings.

Clinical Pearl

Infant Development—Rolling Over

The age at which infants independently roll over has changed because infants now sleep on their back (to reduce the risk of sudden infant death syndrome). Supervised tummy time (infant play in the prone position) helps to stimulate their gross motor development.

A withdrawal of all limbs from a painful stimulus provides a measure of sensory integrity. Other sensory function is not routinely tested.

The patellar tendon reflexes are present at birth, and the Achilles and brachioradial tendon reflexes appear at 6 months of age. When deep tendon reflexes are tested the examiner can use a finger or stethoscope head, rather than the reflex hammer, to

EXAMINATION AND FINDINGS

FIGURE 22-26 Observe purposeful movement such as reaching for the block.

tap the tendon. In each case, expect the muscle attached to the tendon struck to contract. Interpret findings as for adults; however, one or two beats of ankle clonus is common. Infants with sustained ankle clonus should be assessed for neurologic conditions.

The plantar reflex is routinely performed as described in the adult examination on p. 563. A positive Babinski sign, fanning of the toes and dorsiflexion of the great toe, is expected until the infant is 16 to 24 months of age.

The posture and movement of the developing infant are routinely evaluated by the primitive reflexes (Table 22-9). The primitive reflexes appear and disappear in a sequence corresponding with central nervous system development. Symmetry and smoothness of response are important observations. During the assessment observe the posture and movement for any rhythmic twitching of the facial, extremity, and trunk musculature, and for any sustained asymmetric posturing. These signs, especially in paroxysmal episodes, are associated with seizure activity.

Table 22-9   Primitive Reflexes Routinely Evaluated in Infants

Reflex (Appearance)	Procedure and Findings*
Rooting reflex	Touch the corner of the infant's mouth; *when hungry the infant will move the head and open the mouth on the side of stimulation*; present at birth and disappears by 3 to 4 months of age
Palmar grasp (birth)	Making sure the infant's head is in midline, touch the palm of the infant's hand from the ulnar side (opposite the thumb); *note the strong grasp of your finger; sucking facilitates the grasp*; it should be strongest between 1 and 2 months of age and disappear by 3 months.
Plantar grasp (birth)	Touch the plantar surface of the infant's feet at the base of the toes; *the toes should curl downward*; the reflex should be strong up to 8 months of age.
Moro (birth)	With the infant supported in semisitting position, allow the head and trunk to drop back to a 30-degree angle; observe *symmetric abduction and extension of the arms; fingers fan out and thumb and index finger form a C; the arms then adduct in an embracing motion followed by relaxed flexion; the legs may follow a similar pattern of response*; the reflex diminishes in strength by 3 to 4 months and disappears by 6 months.

Table 22-9 Primitive Reflexes Routinely Evaluated in Infants—cont'd

Reflex (Appearance)	Procedure and Findings*
Placing (4 days of age)	Hold the infant upright under the arms next to a table or chair; touch the dorsal side of the foot to the table or chair edge; *observe flexion of the hips and knees and lifting of the foot as if stepping up on the table;* age of disappearance varies
Stepping (between birth and 8 weeks) 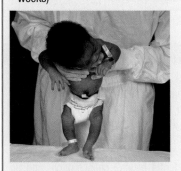	Hold the infant upright under the arms and allow the soles of the feet to touch the surface of the table; *observe for alternate flexion and extension of the legs, simulating walking;* it disappears before voluntary walking.
Asymmetric tonic neck or "fencing" (by 2 to 3 months)	With the infant lying supine and relaxed or sleeping, turn his or her head to one side so the jaw is over the shoulder; observe for *extension of the arm and leg on the side to which the head is turned and for flexion of the opposite arm and leg;* turn the infant's head to the other side, observing the reversal of the extremities' posture; this reflex diminishes at 3 to 4 months of age and disappears by 6 months; be concerned if the infant never exhibits the reflex or seems locked in the fencing position; this reflex must disappear before the infant can roll over or bring the hands to the face.

*Italics indicate expected findings.

Muscle strength and tone are especially important to evaluate in the newborn and infant (see Chapter 21). The newborn's neuromuscular development at the time of birth should be evaluated with the Ballard Clinical Assessment for gestational age (see ⓔ for the Ballard Clinical Assessment).

⚘ Children

Perform the neurologic examination of the young child by observing the neuromuscular developmental progress and skills displayed during the visit. Delay in sitting and walking may be a sign of a cerebellar disorder. Developmental screening tests (e.g., a standardized parent questionnaire) are useful tools to determine if the child is developing as expected with fine and gross motor skills, language, and personal–social skills.

Direct examination of cranial nerves is modified for the age of the child. Often a game is played to elicit the response. Table 22-10 describes these procedures.

Observe the young child at play, noting gait and fine motor coordination. The child beginning to walk has a wide-based gait. The older child walks with feet closer together, has better balance, and recovers more easily when unbalanced. Observe the child's skill in reaching for, grasping, and releasing toys. Expect no tremors or constant overshooting movements.

Heel-to-toe walking, hopping, and jumping are all coordination skills that develop in the young child. Ask the child to show how well they perform each skill, making this a game for the child.

Many of the techniques used in the adult neurologic examination are used for children, with some modifications for the child's level of understanding. Deep tendon reflexes are not always tested in a child who demonstrates appropriate development. When reflexes are tested, use the same techniques described for adults; responses should be the same. Your index finger may take the place of a reflex hammer and be less threatening to a child.

Table 22-10   Cranial Nerve Examination Procedures for Young Children

Cranial Nerves (CN)	Procedures and Observations
CN II	If the child cooperates, the Snellen E, HOTV, or Picture Chart may be used to test vision. Visual fields may be tested, but the child may need the head immobilized.
CN III, IV, and VI	Have the child follow an object with the eyes, immobilizing the head if necessary. Move the object through the cardinal points of gaze to test extraocular muscle movement.
CN V	Observe the child chewing a cookie or cracker, noting bilateral jaw strength. Touch the child's forehead and cheeks with cotton or string and watch the child bat it away.
CN VII	Observe the child's face when smiling, frowning, and crying. Ask the child to show his or her teeth. Demonstrate puffed cheeks and ask the child to imitate.
CN VIII	Observe the child turn to sounds such as a bell or whisper. Whisper a commonly used word behind the child's back and have him or her repeat the word. Perform audiometric testing.
CN IX and X	Elicit gag reflex.
CN XI and XII	Instruct older child to stick out the tongue and shrug the shoulders or raise the arms.

Evaluate light touch sensation by asking the child to close his or her eyes and point to where you touch or tickle. Alternatively, have the child discriminate between hard and soft textures. Use the tuning fork to evaluate vibration sensation, asking the child to point to the area where the buzzing sensation is felt. Superficial pain sensation is not routinely tested in young children because of their fear of pain.

When checking cortical sensory integration, use figures (e.g., circle, square, triangle) rather than numbers to evaluate graphesthesia. Draw each figure twice and ask the child if the figures are the same or different. (Make sure the child understands the terms *same* and *different*.) Practice once with the child's eyes open to improve response.

❀ Pregnant Women

Examination of the pregnant woman is the same as for the adult. Assessment of deep tendon reflexes during the initial examination can serve as a baseline evaluation.

❀ Older Adults

Examination of the neurologic system of the older adult is identical to that of the adult. You may need to allow more time for performing maneuvers that require coordination and movement. Assessing functional status is essential in determining the impact of any illness on the patient.

Medications can impair central nervous system function and cause slowed reaction time, tremors (rhythmic, oscillating, involuntary purposeless movements), and anxiety. Problems may develop because of the dosage, number, or interaction of prescription or nonprescription medications.

The older adult may have diminished smell and taste sensation. Decrease in salty taste acuity is a consistent finding associated with aging (Stewart-Knox et al, 2008). Other common cranial nerve changes include a reduced ability to differentiate colors, reduced upward gaze, slower adjustment to lighting changes, decreased corneal reflex, mid- to high-frequency hearing loss, and a reduced gag reflex (Duthie et al, 2007).

Staying Well

Stroke Prevention

Stroke is a leading cause of death and adult disability. Management of risk factors has been found to reduce the occurrence of a first stroke. Lifestyle modifications that can reduce the risk for stroke include weight reduction, adherence to a diet that is low-fat, low-sodium, and rich in fruits, vegetables, and dairy products, 30 minutes of aerobic exercise daily, moderate alcohol consumption, and no smoking. Treatment of medical conditions such as hypertension, atrial fibrillation, heart disease, diabetes mellitus, hyperlipidemia, and carotid artery stenosis can also reduce the risk for stroke (American Heart Association and American Stroke Association, 2011).

Gait with advancing age is characterized by shorter steps with less lifting of the feet as proprioception declines. Shuffling may occur as speed, balance, and grace decrease with age. Arms are more flexed, and legs may be flexed at the hips and knees (Fig. 22-27). A simple screening test of balance, strength, and cerebellar function includes asking the patient to do the following maneuvers: arising from a chair without using his or her arms, walking normally, standing with the feet together, first with the eyes open and then closed, supporting body weight, first on the heels and then the toes, and then sitting back down (Duthie et al, 2007). See the Functional Assessment box for the Tinetti Balance and Gait Assessment Tool, which can be used for any older adult thought to be at risk for falls or for people who have difficulty performing daily activities (e.g., rising from a chair or performing a task that involves unsupported standing). This tool is useful to monitor changes over time.

Check for fine motor abilities by observing the patient undress and dress without assistance. Tactile and vibratory sensation, as well as position sense, may be reduced in the older adult. These patients may need stronger stimuli to detect sensation.

Changes in deep tendon reflexes occur with aging. The older adult usually has less brisk or even absent reflexes, with response diminishing in the lower extremities before the upper extremities are affected. The Achilles and plantar reflexes may be absent or difficult to elicit in some older adults. The superficial reflexes may also disappear. There is typically an increase in benign essential tremor with aging. Fine motor coordination and agility may be impaired.

FIGURE 22-27 Short, uncertain steps are characteristic of gait with advancing age.

Sample Documentation

History and Physical Examination

Subjective

A 48-year-old man presents for his annual physical examination. No concerns about poor balance, loss of sensation, unsteady gait. History of diabetes mellitus type 1 for 30 years, well-controlled.

Objective

Cranial nerves II to XII grossly intact. Gait is coordinated and even. Romberg negative. Rapid alternating movements are coordinated and smooth. Superficial touch, pain, and vibratory sensation are intact bilaterally in all extremities. Deep tendon reflexes 2+ bilaterally in all extremities. Plantar reflex negative bilaterally. No ankle clonus. Monofilament test reveals decreased sensation on plantar and dorsal surfaces of both feet.

For additional sample documentation, see Chapter 26, pp. 628-631.

Audio: Conducting a Physical Examination of the Neurologic System

FUNCTIONAL ASSESSMENT

Tinetti Balance and Gait Assessment Tool

Balance Tests

Eight positions and position changes are evaluated.

Instructions: The patient is seated in a hard, armless chair. The following maneuvers are tested.

1. Sitting balance	Leans or slides in chair	= 0
	Steady, safe	= 1 _____
2. Arises (ask patient to rise without using arms)	Unable without help	= 0
	Able, uses arms to help	= 1
	Able without using arms	= 2 _____
3. Attempts to arise	Unable without help	= 0
	Able, requires more than one attempt	= 1
	Able to arise, one attempt	= 2 _____
4. Immediate standing balance (first 5 seconds)	Unsteady (swaggers, moves feet, trunk sways)	= 0
	Steady but uses walker or other support	= 1
	Steady without walker or other support	= 2 _____
5. Standing balance (once stance balances)	Unsteady	= 0
	Steady but wide stance (medial heels more than 4 inches apart) or uses cane or other support	= 1
	Narrow stance without support	= 2 _____
6. Nudged (subject at maximum position with feet as close together as possible, examiner pushes lightly on subject's sternum with palm of hand three times)	Begins to fall	= 0
	Staggers, grabs, catches self	= 1
	Steady	= 2 _____
7. Eyes closed (at maximum position, as in 6)	Unsteady	= 0
	Steady	= 1 _____
8. Turning 360 degrees	Discontinuous steps	= 0
	Continuous steps	= 1 _____
	Unsteady (grabs, staggers)	= 0
	Steady	= 1 _____

Continued

FUNCTIONAL ASSESSMENT—cont'd

Tinetti Balance and Gait Assessment Tool

9. Sitting down	Unsafe (misjudges distance, falls into chair)	= 0
	Uses arm or not a smooth motion	= 1
	Safe, smooth motion	= 2 _____

Balance Score: _____ of 16

Gait Tests

Eight components of gait are observed.

Initial instructions: The patient stands with examiner, walks down hallway or across room for at least 10 feet, first at "usual" pace, then back at "rapid but safe" pace (using usual walking aids).

1. Initiation of gait (immediately after being told "go")	Any hesitancy or multiple attempts to start	= 0
	No hesitancy	= 1 _____
2. Step length and height	Right swing foot does not pass left foot with stance	= 0
	Passes left stance foot	= 1 _____
	Right foot does not clear floor completely with step	= 0
	Right foot completely clears floor	= 1 _____
	Left swing foot does not pass right stance foot with step	= 0
	Passes right stance foot	= 1 _____
	Left foot does not clear floor completely with step	= 0
	Left foot completely clears floor	= 1 _____
3. Step symmetry	Right and left step length not equal (estimate)	= 0
	Right and left step length appear equal	= 1 _____
4. Step continuity	Stopping or discontinuity between steps	= 0
	Steps appear continuous	= 1 _____
5. Path (estimated in relation to floor tiles, 12 inches square; observe excursion of one of the subject's feet over about 10 feet of the course)	Marked deviation	= 0
	Mild/moderate deviation or uses walking aid	= 1
	Straight without walking aid	= 2 _____
6. Trunk	Marked sway or uses walking aid	= 0
	No sway, but flexion of knees or back, or spreads arms out	= 1 while walking
	No sway, no flexion, no use of arms, and no use of walking aid	= 2 _____
7. Walking stance	Heels apart	= 0
	Heels almost touching while walking	= 1 _____

Gait Score: _____ of 12

Balance and Gait Score: _____ of 28

- A score below 19 indicates a high risk for falls. A score of 19 to 24 suggests there is a greater chance of falls, but not a high risk.

From Tinetti, 1986.

ABNORMALITIES

Disorders of the central and peripheral nervous systems often fall into groups. A *static* problem may develop at any age and not get better or worse, even though the clinical manifestation may change with time (e.g., cerebral palsy). An individual may have been well until function is lost with a *degenerative* condition (e.g., muscular dystrophy), and it progressively worsens. Some problems are *intermittent* (e.g., seizures), and others are *genetic* (e.g., Huntington chorea), or related to a *metabolic disorder* (vitamin B_{12} deficiency).

NEUROLOGIC SYSTEM

DISORDERS OF THE CENTRAL NERVOUS SYSTEM

Multiple Sclerosis (MS)

A progressive autoimmune disorder characterized by a combination of inflammation and degeneration of the myelin of the brain's white matter, leading to decreased brain mass and obstructed transmission of nerve impulses

Pathophysiology	Subjective Data	Objective Data
• Infectious agents are believed to play a role in triggering MS in susceptible individuals. • Gradual, but unpredictable, progression, with or without remissions; symptom onset between 20 and 40 years of age, and women are affected twice as often as men	• Fatigue • Urinary frequency, urgency, or hesitancy • Sexual dysfunction • Vertigo, weakness, numbness • Blurred vision, diplopia, loss of vision • Emotional changes • Relapse symptoms develop rapidly over hours or days, and symptoms take weeks to recede.	• Muscle weakness, ataxia • Hyperactive deep tendon reflexes • Paresthesia, sensory loss, such as loss of vibration sense • Intention tremor • Optic neuritis • Cognitive changes • Magnetic resonance imaging (MRI) reveals brain lesions that are typically periventricular, ovoid, and perpendicular to the ventricles; spinal cord lesions may also be found.

Seizure Disorder (Epilepsy)

A chronic disorder characterized by recurrent, unprovoked seizures secondary to an underlying brain abnormality

Pathophysiology	Subjective Data	Objective Data
• Episodic abnormal electrical discharges (excessive concurrent firing) of cerebral neurons may be caused by a central nervous system (CNS) disorder, a CNS structural defect, or a disorder that affects functioning of the CNS; examples include brain injury, toxins, stroke, brain tumor, and hypoxic syndromes.	• History of prior seizure • Premonition or aura (headache, mood change, anxiety, irritability, lethargy, changes in appetite, dizziness, and lightheadedness) • Body is stiff and rigid, followed by rhythmic jerking movements. • Eyes roll upward. • Drooling • Loss of bladder or bowel control	• Tonic phase: brief flexion and characteristic cry with contraction of abdominal muscles, followed by generalized extension for 10 to 15 minutes; loss of consciousness for 1 to 2 minutes, eyes deviated upward, and dilated pupils • Clonic phase: contractions alternate with muscle relaxation • Postictal state: coma followed by confusion and lethargy • Common EEG findings of spikes and waves

Encephalitis

Acute inflammation of the brain and spinal cord involving the meninges, often due to a virus

Pathophysiology	Subjective Data	Objective Data
• A virus may be transmitted by the bite of an arthropod or mosquito, such as with West Nile virus, Eastern equine encephalitis, and Japanese encephalitis. Herpes simplex virus may be another cause.	• Mild viral illness with fever • Recovery and quiet stage followed by onset of lethargy, restlessness, and mental confusion	• Altered mental status, confusion, stupor, coma • Photophobia • Stiff neck • Muscle weakness, paralysis, ataxia

ABNORMALITIES

Meningitis

An inflammatory process in the meninges, the membrane around the brain and spinal cord

Pathophysiology

- The bacterial, viral, or fungal organism often colonizes in the upper respiratory tract, invades the bloodstream, and then crosses the blood-brain barrier to infect the cerebrospinal fluid and meninges.

Subjective Data

- Fever, chills
- Headache, stiff neck
- Lethargy, malaise
- Vomiting
- Irritability
- Seizures

Objective Data

- Altered mental status, confusion
- Nuchal rigidity
- Fever
- Brudzinski and Kernig signs may be positive.
- Petechiae and purpura with meningococcal meningitis
- See the Evidence-Based Practice box on p. 566.
- Lumbar puncture and cerebrospinal fluid culture confirm the diagnosis.

Intracranial Tumor

An abnormal growth within the cranial cavity that may be a primary or metastatic cancer

Pathophysiology

- The lesion causes displacement of tissue and pressure, affecting cerebrospinal fluid circulation; function is threatened through compression and destruction of tissues
- The incidence of primary brain tumors peaks between 65 and 79 years (Chandana et al, 2008).

Subjective Data

- Persistent headache, may awaken patient from sleep
- Nausea, early morning vomiting
- Unsteady gait, impaired coordination
- Memory loss and confusion
- Reduced vision acuity or visual loss
- Behavior or personality change
- Seizure
- Other symptoms in children may include irritability, lethargy, weight loss, growth failure, and precocious puberty (Wilne et al, 2007).

Objective Data

- Signs may vary by location of tumor.
- Altered consciousness, confusion
- Papilledema
- Cranial nerve impairment
- Aphasia, language disorder
- Vision loss—hemianopia, nystagmus
- Gait disturbances, ataxia
- Brain imaging by computed tomography (CT) scan or MRI confirms the diagnosis.

Pseudotumor Cerebri

A clinical syndrome of intracranial hypertension that mimics brain tumors

Pathophysiology

- Cause is unknown, but one theory is that an impaired venous outflow leads to increased cerebral blood volume; may be idiopathic (Degnan and Levy, 2011)
- Other potential causes include metabolic disorders, infections, medications (including oral contraceptives and acne medications), hematologic disorders, and brain injury.
- Most common in obese women ages 20 to 44 years; can occur in children (Wall, 2010)

Subjective Data

- Severe daily headache, throbbing, may awaken patient
- Pain behind the eye
- Vomiting
- Short episodes of blurred vision, double vision
- Whooshing sound in ears

Objective Data

- Papilledema
- Inferior nasal vision field defect
- Decreased visual acuity
- Alert, unimpaired consciousness
- Absence of focal neurologic signs
- CT scan or MRI reveals no cause of increased intracranial pressure.

Stroke (Brain Attack or Cerebrovascular Accident)

The sudden interruption of blood supply to a part of the brain or the rupture of a blood vessel, spilling blood into spaces around brain cells

Pathophysiology

- Ischemic strokes (most common cause) occur when a thrombus or embolism interrupts the blood supply, oxygen, and nutrients to the brain, and brain cells die (Fig. 22-28).
- Intracerebral or subarachnoid bleeding causes about 15% of hemorrhagic strokes, often within the distribution of the anterior circulation of the brain (Caulfield and Wijman, 2008); brain cells die due to the bleeding into or around the brain.

Subjective Data

- Sudden numbness or weakness, especially on one side of the body
- Sudden confusion or trouble speaking or understanding speech
- Sudden trouble seeing in one or both eyes
- Sudden trouble with walking, dizziness, or loss of balance or coordination
- Sudden severe headache with no known cause

Objective Data

- Signs vary by part of the brain affected; see Differential Diagnosis table below.
- Elevated blood pressure
- Altered level of consciousness
- Difficulty managing secretions
- Weakness or paralysis of extremities or facial muscles on one or both sides of the body
- Aphasia, receptive or expressive
- Articulation impairment
- Impaired horizontal gaze or hemianopia
- Brain imaging with CT and MRI diagnose the type of stroke.

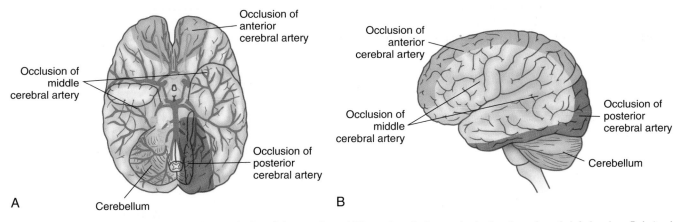

FIGURE 22-28 **Areas of the brain affected by occlusion of the anterior, middle, and posterior cerebral artery branches. A,** Inferior view. **B,** Lateral view. *(Modified from Rudy, 1984.)*

DIFFERENTIAL DIAGNOSIS

Neurologic Signs Associated with Stroke by Artery Affected

Artery Affected	Neurologic Signs
Internal Carotid Artery	
Supplies the cerebral hemispheres and diencephalon by the ophthalmic and ipsilateral hemisphere arteries	Unilateral blindness Severe contralateral hemiplegia and hemianesthesia Profound aphasia
Middle Cerebral Artery	
Supplies frontal lobe, parietal lobe, cortical surfaces of temporal lobe (affecting structures of higher cerebral processes of communication; language interpretation; perception and interpretation of space, sensation, form, and voluntary movement)	Alterations in communication, cognition, mobility, and sensation Contralateral homonymous hemianopia (see Chapter 11) Contralateral hemiplegia or hemiparesis, motor and sensory loss, greater in face and arm than the leg
Anterior Cerebral Artery	
Supplies superior surfaces of frontal and parietal lobes and medial surface of cerebral hemispheres (includes motor and somesthetic cortex serving the legs), basal ganglia, corpus callosum	Emotional lability Confusion, amnesia, personality changes Urinary incontinence Contralateral hemiplegia or hemiparesis, greater in lower than upper extremities
Posterior Cerebral Artery	
Supplies medial and inferior temporal lobes, medial occipital lobe, thalamus, posterior hypothalamus, and visual receptive area	Hemianesthesia Contralateral hemiplegia, greater in face and upper extremities than in lower extremities, cerebellar ataxia, tremor Visual loss—homonymous hemianopia, cortical blindness Receptive aphasia Memory deficits
Vertebral or Basilar Arteries	
Supply the brainstem and cerebellum	Transient ischemic attacks
Incomplete occlusion	Unilateral and bilateral weakness of extremities; upper motor neuron weakness involving face, tongue, and throat; loss of vibratory sense, two-point discrimination, and position sense Diplopia, homonymous hemianopia Nausea, vertigo, tinnitus, and syncope Dysphagia Dysarthria Sometimes confusion and drowsiness

Continued

ABNORMALITIES

DIFFERENTIAL DIAGNOSIS—cont'd

Neurologic Signs Associated with Stroke by Artery Affected

Artery Affected	Neurologic Signs
Anterior portion of pons	"Locked-in" syndrome—no movement except eyelids; sensation and consciousness preserved
Complete occlusion or hemorrhage	Coma Miotic pupils Decerebrate rigidity Respiratory and circulatory abnormalities Death
Posterior Inferior Cerebellar Artery Supplies the lateral and posterior portion of the medulla	Wallenberg syndrome (swallowing difficulty, hoarseness, dizziness, nausea and vomiting, nystagmus, and problems with balance and gait coordination) Ipsilateral anesthesia of face and cornea for pain and temperature (touch preserved) Ipsilateral Horner syndrome (see Chapter 11) Contralateral loss of pain and temperature sensation in trunk and extremities Ipsilateral decompensation of movement
Anterior Inferior and Superior Cerebellar Arteries Supply the cerebellum	Difficulty in articulation, swallowing, gross movements of limbs; nystagmus
Anterior Spinal Artery Supplies the anterior spinal cord	Flaccid paralysis, below level of lesion Loss of pain, touch, temperature sensation (proprioception preserved)
Posterior Spinal Artery Supplies the posterior spinal cord	Sensory loss, particularly proprioception, vibration, touch, and pressure (movement preserved)

DISORDERS OF THE PERIPHERAL NERVOUS SYSTEM

Myasthenia Gravis

An autoimmune disorder of neuromuscular junction involved with muscle activation; autoantibodies directed against the acetylcholine receptors in the neuromuscular junction cause destruction and inflammatory changes in the postsynaptic membranes that lead to muscle dysfunction.

Pathophysiology
- The acetylcholine receptor sites stop transmitting nerve impulses across the neuromuscular junction to direct muscle contraction.
- Confined to ocular muscles in 15% of cases

Subjective Data
- Drooping eyelids
- Double vision
- Difficulty swallowing or speaking
- Fluctuating fatigue or weakness (worse with exercise, improves with rest)
- Inability to work with arms raised above head
- Difficulty walking
- Symptoms are worse later in the day and improve with rest.

Objective Data
- Ptosis that develops within 2 minutes of upward gaze
- Facial weakness when puffing out cheeks
- Hypophonia
- Difficulty managing secretions
- Respiratory compromise or failure
- Weakness of skeletal muscles without reflex, sensory, or coordination abnormalities

Guillain-Barré Syndrome

A postinfectious disorder following a nonspecific gastrointestinal or respiratory infection that causes an acute neuromuscular paralysis

Pathophysiology
- An unusual immune response damages the peripheral nerves
- Results in impaired conduction of nerve impulses between the nodes of Ranvier
- Not associated with an autoimmune or other systemic disorder

Subjective Data
- History of recent illness and recovery
- Progressive weakness, more in the legs than the arms, increased difficulty walking
- Paresthesia
- Pain in the shoulder, back, or posterior thigh
- Double vision

Objective Data
- Distal weakness, usually bilateral and symmetric, and diminished reflexes in ascending pattern
- Ataxia, progressing to flaccid paralysis
- Facial nerve weakness (Bell palsy), diplopia
- Dysphagia, difficulty handling secretions
- Respiratory distress
- Lumbar puncture reveals increased protein in cerebrospinal fluid.

Trigeminal Neuralgia (Tic Douloureux)

Recurrent paroxysmal sharp pain that radiates into one or more branches of the fifth cranial nerve

Pathophysiology
- May be caused by a small artery that chronically compresses the fifth cranial nerve and wears away the nerve's myelin or by irritation of the nerve's afferent portion
- Usual age of onset is 40 to 60 years; women are more commonly affected than men

Subjective Data
- Sharp pain episode on one side of the face that lasts seconds to minutes; pain may rarely be bilateral
- Potential pain triggers are chewing, swallowing, talking, washing the face, brushing the teeth, exposure to cold, and even a breeze across the face.
- Episodes may occur several times a day to several times a month followed by a pain-free period.

Objective Data
- May be normal neurologic findings
- May have slight sensory impairment in the regions of pain
- Pain occurs in the distribution of one or more divisions of the facial nerve.

Bell Palsy

A temporary acute paralysis or weakness of one side of the face

Pathophysiology
- May be caused by an acute inflammation of the facial nerve (cranial nerve VII), such as a viral infection with herpes simplex, which leads to ischemia and demyelination
- Other potential causes include central nervous system lesions (e.g., multiple sclerosis, stroke, or tumor) or structural lesions in the ear or parotid gland.
- Occurs more commonly in patients with diabetes mellitus (Tiemstra and Khatkhate, 2007)

Subjective Data
- Rapidly progressive muscle weakness on one side of face (over 2 to 3 days)
- Feeling of facial numbness (Fig. 22-29)

Objective Data
- Facial creases and nasolabial fold disappear on affected side
- Eyelid will not close on affected side and lower lid sags; leads to eye irritation; eye may tear excessively
- Food and saliva may pool in affected side of mouth
- Facial sensation is intact.

FIGURE 22-29 Characteristic features of Bell palsy. (From Forbes, 2003.)

ABNORMALITIES

Peripheral Neuropathy

A disorder of the peripheral nervous system that results in motor and sensory loss in the distribution of one or more nerves, commonly caused by diabetes mellitus

Pathophysiology	Subjective Data	Objective Data
• Other causes include altered lipid metabolism, vitamin B_{12} or folate deficiency; neuropathy associated with Lyme disease, HIV infection, and diabetic polyneuropathy are believed to have an autoimmune etiology (Vinik et al, 2008). • Impaired blood flow, vasoconstriction, and chronic ischemic changes within the peripheral neuronal fibers lead to the sensory and autonomic nerve function deficits.	• Gradual onset of numbness, tingling, burning, and cramping, most commonly in the hands and feet • Night pain in one or both feet • Early signs may be unusual sensations of walking on cotton, floors feeling strange, or inability to distinguish between coins by feel. • Sensation of burning accompanied by hyperalgesia and allodynia (all sensation is painful)	• Reduced sensation in the foot with the monofilament; loss of pain or sharp touch sensation to the mid-calf level • Distal pulses may be present or diminished. • Diminished or absent ankle and knee reflexes • Decreased or no vibratory sensation below the knees; temperature sensation may be less impaired. • Distal muscle weakness, inability to stand on toes or heels • Skin ulceration or injuries to extremities the patient does not feel

✤ Children

Cerebral Palsy (CP)

A group of permanent disorders of movement and posture development associated with nonprogressive (static) disturbances that occurred in the developing fetal or infant brain

Pathophysiology	Subjective Data	Objective Data
• Major lesions contributing to CP include intracerebral hemorrhage and injury to the immature periventricular white matter in the fetus or premature infant (Johnston, 2011). • Other causes are abnormal brain development of the fetus, intrauterine exposure to maternal infection, kernicterus, and genetic factors (Johnston, 2011). • The incidence is 3.6 per 1000 live births with more males than females affected (Johnston, 2011).	• Delays in gross motor development that become more obvious as the infant ages • Activity limitation, stiff joints and positioning • May have hearing, speech, and language disorders • Feeding difficulties, poor sucking and swallowing coordination • Seizures	• Cognitive impairment or learning disabilities may be present • Spastic CP: hypertonicity, tremors, scissor gait, toe walking • Persistent primitive reflexes, exaggerated deep tendon reflexes • Dyskinetic CP: involuntary slow writhing movements of the extremities; tremors may be present. • Exaggerated posturing, inconsistent muscle tone that varies during the day • Ataxic: abnormalities of movement involving balance and position of trunk and extremities • Intention tremors, past pointing • Increased or decreased muscle tone, may have hypotonia as infant • Instability, wide-based gait

Myelomeningocele (Spina Bifida)

A congenital vertebral defect (commonly at the lumbar or sacral level) that allows spinal cord contents to protrude

Pathophysiology	Subjective Data	Objective Data
• Cause is unknown, but associated with excessive use of alcohol, medications used for seizures and acne, genetic factors, and maternal health conditions (diabetes mellitus, folic acid deficiency, and maternal obesity) • An estimated 1500 infants are born with the condition each year in the United States (Centers for Disease Control and Prevention, 2011).	• May have loss of bowel control or constipation • May have loss of bladder control (incontinence or urinary retention) • Mobility problems	• Exposed meningeal sac filled with fluid and nerves is apparent at birth (Fig. 22-30). • Sensory deficit and paralysis or weakness are dependent on level of defect (the higher the defect, the greater is the neurologic dysfunction); may not be symmetric • Rapidly increasing head circumference (hydrocephalus) • May have hip or foot abnormalities • Learning disabilities and perceptual motor skills

FIGURE 22-30 **Myelomeningocele.** *(From Zitelli and Davis, 1997.)*

Shaken Baby Syndrome

A severe form of child abuse resulting from the violent shaking of infants younger than 1 year of age

Pathophysiology	Subjective Data	Objective Data
• Shaking causes the brain to move around in the skull, stretching and tearing nerve tissue and blood vessels and causing brain damage and a subdural hematoma; the spinal cord may also be damaged as the head is whipped back and forth.	• Fever • Irritability • Lethargy • Decreased food intake • Breathing difficulty or apnea • Seizure • Loss of consciousness	• Altered level of consciousness • Seizures • Bilateral retinal hemorrhages with retinal detachments or folds (see Fig. 11-53) • Absence of visible trauma to the head; fingerprint bruises may be seen on infant's upper arms and body • Bruising, bite marks, or burns may be seen in some infants. • CT scan reveals subdural or subarachnoid hemorrhage. • Signs of old and new fractures of long bones and ribs may be seen on radiographs.

✂ Pregnant Women

Intrapartum Maternal Lumbosacral Plexopathy

A neuropathy that can occur during late pregnancy and delivery

Pathophysiology	Subjective Data	Objective Data
• Occurs when the lumbosacral trunk—and sometimes the superior gluteal and obturator nerves—is compressed between the maternal pelvic rim and the fetal head (a conduction nerve block), leading to motor deficits in a lower extremity (Wilbourne, 2007).	• Intermittent pain that radiates from the buttock into the leg during late pregnancy • Mother may be small and have prolonged labor • Pain subsides after delivery but foot drop may be present.	• Pain radiates from the buttock of the affected extremity in a lumbar 5 distribution • Unilateral foot drop that may take weeks to resolve

✂ Older Adults

Parkinson Disease

A slowly progressive, degenerative neurologic disorder in which deficiency of the dopamine neurotransmitter results in poor communication between parts of the brain that coordinate and control movement and balance

Pathophysiology	Subjective Data	Objective Data
• A history of encephalitis, drug use, or cerebrovascular disease may exist • Genetic, environmental, viral, vascular, toxic, or other factors may be associated with disease onset. • Occurs most often in patients older than 50 years	• Tremors (sometimes unilateral) occur initially at rest and with fatigue, disappearing with intended movement and sleep; progresses to pill-rolling movement of fingers bilaterally and tremor of the head • Slowing of voluntary and automatic movements • Numbness, aching, tingling, and muscle soreness occur in many patients (Fig. 22-31).	• Tremors • Muscular rigidity • Stooped posture, balance and postural instability • Short steps, shuffling, freezing gait • Difficulty swallowing, drooling, voice softening • Slow, slurred monotonous speech • Impaired cognition, dementia

FIGURE 22-31 Characteristic features of Parkinson disease. A, Excessive sweating. **B,** Drooling with excess saliva. **C,** Gait with rapid, short, shuffling steps and reduced arm swinging. *(Modified from Rudy, 1984.)*

Normal Pressure Hydrocephalus

A syndrome simulating degenerative diseases that is caused by noncommunicating hydrocephalus (dilated ventricles with intracranial pressure within expected ranges)

Pathophysiology

- May be due to a slightly elevated baseline cerebrospinal fluid (CSF) and intermittent increased CSF pressure waves (Factora and Luciano, 2006)
- May be a relationship between condition and systemic hypertension (Graff-Radford, 2007)
- Compression of brain tissue and decreased cerebral blood flow lead to signs and symptoms

Subjective Data

- Gait impairment is the first symptom.
- Unsteadiness and difficulty turning
- Forgetfulness, cognitive impairment
- Urinary frequency that progresses to urgency and incontinence over time

Objective Data

- Gait impairment, wide-based stance, short, small steps, and reduced floor clearance
- No tremor
- No sensory impairment
- Cognitive impairment, executive function impaired
- Impaired memory recall for recent events
- CT scan and MRI of the brain reveal enlarged ventricles not attributable to brain atrophy or a congenital problem.

Postpolio Syndrome (Progressive Postpoliomyelitis Muscular Atrophy)

The reappearance of neurologic signs 10 or more years after survival of acute poliomyelitis

Pathophysiology

- During recovery, damaged neurons sent out axonal links to activate muscle fibers that had neurons killed by the poliovirus; the remaining motor neurons activated many more muscle fibers than they were expected to handle; over time, the overloaded damaged neurons died, causing polio symptoms to recur.

Subjective Data

- History of paralytic or nonparalytic polio
- New-onset muscle weakness, muscle cramps
- Increased pain sensitivity
- Fatigue
- Cold intolerance
- Difficulty with swallowing or speaking
- Shortness of breath
- Difficulty sleeping

Objective Data

- Focal and asymmetric muscle weakness and atrophy
- Fasciculations
- Dysphagia, dysarthria
- Sleep apnea, hypoventilation

CHAPTER 23

Sports Participation Evaluation

Each year millions of children, youth, and young adults participate in organized sports and are required by state and local school districts to have a preparticipation physical evaluation (PPE). Rare high-profile cases of death and serious injury on the playing field, usually among college and professional athletes, keep concerns about the risks of sports participation in the public eye.

The overall goal of the PPE is to ensure safe participation in an appropriate physical activity and not to restrict participation unnecessarily. Whether athletes receive the PPE in the context of an ongoing primary care relationship or as a focused preseason checkup, the following goals of the evaluation are universal:

+ To identify conditions that may interfere with a person's ability to participate in a sport
+ To identify health problems that increase the risk of injury or death during sports participation
+ To help select an appropriate sport for a person's particular abilities and physical status

Sports and disciplined physical effort enhance fitness and coordination, increase self-esteem, and provide positive social experiences for participants, including individuals with physical and intellectual disabilities (Box 23-1). Few children and youth have conditions that might limit participation, and most of these conditions are known before the PPE takes place (see Clinical Pearls, "Atlantoaxial Instability" and "Hypertension in the Pediatric Athlete").

A PPE can be performed in many settings. Ideally the PPE occurs in the office of a regular health care provider with whom the individual has a longitudinal relationship and knows the medical and family history. The PPE is individualized and tailored to the specific needs of the particular patient. The PPE may be the only opportunity to assess an athlete's health and safety concerns including issues unrelated to sports participation. Another approach to the PPE is the *stations method*, in which a large number of patients are evaluated in a single session by multiple providers. Each provider takes responsibility for a specific aspect of the evaluation at a station dedicated to that purpose. The stations method can involve providers from a variety of disciplines such as medicine, nursing, athletic training, and physical therapy. Athletes move from one station to the next, with historical and objective information documented throughout on a standard form. A checkout station is critical to the success of this approach. The person in charge of this station reviews the data collected during the evaluation and coordinates any necessary follow-up testing or referrals, communicating directly with the athlete (and parents, if appropriate) and generating a written report. The PPE stations format is not a comprehensive service for addressing issues unrelated to sports participation. The need for patients to concurrently receive routine health maintenance care by their primary care provider should be emphasized at the checkout station.

The PPE should be completed well enough in advance of the planned sports activity so that any needed specialist evaluations, rehabilitation, or therapy can be completed before participation begins. As a general rule, 6 weeks prior to participation is an appropriate time. Primary care providers are often asked to complete a sports participation form based on a recent visit. Because the overall goal of the PPE is to ensure safe participation in sports, explain the importance of scheduling a complete PPE visit to patients and parents. Once an initial, thorough PPE has been completed, subsequent PPEs can be shorter and should focus on interim problems and concerns.

The physical examination component of the PPE should center on high-yield areas, particularly those related to sports participation and issues identified by the history. Items such as auscultation of the lung fields and otoscopy are low-yield—unless the patient is symptomatic at the time of the evaluation. Such findings can distract providers from the more important PPE cardiac and orthopedic examinations.

Recommended components of the PPE are shown in Box 23-2 and followed by the 2010 Physical Examination Form endorsed by the American Academy of Family Physicians, American Academy of Pediatrics, American College of Sports Medicine, American Medical Society for Sports Medicine, American Orthopedic Society for Sports Medicine, and the

SPORTS PARTICIPATION

| Box 23-1 | Special Olympics: Promoting Sports Participation in Individuals with Disabilities |

The Special Olympics offers an opportunity for year-round sports training and athletic competition to approximately 2.5 million individuals with intellectual disabilities (www.specialolympics.org). The official sports include aquatics, track and field, basketball, golf, gymnastics, softball, tennis, and volleyball, among others. Participants must be at least 8 years old. A preparticipation physical evaluation (PPE) is required for admission to the program.

The health care provider should not restrict participation based on a patient's intellectual disability alone. The thorough PPE outlined in this chapter should guide decisions about sports participation clearance, as it does for nondisabled patients. Past experience indicates there is some risk of eye injury in badminton, basketball, floor hockey, handball, soccer, softball, and tennis. An increased risk for those with atlantoaxial instability is associated with alpine skiing, diving, equestrian sports, gymnastics, high jump, soccer, and swimming.

The same care is due for persons seeking to join in the *Paralympic Games*, an opportunity offered by a different organizing group for athletes with a physical disability of a serious nature, such as amputation, cerebral palsy, spinal cord impairment, or visual impairment. These athletes, however, need not have intellectual disability.

Compared to nonparticipants, Special Olympics participants have demonstrated higher self-esteem and greater perceived physical competence and peer acceptance. Parents of child participants perceive better socialization skills and life satisfaction. Considering the physical, emotional, and social benefits of sports participation and physical activity, the American Academy of Pediatrics Council on Children with Disabilities urges pediatric health care providers to promote participation of children with disabilities. Clinicians should help individuals and families overcome barriers to participation and become aware of resources like Special Olympics and the National Center on Physical Activity and Disability (Murphy et al, 2008).

Clinical Pearl

Atlantoaxial Instability

Individuals with Down syndrome are at increased risk of atlantoaxial subluxation. The American Academy of Pediatrics (AAP) previously recommended routine radiologic screening of the cervical spine in asymptomatic children and adolescents. However, because radiographs do not accurately predict which children are at increased risk, the AAP no longer supports this practice (2011). Discuss spinal cord injury risk with parents of children with Down syndrome who will be participating in sports (especially football, soccer, and gymnastics). Inquire about neck or radicular pain, weakness, change in gait, and bowel or bladder function, and perform a careful neurologic examination. You may find increased deep tendon reflexes, a positive Babinski sign, and ankle clonus or a change in tone, strength, or gait. These exam findings require immediate referral to a neurosurgeon with expertise in atlantoaxial instability.

Clinical Pearl

Hypertension in the Pediatric Athlete

Hypertension is the most common cardiovascular condition seen in competitive athletes. Blood pressure measurement is particularly important during the PPE for young athletes. The diagnosis of hypertension is made when blood pressure measurements on three or more occasions are above cutoffs based on the child's gender, age, and height percentile. Stage 1 hypertension is defined as blood pressure measurements in the 95th to 99th percentile plus 5 mm Hg (or higher than 120/80 mm Hg). If the child is asymptomatic, two additional measurements should be taken in the subsequent weeks for confirmation. If the blood pressure is persistently elevated, evaluation for an etiology, comorbid conditions, and end-organ damage is warranted. Lifestyle modification and pharmacotherapy may be indicated. Stage 2 hypertension is defined as blood pressure measurements greater than the 99th percentile. In addition to the evaluation above, make an immediate referral to a pediatric cardiologist. For patients with stage 2 hypertension, temporary restriction from sports participation is based on the cardiovascular demands of a particular sporting activity and the demands of practice and/or preparation. Counsel patients with hypertension to avoid substances known to increase blood pressure (e.g., over the counter supplements, alcohol, tobacco, and highly caffeinated beverages) (American Academy of Pediatrics, 2010).

Evidence-Based Practice in Physical Examination

The Particular Value of a Careful History

The only proven benefit of the preparticipation physical evaluation (PPE) is recognition of athletes at risk for later orthopedic injury. With a careful history, recent or poorly rehabilitated injuries that can become worse with sports participation can be detected. The history provides the most information for the PPE (Bernard and Roberts, 2010). Asthma is a good example. Unless a patient is in respiratory distress when evaluated, it will not be detected during the physical examination. Sudden cardiac death on the playing field is a source of great concern, accounting for 56% to 95% of cases of sudden deaths in young athletes (Barrett, 2012). Other causes of sudden death include blunt chest and head trauma, drug abuse, asthma, heat stroke, and drowning. In a review of 1827 pediatric deaths from the U.S. National Registry of Sudden Death in Young Athletes (1980-2009), it was found that 14% were secondary to traumatic injuries of the head and/or neck (Thomas et al, 2011). Conditions leading to these uncommon events are rarely associated with detectable physical findings. They may, however, be associated with symptoms revealed by a careful medical and family history during the PPE. For adolescent-age patients, it is important to obtain the health history from both the adolescent and the parents. A history and symptom questionnaire is often used and can be very helpful in practice. This is especially important when the PPE is conducted using a station-based screening format (Womack, 2010).

American Osteopathic Academy of Sports Medicine. Many primary care providers are less comfortable with the orthopedic component of the physical examination. In 1977, Garrick developed a "2-minute" screening orthopedic examination. In conjunction with a thorough history, this 14-step musculoskeletal examination continues to be widely used in practice (Fig. 23-1) (Garrick, 2004). The examination consists of observing the athlete in a variety of positions and postures that highlight asymmetries in range of motion, strength, and muscle bulk. These asymmetries serve to identify acute or old, poorly rehabilitated

Box 23-2 | Recommended Components of the Preparticipation Physical Evaluation (PPE)*

General Medical History

- Illnesses or injuries since the last health visit or PPE
- History of having been denied or restricted from participation in sporting activities and reason for restriction
- History of heat illness or muscle cramps
- Current viral illness (patients with mononucleosis may return to play after 3 weeks if no longer symptomatic and no splenomegaly; fever at the time of the exam is an absolute contraindication due to the association with viral myocarditis)
- Sickle cell trait or disease (adequate hydration is necessary and caution should be taken to avoid extreme conditions due to risk of rhabdomyolysis)
- Hospitalizations or surgeries
- All medications used by the athlete (including steroids and nutritional supplements or medications taken to enhance performance)
- Use of any special equipment or protective devices during sports participation
- Allergies (including food-, insect bite–, and exercise-provoked allergies), particularly those associated with anaphylaxis or respiratory compromise
- Absence of paired organs (single-organ athletes may participate if the single organ can be protected and the patient/caregivers understand the risks involved)
- Immunization status, including hepatitis B, varicella, meningococcal, human papillomavirus, and pertussis
- *Height, weight, and body mass index (BMI)*
- *Palpation of lymph nodes*

Cardiac

- Symptoms of exertional chest pain/discomfort
- Unexplained syncope or near-syncope
- Excessive exertional and unexplained dyspnea/fatigue, associated with exercise
- Prior recognition of a heart murmur
- *Elevated systemic blood pressure*
- Family history of premature death (sudden and unexpected, or otherwise) before age 50 years due to heart disease in one or more relatives
- Family history of disability from heart disease in a close relative younger than 50 years
- Specific knowledge of certain cardiac conditions in family members: hypertrophic or dilated cardiomyopathy, long-QT syndrome or other ion channelopathies, Marfan syndrome, or clinically important arrhythmias
- *Heart murmur (auscultation should be performed in both supine and standing positions, or with Valsalva maneuver, to identify murmurs of dynamic left ventricular outflow obstruction); heart rate and rhythm to assess for arrhythmias*
- *Femoral pulses to exclude coarctation of the aorta*
- *Physical stigmata of Marfan syndrome (e.g., arm span greater than height and hyperextensible joints)*

- *Brachial artery blood pressure (sitting position with appropriate size cuff, preferably taken in both arms)*

Respiratory

- Coughing, wheezing, or dyspnea with exercise
- Previous use of asthma medications
- Family history of asthma
- *Lung auscultation*

Neurologic

- History of a head injury with or without symptoms of a concussion (confusion, prolonged headache, memory problems)
- Numbness or tingling in the extremities
- Headaches
- History of seizure
- History of inability to move an extremity after a collision

Vision

- Visual problems
- Glasses or contact lenses
- Previous eye injuries
- *Visual acuity*

Orthopedic

- Previous injuries that have limited sports practice or participation
- Injuries that have been associated with pain, swelling, or the need for medical intervention
- Previous fractures or dislocated joints
- Previous or current use of a brace, orthotic, or other assistive device
- *Screening orthopedic examination*

Psychosocial

- Weight control and body image
- Dietary habits, calcium intake
- Stresses in personal life, at home, or in school
- Feelings of sadness, hopelessness, depression or anxiety
- Use or abuse of recreational drugs, alcohol, tobacco, dietary or performance supplements
- *Attention to signs of eating disorders, including oral ulcerations, decreased tooth enamel, edema*

Genitourinary and Abdominal

- Age at menarche, last menstrual period, regularity of menstrual periods, number of periods in the last year, and longest interval between periods (athletic girls tend to experience menarche at a later age than nonathletic girls).
- *Palpation of the abdomen for organomegaly*
- *Palpation of the testicles*
- *Examination for inguinal hernias*

Dermatologic

- History of rashes, pressure sores, or other skin conditions
- History of boils or MRSA skin infections
- *Skin lesions suggestive of HSV, MRSA or tinea corporis*

From Andrews, 1997; Maron et al, 2007; and 2010 Preparticipation Physical Evaluation History and Physical Examination Forms endorsed by the American Academy of Family Physicians, American Academy of Pediatrics, American College of Sports Medicine, American Medical Society for Sports Medicine, American Orthopedic Society for Sports Medicine, and the American Osteopathic Academy of Sports Medicine.
*Elements of the history and physical examination organized by system. Physical examination items are shown in italics.

■ PREPARTICIPATION PHYSICAL EVALUATION
PHYSICAL EXAMINATION FORM

Name _____ Date of birth _____

PHYSICIAN REMINDERS
1. Consider additional questions on more sensitive issues
   - Do you feel stressed out or under a lot of pressure?
   - Do you ever feel sad, hopeless, depressed, or anxious?
   - Do you feel safe at your home or residence?
   - Have you ever tried cigarettes, chewing tobacco, snuff, or dip?
   - During the past 30 days, did you use chewing tobacco, snuff, or dip?
   - Do you drink alcohol or use any other drugs?
   - Have you ever taken anabolic steroids or used any other performance supplement?
   - Have you ever taken any supplements to help you gain or lose weight or improve your performance?
   - Do you wear a seat belt, use a helmet, and use condoms?
2. Consider reviewing questions on cardiovascular symptoms (questions 5–14).

EXAMINATION			
Height	Weight	□ Male □ Female	
BP / (/) Pulse	Vision R 20/	L 20/	Corrected □ Y □ N

MEDICAL	NORMAL	ABNORMAL FINDINGS
Appearance • Marfan stigmata (kyphoscoliosis, high-arched palate, pectus excavatum, arachnodactyly, arm span > height, hyperlaxity, myopia, MVP, aortic insufficiency)		
Eyes/ears/nose/throat • Pupils equal • Hearing		
Lymph nodes		
Heart[a] • Murmurs (auscultation standing, supine, +/- Valsalva) • Location of point of maximal impulse (PMI)		
Pulses • Simultaneous femoral and radial pulses		
Lungs		
Abdomen		
Genitourinary (males only)[b]		
Skin • HSV, lesions suggestive of MRSA, tinea corporis		
Neurologic[c]		
MUSCULOSKELETAL		
Neck		
Back		
Shoulder/arm		
Elbow/forearm		
Wrist/hand/fingers		
Hip/thigh		
Knee		
Leg/ankle		
Foot/toes		
Functional • Duck-walk, single leg hop		

[a]Consider ECG, echocardiogram, and referral to cardiology for abnormal cardiac history or exam.
[b]Consider GU exam if in private setting. Having third party present is recommended.
[c]Consider cognitive evaluation or baseline neuropsychiatric testing if a history of significant concussion.

□ Cleared for all sports without restriction

□ Cleared for all sports without restriction with recommendations for further evaluation or treatment for _____

□ Not cleared

    □ Pending further evaluation

    □ For any sports

    □ For certain sports _____

        Reason _____

Recommendations _____

I have examined the above-named student and completed the preparticipation physical evaluation. The athlete does not present apparent clinical contraindications to practice and participate in the sport(s) as outlined above. A copy of the physical exam is on record in my office and can be made available to the school at the request of the parents. If conditions arise after the athlete has been cleared for participation, the physician may rescind the clearance until the problem is resolved and the potential consequences are completely explained to the athlete (and parents/guardians).

Name of physician (print/type) _____ Date _____

Address _____ Phone _____

Signature of physician _____, MD or DO

Step 1: Observe the standing athlete from the front for symmetry of trunk, shoulders, and extremities.

Step 2: Observe neck flexion, extension, lateral flexion on each side, and rotation to evaluate range of motion and the cervical spine.

Step 3: Have the athlete shrug the shoulders against resistance from the examiner to evaluate trapezius strength.

Step 4: Have the athlete perform shoulder abduction against resistance from the examiner to assess deltoid strength.

Step 5: Observe internal and external rotation of the shoulder to evaluate range of motion of the glenohumeral joint.

Step 6: Observe extension and flexion of the elbow to assess range of motion.

FIGURE 23-1 The 14-step screening orthopedic examination. The athlete should be dressed so that the joints and muscle groups included in the examination are easily visible—usually gym shorts for males and gym shorts and a T-shirt for females. Keep in mind that one of the most important points to look for in the orthopedic screening examination is symmetry.

Step 7: Observe pronation and supination of the forearm to evaluate elbow and wrist range of motion.

Step 8: Have the athlete clench the fist, then spread the fingers to assess range of motion in the hand and fingers.

Step 9: Observe the standing athlete from the rear for symmetry of trunk, shoulders, and extremities.

Step 10: Have the athlete stand with the knees straight and bend backward from the waist. Discomfort with extension of the lumbar spine may be associated with spondylolysis and spondylolisthesis.

Step 11: Have the athlete stand with the knees straight and flex forward at the waist, first away from the examiner, then toward the examiner, to assess for scoliosis, spine range of motion, and hamstring flexibility.

Step 12: Have the athlete stand facing the examiner with quadriceps flexed to observe symmetry of leg musculature.

Step 13: Have the athlete duck walk four steps to assess hip, knee, and ankle range of motion, strength, and balance.

Step 14: Have the athlete stand on the toes, then the heels to evaluate calf strength, symmetry, and balance.

FIGURE 23-1, cont'd

injuries. The steps pictured in Figure 23-1 help in assessing most of the following:

* Posture and general muscle contour bilaterally
* Patient's duck walk, four steps with knees completely bent
* Spine for curvature and lumbar extension, fingers touching toes with knees straight
* Shoulder and clavicle for dislocation
* Neck, shoulders, elbows, forearms, hands, fingers, and hips for range of motion
* Knee ligaments for drawer sign
    You should also assess the following:
* Gait
* Patient's ability to hop on each foot
* Patient's ability to walk on tiptoes and heels

Once a PPE has been completed, the health care provider can guide the patient with sport selection; plan therapy or rehabilitation of conditions or injuries and, in rare instances, discuss restrictions. The clinician may: (1) provide "clearance" for participation; (2) provide "clearance" for participation with recommendations for further evaluation and/or treatment; (3) restrict participation until further testing is performed; or (4) recommend complete restriction from specific sports or all sports. Decisions are made at the discretion of the clinician, but recommendations to limit participation are not legally binding.

Patients with findings from the PPE may require evaluation by a health care provider with appropriate knowledge and experience to assess the safety of a given sport for the athlete. This is because of the variability of the severity of the disease, the risk of injury among the specific sports in Table 23-1, or both. Box 23-3 discusses guidelines for patients who have experienced a concussion. Two conditions considered absolute contraindications to sports participation are carditis and fever. Carditis (inflammation of the heart) can result in sudden death with exertion, and fever is associated with an increased risk of heat-related illness (Rice, 2008). A good rule: Do not suggest that an athlete "play through" an injury or a problem.

Table 23-1	Classification of Sports According to Contact	
Contact	**Limited-Contact**	**Noncontact**
Basketball	Adventure-racing*	Badminton
Boxing†	Baseball	Bodybuilding‡
Cheerleading	Bicycling	Bowling
Diving	Canoeing or kayaking	Canoeing or kayaking
Extreme sports§	(white water)	(flat water)
Field hockey	Fencing	Crew or rowing
Football, tackle	Field events	Curling
Gymnastics	High jump	Dance
Ice hockey‖	Pole vault	Field events
Lacrosse	Floor hockey	Discus
Martial arts¶	Football, flag or touch	Javelin
Rodeo	Handball	Shot-put
Rugby	Horseback riding	Golf
Skiing, downhill	Martial arts¶	Orienteering#
Ski jumping	Racquetball	Power lifting‡
Snowboarding	Skating	Race walking
Soccer	Ice	Riflery
Team handball	In-line	Rope jumping
Ultimate Frisbee	Roller	Running
Water polo	Skiing	Sailing
Wrestling	Cross-country	Scuba diving
	Water	Swimming
	Skateboarding	Table tennis
	Softball	Tennis
	Squash	Track
	Volleyball	
	Weight lifting	
	Windsurfing or surfing	

From Rice, 2008.

*Adventure-racing has been added since the previous statement was published and is defined as a combination of 2 or more disciplines, including orienteering and navigation, cross-country running, mountain biking, paddling, and climbing and rope skills (AAP, 2001).

†The American Academy of Pediatrics opposes participation in boxing for children, adolescents, and young adults (AAP, 1997).

‡The American Academy of Pediatrics recommends limiting bodybuilding and power lifting until the adolescent achieves sexual rating 5 (Tanner stage V).

§Extreme sports has been added since the previous statement was published.

‖The American Academy of Pediatrics recommends limiting the amount of body checking allowed for hockey players 15 years and younger to reduce injuries.

¶Martial arts can be subclassified as judo, jujitsu, karate, kung fu, and tae kwon do; some forms are contact sports and others are limited-contact sports.

#Orienteering is a race (contest) in which competitors use a map and a compass to find their way through unfamiliar territory.

SPORTS PARTICIPATION

Box 23-3   Sports-Related Concussions

The Centers for Disease Control and Prevention (CDC) estimates that in the United States more than 200,000 patients are treated each year in emergency departments (ED) for concussions and other sports-related traumatic brain injury (TBI) (MMWR, 2011). Sports associated with the greatest number of TBI-related ED visits include football, basketball, soccer, bicycling, and playground activities. The CDC has a number of useful interactive online resources for health care providers, youth, parents, and coaches about recognition, management, and prevention of concussions (www.cdc.gov/concussion). Based on recommendations from the 3rd International Conference on Concussion in Sport, a concussion is defined as "a complex pathophysiological process affecting the brain, induced by traumatic biomechanical forces" (McCrory et al, 2009). The following features relate to the pathophysiologic and clinical characteristics of concussions:

1. Caused by a direct blow to the head, face, neck, or elsewhere on the body with an "impulsive" force transmitted to the head.
2. Typically results in the rapid onset of short-lived impairment of neurologic function that resolves spontaneously.
3. May result in neuropathological changes, but the acute clinical symptoms largely reflect a functional disturbance rather than structural injury
4. Results in a graded set of clinical symptoms that may or may not involve loss of consciousness. Resolution of the clinical and cognitive symptoms typically follows a sequential course with 80% to 90% resolving in 7-10 days.
5. Typically associated with grossly normal structural neuroimaging studies.

A diagnosis of a concussion involves a comprehensive assessment of the following domains: clinical symptoms, physical signs, behavior, balance, sleep, and cognition. These domains are covered in the *SCAT3* form (Fig. 23-2, on next page), which is a standardized tool for evaluating athletes 10 years and older for concussion.

A concussion evaluation should involve a medical assessment (comprehensive history and complete neurological examination), determination of clinical status (i.e., improvement or worsening since the occurrence of the injury), and determination of the need for head imaging. Management of a concussion requires physical and cognitive rest until symptoms resolve followed by a stepwise return to play program. A mental health assessment is also recommended as depressive symptoms are common in athletes.

Return to Play: In general, most patients with concussions will have symptoms that resolve soon after the injury. The following graduated return to play protocol is recommended:

1. No activity, complete physical and cognitive rest. Once asymptomatic, proceed to step 2.
2. Light aerobic exercise; walking, swimming, or stationary cycling, no resistance training
3. Sport-specific exercise without head impact activities (e.g., running drills in soccer)
4. Noncontact training drills (e.g., passing drills in football)
5. Full contact practice after medical clearance
6. Return to play (normal game play)

The patient should only proceed to the next step if he or she is asymptomatic. If symptoms occur, the patient should go back to the previous step and attempt to progress after a 24-hour period of rest. Children and adolescents with concussions may require a longer recovery period than adults. For pediatric patients, cognitive rest may include school modifications and limiting recreational activities like playing video games. Additional factors that may modify return to play recommendations for all patients include prolonged loss of consciousness (longer than 1 minute) and comorbid conditions (e.g., migraine headaches and depression). In these situations, formal neuropsychological assessment, balance assessment, and neuroimaging may be necessary. When possible, concussion management and return to play recommendations should be guided by a multidisciplinary team.

SCAT3™

FIFA®   IIHF   ⬤⬤⬤⬤⬤   iRB   FEI

Sport Concussion Assessment Tool – 3rd Edition

For use by medical professionals only

Name _____

Date/Time of Injury: _____
Date of Assessment: _____

Examiner: _____

What is the SCAT3?[1]

The SCAT3 is a standardized tool for evaluating injured athletes for concussion and can be used in athletes aged from 13 years and older. It supersedes the original SCAT and the SCAT2 published in 2005 and 2009, respectively[2]. For younger persons, ages 12 and under, please use the Child SCAT3. The SCAT3 is designed for use by medical professionals. If you are not qualified, please use the Sport Concussion Recognition Tool[1]. Preseason baseline testing with the SCAT3 can be helpful for interpreting post-injury test scores.

Specific instructions for use of the SCAT3 are provided on page 3. If you are not familiar with the SCAT3, please read through these instructions carefully. This tool may be freely copied in its current form for distribution to individuals, teams, groups and organizations. Any revision or any reproduction in a digital form requires approval by the Concussion in Sport Group.
NOTE: The diagnosis of a concussion is a clinical judgment, ideally made by a medical professional. The SCAT3 should not be used solely to make, or exclude, the diagnosis of concussion in the absence of clinical judgement. An athlete may have a concussion even if their SCAT3 is "normal".

What is a concussion?

A concussion is a disturbance in brain function caused by a direct or indirect force to the head. It results in a variety of non-specific signs and/or symptoms (some examples listed below) and most often does not involve loss of consciousness. Concussion should be suspected in the presence of **any one or more** of the following:

- Symptoms (e.g., headache), or
- Physical signs (e.g., unsteadiness), or
- Impaired brain function (e.g. confusion) or
- Abnormal behaviour (e.g., change in personality).

SIDELINE ASSESSMENT

Indications for Emergency Management

NOTE: A hit to the head can sometimes be associated with a more serious brain injury. Any of the following warrants consideration of activating emergency procedures and urgent transportation to the nearest hospital:

- Glasgow Coma score less than 15
- Deteriorating mental status
- Potential spinal injury
- Progressive, worsening symptoms or new neurologic signs

Potential signs of concussion?

If any of the following signs are observed after a direct or indirect blow to the head, the athlete should stop participation, be evaluated by a medical professional and **should not be permitted to return to sport the same day** if a concussion is suspected.

Any loss of consciousness?		☐ Y ☐ N
"If so, how long?" _____		
Balance or motor incoordination (stumbles, slow/laboured movements, etc.)?		☐ Y ☐ N
Disorientation or confusion (inability to respond appropriately to questions)?		☐ Y ☐ N
Loss of memory:		☐ Y ☐ N
"If so, how long?" _____		
"Before or after the injury?" _____		
Blank or vacant look:		☐ Y ☐ N
Visible facial injury in combination with any of the above:		☐ Y ☐ N

1 Glasgow coma scale (GCS)

Best eye response (E)

No eye opening	1
Eye opening in response to pain	2
Eye opening to speech	3
Eyes opening spontaneously	4

Best verbal response (V)

No verbal response	1
Incomprehensible sounds	2
Inappropriate words	3
Confused	4
Oriented	5

Best motor response (M)

No motor response	1
Extension to pain	2
Abnormal flexion to pain	3
Flexion/Withdrawal to pain	4
Localizes to pain	5
Obeys commands	6

Glasgow Coma score (E + V + M)	of 15

GCS should be recorded for all athletes in case of subsequent deterioration.

2 Maddocks Score[3]

"I am going to ask you a few questions, please listen carefully and give your best effort."
Modified Maddocks questions (1 point for each correct answer)

What venue are we at today?	0	1
Which half is it now?	0	1
Who scored last in this match?	0	1
What team did you play last week/game?	0	1
Did your team win the last game?	0	1
Maddocks score		of 5

Maddocks score is validated for sideline diagnosis of concussion only and is not used for serial testing.

Notes: Mechanism of Injury ("tell me what happened"?):

_____
_____
_____
_____

Any athlete with a suspected concussion should be REMOVED FROM PLAY, medically assessed, monitored for deterioration (i.e., should not be left alone) and should not drive a motor vehicle until cleared to do so by a medical professional. No athlete diagnosed with concussion should be returned to sports participation on the day of Injury.

FIGURE 23-2 SCAT3 Sport Concussion Assessment Tool 3. *(From Consensus Statement: SCAT3 Br J Sports Med 2013; 47:5 259.)*

Continued

SPORTS PARTICIPATION

BACKGROUND

Name: _____ Date: _____

Examiner: _____

Sport/team/school: _____ Date/time of injury: _____

Age: _____ Gender: [ ] M [ ] F

Years of education completed: _____

Dominant hand: [ ] right [ ] left [ ] neither

How many concussions do you think you have had in the past? _____

When was the most recent concussion? _____

How long was your recovery from the most recent concussion? _____

Have you ever been hospitalized or had medical imaging done for a head injury? [ ] Y [ ] N

Have you ever been diagnosed with headaches or migraines? [ ] Y [ ] N

Do you have a learning disability, dyslexia, ADD/ADHD? [ ] Y [ ] N

Have you ever been diagnosed with depression, anxiety or other psychiatric disorder? [ ] Y [ ] N

Has anyone in your family ever been diagnosed with any of these problems? [ ] Y [ ] N

Are you on any medications? If yes, please list: [ ] Y [ ] N

SCAT3 to be done in resting state. Best done 10 or more minutes post excercise.

SYMPTOM EVALUATION

3 How do you feel?

"You should score yourself on the following symptoms, based on how you feel now".

	none	mild		moderate		severe	
Headache	0	1	2	3	4	5	6
"Pressure in head"	0	1	2	3	4	5	6
Neck Pain	0	1	2	3	4	5	6
Nausea or vomiting	0	1	2	3	4	5	6
Dizziness	0	1	2	3	4	5	6
Blurred vision	0	1	2	3	4	5	6
Balance problems	0	1	2	3	4	5	6
Sensitivity to light	0	1	2	3	4	5	6
Sensitivity to noise	0	1	2	3	4	5	6
Feeling slowed down	0	1	2	3	4	5	6
Feeling like "in a fog"	0	1	2	3	4	5	6
"Don't feel right"	0	1	2	3	4	5	6
Difficulty concentrating	0	1	2	3	4	5	6
Difficulty remembering	0	1	2	3	4	5	6
Fatigue or low energy	0	1	2	3	4	5	6
Confusion	0	1	2	3	4	5	6
Drowsiness	0	1	2	3	4	5	6
Trouble falling asleep	0	1	2	3	4	5	6
More emotional	0	1	2	3	4	5	6
Irritability	0	1	2	3	4	5	6
Sadness	0	1	2	3	4	5	6
Nervous or Anxious	0	1	2	3	4	5	6

Total number of symptoms (Maximum possible 22)

Symptom severity score (Maximum possible 132)

Do the symptoms get worse with physical activity? [ ] Y [ ] N

Do the symptoms get worse with mental activity? [ ] Y [ ] N

[ ] self rated   [ ] self rated and clinician monitored

[ ] clinician interview   [ ] self rated with parent input

Overall rating: If you know the athlete well prior to the injury, how different is the athlete acting compared to his/her usual self?

Please circle one response:

no different	very different	unsure	N/A

Scoring on the SCAT3 should not be used as a stand-alone method to diagnose concussion, measure recovery or make decisions about an athlete's readiness to return to competition after concussion. Since signs and symptoms may evolve over time, it is important to consider repeat evaluation in the acute assessment of concussion.

COGNITIVE & PHYSICAL EVALUATION

4 Cognitive assessment
Standardized Assessment of Concussion (SAC)[4]

Orientation (1 point for each correct answer)

What month is it?	0	1
What is the date today?	0	1
What is the day of the week?	0	1
What year is it?	0	1
What time is it right now? (within 1 hour)	0	1
Orientation score		of 5

Immediate memory

List	Trial 1		Trial 2		Trial 3		Alternative word list		
elbow	0	1	0	1	0	1	candle	baby	finger
apple	0	1	0	1	0	1	paper	monkey	penny
carpet	0	1	0	1	0	1	sugar	perfume	blanket
saddle	0	1	0	1	0	1	sandwich	sunset	lemon
bubble	0	1	0	1	0	1	wagon	iron	insect
Total									

Immediate memory score total	of 15

Concentration: Digits Backward

List	Trial 1		Alternative digit list		
4-9-3	0	1	6-2-9	5-2-6	4-1-5
3-8-1-4	0	1	3-2-7-9	1-7-9-5	4-9-6-8
6-2-9-7-1	0	1	1-5-2-8-6	3-8-5-2-7	6-1-8-4-3
7-1-8-4-6-2	0	1	5-3-9-1-4-8	8-3-1-9-6-4	7-2-4-8-5-6
Total of 4					

Concentration: Month in Reverse Order (1 pt. for entire sequence correct)

Dec-Nov-Oct-Sept-Aug-Jul-Jun-May-Apr-Mar-Feb-Jan	0	1

Concentration score	of 5

5 Neck Examination:

Range of motion   Tenderness   Upper and lower limb sensation & strength

Findings: _____

6 Balance examination

Do one or both of the following tests.

Footwear (shoes, barefoot, braces, tape, etc.) _____

Modified Balance Error Scoring System (BESS) testing[5]

Which foot was tested (i.e. which is the **non-dominant** foot)? [ ] Left [ ] Right

Testing surface (hard floor, field, etc.) _____

Condition

Double leg stance:	Errors
Single leg stance (non-dominant foot):	Errors
Tandem stance (non-dominant foot at back):	Errors

And/Or

Tandem gait[6,7]

Time (best of 4 trials): _____ seconds

7 Coordination examination
Upper limb coordination

Which arm was tested: [ ] Left [ ] Right

Coordination score	of 1

8 SAC Delayed Recall[4]

Delayed recall score	of 5

INSTRUCTIONS

Words in *Italics* throughout the SCAT3 are the instructions given to the athlete by the tester.

Symptom Scale

"You should score yourself on the following symptoms, based on how you feel now".

To be completed by the athlete. In situations where the symptom scale is being completed after exercise, it should still be done in a resting state, at least 10 minutes post exercise.
For total number of symptoms, maximum possible is 22.
For Symptom severity score, add all scores in table, maximum possible is 22 x 6 = 132.

SAC[4]
Immediate Memory

"I am going to test your memory. I will read you a list of words and when I am done, repeat back as many words as you can remember, in any order."

Trials 2 & 3:

"I am going to repeat the same list again. Repeat back as many words as you can remember in any order, even if you said the word before."

Complete all 3 trials regardless of score on trial 1 & 2. Read the words at a rate of one per second. **Score 1 pt. for each correct response.** Total score equals sum across all 3 trials. Do not inform the athlete that delayed recall will be tested.

Concentration
Digits backward

"I am going to read you a string of numbers and when I am done, you repeat them back to me backwards, in reverse order of how I read them to you. For example, if I say 7-1-9, you would say 9-1-7."

If correct, go to next string length. If incorrect, read trial 2. **One point possible for each string length**. Stop after incorrect on both trials. The digits should be read at the rate of one per second.

Months in reverse order

"Now tell me the months of the year in reverse order. Start with the last month and go backward. So you'll say December, November ... Go ahead"

1 pt. for entire sequence correct

Delayed Recall

The delayed recall should be performed after completion of the Balance and Coordination Examination.

"Do you remember that list of words I read a few times earlier? Tell me as many words from the list as you can remember in any order."

Score 1 pt. for each correct response

Balance Examination

Modified Balance Error Scoring System (BESS) testing[5]

This balance testing is based on a modified version of the Balance Error Scoring System (BESS)[5]. A stopwatch or watch with a second hand is required for this testing.

"I am now going to test your balance. Please take your shoes off, roll up your pant legs above ankle (if applicable), and remove any ankle taping (if applicable). This test will consist of three twenty second tests with different stances."

(a) Double leg stance:

"The first stance is standing with your feet together with your hands on your hips and with your eyes closed. You should try to maintain stability in that position for 20 seconds. I will be counting the number of times you move out of this position. I will start timing when you are set and have closed your eyes."

(b) Single leg stance:

"If you were to kick a ball, which foot would you use? [This will be the dominant foot] Now stand on your non-dominant foot. The dominant leg should be held in approximately 30 degrees of hip flexion and 45 degrees of knee flexion. Again, you should try to maintain stability for 20 seconds with your hands on your hips and your eyes closed. I will be counting the number of times you move out of this position. If you stumble out of this position, open your eyes and return to the start position and continue balancing. I will start timing when you are set and have closed your eyes."

(c) Tandem stance:

"Now stand heel-to-toe with your non-dominant foot in back. Your weight should be evenly distributed across both feet. Again, you should try to maintain stability for 20 seconds with your hands on your hips and your eyes closed. I will be counting the number of times you move out of this position. If you stumble out of this position, open your eyes and return to the start position and continue balancing. I will start timing when you are set and have closed your eyes."

Balance testing – types of errors

1. Hands lifted off iliac crest
2. Opening eyes
3. Step, stumble, or fall
4. Moving hip into > 30 degrees abduction
5. Lifting forefoot or heel
6. Remaining out of test position > 5 sec

Each of the 20-second trials is scored by counting the errors, or deviations from the proper stance, accumulated by the athlete. The examiner will begin counting errors only after the individual has assumed the proper start position. **The modified BESS is calculated by adding one error point for each error during the three 20-second tests. The maximum total number of errors for any single condition is 10.** If an athlete commits multiple errors simultaneously, only one error is recorded but the athlete should quickly return to the testing position, and counting should resume once subject is set. Subjects that are unable to maintain the testing procedure for a minimum of **five seconds** at the start are assigned the highest possible score, ten, for that testing condition.

OPTION: For further assessment, the same 3 stances can be performed on a surface of medium density foam (e.g., approximately 50 cm x 40 cm x 6 cm).

Tandem Gait[6,7]

Participants are instructed to stand with their feet together behind a starting line (the test is best done with footwear removed). Then, they walk in a forward direction as quickly and as accurately as possible along a 38mm wide (sports tape), 3 meter line with an alternate foot heel-to-toe gait ensuring that they approximate their heel and toe on each step. Once they cross the end of the 3m line, they turn 180 degrees and return to the starting point using the same gait. A total of 4 trials are done and the best time is retained. Athletes should complete the test in 14 seconds. Athletes fail the test if they step off the line, have a separation between their heel and toe, or if they touch or grab the examiner or an object. In this case, the time is not recorded and the trial repeated, if appropriate.

Coordination Examination

Upper limb coordination
Finger-to-nose (FTN) task:

"I am going to test your coordination now. Please sit comfortably on the chair with your eyes open and your arm (either right or left) outstretched (shoulder flexed to 90 degrees and elbow and fingers extended), pointing in front of you. When I give a start signal, I would like you to perform five successive finger to nose repetitions using your index finger to touch the tip of the nose, and then return to the starting position, as quickly and as accurately as possible."

Scoring: 5 correct repetitions in < 4 seconds = 1
Note for testers: Athletes fail the test if they do not touch their nose, do not fully extend their elbow or do not perform five repetitions. **Failure should be scored as 0.**

References & Footnotes

1. This tool has been developed by a group of international experts at the 4th International Consensus meeting on Concussion in Sport held in Zurich, Switzerland in November 2012. The full details of the conference outcomes and the authors of the tool are published in The BJSM Injury Prevention and Health Protection, 2013, Volume 47, Issue 5. The outcome paper will also be simultaneously co-published in other leading biomedical journals with the copyright held by the Concussion in Sport Group, to allow unrestricted distribution, providing no alterations are made.

2. McCrory P et al., Consensus Statement on Concussion in Sport – the 3rd International Conference on Concussion in Sport held in Zurich, November 2008. British Journal of Sports Medicine 2009; 43: i76-89.

3. Maddocks, DL; Dicker, GD; Saling, MM. The assessment of orientation following concussion in athletes. Clinical Journal of Sport Medicine. 1995; 5(1): 32–3.

4. McCrea M. Standardized mental status testing of acute concussion. Clinical Journal of Sport Medicine. 2001; 11: 176–181.

5. Guskiewicz KM. Assessment of postural stability following sport-related concussion. Current Sports Medicine Reports. 2003; 2: 24–30.

6. Schneiders, A.G., Sullivan, S.J., Gray, A., Hammond-Tooke, G. & McCrory, P. Normative values for 16-37 year old subjects for three clinical measures of motor performance used in the assessment of sports concussions. Journal of Science and Medicine in Sport. 2010; 13(2): 196–201.

7. Schneiders, A.G., Sullivan, S.J., Kvarnstrom. J.K., Olsson, M., Yden. T. & Marshall, S.W. The effect of footwear and sports-surface on dynamic neurological screening in sport-related concussion. Journal of Science and Medicine in Sport. 2010; 13(4): 382–386

SPORTS PARTICIPATION

ATHLETE INFORMATION

Any athlete suspected of having a concussion should be removed from play, and then seek medical evaluation.

Signs to watch for

Problems could arise over the first 24–48 hours. The athlete should not be left alone and must go to a hospital at once if they:

- Have a headache that gets worse
- Are very drowsy or can't be awakened
- Can't recognize people or places
- Have repeated vomiting
- Behave unusually or seem confused; are very irritable
- Have seizures (arms and legs jerk uncontrollably)
- Have weak or numb arms or legs
- Are unsteady on their feet; have slurred speech

Remember, it is better to be safe.
Consult your doctor after a suspected concussion.

Return to play

Athletes should not be returned to play the same day of injury.
When returning athletes to play, they should be **medically cleared and then follow a stepwise supervised program,** with stages of progression.

For example:

Rehabilitation stage	Functional exercise at each stage of rehabilitation	Objective of each stage
No activity	Physical and cognitive rest	Recovery
Light aerobic exercise	Walking, swimming or stationary cycling keeping intensity, 70 % maximum predicted heart rate. No resistance training	Increase heart rate
Sport-specific exercise	Skating drills in ice hockey, running drills in soccer. No head impact activities	Add movement
Non-contact training drills	Progression to more complex training drills, eg passing drills in football and ice hockey. May start progressive resistance training	Exercise, coordination, and cognitive load
Full contact practice	Following medical clearance participate in normal training activities	Restore confidence and assess functional skills by coaching staff
Return to play	Normal game play	

There should be at least 24 hours (or longer) for each stage and if symptoms recur the athlete should rest until they resolve once again and then resume the program at the previous asymptomatic stage. Resistance training should only be added in the later stages.

If the athlete is symptomatic for more than 10 days, then consultation by a medical practitioner who is expert in the management of concussion, is recommended.

Medical clearance should be given before return to play.

Scoring Summary:

Test Domain	Score		
	Date:	Date:	Date:
Number of Symptoms of 22			
Symptom Severity Score of 132			
Orientation of 5			
Immediate Memory of 15			
Concentration of 5			
Delayed Recall of 5			
SAC Total			
BESS (total errors)			
Tandem Gait (seconds)			
Coordination of 1			

Notes:

_____
_____
_____
_____
_____
_____
_____
_____
_____
_____
_____
_____
_____

CONCUSSION INJURY ADVICE

(To be given to the **person monitoring** the concussed athlete)

This patient has received an injury to the head. A careful medical examination has been carried out and no sign of any serious complications has been found. Recovery time is variable across individuals and the patient will need monitoring for a further period by a responsible adult. Your treating physician will provide guidance as to this timeframe.

If you notice any change in behaviour, vomiting, dizziness, worsening headache, double vision or excessive drowsiness, please contact your doctor or the nearest hospital emergency department immediately.

Other important points:

- Rest (physically and mentally), including training or playing sports until symptoms resolve and you are medically cleared
- No alcohol
- No prescription or non-prescription drugs without medical supervision. Specifically:
  · No sleeping tablets
  · Do not use aspirin, anti-inflammatory medication or sedating pain killers
- Do not drive until medically cleared
- Do not train or play sport until medically cleared

Clinic phone number

Patient's name _____

Date/time of injury _____

Date/time of medical review _____

Treating physician _____

Contact details or stamp

From McCrory et al, 2009.

Staying Well

The Female Athlete Triad

A trio of problems—*disordered eating, amenorrhea,* and *osteoporosis*—define the female athlete triad. The greatest risk is for athletes whose sport stresses the need to be lean (gymnastics, figure skating, diving, ballet) or to be able to endure (distance running, swimming, cross-country skiing). Early recognition of a possible problem is essential and the sports preparticipation physical evaluation (PPE) is the right time to begin. A review of diet, exercise, and menstrual history should be routine.

Identify an energy deficit, in which calorie expenditure exceeds calorie intake. This may sometimes occur unintentionally but at other times intentionally (e.g., binging and purging, using laxatives, diuretics, and diet pills inappropriately). The body may adapt at first so that the problem may have a subtle onset.

Primary amenorrhea (no onset of menses by 16 years of age), secondary amenorrhea (no periods for 3 cycles in a row or 6 months), or oligomenorrhea (intervals between periods longer than 35 days) are all possibilities in the triad. These findings are not a normal response to exercise. Secondary amenorrhea occurs in approximately 2% to 5% of the general female population. Among female athletes, depending on the sport, secondary amenorrhea occurs in as many as 69% (American College of Sports Medicine, 2007).

More than half of adult bone calcium is deposited during the teenage years, making this a particularly vulnerable time. The prevalence of both menstrual irregularity and disordered eating ranges from 6% to 16% of high school female athletes (Thein-Nissenbaum and Carr, 2011). A too-thin body encourages a low estrogen state and the possibility of menstrual dysfunction and a resultant osteopenia or osteoporosis. The risk of stress fracture increases. The problem needs early recognition as it may be irreversible if discovered too late. The thorough menstrual history is a critical component of the PPE in female athletes.

CHAPTER 24

Putting It All Together

This chapter asks that you integrate all you have learned about interviewing, building a history, and performing the physical examination. It offers a suggested approach and sequence for performing all steps of the physical examination. However, you are encouraged to be flexible and allow for the unique circumstance of each patient and your personal contribution to the process. Knowing yourself, listening carefully to your patients, and ensuring their active participation in their own care will allow you to put it all together.

The relationship with the patient begins with good manners. The relationship becomes well-established through the powerful therapeutic effect of really listening to what the patient says, careful exploration for hidden concerns, and explaining information without patronizing. The enduring message of sound communication is that you care and that the patient is your full partner (Box 24-1).

Building the history and performing the physical examination is subject to your style and comfort. Be flexible in your history-taking routine so that the patient's true story is revealed. Consider starting the interview with "Tell me about yourself," and then listen to hear the story.

The physical examination, the "laying on of hands," is integral to the history, making it possible to understand the objective findings—the disease—but also the great variety of subjective findings that modify the patient's experience with the disease. Technologic expertise is a complement to—but never a substitute for—the skillful physical examination.

At the Start

At the first meeting, tell patients you are a student or explain your level of training, and let them know that you may be more tentative than an experienced health care provider. The pressure and uncertainty you feel about your ability will fade as time, experience, and appropriate supervision help build your self-confidence.

The history and physical examination do not have to be completed in a special sequence or in the same sequence in which you will record them. They can be integrated to meet the needs of the patient or the demands of the moment. Be alert to deviations from the expected. You can ask additional questions to expand on historical information heard earlier or omit steps that may for the moment be unnecessary. In this case you are adapting to circumstance by using clinical judgment. This varies with the nature of the patient's concern, the age and gender of the patient, and even findings during the physical examination.

The patient with a concern and a probable vulnerability may be uneasy, anxious, or even fearful (Box 24-2). It may help to consistently provide an explanation of which part of the examination comes next and to be honest about the potential of uncertainty, discomfort, and/or pain and how long it will last. Be reassuring, but not inappropriately so, and do not offer premature assumptions about potential unexpected findings. Patients evaluate you during the examination and gauge their anxiety by your manner, hesitations in speech, changes in facial expression, and time spent examining a part of the body. Some patients equate the gravity of the situation with the length of time you spend, whereas others equate length of time with thoroughness.

Once you have obtained the basic history, assess urgency, the nature of the concerns, and the body systems involved. Then perform the physical examination, paying particular attention to the body systems of potential concern. You may need to ask more questions or even return to the physical examination to gather all of the needed information. *Do not assume that your initial list of differential diagnoses is certain.* The patient may have an unusual presentation of a common problem, a common presentation of a rare condition, more than one disease process, a confounding emotional or social problem, a new illness superimposed on an existing one, or a combination of any of these factors. Do not ignore any fact or finding that does not fit your initial hypotheses or assume that a single diagnosis exists when two or more may be present. Do not squeeze findings to fit your initial hypotheses regarding the patient's symptoms (see Clinical Pearl, "Respecting Your Instincts"). With all pathophysiologic and psychosocial possibilities in mind and with probabilities and urgency dominant, constantly challenge yourself and resist being tightly bound by your initial impressions (see Chapter 25).

Box 24-1 A Few Reminders for Emphasis

If You Want Effective Relationships with Patients

- Ensure good communication with courtesy and provision of comfort, connection, and confirmation (see Box 1-1, Chapter 1, p. 2).
- Dress neatly and be well groomed.
- Patients are culturally diverse so use the patient's language if possible. It is important for you to be understood, so use colloquialisms if needed. *Do not* use complex medical terminology.
- Avoid distraction and interruption, except for an emergency.
- Adapt to the patient's circumstance. An older adult in a wheelchair is a different challenge than the infant on the parent's lap.
- Be flexible, but be certain at the end that you have made all the necessary observations.
- Make sure the examining table is positioned at a height so you can access the patient from every side.
- Have the patient comfortably draped, paying attention to modesty at every age. Expose the part of the body to be examined appropriately and well, or you may lose the vital finding.
- Always consider the need for a chaperone.
- Keep your hands and stethoscope warm.
- Do not probe too vigorously when examining tender areas.
- Talk but do not chatter; explain as you go, anticipating the patient's concern about what comes next. State the reasons for examining an area and warn of any potential discomfort.
- Ask the patient to do things; never order. Say "please" and "thank you." Occasionally ask if the patient is comfortable or has any questions.
- Observe the patient's demeanor and body language. Apathy, disinterest, or inability to offer a social smile are equally worrisome in adults, infants, and children.
- Be objective as you assess the patient. Make no premature assumptions about what you find.
- Describe first without diagnosing. Do not voice impressions prematurely. For example, a lump in the neck may be a swollen node and not a cyst. Diagnosis can usually wait until all the data are in.
- Use a ruler rather than a coin, piece of fruit, or nut for comparison to describe findings.
- Remember that physical findings have meanings that vary according to age.
- Be reassuring only when you honestly can. Do not make promises you cannot keep.
- Pace the assessment according to the circumstance, the sense of urgency, and the recognition of fatigue and frailty. It is not necessary to do it all at once. Allow for rest and return later to finish up.

Clinical Pearl

Respecting Your Instincts

A reminder: Respect your instinct whenever you come across the unexpected, whenever your sense of what you might call normal has been violated. Pay attention when that happens, even if it does not seem to make sense and/or you cannot explain it easily.

Box 24-2 The Patient We Define as Difficult

Sometimes we find ourselves reacting negatively when patients are:

- Seemingly insatiable in their demands, wanting and feeling entitled to preferential treatment, seeming always on the edge of a lawsuit, and often impressed with their self-determined status in society (the VIP), but really quite dependent
- Denying and being self-destructive, such as by being inattentive to instructions or not following through with treatment regimens
- Rejecting, distrusting, always testing your competency and reliability, expressing pessimism about the efficacy of your effort

It is important to try to understand the patient's needs and insecurities. Show respect and use all available supportive resources. Strategies that may help include: Be clear and precise, keep all promises, set firm limits on what you can do, and try to maintain a compassionate approach. This may enable your partnership to mature, even if it is painful at times. Despite patients' vulnerabilities, they often are inclined to give the health care provider a chance to gain their trust and respect.

Accuracy

You and the patient have responsibility for the reliability of findings and observations, but yours is greater. Take the time with open-ended questions to ensure that the patient has the opportunity to report fully and accurately. Ask follow-up questions as needed. Several things can limit the patient's ability to observe well and to report accurately:

- *Sensory deprivation.* A partial or total loss of any of the senses (e.g., vision, hearing, touch, or smell) is clearly constraining. Do not expect the unaffected senses to be heightened. This may occur with some persons, but not all.
- *Emotional constraints, apparent and unapparent.* Patients who are psychotic, delirious, depressed, or otherwise seriously emotionally affected may confuse you. When you suspect this, carefully and objectively assess mental status during the history and physical examination.
- *Language barriers.* Patients may speak a language different from yours. Translation can be difficult in the best of circumstances, even when using a professional translator. Passing messages among three persons may potentially change the meaning and interpretation of important information, and confusion may be the result. Even using the same language may be a problem if the patient has a limited vocabulary, speaks English as a second language, or cannot read it very well.
- *Cultural barriers.* Consider the probable differences between you and the patient with candor and compassionate inquiry (see Chapter 2, "Cultural Competency"). Gender, race, and ethnicity are obvious differences. Consider other barriers, such as the life experiences among persons who are overweight versus underweight, those with hearing impairment versus normal hearing, gravely ill versus well, and older versus younger. Display respectful curiosity by encouraging conversation about such differences. It is all right to ask how it feels to be too big for an airplane seat designed with uniformity in mind. Uniformity is not part of the human condition.

Identify limitations that may affect accuracy and take the steps to enhance reliability. For example, the patient with a hearing impairment may need a response that facilitates communication such as written questions or lip reading enhanced with good lighting, talking slowly, and keeping your lips visible to the patient. Remember that a person with severe vision impairment cannot see your gestures.

Family, friends, or an emergency medical technician are a frequent resource for information. These suggestions for patient interactions apply equally to them. If possible, make the patient aware that others are providing information. When possible, the patient should set the limits regarding information that can be shared. Autonomy and confidentiality are always in play.

At times patients may be presumed to be "unreliable" because of life situations, limited cognition, indifference, apathy, or personal emotional needs that lead to distortions and overstatements or understatements of reality. Each of these possibilities requires skill and sensitivity to obtain the most accurate information possible. Consider rejecting the descriptor "unreliable" because of its negative connotation.

The Potential for Error

We are all susceptible to error. A practitioner may palpate the same abdomen at different times on the same day and conclude that the liver span is somewhat different each time. Multiple observers may palpate the same abdomen on the same day and report different liver spans. This demonstrates the potential for error in each of us, and the same error may occur with many of the diagnostic tests ordered for our patients (Box 24-3). Every observation has a certain sensitivity (i.e., the assurance that if a patient has an abnormal exam finding that it will be found) and specificity (e.g., the assurance that a healthy patient will not have the abnormal finding). No observation or test has 100% sensitivity and specificity. Remember this potential for error. Candidly question yourself and seek confirmation from others when necessary to minimize your errors.

Uncertainty

The potential of error increases uncertainty and our discomfort. It is more comforting to think in a deterministic or mechanistic fashion, seeking certain and fixed knowledge and avoiding anything subjective as much as possible. We cannot always express our findings in numbers, and probabilities cannot be avoided, but we still try. For example, we use scales (assessment tools) that have several variables requiring a subjective judgment and the assignment of a fixed number to quantify each to arrive at a total score (consider the Glasgow Coma Scale and the Apgar score). That fixed number is really a pseudoquantification, or proxy indicator of severity. There is false comfort in the apparent certainty of numbers. The mature observer is one who is comfortable with probabilities and making decisions with a certain degree of uncertainty.

Examination Sequence

✥ Adults and Adolescents

There is no one right way to perform the physical examination so that the process flows smoothly, minimizes the number of times the patient has to change positions, and conserves patient energy. You need to adapt to the particular setting *and* patient condition *or* abilities. Box 24-4 gives a list of supplies you should have on hand.

Box 24-4 **Equipment Supplies for Physical Examination**

Basic Materials
Cotton balls
Cotton-tipped applicator sticks
Drapes
Examining gloves
Flashlight with transilluminator
Gauze squares
Lubricant
Marking pen
Measuring tape
Nasal speculum
Odorous substances
Ophthalmoscope
Otoscope with pneumatic bulb
Penlight
Percussion hammer
Ruler
Sharp and dull testing implements
Sphygmomanometer
Stethoscope with diaphragm and bell
Taste-testing substances
Thermometer
Tongue blades
Tuning forks
Vaginal speculum
Visual acuity screening charts for near and far vision

Materials for Gathering Specimens
Culture media
Glass slides
KOH (potassium hydroxide)
Occult blood–testing materials
Pap smear spatula/brush/broom, fixative, and container
Saline
Sterile cotton-tipped applicators

Box 24-3 **Humans and Machines**

You can perceive the patient better than any machine by looking, listening, touching, and smelling. Mechanical imaging cannot capture vitality, apathy, or cognitive awareness, but technology can expand our insights. Just like our observations, technologic procedures do not always result in particularly sensitive or specific findings. Other potential limitations include the use of irradiation, potentially toxic contrast agents, and in the case of magnetic resonance imaging, intimidating sound and confinement. Remember that all technologic procedures, as well as all that we do, have a potential cost to the human body, to emotion, and to finances.

FIGURE 24-1 Observe the patient while entering the examining room for manner, dress, interest or apprehension, and mobility.

Modesty matters but do not let it deter examinations essential for appropriate care. Have comfortable gowns and appropriate movable covers available. Always consider the need for a chaperone for the patient, especially for age, gender, and particular examinations (e.g., pelvic and rectal examination and/or a given patient's sensibilities). Health care facilities often have a policy regarding chaperones, so be familiar with the rule. Doors and curtains should be closed. It is also best to leave the room when the patient undresses and prepares for the examination. Do not assume that the patient has the same comfort with the situation that you do.

General Inspection

Begin the inspection as you greet the patient, looking for problematic signs. You can perform parts of your physical examination any time the patient is in your view, during the history or even in the waiting room (Fig. 24-1). If you go there to invite the patient into your examining room, take a moment to observe the appropriateness of dress and grooming, manner of sitting, degree of relaxation, relationship with others in the room, and degree of interest in what is happening in the room. On this first greeting, you can take note of the manner with which you are met and the palm's moistness when you shake hands. Remember not to squeeze too hard when the patient is unknown to you and may have arthritic, painful hands. Observe the gait as the patient walks with you, the luster of the eyes, and the expression of emotion. All of this contributes to your examination, along with the initial assessments of the following:

- Skin color
- Facial expression
- Mobility
  - Use of assistive devices
  - Gait
  - Sitting, rising from chair
  - Taking off coat
- Dress and posture
- Speech pattern, disorders, foreign language
- Difficulty hearing, assistive devices
- Stature and build
- Musculoskeletal deformities
- Vision problems, assistive devices
- Eye contact with examiner
- Orientation, mental alertness
- Nutritional state
- Respiratory problems
- Individuals accompanying patient

Preparation

After completing the interview and respecting modesty, you or an assistant can instruct the patient to empty the bladder, remove as much clothing as is necessary, and put on a gown. Ask for a chaperone if you think it necessary. Modifications in the suggested sequence below are often necessary when the patient has disabilities (Box 24-5).

Measurements

Patient measurements (e.g., height, weight, and temperature) may be taken by an assistant in advance. In some cases you as the examiner will obtain all measurements or repeat certain ones (e.g., blood pressure if the initial measurement was elevated). Height and weight are often measured on the way to the examining room, where the body mass index (BMI) is then calculated. Vital signs (temperature, pulse, respirations, blood pressure, pain assessment, and sometimes oxygen saturation) may be obtained at the start of the physical examination or during the body system assessment. Assessment of distance vision and hearing may be performed by an assistant or at a convenient time during the physical examination.

Patient Seated, Wearing Gown

Patient is seated on examining table; examiner stands in front of patient (Fig. 24-2).

Box 24-5 Examining People with Disabilities

Variations in the approach to physical examination may be required for the patient with disabilities. What body systems are affected? What is the degree of impairment? What specific assistance does the patient require? Be flexible. It may not be necessary for the patient to undress fully, using up energy and time. Removing or rearranging the examination room furnishings will provide the space needed to maneuver a wheelchair. Some patient examination positions can be varied without compromising the quality of the examination (e.g., Alternative Positions for the Pelvic Examination, p. 448-449). Some patients may need just a bit more than usual assistance in getting set for the maneuvers of the examination. Patience and a gentle approach pay off.

FIGURE 24-2 Face the patient who is seated on the examining table.

Head and Face
+ Inspect skin characteristics.
+ Inspect symmetry and external characteristics of eyes and ears.
+ Inspect configuration of skull.
+ Inspect and palpate scalp and hair for texture, distribution, and quantity.
+ Palpate facial bones.
+ Palpate temporomandibular joint while patient opens and closes mouth.
+ Palpate and percuss sinus regions; if tender, transilluminate (while often helpful, the sensitivity and specificity of transillumination are uncertain when considered separately from other findings; see Evidence-Based Practice in Chapter 12, p. 244).
+ Inspect ability to clench teeth, squeeze eyes tightly shut, wrinkle forehead, smile, stick out tongue, puff out cheeks (CN V, VII).
+ Test light-touch sensation of forehead, cheeks, chin (CN V).

Eyes
+ External examination:
    + Inspect eyelids, eyelashes, and palpebral folds.
    + Determine alignment of eyebrows.
    + Inspect sclera, conjunctiva, and iris.
    + Palpate lacrimal apparatus.
    + Near vision screening: Rosenbaum chart (CN II)
+ Eye function:
    + Test pupillary response to light and accommodation.
    + Perform cover-uncover test and corneal light reflex.
    + Test extraocular eye movements (CN III, IV, VI).
    + Assess visual fields (CN II).
    + Test corneal reflexes (CN V), if indicated.
+ Ophthalmoscopic examination:
    + Test red reflex.
    + Inspect lens.
    + Inspect disc, cup margins, vessels, and retinal surface.

Ears
+ Inspect alignment and placement.
+ Inspect surface characteristics.
+ Palpate auricle.
+ Screen hearing with whisper test (CN VIII).
+ Perform otoscopic examination.
    + Inspect canals.
    + Inspect tympanic membranes for landmarks, deformities, and inflammation.
+ Perform Rinne and Weber tests.

Nose
+ Note structure, position of septum.
+ Determine patency of each nostril.
+ Inspect mucosa, septum, and turbinates with nasal speculum.
+ Assess olfactory function: Test sense of smell (CN I) when clinically necessary.

Mouth and Pharynx
+ Inspect lips, buccal mucosa, gums, hard and soft palates, and floor of mouth for color, surface characteristics, and any other apparent abnormalities.
+ Inspect oropharynx. Note anteroposterior pillars, uvula, tonsils, posterior pharynx, and mouth odor.
+ Inspect teeth for color, number, and surface characteristics.
+ Inspect tongue for color, characteristics, symmetry, and movement (CN XII).
+ Test gag reflex and soft palate rising with "ah" (CN IX, X).
+ Perform taste test (CN VII, IX) when clinically necessary.

Neck
+ Inspect for symmetry and smoothness of neck and thyroid.
+ Inspect for jugular venous distention (also when patient is supine).
+ Inspect and palpate range of motion; test resistance against examiner's hand.
+ Test shoulder shrug (CN IX).
+ Palpate carotid pulses, one at a time (also when patient is supine).
+ Palpate tracheal position.
+ Palpate thyroid.
+ Palpate lymph nodes: preauricular, postauricular, occipital, tonsillar, submaxillary, submental, superficial cervical chain, posterior cervical, deep cervical, supraclavicular, and infraclavicular.
+ Auscultate carotid arteries and thyroid.

Upper Extremities
+ Inspect skin and nail characteristics.
+ Inspect symmetry of muscle mass.
+ Observe and palpate hands, arms, and shoulders, including epitrochlear nodes, note musculoskeletal deformities.
+ Assess joint range of motion and muscle strength: fingers, wrists, elbows, and shoulders.
+ Assess pulses: radial, brachial.

FIGURE 24-3 Examine the patient's back without the gown.

FIGURE 24-4 Examine the patient's anterior chest while exposed.

Patient Seated, Back Exposed

Patient is still seated on examining table. Gown is pulled down to the waist for males so the entire chest and back are exposed; for females, back is exposed, but breasts are covered (Fig. 24-3). Examiner stands behind the patient.

Back and Posterior Chest
+ Inspect skin and thoracic configuration.
+ Inspect symmetry of shoulders, musculoskeletal development.
+ Inspect and palpate the scapula and spine.
+ Palpate and percuss costovertebral angle.

Lungs
+ Inspect respiration: excursion, depth, rhythm, and pattern.
+ Palpate for expansion and tactile fremitus.
+ Palpate scapular and subscapular nodes.
+ Percuss posterior chest and lateral walls systematically for resonance.
+ Percuss to measure diaphragmatic excursion.
+ Auscultate systematically for breath sounds. Note characteristics and adventitious sounds.

Patient Seated, Chest Exposed

Examiner moves around to the front of the patient (Fig. 24-4). The gown is lowered in females to expose the anterior chest.

Anterior, Chest, Lungs, and Heart
+ Inspect skin, musculoskeletal development, and symmetry.
+ Inspect respirations: patient posture, respiratory effort.
+ Inspect for pulsations or heaving.
+ Palpate chest wall for stability, crepitation, and tenderness.
+ Palpate precordium for thrills, heaves, and pulsations.
+ Palpate left chest to locate apical impulse.
+ Palpate for tactile fremitus.
+ Palpate axillary lymph nodes.
+ Percuss systematically for resonance.
+ Auscultate systematically for breath sounds.
+ Auscultate systematically for heart sounds: aortic, pulmonic, second pulmonic, mitral, and tricuspid areas.

Female Breasts
+ Inspect in the following positions: patient's arms hanging loosely at the sides, extended over head or flexed behind the neck, pushing hands on hips, leaning forward from the waist.
+ Perform chest wall sweep and bimanual digital palpation.
+ Palpate axillary, supraclavicular, and infraclavicular lymph nodes (if not already performed).

Male Breasts
+ Inspect breasts and nipples for symmetry, enlargement, and surface characteristics.
+ Palpate breast tissue.
+ Palpate axillary, supraclavicular, and infraclavicular lymph nodes.

Patient Reclining 45 Degrees

Assist the patient to a reclining position at a 45-degree angle (Fig. 24-5). Examiner stands to the side of the patient that allows the

FIGURE 24-5 Examine the patient while reclining with chest exposed.

best approach for necessary examination and comfort for patient and examiner.

+ Inspect chest in recumbent position.
+ Inspect jugular venous pulsations and measure right jugular venous pressure.

Patient Supine, Chest Exposed

Assist the patient into a supine position. If the patient cannot tolerate lying flat, maintain head elevation at 30-degree angle if possible. Uncover the chest while keeping the abdomen and lower extremities draped.

Female Breasts

+ Palpate all areas of breast tissue systematically using light, medium, and deep palpation with the patient's arm over her head.
+ Depress nipple into well behind the areola.

Heart

+ Palpate the chest wall for thrills, heaves, and pulsations.
+ Auscultate systematically; you can turn the patient slightly to the left side and repeat auscultation.

Patient Supine, Abdomen Exposed

Patient remains supine. Cover the chest with the patient's gown. Arrange draping to expose the abdomen from pubis to epigastrium (Fig. 24-6).

Abdomen

+ Inspect skin characteristics, contour, pulsations, and movement.
+ Auscultate all quadrants for bowel sounds.
+ Auscultate the aorta and renal, iliac, and femoral arteries for bruits or venous hums.
+ Percuss all quadrants for tone.
+ Percuss liver borders and estimate span.
+ Percuss left midaxillary line for splenic dullness.
+ Lightly palpate all quadrants.
+ Deeply palpate all quadrants.
+ Palpate right costal margin for liver border.
+ Palpate left costal margin for spleen.
+ Palpate laterally at the flanks for right and left kidneys.
+ Palpate midline for aortic pulsation.
+ Test abdominal reflexes.

+ Have patient raise the head as you inspect the abdominal muscles.

Inguinal Area

+ Palpate for lymph nodes, pulses, and hernias.

External Genitalia, Males

+ Inspect penis, urethral meatus, scrotum, and pubic hair.
+ Palpate scrotal contents.
+ Test cremasteric reflex.

Patient Supine, Legs Exposed

Patient remains supine. Arrange drapes to cover the abdomen and pubis and to expose the lower extremities (Fig. 24-7).

Feet and Legs

+ Inspect for skin characteristics, hair distribution, muscle mass, and musculoskeletal configuration.
+ Palpate for temperature, texture, edema, and pulses (dorsalis pedis, posterior tibial, popliteal).
+ Test range of motion and strength of toes, feet, ankles, and knees.

Hips

+ Palpate hips for stability.
+ Test range of motion and strength of hips.

Patient Sitting, Lap Draped

Assist the patient to a sitting position. The patient should have the gown on with a drape across the lap (Fig. 24-8).

Musculoskeletal.

+ Observe patient moving from lying to sitting position.
+ Note coordination, use of muscles, and ease of movement.

Neurologic.

+ Test sensory function: dull and sharp sensation of forehead, paranasal sinus area, lower arms, hands, lower legs, and feet.
+ Test vibratory sensation of wrists and ankles.
+ Test two-point discrimination of palms, thighs, and back.
+ Test stereognosis and graphesthesia.
+ Test upper extremity fine motor function and coordination. Ask the patient to perform the following tasks:
  + Touch the nose with alternating index fingers.

FIGURE 24-6 Examine the patient while reclining with abdomen exposed.

FIGURE 24-7 Examine the patient in supine position with legs exposed.

FIGURE 24-8 Examine the patient seated with a drape across the lap.

+ Rapidly alternate fingers to thumb.
+ Rapidly move index finger between the patient's nose and the examiner's finger.
+ Test lower extremity fine motor function and coordination, asking the patient to do the following:
    + Run heel down tibia of opposite leg.
    + Alternately and rapidly cross leg over opposite knee.
+ Test position sense of upper and lower extremities.
+ Test deep tendon reflexes and compare bilaterally: biceps, triceps, brachioradial, patellar, and Achilles.
+ Test plantar reflex bilaterally.

Patient Standing

Assist patient to a standing position (Fig. 24-9). Examiner stands next to patient.

Spine

+ Inspect and palpate spine as patient bends over at waist.
+ Test range of motion: flexion, hyperextension, lateral bending, rotation of upper trunk.

FIGURE 24-9 Examine the patient while standing.

Neurologic

+ Observe gait.
+ Test proprioception and cerebellar function.
+ Assess Romberg test.
+ Ask the patient to walk heel to toe.
+ Ask the patient to stand on one foot, then the other, with eyes closed.
+ Ask the patient to hop in place on one foot, then the other.

Abdominal/Genital

+ Test for inguinal and femoral hernias.

Female Patient, Lithotomy Position

Assist female patients into lithotomy position and drape appropriately (Fig. 24-10). Examiner is seated.

External Genitalia

+ Inspect pubic hair, labia, clitoris, urethral opening, vaginal opening, perineal and perianal areas, and anus.
+ Palpate labia and Bartholin glands; milk Skene glands.

Internal Genitalia

+ Perform speculum examination:
    + Inspect vagina and cervix.
    + Collect Pap smear/human papillomavirus (HPV) and other necessary specimens.
+ Perform bimanual palpation to assess for characteristics of vagina, cervix, uterus, and adnexa. Examiner is standing.
+ Perform rectovaginal examination to assess rectovaginal septum and broad ligaments.
+ Perform rectal examination:
    + Assess anal sphincter tone and surface characteristics; palpate circumferentially for rectal mass.
    + Obtain rectal culture if needed.
    + Note characteristics of stool when gloved finger is removed.

FIGURE 24-10 Examining the female patient in lithotomy position, appropriately draped.

Male Patient, Bending Forward (Lateral Decubitus or Knee-Chest Positions Are Also Possible)

Assist male patients in leaning over examining table (or into knee-chest position or lateral decubitus position if preferred) (Fig. 24-11). Examiner is behind patient. Ask the patient, unlike

FIGURE 24-11 Examining the male patient while bending over the examining table.

in this illustration, to point his toes inward and to put his arms and chest on the table to help relax the buttocks and make the examination easier.

- Inspect sacrococcygeal and perianal areas.
- Perform rectal examination:
  - Palpate sphincter tone and surface characteristics; palpate circumferentially for rectal mass.
  - Obtain rectal culture if needed.
  - Palpate prostate gland and seminal vesicles.
  - Note characteristics of stool when gloved finger is removed. Test for occult blood.

In the ambulatory setting, upon concluding the examination, you may excuse yourself to allow the patient to get dressed. When you return, discuss your findings and your interpretations to the extent that you can, and ask any needed additional questions. Make sure the patient's accompanying family member is included in this discussion, if appropriate. This is a final time during the visit for review, reflection, and an opportunity to address questions, concerns, or stressful matters. You must be sure that the patient has a clear understanding of the situation or plan going forward.

If the patient is examined in a hospital bed, remember to put everything back in order when you are finished. Make sure the patient is comfortably settled in an appropriate manner, with the bed lowered and the side rails up if the clinical condition warrants, and nursing call buttons within easy reach.

✤ Infants

Newborns

The newborn has greater risk and a better potential for health than patients of other ages. The Apgar score (see Chapter 13, p. 280), taken at 1 and 5 minutes of age, provides insight to the baby's in utero, intrapartum, and immediate postnatal experience. A low score for several of the variables—color, heart rate, respirations, muscle tone, and reflex irritability—is evidence of difficulty. The Apgar score does not identify the problems that are suggested by cyanosis, increased irritability, tachypnea,

tachycardia, or loss of muscle tone. The score should not be interpreted as an actual quantitative measure. It is an assessment of combined objective and subjective observations, and it allows communication from one observer to the next over time.

Because menstrual histories are often inaccurate, more objective means of estimating the newborn's gestational age are required. The Ballard Gestational Age Assessment Tool contains six physical and six neuromuscular newborn characteristics that should be evaluated within 36 hours of birth to establish or confirm the preterm newborn's gestational age (see Chapter 6, and the full-term newborn (40 weeks' gestation) commonly has the following physical characteristics: many creases on the sole of the foot, the breast nodule of 4 mm diameter, cartilage present in the helix of the ear, and the testes descended into the scrotum covered with rugae. Increasing muscle tone with a posture of predominantly flexed extremities is another sign of increased maturity.

Major congenital anomalies are usually obvious, but there are exceptions, such as a life-threatening diaphragmatic hernia. Maintain a high index of suspicion. Search for clues from information about the newborn's intrauterine life, the mother's labor and delivery experience, and the family history. For example, if the mother has a fever during or after delivery, or if she has herpetic lesions about the mouth or genitalia, the infant may be at risk. The mother's use of drugs—prescribed, over the counter, or illicit—may have an impact. Some may have teratogenic effects. The mother's frequent use of sedatives or opioids may cause irritability, jitteriness, poor sucking, and other problems as the newborn goes through withdrawal (neonatal withdrawal syndrome). Problems with earlier pregnancies may be relevant to the newborn's intrauterine life. The fate of siblings may suggest the fate of your present patient.

As with all patients, it is important to look at the baby first. You can learn a lot before touching, without abruptly handling or using an instrument. Note the baby's degree of awareness or apathy; the posture, and whether unusual flaccidity, tension, or spasticity is present; skin color; and unexpected gross deformities, or unusual facies. The responsive, eager infant with a strong suck is reassuring. Note the presence or absence of spontaneity in the baby's behavior, and always keep track of the interaction between parents and between parent and infant. Observing a feeding is informative, often the baby demonstrates interest in life by latching on to the breast or bottle eagerly and with strength.

When you begin the physical examination, palpate the head and fontanels (best done with baby upright), then the extremities and abdomen, and finally examine the rest of the baby. Use a gentle touch that will not obscure unusual findings. Chest percussion is generally of little value because of the relatively small chest and the examiner's relatively large hands and fingers. Abdominal percussion may have value, especially when the abdomen is distended.

Older Infants

With no best sequence for the physical examination, vary the sequence depending on the infant's age and whether awake or asleep at the start. Aim for cooperation by the infant for as long as possible. Again, observe as much as you can before touching (e.g., the quality and rate of respiration, flaring of the alae nasi, skin color, even the visible apical thrust). Defer to the end anything invasive (e.g., examination of the ears, throat, and eyes).

Take advantage of opportunities presented throughout the examination. The sleeping infant offers a wonderful chance to auscultate the heart, lungs, and abdomen and to observe the infant's position at rest. All is not lost when the infant is crying. Evaluate the quality or lustiness of the cry, tactile fremitus, lung excursion, and facial symmetry. The mouth and pharynx can be assessed for integrity of the soft palate and cranial nerves IX, X, and XII. Is stridor or hoarseness present? The crying infant needs to take a breath, so be ready to listen to the heart and lungs each time a breath is taken. Over several intervals of breathing, you can hear enough of the heart and lung sounds. A crying baby may keep the eyes tightly shut, but the parent can stand and hold the infant over the shoulder while you stand behind the parent. At this point, the child will often stop crying for a moment and open the eyes. If you are poised with ophthalmoscope, you can quickly make some assessment (e.g., red reflex, corneal light reflex, and even pupillary response to light). Observe the infant during feeding to evaluate sucking and swallowing coordination, cranial nerve XII, and alertness and responsiveness. Seizing these advantages often requires a change in the examination sequence to suit the moment. Give the older infant less than a year of age something to hold in each hand. You may be able gauge the infant's interest in the objects, and also have some freedom to use the stethoscope without having it grabbed.

Examination Sequence with Infants

The following is a guideline for the examination sequence of the newborn or young infant. The infant's temperature, weight, length, and head circumference are usually measured first. Weight, length, and head circumference are plotted on a growth curve for the infant's age and gender.

General Inspection

Inspect the undressed, supine newborn on a warming table; inspect the older infant preferably on a parent's lap (Fig. 24-12).

+ Assess positioning or posture at rest: symmetry and size of extremities, the newborn's assumption of in utero position, flexion of extremities, unusual flaccidity or spasticity, any difference in positioning between upper and lower extremities.
+ Lift infant and test Moro reflex with a sudden dropping motion.
+ Note voluntary movement of extremities.
+ Inspect the skin: color, meconium staining, and vernix in newborn.
+ Note the presence of tremors.
+ Assess for any apparent anomalies.
+ Inspect the face: symmetry of features, spacing and position of features (e.g., intercanthal distance, presence and characteristics of the philtrum).
+ Inspect configuration and movement of the chest.
+ Inspect shape of the abdomen, movement with respiration.

FIGURE 24-12 Infants are often more comfortable when examined on a parent's lap.

FIGURE 24-13 Examining the chest of an infant on the parent's lap.

Chest, Lungs, and Heart

+ Inspect the following: chest structure, symmetry of expansion with respiration; presence of retractions, heaves, or lifts (Fig. 24-13).
+ Note quality of respirations; count the rate.
+ Inspect the breasts for nipple and tissue development.
+ Palpate the chest and precordium. Locate the apical impulse (point of maximal impulse); note any thrills; note tactile fremitus in crying infant.
+ Auscultate entire anterior and lateral chest for breath sounds; note any bowel sounds.
+ Auscultate each cardiac listening area for S1 and S2, splitting, murmurs.
+ Count the apical pulse rate.
+ Percussion is not always performed, but may be necessary at times.

Abdomen

+ Inspect shape and configuration. Note scaphoid or distended appearance.
+ Inspect the umbilicus. Inspect the newborn cord stump, count the vessels, note oozing of blood. If the stump has fallen off, inspect the area for lesions, erythema, drainage, and foul odor.
+ Auscultate each quadrant for bowel sounds.
+ Lightly palpate all areas. Note size of liver, muscle tone, bladder, and spleen tip (Fig. 24-14).
+ Palpate more deeply for kidneys, any masses, note any muscle rigidity or tenseness.

FIGURE 24-14 Examining the infant's abdomen while reclining on parent's lap.

FIGURE 24-15 Inspect and palpate the infant's face.

+ Percuss each quadrant.
+ Check skin turgor.
+ Palpate the inguinal area for femoral pulses and lymph nodes.

Head and Neck. Inspection and palpation can be done before or simultaneously with use of invasive instruments (Fig. 24-15).

+ Inspect head shape. Note molding, swelling, scalp electrode site, and hairline.
+ Palpate the head: anterior and posterior fontanels, sutures, areas of swelling or asymmetry. Measure fontanels in two dimensions.
+ Transilluminate newborn's skull, if clinically necessary.
+ Inspect ears. Note shape, position, and alignment of auricles; pits, sinuses.
+ Perform otoscopic examination; assess patency of auditory canals and characteristics of the tympanic membranes.
+ Evaluate hearing.
+ Inspect eyes:
    + Swelling of eyelids and discharge, size, shape, position, epicanthal folds, conjunctivae, pupils
    + Pupillary response to light
    + Corneal light reflex
    + Red reflex; ophthalmoscopic examination when age and cooperation permit
    + Inspect eye movement: nystagmus, tracking a light or following a moving picture or face
+ Evaluate vision.
+ Inspect nose:
    + Flaring, discharge, size, and shape
    + Nasal mucosa, alignment of septum
+ Check patency of choanae. Observe respiratory effort while alternately occluding each naris.
+ Inspect mouth: lips, gums, hard and soft palates; size of tongue; excessive secretions in the newborn, drooling in the infant; presence of teeth, lesions.
+ Palpate mouth. Insert gloved small finger into mouth, palpate hard and soft palates with fingerpad, evaluate suck.
+ Stimulate gag reflex.
+ Stroke each side of mouth to evaluate rooting reflex.
+ Lift infant's trunk, allowing head to fall back and rest against the table, slightly hyperextended. Inspect and palpate the position of the trachea.
+ Inspect for alignment of head with neck.

+ Inspect for webbing, excess skinfolds.
+ Palpate for masses, thyroid, muscle tone.
+ Palpate lymph nodes: anterior and posterior cervical, preauricular, postauricular, submental, sublingual, tonsillar, supraclavicular.
+ Palpate the clavicles for integrity, crepitus.
+ Rotate head to each side for passive range of motion.
+ Observe the asymmetric tonic neck reflex.

Upper Extremities

+ Inspect and palpate arms.
+ Move arms through range of motion.
+ Palpate brachial or radial pulses; compare quality and timing with femoral pulses.
+ Open the hands: Inspect nails and palmar and phalangeal creases; count fingers.
+ Place a finger in infant's palms to evaluate palmar grasp reflex.
+ Keeping fingers in infant's hands, pull the infant slowly to sitting position, evaluate grasp and arm strength; evaluate head control.

Lower Extremities

+ Inspect the legs and feet for alignment and symmetry of skinfolds (Fig. 24-16).
+ Palpate the bones and muscles of each leg.
+ Move legs through range of motion; adduct and abduct the hips.
+ Palpate the femoral and dorsalis pedis pulses.
+ Count the toes.
+ Elicit the plantar, patellar, and Achilles reflexes.
+ Measure blood pressure in absence of femoral pulse or if otherwise clinically indicated.

FIGURE 24-16 Examine the infant's lower extremities.

Genitals and Rectum

+ Females
    + Inspect external genitalia, noting size of clitoris, any discharge, hymenal opening, and any ambiguity of structures.
    + Observe voiding for strength of stream.
+ Males
    + Inspect placement of urethral opening without fully retracting the foreskin.
    + Inspect scrotum for rugae and presence of contents; note any ambiguity of structures.
    + Palpate scrotum for the testes, presence of hernia or hydrocele.
    + Transilluminate the scrotum when a mass other than testes is noted.
    + Observe voiding for strength of stream.
+ Inspect rectum. Assess sphincter tone; if newborn has not passed meconium within 24 hours of birth, evaluate rectal patency with a soft catheter.

Neurologic.

Hold the infant in vertical suspension, facing you with your hands under the axillae.

+ Observe for the sunsetting sign as the baby's eyes open.
+ Perform the doll's eyes maneuver.
+ Evaluate general body strength. Without gripping the infant's chest, keep your hands under the infant's axillae, and note whether the baby begins to slip through your hands or maintains its position.
+ Elicit the stepping and placing reflexes, if indicated.

Back.

Position the newborn prone on the warming table or have the parent hold the infant upright over the shoulder (Fig. 24-17).

+ Inspect spine: Observe for alignment, symmetry of muscle development, any masses, tufts of hair, dimples, skin pigmentation or discoloration, or defects over lower spine.
+ Palpate each spinal process for defect.
+ Auscultate posterior chest for breath sounds, any heart sounds.
+ Inspect symmetry of gluteal folds.

FIGURE 24-17 Examining the infant's back while held by the parent.

Behavior.

Throughout examination of the newborn, note the alertness, ability to be quieted or consoled, and the response to handling. With an older infant, note alertness, responsiveness to the parent or other adult caregivers, and the ability of the parent to sense and respond to the infant's need for consolation. The child's ability at any age to react socially offers clues to physical and emotional well-being. The classic example is the "social smile"—the smile meant for you that we learn to expect from infants by the time they are 2 to 3 months old. Consider each of the following as you evaluate the infant's behavior:

+ Is that smile real and meant for you?
+ Is the infant playful, alert, and responsive or is there dullness and apparent apathy?
+ If the infant is fearful, does your soothing effort help to ease the fear?
+ Does the infant move freely, show interest in the immediate environment, reach for toys, and ask questions?
+ Note the responses to voices or noise: quieting, stopping movement, turning toward sounds.

❧ Children

For children small enough, the parent's lap is a splendid examining table. It is helpful during the interview to keep the child and parent together and to observe their interaction. How they feel about each other is conveyed through touch, soothing and reassuring gestures, and the child's response. Take note of the obvious and subtle ways in which children and parents communicate with each other. Excessive parental indulgence may indicate a smothering relationship. If interaction is minimal and the child does not look to the parent for help, the family dynamics may be devoid of warmth and affection. Ask the parent to be present if you need to perform procedures (e.g., venipuncture) as this is will be reassuring to the child. Most parents accept, and the reaction to your request gives you more information about family dynamics and emotional resources.

With the young child, you will often build a history and help prepare the child for the physical examination at the same time. For example, you may start with the history while establishing some reassuring contact. For example, playing with the child (providing a ball or age-appropriate book) may reveal developmental progress, and help win cooperation. A few pleasant words, relaxed moments, and patience can break the ice. Children do not know your routine. Often you are a stranger, and the environment may be frightening. Not every child will be smiling and happy about an examination.

Flexibility is important when examining young children. Avoid rushing, and do not persist if the child is anxious. Be thorough, but unless there is urgency, you may defer some aspects of the examination for when the child is more relaxed and less afraid of you. Children may be fearful because they have had procedures that hurt, or they do not want to be separated from a trusted, familiar figure. In some cases the child has been abused at home or in other settings. Some children have learned that perverse behavior can manipulate and get a rise out of adults. It is important to respect the child's fear; to explain what is going on; and to be honest, firm, unapologetic, and gently expeditious. You also need to develop comfort in working in the presence of

PUTTING IT ALL TOGETHER

Box 24-6   Some Tips for Examining a Young Child

- Telling a story or asking about the child's experience (e.g., school, games, or friends) can help to attract attention or, at times, to distract.
- Restraining the child and having adults looming over the examining table increases the child's apprehension and decreases cooperation. If the child's arms and head must be kept still (e.g., to look at the ears), the child is often less distressed if seated on the parent's lap and held by the parents' arms.
- Use the tongue blade only at the end of the examination if it must be used. Ease the tendency to gag by moistening it first with warm water.
- Ask a child to "blow out" your flashlight as a way to introduce your instruments. Offer them as toys (they will not break), or draw a doll's face on a tongue blade. You might even get down on the floor with the child, or use your own lap as an examining table. Anything goes (within bounds of propriety) to get the information you need.
- Enlist the help of the ticklish child. Place your hand on top of the child's to gently probe the abdomen or the axilla. The diaphragm of your stethoscope can also serve as a probe.
- Hold babies; feed them. You will know each other better.
- Be patient with discomfort or resistance. If the situation allows, come back to that portion of the examination later when calm may be restored.
- Use brief, specific, polite directions. Do not ask the child's permission for each step. It is better to say, "Please open your mouth" rather than "Do you want to open your mouth?" After all, what will you do next if the answer is "no?"

---

a parent who is sharply observant, sometimes tentative, or sometimes hostile. Do not separate the child from the parent for the sole purpose of improving your personal comfort.

General Inspection

General inspection may begin in the waiting room or as the child enters the examining room. The temperature, weight, length or height, and head circumference (up to age 2 years) are usually obtained earlier. Offer toys or paper and crayons to entertain the child, to develop rapport, and to evaluate development and neurologic status. The parent should have already completed a developmental screening questionnaire to provide information about the child's language, motor coordination, and social skills. Evaluate mental status as the child interacts with you and with the parent. Take seriously and investigate any sense of possible stress in the parent–child relationship and any parental report of a developmental issue.

The following sequence is a guideline. Take advantage of opportunities the child presents during the examination to make your observations. You will find that the sequence of examination may vary with each child (Box 24-6).

Child Playing

The child playing on the floor offers an opportunity to evaluate both the musculoskeletal and neurologic systems while developing a rapport with the child (Fig. 24-18).

FIGURE 24-18 Provide toys or other items to observe the child's development.

FIGURE 24-19 Young children can also be examined on the parent's lap.

- Observe the child's spontaneous activities.
- Ask the child to demonstrate some skills: turning pages in a book, building block towers, drawing geometric figures, or coloring.
- Evaluate gait, jumping, hopping, and range of motion.
- Muscle strength: Observe the child climbing on the parent's lap, stooping, and recovering.

Child on Parent's Lap

The parent's lap is a fine and helpful examining table. Begin with the child sitting and undressed except for the diaper or underpants (Fig. 24-19).

Upper Extremities.

- Inspect arms for movement, size, shape, and skin lesions. Observe use of the hands; inspect hands for number and configuration of fingers and palmar creases.
- Palpate radial pulses.
- Elicit biceps and triceps reflexes when the child cooperates.
- Take blood pressure at this point or later, depending on child's comfort with the examination.

Lower Extremities. Child may stand for much or part of the examination.

- Inspect legs for movement, size, shape, alignment, and lesions.
- Inspect feet for alignment, longitudinal arch, and number of toes.
- Palpate dorsalis pedis pulse.
- Elicit plantar reflex and, if cooperative, the Achilles and patellar reflexes.

FIGURE 24-20 Inspect and palpate the child's head and neck.

FIGURE 24-21 Examine the child while standing and bending to touch the toes.

FIGURE 24-22 In some children, it is better to postpone the use of instruments until the end of the examination.

Head and Neck.
+ Inspect head (Fig. 24-20):
    + Inspect shape, hairline, and hair.
    + Inspect eyelids, palpebral folds, conjunctivae, sclerae, and irides.
    + Inspect position of auricles.
+ Palpate the skull for irregularities and depressions; hair for texture.
+ Inspect neck for alignment, webbing, and voluntary movement.
+ Palpate neck noting trachea and its position, thyroid, muscle tone, and lymph nodes.

Chest, Heart, and Lungs.
+ Inspect the chest for respiratory movement, size, shape, precordial movement, deformity, and nipple and breast development.
+ Palpate the anterior chest, locate the point of maximal impulse; note tactile fremitus in the talking or crying child.
+ Auscultate the anterior, lateral, and posterior chest for breath sounds; count respirations.
+ Auscultate all cardiac listening areas for S1 and S2, splitting, and murmurs; count apical pulse.

Child Relatively Supine, Still on Lap, Diaper Loosened
+ Inspect abdomen.
+ Auscultate for bowel sounds.
+ Palpate the abdomen. Identify size of the liver and any other palpable organs or masses.
+ Percuss the abdomen.
+ Palpate the femoral pulses, compare to radial pulses.
+ Palpate for inguinal lymph nodes.
+ Inspect the external genitalia.
+ Males: Palpate scrotum for descent of testes and other masses.

Child Standing
+ Inspect spinal alignment as the child bends slowly forward to touch toes (Fig. 24-21).
+ Observe posture from anterior, posterior, and lateral views.
+ Observe gait.

Child Returns to Parent's Lap
Reduce the child's fear of the funduscopic, otoscopic, oropharyngeal examinations by permitting the child to handle the instruments, "blow out" the light, or use them on a doll or the parent. Attempt to gain the child's cooperation, even if it takes more time (Fig. 24-22). If successful in gaining cooperation future visits will be more pleasant for the child and for you. Only as a last resort restrain the child for these examinations. After finishing these preliminary maneuvers, perform the following:
+ Inspect the eyes: pupillary light reflex, red reflex, corneal light reflex, and extraocular movements. Vision screening with the Snellen E or HOTV chart should begin by about age 3 years (see Chapter 11, pp. 221-222).
+ Perform funduscopic examination.
+ Perform otoscopic examination.
+ Evaluate hearing.
+ Inspect nasal mucosa.
+ Inspect mouth and pharynx.

By the time the child is school age, it is usually possible to use an examination sequence very similar to that for adults.

❀ Pregnant Women
Pregnancy requires frequent abdominal and pelvic evaluation to assess the mother's status and fetal well-being. Late in pregnancy the woman may find it difficult to assume the supine position without experiencing hypotension. Ask for this position only when necessary, and provide alternatives by elevating the backrest or by supplying pillows to allow the side-lying position. Abdominal assessment is more comfortable for the woman and more

accurate if the bladder is empty. Urinary urgency and frequency are common during pregnancy.

The baseline physical examination is important. A healthy woman may not have had a recent examination before becoming pregnant. Baseline vital signs, height, current weight, and prepregnancy weight should be recorded. The examination may be performed in the same sequence used for other adults with special attention paid to the abdomen and pelvic examination. All physical findings that may be significant later in pregnancy or potentially affect the fetus should be addressed and documented (e.g., cervical abnormalities, hyperthyroidism, cardiac problems, hypertension, and infections) (Gregory et al, 2012).

⚘ Older Adults

Physical examination of the older adult may require some changes from the usual adult process. Patients who are older and/or frail have difficulty assuming the lithotomy and knee-chest positions. Some patients will need a little extra assistance from you, but sometimes an alternate position is required (see Chapter 18, pp. 447-449). The quality of clinical data is not compromised with these changes. Your skill and patience are far more important in ensuring accuracy. A hurried pace or impatience may fluster or confuse an older patient. In neurologic testing, reaction time may be longer or may require more intense stimuli.

Functional assessment (see Chapter 1, p. 19) is an essential examination of every older adult, whether it is one who is well or is not coping well in the community environment. Consider how the patient walks, follows instructions, undresses, and maneuvers to the examining table. This tells you about mobility, balance, fine motor skills (e.g., unbuttoning clothes), and range of motion, as well as some clues about perceptual abilities and mental status. Some older adults have a variety of conditions that suggest poor health. For many, the bottom line is not a physical defect, but something else that gets in the way of successful daily living.

That "something else" may be perceptions of ill health that may suggest physical disease when another problem exists. Examples include the loss or impairment of a significant relationship (e.g., illness, death, divorce, or just moving to a new city), inadequate understanding about one's problems, poor self-image, or substance abuse. Secondary gains from complaining (e.g., indulgent family response by providing extra comforts or attention, or distraction from other problems) may also be involved.

Functional assessment, then, is the determination of the extent to which patients can deal with the consistent demands of life. This includes self-care activities and daily living activities such as the ability to drive a car, use public transportation, prepare a meal, and even tap the numbers on a telephone. It includes a comprehensive history, physical examination, and social assessment. In particular:

+ Detailed listing of all medications (e.g., prescribed and over the counter drugs, especially hypnotics, sedatives, and laxatives). Try the "brown bag approach." Ask the patient to bring in all medications, prescribed by all health care providers and all nonprescribed medications, including herbs, vitamins, and other complementary and alternative therapies.
+ Review function, including activities of daily living (ADLs), evaluating the degree of independence versus need for caretaker assistance:
  + *Basic ADLs:* bathing, dressing, toileting, ambulation, feeding
  + *Instrumental ADLs:* housekeeping, grocery shopping, meal preparation, medication adherence, communication skills, money management
  + Use of assistive devices for ambulation and function: cane, walker, commode chair, hospital bed
+ Systems review, particularly common geriatric problems:
  + Nutritional status, evidence of malnutrition
  + Urinary incontinence
  + Memory changes, signs of dementia
  + Depression
  + Medication-induced delirium
  + Prior falls or fear of falling
+ Social situation:
  + Identification of caretakers and probable caretakers, including those who maintain the home environment
  + Assessment of caretaker abilities
  + Assessment of financial resources and health insurance, with particular attention to long-term services not ordinarily covered: personal grooming, home care, medication supervision
  + Existence of advance directives and an assigned health care agent (durable power of attorney for health care decisions by a family member or trusted person)
+ Physical examination with particular focus on the following:
  + Mental status with specific attention to cognition, memory, and mood
  + Respiratory examination for dyspnea on exertion
  + Blood pressure for orthostatic hypotension
  + Musculoskeletal evaluation of strength with special attention on ability to independently rise from the bed and a chair
  + Neurologic examination of balance, coordination, gait
  + Skin for signs of decubitus ulcers or venous stasis ulcers

The Closing Discussion

Each interaction with a patient is unique. You will at times be worried, rushed, and tired. Because you are human, you may respond differently to people who will live and to those who are dying, to children and older adults, to men and women, or to persons of different cultural groups. Be aware of your biases and constrain them (see Box 24-7).

You are at the point of organizing the information you have assembled into a usable whole, ready for providing care, caring, and problem solving. Be disciplined enough to pursue complete information, even when the solution seems obvious (because sometimes the obvious is wrong), and courageous enough to make the decision for urgency when the data are incomplete. Following analysis of all findings and initial impressions from the history and physical examination, clinical judgment will guide

Box 24-7 How Are You Doing?

You should constantly assess how you communicated while building the history and doing the physical examination:
- Were you courteous?
- Did you provide comfort?
- Did you connect with the patient?
- Did you confirm your understanding and the patient's understanding of what happened?

Did You at the Start?
- Say "hello," and appropriately greet the patient and others present.
- Introduce yourself and ask others present how they are related to the patient.
- Give attention to everyone's comfort.
- Minimize noise as much as possible.
- Explain your approach to the history and physical examination.
- Assess the patient's approach and understanding.
- Begin with a comfortable, open-ended question, such as, "How can I be of help?"

Did You, as You Talked with the Patient?
- Make it easy for the patient to talk.
- Move appropriately from open-ended questions to specific questions.

- Clarify what was unclear as well as you could.
- Steer the course of the interview unobtrusively.
- Ask one question at a time, leaving time for the answer.
- Offer occasional repetition of what you have heard to let the patient know you are really listening.

Did You, Throughout?
- Maintain appropriate eye contact.
- Sit comfortably.
- Pace the conversation, allowing enough time for the patient's comments, expressions, thoughts, and feelings.
- Empathize when appropriate.
- Restate your willingness to help when appropriate.
- Confirm that you and the patient are allies, working together to find appropriate outcomes.
- Ensure the necessary understandings between you and the patient.

Did You, at the Finish?
- Summarize and recheck for accuracy.
- Ask if there were any other questions or concerns.
- Appropriately indicate next steps.
- Say "thank you" with appreciation and with an appropriate "good-bye."

the identification of the diagnosis or need for additional diagnostic testing (see Chapter 25). Make sure that information is well-documented to ensure competent care to the patient and for protection should there ever be a legal challenge to your care (see Chapter 26).

Summary information is shared with the patient in this health care visit. Follow guidelines for effective communication and partnership with the patient when having this discussion. When bad news must be shared, plan how to do this effectively (Box 24-8).

Serving the whole patient—the physical, emotional, and social needs—demands discipline and flexibility within that discipline. Contrary to the view of some, the building of a history and the performance of a physical examination are still and will remain the heart, soul, and mind of an alliance with the patient.

Box 24-8 The Stressful Moment

For patients of any age and those who support them, certain principles are guides when disturbing or bad news must be communicated. First, turn off your pager and cell phone and arrange a quiet setting as free as possible of ambient noise and distraction.
- If you do not know the patient well, try to involve family members or other trusted persons who are essential for emotional and practical support. Consider their base of knowledge, experience, and understanding of the situation.
- Be specific in all details, providing information in a deliberate flow adjusted to the needs of the patient, allowing time for questions and for frequent repetition whenever necessary.
- Use jargon-free language adapted to the patient's understanding.
- Inform the patient immediately unless, for example, the sensorium is clouded. Otherwise, there is seldom, if any, justification for delay in offering information.

CHAPTER 25

Taking the Next Steps: Critical Thinking

Critical thinking is the process by which the information gathered from the history and physical examination is merged with clinical knowledge, experience, and the current best evidence to formulate the next steps in patient care—development of the diagnostic and management plans. Critical reflection involves thinking through the reasoning for these decisions. This reflection can help you progress from rote decision making to critical thinking.

evolve *http://evolve.elsevier.com/Seidel*
• NCLEX Review Questions

The Clinical Examination

Thus far, we have been concerned with the initial patient interaction, establishment of respectful rapport, and information-gathering processes (i.e., history and physical examination). Organizing, integrating, and analyzing information represent the next step in caring for patients. This process, called *critical thinking*, leads to the development of potential diagnoses, workup priorities, and management plans (Box 25-1). Formulating management plans should occur in partnership with patients and their families. Working with the patient to determine the best course of action is often called *shared decision making* or *patient-centered care*.

Critical Thinking

Assessment, Judgment, and Evidence

Critical thinking involves bringing knowledge of the patient, clinical experience, and decision-making skills together with the current best evidence regarding the issues involved. The best available evidence must be carefully obtained from the volumes of information available in books, journals, and online. Use of evidence in decision making is called *evidence-based practice*.

The first step in critical thinking is to assess what has been learned from the patient and to determine its value and significance. Priorities are then assigned to information that might influence clinical judgment as management plans and clinical impressions are created.

Further assessment depends on health care provider, patient, and family preferences, which may be influenced by feelings, attitudes, and values. By using critical reflection, you can think through your own beliefs, values, cultural practices, and attitudes for potential bias affecting the decision-making process. Clinical impressions help direct further assessment, which must be balanced by advantage and risk to the patient, cost considerations, and use of available resources. Given this as well as the leading diagnoses, a potential management plan for immediate and ongoing care can be formulated using shared decision making.

Problem Identification

A problem may be defined as anything that will need further evaluation and/or attention. It may be related to one or more of the following:

+ An uncertain diagnosis
+ New symptoms or physical examination findings related to a previous diagnosis
+ New symptoms or findings of unknown etiology
+ Unusual findings revealed in the clinical examination or by laboratory tests
+ Personal or social difficulties

Formulate problems as specifically as possible. Identify and list the signs and symptoms associated with each of the patient's concerns as well as abnormalities discovered during the physical examination. This listing of findings, the problem list, is key to developing a complete understanding of a patient's concern. This list is used to form hypotheses based on the available information (Box 25-2). Review the list and note the absence of findings that you might expect in support of your hypotheses. Think through the patient's verbal and nonverbal communication, and determine whether there are questions you may have neglected to ask or information you did not fully understand. Gather additional information from the patient to fill in these gaps. Beware of "red herrings," the bits of information that are distracting and draw your thinking away from central issues (Box 25-3). Critically evaluate unexpected or unusual findings, but do not let them distort full consideration of all you have learned.

After a match between the data (both subjective and objective) and a presumed diagnosis is made, consider the appropriate laboratory or radiologic studies to confirm the diagnosis.

Box 25-1   Steps for Critical Thinking

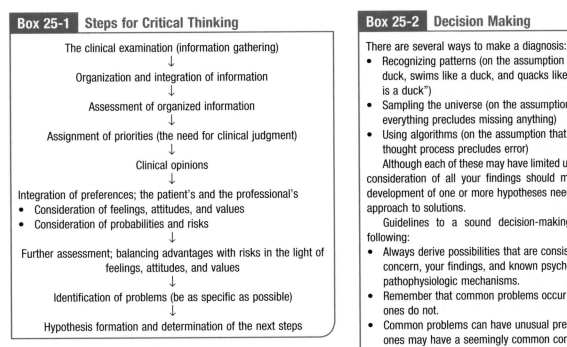

The clinical examination (information gathering)
↓
Organization and integration of information
↓
Assessment of organized information
↓
Assignment of priorities (the need for clinical judgment)
↓
Clinical opinions
↓
Integration of preferences; the patient's and the professional's
- Consideration of feelings, attitudes, and values
- Consideration of probabilities and risks
↓
Further assessment; balancing advantages with risks in the light of feelings, attitudes, and values
↓
Identification of problems (be as specific as possible)
↓
Hypothesis formation and determination of the next steps

Box 25-2   Decision Making

There are several ways to make a diagnosis:
- Recognizing patterns (on the assumption that "If it walks like a duck, swims like a duck, and quacks like a duck—it most likely is a duck")
- Sampling the universe (on the assumption that including everything precludes missing anything)
- Using algorithms (on the assumption that a rigidly defined thought process precludes error)

Although each of these may have limited use in specific situations, consideration of all your findings should most often result in the development of one or more hypotheses needing an evidence-based approach to solutions.

Guidelines to a sound decision-making process include the following:
- Always derive possibilities that are consistent with the chief concern, your findings, and known psychosocial and pathophysiologic mechanisms.
- Remember that common problems occur commonly, and rare ones do not.
- Common problems can have unusual presentations and rare ones may have a seemingly common concern.
- Rare problems that have an available treatment should be considered.
- Do not rush to a diagnosis with no available treatment, and do not pursue a line of reasoning that will not alter your course of action.
- Do not undertake procedures that are not related to your hypotheses.
- Always consider potential harm and cost as well as benefit when determining the need for a test or action.
- Consider whether the risk is worth the potential gain in information, invoking the ethical principle of nonmaleficence; *Primum non nocere:* "first, do no harm."
- Recognize that your leading hypotheses may not be valid. Remain open in your thinking and be ready to discard or modify your hypotheses when necessary; avoid the tendency to discount information that may invalidate your favorite thoughts.
- Try to have a single process explain all or most of your data, but do not be rigid in this regard. After all, a patient with many concerns and problems may have more than one disease; two common diseases may occur simultaneously more often than one rare disease alone.
- Probability and utility should always be your guides to sequencing your actions unless a life-threatening situation exists. A conscientious estimate of probability is the best way to define the limits of uncertainty and the best way to establish priorities.

Specialty consultation may be needed before establishing the diagnosis.

Valid Hypotheses

Critical thinking allows you to consider and discard the variety of possible diagnoses—from the common to the rare—before settling on the best match between the patient's signs and symptoms and a specific disorder. It has been said (Kopp, 1997) that there are at least three diagnoses for every disease: the one that unifies what you have learned, the one you cannot afford to miss, and the one that it actually is. Sometimes they are the same one, but usually not. Do not be hasty. Do not let first thoughts narrow the focus of questions during the interview. In other words, do not jump to conclusions.

One of the clichés of clinical practice is that all findings should be unified into one diagnosis, Occam's razor or lex parsimoniae ("law of parsimony" or "law of succinctness") (Thorburn, 1918). Although you should strive to look for the fewest possible causes that will account for all the symptoms, this may not always be possible. More than one disease process can exist at one time in the same person, an acute illness can occur in the context of a chronic one, and a chronic disease can cycle through remission and relapse. Carefully chosen laboratory or radiologic studies can often help validate your observations and confirm your clinical impressions (Box 25-4).

Possible Barriers to Critical Thinking

Illness evolves from disease and is almost always multifaceted. Not all of the findings can be explained on a pathophysiologic level because sometimes physical symptoms are inseparable from emotional symptoms. Therefore, avoid being misled into believing that, given a pathophysiologic conclusion, management targeted to that finding will necessarily solve the problem. You must consider the full range of issues—from the physical to the

Box 25-3   Red Herrings

A patient with swollen cervical nodes and fever owns a cat, which had claws, but the patient did not have cat scratch disease. The too-obvious apparent source of the problem, a "red herring," delayed the ultimate diagnosis of non-Hodgkin lymphoma.

| Box 25-4 | "A Patient Can Have as Many Diagnoses as He Darn Well Pleases" |

Hilliard and colleagues have reminded us that common problems happen commonly and even at the same time (Hilliard, 2004). They noted that C.F.M. Saint stated several decades ago that more than one disease may be responsible for a patient's signs and symptoms when he could find no pathophysiologic explanation for the coexistence of hiatal hernia, gallbladder disease, and diverticulosis in one of his patients. That, they added, was the same point made by Hickam's dictum: "A patient can have as many diagnoses as he darn well pleases." It was William Osler, however, who invoked the competing fourteenth-century philosophy of William of Occam: "Plurality must not be posited without necessity." In other words, do not consider more than one diagnosis unless you really have to, and, "among competing hypotheses, favor the simplest one." Thus, we are given the term "Occam's razor" to signify this.

But, suppose Occam's razor doesn't always work. As Hilliard writes, "As the population continues to age—and as diagnostic studies increase in number and sophistication—the dulling of Occam's razor is certain to continue." What are you to think, then? We suggest that you think critically about Saint or Occam and use their hypotheses for appropriate balance as you make your clinical judgments.

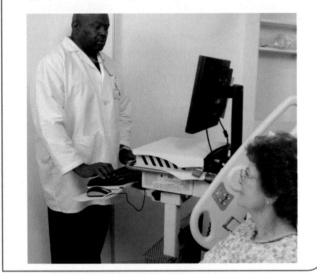

emotional, social, and economic—that might affect the expected outcomes. The pitfall is that in allowing yourself to be lost in physical detail you lose the context of the broader view.

Feelings, Attitudes, and Values. Critical thinking becomes complex because of emotions in both patient and provider. Feelings, attitudes, and values may be strong enough that our decision making may be impaired. If these feelings are to be given a proper context, you must know yourself and take time for personal reflection (see Chapter 2, p. 22 for a discussion of self-awareness). Critical reflection involves thinking through the reasoning for these decisions. The questioning must be relentless: "What is really happening?" "Have my feelings overtaken logic?" "Have ethical concepts been ignored?" "What are the issues that matter?" "What should take precedence?" "Do I understand my contribution to the interaction?" "Do I understand the patient?" "How do I feel about all this?" "How does the patient feel about it?"

The Ethical Context. Ethics does not provide answers. Consideration of ethical principles provides the framework for respectful, flexible discussion and disciplined approach to decision making. For example, given a problem, a perceived necessary violation of confidentiality, several concepts must be considered.

- *Autonomy:* The patient's need for self-determination. Autonomy suggests that choices exist and a patient may choose between alternatives. Uncertainty exists when the patient is a child or is in some way impaired. Parents, guardians, family, or other significant persons may then be included, and the boundaries of that participation must be clearly set, sometimes by an advance directive from the patient. Competency is not always easily determined, and there may be disagreement. Both the mental status examination (see Chapter 5) and consultation with individuals who know the person well can assist.
- *Beneficence:* Do good for the patient. This may be too eagerly pursued and may result in a paternalism that might smother autonomy. "Father" or "mother" may sometimes know best, but not always. However, paternalism need not be a "no-no" when used with constraint and respect for autonomy.
- *Nonmaleficence:* Do no harm to the patient.
- *Utilitarianism:* Consider appropriate use of resources with concern for the greater good of the larger community.
- *Fairness and justice:* Recognize the balance between autonomy and competing interests of the family and community.
- *Deontologic imperatives:* Our responsibilities for offering care are established by tradition and in cultural contexts. Because cultures vary, these may not be universally binding.
- Ethical principles can come into conflict in any given circumstance. If it is difficult to make a decision, consider the following:
  - Is the problem one of ethics and not of poor communication, internal family conflict, money problems, legal confusion, or cultural or personality conflict?
  - Are the facts clearly stated and the attitudes of patients and/or their representatives clearly communicated?
  - Is there a reasonable chance for a satisfactory health or medical care outcome?

In the end, the patient's point of view might well prevail without a compelling argument to do otherwise.

Mechanism and Probabilism. Mechanistic (deterministic) thinking is governed by a sense that knowledge must be certain and not subject to attributes of the observer. Knowledge is to be free of belief, attitudes, and values. Our decision making must have a balance between mechanism and probabilism (certainty in knowledge is impossible). There are variables in the decision-making process such as the individual patient, our age and experience, and fatigue. Accepting the inevitability of probability simply recognizes that the certainty of truth, whatever that may be, is hard to achieve. Why is this so?

- Causes may act or interact differently at different times.
- The same effect may not always have the same cause.
- The effect of a given cause cannot be isolated with certainty.

Causes, effects, and our interpretations of them change probabilistically with time. They involve uncertainty, conjecture, and chance. Dependence on the purely scientific and technical offers an unrealistic comfort (Box 25-5). Acknowledging this may be viewed as gambling. A high probability diminishes uncertainty; a low probability does not.

Do not be dominated by the mechanistic assumption that there is a precise and discoverable cause for every event. Make judgments on the basis of well-informed probabilities and recognize the complexity of the decision-making process. Critical thinking does not require a compulsive listing of all of the possible options in diagnosis and management. Rather, it is dominated by hypothesis development; asking whether a particular diagnosis should be made depending on its probability; and whether a test may be indicated, depending on the likelihood suggested by its sensitivity and specificity.

Validity of the Clinical Examination

We practice in a time when there is considerable effort to reduce health care cost. Recognize that the majority of diagnoses can be achieved with information from a competent history and physical examination, and then limit indiscriminate use of unnecessary technology.

Keep the following definitions in mind (see Fig. 25-1):

+ Sensitivity: the ability of an observation to identify correctly those who have a disease
+ Specificity: the ability of an observation to identify correctly those who do not have the disease
+ True positive: an expected observation that is found when the disease characterized by that observation is present
+ True negative: an expected observation that is not found when the disease characterized by that observation is not present
+ False positive: an observation made that suggests a disease when that disease is not present
+ False negative: an observation that suggests a disease is not present when in fact it is (e.g., absence of cough or respiratory findings when lung cancer is present). Positive predictive value: the proportion of persons with an observation characteristic of a disease who have it (e.g., when an observation is made 100 times, and on 95 of those occasions that observation proves to be consistent with the ultimate diagnosis, the positive predictive value of the observation is 95%)
+ Negative predictive value: the proportion of persons with an expected observation who ultimately prove not to have the expected condition (e.g., if 100 observations are made expecting a disease, and 95 times that observation is not found and the condition proves not to have been the diagnosis, the negative predictive value of the observation is 95%)

Bayes Theorem

As a critical thinker, you will discover that the likelihood of your diagnosis being related to your findings depends on:

1. The probability of those findings being associated with that diagnosis
2. The prevalence of both that particular diagnosis and that combination of findings in the community in which you are serving

---

> ### Box 25-5 The Electronic Environment
>
> The electronic environment provides remarkable resources. Patients now come to health care providers with a wealth of information, myths that need to be demystified, and false information. The Internet can be a terrific source of patient education information but knowing which websites have accurate and valid information is challenging. It can remind you about unrecognized diagnostic possibilities and can place all the patient information at your fingertips. Still, it can be considered a threat. There is an unacceptable temptation at times to substitute electronic support for critical thinking and judgment. As sophisticated and accessible as the electronic environment has become, the most advanced software coupled with the sleekest hardware still has no sense of the subtleties of the human dimension. It is your responsibility to artfully merge subjective and objective data with best evidence, and your knowledge and experience to make a clinical judgment.

	Has disease	Does not have disease	
Test positive	True positive (TP)	False positive (FP)	Positive Predictive Value (people with positive test who have disease) (TP/ (TP+ FP)
Test negative	False negative (FN)	True negative (TN)	Negative Predictive Value (people with negative test who do NOT have disease) (TN/ (TN + FN)
	Sensitivity: people with disease who test positive (true positive rate) TP/ (TP = FN)	Specificity: people without disease who test negative (true negative rate) TN/ (FP + TN)	

FIGURE 25-1 Sensitivity and specificity, true positive/negative, and positive/negative predictive values.

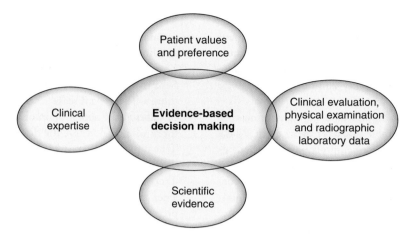

FIGURE 25-2 Evidenced-based decision making.

These considerations have been formalized as Bayes theorem. This juggling of probabilities is implicit during diagnostic decision making. We do not think consciously of Bayes theorem most of the time, but we are using it at some level all of the time.

We have stressed that diagnostic decision making is generally best served by the development of hypotheses that will provide a disciplined approach to solutions. If you are uncertain about an observation, never hesitate to recheck its validity. That is vital to critical thinking. Much as you strive to be scientific and base what you do on the disciplined principles of science, at times you will make undeniable intuitive judgments. Intuition, however, must be as fully subject to critical thinking as any other aspect of your effort.

Evidence-Based Practice

Evidence-based practice (EBP) is a system that incorporates the best available scientific evidence to clinical decision making, in the care of the individual patient. EBP balances the strength of the evidence, the risks and benefits of treatment (including lack of treatment), and diagnostic tests while integrating clinical expertise. Evidence-based decision making is the intersection of your clinical observations from the history and physical examination clinical expertise, patient values and preferences, and the best evidence (see Fig. 25-2) and translating this decision-making process to critical thinking.

Evaluation and Management Plan and Setting Priorities

You decide what you think is going on (the diagnosis) and what you are going to do about it (the management plan). You often need to investigate further, deciding on which of the available laboratory and imaging techniques you might use and who might help you with them. Having thought critically (using shared decision making), you can arrive jointly at an approach that may include the following:

+ Laboratory and radiologic studies
+ Subspecialty consultation
+ Medications prescribed, equipment (e.g., walker or wheelchair), or assistive technology (e.g., IV pumps, ventilator)

+ Special care (e.g., home nursing, physical therapy, respiratory therapy)
+ Diet modification
+ Activity modification
+ Follow-up visit
+ Patient education

In addition, you need to decide the degree of urgency, the next step, and what underlies the issues in terms of the social, economic, and pathophysiologic considerations. Priorities must be set. The following is only a partial guide:

+ What is the patient's physical condition?
    + Is something going on that overrides every other consideration (e.g., a problem with the central nervous system, heart, kidneys, pain, a change in mental status) and needs immediate attention?
    + Are there abnormal laboratory values or radiologic findings that need immediate attention?
+ What is the patient's social circumstance?
    + Will a job be threatened if there is an absence from work?
    + Are there small children at home for whom no other caretaker is available?
    + Is there available and convenient transportation to and from services and care?
+ What is the patient's economic circumstance?
    + Is there adequate insurance coverage?
    + Is the cost of care going to compromise other areas of the patient's life?

These considerations suggest the kind of critical judgment that helps to set priorities and develop a management plan in collaboration with the patient. Perhaps, without risk, in some cases tests, treatments, or therapies can be delayed. Perhaps, alternatively, there might be a sequence of steps that meets priority needs, some that need to be done now and some that might await the information gleaned from an earlier step or the result of a first therapeutic attempt.

Certainly, the patient's subsequent behavior is a major variable in their health status (e.g., smoking cessation) or therapy (e.g., medication adherence). The patient must be actively and positively involved for an optimal outcome. Does the patient want to take the necessary steps? Behavior change is a process involving progress through a series of stages. The Transtheoretical Model of Behavior Change assesses an individual's readiness to change; (Table 25-1). What is the extent of the patient's commitment and recognition that the benefits of action outweigh any possible disadvantages? What is the patient's ability to sustain the effort?

Developing a sequence for your critical thinking can be facilitated by careful attention to Chapter 26, pp. 628-631, and its consideration of the problem-oriented medical record. Careful attention to recording the findings in the history and physical examination will aid in organizing your thoughts and lead to critical thinking.

Table 25-1	Stages of Change
Stage of Change	**Description**
Precontemplation	Not yet admitting there is a problem behavior that needs to be changed, or not intending to take action
Contemplation	Admitting that there is a problem but not yet ready or sure of wanting to make a change, starting to think about pros and cons for continued action
Preparation	Intending to take action in the immediate future, beginning to take small steps toward change
Action	Changing behavior, overt modification in behavior
Maintenance	Being able to sustain action and working to prevent relapse
Termination	No temptation and confidence in not returning to old behavior
Relapse	Not considered a stage in itself but rather the shift from Action or Maintenance to an earlier stage (Precontemplation or Contemplation)

Prochaska and Velicer, 1997.

CHAPTER 26

Recording Information

After performing the history and physical examination, the health care provider must organize, synthesize, and record the data along with the problems identified, diagnostic evaluation, and plan of care. The information in the patient's record enables you and your colleagues to care for the patient by identifying health problems, making diagnoses and judgments of diagnostic testing needed, planning appropriate care, and monitoring the patient's responses to treatment. The patient's record is only as good as the accuracy, depth, and detail provided. Additionally, as the Electronic Medical Record (EMR) becomes more widely utilized, it is even more critical to maintain standards of documentation excellence.

evolve *http://evolve.elsevier.com/Seidel*
• NCLEX Review Questions

The patient's record is a legal document, and any information contained in it may be used in court and in other legal proceedings, as well as to make health care payment determinations. Your documentation will be read by many individuals (including possibly the patient and family members). It is your responsibility to document the facts of the history and your physical examination findings *legibly* and accurately. All entries should be dated and timed. Recorded information should not be erased. If using a paper chart, make necessary changes by lining out data, leaving crossed-out data legible. Initial and date the changes. When using an EMR, include an addendum to correct or update your documentation. Any portion of the examination that has been deferred or omitted should be so noted, rather than neglecting to mention particular findings. It is appropriate in some circumstances to defer a portion of an examination while stating the reason for that deferral. A clear, exact record of your assessment, an analysis of the problem, and a management plan are vital for communicating with consultants and for your protection in case there is ever a question relevant to your care of the patient.

General Guidelines

It is certainly permissible to take brief notes about the patient's concerns and your findings during the course of the interview and physical examination. It is respectful to request permission and inform the patient you will be taking notes or recording information in the patient's record.

You should record certain data as you obtain it, specifically the vital signs and any measurements. Do not try to record all the details during the visit, because writing or typing must not distract your attention from the patient. Jotting down simple notes should be sufficient in preparation for the subsequent write-up, dictation or EMR entry. This allows you to gather, reflect, and organize all the data appropriately before making the record final. It is essential to complete data recording as soon as possible after the examination while your memory for detail is fresh. Resist going on to other patients before completing the first patient's record. Although this is sometimes unavoidable, you can easily become confused about which patient had a particular finding or even forget to record an important finding.

It is unacceptable to copy other providers' documented work (e.g., history taken, exam performed, or thought processes outlined) and enter it into your own documentation as if you did the work. Text copied from another person's note must always be attributed to the source. Information integrity refers to the dependability of information and is further defined as the accuracy, consistency, and reliability of information content, processes, and systems. This is not only an important concept in a legal proceeding, but is critical for safe patient care. Hospital care is often fragmented, and handoffs and cross coverage prevail. Providers need to be able to trust the documentation upon which they will base clinical decisions at the point of care.

Be concise! Use an outline form to avoid the repetition of phrases such as, "patient states." Avoid the use of abbreviations and symbols as much as possible because meanings may differ among health professionals (Box 26-1 and Table 26-1). Similarly, avoid the use of words such as normal, good, poor, and negative, because these words are open to various interpretations by other examiners.

Document what you observe and what the patient tells you, rather than the conclusions you interpret or infer. Use direct quotes from the patient when a description is particularly vivid. Keep subjective and symptomatic data in the history, making sure none gets woven into the physical findings. Physical examination findings should be the result of your observation and

RECORDING INFORMATION

Box 26-1 — Abbreviations and Acronyms: The Initial Challenge to Reliability

There was a time when recorded histories and physical examinations contained few, if any, acronyms. After World War II, the use of initials began to proliferate. Today, it is a compulsive problem leading to misunderstanding that is at times inconvenient and at times dangerous.

When our interprofessional languages are obscured by acronyms, communication suffers and the safety of patients may be compromised. For example, ROM has many different meanings. The obstetrician uses ROM for rupture of membranes. The pediatrician uses ROM for right otitis media. The physiatrist uses ROM for range of motion. To show you how bad this can get, try interpreting the following statement seen in a hospital chart:

67yo CM who CVA, CABG×2, GERD, CRI on HD, n POD #5 - Ex Lap for MVC with OA, s for WO, & R F C O A W.

Table 26-1 — Prohibited Abbreviations

The Joint Commission has identified "improving communications among caregivers" as a patient safety goal. Certain abbreviations have been placed on a "do not use" list when an error in misreading the abbreviation could cause harm.

When considering the use of initials, abbreviations, and acronyms to get things said and written in a hurry, resist the temptation.

Official "Do Not Use" List[1]

Do Not Use	Potential Problem	Use Instead
U (unit)	Mistaken for "0" (zero), the number "4" (four) or "cc"	Write "unit"
IU (International Unit)	Mistaken for IV (intravenous) or the number 10 (ten)	Write "International Unit"
Q.D., QD, q.d., qd (daily)	Mistaken for each other	Write "daily"
Q.O.D., QOD, q.o.d, qod (every other day)	Period after the Q mistaken for "I" and the "O" mistaken for "I"	Write "every other day"
Trailing zero (X.0 mg)*	Decimal point is missed	Write X mg
Lack of leading zero (.X mg)		Write 0.X mg
MS	Can mean morphine sulfate or magnesium sulfate	Write "morphine sulfate"
MSO_4 and $MgSO_4$	Confused for one another	Write "magnesium sulfate"

The Joint Commission.

[1]Applies to all orders and all medication-related documentation that is handwritten (including free-text computer entry) or on pre-printed forms.

*Exception: A "trailing zero" may be used only where required to demonstrate the level of precision of the value being reported, such as for laboratory results, imaging studies that report size of lesions, or catheter/tube sizes. It may not be used in medication orders or other medication-related documentation.

---

interpretation of the patient's description. For example, when a patient reports pain (a symptom) during palpation, you should note tenderness (a sign) in the record, and report the patient's reaction to pain, such as crying, withdrawal, rigid posturing, or facial expression. Record expected and unexpected findings; both what the patient tells you and what you observe. Detectable changes can then be better compared and documented in the future. Clues about health changes over time are lost if such details are not recorded in the patient's record.

EMR Replicating Functions

Although potentially being a very effective tool, the ability to easily copy and paste or carry forward (CPCF) text from one note to another has become the latest hazard in electronic medical documentation (Box 26-2). Whereas legibility is no longer an issue with electronic records, copy and paste is now looming as the greatest patient safety, legal, and regulatory challenge for EMRs. When CPCF is used inappropriately (Box 26-3), it can impact patient safety by rendering meaningless an essential communication tool relied upon at the point of care. Any copied information must be verified, and subsequently edited or removed if necessary, to ensure that it is not erroneous or out of date. Text copied from another health care professional's note must always be attributed to the source.

Organization of the Note

Most health care providers use a customary organization of information from the interview and physical examination. Health care facilities often incorporate the information in standardized

---

Box 26-2 — Use and Misuse of CPCF

Although text replication is generally discouraged, it can improve efficiency, decrease information drop-off, and decrease typing errors, and thus there may be some uses that are potentially acceptable.

Potentially Acceptable Uses of CPCF

1. The author's previously documented assessment and plan on a given patient that has carried forward to subsequent notes, subject to editing for relevance and accuracy.
2. Auto populated, presumably static information (e.g., PMH and FH) entered by other providers and carried forward into new documents, subject to confirmation and editing if needed
3. Cumulative, dated information that carries forward to create a running log of daily hospital events
4. Copying and pasting important lists or information (e.g., medication lists), which can prevent potential clinically relevant retyping errors

Unacceptable Uses of CPCF

1. Copying previous providers' documented work (e.g., history, exam, or thought processes) and entering it into a new note unedited (or minimally edited) as if the new author did the work
2. Unedited text carried forward from other notes (including the author's) that results in conflicting or inaccurate information
3. Unedited or minimally edited notes carried forward from day to day that do not allow readers to determine changes in clinical course

RECORDING INFORMATION

Box 26-3 | **Implications of Misuse of CPCF**

1. Copying subjective information obtained by other providers without appropriate editing degrades patient narratives, which form the basis for complex decision making.
2. Perpetuation of inaccurate data or diagnoses cloned from previous notes can result in poor patient care decisions.
3. Incorporating (or not removing) redundant or irrelevant information lengthens the document, dwarfs the information that is most important at the time, and makes it difficult to determine what is old and new. When urgent information is needed at the point of care, patient safety can suffer.
4. Unless edited and reorganized daily, copied assessments and plans may not reflect changes in a patient's status or clinical course (e.g., "pulmonary" is always on top though may not be currently relevant); in handwritten notes, providers usually filter and organize pieces of information that are most relevant to the patient's care at the time.
5. When providers authenticate their notes containing large amounts of text from previous providers, it can appear as though they did not do the work (e.g., take the history, formulate the plan) themselves. Attributing authorship to parts of a note that one did not create is not only unethical, it can result in mistrust of the entire document by the legal system and be considered fraud by payers and regulators such as The Joint Commission.
6. When copied text is not edited appropriately, conflicting information or improper time representation can call into question the reliability of the entire note.

Source: The Johns Hopkins Health System: *Guidelines and principles for proper use of the EMR*, 2013.

---

forms or templates within an EMR. Following this customary outline of information enables all providers in an integrated system to find and use the patient information more efficiently. The problem-oriented medical record (POMR) with SOAP (**S**ubjective, **O**bjective, **A**ssessment, and **P**lan) notes is one such system. The POMR can also be created in the APSO (**A**ssessment, **P**lan, **S**ubjective, and **O**bjective) format.

Organizing the Patient's Health Record with SOAP Notes

S Subjective data—the information, including the absence or presence of pertinent symptoms, that the patient tells you

O Objective data—your direct observations from what you see, hear, smell, and touch

A Assessment—your interpretations and conclusions, your rationale, the diagnostic possibilities, and present and anticipated problems

P Plan—diagnostic testing, therapeutic modalities, need for consultants, and rationale for these decisions

Subjective Data

Subjective data are the information that patients offer about their condition.

Describe the patient's concerns or unexpected findings by their quality or character. For example, indicating the presence

of pain without providing characteristics (e.g., timing, location, severity, and quality) is not useful, either for determining the extent of the present problem or for future comparison. Record the severity of pain using the patient's response or score on a pain scale. Be sure to name the pain scale in the record. The severity of pain may also be described by its interference with activity. Note whether the patient is able to continue regular activity despite pain or whether it is necessary to decrease or stop all activity until pain subsides (see Chapter 4, Vital Signs and Pain Assessment). Similar detail should be provided for other signs. A very useful way to record expected findings is to indicate the absence of symptoms (e.g., "no vomiting, diarrhea, or constipation").

Objective Data

Objective data are the findings resulting from direct observation—what you see, hear, and touch.

Relate physical findings to the processes of inspection, palpation, auscultation, and percussion, making clear the process of detection so confusion does not occur. For example, "no masses on palpation" may be stated when recording abdominal findings. Include details about expected objective findings, such as "tympanic membranes pearly gray, translucent, light reflex and bony landmarks present, mobility to positive and negative pressure bilaterally." Also provide an accurate description of unexpected objective findings. Suggestions for recording the character and quality of objective findings follow.

Location of Findings. Use topographic and anatomic landmarks to add precision to your description of findings. Indicating the liver span measurement at the midclavicular line enables future comparison, because measurement at this location can be replicated. The location of the apical impulse is commonly described by both a topographic landmark (the midsternal line) and an anatomic landmark (a specific intercostal space); for example, "the apical impulse is 4 cm from the midsternal line at the fifth intercostal space."

In some cases, location of a finding on or near a specific structure (e.g., tympanic membrane, rectum, vaginal vestibule) may be described by its position on a clock. It is important that others recognize the same landmarks for the 12-o'clock reference point. For rectal findings use the anterior midline, and for vaginal vestibule findings (e.g., Bartholin glands, episiotomy scar) use the clitoris.

Incremental Grading. Findings that vary by degrees are customarily graded or recorded in an incremental scale format. Pulse amplitude, heart murmur intensity, muscle strength, and deep tendon reflexes are findings often recorded in this manner. In addition, retinal vessel changes and prostate size are sometimes graded similarly. See the chapters in which these examination techniques are discussed for the grading system used to describe the findings.

Organs, Masses, and Lesions. For organs, any type of mass (e.g., an enlarged lymph node), or skin lesion, describe the following characteristics noted during inspection and palpation:

- Texture or consistency: smooth, soft, firm, nodular, granular, fibrous, matted
- Size: recorded in centimeters on two dimensions, plus height if the lesion is elevated. Future changes in the lesion size can then be accurately detected. (This is more precise than comparing the lesion's size to fruit or nuts, which have different dimensions.)
- Shape or configuration: annular, linear, tubular, elliptical
- Mobility: moves freely under skin or fixed to overlying skin or underlying tissue
- Tenderness
- Induration
- Heat
- Color: hyperpigmentation or hypopigmentation, redness or erythema, or the specific color of the lesion
- Location
- Other characteristics, for example, oozing, bleeding, discharge, scab formation, scarring, excoriation

Discharge. Regardless of the site, describe discharge by color and consistency (e.g., clear, serous, mucoid, white, green, yellow, purulent, bloody, or sanguineous), odor, and amount (e.g., minimal, moderate, copious).

Illustrations

Drawings can sometimes provide a better description than words and should be used when appropriate. You do not have to be an artist to communicate information. Illustrations are particularly useful in describing the origin of pain and where it radiates and the size, shape, and location of a lesion (Fig. 26-1). Stick figures are useful to compare findings in extremities, such as pulse amplitude and deep tendon reflex response (Fig. 26-2). Photographs included in the chart can provide very useful information, though you need to be aware of any institutional consent policies that apply to this practice.

FIGURE 26-1 Illustration of the location of a breast mass.

FIGURE 26-2 Illustration of a stick person.

Problem-Oriented Medical Record

The POMR is a commonly used process to organize patient data gained during the history and physical examination. After the history and physical examination are completed, the POMR provides a format for collecting and recording your thoughts that assists with critical thinking and clinical decision making—determining the patient's problems as well as the possible and probable diagnoses.

After the subjective and objective data are documented, along with the problems identified, the diagnostic and therapeutic plan is made with the patient as a full participant. The written record describes plans made and actions taken to address these problems, lists the information and education provided to the patient, and describes the patient's response to care provided.

The record must be well organized and written precisely, legibly, and concisely to facilitate your thinking and the thinking of your colleagues who may need to care for the patient. The consistent recording format enables more effective communication and coordination among professionals caring for the patient.

There are six components of the POMR:
- Comprehensive health history
- Complete physical examination
- Problem list
- Assessment and plan
- Baseline and problem-directed laboratory and radiologic imaging studies
- Progress notes

Comprehensive Health History and Physical Examination

All relevant data regarding the comprehensive health history should be recorded, including both absence and presence of pertinent findings that contribute directly to your assessment. Arrange the history in chronologic order, starting with the current episode and then filling in relevant background information. Arrange the physical examination findings in a consistent order and style. This allows future readers, and you, to find specific points of information. It also enables you to quickly remember key components for assessment on each encounter.

Make your headings clear, using indentations and spacing to accentuate the organization of your documentation. Be concise yet complete! Avoid abbreviations as much as possible.

Problem List

The problem list is created after the subjective and objective information has been organized. All pertinent data and examination findings, laboratory data, and prior diagnoses are reviewed to develop a problem list in the form of a running log with the following information: problem number, date of onset, description of problem, and date problem was resolved or became an inactive concern.

A problem may be defined as anything that will require further evaluation or attention. Problems arise in many varieties, for example, the questions regarding diagnosis, the availability of diagnostic and therapeutic resources, ethical issues, and factors in the patient's life—social, emotional, monetary or insurance related, work related, school related, family related, and even the availability of caretakers. A problem may be related to any of the following:

+ A firmly established diagnosis (e.g., diabetes mellitus, hypertension)
+ A new symptom or physical finding of unknown etiology or significance (e.g., right knee effusion)
+ Unexpected and new findings revealed by laboratory tests (e.g., microcytic anemia)
+ Personal or social difficulties (e.g., unemployment, homelessness)
+ Risk factors for serious conditions (e.g., smoking, family history of coronary artery disease)
+ Factors crucial to remember long term (e.g., allergy to penicillin)

You may list problems in separate lists, for example, diagnostic issues, care and therapeutic issues, and long-range issues, or you may make one list. The needs of a particular patient and the resources available to you will influence your judgment and your ultimate approach. The nature of the patient's problems determines the sequence in which you list them. Problems may be listed in chronologic order, listed according to the severity of problem, or listed in the order of chronologic presentation. Some controlling variables with regard to the sequencing of listed problems include the following:

+ Possibility that the diagnosis is life threatening and needs immediate attention; the relative gravity of the problem
+ Probability/possibility ratio: priority given to the probable diagnoses or therapeutic actions
+ Likelihood of the probabilities in a differential diagnosis—the more probable taking precedence
+ Availability and cost of the diagnostic, therapeutic, and caretaking resources; cost relative to need and availability
+ Time sequence in which the problems arose and the time sequence dictated by their relative urgency

This list enables all health care providers to quickly assess the patient's history by the summary presented on this list. When a problem is resolved, the date of resolution should be entered and this item can then be removed from the active problem list. Surgical correction of a condition and recovery from an acute infectious process are examples of resolved problems.

Assessment

The assessment section is composed of your interpretations and conclusions, their rationale, the diagnostic strategy, present and anticipated problems, and the needs of ongoing as well as future care—what you think (see Chapter 25, Taking the Next Steps: Critical Thinking).

Develop an assessment for each problem on the problem list. Begin the process of making a differential diagnosis by discussing and giving priority to possible causes and contributing factors for a problem or symptom. Present the rationale for the potential causes and validate the assessment from data contained in the comprehensive health history, physical examination, consultations, and any laboratory data available. When a serious potential cause is no longer under consideration, explain why.

Describe any pertinent absence of information when other portions of the history or physical examination suggest that an abnormality might exist or develop in an area (e.g., absence of wheezing in someone with dyspnea). Avoid the use of words such as "normal" or phrases such as "within normal limits" because they do not describe what is inspected, palpated, percussed, or auscultated. Be as objective as possible. Assessment may include anticipated potential problems such as complications or progression of the disease.

Plan

The plan describes the need to invoke diagnostic resources, therapeutic modalities, other professional resources, and the rationale for these decisions—what you intend to do.

Develop a plan for each problem on the problem list. The plan is divided into three sections: diagnostics, therapeutics (if known), and patient education:

+ **Diagnostics.** List the diagnostic tests to be performed or ordered.
+ **Therapeutics.** Describe the therapeutic treatment plan. Provide a rationale for any change or addition to an established treatment plan. List any referrals initiated, with their purpose and to whom the referral is made. State the target date for reevaluating the plan.
+ **Patient education.** Describe health education provided or planned. Include materials dispensed and evidence of the patient's understanding or lack thereof.

SOAP Notes

The organization of the patient data within the POMR, especially for care beyond the initial evaluation, is often recorded in a series of SOAP notes. Each problem is recorded separately. Subjective and objective data relevant to each problem are clustered together, followed by the assessment and the plan (Box 26-4). Alternatively, all of the subjective and objective data can be recorded in totality. Then the list of problems with the assessment and plan for each are written.

Box 26-4 Governing Principles for Using POMR, APSO, and SOAP

- Record legibly the information you judge is needed; you will write more early in your career, but as time goes by, you will learn to edit with experience and wisdom, especially under the time pressures you will face.
- Organize! Tell the unique story of your patient chronologically and precisely, including positive as well as relevant negative information.
- Use clear headings.
- Precision requires exact description, for example use a tape measure to measure the size of swelling.
- Be terse. An "erythematous" throat may also be described as "red" and a bulge in an "eardrum" is as well understood as "tympanic membrane."

APSO Notes

In the setting of broader implementation of the EMR, one consequence that has occurred is an increased amount of data that can be incorporated in the note. The busy health care provider will be challenged to quickly find the most clinically useful information, the assessment and plan. In the SOAP format one may be required to scroll or click through multiple screens before locating this. With the APSO format the assessment and plan are moved to the beginning of the document, with all remaining data available in the remainder of the note.

Notes from Subsequent Evaluations

Whether it is during each of the hospital days following an inpatient admission (progress notes) or subsequent outpatient visits for episodic illness or preventative care (ambulatory care notes), the encounter is recorded within the medical record. Because there exists in the record an established amount of baseline information, recording of the POMR can be focused primarily on updating information.

An interval history—including subjective status of the problem, current medications, and review of systems related to the problem—is presented in the subjective portion of the note. The objective portion includes vital signs, a record of any physical examination performed at the time of the visit, and results of laboratory data or radiographic studies performed since the last visit.

The assessment section includes your evaluation of the problem status. If the problem was formerly a symptom, such as shortness of breath, you may have enough data to make a diagnosis. The rationale for the diagnosis is presented in this section, and the problems, allergies, and medications list is updated accordingly.

Similar to the comprehensive health history and exam documentation, plans are presented in three components: diagnostic, therapeutic, and patient education.

Problem-Oriented Medical Record Format

The History

The patient's history, especially for an initial visit, provides a comprehensive database. The following organized sequence will guide you in creating a POMR.

Identifying Information. The patient's name, date of birth, and an assigned medical record number are the first items of information recorded. Most health agencies have forms or EMR templates with headings for each category of information to be recorded. This information should be contained on every page of documentation.

Problems, Allergies, Medications, and Immunizations (PAMI) List. Although the PAMI list itself is added to the record after the subjective and objective information has been organized, the printed POMR form provides space for this information at the beginning of the record, where it can be reviewed at a glance by medical personnel. The PAMI list is an ongoing record of a patient's medical problems, allergies with associated reactions, medications with dosages and instructions of how these are administered, and past immunizations. This list should be reviewed, reconciled, and updated with the patient at each visit and when admitted to the hospital.

For each entry, the date of onset or initiation is recorded and space is also provided to record the date that the problem was resolved, the medication discontinued, or the date and route that an immunization was given.

General Patient Information. Additional identifying information for each patient includes address, home and/or cell phone number, employer, position or title, work address and telephone number, e-mail address, gender, marital status, and health insurance status, plan name, and member identification number.

Source and Reliability of Information. Document the historian's identity: that is, the patient or the person's relationship to the patient. State your judgment about the reliability of the historian's information. Indicate when the history is taken from the patient's medical record.

Chief Concern/Presenting Problem/Reason for Seeking Care. The chief concern or presenting problem is a brief description of the patient's main reason for seeking care. The information may be stated verbatim in quotation marks. Always include the duration of the chief concern or problem.

History of Present Illness. This section contains a detailed description of all symptoms that may be related to the chief concern, and it describes the concern or problem chronologically, dating events and symptoms. When describing the present illness, it is important for the examiner to record the absence of certain symptoms commonly associated with the particular area, or system, involved. Also inquire about anyone in the household with the same symptoms or possible exposure to infectious or toxic agents. If pertinent to the present illness, include relevant information from the review of systems, family history, and personal/social history. When more than one problem is identified, address each problem in a separate paragraph. Include the following details of each symptom's occurrence, described in narrative form by categories:

- Onset: when the problem or symptom first started; chronologic order of events; setting and circumstances (e.g., while exercising, sleeping, working); manner of the onset (sudden versus gradual)
- Location: exact location of pain (localized, generalized, radiation patterns)
- Duration: length of problem or episode; if intermittent, duration of each episode
- Character: nature of pain (e.g., stabbing, burning, sharp, dull, gnawing)
- Aggravating and associated factors: food, activity, rest, certain movements; nausea, vomiting, diarrhea, fever, chills
- Relieving factors and effect on the problem: food, rest, activity, position, prescribed and/or home remedies, alternative or complementary therapies

+ Temporal factors: frequency of occurrence (single attack, intermittent, chronic); describe typical attack; change in symptom intensity, improvement or worsening over time
+ Severity of the symptoms: 0 to 10 scale, effect on lifestyle, work performance

Recording the History of the Present Illness: OLD-CARTS. The OLDCARTS mnemonic helps make sure all characteristics of a problem are described in the history of present illness (HPI) to ensure a comprehensive presentation. The order of recording these characteristics does not need to be consistent.

O Onset
L Location
D Duration
C Character
A Aggravating/associated factors
R Relieving factors
T Temporal factors
S Severity of symptoms

Past Medical History. The past medical history (PMH) includes general health over the patient's lifetime, as well as disabilities and functional limitations, as the patient perceives them. List and describe each of the following with dates of occurrence and any specific information available:

+ Hospitalizations and/or surgery (including outpatient surgery): dates, hospital, diagnosis, complications, injuries, disabilities
+ Major childhood illnesses: measles, mumps, pertussis, varicella, scarlet fever, rheumatic fever
+ Major adult illnesses: tuberculosis, hepatitis, diabetes mellitus, hypertension, myocardial infarction, tropical or parasitic diseases, other infections
+ Serious injuries: traumatic brain injury, liver laceration, spinal injury, fractures
+ Immunizations: polio, diphtheria, pertussis, tetanus toxoid, hepatitis B, measles, mumps, rubella, *Haemophilus influenzae*, varicella, influenza, hepatitis A, meningococcal, human papillomavirus, pneumococcal, zoster, cholera, typhus, typhoid, anthrax, smallpox, Bacille Calmette-Guérin (BCG), last PPD or other skin tests, unusual reaction to immunizations
+ Medications: past, current, and recent medications (dosage, nonprescription medications, vitamins); complementary and herbal therapies
+ Allergies: drugs, foods, environmental allergens, along with the allergic reaction (e.g., rash, anaphylaxis)
+ Transfusions: reason, date, and number of units transfused; reaction, if any
+ Mental health: mood disorders, psychiatric therapy, or medications
+ Recent laboratory tests: glucose, cholesterol, Pap smear/HPV, HIV, mammogram, colonoscopy or fecal occult blood test (FOBT), prostate specific antigen (PSA)

Family History. Include a pedigree (with at least three generations). An example is shown in Figure 26-3. If it is not part of the pedigree, include a family history (FH) of major health or genetic disorders (e.g., hypertension, cancer, cardiac, respiratory, kidney disease, strokes, or thyroid disorders; asthma or other allergic manifestations; blood dyscrasias; psychiatric illness; tuberculosis; rheumatologic diseases; diabetes mellitus; hepatitis; or other familial disorders). Spontaneous abortions and stillbirths suggest genetic problems. Include the age and health of the spouse and children.

Personal and Social History. The information included in this section varies according to the concerns of the patient and the influence of the health problem on the patient's life.

+ Cultural background and practices, birthplace, where raised, home environment as youth, education, position in family, marital status or same-sex partner, general life satisfaction, hobbies, interests, sources of stress, religious preference (religious or cultural proscriptions concerning medical care)
+ Home environment: number of individuals in household, pets, economic condition
+ Occupation: usual work and present work if different, list of job changes, work conditions and hours, physical or mental strain, duration of employment; present and past exposure to heat and cold, industrial toxins; protective devices required or used; military service
+ Environment: home, school, work, structural barriers if physically disabled, community services utilized; travel and other exposure to contagious diseases, residence in tropics; water and milk supply, other sources of infection when applicable
+ Current health habits and/or risk factors: exercise; smoking (packs per day times duration); salt intake; obesity/weight control; diet; alcohol intake: beer, wine, hard liquor (amount/day), duration; CAGE (see Box 1-3, p. 8) or TACE (see Box 1-4, p. 8) question responses; blackouts, seizures, or delirium tremens; drug or alcohol treatment program or support group; illicit drugs used (e.g., marijuana, cocaine, heroin, LSD, PCP, methamphetamine) and methods (e.g., injection, ingestion, sniffing, smoking, or use of shared needles)
+ Exposure to chemicals, toxins, poisons, asbestos, or radioactive material at home or work and duration; caffeine use (cups/glasses/day)
+ Sexual activity: contraceptive or barrier protection method used; past sexually transmitted infection (e.g., syphilis, gonorrhea, chlamydia, pelvic inflammatory disease, herpes, warts); treatment
+ Concerns about cost of care, health care coverage

Review of Systems

+ General constitutional symptoms: fever, chills, malaise, easily fatigued, night sweats, weight (average, preferred, present, change over a specified period and whether this change was intentional)
+ Skin, hair, and nails: rash or eruption, itching, pigmentation or texture change; excessive sweating, unusual nail or hair growth
+ Head and neck: frequent or unusual headaches, their location, dizziness, syncope; brain injuries, concussions, loss of consciousness (momentary or prolonged)

FIGURE 26-3 A, Common pedigree symbols. **B,** Sample pedigree for autosomal recessive condition.

- Eyes: visual acuity, blurring, double vision, light sensitivity, pain, change in appearance or vision; use of glasses/contacts, eye drops, other medication; history of trauma, glaucoma, familial eye disease
- Ears: hearing loss, pain, discharge, tinnitus, vertigo
- Nose: sense of smell, frequency of colds, obstruction, nosebleeds, postnasal discharge, sinus pain
- Throat and mouth: hoarseness or change in voice; frequent sore throats, bleeding or swelling of gums; recent tooth abscesses or extraction; soreness of tongue or buccal mucosa, ulcers; disturbance of taste
- Lymphatic: enlargement, tenderness, suppuration
- Chest and lungs: pain related to respiration, dyspnea, cyanosis, wheezing, cough, sputum (character and quantity), hemoptysis, night sweats, exposure to tuberculosis; last chest radiograph
- Breasts: development, pain, tenderness, discharge, lumps, galactorrhea, mammograms (screening or diagnostic)
- Heart and blood vessels: chest pain or distress, precipitating causes, timing and duration, relieving factors, palpitations, dyspnea, orthopnea (number of pillows), edema, hypertension, previous myocardial infarction, exercise tolerance (flights of steps, distance walking), past electrocardiogram and cardiac tests
- Peripheral vasculature: claudication (frequency, severity), tendency to bruise or bleed, thromboses, thrombophlebitis
- Hematologic: anemia, any known blood cell disorder

- Gastrointestinal: appetite, digestion, intolerance of any foods, dysphagia, heartburn, nausea, vomiting, hematemesis, bowel regularity, constipation, diarrhea, change in stool color or contents (clay, tarry, fresh blood, mucus, undigested food), flatulence, hemorrhoids, hepatitis, jaundice, dark urine; history of ulcer, gallstones, polyps, tumor; previous radiographic studies, sigmoidoscopy, colonoscopy (where, when, findings)
- Diet: appetite, likes and dislikes, restrictions (because of religion, allergy, or other disease), vitamins and other supplement, caffeine-containing beverages (coffee, tea, cola); food diary or daily listing of food and liquid intake as needed
- Endocrine: thyroid enlargement or tenderness, heat or cold intolerance, unexplained weight change, polydipsia, polyuria, changes in facial or body hair, increased hat and glove size, skin striae
  - Males: puberty onset, erections, emissions, testicular pain, libido, infertility
  - Females: menses onset, regularity, duration, amount of flow; dysmenorrhea; last period; intermenstrual discharge or bleeding; itching; date of last Pap smear/HPV test; age at menopause; libido; frequency of intercourse; sexual difficulties
  - Pregnancy: infertility; gravidity and parity (G = number of pregnancies, P = number of childbirths, A = number of abortions/miscarriages, L = number of living children); number and duration of each pregnancy, delivery method;

complications during any pregnancy or postpartum period; use of oral or other contraceptives

- Genitourinary: dysuria, flank or suprapubic pain, urgency, frequency, nocturia, hematuria, polyuria, hesitancy, dribbling, loss in force of stream, passage of stone; edema of face, stress incontinence, hernias, sexually transmitted infection
- Musculoskeletal: joint stiffness, pain, restriction of motion, swelling, redness, heat, bony deformity, number and pattern of joint involvement
- Neurologic: syncope, seizures, weakness or paralysis, problems with sensation or coordination, tremors
- Mental health: depression, mania, mood changes, difficulty concentrating, nervousness, tension, suicidal thoughts, irritability, sleep disturbances

Physical Examination Findings

Record the objective data by body systems and anatomic location. Begin with a general statement about the overall health status of the patient. All observations of physical signs should be described in the appropriate body system or region, usually organized in sequence from head to toe. Take care to describe findings in detail rather than make diagnostic statements. The findings generally included in each category follow.

General Statement

- Age, race, gender, general appearance
- Weight, height, body mass index
- Vital signs: temperature, pulse rate, respiratory rate, blood pressure, orthostatic (lying, sitting, and standing) pulse and blood pressure when appropriate

Mental Status

- Physical appearance and behavior
- Cognitive: consciousness level, response to questions, reasoning or judgment, arithmetic ability, memory, attention span; specific mental test scores
- Emotional stability: depression, anxiety, disturbance in thought content, hallucinations
- Speech and language: voice quality, articulation, coherence, comprehension

Skin

- Color, uniformity, integrity, texture, temperature, turgor, hygiene, tattoos, scars
- Presence of edema, moisture, excessive perspiration, unusual odor
- Presence and description of lesions (size, shape, location, configuration, blanching, inflammation, tenderness, induration, discharge), trauma
- Hair texture, distribution, color, quality
- Nail configuration, color, texture, condition, nail base angle for clubbing, ridging, beading, pitting, peeling, nail plate firmness, adherence to nail bed

Head

- Size and contour of head, scalp appearance, head position
- Symmetry and spacing of facial features, tics, characteristic facies
- Presence of edema or puffiness
- Temporal arteries: pulsations, thickening, hardness, tenderness, bruits

Eyes

- Visual acuity (near, distant), visual fields
- Appearance of orbits (edema, sagging tissue, puffiness), color of conjunctivae and sclerae, eyelids (redness, flakiness, fasciculations, ptosis), eyebrows
- Extraocular movements, corneal light reflex, cover-uncover test, nystagmus
- Pupillary shape, size, consensual response to light and accommodation, depth of anterior chamber
- Ophthalmoscopic findings of cornea, lens, retina, red reflex, optic disc and macular characteristics, retinal vessel size, caliber, and arteriovenous (AV) crossings, arteriole-venule ratio, exudates, hemorrhages

Ears

- Configuration, position, and alignment of auricles; nodules; tenderness of auricles, or in mastoid area
- Otoscopic findings of canals (cerumen, lesions, discharge, foreign body) and tympanic membranes (integrity, color, bony landmarks, light reflex, mobility, bulging, retraction), fluid, air bubbles
- Hearing: Weber and Rinne tests, whispered voice, conversation

Nose

- Appearance of external nose, nasal patency
- Presence of discharge, crusting, flaring, polyp
- Appearance of turbinates, alignment of septum
- Presence of sinus tenderness, swelling
- Discrimination of odors

Throat and Mouth

- Number, occlusion, and condition of teeth; missing teeth; presence of dental appliances
- Characteristics of lips, tongue, buccal and oral mucosa, and floor of mouth (color, moisture, surface characteristics, symmetry, induration)
- Appearance of oropharynx, palate, and tonsils; tonsil size
- Symmetry and movement of tongue, soft palate, and uvula; gag reflex
- Voice quality
- Discrimination of taste

Neck

- Fullness, mobility, suppleness, and strength
- Position of trachea, tracheal tug, movement of hyoid bone and cartilages with swallowing
- Thyroid size, shape, nodules, tenderness, bruits
- Presence of masses, webbing, skinfolds

Chest

- Size and shape of chest, anteroposterior versus transverse diameter, symmetry of movement with respiration, superficial venous patterns
- Tenderness over ribs, bony prominences
- Presence of retractions, use of accessory muscles
- Diaphragmatic excursion

Lungs

- Respiratory rate, depth, regularity, quietness or ease of respiration
- Palpation findings: symmetry and quality of tactile fremitus

- Percussion findings: quality and symmetry of percussion notes
- Auscultation findings: characteristics of breath sounds (intensity, pitch, duration, quality), phase and location where audible
- Characteristics of cough, stridor
- Presence of friction rub, egophony, bronchophony, whispered pectoriloquy, vocal resonance

Breasts
- Size, contour, symmetry, supernumerary nipples, venous patterns, lesions
- Tissue consistency, presence of masses, scars, tenderness, thickening, retractions or dimpling
- Characteristics of nipples and areolae (inversion, eversion, retraction), discharge

Heart
- Anatomic location of apical impulse, pulsations
- Heart rate, rhythm
- Palpation findings: thrills, heaves, or lifts
- Auscultation findings: characteristics of S_1 and S_2 (location, intensity, pitch, timing, splitting, systole, diastole)
- Presence of murmurs, clicks, snaps, S_3 or S_4; description by timing, location, radiation, intensity, pitch, quality, variation with respiration

Blood Vessels
- Amplitude, symmetry of pulses in extremities
- Jugular vein pulsations and distention, pressure measurement; jugular vein and carotid artery pulse waves
- Presence of bruits over abdominal aorta and carotid, temporal, renal, iliac, and femoral arteries
- Temperature, color, hair distribution, skin texture, muscle atrophy, nail beds of lower extremities
- Presence of edema, swelling, vein distention, varicosities, circumference of extremities
- Tenderness of lower extremities or along superficial vein

Abdomen
- Shape, contour, visible aorta pulsations, surface motion, venous patterns, scars, hernia or separation of muscles, peristalsis
- Auscultation findings: presence and character of bowel sounds, friction rub over liver or spleen
- Palpation findings: aorta, organs, feces, masses; location, size, contour, consistency, tenderness, muscle resistance
- Percussion findings: tone in each quadrant, areas of different percussion notes, costovertebral angle (CVA) tenderness, liver span

Male Genitalia
- Appearance of external genitalia, penis (symmetry, circumcision status, unusual thickening, color, texture, location and size of urethral opening, discharge), urethral discharge with stripping, lesions, distribution of pubic hair
- Palpation findings: penis, testes, epididymides, vasa deferentia, contour, consistency, tenderness
- Presence of hernia or scrotal swelling, transillumination findings

Female Genitalia
- Appearance of external genitalia and perineum, distribution of pubic hair, tenderness, scarring, discharge, inflammation, irritation, lesions, caruncle, polyps
- Internal examination findings: appearance of vaginal mucosa, cervix (color, position, surface characteristics, shape of os), discharge, odor
- Bimanual examination findings: size, contour, and position of uterus, tenderness and mobility of cervix, uterus, adnexa, and ovaries (size, shape, consistency, tenderness)
- Rectovaginal examination findings
- Urinary incontinence when patient bears down

Anus and Rectum
- Perianal area: appearance, presence of hemorrhoids, fissures, skin tags, pilonidal dimpling, hair tufts, inflammation, excoriation
- Rectal wall contour, tenderness, sphincter tone and control
- Prostate size, contour, consistency, mobility
- Color and consistency of stool

Lymphatic System
- Presence of lymph nodes in head, neck, submandibular, supraclavicular, infraclavicular, epitrochlear, axillary, or inguinal areas
- Size, shape, warmth, tenderness, mobility, consistency (matted or discreteness of nodes)
- Redness or streaks in localized area

Musculoskeletal System
- Posture: alignment of extremities and spine, symmetry of body parts
- Symmetry of muscle mass, tone, fasciculation, spasms
- Range of motion (active and passive)
- Appearance of joints: presence of deformities, tenderness, crepitus, swelling
- Muscle strength

Neurologic System
- Cranial nerves: specific findings for each or specify those tested if findings are recorded in head and neck sections.
- Gait (posture, rhythm, sequence of stride and arm movements)
- Balance, coordination with rapid alternating motions
- Sensory function: presence and symmetry of response to pain, touch, vibration, temperature stimuli; monofilament test
- Superficial and deep tendon reflexes: symmetry, grade, plantar reflex, ankle clonus

Assessment (for Each Problem on Problem List)

The diagnosis with rationale, derived from the subjective and objective data, is stated. If a diagnosis cannot yet be made, differential diagnoses are prioritized. Assessment includes anticipated potential problems, if appropriate (e.g., complications, progression of disease, sequelae).

Plan (for Each Problem on Problem List)

- Diagnostic tests performed or ordered
- Therapeutic treatment plan, including changes or additions to the established treatment plan, with rationale
- Patient education: health education provided or planned; materials such as websites provided, handouts/pamphlets dispensed; evidence of patient's understanding (or lack of understanding); counseling

- Referrals initiated (including to whom the patient is referred and the purpose)
- Target dates for reevaluating the results of the plan

�֍ Infants

The organizational structure for recording the history and physical examination of newborns and infants is the same as for adults. The recorded information varies from the adult's primarily because of the developmental status of the infant. With newborns the focus is on their transition to extrauterine life and the detection of any congenital anomalies. Specific additions to the history and physical examination follow.

History

Present Problem. For older infants, record information as for adults; however, for newborns include the details of the mother's pregnancy and any untoward events occurring since birth.

Details of Pregnancy. Mother's health during pregnancy, age, specific conditions (e.g., hypertension, diabetes, lupus, seizures, bleeding, proteinuria, preeclampsia); infectious illnesses (gestational month of infection); radiation exposure; medications taken; use of tobacco, alcohol, or illicit drugs

Prenatal care: weight gained, planned pregnancy, attitude toward pregnancy, duration of pregnancy, support from partner and family members

Labor and delivery: spontaneous, induced, duration, analgesia or anesthesia, complications, presentation, forceps, vacuum extraction, vaginal or cesarean section.

Infant's Status at Birth. Birth weight, respiratory status, color, Apgar scores at 1 and 5 minutes if known; newborn's condition and duration of hospital stay, nutrition; congenital anomalies, meconium staining, bilirubin phototherapy, bleeding, convulsions, prescriptions (e.g., antibiotics)

First Month of Life. Jaundice, bleeding, seizures, other evidence of illness

Past Medical History. Birth history represents the newborn's past medical history. Older infants should have general health as well as prenatal and neonatal events added to this category unless this information is directly related to the present problem.

Family History. Focus on the number of miscarriages, number of deceased children, congenital anomalies, and hereditary disorders in the family.

Personal and Social History. Focus on the newborn's and infant's family and household structure, number of siblings, other children in the home, presence of both parents in the home, other adult caregivers, financial stressors, housing situation, arrangements for child care, and mother's plans to return to work.

Growth and Development. Placement of this information is according to the purpose of the examination. For the infant with no growth or development problems, it may be recorded as either history or review of systems, or it may be a separate category. When a problem with growth or development is apparent, the information will be recorded in the section for the present problem. Passing or failing of a developmental screening tool would be recorded with objective data.

Developmental Milestones. List developmental milestones with the age at which they are attained (e.g., holds head erect while in sitting position, rolls over front to back and back to front, sits unsupported, stands and walks without support, first words and sentences, dresses self).

Injury Prevention. List parents' efforts to consistently prevent injuries based on infant's chronologic and developmental age (e.g., use of car safety seat, stair gates).

Diet. Placement of this information varies by health care facility; it may appear in the present illness or review of systems, or it may be a separate category.

Breast-Fed Infants. Note the frequency; use of supplemental formula and vitamin D supplementation; mother's diet, fluid intake, concern with milk supply, any problems with nipple soreness, cracking, or infections; and age weaned.

Formula-Fed Infants. Note the specific formula and preparation method; concentration and amount of water added; frequency of feeding; amount per feeding; total ounces per day; and whether juice, water, or vitamins are given.

Solid Foods. Note the age at which cereal and other foods were introduced; specifics about feeding methods, amount, food preparation; and the response of infant to foods.

Physical Examination Findings

General
- Age in hours, days, weeks, or months; gender; race
- Gestational age
- Length, weight, and head circumference with percentiles; for newborns, percentiles for gestational age

Mental Status
- Infant state during examination (irritable, crying, sleeping, alert, quiet)

Skin
- Color, texture, presence of lanugo or vernix, Mongolian spot, nails
- Presence of hemangiomas, nevi, telangiectasia, milia

Lymphatics
- Visible or palpable lymph nodes

Head
- Shape, molding, forceps or electrode marks
- Fontanel size, dysmorphic facial features, swelling

Eyes
- Red reflex, corneal light reflex, follows object with eyes
- Swelling of lids, discharge

Ears
- Shape and alignment of auricles, presence of skin tags or pits
- Startle to noise or response to voice

Nose
- Patency of nares, nasal flaring, discharge

Mouth
- Palate and lip integrity
- Presence and number of teeth
- Strength of sucking, coordinated sucking, and swallowing

Neck
- Head position, neck control
- Presence of masses, webbing, excess skinfolds

Chest and Lungs

+ Symmetry of shape, circumference
+ Breast swelling or discharge
+ Abdominal or thoracic breathing
+ Presence of retractions (intercostal, supraclavicular, substernal), presence of grunting or stridor
+ Quality of cry

Heart and Blood Vessels

+ Recording as for adults, but with peripheral vascular findings integrated in this section

Abdomen

+ Number of umbilical arteries and veins, stump dryness, color, odor
+ Any bulging or separation of abdominal wall
+ Apparent peristaltic waves

Male Genitalia

+ Appearance of penis, scrotum; position of urethra
+ Location of testes: descended, descendible, not descended, not palpable
+ Urinary stream
+ Presence of hernia or hydrocele

Female Genitalia

+ Appearance of labia, presence of discharge

Anus, Rectum

+ Perforate, sphincter control
+ Character of meconium or stool, if observed
+ Presence of sacral dimple, skin pigmentation or hair tuft

Musculoskeletal System

+ Alignment of limbs and spine
+ Presence of joint deformity, fixed or flexible; integrity of clavicles
+ Symmetry of movement in all extremities, hip abduction
+ Number of fingers and toes, webbing or extra digits, palmar creases

Neurologic System

+ Presence and symmetry of primitive reflexes
+ Consolability, presence of tremors or jitteriness
+ Gross and fine motor development

❈ Children and Adolescents

As during infancy, some adaptations in the recorded history reflect the developmental progress of the child. Such modifications in recording the child's history are discussed next.

History

Past Medical History. Prenatal and neonatal history is less important as the child gets older. Birth weight and major neonatal problems are generally included in the history of an initial examination until the child reaches school age. If a health problem can be related to birth events, more detail is recorded, often summarized from previous records, because the mother's recall may not be as accurate as time elapses.

Personal and Social History. Record how the child gets along with parents and other adult caregivers, siblings, and other children; his or her behavior in group situations; and any evidence of family problems. Include the principal caretaker, parents' relationship (e.g., married, divorced, separated, single parent, foster parent), education attainment of parents, involvement with social service agencies. Describe injury prevention strategies used by family.

For older children, record school performance: grade level, progress, adjustment to school, and parents' attitude toward education. Note any habits of the child, such as nail biting or thumb sucking; note hobbies, sports participation, clubs, and temperament.

For adolescents, add peer group activities, conflicts, relationships, sexual activity, alcohol or illicit drug use, concerns with gender identity and independence, self-esteem, favorite activities, type of job, and potential hazards. This may be summarized with the HEEADSSS tool (see Box 1-12, p. 17).

Growth and Development. For toddlers and young children, list motor skills and language milestones attained, age toilet trained, and age weaned from bottle.

Physical Examination Findings.
The physical findings are recorded in the same format used for adults and infants. Some additional notations related to development include the following:

Mental Status. Record mental status and cognitive development status.

Breasts. For females, record the Tanner stage of breast development.

Genitalia. Record the Tanner stage of pubic hair and genital development as appropriate. Record the sexual maturity rating.

Neurologic System. Findings should indicate developmental expectations of cerebellar function, cranial nerves, and deep tendon reflexes.

❈ Pregnant Women

The organizational structure of the record does not vary from that of other adults; however, information about the pregnancy is added, and some aspects of the examination are modified.

History

History of Present Illness. List the gravidity and parity, last menstrual period, and expected delivery date. Is it a planned pregnancy? Describe details about specific problems such as bleeding or spotting, nausea, vomiting, fatigue, edema, illness, injury, surgery, or exposure to drugs, chemicals, radiation, or infections since conception.

Obstetric History. This additional history category should provide information on previous pregnancies, type of delivery, length of labor, complications in pregnancy, labor, postpartum; weight and gender of newborn; and previous abortions.

Menstrual and Gynecologic History. Age at menarche, characteristics of cycle, unusual bleeding, use of contraceptives, sexual history, most recent Pap smear/HPV test, infertility.

Personal and Social History. In addition to the information usually obtained, include the adjustment to the pregnancy by the woman and her significant other, information about whether pregnancy was planned, acceptance by the father and family, any history of partner violence, and father's role or other support available to the mother and child after delivery.

Physical Examination Findings

Abdomen

*   Status of the pregnancy, fundal height in relation to dates
*   Fetal heart rate, position, well-being, movement
*   Contractions

Pelvic Region

*   Pelvic measurements
*   Uterine size
*   During late pregnancy and labor: centimeters of dilation and effacement, station of the fetus, position of the fetal head or presenting part
*   Leaking of fluid or rupture of membranes

⚕ Older Adults

The organizational structure, again, does not vary from that recorded for other adults. A few modifications in aspects of the history and physical examination are made, as described in the following.

History

Personal and Social History. Describe the community and family support systems. Add the functional assessment of ability to prepare meals, manage personal affairs, and engage in social and other meaningful activities. Identify plans for advance directives and power of attorney for health care decisions.

Physical Examination Findings

General Assessment

*   Extra time to assume positions for physical examination
*   Position modifications needed for specific systems

Mental Status

*   Functional assessment of cognitive function, memory, and reasoning and calculation

Skin

*   Presence of common lesions of older age
*   Turgor, resilience of skin
*   Condition and thickness of nails, especially toenails
*   Character and color of hair, baldness patterns

Chest and Lungs

*   Change in chest shape and percussion tones
*   Effect of chest shape on respiratory status

Heart and Blood Vessels

*   Location of the apical pulse
*   Characteristics of superficial vessels and distal pulses

Musculoskeletal System

*   Posture and muscle mass changes
*   Functional assessment of mobility and muscle strength

Neurologic System

*   Functional assessment of fine motor movements
*   Gait and balance, sensation

Sample Records

Information must be recorded as precisely as possible. Colorful language or expressive metaphors can be used, but select words for the patient's history carefully, because some words may have different implications. Health care providers have commonly used the term *denies* when a patient reports that no symptom has occurred. The term *denies* may imply a confrontational or unproductive relationship. It is better to write either "reports no" or "indicates no" symptoms, statements that more positively record the patient's cooperation in providing needed information.

Inpatient Admission Note

The following is an example of a written admission note.

Identifying Information: R.S. is a 68-year-old man admitted to the hospital on September 3, 2013. The history is obtained from the patient and he is considered to be a reliable historian.

    Chief Concern: "Having a hard time catching my breath."

History of Present Illness

The patient is a 68-year-old man with type 2 diabetes mellitus and hypertension who presented to the Emergency Department on 9/3/13 with 5 days of increasing difficulty in breathing. At that time he began to note increasing difficulty breathing when he would go up the steps in his home. This became progressively worse over the next several days to the point where he was feeling uncomfortable breathing even at rest. In that time he also has been having increasing difficulty sleeping at night, having to prop himself up on 4 pillows and waking up short of breath over the last 3 nights. He had to spend the entire night prior to his admission sitting up in a chair because he couldn't lie down without becoming short of breath. Finally, when he "couldn't talk without losing [his] breath," he called 911 and was transported to the hospital.

    R.S. has no prior history of these episodes, and reports no prior history of cardiac or pulmonary disease. He reports no chest pain. Prior to the onset of these symptoms 5 days ago, he would go for daily walks

with his dog and have no dyspnea or chest pain. He does report swelling developing in his ankles and feet over the last several days. He has also noticed a weight gain over the last several days of about 8 pounds, despite having a poor appetite. As far as he knows, his diabetes and hypertension have been well controlled and he last saw his physician 2 months ago. He has had no cough, sputum production, hemoptysis, wheezing, fever, or chills. He does not report a history of hyperlipidemia or smoking, but does report a family history (FH) of coronary artery disease in his mother and brother.

Past Medical History

Childhood Illnesses: Reports having all "usual childhood illnesses"; unable to recall specific ones.

Adult Illnesses

1. Hypertension—diagnosed in 1999, on medication since 2001 and reportedly well controlled
2. Diabetes mellitus (type II)—diagnosed in 1999, on oral medicine since time of diagnosis. Last hemoglobin A1c 7.2% 2 months ago. No history of retinopathy, nephropathy, or peripheral neuropathy.
3. Hypothyroidism—diagnosed 2003, last TSH (thyroid stimulating hormone) was 1.05 in 2012

Prior Surgery

1. Appendectomy—1950
2. Inguinal hernia repair, left side—1963
3. Sigmoid colectomy for sessile villous adenoma, 1997—last colonoscopy was 2009 and was without pathology

Medications on Admission

Hydrochlorothiazide 25 mg by mouth each day (hypertension)
Lisinopril 20 mg by mouth each day (hypertension)
Metformin 1000 mg by mouth twice daily (diabetes)
L-Thyroxine 100 mcg by mouth each day (hypothyroidism)
Acetaminophen as needed (used rarely for knee pain)
Multivitamin (Centrum Silver) one by mouth each day
No herbal medicines or other over the counter medicines

Allergies

Penicillin: causes hives, no history of anaphylaxis
No known environmental or food allergies

Family History

The patient's parents are deceased. His father died at age 61 of complications of colon cancer. He also had type 2 diabetes mellitus. His mother died at age 72 of a myocardial infarction. She also had an ischemic stroke at age 68. She was a smoker and had hypertension as well as hypothyroidism. The patient has one living brother at age 70 who has coronary artery disease and had a coronary artery bypass graft last year. He also has type 2 diabetes, is a smoker, and has mild chronic obstructive lung disease (COPD). He has one brother who died in a motor vehicle accident at age 20. He had no prior medical problems. He has one sister who died at age 54 of breast cancer, without other medical problems. The patient has three children (two sons ages 46 and 44 and a daughter age 41), two of whom are in good health. One of his sons was diagnosed with hypertension at age 37. There is no other family history of heart disease, diabetes, or cancer. He has no history of anyone in his family having a similar presentation to his current illness.

Social History

The patient was born in Louisville, KY. He completed school through the tenth grade and then joined the military for 5 years. After his military service, he moved to Baltimore and worked at City Marine Terminal for his entire career. He retired at age 60. He was exposed to asbestos and a variety of chemical agents through much of his career, but couldn't specify. He is now retired and spends time with his grandchildren and working on his house.

He was married at age 20. He and his wife were together for 44 years until her death 4 years ago due to lung cancer. He has three children, all of whom live in the area, and five grandchildren, and reports a good relationship with them. He is still grieving his wife's death, but feels that things are getting easier. He lives independently in the same house in which he and his wife raised their children.

He is not currently sexually active and has not been since his wife's death. He has no prior history of sexually transmitted infections. He has never smoked, and he drinks one to two beers a month. He reports that he used to drink heavily during his military service, but has not since that time. He reports no illicit drug use.

The patient does not get regular exercise other than walking his dog for about 30 to 40 minutes each morning. He does not watch his diet as closely as he thinks he should, but does try to avoid sweets because of his diabetes.

Review of Systems

Constitutional: weight as per HPI; no weakness, fatigue, fever, or night sweats
Eyes: He does wear glasses for reading only. He has no blurred vision, eye pain, redness, tearing, diplopia, or flashing lights.
Ears: no hearing loss, tinnitus, discharge
Nose: no nasal congestion, epistaxis
Mouth and throat: wears upper dentures, last saw dentist 4 months ago, no mouth dryness, throat pain, hoarseness
Neck: no lumps or swollen glands, pain, or neck stiffness
Respiratory: as per HPI
Cardiac: as per HPI
Gastrointestinal: No dysphagia, heartburn, dyspepsia, nausea, vomiting. He does report constipation over the last 5 to 6 years, no change recently. No blood in stool or black tarry stool. No abdominal pain, or diarrhea.
Genitourinary: Urinary frequency and nocturia over the last year, 6 times per night. No hesitancy, urgency, dysuria, or hematuria. No penile discharge or pain, no testicular pain. He has not been able to have an erection for 3 years.
Peripheral vascular: no intermittent claudication, no leg cramps
Musculoskeletal: mild bilateral knee pain with extended ambulation, stable over the last 1 to 2 years; no other joint pain, stiffness, swelling, or muscle pain
Hematologic: no easy bruising, bleeding, or history of blood clots; no prior blood transfusions
Endocrine: as per HPI and PMH
Skin: no rashes, dryness, color change, or abnormalities of hair or nails
Neurologic: no headaches, head injuries, lightheadedness, vertigo, syncope, seizures, focal weakness, numbness, paresthesias, tremor, gait instability or falls, or declining memory
Mental health: Despite experiencing grief over his wife's death at times, he expressed no pervasive sadness or worry, and feels optimistic about the future. Prior to this current illness, he had good energy, and reports good memory, concentration, and interest in activities.

Physical Exam

General appearance: This is a well-developed white man appearing his stated age, in no respiratory distress sitting up in bed. He is alert and cooperative with the exam.
Vital signs: heart rate 68 beats per minute, blood pressure (left arm, regular adult cuff) 135/70, temperature (oral) 37° C, respiratory rate 18 per minute, Pain 0/10, Weight 65 kg
HEENT: Head is normocephalic without scalp or facial tenderness. Eyes: Conjunctivae are pink and sclerae are without injection or jaundice. Bilateral arcus senilis is present. Pupils are equal in size and react equally (4-2 mm) to light. Fundi showed sharp disc margins, and arteriole/venous nicking was present. No hemorrhages or exudates seen. Ears: External auditory canals had moderate cerumen (left greater than right). Tympanic membranes were intact and without erythema. Hearing was grossly intact. Nasopharynx mucosa was pink with slight septal deviation from left to right. The oropharynx had no lesions or exudates, and the mucus membranes were moist. Upper dentures were present, lower teeth were in good repair.

Continued

Neck: Trachea was midline, the thyroid was not palpable. Jugular venous distention was present (approximately 9 cm). Hepatojugular reflux was present. Carotid upstrokes were strong without bruits. No meningismus.

Lymph nodes: No cervical or axillary lymph nodes were palpable. Small, shoddy, rubbery, mobile, nontender inguinal nodes were present bilaterally, all approximately 5 mm in size.

Chest: Thoracic expansion was symmetric. There was dullness to percussion at both bases. Diaphragmatic excursion was difficult to assess due to dullness to percussion at the bases. Breath sounds were remarkable for crackles up to the angle of scapula bilaterally. No rhonchi, wheezes, or stridor. No egophony, bronchophony, or tactile fremitus.

Cardiac: Point of maximal impulse is noted in the fifth intercostal space 4 cm laterally from the midclavicular line. Regular rate and rhythm. S_1 normal, S_2 physiologically split. S_3 is present, no S_4. A II/VI blowing, holosystolic murmur was present at the apex radiating into the axilla.

Abdomen: Nondistended, no tenderness to palpation. Bowel sounds were present but hypoactive. No masses were palpable. The liver span percussed to 8 cm and the edge was smooth and palpable 2 cm below the right costal margin. The spleen was not palpable.

GU: Penis and testicles are without lesions. No inguinal hernias are present. Rectal exam had intact tone. Moderately enlarged, firm, symmetric, nontender prostate without nodules.

Extremities: No cyanosis or clubbing. 1+ pitting edema was present in the lower extremities up to the knees and was symmetrical. Peripheral pulses at the dorsalis pedis and posterior tibial positions were palpable and strong bilaterally.

Musculoskeletal: Hands were without joint deformities with good finger curl and wrist movement. Bilateral knees showed mild hypertrophic joint deformity with reduced range of motion in extension bilaterally (to about 160 degrees). No erythema, warmth, tenderness, or effusion. Bulge sign negative. Other joints unremarkable.

Skin: Warm and dry, no rashes. Tattoo present on right shoulder. Well-healed incisions over abdomen in the left inguinal region and right lower quadrant. Hair with male-pattern baldness. No skin or nail lesions.

Neurologic

1. Mental status—Awake, alert and attentive. Oriented in all spheres. Speech fluent and repetition intact, able to point way out of room. Mood is euthymic and affect is appropriate to situation with full range. Thoughts are appropriate; no evidence of disordered thinking.
2. Cranial nerves—II-XII are intact: visual acuity 20/20 with correction, visual fields intact, extraocular movements intact, facial sensation and movement—intact, hearing intact, soft palate—elevates well, tongue protrudes in midline, intact shoulder shrug.
3. Motor—Intact and symmetric; no pronator drift; strength 5/5 in deltoids, finger extensors, hip flexors, and foot dorsiflexion bilaterally
4. Sensory—Intact to monofilament and fine touch, fingers, mid-thighs, toes—bilaterally. Vibratory sense intact of great toes bilaterally. Proprioception in toes intact.
5. Reflexes—2+ and symmetric in biceps and patella. Babinski reflex negative.
6. Coordination/gait—Intact finger to nose bilaterally. Intact rapid alternating movement. Stands and walks 10 feet without difficulty. Romberg negative; tandem walk, heel walk, toe walk intact.

Assessment

R.S. is a 68-year-old man who presents with new-onset dyspnea on exertion, orthopnea, and paroxysmal nocturnal dyspnea of 5 days' duration. His physical exam is significant for the presence of jugular venous distention, hepatojugular reflux, a displaced point of maximal impulse with an S_3 and a holosystolic murmur, and peripheral edema. The most likely etiology for his illness is congestive heart failure. Other etiologies for the progressive dyspnea include pneumonia, pulmonary embolus, pneumothorax, pleural effusion, and pericardial effusion. However, the history and findings are most consistent with congestive heart failure and the absence of fever and constitutional symptoms argues against pneumonia. His physical exam is not consistent with a pneumothorax or pulmonary embolus. He likely does have pleural effusions present based on his exam, but this is most likely secondary to congestive heart failure.

In this patient the most likely explanation for congestive heart failure is coronary artery disease given his multiple risk factors, with the possibility of a silent myocardial infarction in the setting of diabetes. Other etiologies to consider would be primary valvular disease given a murmur consistent with mitral regurgitation, but the rapidity with which his symptoms developed argues against this being the sole answer. He could have a primary cardiomyopathy either from long-standing hypertension, hypothyroidism, or alcohol (although his use is limited, unless he is underreporting his current use). Much less likely would be an occupational exposure such as to heavy metals given his work in the shipyard.

Plan

1. Cardiac: Obtain chest radiograph, complete metabolic panel and complete blood count, and an electrocardiogram.
   - Perform serial cardiac enzyme screening to evaluate for myocardial infarction.
   - Obtain echocardiogram to assess chamber size, valvular and left ventricular function.
   - Give oxygen 2 L/min and begin diuresis with furosemide, 20 mg IV every 12 hours.
   - Monitor intake/urine output, daily weight, and electrolytes.
   - Consider further assessment for coronary artery disease pending results of data above.
2. Endocrine: Hold metformin while in the hospital if contrast studies needed. Monitor finger sticks with sliding scale insulin for glucose control. Obtain hemoglobin A1c and thyroid stimulating hormone.
3. Ophthalmology: Continue current eye drops for glaucoma.
4. Musculoskeletal: As needed acetaminophen for likely bilateral osteoarthritis of his knees.
5. Health maintenance: Consider Pneumovax given diabetes. Consider influenza and zoster vaccine. Up to date with cancer screening.

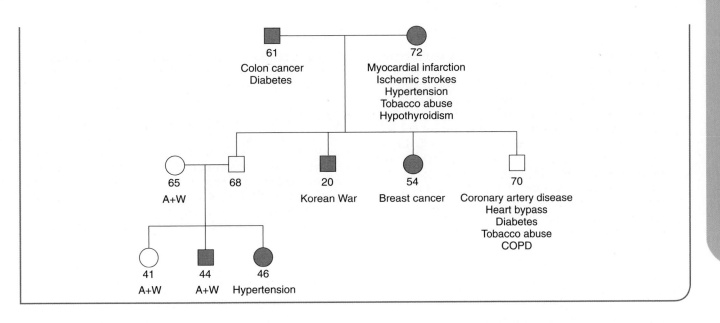

Summary

As you begin to examine patients, it is often difficult to determine how to cluster information that will lead to a diagnosis. As a result, all collected information is initially part of the puzzle. With experience, you will be able to identify appropriate groupings of information, enabling you to better organize and synthesize the raw data. Your first attempts to write a complete history and physical examination will be lengthy and perhaps disorganized, but clinical experience will eventually lead to a more concise and organized record.

CHAPTER **27**

Emergency or Life-Threatening Situations

An emergency situation, whether it is unresponsiveness, an acute medical condition, drug intoxication, or trauma, requires a change in the usual sequence of history taking and examination. Life-threatening conditions, such as airway obstruction, cardiac arrest, hypovolemic shock, and respiratory failure, must be rapidly identified and managed. The steps to complete the assessment for life-threatening conditions take seconds, not minutes. The rapid sequential assessment process focuses on patient physiology to identify priority lifesaving interventions.

In an emergency patients are assessed and treatment priorities are established based on the presenting physiology, with a goal of stability of vital signs rather than on a specific diagnosis. National organizations such as the American College of Surgeons Committee on Trauma and the American Heart Association have defined an approach for the emergency assessment of patients with trauma and cardiac arrest. Using this approach, the patient's vital functions are determined quickly through a rapid primary assessment with resuscitation of vital functions as necessary (see Box 27-1 for the basic life support assessment sequence).

Emergency Assessment of the Injured Patient

The Primary Survey

The primary survey or initial assessment is completed very rapidly. With a stable patient it may take only 30 seconds. However, it may take several minutes when a mechanism of injury or the patient's physiologic responses make you suspect a potential critical condition. The patient history obtained during the primary survey is often limited to the chief concern (e.g., the mechanism of injury). The initial assessment for the patient with an emergency medical condition varies somewhat from the primary survey for the injured patient (see pp. 639-640).

Airway and Cervical Spine. The patency of the upper airway is assessed at the start by asking the patient a question. If the patient answers, the patient is responsive and the airway is

open at this time (Box 27-2). Keep the patient talking so that you know the airway is maintained. Have suction equipment readily available to prevent aspiration in case the patient vomits.

If the patient does not respond, place your ear close to the patient's nose and mouth to detect any air movement (Fig. 27-1). Look for any blood, vomitus, teeth, or any foreign bodies that may be obstructing the airway. Determine if any fractures of the mandible, face, or larynx could be obstructing the airway.

If the airway is obstructed and the patient is supine, use a chin lift or jaw thrust (if any potential injury to the cervical spine has occurred) to raise the tongue (the most common cause of airway obstruction) out of the oropharynx (Fig. 27-2). Do not hyperextend, hyperflex, or rotate the patient's head and neck to establish or maintain an airway. Remove blood, vomitus, or foreign bodies from the airway by suction. Endotracheal intubation is sometimes needed to control and protect the airway.

The cervical spine must be stabilized when performing any airway maneuvers or moving the patient in cases of multisystem injury or trauma above the clavicles. Excessive movement of the cervical spine can convert a fracture or dislocation without neurologic damage to one with neurologic injury. Stabilize the cervical spine by manually maintaining the neck in a neutral position, in alignment with the body (Fig. 27-3). Once the patient's vital functions are more stable, radiologic imaging of all seven cervical vertebrae is often obtained to diagnose the presence or absence of cervical spine injury.

Breathing. Expose the patient's chest to assess breathing effort and to observe for a paradoxical chest movement (entire chest does not rise and fall in synchrony), open chest wounds, and bruising. Note the approximate rate and depth of respirations rather than taking the time to count the respiratory rate. Bilateral chest movement should be synchronized with breathing. Use the stethoscope to auscultate for the presence of breath sounds. Note any signs of respiratory distress such as retractions, tachypnea, and cyanosis. Apply a pulse oximeter if available.

Palpate the upper chest and neck for crepitation, a sign of air leakage into soft tissue. Bruising should alert you to the possibility of a *pulmonary contusion* (bruising of the lung tissue caused by the energy of an external impact transmitted through the chest wall). This injury may result in a pneumothorax.

| Box 27-1 | Basic Life Support Survey for an Unconscious Patient |

First: Check for responsiveness and for abnormal or absent breathing (chest movement).

Second: Call for emergency responders and get a defibrillator if one is available, or send someone to do this.

Third: Check for the carotid pulse for 10 seconds.
- If no pulse, begin cardiopulmonary resuscitation. Perform chest compressions at a rate of 100 per minute, interrupting after 30 compressions to give 2 breaths. Repeat cycles of 30 compressions and 2 breaths.
- If a pulse is present, begin rescue breathing at 10 to 12 breaths per minute

Fourth: If no pulse, use the defibrillator when it arrives to check for a shockable rhythm.
- Provide shocks as indicated.
- Resume cardiopulmonary resuscitation immediately after each shock.

From Sinz and Navarro, 2011.

FIGURE 27-1 Look, listen, and feel for adequate breathing to assess patency of the upper airway.

FIGURE 27-2 Use a chin lift to lift the tongue out of the oropharynx and ensure an open airway.

| Box 27-2 | Assessment of Airway Patency |

Signs of Obstruction
- Hoarse voice and/or cough, sometimes characterized as a "bark"
- Apprehension: tense, deeply worried facial expression
- Stridor: severity related to extent of obstruction and the patient's respiratory effort
  - Inspiratory: obstruction at the glottis, epiglottis
  - Expiratory: obstruction below the glottis (wheezing)
- Retraction
  - Suprasternal notch: obstruction at or above trachea
  - Intercostal and subcostal, below suprasternal notch: obstruction in bronchial tree or below
- Altered mental status
- Drooling (difficulty swallowing): obstruction at glottis or above
- Bleeding from mouth or nose
- Subcutaneous emphysema, particularly with trauma
- Facial or mandible fracture, often palpable

Symptoms of Obstruction
- Respiratory distress: dyspnea, tachypnea
- Difficulty swallowing
- Pain, such as a sore throat
- Cough and associated strain or change in voice
- Behavior change: restlessness or lethargy

FIGURE 27-3 Properly position both hands to stabilize and maintain the head and neck in a neutral position, in alignment with the body.

Provide 100% oxygen and ventilatory assistance with a bag-valve-mask as needed before continuing with the primary survey. Cover open chest wounds immediately with a hand to minimize the entry of atmospheric air into the chest until definitive treatment is available, then apply an occlusive dressing taped on three sides. Paradoxical chest movement may be associated with fractured ribs or a flail chest (a section of the chest is disconnected from the bony structure, as may occur with multiple rib fractures). A flail chest also indicates an underlying lung injury (pulmonary contusion).

Circulation. Adequate circulation is needed to oxygenate the brain and other organs. Circulation can be impaired because of cardiac conditions, hemorrhage, dehydration, and other medical conditions. To assess circulation, note level of responsiveness, the skin color, and the presence, quality, and rate of the carotid or femoral pulses (Fig. 27-4). Use the capillary refill time to assess the adequacy of tissue perfusion. Press firmly over a nail bed or bony prominence (e.g., chin, forehead, or sternum) until the skin blanches. Remove the pressure and count the seconds it takes for color to return. A capillary refill time in excess of 2 seconds indicates poor perfusion unless an extremity is cold. Perform a quick total body appraisal for bleeding sites, being especially careful to look and feel for dampness in dark clothing that may hide hemorrhage. Consider the possibility of internal hemorrhage with some mechanisms of injury. Hypovolemic shock can occur with significant blood loss, either by external bleeding or by internal bleeding into the thoracic and abdominal cavities (see p. 643).

Control visible bleeding with manual pressure before continuing the primary survey, and estimate the amount of blood loss.

A tourniquet around an extremity may be used in cases of extreme bleeding. Replacement of intravascular volume is initiated with warmed intravenous fluids.

Disability. A brief neurologic evaluation is performed to identify significant disability. Assess the patient's responsiveness with AVPU or level of consciousness with the Glasgow Coma Scale (Table 27-1). This tool allows numeric scoring of the patient's verbal, motor, and eye opening responses to specific stimuli to assess the cerebral cortex and brainstem function. Versions are available for the adult, infant, and young child. The Glasgow Coma Scale score is repeated at intervals to detect changes in the patient's level of consciousness. A decrease in the level of consciousness may indicate hypoxemia or hypovolemic shock, necessitating a reevaluation of the patient's ABCs. See Table 5-1 on p. 67 for common causes of unresponsiveness. Additional neurologic assessments to be performed include the pupillary size and reactivity, lateralizing signs, or spinal cord injury level. See Clinical Pearl, "Mnemonic AVPU."

FIGURE 27-4 Check the carotid pulse to confirm circulation, one side at a time.

Clinical Pearl

Mnemonic AVPU

A quick way to initially assess a patient's level of responsiveness is with the mnemonic AVPU:

A Alert: no stimuli needed
V Verbal stimuli: responsive to
P Painful stimuli: responsive to
U Unresponsive to verbal and pain stimuli

Table 27-1   Glasgow Coma Scale

Assessed Behavior	Adult Criteria	Infant and Young Child Criteria	Score
Eye opening	Spontaneous opening	Spontaneous opening	4
	To verbal stimuli	To loud noise	3
	To pain	To pain	2
	No response	No response	1
Verbal response	Oriented to appropriate stimulation	Smiles, coos, cries	5
	Confused	Irritable, cries	4
	Inappropriate words	Inappropriate crying	3
	Incoherent	Grunts, moans	2
	None	No response	1
Motor response	Obeys commands	Spontaneous movement	6
	Localizes pain	Withdraws to touch	5
	Withdraws from pain	Withdraws to pain	4
	Flexion to pain (decorticate)	Abnormal flexion (decorticate)	3
	Extension to pain (decerebrate)	Abnormal extension (decerebrate)	2
	None	No response	1

The patient's best response in each category is matched to the criteria for scoring. Appropriate verbal stimuli are questions eliciting the patient's level of orientation to person, place, and time. Painful stimuli are used when necessary to obtain eye opening and motor responses. Begin with less painful stimuli (e.g., pinching the skin) and progress to squeezing muscle mass or tendons if there is no response. Three scores are summed for the total GCS score. A maximum score of 15 indicates the optimal level of consciousness, and the minimal score of 3 indicates deepest coma.

Modified from Teasdale and Jennett, 1974; and James, 1986.

Exposure and Environmental Control. In cases of trauma, the patient should be as completely undressed as possible to facilitate a brief body search for major injuries that may have been missed during the prior steps of the primary survey. Hypothermia is a concern, so use warm blankets, warmed intravenous fluids, and a warm environment to maintain the patient's body temperature. See Clinical Pearl, "A Reminder for Resuscitation."

Clinical Pearl

Delay Secondary Assessment to Resuscitate

Life-saving measures—chest compressions, airway management, defibrillation, oxygen, assisted ventilation, intravenous fluids, and medications—are initiated as soon as the problem is identified, rather than after completion of the assessment. Once the life-threatening problem is stabilized, the initial assessment can be continued. Only when all vital functions have been assessed and treated is an effort made to identify the cause or diagnose the emergency condition through a more detailed assessment and history.

Secondary Assessment of the Injured Patient

Assess the vital signs before beginning the head-to-toe survey of the body to identify additional injuries. Count the heart and respiratory rates and obtain blood pressure. Monitor oxygen saturation level. Compare the vital sign values for the patient with those expected. Recognize that vital sign values above or below those expected for the person's age may indicate physiologic derangement or preexisting health conditions. Remember, the blood pressure is not a good predictor of tissue perfusion because the patient may compensate for hypovolemia until up to 30% of blood volume has been lost (American College of Surgeons, 2012).

History. Usually someone other than the examiner obtains an abbreviated history from the patient, family, emergency medical technicians, or scene bystanders. Pertinent information is then shared with the examiner during the assessment process. See Clinical Pearl, "Mnemonic AMPLE."

Clinical Pearl

Mnemonic AMPLE

This abbreviated history focuses on information relevant to the emergency condition. Use the mnemonic AMPLE to remember the key categories of this history.

A   Allergies
M   Medications or drugs of any type currently being taken by the patient
P   Past illnesses (e.g., diabetes, epilepsy, hypertension); Pregnancy
L   Last meal
E   Events preceding the precipitating event; Environment related to the injury

---

Identify the mechanism of injury that describes the nature and force of the energy transmitted to the body. Because the mechanism of injury is associated with patterns of injury, it provides important clues about physiologic responses and interventions needed (see pp. 636-637). It is also important to identify potential exposure to hazardous materials, for example, chemicals or toxins.

Head and Neck. Inspect and palpate the face, head, and scalp, looking for any depressions, bone instability, crepitus, lacerations, contusions, penetrating injuries, or drainage from the ears or nose. Clear or amber-colored drainage from the nose or ears may indicate a basilar skull fracture. Use an otoscope to inspect the tympanic membranes for blood in the middle ear. Note any bruising around the eyes (raccoon eyes) or behind the ears (Battle sign), indicating a basilar skull fracture (Fig. 27-5). Assess facial structures for any fractures.

Examine the eyes for pupillary size and responsiveness to light. Examine the retinas and conjunctivae for hemorrhage and the lens for dislocation. A quick visual examination of both eyes is performed by asking a conscious patient to read the words on the side of any container. Extraocular movements are also examined.

Inspect the neck for unexpected findings such as penetrating injury, bruising (e.g., seatbelt mark), and tracheal deviation from the midline. Palpate for deformity and crepitus. Auscultate the carotid arteries for bruits. Be certain that the neck is manually maintained in neutral position until radiographic studies confirm the absence of cervical injury.

Chest. Inspect the anterior and posterior chest for bruising and obvious signs of deformity. Palpate the sternum, each rib, and clavicle. Note pain and dyspnea. Blunt sternal pressure will be painful if any attached ribs are fractured. Patterns of bruising may indicate the mechanism of injury, such as a steering wheel or tire track, and may signal a possible pulmonary contusion.

Auscultate breath sounds at the apex, base, and midaxillary areas. Note any diminished or absent breath sounds, which may indicate a pneumothorax or hemothorax. Auscultate the heart for clarity of heart sounds. Distant, muffled heart sounds may indicate cardiac tamponade, a life-threatening condition; however, heart sounds may be difficult to hear in a noisy environment. Distended neck veins (increased jugular venous pressure) may indicate cardiac tamponade, pneumothorax, or any problem that causes obstruction of the cardiovascular system. However, hypovolemia may prevent distention of neck veins. A tension pneumothorax may manifest with decreased breath sounds, hyperresonance to percussion, and shock. Chest imaging is often ordered to confirm examination findings.

Abdomen. Inspect the abdomen for bruising and distention. Gently palpate the abdomen, noting guarding and pain. Hollow organs in the abdomen are often ruptured with blunt trauma and result in occult hemorrhage; pain and distention may indicate an underlying hemorrhage (see Fig. 27-5). Peritoneal lavage or diagnostic imaging may be performed.

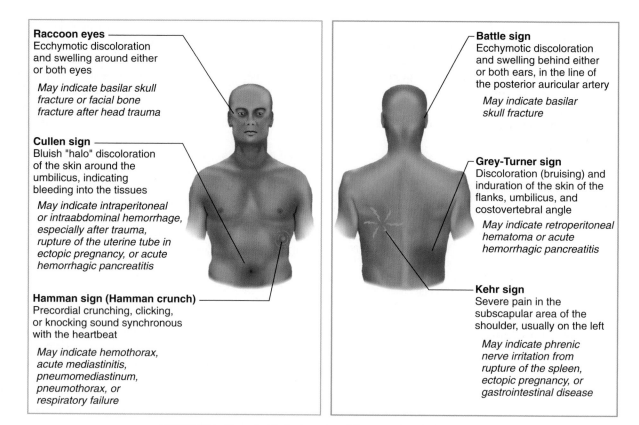

Raccoon eyes
Ecchymotic discoloration
and swelling around either
or both eyes

*May indicate basilar skull
fracture or facial bone
fracture after head trauma*

Cullen sign
Bluish "halo" discoloration
of the skin around the
umbilicus, indicating
bleeding into the tissues

*May indicate intraperitoneal
or intraabdominal hemorrhage,
especially after trauma,
rupture of the uterine tube in
ectopic pregnancy, or acute
hemorrhagic pancreatitis*

Hamman sign (Hamman crunch)
Precordial crunching, clicking,
or knocking sound synchronous
with the heartbeat

*May indicate hemothorax,
acute mediastinitis,
pneumomediastinum,
pneumothorax, or
respiratory failure*

Battle sign
Ecchymotic discoloration
and swelling behind either
or both ears, in the line of
the posterior auricular artery

*May indicate basilar
skull fracture*

Grey-Turner sign
Discoloration (bruising) and
induration of the skin of the
flanks, umbilicus, and
costovertebral angle

*May indicate retroperitoneal
hematoma or acute
hemorrhagic pancreatitis*

Kehr sign
Severe pain in the
subscapular area of the
shoulder, usually on the left

*May indicate phrenic
nerve irritation from
rupture of the spleen,
ectopic pregnancy, or
gastrointestinal disease*

FIGURE 27-5 Signs that indicate serious injury associated with trauma.

Extremities and Back. Inspect and palpate all extremities for signs of fractures or deformities, crepitus, pain, and lack of spontaneous movement. Palpation of the bones with rotational or three-point pressure along the shaft helps identify fractures where alignment has been maintained. Note any wounds over the site of a suspected fracture, the possible indication of an open fracture. Palpate all peripheral pulses. It is particularly important to document skin temperature, capillary refill time, and the presence of distal pulses in extremities with a suspected fracture.

Maintain cervical spine stabilization and alignment of the thoracic and lumbar spine when inspecting the back. Use three persons to log-roll the patient.

Suspect pelvic fractures if bruising is seen over the iliac wings, pubis, labia, or scrotum and by pain on palpation. If the patient is unconscious, an experienced examiner should test for mobility of the pelvic ring by placing gentle anterior and posterior pressure against the iliac wings and symphysis pubis with the heels of the hands. The maneuver is not repeated as it can cause additional bleeding. Pelvic fractures are associated with occult hemorrhage, which may become a life-threatening condition.

Rectum and Perineum. Inspect the peritoneum for bruising, lacerations, or urethral bleeding. Perform rectal examination to detect blood within the bowel lumen, a high-riding prostate, pelvic fractures, the integrity of the abdominal wall, and the quality of sphincter tone. A vaginal examination is sometimes performed for bleeding and lacerations.

Neurologic Examination. Perform a more complete neurologic evaluation once the patient's condition has been stabilized. Reassess the patient's Glasgow Coma Scale score (Table 27-1) as well as pupillary size and reactivity. Then perform a more detailed motor and sensory evaluation. Note any paralysis or paresis, which suggests major injury to the spinal column or peripheral nervous system. Pain should be noted, its location, and the degree of its intensity recorded whenever possible.

Reevaluate the Patient. The patient must be reevaluated frequently so that any new signs and symptoms are not overlooked. Perform the primary survey every 5 minutes and compare the results with those obtained in previous assessments. Monitor vital signs continuously. Frequently monitor the patient's level of consciousness to detect deterioration in neurologic functioning. As life-threatening conditions are managed, other equally life-threatening problems may develop, and less severe conditions may become evident. A high index of suspicion and constant alertness during examination may lead to early recognition and management.

Injury Mechanisms

When the patient has been injured, a history of the injury and identification of the injury mechanism help determine the severity of injury.

Blunt Trauma

Blunt trauma mechanisms include motor vehicle crashes, falls, being struck by an object, and various recreational or sports activities. The force, surface struck, direction of impact, and body part affected determine the severity and pattern of injuries. For example, motor vehicle crashes account for the majority of severe blunt trauma cases. Emergency personnel at the scene should describe the appearance of the vehicle and the damage sustained to the passenger compartment. From that information the emergency trauma team can identify the areas of the body that absorbed the greatest transfer of energy and suspect specific injuries. The following are some examples (American College of Surgeons, 2012):

+ A bent steering wheel may be associated with an anterior flail chest, pneumothorax, aortic disruption, myocardial contusion, and fractured spleen or liver.
+ A bull's-eye fracture of the windshield may be associated with a cervical spine injury and brain injury. The delta V (change in force) associated with deceleration of the brain's movement within the skull has a relationship with the severity of the brain injury. The initial impact (*coup* injury) is that closest to the point of impact. The brain then moves and is again injured as it impacts the opposite side of the skull (*contrecoup*) during deceleration.
+ Side impact may be associated with contralateral neck sprain or cervical fracture, lateral flail chest, pneumothorax, aortic disruption, ruptured diaphragm, fractured spleen, kidney, or liver (depending on the side of impact), and fractured pelvis or acetabulum.
+ Rear impact collision can result in cervical spine injury or soft tissue injury of the neck.
+ Persons ejected from a vehicle are at high risk for multiple severe injuries.

Penetrating Trauma

Penetrating trauma mechanisms include firearm injuries, stabbings, and impalement. Two factors help determine the type of injury and subsequent management:

+ The region of the body and organs in the path of the penetrating object
+ The transfer of energy is determined by the force of impact by the penetrating object, such as the velocity of the missile, caliber, and distance from the source. Energy transfer is also determined by the rate or change in speed once the missile is inside the patient's body.

Burns

Burns should alert the examiner to the possibilities of smoke, heat, and toxic chemical inhalation and carbon monoxide poisoning causing airway inflammation. Anticipate airway obstruction in all cases of burns to the face, inhalation injury, hoarseness, and carbon deposits in the mouth or nose. Suspect and assess for additional injuries if the patient was injured in an explosion or might have fallen while attempting to escape a fire. The body surface area and burn depth are determined (Fig. 27-6).

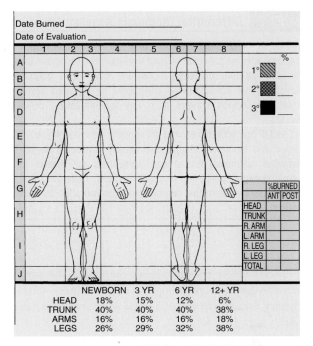

FIGURE 27-6 To estimate to total body surface area burned, mark the areas of the patient's burns on the chart. Then estimate the area of each body part burned, using the percentage of body surface area for each body part according to the age of the patient. Insert the percentages into the chart and sum to obtain the total body surface area burned. *ANT,* Anterior; *POST,* posterior.

Assessment of an Acute Medical Emergency

Advanced Cardiac Life Support Survey

Once the basic life support survey has been completed and the patient is conscious, additional assessment is needed. Perform a systematic rapid examination of the patient's vital functions and physiologic status in a sequence known as the ABCs (*Airway, Breathing, Circulation*). This rapid assessment process is also known as the primary survey or initial assessment. The immediate goal is to identify life-threatening conditions such as airway obstruction, impaired ventilation and hypoxemia, or impaired cardiac function and circulation—the physiologic responses to an acute medical emergency.

+ **Airway:** Identify an obstructed airway or need for an airway management device (e.g., endotracheal tube).
+ **Breathing:** Identify the adequacy of ventilation and oxygenation, including oxygen saturation.
+ **Circulation:** Identify the presence of the carotid pulse to determine if chest compressions are needed. Attach a cardiac monitor or defibrillator to identify the cardiac rhythm and potential need for defibrillation.
+ **Differential diagnosis:** This is the beginning of the physical examination to find and treat reversible causes of the emergency (Box 27-3).

As with serious injuries, the advanced cardiac life support survey is interrupted to manage a life-threatening physiologic condition as soon as it is detected. For example, if a patient is not breathing, rescue breaths, oxygen, and assisted ventilation must

---

Box 27-3 | **Differential Diagnosis Assessment**

An in-depth, head-to-toe examination to identify anatomic problems or reasons why the patient developed the emergency condition begins only after all life-threatening conditions have been adequately addressed. This examination is interrupted for repeated advanced cardiac life support surveys or if any life-threatening condition develops.

Special procedures required for patient assessment, such as imaging and laboratory studies, are usually conducted during the differential diagnosis assessment. Sometimes the reason for a medical emergency may not be readily evident. Table 27-2 defines eight primary symptoms that may be associated with a life-threatening condition.

---

be provided before the assessment continues. The survey is repeated frequently—for example, every 5 minutes—during an emergency because the patient's physiologic status may change rapidly.

✂ Assessment of Infants and Children

A smaller anatomy and differing physiologic responses to injury and acute illness are important considerations when examining infants and children during an emergency (Box 27-4 on p. 640). For example, the force of injury is more widely distributed through the body of children as compared to adults, resulting in a greater likelihood of multiple injuries (Avarello and Cantor, 2007). Additionally, cardiac arrest is rarely a primary event in children as it is in adults; however some children do experience ventricular fibrillation and cardiac arrest. The child more commonly experiences respiratory and ventilatory failure or shock that progresses to respiratory arrest and subsequent cardiac arrest (Chameides et al, 2011). For this reason, repeated primary assessment of the child with respiratory distress is essential so that deterioration to respiratory failure is prevented (see Physical Variations, "Pediatric Priorities").

Physical Variations

Pediatric Priorities

The assessment sequence and assessment priorities for the infant and child are the same as for adults. The child's size, blood volume, and fluid requirements may be smaller, and the disease or the mechanism of injury may be different, but the airway, breathing, and circulation must be ensured. Remember to keep the infant or child warm and to involve the parents as much as possible every step of the way.

During respiratory failure, carbon dioxide is not effectively exhaled, resulting in hypoxia. In the event of hypovolemic shock (poor tissue perfusion), blood is shunted to the vital organs, allowing the child a short period of physiologic compensation. Progression to hypoxemia, acidosis (low blood pH), and tissue acidosis occur if hypoxia and poor tissue perfusion are not reversed. Early intervention usually prevents progression to cardiac arrest.

Considerations in the emergency assessment of the infant and child include the following:

+ A crying or talking child has, at that moment, a patent airway.
+ Assessment with AVPU level of responsiveness (see p. 634) is as helpful with children as with adults.
+ If the child is responsive, attempt to establish rapport with the child consistent with the situation. Try to get as much information as possible when the child will communicate, such as, "Please use one finger to show me where it hurts."
+ The approximate expected systolic blood pressure for a child older than 1 year: 80 + (2 × child's age in years). This estimated value can be used until the child is stabilized when comparison can be made with the actual norms for the child's age, gender, and height percentile.
+ Capillary refill time longer than 2 seconds is a marker for poor tissue perfusion, just as for adults.
+ Because of the young child's large body surface area, exposure of the body for assessment causes significant heat loss. Try to keep an infant or child warm with heat lamps or a radiant warmer during assessment and treatment.
+ The mnemonic AMPLE (p. 635) is also useful for remembering the key elements of the child's history of the emergency. If an infant is only a few weeks old, add questions about the due date, the mother's pregnancy, delivery, and any health problems.
+ Evaluate the meaning of signs and symptoms with deliberate speed (Table 27-3 on p. 641).
+ The child's weight in kilograms is essential for calculating resuscitation medication dosages and intravenous fluid volumes. Parents usually know the child's weight in pounds. The conversion factor is 2.2 lb = 1 kg. If the weight is not known, a length-based resuscitation tape provides a reasonably close estimate of weight, and can guide decisions about the size of equipment, fluid volume, and drug doses appropriate for the child.

✂ Assessment of Older Adults

Older adults have organ system changes with aging that impact their physiologic reserves during an emergency. Examples include heart disease and high blood pressure as well as decreases in brain mass, respiratory vital capacity, cardiac stroke volume and heart rate, and renal function (American College of Surgeons, 2012). Older adults usually have multiple chronic health conditions that may limit their physiologic response to injuries (Chang and Schecter, 2007).

Although the primary and secondary assessments follow the same sequence, considerations in the emergency assessment of an older adult include (Birnbaumer, 2009a; Birnbaumer, 2009b):

+ Arthritic changes may limit mobility of the neck and temporomandibular joint and make it more difficult to open the mouth and obtain an airway.
+ The muscles in the upper airway weaken with age, leading to weaker cough and gag reflexes. The older adult has a higher potential for aspiration and obstruction.

Text continued on p. 641.

Table 27-2 Symptoms and Risks of Serious and Life-Threatening Conditions

Primary Symptoms	Possible Accompanying Symptoms	Possible Diagnosis	Risk
Vomiting blood or black or dark brown material that resembles coffee grounds	Recurrent bouts of gnawing pain in the upper part of the abdomen Black or tarlike stool Weakness Pallor Progressive fatigue Increased awareness of a rapid heartbeat (palpitations)	Bleeding ulcer of the stomach or duodenum, bleeding from esophageal varices	Possibly fatal hemorrhage
Crushing pain in the center of the chest	Radiation of the pain to the left arm, neck, jaw, shoulder Sweating Nausea and vomiting Unrelenting indigestion Shortness of breath Cool, clammy skin Fainting Feeling of impending doom	Myocardial infarction	Many deaths occur within minutes or hours of the attack, so the speed of treatment is crucial.
Severe throbbing pain in and around one bloodshot eye	Blurred or acute loss of vision in the affected eye Pain, headache Eyeball is both tender and firm to the touch Abnormal sensitivity to light (photosensitivity) Fixed and dilated pupil	Acute glaucoma	Delay in treatment can result in permanent blindness in affected eye. In many cases vision loss occurs very quickly.
Flashes of light in the field of vision of one eye	Absence of pain in the affected eye Black cobweb-like floating spots Partial loss of vision spreading as a curtain-like shadow from the top or one side of the eye	Retinal detachment	Extension of detachment with delayed treatment leading to permanent loss of peripheral or central vision depending on area of detachment.
Sudden and progressively more severe abdominal pain	Nausea and vomiting Swollen or tender abdomen Severe constipation Temperature above 100° F (38° C)	Acute abdomen (e.g., appendicitis, intestinal obstruction)	Delayed treatment can result in rupture or ischemic destruction of the involved organ and peritonitis.
Sudden feeling of weakness and unsteadiness that may result in momentary loss of consciousness	Weakness or paralysis of arm(s) or leg(s) Numbness and/or tingling in any part of the body Excruciating headache Confusion Difficulty speaking Blurred or double vision, or loss of vision in one eye	Transient ischemic attack (TIA) or stroke (brain attack)	TIA: Signs last 24 hours, but it may signal an impending stroke. Stroke: The outcome depends on the location and extent brain deprived of blood supply. (See Fig. 22-28 on p. 575.) Some are fatal, some cause permanent disability, some have no long-lasting effect.
Sudden onset of difficulty breathing (often in the middle of the night) and worsens rapidly	Restlessness, anxiety, and sense of doom Increased distress when lying down Swollen ankles Cough producing frothy pink or brownish, blood-flecked sputum Audible bubbling sound when breathing Crackles on auscultation Bluish lips and nail beds Profuse sweating	Pulmonary edema, related to sudden left-sided heart failure	Delayed treatment can be fatal.

Box 27-4 Ways in Which Children Differ Physically from Adults

Although children differ physically from adults, the closer they are in age to an adult, the more like an adult they become.

Characteristics of Young Children

Skin
- The skin is thinner, with less subcutaneous fat, and is less protective against burns and more likely to develop hypothermia.

Head
- Until about age 4 years, the head is larger and heavier relative to the rest of the body.
- The bones of the skull are softer and are separated by fibrous tissue and cartilage until about age 5 years; this is somewhat protective against increased intracranial pressure, at least for a short time.
- The developing brain, particularly to age 5 years, is more vulnerable to injury, infection, and poisons. The dura, very firmly attached to the skull, has bridging veins to the brain, which are apt to tear and bleed with inflicted injury, such as shaken baby syndrome.

Airway
- Nasal passages are relatively smaller and more easily obstructed with discharges or foreign bodies. Because newborns and young infants are obligate nose breathers, they are particularly vulnerable.
- The tongue is relatively larger and more easily able to obstruct the upper airway.
- The trachea is narrower and its cartilage more elastic and collapsible, and is therefore more vulnerable to edema, pressure, and inflammation; hyperextension or flexion can crimp and obstruct.
- The larynx is higher and more anterior, and is therefore more "available" for aspiration.

Chest and Lungs
- The rib cage is more elastic and flexible, less vulnerable to fracture, and more apt to allow retraction during increased respiratory distress.

- The mediastinum is more mobile and more vulnerable to tension pneumothorax.
- Chest muscles are not well developed. Their use, in addition to the expected diaphragmatic effort, suggests respiratory distress; they tire more easily with prolonged effort.
- The higher metabolic rate and greater oxygen requirement increase vulnerability to hypoxemia.

Heart and Circulation
- Infants and children have a smaller total circulating blood volume but will lose as much blood as an adult from a similar laceration.
- When a significant blood or fluid volume is lost, children compensate and maintain their blood pressure longer than adults do, even to the point of cardiac arrest.
- Bradycardia, usually the initial response to hypoxemia in neonates, may herald cardiac arrest.

Abdomen
- The liver and spleen are relatively larger and more vascular and are less protected by the ribs and abdominal muscles making them more susceptible to injury.

Extremities
- Bones are not fully calcified and are softer than bones of adults until puberty; more vulnerable to fracture.

Nervous System
- An infant is able to feel pain anywhere in the body but cannot always localize or isolate it; older infants and toddlers can push your hand away from a painful location.
- Children who appear passive in stressful situations and do not seek comforting reassurance from parents may have an altered, depressed level of consciousness or, if alert, may be providing a clue to child abuse.

Head proportionately larger and heavier; prone to head injury

Short neck

Healthy heart, faster heart rate

Bones are softer, bend, and may fracture more easily

Abdominal breathing

Fontanel and open sutures palpable

Small nasal and oral airway passages, large tongue

Shorter, narrower trachea; collapsible tracheal rings

Faster respiratory rate; muscles fatigue easily in cases of respiratory distress

Spleen and liver more exposed to trauma

Large body surface area; prone to hypothermia

Modified from American Academy of Pediatrics, 2006; Ball and Bindler, 2008, p. 147.

Table 27-3	Assessment Findings that Indicate a Sense of Urgency in Infants and Children
Physiology Affected	**Signs and Symptoms of Concern**
Responsiveness	• Combative or inconsolable • Decreased responsiveness, lethargy • Poor muscle tone • Weak or high-pitched cry, moaning • Personality change, failure to make eye contact, glassy-eyed stare, lack of interest in play or interaction • Does not recognize parents
Airway and Breathing	• Respiratory rate greater than 60 breaths per minute, sustained, especially with oxygen administration • Respiratory rate less than 20 breaths per minute, especially in the presence of acute illness or with injury to the chest or abdomen • Respiratory distress, nasal flaring, retractions (intercostal, supraclavicular, and sternal) • Airway sounds: stridor, muffled speech, grunting, signs of obstruction • Head bobbing with each breath: impending respiratory failure • Position: tripod, refusing to lie down • Asymmetric chest movements or see-saw respirations (chest rises as abdomen falls and vice versa)
Circulation	• Pale, cool skin—mottling, pallor, and peripheral cyanosis are indicators of poor tissue perfusion or respiratory distress • Pulses—absence of peripheral pulses indicates poor tissue perfusion; absent central pulse is an ominous sign • Capillary refill time—greater than 2 seconds indicates poor tissue perfusion, hypothermia, constricted blood flow (e.g., tight cast) • Sunken fontanel, doughy skin texture, dry mucous membrane may indicate hypovolemia due to dehydration • Heart rate—greater than 160 or less than 80 per minute in child under age 5 years; greater than 140 per minute in child 5 years and older • Bradycardia—sign of impending cardiac arrest • Sustained sinus tachycardia—indicates hypovolemia • Blood pressure—hypotension is a late sign of hypovolemia, indicates cardiovascular decompensation (a decrease of 10 mm Hg is significant) • Oliguria

* Increased stiffness of the rib cage may lead to an increased rate of rib fractures and pulmonary contusion in cases of chest wall injuries.
* Older adults have a decreased energy reserve, and the increased work of breathing may lead to respiratory failure more quickly than in younger adults.
* Cardiovascular changes include coronary artery stenosis, changes in the conduction system dysrhythmias, and decreased ventricular filling associated with a lower cardiac output.
* Hypotension and hypovolemia increase the risk for myocardial ischemia. The older adult is less able to compensate quickly for low perfusion states. Knowledge of the older adult's usual blood pressure reading is important when assessing for a falling blood pressure and shock.
* Patients taking beta-blocker medications are unable to compensate and increase their heart rate in cases of shock or dehydration.
* Patients on anticoagulation therapy will have increased bleeding.
* Nerve endings deteriorate and perception of pain may be reduced.
* Chronic mental status changes may be present in an older adult making assessment of responsiveness difficult.
* The skin has thinner subcutaneous fat and is injured more easily. Hypothermia is also a greater risk in older adults.

Legal Considerations

Records

Medical and legal problems may arise during emergency situations, and precise records of what you observed, evaluated, ordered, and performed are essential. Pertinent negatives are as important as pertinent positives. Flow sheets that enable chronologic recording of assessments and care provided are useful in emergency situations.

Consent for Treatment

Written informed consent for procedures and health care is usually obtained before treatment. In life-threatening emergencies, when the patient is unconscious or incapacitated, the needed emergency assessment and treatment are provided. Implied consent for treatment is based on the principle that a reasonably competent person would have consented for treatment, and delay in care could cause death or irreparable harm to the patient (Bitterman, 2009).

Trauma Due to Violence

If the patient's injury could be associated with violence or sexual assault, health care providers must preserve evidence. Any such injuries must be reported to legal authorities. All items, such as bullets and clothing, must be saved for law enforcement personnel, with a documented chain of possession by health professionals.

Medical Orders for Life-Sustaining Treatment

Make a conscientious effort to learn whether a patient has made an advance directive, a formal statement of desired medical care in the event of a catastrophic injury or illness. Such a document states conditions under which a patient wants specific medical interventions used, limited, or forbidden when unable to make health care decisions. Each state has a name for an advance directive, such as durable or medical power of attorney or designated health care agent. A close relative or other trusted person is designated to make health care decisions when the patient is unable to. Both documents are especially important if the illness or injury results in a cognitive impairment that prevents participation in medical decision making. A central concern is the extent to which life-sustaining measures should be instituted.

Summary

In contrast to most health care situations, in an emergency situation diagnosis is not made before the initiation of treatment. Rather, the life-threatening physiologic signs of disease or trauma are identified rapidly and treated immediately. The diagnosis causing the physiologic signs is investigated after the patient's condition is stabilized, and a thorough examination can then be performed.

ABNORMALITIES

Upper Airway Obstruction

Compromise of the airway space, resulting in impaired respiratory exchange

Pathophysiology	Subjective Data	Objective Data
• Several potential causes include the following: aspirated foreign body or chemicals; inflammation of the airway due to smoke or other chemical inhalation; infection such as laryngotracheitis (croup) or retropharyngeal abscess; trauma to the neck or face; and tumor or goiter.	• History of a choking episode or exposure to chemicals or smoke • History of infection with fever • Fatigue • Shortness of breath • Sore throat	• Patient may grasp neck with inability to speak • Apnea • Severe dyspnea and tachypnea • Stridor or hoarseness • Dysphagia, drooling • Extreme anxiety progressing to altered mental status (lethargy to coma) • Tripod positioning

Hypoxemia

Severely reduced blood oxygen levels in major organs

Pathophysiology	Subjective Data	Objective Data
• Results from conditions (e.g., upper airway obstruction, asthma, and hypovolemic shock) that cause respiratory distress, poor tissue perfusion, or ventilatory failure or from severe lung injury (e.g., pulmonary contusion) with increased permeability of alveoli	• History of choking episode, reactive airway disease (asthma), or chronic respiratory condition • Thoracic injury • Shortness of breath • Fatigue	• Severe dyspnea and tachypnea • Pallor, mottling, or cyanosis • Altered mental status (lethargy to coma; anxiety and combativeness may precede lethargy) • Tachycardia

Shock State

An abnormality of the circulatory system that results in inadequate organ perfusion and tissue oxygenation

Pathophysiology	Subjective Data	Objective Data
• Hypovolemic shock common causes include hemorrhage associated with injury or gastrointestinal bleeding, dehydration, or fluid loss associated with burn injury. • Septic shock is caused by several different organisms, leading to a systemic inflammatory response syndrome that impairs circulatory functioning and clotting functioning. • Shock may result from an injury above the diaphragm causing poor cardiac functioning (e.g., myocardial contusion or tension pneumothorax). • Injury to the spinal cord may cause a shock state when loss of sympathetic nervous system tone causes blood to pool in the extremities.	• History and mechanism of injury with potential for hypovolemia or circulatory system impairment or of overwhelming infection • Vomiting and diarrhea • Black, tarry stools • Abdominal pain • Rapid heart rate • Shortness of breath • Fatigue • Feels cold • Fever	• Anxiety • Pallor, cold extremities • Diaphoresis • Coma (or altered mental status) • Tachycardia • Decreasing systolic blood pressure or hypotension • Delayed capillary refill time • Tachypnea, respiratory distress • Oliguria • Circulatory collapse • In septic shock in adults, the systolic blood pressure is less than 90 mm Hg or less than 40 mm Hg from baseline, or mean arterial pressure less than 70 mm Hg, despite adequate fluid resuscitation (Catenacci and King, 2008).

Ventilatory Failure

Compromised exhalation of carbon dioxide because of alveolar hypoventilation

Pathophysiology	Subjective Data	Objective Data
• Numerous disorders can cause or progress to ventilatory failure if not managed, including upper airway obstruction, central nervous system disorder, increased intracranial pressure, Guillain-Barré syndrome, drug overdose, pulmonary contusion, flail chest, or severe kyphoscoliosis.	• History or mechanism of injury placing individual at risk • Headache • Respiratory distress • Apprehension	• Altered mental status—confusion or lethargy progressing to coma (may be subtle if the process is chronic) • Slowed respiratory rate • Paradoxical respirations • Blood gases reveal hypoxemia and hypercapnia.

Increased Intracranial Pressure

An increase in volume of brain tissue, blood, or cerebrospinal fluid (CSF) within the closed space of the skull that results in elevated pressure

Pathophysiology	Subjective Data	Objective Data
• Intracranial causes include brain trauma (cerebral edema, hematoma), tumor, ischemic stroke, brain abscess, or hydrocephalus • Extracranial causes include hypoxia or hypercarbia, seizure, metabolic or drug induced, or hyperpyrexia (Rangel-Castillo et al, 2008).	• History of brain injury, seizure, stroke, or other condition • Headache • Nausea and vomiting	• Changes in mental status, lethargy, irritability, slowed responsiveness; may progress to stupor or coma • Seizures or syncope • Papilledema • Cranial nerve palsy, particularly VI (abducens paralysis) • Cushing triad: bradycardia, rising blood pressure, and irregular respirations • Also in infants: bulging fontanel, irritable or high-pitched cry, inconsolable, change in vital signs • Radiographic studies may reveal a mass, generalized edema, or excessive cerebrospinal fluid.

ABNORMALITIES

Pulmonary Embolism

Migration of a blood clot from the deep veins of the legs or pelvis to the lung vasculature

Pathophysiology	Subjective Data	Objective Data
• Venous stasis and endothelial injury can lead to adhesion of platelets and clot formation. • Certain individuals may be predisposed due to hematologic disease, such as those with clotting abnormalities. • Family history of deep vein thrombosis	• History of reduced mobility or bed bound, surgery in past month, long airplane trip • Shortness of breath • Chest pain, stabbing and sharp that worsens with breathing or coughing • Cough, coughing up blood • Palpitations • Anxiety • Leg pain and swelling	• Tachycardia • Diaphoresis • Tachypnea • Pain with deep leg vein palpation, unilateral swelling • Syncope • Cough, hemoptysis • A ventilation/perfusion lung scan may diagnose the condition

Severe Asthma Episode (Status Asthmaticus)

An acute severe asthma exacerbation that does not respond to usual treatment in the emergency department

Pathophysiology	Subjective Data	Objective Data
• Chronic inflammation of the airway is present in asthma, and a variety of physical, chemical, and pharmacologic stimuli trigger bronchospasm and mucus obstruction of the intrapulmonary airways.	• History of dyspnea and increasing use of medication over a period of many days, or sudden onset of symptoms • Shortness of breath • Wheezing • Coughing • Fatigue	• Ability to say only a few words between breaths • Tachycardia (often more than 130 beats/min in adults) • Tachypnea (may be variable) • Hypertension • Dyspnea • Hypoxemia • Wheezing (unless airflow is so diminished that it obscures wheezing) • Pulsus paradoxus greater than 20 mm Hg • Altered mental status may be present.

Status Epilepticus

A prolonged seizure or series of seizures that occur without recovery of consciousness

Pathophysiology	Subjective Data	Objective Data
• May occur in patients with various seizure disorders, including generalized and partial seizures • May occur in association with an acute illness, a febrile illness, progressive central nervous system (CNS) disorder, or prior history of a CNS insult (Riviello et al, 2006)	• History of seizures, neurologic disorder, or injury • Shaking movements • Loss of consciousness and unresponsive for longer than usual	• Tonic-clonic movements with unresponsiveness, prolonged as much as 30 to 60 minutes (movements may be diminished by drugs used to manage the seizures) • Hypotension • Cardiac dysrhythmias • Fever • Pallor to cyanosis • Hypoxemia may result from impaired respirations during tonic stage • Hypoglycemia due to increased metabolic rate

Photo and Illustration Credits

400 Self-assessment picture tests in clinical medicine, Chicago, 1984, Year Book.

American Academy of Dermatology: Available at http://www.aad.org. Accessed January 2006.

American College of Rheumatology: *Clinical slide collection on the rheumatic diseases*, Atlanta, 1991, American College of Rheumatology.

American Journal of Obstetrics and Gynecology: *Tailoring radicality in demolitive surgery for deeply infiltrating endometriosis*, 2005, 114-117.

Andrews JS: Making the most of the sports physical, *Contemp Pediatr* 14(3):196-197, 1997.

Ansell BM, et al: *Color atlas of pediatric rheumatology*, London, 1992, Mosby-Wolfe.

Baggish MS: *Colposcopy of the cervix, vagina, and vulva: a comprehensive textbook*, Philadelphia, 2003, Mosby.

Ball JW, Bindler R: *Pediatric nursing: caring for children*, ed 4, Upper Saddle River, NJ, 2008, Prentice Hall Health.

Baran R, et al: *Color atlas of the hair, scalp, and nails*, St Louis, 1991, Mosby.

Beaty JH, Canale ST, editors: *Campbell's operative orthopaedics*, ed 10, St. Louis, 2003, Mosby.

Beeching NJ, Nye FJ: *Diagnostic picture tests in clinical infectious disease*, London, 1996, Mosby-Wolfe.

Berne RM, Levy MN: *Principles of physiology*, ed 2, St Louis, 1996, Mosby.

Bingham BJG, et al: *Atlas of clinical otolaryngology*, St Louis, 1992, Mosby.

Burke B: The dietary history as a tool in research, *J Am Diet Assoc* 23:1044-1046, 1947.

Busam KJ: *Dermatopathology: a volume in the series foundations in diagnostic pathology*, Philadelphia, 2009, Saunders.

Callen JP, et al: *Color atlas of dermatology*, Philadelphia, 2000, Saunders.

Canobbio MM: *Cardiovascular disorders*, St Louis, 1990, Mosby.

Carey WD, *Current Clinical Medicine*, ed 2, Philadelphia, 2010, Saunders.

Centers for Disease Control and Prevention, National Center for Infectious Disease, Atlantita.

Chessell GSJ, et al: *Diagnostic picture tests in clinical medicine*, London, 1984, Wolfe Medical Publications.

Chung KC: *Hand and Upper Extremity Reconstruction with DVD: A Volume in the Procedures in Reconstructive Surgery Series*, Philadelphia, 2009, Saunders.

Cohen BA: *Atlas of pediatric dermatology*, St Louis, 1993, Mosby.

Cummings CW, et al: *Cummings otolaryngology: head and neck surgery*, ed 4, St. Louis, 2005, Mosby.

Davidson MA: Developmental Disabilities, Part I Primary Care for Children and Adolescents with Down Syndrome, *Pediatr Clin North Am* 55:1099-1111, 2008.

Donaldson DD: *Atlas of the eye: the crystalline lens*, (vol v), St Louis, 1976, Mosby.

Doughty DB, Jackson DB: *Gastrointestinal disorders*, St Louis, 1993, Mosby.

Leifer G: *Introduction to maternity & pediatric Nursing*, ed 6, St Louis, 2011, Suanders.

Edge V, Miller M: *Women's health care*, St Louis, 1994, Mosby.

Errico T: *Surgical management of spinal deformities*, Philadelphia, 2009, Saunders.

Farrar WE, et al: *Infectious diseases*, ed 2, London, 1992, Gower.

Fedele L, et al: Tailoring radicality in demolitive surgery for deeply infiltrating endometriosis, *Am J Obstet Gynecol* 193:114-117, 2005.

Feldt KS: The checklist of non-verbal pain indicators (CNPI), *Pain Manag Nurs* 1(1):13-21, 2000.

Folstein MF, et al: "Mini-mental state": a practical method for grading the cognitive state of patients for the clinician, *J Psychiatr Res* 12:189, 1975.

Forbes CD, Jackson WF: *Color atlas and text of clinical medicine*, ed 3, London, 2003, Mosby Ltd.

Frisch RE: Growth Diagrams 1965 Netherlands: Second National Survey on 0-24-Year-Olds, by Van Wieringen JC, Wafelbakker F, Verbrugge HP, DeHaas JH. Groningen: Wolters-Noordhoff Publishing, *Pediatrics* 68, 1971.

Gallager HS, et al: *The breast*, St Louis, 1978, Mosby.

Goldman L, Ausiello DA: *Cecil medicine*, ed 23, Philadelphia, 2008, Saunders.

Goldman MP, Fitzpatrick RE: *Cutaneous laser surgery: the art and science of selective photothermolysis*, St Louis, 1994, Mosby.

Grimes D: *Infectious diseases*, St Louis, 1991, Mosby.

Guzzetta CD, Dossey BM: *Cardiovascular nursing: holistic practice*, St Louis, 1992, Mosby.

Habif TP: *Clinical dermatology*, ed 4, St Louis, 2004, Mosby.

Hochberg MC, et al: *Rheumatology*, ed 3, St Louis, 2008, Mosby.

Harris JA, et al: *The measurement of man*, Minneapolis, 1930, University of Minnesota Press.

Hockenberry MJ, Wilson D: *Wong's essentials of pediatric nursing*, ed 8, St Louis, 2009, Mosby.

Hockenberry MJ, Wilson D: *Wong's essentials of pediatric nursing*, ed 9, St Louis, 2013, Mosby.

Hughes JG: *Synopsis of pediatrics*, ed 6, St Louis, 1984, Mosby.

Ignatavicius D: *Medical-Surgical Nursing: Critical Thinking for Collaborative Care*, St Louis, 2006, Mosby.

James WD, Berger TG, Elston DM: *Andrew's diseases of the skin: clinical dermatology*, ed 10, London, 2006, WB Saunders.

Johr RH, et al: *Dermoscopy*, London, 2004, Mosby.

Kumar V, et al: *Robbins and Cotran pathologic basis of disease*, ed 7, Philadelphia, 2006, Saunders.

LaFleur Brooks M: *Exploring medical language*, ed 7, St Louis, 2009, Mosby.

Lawrence CM, Cox NH: *Physical signs in dermatology: color atlas and text*, St Louis, 1993, Mosby.

Lemmi FO, Lemmi CAE: *Physical assessment findings CD-ROM*, Philadelphia, 2000, Saunders.

Lemmi FO, Lemmi CAE: *Physical assessment findings CD-ROM*, Philadelphia, 2009, Saunders.

Lloyd-Davies RW, et al: *Color atlas of urology*, ed 2, London, 1994, Mosby.

Lowdermilk DL, et al: *Maternity and women's health care*, ed 6, St Louis, 1997, Mosby.

Lowdermilk DL, Perry SE: *Maternity and women's health care*, ed 8, St Louis, 2007, Mosby.

Mansel R, Bundred N: *Color atlas of breast disease*, St Louis, 1995, Mosby.

McCance KM, Huether SE: *Pathophysiology: the biologic basis for disease in adults and children*, ed 5, St Louis, 2006, Mosby.

McCrory P, et al: The SCAT card, *Brit J Sports Med* (vol 39), 2005.

Medcom: *Selected topics in ophthalmology: Medcom clinical lecture guides*, Garden Grove, Calif, 1983, Medcom.

Meheus A, Ursi JP: *Sexually transmitted diseases*, Kalamazoo, Mich, 1982, Upjohn.

Merkel SI, et al: FLACC behavioral pain assessment scale, *Pediatr Nurs* 23(3):293-297, 1997.

Miller RD: *Miller's anesthesia*, ed 7, Philadelphia, 2010, Churchill Livingston.

Morison M, Moffatt C: *A colour guide to the assessment and management of leg ulcers*, ed 2, St Louis, 1994, Mosby.

Morse SA, et al: *Atlas of sexually transmitted diseases and AIDS*, ed 3, St Louis, 2003, Mosby.

Newell FW: *Ophthalmology: principles and concepts*, ed 8, St Louis, 1996, Mosby.

Ortholutions. http://www.ortholutions.com/scoliometer.html. Accessed March 2013.

Patzelt J: *Basics augenheilkunde*, ed 2, Germany, 2009, Urban & Fischer.

Palay DA, Krachmer JH: *Ophthalmology for the primary care physician*, St Louis, 1997, Mosby.

Patton KT, Thibodeau GA: *Anatomy and physiology*, ed 7, St Louis, 2010, Mosby.

Rudy EB: *Advanced neurological and neurosurgical nursing*, St Louis, 1984, Mosby.

Saha S, Beach MC, Cooper LA: Patient centeredness, cultural competence and healthcare quality, *J Natl Med Assoc* 100(11):1275-1285, 2008.

Salvo S: *Mosby's pathology for massage therapists*, ed 3, St Louis, 2009, Mosby.

Sheikh JI, Yesavage JA: Geriatric depression scale: recent evidence and development of a shorter version, *Clin Gerontol* 5:165-172, 1986.

Sigler BA, Schuring LT: *Ear, nose, and throat disorders*, St Louis, 1993, Mosby.

Skarin AT: *Atlas of diagnostic oncology*, ed 2, London, 1996, Mosby-Wolfe.

Skirven TM, et al: *Rehabilitation of the Hand and Upper Extremity*, ed 6, Philadelphia, 2011, Mosby.

Spicknall KE, et al: Clubbing: An update on diagnosis, differential diagnosis, pathophysiology, and clinical relevance, *J Am Acad Dermatol* 1020-1028, 2005.

Stein HA, et al: *The ophthalmic assistant: fundamentals and clinical practice*, ed 5, St Louis, 1988, Mosby.

Stein HA, et al: *The ophthalmic assistant: fundamentals and clinical practice*, ed 6, St Louis, 1994, Mosby.

Stenchever M, et al: *Comprehensive gynecology*, ed 4, St Louis, 2001, Mosby.

Swartz MH: *Textbook of physical diagnosis*, ed 6, Philadelphia, 2009, Saunders.

Symonds EM, Macpherson MBA: *Color atlas of obstetrics and gynecology*, St Louis, 1994, Mosby.

Talley NJ, O'Connor S: *Clinical examination: a systematic guide to physical diagnosis*, ed 6, Australia, 2010, Churchill.

Thibodeau GA, Patton KT: *Anatomy and physiology*, ed 5, St Louis, 2003, Mosby.

Thompson JM, et al: *Mosby's clinical nursing*, ed 4, St Louis, 1997, Mosby.

Thompson JM, Wilson SF: *Health assessment for nursing practice*, St Louis, 1996, Mosby.

U.S. Department of Agriculture: ChooseMyPlate, 2011, http://www.choosemyplate.gov. Accessed March 2013.

Van Tuijl JH, Schmid A, Van Kranen-Mastenbroek VH, et al: Isolated spinal accessory neuropathy in an adolescent: a case study, *Eur J Paediatr Neurol* 10:83-85, 2006.

Van Wieringen JC, Wafelbakker F, Verbrugge HP, DeHaas JH: Groningen: Noordhoff Uitgevers BV: *Growth diagrams 1965 Netherlands: second national survey on 0-24-year-olds*, The Netherlands.

Weston WL, Lane AT: *Color textbook of pediatric dermatology*, St Louis, 1991, Mosby.

Weston WL, et al: *Color textbook of pediatric dermatology.* ed 2, 1996, Mosby, St Louis.

Weston WL, et al: *Color textbook of pediatric dermatology*, ed 4, St Louis, 2007, Mosby.

White GM: *Color atlas of regional dermatology*, St Louis, 1994, Mosby.

White GA, Cox NH: *Diseases of the Skin: A Color Atlas and Text*, ed 2, St Louis, 2006, Mosby.

Wilson SF, Giddens J: *Health assessment for nursing practice*, ed 4, St Louis, 2009, Mosby.

Wilson SF, Giddens J: *Health assessment for nursing practice*, ed 5, St Louis, 2013, Mosby.

Wilson SF, Thompson JM: *Respiratory disorders*, St Louis, 1990, Mosby.

Wong DL, et al: *Whaley and Wong's nursing care of infants and children*, ed 6, St Louis, 1999, Mosby.

Wood NK, Goaz PW: *Differential diagnosis of oral lesions*, ed 4, St Louis, 1991, Mosby.

Yannuzzi LA, et al: *The retina atlas*, St Louis, 1995, Mosby.

Zaoutis LB, Chiang VW: *Comprehensive pediatric hospital medicine*, Philadelphia, 2007, Elsevier.

Zitelli BJ, Davis HW: *Atlas of pediatric physical diagnosis*, ed 3, St Louis, 1997, Mosby.

Zitelli BJ, Davis HW: *Atlas of pediatric physical diagnosis*, ed 5, St Louis, 2007, Mosby.

Zitelli BJ, Davis HW: *Atlas of pediatric physical diagnosis*, ed 6, St Louis, 2012, Mosby.

ILLUSTRATION CREDITS

References and Readings

Aalberts JJJ, van den Berg MP, Bergman JEH, et al: The many faces of aggressive aortic pathology: Loeys-Dietz syndrome, *Neth Heart J* 16(9):299-304, 2008.

Aaron SD, Vandemheen KL, Boulet LP, et al: Overdiagnosis of asthma in obese and nonobese adults, *CMAJ* 179:1121, 2008.

Abbassi V: Growth and normal puberty, *Pediatrics* 102(2 pt 3): 507-511, 1998.

Abeloff MD, Armitage JO, Niederhuber JE, et al: *Abeloff's Clinical Oncology*, ed 4, St Louis, 2008, Elsevier.

Aboyans V, et al: Risk factors for progression of peripheral arterial disease in large and small vessels, *Circulation* 113(22):2623, 2006.

Abrams B, Pickett K: Maternal nutrition. In Creasey RK, Resnik R, editors: *Maternal-fetal medicine*, ed 4, Philadelphia, 1999, WB Saunders.

Adams JA: Evolution of a classification scale: medical evaluation of suspected child sexual abuse, *Child Maltreat* 6(1):31-36, 2001.

Adams LA, Lindor KD: Nonalcoholic fatty liver disease, *Ann Epidemiol* 17(11):863-869, 2007.

Adams MS, Niswander JD: Birth weight of North American Indians: a correlation and amplification, *Hum Biol* 45:351, 1973.

Adelman WP: Nicotine replacement therapy for teenagers, *Arch Pediatr Adolesc Med* 158:205-206, 2004.

Agarwal PK, et al: Retractile testis—is it really a normal variant? *J Urol* 175:1496-1499, 2006.

Age-Related Eye Disease Study Research Group: A randomized, placebo-controlled clinical trial of high-dose supplementation with vitamins C and E, beta carotene, and zinc for age-related macular degeneration and vision loss, *Arch Ophthalmol* 119:1417, 2000.

Ahmadi H, et al: Age-related changes in normal sagittal relationship between globe and orbit, *J Plast Reconstr Aesthet Surg* 60:246-250, 2007.

Ailawadi G, et al: Current concepts in the pathogenesis of abdominal aortic aneurysm, *J Vasc Surg* 38(3):584-588, 2003.

Alikhan R, et al: Risk factors for venous thromboembolism in hospitalized patients with acute medical illness: analysis of the MEDENOX study, *Arch Intern Med* 164(9):963-968, 2004.

American Academy of Family Physicians, Summary of Recommendations for Clinical Preventive Services, September 2012, http://www.aafp.org/online/etc/medialib/aafp_org/documents/clinical/cps/rcps08-2005.par.0001.file.tmp/june2010.pdf.

American Academy of Ophthalmology: *Preferred practice pattern: pediatric eye evaluations*, San Francisco, 2003, American Academy of Ophthalmology.

American Academy of Ophthalmology Pediatric Ophthalmology/Strabismus Panel: *Preferred Practice Pattern® Guidelines. Pediatric eye evaluations*, San Francisco, CA, 2007.

American Academy of Pediatrics, Committee on Child Abuse and Neglect: Guidelines for the evaluation of sexual abuse of children: subject review, *Pediatrics* 103(1):186-191, 1999.

American Academy of Pediatrics, Committee on Sports Medicine and Fitness: Medical conditions affecting sports participation, *Pediatrics* 107(5):1205-1209, 2001.

American Academy of Pediatrics, Committee on Sports Medicine and Fitness: Participation in boxing by children, adolescents, and young adults, *Pediatrics* 99(1):134-135, 1997.

American Academy of Pediatrics, Committee on Infectious Disease: *Red book: report of the Committee on Infectious Disease*, ed 26, Elk Grove Village, Ill, 2003, American Academy of Pediatrics.

American Academy of Pediatrics Committee on Quality Improvement, Subcommittee on Developmental Dysplasia of the Hip: Clinical practice guideline: early detection of developmental dysplasia of the hip, *Pediatrics* 105(4):896-905, 2000.

American Academy of Pediatrics, Committee on Sports Medicine and Fitness: Medical conditions affecting sports participation, *Pediatrics* 94(5):757, 2001.

American Academy of Pediatrics: Eye examination in infants, children and young adults by pediatricians, *Pediatrics* 111(4):902-907, 2003.

American Academy of Pediatrics: Management of Hyperbilirubinemia in the Newborn Infant 35 or More Weeks of Gestation, *Pediatrics* 114(1):297-316, 2004.

American Academy of Pediatrics: *Pediatric education for prehospital of providers*, ed 2, Sudbury, Mass, 2006, Jones & Bartlett Publishers, pp 2-31.

American Academy of Pediatrics Committee on Practice and Ambulatory Medicine and Section on Ophthalmology: Use of Photoscreening for Children's Vision Screening, *Pediatrics* 109(3):524-525, 2002.

American Academy of Pediatrics: Male Circumcision, *Pediatrics* 130(3):e756–e785, 2012, (doi: 10.1542/peds.2012-1990).

American Academy of Pediatrics, Marilynn J: Bull and the Committee on Genetics: Health supervision for children with Down syndrome, *Pediatrics* 128:393-406, 2011.

American Academy of Pediatrics, Rebecca A, Demorest Reginald L: Washington and the Council on Sports Medicine and Fitness: Athletic participation by children and adolescents who have systemic hypertension, *Pediatrics* 125(6):1287-1294, 2010.

American Academy of Pediatrics, Section on Ophthalmology, American Academy of Ophthalmology, American Association for

Pediatric Ophthalmology and Strabismus: Screening examination of premature infants for retinopathy of prematurity, *Pediatrics* 117(2):572-576, 2006.

American Academy of Pediatrics, Section on Sports Medicine and Fitness: Female athlete triad, *Sports Shorts* 8(July), 2002.

American Academy of Pediatrics: Sports preparticipation examination. In Dyment PG, editor: *Sports medicine: health care for young athletes*, ed 2, Elk Grove Village, Ill, 1991, American Academy of Pediatrics.

American Cancer Society: 2012, (http://www.cancer.org/Cancer/ColonandRectumCancer/DetailedGuide/colorectal-cancer-risk-factors).

American Cancer Society: *Breast Cancer Facts & Figures 2011-2012*, Atlanta, 2014, American Cancer Society, Inc.

American Cancer Society: *Oral cavity and oropharyngeal cancers*, 2012, Retrieved from http://www.cancer.org/Cancer/OralCavityand OropharyngealCancer/DetailedGuide/oral-cavity-and-oropharyngeal-cancer-risk-factors.

American Cancer Society (ACS): www.cancer.org, 2012; accessed May 29, 2012.

American Cancer Society: *What are the risk factors for cervical cancer?* http://www.cancer.org/Cancer/CervicalCancer/MoreInformation/CervicalCancerPreventionandEarlyDetection/cervical-cancer-prevention-and-early-detection-cervical-cancer-risk-factors. Last Revised: 03/14/2012.

American Cancer Society: *What are the risk factors for ovarian cancer?* http://www.cancer.org/Cancer/OvarianCancer/DetailedGuide/ovarian-cancer-risk-factors. Last Revised: 07/27/2012.

American Cancer Society: *What are the risk factors for endometrial cancer?* http://www.cancer.org/Cancer/EndometrialCancer/DetailedGuide/endometrial-uterine-cancer-risk-factors. Last Revised: 07/25/2012.

American Cancer Society: *American Cancer Society Guidelines for the Early Detection of Cancer*, http://www.cancer.org/Healthy/FindCancerEarly/CancerScreeningGuidelines/american-cancer-society-guidelines-for-the-early-detection-of-cancer. Last Revised: 06/15/2012.

American Cancer Society: *What are the risk factors for testicular cancer?* http://www.cancer.org/Cancer/testicularcancer/detailedguide/testicular-cancer-risk-factors. Last Revised: 05/14/2012.

American Cancer Society: *What are the risk factors for penile cancer?* http://www.cancer.org/cancer/penilecancer/detailedguide/penile-cancer-risk-factors. Last Revised: 05/02/2012.

American Cancer Society: *Prostate cancer*, http://www.cancer.org/cancer/prostatecancer/detailedguide/prostate-cancer-risk-factors. Last Revised: 09/04/2012.

American Cancer Society: *Anal cancer*, http://www.cancer.org/cancer/analcancer/detailedguide/anal-cancer-risk-factors. Last Revised: 01/05/2012.

American Cancer Society: *American Cancer Society recommendations for the early detection of prostate cancer*, http://www.cancer.org/cancer/prostatecancer/detailedguide/prostate-cancer-detection. Last Revised: 09/04/2012.

American College of Allergy, Asthma and Immunology (ACAAI): *Latex allergies*. Available at www.acaai.org/public/linkpages/latex.htm.

American College of Gastroenterology: *American College of Gastroenterology colon cancer resource kit for physicians and patients*, 2004. Available at www.acg.gi.org.

American College of Sports Medicine: The female athlete triad, *Med Sci Sports Exerc* 39(10):1867-1882, 2007.

American College of Surgeons Committee on Trauma: *Advanced Trauma Life Support*, ed 9, Chicago, IL, 2002.

American Heart Association and American Stroke Association: *About stroke: Understanding the risk*, Retrieved from http://www.strokeassociation.org/STROKEORG/AboutStroke/UnderstandingRisk/Understanding-Stroke-Risk_UCM_308539_SubHomePage.jsp, 2011.

American Optometric Association: *Pediatric eye and vision examination reference guide for clinicians*, ed 2, St Louis, 2002, American Optometric Association.

American Psychiatric Association: *Diagnostic and statistical manual of mental disorders*, ed 4, Washington, DC, 1994, APA.

American Speech and Language Association: *How does your child hear and talk?* Retrieved from http://www.asha.org/public/speech/development/chart.htm, 2011.

American Speech Language and Hearing Association: *How Does Your Child Hear and Talk*, 2012, Retrieved from http://www.asha.org/public/speech/development/01.htm.

Amichai B, Grunwald MH: Pigmentary demarcation lines of pregnancy, *Eur J Obstet Gynecol Reprod Biol* 131(2):239-240, 2007.

Aminzadeh Z, Roudgari A: Jolt accentuation of headache in diagnosis of acute meningitis, *Iran J Clin Infect Dis* 5(2):106-109, 2010.

Anand SS, et al: Does this patient have deep vein thrombosis? *JAMA* 279:1094, 1998.

Anderson DJ, Kaye KS: Skin and soft tissue infections in older adults, *Clin Geriatr Med* 3(3):595-613, 2007.

Andrews JS: Making the most of the sports physical, *Contemp Pediatr* 14(3):182-205, 1997.

Andrews MD, Burns M: Common tinea infections in children, *Am Fam Physician* 77(10):1415-1420, 2008.

Andriole GL, et al: for the PLCO Project Team: Mortality results from a randomized prostate-cancer screening trial, *N Engl J Med* 360:1310-1319, 2009.

Andriole GL, Crawford ED, Grubb RL III, et al: for the PLCO Project Team, Prostate Cancer Screening in the Randomized Prostate, Lung, Colorectal, and Ovarian Cancer Screening Trial: Mortality Results after 13 Years of Follow-up, *JNCI J Natl Cancer Inst* 104(2):125-132, 2012.

Angell M: Privilege and health: what is the connection? *N Engl J Med* 329(2):126-127, 1993.

Anthony KK, Schanberg LE: Pediatric pain syndromes and management of pain in children and adolescents with rheumatic disease, *Pediatr Clin North Am* 52:611-639, 2005.

Appelbaum PS: Assessment of patient's competence to consent to treatment, *N Engl J Med* 357:1834-1840, 2007.

Arab L, Wesseling-Perry K, Jardack P, et al: Eight self-administered 24-hour dietary recalls using the Internet are feasible in African Americans and Whites: the energetics study, *J Am Diet Assoc* 110(6):857-864, 2010.

Armitage J: Approach to the Patient With Lymphadenopathy and Splenomegaly. In Goldman L, Safer AI, editors: *Goldman's Cecil Medicine*, ed 24, Philadelphia, 2012, Saunders Elsevier.

Aronow WS: Hypertension in the elderly, *Clin Geriatr Med* 25:579-590, 2009.

Arosarena OA: Cleft lip and palate, *Otolaryngol Clin North Am* 40:27-60, 2007.

Arvidson CR: The adolescent gynecologic exam, *Pediatr Nurs* 25(1):71-74, 1999.

Ashwell M, Gunn P, Gibson S: Waist-to-height ratio is a better screening tool than waist circumference and BMI for adult cardiometabolic risk factors: systematic review and meta-analysis, *Obes Rev* 13(3):275-286, 2012.

Athey J, Moody-Williams J: *Serving disaster survivors: achieving cultural competence in crisis counseling,* Washington, DC, 2000, Emergency Services and Disaster Relief Branch, Center for Mental Health Services, Substance Abuse and Mental Health Services Administration.

Atroshi I, et al: Prevalence of carpal tunnel syndrome in a general population, *JAMA* 282(2):153-158, 1999.

Attia J, et al: Does this patient have acute meningitis? *JAMA* 282(2):175-181, 1999.

Augustyn M, et al: Silent victims: children who witness violence, *Contemp Pediatr* 12:35, 1995.

Auster S: *Spirituality and medicine.* Personal communication [from the Uniformed Services University of the Health Sciences], January 6, 2004.

Autotte PA: Folk medicine, *Arch Pediatr Adolesc Med* 149(9):949-950, 1995.

Avarello JT, Cantor RM: Pediatric major trauma: an approach to evaluation and management, *Emerg Med Clin North Am* 25:803-836, 2007.

Azoulay E: Pleural effusions in the intensive care unit, *Curr Opin Pulm Med* 9(4):291-297, 2003.

Bachmann LM, Kolb E, Koller MT, et al: Accuracy of Ottawa Ankle Rules to exclude fractures of the ankle and mid-foot: systematic review, *BMJ* 326(7386):417, 2003.

Badgett RG, et al: Can the clinical examination diagnose left-sided heart failure in adults? *JAMA* 277(21):1712-1719, 1997.

Ball JW, Bindler RC: *Pediatric nursing: caring for children,* ed 4, Upper Saddle River, NJ, 2008, Pearson Prentice Hall, p 147.

Ballock RT, Richards BS: Hip dysplasia: early diagnosis makes a difference, *Contemp Pediatr* 14:108, 1997.

Bamji M, et al: Palpable lymph nodes in healthy newborns and infants, *Pediatrics* 78(4):573-575, 1986.

Barkun AN, Grover SA: Update: Splenomegaly. In Simel DL, Rennie D, editors: *The Rational Clinical Examination Evidence-Based Clinical Diagnosis,* New York, 2009, McGraw Hill.

Barlow SE: the Expert Committee: Expert Committee Recommendations Regarding the Prevention, Assessment, and Treatment of Child and Adolescent Overweight and Obesity: summary report, *Pediatrics* 120:S164–S192, 2007.

Barone M, et al: *Material prepared for pediatric communication seminars,* at the Johns Hopkins School of Medicine, Baltimore, Md, 2003.

Barrett MJ, Ayub B, Martinez MW: Cardiac auscultation in sports medicine: strategies to improve clinical care, *Curr Sports Med Rep* 11(2):78-84, 2012.

Barretto RL, Mathog RH: Orbital measurement in black and white populations, *Laryngoscope* 109(7):1051-1054, 1999.

Barton M, Harris R MD, MPH: Does This Patient Have Breast Cancer? The Screening Clinical Breast Examination: Should It Be Done? How? In Simel DL, Rennie D, editors: *The rational clinical examination: evidence based clinical diagnosis,* 2009, McGraw-Hill, pp 87-98.

Ben-Shlomo A, Melmed S: Acromegaly, *Endocrinol Metab Clin North Am* 37:101-122, 2008.

Berde CB, Sethna NF: Analgesics for the treatment of pain in children, *N Engl J Med* 347:1094-1103, 2002.

Berenson A, et al: Inadequate weight gain among pregnant adolescents: risk factors and relationship to infant birth weight, *Am J Obstet Gynecol* 176:1220, 1997.

Bernius M, Perlin D: Pediatric ear, nose, and throat emergencies, *Pediatr Clin North Am* 53:195-214, 2006.

Bertakis KD, Azari R: Patient-centered care: the influence of patient and resident physician gender and gender concordance in primary care, *J Womens Health* 21(3):326-333, 2012.

Bhattacharyya I, Chehal HK: White lesions, *Otolaryngol Clin North Am* 44:109-131, 2011.

Birnbaumer DM: The Elder Patient. In Marx JA, Hockberger RS, Walls RM, et al, *Rosen's Emergency Medicine,* ed 7, Philadelphia, PA, 2009a, Elsevier Mosby, pp 2348-2352.

Birnbaumer DM: Geriatric trauma. In Marx JA, Hockberger RS, Walls RM, et al, editors: *Rosen's Emergency Medicine,* ed 7, Philadelphia, PA, 2009, Elsevier Mosby, pp 281-285.

Binns HJ, et al: Growth of Chicago-area infants 1985 through 1987: not what the curves predict, *Arch Pediatr Adolesc Med* 150:842, 1996.

Birklein F: Complex regional pain syndrome, *J Neurol* 252:131-138, 2005.

Biro FM, Galvez MP, Greenspan LC, et al: Pubertal assessment method and baseline characteristics in a mixed longitudinal study of girls, *Pediatrics* 126(3):e583–e590, 2010.

Bitterman RA: Medicolegal issues and risk management. In Marx JA, Hockberger RS, Walls RM, et al, *Rosen's Emergency Medicine,* ed 7, Philadelphia, PA, 2009, Elsevier Mosby, pp 2582-2599.

Blackhall LJ, et al: Ethnicity and attitudes toward patient autonomy, *JAMA* 274:820, 1996.

Blakeley JA, Ribeiro VES: Glucosamine and osteoarthritis, *Am J Nurs* 104(2):54-59, 2004.

Blatt SD, Simms M: Foster care: special children, special needs, *Contemp Pediatr* 14:109-129, 1997.

Bliss M: *William Osler, a life in medicine,* New York, 1999, Oxford University Press, p 83.

Boekeloo BO, et al: Young adolescents' comfort with discussion about sexual problems with their physicians, *Arch Pediatr Adolesc Med* 150(11):1146-1152, 1996.

Borowsky IW, et al: Adolescent suicide attempts: risks and protectors, *Pediatrics* 107:485-492, 2004.

Borson S, et al: The Mini-Cog: a cognitive "vital signs" measure for dementia screening in multi-lingual elderly, *Int J Geriatr Psychiatry* 15(11):1021-1027, 2000.

Botash A: *Pediatrics, child sexual abuse,* January 9, 2004. Available at www.emedicine.com.

Boustani M, et al: Screening for dementia in primary care: a summary of the evidence for the U.S. Preventive Services Task Force, *Ann Intern Med* 138:927-937, 2003.

Boyars MC: Chest auscultation: how to maximize its diagnostic value in lung disease, *Consultant* 37(2):415-427, 1997.

Bowditch MG, et al: The significance of an absent ankle reflex, *J Bone Joint Surg Br* 78(2):276-279, 1996.

Brace RA, Resnik R: Maternal dynamics and disorders of amniotic fluid. In Creasey RK, Resnik R, editors: *Maternal-fetal medicine,* ed 4, Philadelphia, 1999, WB Saunders.

Brady T, et al: Pediatric hypertension, *Contemp Pediatr* 25(11):46-56, 2008. Available at contemporarypediatrics.com.

Brandt MM, Wahl WL: Liberal use of CT scanning helps to diagnose appendicitis in adults, *Am Surg* 69(9):727-731, 2003.

Branski SH: Delirium in hospitalized geriatric patients, *Am J Nurs* 98(4):16D–16L, 1998.

Brooke P, Bullock R: Validation of a 6-item cognitive impairment test with a view to primary care, *Int J Geriatr Psychiatry* 14(11):936-940, 1999.

REFERENCES AND READINGS

Borkan JM, Culhane-Pera KA, Goldman RE: Towards Cultural Humility in Healthcare for a Cultrually Diverse Rhode Island, *Med Health: R I* 91(12), 2008.

Brosman SA: *Penile cancer, emedicine from WebMD*, 2008. Available at http://emedicine.medscape.com/article/446554 -overview.

Brothwell DR, et al: Congenital absence of teeth in human populations. In Brothwell DR, editor: *Dental anthropology*, Tarrytown, NY, 1963, Pergamon Press.

Brown JE, Carlson M: Nutrition and multi-fetal pregnancy, *J Am Diet Assoc* 100(3):343-348, 2000.

Brown MS, Hurlock JT: Preparation of the breast for breast feeding, *Nurs Res* 24:448, 1975.

Brown-Jones LC, Orr OP: Enlisting parents as allies against depression, *Contemp Pediatr* 13:6, 1996.

Bruckenthal P, D'Arcy YM: Assessment and management of pain in older adults: a review of the basics, *Top Adv Pract Nurs eJ* 7(1), 2007. Available at http://www.medscape.com/viewarticle/556382.

Brzoza Z: Pruritic urticarial papules and plaques of pregnancy, *J Midwif Womens Health* 52(1):44-48, 2007.

Bukutu C, et al: Complementary, holistic, and integrative medicine: therapies for acute otitis media, *Pediatr Rev* 29(6):193-199, 2008.

Bundy DG, et al: Does this child have appendicitis? *JAMA* 298(4):438-451, 2007.

Burchard KW, Rowland-Morin PA: A new method of assessing the interpersonal skills of surgeons, *Acad Med* 65(4):274-276, 1990.

Burrow GN, Duffy TP: *Medical complications during pregnancy*, ed 6, Philadelphia, 2004, WB Saunders.

Bynum DT: Clinical snapshot: gout, *Am J Nurs* 97(7):36-37, 1997.

Cadarette SM, et al: Development and validation of the Osteoporosis Risk Assessment Instrument to facilitate selection of women for bone densitometry, *Can Med Assoc J* 162(9):1289-1294, 2000.

Callahan CM: The benefit of the doubt, *JAMA* 264:341, 1990.

Campinha-Bacote J: Delivering Patient-Centered Care in the Midst of a Cultural Conflict: The Role of Cultural Competence, *OJIN: Online J Issues Nurs* 16(2):Manuscript 5, 2011.

Campinha-Bacote J: *The Process of Cultural Competency in the Delivery of Healthcare Services: A Culturally Competent Model of Care*, OH, 2003, Transcultural C.A.R.E. Associates.

Caputo GM, et al: Assessment and management of foot disease in patients with diabetes, *N Engl J Med* 331(13):854-860, 1994.

Carli P, et al: Dermoscopy as a second step in the diagnosis of doubtful pigmented skin lesions: how great is the risk of missing a melanoma? *J Eur Acad Dermatol Venereol* 15(1):24, 2001.

Carlson MC, Xue Q, Zhou J, et al: Executive decline and dysfunction precedes declines in memory: The Women's Health and Aging Study II, *J Gerontol* 64A(1):110-117, 2009.

Carrese JA, Rhodes LA: Western bioethics on the Navajo reservation: benefit or harm? *JAMA* 274:826, 1995.

Cartwright SL, Knudson MP: Evaluation of acute abdominal pain in adults, *Am Fam Physician* 77(7):971-978, 2008.

Castallani RJ, Rolston RK, Smith MA: Alzheimer disease, *Dis Month* 56(9):484-546, 2010.

Castiglia PT: Depression in children, *J Pediatr Health Care* 14(2):73-75, 2000.

Catenacci MH, King K: Severe sepsis and septic shock: improving outcomes in the emergency department, *Emerg Med Clin North Am* 26:603-623, 2008.

Caulfield AF, Wijman CAC: Management of acute ischemic stroke, *Neurol Clin* 26:345-371, 2008.

Centers for Disease Control and Prevention: *National diabetes fact sheet: national estimates and general information on diabetes and prediabetes in the United States, 2011.* Atlanta, GA, 2011, U.S. Department of Health and Human Services, Centers for Disease Control and Prevention.

Center for Disease Control and Prevention, Division of Nutrition, Physical Activity, and Obesity: *Overweight and Obesity*, retrieved from http://www.cdc.gov/obesity/index.html, 2012.

Centers for Disease Control: *Guide to Taking a Sexual History.* CS120957, CDC Publication: 99-8445. www.cdc.gov/std/treatment/SexualHistory.pdf.

Centers for Disease Control and Prevention: Sexually transmitted diseases treatment guideline, 2010, *MMWR* December 17, 2010 / Vol. 59 / No. RR-12, 2010. Available at http://www.cdc.gov/std/treatment/2010/STD-Treatment-2010-RR5912.pdf.

Centers for Disease Control and Prevention: *Food borne illness*, 2005. Available at www.cdc.gov/ncidod/dbmd/diseaseinfo/foodborneinfections_g.htm.

Centers for Disease Control and Prevention: *Hepatitis.* Available at www.cdc.gov/ncidod/diseases/hepatitis/index.htm, revised 12/1/05.

Centers for Disease Control: *HPV Vaccine Information for Clinicians—Fact Sheet*, http://www.cdc.gov/std/hpv/STDFact-HPV-vaccine-hcp.htm; Last updated July 12, 2012.

Centers for Disease Control and Prevention: *MMWR* 2011. CDC Health Disparities and Inequalities Report—United States, 2011 Supp/Vol 60.

Centers for Disease Control and Prevention MMWR (January 14, 2011) CDC Health Disparities and Inequalities Report—United States, 2011 Supp/Vol 60.

Centers for Disease Control and Prevention: Recommended adult immunization schedule—United States, 2012, *Morb Mortal Wkly Rep* 61(4):1-7, 2012.

Centers for Disease Control and Prevention: *Public health emergency preparedness and response.* Available at www.bt.cdc.gov/Agent/Agentlist.asp, 2004.

Centers for Disease Control and Prevention: *Spina bifida: Data and statistics in the United States.* Retrieved from http://www.cdc.gov/ncbddd/spinabifida/data.html, 2011.

Centers for Disease Control and Prevention: *Standard Precautions.* Available at www.cdc.gov/ncidod/dhqp/guidelines.html, updated September 2005.

Centers for Disease Control and Prevention: *Transmission-based precautions.* www.cdc.gov/ncidod/dhqp/gl_isolation.html, updated April 2005.

Centers for Disease Control and Prevention: *Travelers' diarrhea*, 2009. Available at www.cdc.gov/travel/yellowbook/2010/chapter2/travelers-diarrhea.aspx.

Centers for Disease Control and Prevention: *Vaccines and preventable diseases*, 2008. Available at http://www.cdc.gov/vaccines/vpd-vac/default.htm.

Center for Substance Abuse Treatment: *Substance Abuse Treatment: Addressing the Specific Needs of Women.* Treatment Improvement Protocol (TIP) Series 51. HHS Publication No. (SMA) 09-4426. Rockville, MD, 2009, Substance Abuse and Mental Health Services Administration.

Chameides L, Samson RA, Schexnayder SM, et al: *Pediatric Advanced Life Support*, Dallas, TX, 2011, American Heart Association.

Chandana SS, et al: Primary brain tumors in adults, *Am Fam Physician* 77(10):1423-1430, 2008.

Chang TT, Schecter WP: Injury in the elderly and end-of-life decisions, *Surg Clin North Am* 87:229-245, 2007.

Chapman IM: The anorexia of aging, *Clin Geriatr Med* 23:735-756, 2007.

Charoenkwan K, Ninunanahaeminda K, Khunamornpong S, et al: Effects of gel lubricant on cervical cytology, *Acta Cytol* 52(6):654-658, 2008.

Chaux A, Cubilla AL: The role of human papillomavirus infection in the pathogenesis of penile squamous cell carcinomas, *Semin Diagn Pathol* 29(2):67-71, 2012.

Chawarska K, Campbell D, Chen L, et al: Early generalized overgrowth in boys with autism, *Arch Gen Psychiatry* 68(10):1021-1031, 2011.

Chernick V, editor: *Kendig's disorders of the respiratory tract in children*, ed 5, Philadelphia, 1990, WB Saunders.

Chiao EY, et al: Screening HIV-infected individuals for anal cancer precursor lesions: a systematic review, *HIV/AIDS* 43:223-233, 2006.

Chiesa R, et al: Chronic venous disorders: correlation between visible signs, symptoms, and presence of functional disease, *J Vasc Surg* 46(2):322-330, 2007.

Chobanian AV, Bakris GL, Black HR, et al: Seventh report of the Joint Committee on prevention, detection, evaluation, and treatment of high blood pressure, *Hypertension* 42:1206, 2003.

Chopard G, Pitard A, Ferreira S, et al: Combining the Memory Impairment Screen and the Isaacs Set Test: A practical tool for screening dementias, *J Am Geriatr Soc* 55(9):1426-1430, 2007.

Chou R, et al: Diagnosis and treatment of low back pain: a joint clinical practice guideline from the American College of Physicians and the American Pain Society, *Ann Intern Med* 147(7):478-491, 2007.

Christensen FC, Rayburn WF: Fetal movement counts, *Obstet Gynecol Clin North Am* 26(4):607-621, 1999.

Christianson RE, et al: Incidence of congenital anomalies among white and black live births with long-term follow-up, *Am J Public Health* 71:1333, 1981.

Chumlea W, et al: Age at menarche and racial comparisons in U.S. girls, *Pediatrics* 111:110-113, 2003. Available at www.pediatrics.org/cgi/content/full/111/1/110.

Churgay CA: Diagnosis and treatment of pediatric foot deformities, *Am Fam Physician* 47(4):883-889, 1993.

Clemmons DR: Value of insulin-like growth factor system markers on the assessment of growth hormone status, *Endocrinol Metab Clin North Am* 36:109-129, 2007.

Collins JW Jr, David RJ: Differential survival rates among low birth weight black and white infants in a tertiary care hospital, *Epidemiology* 1:16, 1990.

Committee on Genetics, Section on Endocrinology and Section on Urology: Evaluation of the newborn with developmental anomalies of the external genitalia, *Pediatrics* 106:138-142, 2000. Available at http://www.pediatrics.org/cgi/content/full/106/1/138.

Conen D, et al: Metabolic syndrome, inflammation, and risk of symptomatic peripheral artery disease in women: a prospective study, *Circulation* 120(12):1041, 2009.

Connelly JE: Emotions and clinical decisions, *SGIM News* 13:1, 1990.

Consensus Document of the International Society of Lymphology: the diagnosis and treatment of peripheral lymphedema, *Lymphology* 36(2):84-91, 2003.

Council on Cardiovascular Disease in the Young, Committee on Rheumatic Fever, Endocarditis, and Kawasaki Disease, American Heart Association: Diagnostic guidelines for Kawasaki disease, *Circulation* 103:335-336, 2001.

Cote BM, Allen PJ: The developmental origins of health and disease hypothesis, *Pediatr Nurs* 36(3):157-167, 2010.

Crane BT, Schessel DA, Nedzelski J, et al: Peripheral vestibular disorders. In Flint PW, Haughey BH, Lund VJ, et al, editors: *Cummings Otolaryngology Head & Neck Surgery*, ed 5, Philadelphia, 2010, Mosby Elsevier, pp 2328-2345.

Criddle LM, et al: Standardizing stroke assessment using the National Institutes of Health Stroke Scale, *J Emerg Nurs* 26(6):541-546, 2003.

Criqui MH, et al: Risk factors for chronic venous disease: the San Diego Population Study, *J Vasc Surg* 46(2):331-337, 2007.

Criqui MH, et al: Ethnicity and peripheral arterial disease: the San Diego Population Study, *Circulation* 112(17):2703-2707, 2005.

Cromer, B: Adolescent physical and social development. In Kleigman RM, Stanton BF, St. Geme JW, et al, editors: *Nelson Textbook of Pediatrics*, ed 19, Philadelphia, PA, 2011, Elsevier Saunders, pp 649-654.

Crowell DH, et al: Race, ethnicity and birth-weight: Hawaii 1983 to 1986, *Hawaii Med J* 51:242, 1992.

Cuellar NG, Brennan AM, Vito K, et al: Cultural competence in the undergraduate nursing curriculum, *J Prof Nurs* 24(3):143-149, 2008. Review.

Cugell DW: Lung sound nomenclature, *Am Rev Respir Dis* 136:1016, 1987.

Curlin FA, et al: Religion, conscience and controversial clinical practices, *N Engl J Med* 356:593-600, 2007.

Culture and chronic illness: raising children with disabling conditions in a culturally diverse world: proceedings of a conference, *Pediatrics* 91(5 Pt 2):1025-1081, 1993.

Cunningham G, et al: *Williams obstetrics*, ed 22, Columbus, Ohio, 2005, McGraw-Hill.

Curative Health Services: *The curative footsense 5.07 monofilament*, East Setauket, NJ, 1996, Curative Health Services.

D'Arcy CA, McGee S: Does this patient have carpal tunnel syndrome? *JAMA* 283(23):3110-3117, 2000.

D'Arcy CA, McGee S: The rational clinical examination: does this patient have carpal tunnel syndrome? *JAMA* 283(23):3110-3117, 2000.

Dains JE, et al: Common problems of the musculo skeletal system. In Dains JE, Baumann LC, Scheibel P, editors: *Advanced health assessment and clinical diagnosis in primary care*, St Louis, 1998, Mosby.

Dains JE, et al: *Health assessment and clinical diagnosis in primary care*, ed 3, St Louis, 2007, Mosby.

Danford DA: Effective use of the consultant, laboratory testing, and echocardiography for the pediatric patient with heart murmur, *Pediatr Ann* 29(8):482-488, 2000.

Daniels SR, Greer FR; the Committee on Nutrition: Lipid screening and cardiovascular health in childhood, *Pediatrics* 122:198-208, 2008.

Daniels SR, et al: The utility of body mass index as a measure of body fatness in children and adolescents: differences by race and gender, *Pediatrics* 99(6):804-807, 1997.

Davies T, Mills C: *Personal communication*, September 15, 1997.

Defer TM: An evidence-based approach to low back pain in primary care, *Adv Stud Med* 4(3):135-148, 2004.

Delves PJ, Roitt IM: The immune system, *N Engl J Med* 343:108-116, 2000.

DeMuri GP, Wald ER: Acute sinusitis: Clinical manifestations and treatment options, *Pediatr Ann* 39(1):34-40, 2010.

Degnan AJ, Levy LM: Pseudotumor Cerebri: Brief Review of Clinical Syndrome and Imaging Findings, *Am J Neuroradiol* 32:1986-1993, 2011.

Department of Health and Human: *2008 Physical Activity Guidelines for Americans*. http://www.health.gov/paguidelines/default .aspx.

Department of Health and Human Services (U.S.), Centers for Disease Control and Prevention: Non-fatal sports- and recreation-related traumatic brain injuries treated in emergency departments: United States, 2001-2005, *Morbid Mort Wkly Rep* 56(29):733-737, 2007.

Department Health and Human Services, National Institute for Occupational Safety and Health: *Latex Allergy A Prevention Guide*, Publication Number 98-113, 1998, http://www.cdc.gov/niosh/docs/98-113/.

Des Jardin T, Burton GG: *Clinical manifestations and assessment of respiratory disease*, ed 3, St Louis, 1995, Mosby.

DeSwiet MD: The respiratory system. In Hytten F, Chamberlain G, editors: *Clinical physiology in obstetrics*, ed 2, Boston, 1991, Blackwell Scientific.

Dattner AM: *Seborrheic Dermatitis in Rakel: Integrative Medicine*, ed 3, Philadelphia, 2012, Elsevier Saunders.

DeVore ER, Ginsburg KR: The protective effects of good parenting on adolescents, *Curr Opin Pediatr* 17(4):460-465, 2005.

Dew P: Is tympanic membrane thermometry the best method for recording temperature in children? *J Child Health Care* 10:96, 2006.

DiClemente C, Prochaska J: Toward a comprehensive transtheoretical model of change. In Miller WR, Healther N, editors: *Treating addictive behaviors*, New York, 1998, Plenum Press.

Dietary Guidelines for Americans: 2005. Available at www.health.gov/dietaryguidelines/dga2005/document/.

DiFrancesco E: Getting teens to talk to you, *Pediatr News* Aug 19, 1992.

Dillon MJ: Investigation and management of hypertension in children: a personal perspective, *Pediatr Nephrol* 1(1):59-68, 1987.

Dimberg EL, Burns TM: Management of common neurologic conditions in sports, *Clin Sports Med* 21:637-662, 2005.

Dodd V: Gestational age assessment, *Neonatal Netw* 15(1):27-36, 1996.

Doerflinger DMC: The Mini-Cog, *Am J Nurs* 107(12):62-71, 2007.

Donnelly WJ: Medical language as symptoms: doctor talk in teaching hospitals, *Perspect Biol Med* 30:81, 1986.

Doty RL: Disturbances of smell and taste. In Daroff RB, Fenichel GM, Jankovic J, et al, editors: *Bradley's Neurology in Clinical Practice*, ed 6, Philadelphia, PA, 2012, Elsevier Saunders, pp 197-204.

Dowd R, Cavalieri RJ: Help your patient live with osteoporosis, *Am J Nurs* 99(4):55, 57-60, 1999.

Dowling S, Spooner CH, Liang Y, et al: Accuracy of Ottawa Ankle Rules to exclude fractures of the ankle and midfoot in children: a meta-analysis, *Acad Emerg Med* 16(4):277-287, 2009. Doi: 10.1111/j.1553-2712.2008.00333.x. Epub 2009 Feb 2.

Drago F, Broccolo F, Rebora A: Pityriasis rosea: An update with a critical appraisal of its possible herpesviral etiology, *J Am Acad Dermatol* 61(2), 2009.

Drazner MH, et al: Prognostic importance of elevated jugular venous pressure and a third heart sound in patients with heart failure, *N Engl J Med* 345(8):574-581, 2001.

Drolett B, et al: The hair collar sign: marker for cranial dysraphism, *Pediatrics* 96(2 Pt 1):309-313, 1995.

Druzin ML, et al: Antepartum fetal evaluation. In Gabbe SG, Niebyl JR, Simpson JL, editors: *Obstetrics: normal and problem pregnancies*, ed 4, London, 2002, Churchill Livingstone.

Duklewski AK, Aronson AA: Ovarian cysts, *Emedicine* Jun 18, 2007. Available at http://www.emedicine.com/EMERG/topic352.htm.

Duthie EH: History and physical examination. In Duthie EH, Katz PR, Malone ML, editors: *Practice of Geriatrics*, ed 4, Philadelphia, 2007, Saunders Elsevier, pp 3-15.

Ebell MH: Diagnosis of appendicitis: part 1. History and physical examination, *Am Fam Physician* 15(6):828-830, 2008.

Ebell MH, Smith MA, Barry HC, et al: Does this patient have strep throat? In Simel DL, Rennie D, editors: *The Rational Clinical Examination: Evidence-Based Clinical Diagnosis*, New York, NY, 2009, McGraw Hill Medical, pp 615-622.

Eddy DM: The anatomy of a decision, *JAMA* 263:441, 1990.

Edge V, Miller M: *Women's health care*, St Louis, 1994, Mosby.

Eichelberger MR, et al: *Pediatric emergencies: a manual for prehospital care providers*, Englewood Cliffs, NJ, 1998, Brady.

Emanuel EJ, Emanuel LL: Four models of the physician-patient relationship, *JAMA* 267:2221, 1992.

Emergency Cardiovascular Care Committee, American Heart Association: Response to cardiac arrest and selected life-threatening medical emergencies: the medical emergency response plan for schools, *Pediatrics* 113:155-168, 2004.

Escobar-Chaves SL, et al: Impact of the media on adolescent sexual attitudes and behaviors, *Pediatrics* 116:303-326, 2005.

Esteban-Santillan C, et al: Clock drawing test in very mild Alzheimer's disease, *J Am Geriatr Soc* 46(10):1266-1269, 1998.

Euling SY, Herman-Giddens ME, Lee PA, et al: Examination of U.S. Puberty-Timing Data from 1940 to 1994 for Secular Trends: panel Findings, *Pediatrics* 121:S172, 2008. DOI 10.1542/peds.2007-1813D.

Euling SY, Herman-Giddens ME, Lee PA, et al: Examination of U.S. Puberty-Timing Data from 1940 to 1994 for Secular Trends: Panel Findings, *Pediatrics* 121:S172–S191, 2008.

European Stroke Organisation, et al: ESC Guidelines on the diagnosis and treatment of peripheral artery diseases: Document covering atherosclerotic disease of extracranial carotid and vertebral, mesenteric, renal, upper and lower extremity arteries: the Task Force on the Diagnosis and Treatment of Peripheral Artery Diseases of the European Society of Cardiology (ESC), *Eur Heart J* 32(22):2851, 2011.

Ewing JA: Detecting alcoholism, the CAGE questionnaire, *JAMA* 252:1905, 1984.

Expert Panel on Integrated Guidelines for Cardiovascular Health and Risk Reduction in Children and Adolescents: Summary Report, *Pediatrics* 128(Suppl 5):213-256, 2011.

Factora R, Luciano M: Normal pressure hydrocephalus: diagnosis and new approaches to treatment, *Clin Geriatr Med* 22:645-657, 2006.

Fai FV, et al: Assessment of fetal health should be based on maternal perception of clusters rather than episodes of fetal movements, *J Obstet Gynecol Res* 22:299, 1996.

Falkner G, Tanner J: *Human growth, I: principles and prenatal growth*, New York, 1978, Plenum Press.

FAO/WHO/UNU: Energy and protein requirements. Report of a joint FAO/WHO/UNU expert consultation, *World Health Organ Tech Rep Ser* 724:1-206, 1985.

Fashner J, Ericson K, Werner S: Treatment of the common cold in children and adults, *Am Fam Physician* 86(2):153-159, 2012.

FDA *approves technetium (99m Tc) Fanolesomab, NeutroSpec (murine monoclonal antibody to CD15) for the scintigraphic imaging of patients with equivocal signs and symptoms of appendicitis who are five years of age or older*, July 7, 2004. Available at www.fda.gov/cder/previous_news.htm.

Fedarko NS: The Biology of Aging and Frailty, *Clin Geriatr Med* 27:27-37, 2011. doi:10.1016/j.cger.2010.08.006.

Fedullo PF, Tapson VF: The evaluation of suspected pulmonary embolism, *N Engl J Med* 349:1247-1256, 2003.

Feero WG, Green ED: Genomics education for healthcare professions in the 21st century, *JAMA* 306(9):989-990, 2011.

Feigelman S: Overview and assessment of variability. In Kliegman RM, Behrman RE, Jenson HB, et al, editors: *Nelson textbook of pediatrics*, ed 18, Philadelphia, 2007, Saunders Elsevier, pp 33-40.

Feldhaus KM, et al: Accuracy of 3 brief screening questions for detecting partner violence in the emergency department, *JAMA* 277(17):1400-1401, 1997.

Feldmann J, Middleman A: Adolescent sexuality and sexual behavior, *Curr Opin Obstet Gynecol* 14(5):489-493, 2002.

Feldt KS: The checklist of nonverbal pain indicators (CNPI), *Pain Manag Nurs* 1(1):13-21, 2000.

Felix HC, Adams B, Fausett JK, et al: Calculating reach of evidence-based weight loss and memory improvement interventions among older adults attending Arkansas senior centers, 2008-2011, *Prev Chronic Dis* 9:110141, 2012. DOI: http://dx.doi.org/10.5888/pcd9.110141.

Fenton TR: *A new growth chart for preterm babies: Babson and Benda's chart updated with recent data and new format, BMC Pediatr* December 13, 2003. Available at http://www.biomedcentral.com/1471-2431/3/13.

Fernandez ID, et al: Discordance in the assessment of prepregnancy weight status of adolescents: a comparison between the Centers for Disease Control and Prevention sex- and age-specific body mass index classification and the Institute of Medicine–based classification used for maternal weight gain guidelines, *J Am Diet Assoc* 108:998-1002, 2008.

Ferreyra S, Hughes K: *Table manners: a guide to the pelvic examination for disabled women and health care providers*, Alameda/San Francisco, 1982, Planned Parenthood.

Ferrieri P: for the Jones Criteria Working Group: Proceedings of the Jones Criteria Workshop, *Circulation* 106:2521-2523, 2002.

Ferrini R, Woolf S: Screening for prostate cancer in American Men, American College of Preventive Medicine Practice Policy Statement, *Am J Prevent Med* 15:18-84, 1998.

Ferris M: Pain in the cognitively impaired elderly: guidance for clinicians, *Top Adv Pract Nurs eJ* 2008. Available at http://www.medscape.com/viewarticle/573642.

Ferro RT, et al: A nonoperative approach to shoulder impingement syndrome, *Adv Stud Med* 3(9):518-528, 2003.

Fiegelman S: The first year. In Kliegman RM, Stanton BF, St. Geme JW, et al, editors: *Nelson Textbook of Pediatrics*, ed 19, Philadelphia, PA, 2011, Elsevier Saunders, pp 26-31.

Fisher B, et al: Tamoxifen for prevention of breast cancer: report of the National Surgical Adjuvant Breast and Bowel Project P-1 Study, *J Natl Cancer Inst* 16;90(18):1371-1388, 1998.

Flegal KM, Carroll MD, Ogden CL, et al: Prevalence and trends in obesity among U.S. adults, 1999-2008, *J Am Med Assoc* 303(3):235-241, 2010.

Flores G: The impact of medical interpreter services on the quality of health care: a systematic review, *Med Care Res Rev* 62(3):255-299, 2005.

Flores G: Committee On Pediatric Research: Technical report—racial and ethnic disparities in the health and health care of children, *Pediatrics* 125(4):e979–e1020, 2010. Epub 2010 Mar 29.

Folstein M, et al: The meaning of cognitive impairment in the elderly, *J Am Geriatr Soc* 33:228, 1985.

Folstein MF, et al: "Mini-Mental State": a practical method for grading the cognitive state of patients for the clinician, *J Psychiatric Res* 12:189, 1975.

Ford CA, Millstein SG: Delivery of confidentiality assurances to adolescents by primary care physicians, *Arch Pediatr Adolesc Med* 151(5):505-509, 1997.

Forrest J, et al: Recognizing quiet delirium, *Am J Nurs* 107(4):35-39, 2007.

Fosarelli P: Children and the development of faith: implications for pediatric practice, *Contemp Pediatr* 20:85-98, 2003.

Fox GN: Teaching first trimester uterine sizing, *J Fam Pract* 21(5): 400-401, 1985.

Franklin SS, et al: Is pulse pressure useful in predicting risk for coronary heart disease? *Circulation* 100:354, 1999.

Freeman JM: The three-cent neurologic exam and other tools for an era of managed care, *Contemp Pediatr* 14:153, 1997.

Freudenreich O, Weiss AP, Goff DC: Psychosis and schizophrenia. In Stern TA, Rosenbaum JF, Fava M, et al, editors: *Massachusetts General Hospital Comprehensive Clinical Psychiatry*, ed 1, Philadelphia, PA, 2008, Elsevier Mosby, pp 371-389.

Friedman RA: Uncovering an epidemic: screening for mental illness in teens, *N Engl J Med* 355:2717-2719, 2006.

Frisancho A: New norms of upper limb fat and muscle areas for assessment of nutritional status, *Am J Clin Nutr* 34:2540, 1981.

Frisancho AR: New standards of weight and body composition by frame size and height for assessment of nutritional status of adults and the elderly, *Am J Clin Nutr* 40:808, 1984.

Froehling DA, et al: Does this dizzy patient have a serious form of vertigo? *JAMA* 271(5):385-388, 1994.

Frommelt MA: Differential diagnosis and approach to a heart murmur in term infants, *Pediatr Clin North Am* 51(4):1023-1032, 2004.

Gabbe SG, et al: *Obstetrics: normal and problem pregnancies*, ed 6, Philadephia, 2012, Saunders Elsevier.

Gabbe SG, Niebyl JR, Simpson JL, et al: *Obstetrics: Normal and Problem Pregnancies*, ed 6, Philadelphia, PA, 2012, Elsevier Saunders, pp 42-65.

Galioto NJ: Peritonsillar abscess, *Am Fam Physician* 77(2):199-202, 2008.

Gallagher RP, et al: Melanocytic nevus density in Asian, indo-Pakistani, and white children: the Vancouver Mole Study, *J Am Acad Dermatol* 25(3):507, 1991.

Gallagher-Allred CR: *Implementing nutrition screening and intervention strategies*, Washington, DC, 1993, Nutrition Screening Initiative.

Gallo AM: Osteoporosis and children at risk with genetic hypercalciuria, *Image J Nurs Sch* 28:368, 1996.

Garrick JG: Preparticipation orthopedic screening evaluation, *Clin J Sport Med* 14(3):123-126, 2004.

Gates GA, et al: Screening for handicapping hearing loss in the elderly, *J Fam Pract* 52(1):56-62, 2003.

Geda YE, Topazian HM, Lewis RA, et al: Engaging in cognitive activities, aging, and mild cognitive ampairment: A population-based study, *J Neuropsychiatry Clin Neurosci* 23(2):149-154, 2011.

George A, Shamim S, Johnson M, et al: Periodontal treatment during pregnancy and birth outcomes: a meta-analysis of randomised trials, *Int J Evid Based Healthc* 9(2):122-147, 2011. doi: 10.1111/j.1744-1609.2011.00210.x.

Gholve PA, Cameron DB, Millis MB: Slipped capital femoral epiphysis update, *Curr Opin Pediatr* 21(1):39-45, 2009. Doi: 10.1097/MOP.0b013e328320acea.

Gilchrist J, Thomas KE, Xu L, et al: Nonfatal sports and recreation related traumatic brain injuries among children and adolescents treated in emergency departments in the United States, 2001-2009, *MMWR* 60(39):1337-1342, 2011.

Gilron I, et al: Neuropathic pain: a practical guide for the clinician, *Canad Med Assoc J* 175(3):265-275, 2006.

Gilson M, Desai A, Cardoza-Favarato G, et al: Does gel affect cytology or comfort in the screening papanicolaou smear? *J Am Board Fam Med* 19(4):340-344, 2006.

Gilchrist J, Thomas KE, Xu L, et al: Nonfatal sports and recreation related traumatic brain injuries among children and adolescents treated in emergency departments in the United States, 2001-2009, *MMWR* 60(39):1337-1342, 2011.

Gjerdingen D, Crow S, McGovern P, et al: Postpartum Depression Screening at Well-Child Visits: Validity of a 2-Question Screen and the PHQ-9, *Ann Fam Med* 7(1):63-70, 2009. doi: 10.1370/afm.933.

Glascoe FP, Macias MM: How you can implement the AAP's new policy on developmental and behavioral screening? *Contemp Pediatr* 20:85-102, 2003.

Global strategy for the diagnosis, management, and prevention of chronic obstructive pulmonary disease: Revised 2011. Global Initiative for Chronic Obstructive Lung Disease (GOLD). www.goldcopd.org (Accessed on September 10, 2012).

Gluckman PD, Hanson MA, Cooper C, et al: Effect of in utero and early-life conditions on adult health and disease, *NEJM* 359(1):61-73, 2008.

Gold A: Physicians' "Right of Conscience"—Beyond Politics, *J Law Med Ethics* 38:134-142, 2010. doi: 10.1111/j.1748-720X.2010.00473.x.

Goldberg B, et al: Preparticipation sports assessment: an objective evaluation, *Pediatrics* 66(5):736, 1980.

Goldenberg N, Barkan A: Factors regulating growth hormone secretion in humans, *Endocrinol Metab Clin North Am* 36:37-55, 2007.

Goldenring JM, Rosen DS: Getting into adolescent heads, an essential update, *Contemp Pediatr* 21:64-90, 2004.

Goldstein MA, Silverman ME: Neuropsychiatric assessment, *Psychiatric Clin North Am* 28:507-547, 2005.

Gonsalves WG, et al: Common oral lesions: part II. Masses and neoplasms, *Am Fam Physician* 75:509-512, 2007.

Goodacre S, et al: Meta-analysis: the value of clinical assessment in the diagnosis of deep venous thrombosis, *Ann Intern Med* 143(2):129-139, 2005.

Goodenough-Harris Drawing Test, Psychological Corporation. Available at http://www.psychcorp.co.uk/product.aspx?n=1316&s=1319&cat=1992&skey=2314&mode=Producthomeandpricelist.

Gorman WP, et al: ABC of arterial and venous disease. Swollen lower limb 1: general assessment and deep vein thrombosis, *BMJ* 320(7247):1453-1456, 2000.

Gotzsche PC, Olsen O: Is screening for breast cancer with mammography justifiable? *Lancet* 355(9198):129-134, 2000.

Graff-Radford NR: Normal pressure hydrocephalus, *Neurol Clin* 25:809-832, 2007.

Grant A: *Nutritional assessment guidelines*, ed 2, Seattle, 1979, Author.

Greenberg SA: The Geriatric Depression Scale: Short form, *Am J Nurs* 107(10):60-69, 2007.

Gregory KD, Niebyl JR, Johnson TRB: Preconception and Prenatal Care: Part of the Continuum. In Gabbe SG, Niebyl JR, Simpson JL, et al, editors: *Obstetrics: Normal and Problem Pregnancies*, ed 6, Philadelphia, PA, 2012, Elsevier Saunders, pp 101-124.

Gregory KD, Niebyl JR, Johnson TRB: Preconception and prenatal care: Part of the continuum. In Gabbe SG, Niebyl JR, Simpson JL,

et al, editors: *Obstetrics: Normal and Problem Pregnancies*, ed 6, Philadelphia, PA, 2012, Elsevier Saunders, pp 102-124.

Griffith WF, Stuart GS, Gluck KL, et al: Vaginal speculum lubrication and its effects on cervical cytology and microbiology, *Contraception* 72(1):60-64, 2005. 2005 Jul.

Gross E: Congenital neck lesions, *Surg Clin North Am* 86(2):383-392, 2006.

Gross RH: The pediatric orthopaedic examination. In Morrissy RT, Weinstein SL, editors: *Lovell & Winter's pediatric orthopaedics*, ed 4, Philadelphia, 1996, Lippincott-Raven.

Grummer-Strawn LM, Reinold C, Krebs NF: Use of World Health Organization and CDC growth charts for children aged 0-59 months in the United States, *Morb Mortal Wkly Rep* 59(rr09):1-15, 2010.

Grundy S, et al: Implications of recent clinical trials for the National Cholesterol Education Program Adult Treatment Panel III Guidelines, *Circulation* 110:227-239, 2004. Available at http://www.circulationaha.org.

Guidelines for the diagnosis of rheumatic fever. Jones criteria, 1992 update, *JAMA* 21(15):2069-2073, 1992.

Guilbert TW, Taussig LM: Doctor, he's been coughing for a month: is it serious? *Contemp Pediatr* 15:155-172, 1998.

Gunasekera H, et al: The global burden of otitis media and hearing impairment: a systematic review, *Pediatrics* 121(1):S107, 2008.

Guo SS, et al: Weight-for-length reference data for preterm, low-birth-weight infants, *Arch Pediatr Adolesc Med* 150:964-970, 1996.

Guzzetta CD, Dossey BM: *Cardiovascular nursing: holistic practice*, St Louis, 1992, Mosby.

Habif TP: *Clinical dermatology*, ed 4, 2004, Mosby, inc. Available at www.mdconsult.com, http://www.emedicine.com/derm/TOPIC159.HTM.

Habif TP: *Clinical Dermatology, a color guide to diagnosis and therapy*, ed 5, St Louis, 2010, Elsevier.

Hahn BA: Children's health: racial and ethnic differences in the use of prescription medications, *Pediatrics* 95(5):727-732, 1995.

Haidet P, Paterniti DA: "Building" a history rather than "taking" one, *Arch Intern Med* 163:1134-1140, 2003.

Haidet P: Patient-centredness and its challenge of prevailing professional norms, *Med Educ* 44:643-644, 2010.

Haka-Ikse K, Mian M: Sexuality in children, *Pediatr Rev* 14:10, 1993.

Harawa NT, Ford CL: The foundation of modern racial categories and implications for research on black/white disparities in health, *Ethn Dis* 19:209e217, 2009.

Hardie GE, et al: Ethnic differences: word descriptors used by African-American and white asthma patients during induced bronchoconstriction, *Chest* 117(4):935-943, 2000.

Hardin DM Jr: Acute appendicitis: review and update, *Am Fam Physician* 60(7):2027-2034, 1999.

Harer WBJ, Valenzuela G, Lebo D: Lubrication of the vaginal introitus and external speculum had no effect on papanicolaou smear interpretation/Commentary, *Evid Based Med* 8(3):79, 2003.

Harrison D, Bueno M, Yamada J, et al: Analgesic effects of sweet-tasting solutions for infants: Current state of equipoise, *Pediatrics* 126(5):894-902, 2010.

Hartmann LC, et al: Efficacy of bilateral prophylactic mastectomy in BRCA1 and BRCA2 gene mutation carriers, *J Natl Cancer Inst* 93(21):1633-1637, 2001.

Harvey AM, et al: *The principles and practice of medicine*, ed 22, Norwalk, Conn, 1988, Appleton & Lange.

Harvey WP: *Cardiac pearls*, Newton, NJ, 1943, Laennec Publishing, pp 62-64.

Hastriter EV, Olsson JM: Hoarseness, *Pediatr Rev* 27(6):e47–e48, 2006.

Hatala R, Attia J, Wong JG: Update: Meningitis, adult. In Simel DL, Rennie D, editors: *The Rational Clinical Examination: Evidence-Based Clinical Diagnosis*, New York, NY, 2009, McGraw Hill Medical, pp 402-406.

Hawker K, Frohman E: Multiple sclerosis, *Prim Care Clin Office Pract* 31:201-226, 2004.

Hedley AA, et al: Prevalence of overweight and obesity among U.S. children, adolescents, and adults, 1999-2002, *JAMA* 291(23):2847-2850, 2004.

Henderson DA, et al: Smallpox as a biological weapon: medical and public health management, Working Group on Civilian Biodefense, *JAMA* 281(22):2127-2137, 1999.

Hendrick RE, Helvie MA: United States Preventive Services Task Force Screening Mammography Recommendations: Science Ignored, *Am J Roentgenol* 196, 2011. DOI:10.2214/AJR.10.5609.

Hennigan L, et al: Methods for managing pelvic examination anxiety: individual differences and relaxation techniques, *J Pediatr Health Care* 14(1):9-12, 2000.

Henry SG, Fuhrel-Forbis A, Rogers MAM, et al: Association between nonverbal communication during clinical interactions and outcomes: A systematic review and meta-analysis, *Patient Educ Couns* 86:297-315, 2012.

Hermann-Giddens ME, Bourdony CJ, Dowshen SA, et al: *Assessment of sexual maturity stages in girls and boys*. Elk Grove Village, IL, 2011, American Academy of Pediatrics.

Herr K, et al: Pain assessment in the nonverbal patient: position statement with clinical practice recommendations, *Pain Manag Nurs* 7(2):44-52, 2006.

Hershko DD, et al: The role of selective computed tomography in the diagnosis and management of suspected acute appendicitis, *Am Surg* 68(11):1003-1007, 2002.

Hilliard AA, et al: Occam's razor versus saint's triad, *N Engl J Med* 350:599-603, 2004.

Hirsch AT, et al: Peripheral arterial disease detection, awareness, and treatment in primary care, *JAMA* 286(11):1317-1324, 2001.

Hirsch ED Jr: *Cultural literacy: what every American needs to know*, Boston, 1987, Houghton Mifflin.

Hitchcock JM, Wilson HS: Personal risking: lesbian self-disclosure of sexual orientation to professional health care providers, *Nurs Res* 41:178, 1992.

Hoberman A, Paradise JL: Acute otitis media: diagnosis and management in the year 2000, *Pediatr Ann* 29(10):609-620, 2000.

Hockenberry MJ, et al: *Nursing care of infants and children*, ed 7, St Louis, 2003, Mosby.

Hockenberry MJ: *Wong's essentials of pediatric nursing*, ed 7, St Louis, 2005, Mosby.

Hodgson SF, Johnston CC: *AACE clinical practice guidelines for the prevention of postmenopausal osteoporosis*, Brandamore, Pa, 1998, Herrin Communications.

Hoekelman RA, et al: *Primary pediatric care*, ed 3, St Louis, 1997, Mosby.

Holzberg M: Common nail disorders, *Dermatol Clin* 24(3):349-354, 2006.

Horner G: Sexual behavior in children. Normal or not? *J Pediatr Health Care* 18(2):57-64, 2004.

Hubert PM: Revealing patient concerns, *Am J Nurs* 98:16H–116L, 1998.

Huether SE: Pain, temperature, regulation, sleep, and sensory function. In McCance KL, Huether SE, Brashers VL, et al, editors: *Pathophysiology: The Biologic Basis for Disease in Adults and Children*, ed 6, St Louis, MO, 2009, Elsevier Mosby, pp 451-524.

Hulsey TC, et al: Birth weights of infants of black and white mothers without pregnancy complications, *Am J Obstet Gynecol* 164(part 1):1299, 1991.

Iams JD: Preterm birth. In Gabbe SG, Niebyl JR, Simpson JL, editors: *Obstetrics: normal and problem pregnancies*, ed 4, London, 2002, Churchill Livingstone.

Iavazzo C, Madhuri K, Essapen S, et al: Sister Mary Joseph's Nodules as a First Manifestation of Primary Peritoneal Cancer. Case Rep Obstet Gynecol 2012; Article ID 467240.

Ikegami N: Functional assessment and its place in health care, *N Engl J Med* 332(9):598-599, 1995.

Infant Nutrition and Feeding: *A guide for use in the WIC and CSF programs*, U.S. Department of Agriculture Food and Nutrition Service Special Supplemental Food Programs, September 2008. Available at www.nal.usda.gov.

Inglesby TV, et al: Anthrax as a biological weapon: medical and public health management. Working Group on Civilian Biodefense, *JAMA* 281(18):1735-1745, 1999.

Institute of Medicine: *Crossing the quality chasm: a new health system for the 21st century*, Washington (DC), 2001, National Academies Press.

Institute of Medicine and National Research Council: *Weight gain during pregnancy: Reexamining the guidelines*, Washington, DC, 2009, The National Academies Press, retrieved from http://www.nap.edu/catalog.php?record_id=12584.

International Society Lymphology: The Diagnosis And Treatment Of Peripheral Lymphedema Consensus Document of the International Society of Lymphology, *Lymphology* 36:84-91, 2003.

Isaacs B, Akhtar AJ: The Set Test: a rapid test of mental function in old people, *Age Ageing* 1(4):222-226, 1972.

Isaacson G: Sinusitis in childhood, *Pediatr Clin North Am* 43:1297, 1996.

Isaacson G: Diagnosis of pediatric cholesteatoma, *Pediatrics* 120(3):603-608, 2007.

Jackson JL, et al: Evaluation of acute knee pain in primary care, *Ann Intern Med* 139(7):575-588, 2003.

Jacobson A: Research for practice: saving limbs with Semmes-Weinstein monofilament, *Am J Nurs* 99(2):76, 1999.

Jacobson RD: Approach to the child with weakness or clumsiness, *Pediatr Clin North Am* 45(1):145-168, 1998.

Jalili M, Gharebaghi H: Validation of the Ottawa Knee Rule in Iran: a prospective study, *Emerg Med J* 27(11):849-851, 2010. Doi: 10.1136/emj.2009.080267. Epub 2010 Apr 8.

James HE: Neurologic evaluation and support of the child with acute brain insult, *Pediatr Ann* 15(1):17, 1986.

James WD, Carter JM, Rodman OG: Pigmentary demarcation lines: A population survey, *J Am Acad Dermatol* 16(3 Part 1):584-590, 1987.

James WD, Meltzer MS, Guill MA, et al: Pigmentary demarcation lines associated with pregnancy, *J Am Acad Dermatol* 11(3):438-4403, 1984.

Jantz JW, et al: A motor milestone change noted with a change in sleep position, *Arch Pediatr Adolesc Med* 151:565, 1997.

Jauhar S: The demise of the physical exam, *N Engl J Med* 354:548-551, 2006.

Jecker NS, et al: Caring for patients in cross-cultural settings, *Hastings Center Rep* 25:6, 1995.

Jerant AF, et al: Early detection and treatment of skin cancer, *Am Fam Physician* 62(2):357-368, 375-376, 2000.

Jessop S: HIV associated Kaposi sarcoma, *Dermatol Clin* 24(4):509-520, 2006.

Johns Hopkins University Center for Civilian Biodefense Studies: 2001. Available at www.hopkins-biodefense.org/index .html.

Johnston MV: Cerebral palsy. In Kleigman RM, Stanton BF, St Geme JW, et al, editors: *Nelson Textbook of Pediatrics*, ed 19, Philadelphia, PA, 2011, Elsevier Saunders, pp 2061-2065.

Joint Commission: Preventing pediatric medication errors, *Sentinel Event Alert* 39, 2008. Retrieved from http://www.jointcommission. org/assets/1/18/SEA_39.PDF.

Joint Commission: Facts about pain management, 2013, Retrieved from http://www.jointcommission.org/pain_management/.

Jones AK: Primary care management of acute low back pain, *Nurse Pract* 22:50, 1997.

Jones DW, et al: Measuring blood pressure accurately: new and persistent challenges, *JAMA* 289(8):1027-1030, 2003.

Jones WS, Kaleida PH: How helpful is pneumatic otoscopy in improving diagnostic accuracy? *Pediatrics* 112(3):510-513, 2003.

Juarez JA, Marvel K, Brezinski KL, et al: Bridging the gap: a curriculum to teach residents cultural humility, *Fam Med* 38(2):97-102, 2006.

Kain CD, et al: The older adult: a comparative assessment, *Nurs Clin North Am* 25:833, 1990.

Kahn JA, Emans SJ: Gynecologic examination of the prepubertal girl, *Contemp Pediatr* 16(3):148-159, 1999.

Kahn MW: Etiquette-based medicine, *N Engl J Med* 358:1988-1989, 2008.

Kalantri S, et al: Accuracy and reliability of physical signs in the diagnosis of pleural effusion, *Respir Med* 101(3):431-438, 2007.

Kanwar VS, Jorgensen S: *Lymphadenopathy*, WebMD, emedicine, November 8, 2007. Available at http://www.emedicine.com/PED/ topic1333.htm.

Kaplowitz PB: Delayed puberty, *Pediatr Rev* 31(5):189-195, 2010.

Kaplowitz PB: Link between body fat and timing of puberty, *Pediatrics* 121(Suppl 3):S208–S217, 2008.

Kass-Wolff J, Wilson E: Pediatric gynecology: assessment strategies and common problems, *Semin Reprod Med* 21(4):329-338, 2003.

Katbamna B, Crumpton T, Patel DR: Hearing impairment in children, *Pediatr Clin North Am* 55:1175-1188, 2008.

Katz ER, DeMaso DR: Chapter 21, Enuresis. In Kleigman RM, Stanton BF, St. GemeIII JW, et al, editors: *Nelson Textbook of Pediatrics*, ed 19, Philadelphia, 2011, Saunders Elsevier Inc.

Katz VL: Postpartum care. In Gabbe SG, Niebyl JR, Simpson JL, et al, editors: *Obstetrics: Normal and Problem Pregnancies*, ed 6, Philadelphia, PA, 2012, Elsevier Saunders, pp 517-532.

Kavey RW, Daniels SR, Flynn JT: Management of high blood pressure in children and adolescents, *Cardiol Clin North Am* 28:597-607, 2010.

Keane V: Assessment of growth. In Kleigman RM, Stanton BF, St. Geme JW, et al, editors: *Nelson Textbook of Pediatrics*, ed 19, Philadelphia, PA, 2011, Elsevier Saunders, pp 39e1-39e6.

Keisler BD, Hosey RG: Ergogenic aids: an update on ephedra, *Curr Sports Med Rep* 4(4):231-235, 2005.

Keith NM, et al: Some different types of essential hypertension: their course and prognosis, *Am J Med Sci* 197:337, 1939.

Keller C, Stevens KR: Childhood obesity: measurement and risk assessment, *Pediatr Nurs* 22:494, 1996.

Kellogg N, the Committee on Child Abuse and Neglect: American Academy Of Pediatrics, *Eval Sex Abus Child Pediatr* 116(2), 2005.

Kelly DP, Natale MJ: Neurodevelopmental function and dysfunction in the school-aged child. In Kleigman RM, Stanton BF, St. Geme JW, et al, editors: *Nelson Textbook of Pediatrics*, ed 19, Philadelphia, PA, 2011, Elsevier Saunders, pp 108-112.

Kemper KJ, Rivara FP: Parents in jail, *Pediatrics* 92(2):261-264, 1993.

Kennedy RM, Lulmann J, Zempsky WT: Clinical implications of unmanaged needle-insertion pain and distress in children, *Pediatrics* 122(Suppl 3):S130–S133, 2008.

Kerber AK, Baloh RW: Neuro-otolaryngology: Diagnosis and management of neuro-otological disorders. In Daroff RB, Fenichel GM, Jankovic J, et al, editors: *Bradley's Neurology in Clinical Practice*, ed 6, Philadelphia, PA, 2012, Elsevier Saunders, pp 644-667.

Kerchner K: Lower extremity lymphedema update: pathophysiology, diagnosis, and treatment guidelines, *J Am Acad Dermatol* 59(2):324-331, 2008.

Kerker BD, et al: Identification of violence in the home, *Arch Pediatr Adolesc Med* 154:457-462, 2000.

Khan NA, et al: Does the clinical examination predict lower extremity peripheral arterial disease? *JAMA* 295(5):536, 2006.

Khandker RK, et al: A decision model and cost-effectiveness analysis of colorectal cancer screening and surveillance guidelines for average-risk adults, *Int J Technol Assess Health Care* 16(3):799-810, 2000.

Khera P, et al: Diffuse gingival enlargement, *J Am Acad Dermatol* 52(3):491-499, 2005.

Kim CH, Younossi ZM: Nonalcoholic fatty liver disease: a manifestation of the metabolic syndrome, *Cleve Clin J Med* 75(10):721-728, 2008.

Kim HK: Pathophysiology and new strategies for the treatment of Legg-Calvé-Perthes disease, *J Bone Joint Surg Am* 94(7):659-669, 2012. Doi: 10.2106/JBJS.J.01834.

King D, Avner JR: Altered mental status, *Clin Pediatr Emerg Med* 4:171-178, 2003.

Kippenberger S, Havlíček J, Bernd A, et al: 'Nosing Around' the human skin: What information is concealed in skin odour? *Exp Dermatol* 21:9, 655-659, 2012, doi.org/10.1111/j.1600-0625. 2012.01545.x.

Kipper SL, et al: Neutrophil-specific 99mTc-labeled anti-CD15 monoclonal antibody imaging for diagnosis of equivocal appendicitis, *J Nucl Med* 41:447-455, 2000.

Klein S, Allison DB, Heymsfield SB, et al: Waist Circumference and Cardiometabolic Risk: a Consensus Statement from Shaping America's Health: Association for Weight Management and Obesity Prevention; NAASO, the Obesity Society; the American Society for Nutrition; and the American Diabetes Association, *Obesity (Silver Spring)* 15(5):1061-1067, 2007.

Kliegman RM, Stanton BF, St. Geme JW III, et al: *Nelson Textbook of Pediatrics*, ed 19, Philadelphia, 2011, Saunders Elsevier.

Kliegman RM, Stanton BF, St. Geme JW III, et al, editors: *Nelson Textbook of Pediatrics*, ed 19, Phihladelphia, 2011, Saunders Elsevier Inc.

Kleinman A, et al: Clinical lessons from anthropological and cross-cultural research, *Ann Intern Med* 88:251, 1978.

Kluckhohn C: *Culture and behavior*, New York, 1962, The Free Press.

Kluckhohn F: Dominant and variant value orientation. In Brink P, editor: *Transcultural nursing: a book of readings*, Englewood Cliffs, NJ, 1976, Prentice-Hall.

Knight JR, et al: Reliabilities of short substance abuse screening tests among adolescent medical patients, *Pediatrics* 105(4 Pt 2):948-953, 2000.

Knight JR, et al: Validity of the CRAFFT substance abuse screening test among adolescent clinic patients, *Arch Pediatr Adolesc Med* 156:607-614, 2002.

Knowles SR: Recognition and management of severe cutaneous drug reactions, *Dermatol Clin* 25(2):245-253, 2007.

Kokotos F, Adam HM: Vulvovaginitis, *Pediatr Rev* 27:116-117, 2006.

Konstantinou K, Dunn KM: Sciatica: review of epidemiological studies and prevalence estimates, *Spine* 33(22):2464-2472, 2008.

Koop CE: *The Surgeon General's letter on child sexual abuse*, Rockville, Md, 1988, U.S. Department of Health and Human Services, Public Health Service.

Koplan JP, et al, editors: *Progress in preventing childhood obesity*, Washington, DC, 2007, National Academies Press, pp 24-25.

Kopp VJ: Diagnoses [letter to the editor], *N Engl J Med* 337:941-942, 1997.

Koutures CG, Landry GL: The acutely injured knee, *Pediatr Ann* 26:50, 1997.

Köşüş A, Köşüş N, Duran M, et al: Effect of liquid-based gel application during speculum examination on satisfactory level of smear examination, *Arch Gynecol Obstet* 285:1599-1602, 2012.

Krebs NF, et al: Assessment of child and adolescent overweight and obesity, *Pediatrics* 120(Suppl 4):S193–S228, 2007.

Krugger KW: Cerebral palsy: an overview, *Am Fam Physician* 73(1):91-100, 2006.

Kuo DZ, O'Connor KG, Flores G, et al: Paediatricians' use of language services for families with limited English proficiency, *Pediatrics* 119(4):e920-927, 2007.

Kuczmarski MF, et al: Descriptive anthropometric reference data for older Americans, *J Am Diet Assoc* 100:59-66, 2000.

Kumar V, et al: *Robbins and Cotran Pathologic basis of disease*, ed 7, Philadelphia, 2005, Elsevier Saunders.

Kuschner SH, et al: Tinel's sign and Phalen's test in carpal tunnel syndrome, *Orthopedics* 15(11):1297-1302, 1992.

Labuguen RH: Initial evaluation of vertigo, *Am Fam Physician* 73(2):244-251, 2006.

Lanham DM, et al: Accuracy of tympanic temperature readings in children under 6 years of age, *Pediatr Nurs* 25(1):39-42, 1999.

Lapinsky S: Cardiopulmonary changes in pregnancy: what you need to know, *Womens Health Prim Care* 2:353, 1999.

La Rue A: Healthy brain aging: Role of cognitive reserve, cognitive stimulation, and cognitive exercises, *Clin Geriatr Med* 26:99-111, 2010.

Lederle FA: In the clinic. Abdominal aortic aneurysm, *Ann Intern Med* 150(9), 2009.

Lederle FA, Simel DL: The rational clinical examination. Does this patient have abdominal aortic aneurysm? *JAMA* 281(1):77-82, 1999.

Lee JM, et al: Weight status in young girls and the onset of puberty, *Pediatrics* 119:e624–e630, 2007.

Lembo NJ, et al: Bedside diagnosis of systolic murmurs, *N Engl J Med* 318:1572, 1988.

Leung RS, Katial R: The diagnosis and management of acute and chronic sinusitis, *Prim Care: Clin Off Pract* 35:11-24, 2008.

Levin B, et al: American Cancer Society Colorectal Cancer Advisory Group; U.S. Multi-Society Task Force; American College of Radiology Colon Cancer Committee: Screening and surveillance for the early detection of colorectal cancer and adenomatous polyps, 2008: a joint guideline from the American Cancer Society, the U.S. Multi-Society Task Force on Colorectal Cancer, and the American College of Radiology, *Gastroenterology* 134(5):1570-1595, 2008.

Levin J: When doctors question kids [letter to editor], *N Engl J Med* 323:1569, 1990.

Lichtenstein D, et al: Comparative diagnostic performances of auscultation, chest radiography, and lung ultrasonography in acute respiratory distress syndrome, *Anesthesiology* 100(1):9-15, 2004.

Light RW: Clinical practice. Pleural effusion, *N Engl J Med* 346(25):1971-1977, 2002.

Lively MW: Making sure young athletes are fit to compete in Special Olympics, *Contemp Pediatr* 20:101-107, 2003.

Lobo RA: Primary and secondary amenorrhea and precocious puberty: Etiology, diagnostic evaluation, management. In Lentz GM, Lobo RA, Gershenson DM, et al, editors: *Comprehensive Gynecology*, ed 6, St Louis, MO, 2012, Elsevier Mosby, pp 815-836.

Low MJ: Neuroendocrinology. In Melmed S, Polonsky KS, Larsen PR, et al, editors: *Williams Textbook of Endocrinology*, ed 12, Philadelphia, 2011, Elsevier Saunders, pp 103-174.

Lowdermilk DL, Perry SE: *Maternity and women's health care*, ed 8, St Louis, 2004, Mosby.

Lowrey GH: *Growth and development of children*, ed 8, Chicago, 1986, Mosby.

Luba KM, Stulberg DL: Chronic plaque psoriasis, *Am Fam Physician* 73(4):636-644, 2006.

Lussier M-T, Richard C: Self-disclosure during medical encounters, *Can Fam Physician* 53(3):421-422, 2007.

Lynch SH: Elder abuse: what to look for and how to intervene, *Am J Nurs* 97:27-32, 1997.

Lyon RM, Street CC: Pediatric sports injury: when to refer or x-ray, *Pediatr Clin North Am* 45(1):221-244, 1998.

Mace SE: Acute bacterial meningitis, *Emerg Med Clin North Am* 38:281-317, 2008.

Mackie RM, et al: The use of the dermatoscope to identify early melanoma using the three-colour test, *Br J Dermatol* 146(3):481, 2002.

Magauran BG: Risk Management for the Emergency Physician: Competency and Decision-Making Capacity, Informed Consent, and Refusal of Care Against Medical Advice, *Emerg Med Clin N Am* 27:605-614, 2009. doi:10.1016/j.emc.2009.08.001.

Makadon HJ: Ending LGBT invisibility in health care: the first step in ensuring equitable care, *Cleve Clin J Med* 78(4):220-224, 2011. http://www.ccjm.org/content/78/4/220.full. doi: 10.3949/ccjm.78gr.10006.

Mallants C, Casteels K: Practical approach to childhood masturbation—a review, *Eur J Pediatr* 167(10):1111-1117, 2008.

Mallory MD, et al: Bronchiolitis management preferences and the influence of pulse oximetry and respiratory rate on the decision to admit, *Pediatrics* 111:e45–e51, 2003.

Mandell GL, et al: *Principles and practice of infectious diseases*, ed 6, Philadelphia, 2005, Elsevier Churchill Livingstone.

Mankin KP, Zimbler S: Gait and leg alignment: what's normal and what's not, *Contemp Pediatr* 14(11):41-70, 1997.

Mann JM: Medicine and public health, ethics and human rights, *Hastings Cent Rep* May-June:6-13, 1997.

Manning ML: Health assessment of the early adolescent, *Nurs Clin North Am* 25:923, 1990.

Marcus CL: Does your child snore? *Contemp Pediatr* 15(2):101-115, 1998.

Marder MZ: The standard of care for oral diagnosis as it relates to oral cancer, *in Compendium* 19:569-582, 1998.

Margileth AM, Hadfield TL: A new look at old cat-scratch, *Contemp Pediatr* 7:25, 1990.

Marin JR, Alpern ER: Abdominal pain in children, *Emerg Med Clin North Am* 29(2):401-428, ix–x, 2011.

Marinis A, Yiallourou A, Samanides L, et al: Intussusception of the bowel in adults: a review, *World J Gastroenterol* 15(4):407, 2009.

Maron BJ, et al: Recommendations and considerations related to preparticipation screening for cardiovascular abnormalities in competitive athletes: update 2007. A Scientific Statement from the American Heart Association, Nutrition, Physical Activity and Metabolism Council, *Circulation* 115:1643-1655, 2007.

Martin HA, et al: Shaken baby syndrome, *Crit Care Clin North Am* 18:279-286, 2006.

Maslow K, Mezey M: Recognition of dementia in hospitalized older adults, *Am J Nurs* 108(1):40-49, 2008.

Matthews C: Perspective: Screening for HPV- associated anal dysplasia, *Top HIV Med* 11(2):45-49, 2003.

Mattson JE: The language of pain, *Reflect Nurs Leadersh* 4th quarter:11-14, 2000.

Maynard CK: Differentiate depression from dementia, *Nurse Pract* 28(3):18-27, 2003.

McCance KL, Huether SE, Brashers VL, et al: *Pathophysiology: The biologic basis for disease in adults and children*, ed 6, St Louis, MO, 2011, Elsevier Mosby.

McCance KL, Huether SE, Brashers VL, et al: *Pathophysiology: The biologic basis for disease in adults and children*, ed 6, St Louis, MO, 2010, Elsevier Mosby.

McCarthy PL, et al: History and observation variables in assessing febrile children, *Pediatrics* 65:1090, 1985.

McCarty DJ: *Arthritis and allied conditions: a textbook of rheumatology*, ed 2, Philadelphia, 1993, Lea & Febiger.

McClain N, et al: Evaluation of sexual abuse in the pediatric patient, *J Pediatr Health Care* 14(3):93-102, 2000.

McCrory P, Meeuwisse W, Johnston K, et al: Consensus statement on concussion in sport—The 3rd International Conference on concussion in sport, held in Zurich, November 2008, *J Clin Neurosci* 16:755-763, 2009.

McDermott MM, et al: Leg symptoms in peripheral arterial disease: associated clinical characteristics and functional impairment, *JAMA* 286(13):1599-1606, 2001.

McDermott TD, et al: A comparison of conventional percussion and auscultation percussion in the detection of pleural effusions of hospitalized patients, *J Am Acad Nurse Pract* 9(10):483-486, 1997.

McDowell JD: An overview of the epidemiology and common risk factors for oral squamous cell carcinoma, *Otolaryngol Clin North Am* 39:277-294, 2006.

McGee S: *Evidence-based physical diagnosis*, Philadelphia, 2001, WB Saunders.

McGee S: *Evidence based physical diagnosis*, ed 3, Philadelphia, PA, 2012, Elsevier Saunders, pp 43-47.

McGee SR: Percussion and physical diagnosis: separating myth from science, *Dis Mon* 41(10):641-692, 1995.

McGee SR, Boyko EJ: Physical examination and chronic lower-extremity ischemia: a critical review, *Arch Intern Med* 158(12):1357-1364, 1998.

McGibbon A, Chen GI, Peltekian KM, et al: An evidence-based manual for abdominal paracentesis, *Dig Dis Sci* 52(12):3307-3315, 2007.

McMillan JA, et al: *The whole pediatric catalogue* (vol 3), Philadelphia, 1982, WB Saunders.

McNair C, et al: Postoperative pain assessment in the neonatal intensive care unit, *Arch Dis Child Fetal Neonatal Ed* 89:F537–F541, 2004.

Meadows TA, et al: Ethnic differences in the prevalence and treatment of cardiovascular risk factors in U.S. outpatients with peripheral arterial disease: insights from the reduction of atherothrombosis for continued health (REACH) registry, *Am Heart J* 158(6):1038, 2009.

Meberg A, et al: First Day of Life pulse oximetry screening to detect congenital heart defects, *J Pediatr* 152(6):761-765, 2008.

Medina LS, et al: Children with headache: clinical predictors of surgical space-occupying lesions and the role of neuroimaging, *Radiol* 202(3):819-824, 1997.

Mell HK: Management of oral and genital herpes in the emergency department, *Emerg Med Clin North Am* 26(2):457-473, 2008.

Melmed S, Kleinberg D: Physiology and disorders of pituitary hormone axes. In Kronenberg HM, et al, editors: *Williams Textbook of endocrinology*, ed 11, Philadelphia, 2008, Saunders Elsevier, pp 180-234.

Mendelson M, Lang R: Pregnancy and cardiovascular disease. In Barron WM, Lindheimere MD, Davison JM, editors: *Medical disorders during pregnancy*, St Louis, 2000, Mosby.

Merkel S, Voepel-Lewis T, Shayevitz JR, et al: The FLACC: A behavioral scale for scoring postoperative pain in young children, *Pediatr Nurs* 23(2):293-297, 1997.

Metlay JP, et al: Does this patient have community-acquired pneumonia? Diagnosing pneumonia by history and physical examination, *JAMA* 278(17):1440-1445, 1997.

Merriam-Webster: http://www.merriam-webster.com/dictionary, 2012.

Meuller DH, Burke F: Vitamin and mineral therapy. In Morrison G, Hark L, editors: *Medical nutrition and disease*, Cambridge, 1996, Blackwell Science.

Migliori ME, Gladstone GJ: Determination of the normal range of exophthalmometric values for black and white adults, *Am J Ophthalmol* 98:438, 1984.

Modigliani RM: Gastrointestinal and pancreatic disorders. In Barron WM, Lindheimer MD, editors: *Medical disorders during pregnancy*, ed 3, St Louis, 2000, Mosby.

Miranda J, Cooper LA: Disparities in care for depression among primary care patients, *J Gen Intern Med* 19(2):120-126, 2004.

Molitch M: Pituitary, thyroid, adrenal, and parathyroid disorders. In Barron WM, Lindheimer MD, editors: *Medical disorders during pregnancy*, ed 3, St Louis, 2000, Mosby.

Moody CW: Male child sexual abuse, *J Pediatr Health Care* 13(3 Pt 1):112-119, 1999.

Morash D, Fowlder K: An evidence-based approach to changing practice: using sucrose for infant analgesia, *J Pediatr Nurs* 19(5):366-370, 2004.

Moreno MA: *Premenstrual syndrome*, e-medicine, May 22, 2006. Available at http://www.emedicine.com/ped/topic1890.htm.

Morrow M: The evaluation of common breast problems, *Am Fam Physician* 61(8):2371-2378, 2000.

Moser SJ, et al: Rett syndrome: Clinical and electrophysiologic aspects, *Pediatr Neurol* 36:95-100, 2007.

Mounsey AL, et al: Diagnosis and management of endometriosis, *Am Fam Physician* 74(4):N594–N601, 2006.

Moyer VA; on behalf of the U.S: Preventive Services Task Force. Screening for Cervical Cancer: U.S. Preventive Services Task Force Recommendation Statement, *Ann Intern Med* 2012 Mar 14.

Mower WR: Pulse oximetry as a fifth pediatric vital sign, *Pediatrics* 99(5):681-686, 1997.

Mower WR: Pulse oximetry as a fifth vital sign in emergency geriatric assessment, *Acad Emerg Med* 5(9):858-865, 1998.

Moyer LA, et al: Hepatitis C: part II. Prevention counseling and medical evaluation, *Am Fam Physician* 59(2):349-354, 357, 1999.

Murabito JM, et al: Prevalence and clinical correlates of peripheral arterial disease in the Framingham Offspring Study, *Am Heart J* 143(6):961-965, 2002.

Murphy NA, Carbone PS; the Council on Children with Disabilities: Promoting the participation of children with disabilities in sports, recreation and physical activities, *Pediatrics* 121(5):1057-1061, 2008.

Muzik M, Marcus SM, Heringhausen JE, et al: When depression complicates childbearing: Guidelines for screening and treatment during antenatal and postpartum obstetric care, *Obstet Gynecol Clin North Am* 36:771-788, 2009.

Nakama T, Hashikawa K, Higuchi M, et al: Pigmentary demarcation lines associated with pregnancy, *Clin Exp Dermatol* 34:e573–e576, 2009. doi: 10.1111/j.1365-2230.2009.03247.x.

National Academy of Sciences, institute of Medicine, Food and Nutrition Board: *Dietary reference intakes for energy, carbohydrate, fiber, fat, fatty acids, cholesterol, protein, and amino acids (macronutrients)*, 2005. Available at www.nap.edu.

National Asthma Education and Prevention Program: *Expert panel report III: Guidelines for the diagnosis and management of asthma*, Bethesda, MD, 2007, National Heart, Lung, and Blood Institute, (NIH publication no. 08-4051). www.nhlbi.nih.gov/guidelines/asthma/asthgdln.htm (Accessed on January 05, 2012).

National Cancer Institute: *Breast Cancer Prevention (PDQ®)*. www.cancer.gov/cancertopics/pdq/prevention/breast/HealthProfessional/page1/AllPages#Section_175, 3/29/2012.

National Cancer Institute: *Familial testicular cancer.* http://familial-testicular-cancer.cancer.gov/index.html. Accessed 1/24/2013.

National Cancer Institute and the National Surgical Adjuvant Breast and Bowel Project: *Breast Cancer Risk Assessment Tool.* Available at http://www.cancer.gov/brisktool/.

National Cancer Institute: *Melanoma Cancer Risk.* http://www.cancer.gov/melanomarisktool/melanoma-cancer-risk.html. Last modified date: 09/10/2008; accessed Nov 10, 2012.

National Cancer Institute: *Oral Cancer Prevention PDQ®*, 2012. Retrieved from http://www.cancer.gov/cancertopics/pdq/prevention/oral/HealthProfessional#Section_121.

National Cancer Institute: *Cervical Cancer Prevention (PDQ®)*. http://www.cancer.gov/cancertopics/pdq/prevention/cervical/HealthProfessional. Last Modified: 01/13/2012.

National Cancer Institute: *Genetics of Breast and Ovarian Cancer (PDQ®)*. http://www.cancer.gov/cancertopics/pdq/genetics/breast-and-ovarian/HealthProfessional#Section_339. Last Modified: 08/08/2012.

National Cancer Institute: *Endometrial Cancer Prevention (PDQ®)*. http://www.cancer.gov/cancertopics/prevention-genetics-causes/endometrial. Last Modified: 01/25/2012.

National Cancer Institute: *Cervical Cancer Screening (PDQ®)*. http://www.cancer.gov/cancertopics/pdq/screening/cervical/HealthProfessional. Last Modified: 06/01/2012.

National Cancer Institute: *Colorectal Cancer Prevention (PDQ®)*. http://www.cancer.gov/cancertopics/pdq/prevention/colorectal/HealthProfessionalal. Last Modified: 06/01/2012.

National Cancer Institute: *Prostate Cancer Prevention (PDQ®)*. http://www.cancer.gov/cancertopics/pdq/prevention/prostate/healthprofessional. Last Modified: 3/29/2012.

National Center for Health Statistics: *National Health and Nutrition Examination Survey III (1988-1994)*, 1996. Available at www.cdc.gov/nchs/about/major/nhanes/datalink.htm.

National Center for Infectious Diseases: *Epidemiology and prevention of viral hepatitis A to E, online slide set.* Available at www.cdc.gov/ncidod/diseases/hepatitis/slideset/httoc.htm.

National Center for Infectious Diseases: *Hepatitis fact sheets.* Available at www.cdc.gov/ncidod/diseases/hepatitis/hepatitis.htm.

National Cholesterol Education Program (NCEP): Expert Panel on Detection, Evaluation, and Treatment of High Blood Cholesterol in Adults (Adult Treatment Panel III): Executive summary of the third report, *JAMA* 285(19):2486-2497, 2001.

National Heart, Lung, and Blood Institute: *Blood pressure tables for children and adolescents from the fourth report on the diagnosis, evaluation, and treatment of high blood pressure in children and adolescents.* 2004. Retrieved from http://www.nhlbi.nih.gov/guidelines/hypertension/child_tbl.htm, accessed 6/11/2004.

National High Blood Pressure Education Program Working Group on High Blood Pressure in Children and Adolescents: The fourth report on the diagnosis, evaluation, and treatment of high blood pressure in children and adolescents, *Pediatrics* 114(2):555-576, 2004.

National Institutes of Health: *The seventh report of the Joint National Committee on Prevention, Detection, Evaluation, and Treatment of High Blood Pressure (JNC7)*, Bethesda, Md, 2004, National Heart, Lung, and Blood Institute, NIH publication No. 04-5230.

National Institute of Neurological Disorders and Stroke: *Neurofibromatosis.* http://www.ninds.nih.gov/disorders/neurofibromatosis/detail_neurofibromatosis.htm Last updated January 13, 2012; accessed Jun 14, 2012.

National Pressure Ulcer Advisory Panel, 2007. http://www.npuap.org/resources/educational-and-clinical-resources/npuap-pressure-ulcer-stagescategories/; accessed August 24, 2013.

National Pressure Ulcer Advisory Panel: http://www.npuap.org/pr2.htm; accessed June 2, 2021.

Nawaz H, et al: Concordance of clinical findings and clinical judgment in the diagnosis of streptococcal pharyngitis, *Acad Emerg Med* 7(10):1104-1109, 2000.

Nelson HD, Peggy Nygren P, McInerney Y: *Screening for Family and Intimate Partner Violence. Evidence Synthesis No. 28. AHRQ Contract No. 290-97-0018*, Rockville, MD, 2004, Agency for Healthcare Research and Quality.

Nelson HD, Bougatsos C, Blazina I: *Screening Women for Intimate Partner Violence and Elderly and Vulnerable Adults for Abuse: Systematic Review to Update the 2004 U.S. Preventive Services Task Force Recommendation. Evidence Synthesis No. 92. AHRQ Publication No. 12-05167-EF-1*, Rockville, MD, 2012, Agency for Healthcare Research and Quality.

Neuman LK, et al: The diagnosis of Cushing's syndrome: an Endocrine Society clinical practice guideline, *J Clin Endocrinol Metab* 93(5):1526-1540, 2008.

Nirupama K, DeSilva NK, Merritt DF: Chapter 545—Breast Concerns, In Kliegman RM, et al, editors: *Nelson Textbook of Pediatrics*, ed 19, Philadelphia, 2011, Saunders Elsevier.

Noble J, editor: *Textbook of primary care medicine*, ed 3, *Psoriasis and other papulosquamous diseases*, St Louis, 2001, Mosby. Available at www.mdconsult.com.

Nuss R, Manco-Johnson MJ: Venous thrombosis: issues for the pediatrician, *Contemp Pediatr* 17:75, 2000.

Obel J: Losing the touch: as technology and medical education change, doctors may lose the ability to perform physical exams, *Wash Post* June 17, 2003.

O'Connor NR, et al: Newborn skin: part I. Common rashes, *Am Fam Physician* 77(1):47-52, 2008.

Ogden CL, Carroll MD, Curtin LR, et al: Prevalence of high body mass index in U.S. children and adolescents, 2007-2008, *JAMA* 303(3):242-249. 2010.

Ogden CL, Carroll MD, Kit BK, et al: *Prevalence of Obesity in the United States, 2009-2010, NCHS Data Brief*, 82, 2012, retrieved from http://www.cdc.gov/nchs/data/databriefs/db82.pdf.

O'Hanlon-Nichols T: Basic assessment series: a review of the adult musculoskeletal system, *Am J Nurs* 98(6):48-52, 1998.

O'Hara MW, Stuart S, Watson D, et al: Brief Scales to Detect Postpartum Depression and Anxiety Symptoms, *J Womens Health (Larchmt)* 2012 [Epub ahead of print]

Olson AL, et al: Brief maternal depression screening at well-child visits, *Pediatrics* 118:207-216, 2006.

Olson LM, et al: At what age can children report dependably on their health status? *Pediatrics* 119:135, 2007.

Omnibus Budget Reconciliation Act [OBRA] of 1990 [Federal Patient Self-Determination Act], 1990 U.S.C. 135cc a Subpart E, Sections 4206 and 4751.

Papiernik E, et al: Ethnic differences in duration of pregnancy, *Ann Hum Biol* 13:259, 1986.

Park MK, et al: Comparison of auscultatory and oscillometric blood pressures, *Arch Pediatr Adolesc Med* 155:50-54, 2001.

Patrick D, et al: Increased CT scan utilization does not improve the diagnostic accuracy of appendicitis in children, *J Pediatr Surg* 38(5):659-662, 2003.

Pasero C, McCaffery M: *Pain assessment and pharmacologic management*, St Louis, MO, 2011, Elsevier Mosby.

Pawson EG, Petrakis NL: Comparisons of breast pigmentation among women of different racial groups, *Hum Biol* 47:441, 1975.

Peck J, Cusack C, Abdelmale M: Pigmentary demarcation lines, *J Am Acad Dermatol* 64(2 Suppl 1), 2011.

Pedigree Standardization Task Force of the National Society of Genetic Counselors, Bennett RL, et al: Recommendations for standardized human pedigree nomenclature, *Am J Hum Genet* 56:745-752, 1995.

Penninger J: Urinary incontinence: new approaches to age-old problems, *Gt Houst Nurs* 1:2, 1993.

Perez J, et al: Liberal use of computed tomography scanning does not improve diagnostic accuracy in appendicitis, *Am J Surg* 185(3):194-197, 2003.

Perkins HS, et al: Cultural differences among health professionals, *J Clin Ethics* 9:108-117, 1998.

Perniciano J: Development, behavior, and mental health. In Tschudy MM, Arcara KM, editors: *The Harriet Lane Handbook*, ed 19, Philadelphia, PA, 2012, Elsevier Mosby, pp 226-242.

Persing J, et al: Prevention and management of positional skull deformities in infants, *Pediatrics* 112:199-202, 2003.

Peters R, Flack M: Hypertensive disorders of pregnancy, *J Obstet Gynecol Neonat Nurs* 33:209, 2004.

Petit J, Barkhaus PE: Evaluation and management of polyneuropathy: a practical approach, *Nurse Pract* 22:131, 1997.

Piccoli M, et al: Bedside diagnosis and follow-up of patients with pleural effusion by a hand-carried ultrasound device early after cardiac surgery, *Chest* 128(5):3413-3420, 2005.

Pickering TG, et al: Recommendations for blood pressure measurement in humans: an AHA scientific statement from the Council on High Blood Pressure Research Professional and Public Education Subcommittee, *J Clin Hypertens* 7:102, 2005.

Pickett-Blakely O, Bleich SN, Cooper LA: Patient-physician gender concordance and weight-related counseling of obese patients, *Am J Prev Med* 40(6):616-619, 2011.

Pies R, Rogers D: *The recognition and treatment of depression: a review for the primary care clinician*, 2005. Available at http://www.medscape.com/viewprogram/4572_pnt.

Pinto S, et al: Treatments for dysarthria in Parkinson's disease, *Lancet Neurol* 3:547-566, 2004.

Plant SM: Boundary violations in professional-client relationships: overview and guidelines for prevention, *Sexual Marital Ther* 12:79, 1997.

Pow-Sang MR, Ferreira U, Pow-Sang JM, et al: Epidemiology and Natural History of Penile Cancer, *Urology* 76(2 Suppl 1), 2010.

Prazor GE, Friedman SB: An office-based approach to adolescent psychosocial issues, *Contemp Pediatr* 14:59, 1997.

President's Commission for the Study of Ethical Problems in Medicine and Biomedical and Behavioral Research: *The ethical and legal implications of informed consent in the patient-practitioner relationship. Making health care decisions, vol. 1, Report*, Washington, DC, 1982, U.S. Government Printing Office.

Puchalski CM, Romer AL: Taking a spiritual history allows clinicians to understand patients more fully, *J Palliat Med* 3:129-137, 2000.

Purnell LD, Paulanka BJ, editors: *Transcultural health care: A culturally competent approach*, ed 2, Philadelphia, 2008, E. A. Davis.

Pyeritz RE: The family history: the first genetic test, and still useful after all those years? *Genet Med* 14:3-9, 2012. doi:10.1038/gim.0b013e3182310bcf.

Qaseem A, et al: Current diagnosis of venous thromboembolism in primary care: a clinical practice guideline from the American Academy of Family Physicians and the American College of Physicians, *Ann Intern Med* 146(6):454-458, 2007.

Quality Standards Subcommittee of the American Academy of Neurology: The management of concussion in sports (practice parameter), *Neurology* 48:581-585, 1997.

Quant JR, Woo GC: Normal Values of Eye Position in the Chinese Population of Hong Kong, *Optom Vis Sci* 69(2):152-158, 1992.

Quill TE: Recognizing and adjusting to barriers in doctor-patient communication, *Ann Intern Med* 112:51, 1989.

Rabinowitz PM: Pet-related infections, *Am Fam Physician* 76(9):1314-1322, 2007.

Rabins PV: Research update: mild cognitive impairment (MCI)– definition, diagnosis, and treatment possibilities, *Adv Stud Med* 4(6):290-296, 2004.

RADAR: *A domestic violence intervention*, Waltham, Mass, 1992, Massachusetts Medical Society.

Rademaker J: Hodgkin's and non-Hodgkin's lymphomas, *Radiol Clin North Am* 45(1):69-83, 2007.

Rahhal RM, et al: A child with an abdominal mass, *Hosp Physician* 2006.

Raj GV, Wiener JS: Varicoceles in adolescents: when to observe, when to intervene, *Contemp Pediatr* 21:39, 2004.

Rampen FH: Nevocytic nevi and skin complexion, *Dermatologica* 176(3):111-114, 1988.

Rampen FH, de Wit PE: Racial differences in mole proneness, *Acta Derm Venereol* 69(3):234-236, 1989.

Ramsburg KL: Rheumatoid arthritis, *Am J Nurs* 100(11):40-43, 2000.

Rangel-Castillo L, et al: Management of intracranial hypertension, *Neurol Clin* 26:521-541, 2008.

Rapini D: The skin and pregnancy. In Creasey RK, Resnik R, editors: *Maternal-fetal medicine*, ed 4, Philadelphia, 1999, WB Saunders.

Rathore SS, et al: Sex-based differences in the effect of digoxin for the treatment of heart failure, *N Engl J Med* 347:1403-1410, 2002.

Raviola G, Gosselin GJ, Walter HJ, et al: Pervasive developmental disorders and childhood psychosis. In Kleigman RM, Stanton BF, St. Geme JW, et al, editors: *Nelson Textbook of Pediatrics*, ed 19, Philadelphia, PA, 2011, Elsevier Saunders, pp 100-107.

Ravussin E, Tataranni PA: Dietary fat and human obesity, *J Am Diet Assoc* 97:S42, 1997.

Ravussin E, Tataranni PA: Dietary fat and human obesity. In Williams CL, Williams GM, editors: *Reducing dietary fat: putting theory into practice*, Chicago, 1997, American Dietetic Association.

Rawlings AV: Ethnic skin types: are there differences in skin structure and function? *Int J Cosmet Sci* 28(2):79-93, 2006.

Reddel HK, Taylor DR, Bateman ED, et al: An official American Thoracic Society/European Respiratory Society statement: asthma control and exacerbations: standardizing endpoints for clinical asthma trials and clinical practice, *Am J Respir Crit Care Med* 180:59, 2009.

Reifsnider E, Gill S: Nutrition for the childbearing years, *J Obstet Gynecol Neonat Nurs* 29(1):43-55, 2000.

Reinold C, Dalenius K, Brindley P, et al: *Pregnancy Nutrition Surveillance 2009 Report*, Atlanta, 2011, U.S. Department of Health and Human Services, Centers for Disease Control and Prevention; retrieved from http://www.cdc.gov/pednss/pdfs/PNSS_2009_text_only.pdf.

Reiter EO, Rosenfield RG: Endocrine regulation of growth. In Kronenberg HM, Melmed S, Polonsky KS, et al, editors: *Williams textbook of endocrinology*, ed 11, Philadelphia, 2008, Saunders Elsevier, pp 857-879.

Relethford JH: Race and global patterns of phenotypic variation, *Am J Phys Anthropol* 139:16-22, 2009.

Rennard SI: Looking at the patient—approaching the problem of COPD, *N Engl J Med* 350:965-966, 2004.

Revere C, Hasty R: Diagnostic and characteristic signs of illness and injury, *J Emerg Nurs* 19(2):137-139, 1993.

Rhodes LA: Norms of culture in a "culture" of norms, *Arch Pediatr Adolesc Med* 157:1155-1156, 2003.

Rice SG; American Academy of Pediatrics Council on Sports Medicine and Fitness: Medical conditions affecting sports participation, *Pediatrics* 121(4):841-848, 2008.

Rice VH, Stead LF: Nursing interventions for smoking cessation. Cochrane Database Syst Rev (1):CD001188, 2008.

Rich EC, et al: Reconsidering the family history in primary care, *J Gen Intern Med* 19:273-280, 2004.

Riggs SR, Alario A: *RAFFT questions: project ADEPT manual*, Providence, RI, 1987, Brown University.

Risch N: Dissecting racial and ethnic differences, *N Engl J Med* 26;354(4):408-411, 2006.

Risser AL, Mazur LJ: Use of folk remedies in a Hispanic population, *Arch Pediatr Adolesc Med* 149(9):978-981, 1995.

Rivara FP, Wasserman AL: Teaching psychosocial issues to pediatric house officers, *J Med Educ* 59:45, 1984.

Riviello JJ, et al: Practice parameter: diagnostic assessment of the child with status epilepticus (an evidence-based review), *Neurology* 67:1542-1550, 2006.

Robinson CH, et al, editors: *Basic nutrition and diet therapy*, ed 7, Upper Saddle River, NJ, 1993, Prentice Hall.

Rockwood K, Mitnitski A: Frailty Defined by Deficit Accumulation and Geriatric Medicine Defined by Frailty, *Clin Geriatr Med* 27:17-26, 2011. doi:10.1016/j.cger.2010.08.008.

Rose LC: Recognizing neoplastic skin lesions: a photo guide, *Am Fam Physician* 58(4):873-884, 887-888, 1998.

Rose VL: CDC issues new recommendations for the prevention and control of hepatitis C virus infection, *Am Fam Physician* 59(5):1321-1323, 1999.

Rossi BV, Ference EH, Zurakowski D, et al: The clinical presentation and surgical management of adnexal torsion in the pediatric and adolescent population, *J Pediatr Adolesc Gynecol* 25(2):109-113, 2012.

Ryan C, Futterman D: Caring for gay and lesbian teens, *Contemp Pediatr* 15:107-130, 1998.

Sackett DL, et al: Evidence-based medicine: what it is and what it isn't, *Br Med J* 312:71, 1996.

Saha S, Beach MC, Cooper LA: Patient centeredness, cultural competence and healthcare quality, *J Natl Med Assoc* 100(11):1275-1285, 2008.

Saksouk FA: *Cervix cancer. emedicine.* Available at http://www.emedicine.com/radio/topic140.htm.

Sam S, Frohman LA: Normal physiology of hypothalamic pituitary regulation, *Endocrinol Metab Clin North Am* 37:1-22, 2008.

Samiy AH, et al: *Textbook of diagnostic medicine*, Philadelphia, 1987, Lea & Febiger.

Sapar JR: *Headache disorders: current concepts and treatment strategies*, Boston, 1983, PSG Publishing.

Saphis J: Human genetics: constructing a family pedigree, *Am J Nurs* 102(7):44-49, 2002.

Sargent-Cox K, Cherbuin N, Sachdev P, et al: Subjective Health and Memory Predictors of Mild Cognitive Disorders and Cognitive Decline in Ageing: The Personality and Total Health (PATH) through Life Study, *Dement Geriatr Cogn Disord* 31:45-52, 2011.

Saslow D, et al: for the American Cancer Society Breast Cancer Advisory Group: American Cancer Society Guidelines for Breast Screening with MRI as an Adjunct to Mammography, *CA Cancer J Clin* 57:75-89, 2007.

Satter EK: *Folliculitis. emedicine*, Apr 17, 2008. Available at www.emedicine.com.medscape.com/article/1070456-overview.

Schairer C, et al: Menopausal estrogen and estrogen-progestin replacement therapy and breast cancer risk, *JAMA* 283(4):485-491, 2000.

Schröder FH, et al, for the ERSPC Investigators: Screening and prostate-cancer mortality in a randomized European study, *N Engl J Med* 360:1320-1328, 2009.

Schroeder AR, et al: Impact of pulse oximetry and oxygen therapy on length of stay in bronchiolitis hospitalizations, *Arch Pediatr Adolesc Med* 158:527-530, 2004.

Schroder FH, Hugosson J, Roobol MJ, et al: Prostate-cancer mortality at 11 years of follow-up, *N Engl J Med* 366:981-990, 2012.

Schwartz RA, et al: Kaposi sarcoma: a continuing conundrum, *J Am Acad Dermatol* 59(2):179-206, 2008.

Schwartz RH: Pneumatic otoscopy: an old diagnostic tool revisited, *Infect Dis Child* 20(6):9-11, 2007.

Schwartz SJ, Weisskirch RS, Zamboanga BL, et al: Dimensions of acculturation: associations with health risk behaviors among college students from immigrant families, *J Couns Psychol* 58(1):27-41, 2011.

Scott M, Gelhot AR: Gastroesophageal reflux disease: diagnosis and management, *Am Fam Physician* 59(5):1161-1169, 1199, 1999.

Seeleman C, Suurmond J, Stronks K: Cultural competence: a conceptual framework for teaching and learning, *Med Educ* 43(3):229-237, 2009.

Seidel HM: On paternalism, *Pediatr Ann* 21:295, 1992.

Seth R, et al: How far is the sternal angle from the mid-right atrium? *J Gen Intern Med* 17(11):852-856, 2002.

Shah S, et al: Risk of bacteremia in young children with pneumonia treated as outpatients, *Arch Pediatr Adolesc Med* 157:389-393, 2003.

Shaper A: Obesity and cardiovascular disease. In Chadwick D, Cardew G, editors: *The origins and consequences of obesity*, Chichester, 1996, CIBA Foundation Symposium 201.

Shapiro W: *Hemolytic uremic syndrome*. Available at www.emedicine.com.

Shaw BA, et al: Avoiding the pitfalls of orthopedic disorders, *Contemp Pediatr* 15(6):122-135, 1998.

Shay DK, et al: Bronchiolitis-associated mortality and estimates of respiratory syncytial virus—associated deaths among U.S. children, *J Infect Dis* 183:16-22, 2001.

Sherin KM, et al: HITS: A short domestic violence screening tool for use in a family practice setting, *Fam Med* 30(7):508-512, 1998.

Shinitzky HE, Kub J: The art of motivating behavioral change: the use of motivational interviewing to promote health, *Public Health Nurs* 18(3):178-185, 2001.

Shipman JJ: *Mnemonics and tactics in surgery and medicine*, ed 2, Chicago, 1984, Mosby.

Shoaf SC: What your patient's mouth may be telling you, *Clin Rev* 13(8):41-48, 2003.

Siccoli M, et al: Facial pain: Clinical differential diagnosis, *Lancet Neurol* 5:257-267, 2006.

Siebert JW, Danner CJ: Eustachian tube function and the middle ear, *Otolaryngol Clin North Am* 39:1221-1235, 2006.

Siegel GB, et al: Managing anemia in pediatric office practice: Part 1, *Pediatr Rev* 23:75, 2002.

Siegel JD, et al: and the Healthcare Infection Control Practices Advisory Committee: *2007 Guideline for isolation precautions: preventing transmission of infectious agents in healthcare settings*, June 2007. Available at http://www.cdc.gov/ncidod/dhqp/pdf/isolation2007.pdf.

Siegel JD, Rhinehart E, Jackson M, et al: 2007 Guideline for isolation precautions: preventing transmission of infectious agents in healthcare settings, June 2007. Retrieved from http://www.cdc.gov/ncidod/dhqp/pdf/isolation2007.pdf.

Siegler R: *Children's thinking*, Englewood Cliffs, NJ, 1991, Prentice-Hall.

Simel DL: The clinical examination: an agenda to make it more rational, *JAMA* 277:572, 1997.

Simel DL, Williams JW: Update: Sinusitis. In Simel DL, Rennie D, editors: *The rational clinical examination: Evidence-based clinical diagnosis*, New York, NY, 2009, McGraw Hill Medical, pp 601-602.

Simel DL: Update: Ascites. In Simel DL, Rennie D, editors: *The Rational Clinical Examination Evidence-Based Clinical Diagnosis*, New York, 2009, McGraw Hill.

Siminoski K: Does this patient have a goiter? *JAMA* 273:813, 1995.

Sin DD, et al: The relationship between birthweight and childhood asthma, *Arch Pediatr Adolesc Med* 158:60-64, 2004.

Singh-Manoux A, Kivimaki M, Glymour MM, et al: Timing of onset of cognitive decline: Results from Whitehall II prospective cohort study, *Br Med J* 344:d7622, 2012.

Singer P: *A darwinian left: politics, evolution and cooperation*, New Haven, Conn, 1999, Yale University Press.

Sinhal, A: Early Nutrition and Long-Term Cardiovascular Health, *Nutrition Reviews*, 64(5):S44–S49, 2006.

Sinz, E, Navarro, K, editors: *Advanced Cardiac Life Support*, Dallas, TX, 2011, American Heart Association.

Sloan RP, et al: Should physicians prescribe religious activities? *N Engl J Med* 342:1913-1916, 2000.

Smith DM, et al: *Preparticipation physical evaluation*, ed 2, Minneapolis, 1997, McGraw-Hill.

Smith J, Serafi J: Delirium and dementia. In Marx JA, Hockberger RS, Walls RM, et al, editors: *Rosen's Emergency Medicine*, ed 7, Philadelphia, PA, 2009, Elsevier Saunders, pp 1367-1378.

Smith M, Buckwalter K: Behaviors associated with dementia, *Am J Nurs* 105(7):40-51, 2005.

Smith RA, Cokkinides V, Brawley OW: Cancer screening in the United States, 2012, *CA Cancer J Clin* 62:2, 129-142, 2012. DOI: 10.3322/caac.20143.

Smith W: Fibromyalgia syndrome, *Nurs Clin North Am* 33(4):653-668, 1998.

Smith-Alnimer M, Watford MF: Alcohol withdrawal and delirium tremens, *Am J Nurs* 104(5):72a–72g, 2004.

Snyder DR, Christmas C, editors: *Geriatric education for emergency medical services*, Sudbury, Mass, 2003, Jones & Bartlett.

Snyderman D, Rovner BW: Mental status examination in primary care: A review, *Am Fam Physician* 80(8):809-814, 2009.

Sokol RJ, et al: The TACE questions: practical prenatal detection of risk drinking, *Am J Obstet Gynecol* 160:863, 1989.

Solomon DH, et al: The rational clinical examination. Does this patient have a torn meniscus or ligament of the knee? Value of the physical examination, *JAMA* 286(13):1610-1620, 2001.

Special Writing Group of the Committee on Rheumatic Fever, Endocarditis, and Kawasaki Disease of the Council on Cardiovascular Disease in the Young of the American Heart Association.

Sprague J: Vision screening. In Krajicek M, Tomlinson AIT, editors: *Detection of developmental problems in children*, ed 2, Baltimore, 1983, University Park Press.

Starr NB, et al: Malocclusion: how important is that bite? *J Pediatr Health Care* 13:245-247, 1999.

Stashwick C: When you suspect an eating disorder, *Contemp Pediatr* 13:124, 1996.

Stavroudis L: Medical malpractice grand rounds presentation, *Johns Hopkins Child Center* May 31, 2004.

Stead LF, Bergson G, Lancaster T: Physician advice for smoking cessation, *Cochrane Database Syst Rev* (2):CD000165, 2008.

Stellwagen LM, et al: Look for the "stuck baby" to identify congenital torticollis, *Contemp Pediatr* 21:55, 2004.

Stephens B: The premature infant pain profile: Evaluation 13 years after development, *Clin J Pain* 26(9):813-830, 2010.

Stern TA, Rosenbaum JF, Fava M, et al, editors: *Massachusetts General Hospital Comprehensive Clinical Psychiatry*, ed 1, Philadelphia, PA, 2008, Elsevier Mosby, pp 231-246.

Stevens B: The premature infant pain profile: evaluation 13 years after development, *Clin J Pain* 26(9):813-830, 2010.

Stewart-Knox BJ, Simpson EEA, Parr1 H, et al: Taste acuity in response to zinc supplementation in older Europeans, *Br J Nutr* 99:129-136, 2008.

Stiell IG, et al: Decision rules for the use of radiography in acute ankle injuries: refinement and prospective validation, *JAMA* 269(9):1127-1132, 1993.

Stiell IG, et al: Prospective validation of a decision rule for the use of radiography in acute knee injuries, *JAMA* 275(8):641-642, 1996.

Steis MR, Schrauf RW: A review of translations and adaptations of the Mini-Mental State Examination in languages other than English and Spanish, *Res Gerontol Nurs* 2(3):214-224, 2009.

Stocker JT: Clinical and pathologic differential diagnosis of selected potential bioterrorism agents of interest to pediatric health care providers, *Clin Lab Med* 26(2):329-344, viii, 2006.

Studdiford J, Lamb K, Horvath K, et al: Development of unilateral cervical and supraclavicular lymphadenopathy after human papilloma virus vaccination, *Pharmacotherapy* 28(9):1194-1197, 2008.

Stone J, Moskowitz GB: Non-conscious bias in medical decision making: what can be done to reduce it? *Med Educ* 45(8):768-776, 2011.

Stulc DM: The family as a bearer of culture. In Cookfair JM, editor: *Nursing process and practice in the community*, St Louis, 1991, Mosby.

Subcommittee on the Tenth Edition of the RDAs, Food and Nutrition Board: *Recommended dietary allowances*, ed 10, Washington, DC, 1989, National Academy Press.

Subha ST, Raman R: Role of impacted cerumen in hearing loss, *Ear Nose Throat J* 85(10):650-653, 2006.

Suchman AL, et al: A model of empathic communication in the medical interview, *JAMA* 277:678-682, 1997.

Tachdjian MO: *Clinical pediatric orthopedics: the art of diagnosis and principles of management*, Stamford, Conn, 1997, Appleton & Lange.

Taddio A, Shah V, Hancock R, et al: Assessing postoperative pain in neonates: A multicenter observational study, *Pediatrics* 118(4):e992–e1000, 2008.

Tamariz LJ, et al: Usefulness of clinical prediction rules for the diagnosis of venous thromboembolism: a systematic review, *Am J Med* 117(9):676-684, 2004.

Tanner JM, Davies PS: Clinical longitudinal standards for height and height velocity for North American children, *J Pediatr* 107(3):317-329, 1985.

Taylor L, Willies-Jacobo LJ: The culturally competent pediatrician: respecting ethnicity in your practice, *Contemp Pediatr* 20:83-105, 2003.

Teasdale G, Jennett B: Assessment of coma and impaired consciousness: a practical scale, *Lancet* 2:81-84, 1974.

Teoh TG, Fisk NM: Hydramnios, oligohydramnios. In James DK, et al, editors: *High risk pregnancy: management options*, ed 2, Philadelphia, 1999, WB Saunders.

The Joint Commission: *History tracking report: 2009 to 2008 requirements, accreditation program: hospital: chapter: rights and responsibilities of the individual*, 2008. Available at http://search .jointcommission.org/search?q=pain&site=Entire-Site&client =jcaho_frontend&output=xml_no_dtd&proxystylesheet=jcaho _frontend.

Thein-Nissenbaum JM, Carr KE: Female athlete triad syndrome in the high school athlete, *Phys Ther Sport* 12(3):108-116, 2011.

Theophilopoulos EP, Barrett DJ: Getting a grip on the pediatric hip, *Contemp Pediatr* 15(11):43-65, 1998.

Thibodeau GA, Patton KT: *Anatomy and physiology*, ed 5, St Louis, 2003, Mosby.

Thomas DB, et al: Randomized trial of breast self-examination in Shanghai: final results, *J Natl Cancer Inst* 94(19):1445-1457, 2002.

Thomas KE, et al: The diagnostic accuracy of Kernig's sign, Brudzinski's sign, and nuchal rigiditiy in adults with suspected meningitis, *Clin Infect Dis* 35:46-52, 2002.

Thomas M, Haas TS, Doerer JJ, et al: Epidemiology of sudden death in young, competitive athletes due to blunt trauma, *Pediatrics* 128(1):e1-8, 2011.

Thomas SP: Anger: the mismanaged emotion, *Dermatol Nurs* 15:351-357, 2003.

Thompson JK, Cohen ME: Studies on the normal circulation in normal pregnancy: II, vital capacity observations in normal pregnant women, *Surg Gynecol Obstet* 66:591, 1938.

Thompson M: Deriving temperature and age appropriate heart rate centiles for children with acute infections, *Arch Dis Child* 94(5):361-365, 2009.

Thomson M: Heavy birthweight in Native Indians of British Columbia, *Can J Public Health* 81:443, 1990.

Thorburn WM: The myth of Occam's razor, *Mind* 27(107):345-353, 1918.

Thurman DJ, et al: Practice parameter: assessing patients in a neurology practice for risk of falls (an evidence-based review), *Neurology* 70:473-479, 2008.

Tiemstra JD, Khatkhate N: Bells's palsy: diagnosis and management, *Am Fam Physician* 76(7):997-1002, 2007.

Tinetti ME: Performance-oriented assessment of mobility problems in elderly patients, *J Am Geriatr Soc* 34(2):119-126, 1986.

Trotter TL, Martin HM: Family history in pediatric primary care, *Pediatrics* 120(Suppl 2):560-565, 2007.

Tunzi M, Gray GR: Common skin conditions during pregnancy, *Am Fam Physician* 75(2):211-218, 2007.

Twycross A, Dowden SJ, Bruce E, editors: *Managing pain in children*, United Kingdom, 2009, Wiley-Blackwell.

U.S. Cancer Statistics Working Group: *United States Cancer Statistics: 1999-2007 Incidence and Mortality Web-based Report*, Atlanta (GA), 2010, Department of Health and Human Services, Centers for Disease Control and Prevention, and National Cancer Institute.

U.S. Department of Agriculture and U.S. Department of Health and Human Services: *Dietary Guidelines for Americans*, ed 7, Washington, DC, 2010, U.S. Government Printing Office.

U.S. Department of Health and Human Services: *Your Guide to Lowering Your Cholesterol with TLC*. December 2005. found at http://www.nhlbi.nih.gov/health/public/heart/chol/chol_tlc.pdf.

U.S. Department of Agriculture, Center for Nutrition and Promotion: *MyPyramid*, 2009. Available at www.Mypyramid.gov.

U.S. Preventive Health Services Task Force: Screening for dementia: recommendations and rationale, *Am J Nurs* 103(9):87-95, 2003.

U.S. Preventive Services Task Force: Screening for Abdominal Aortic Aneurysm, *Ann Intern Med* 142:198-202, 2005.

U.S. Preventive Services Task Force Recommendation Statement: Screening for Breast Cancer, *Ann Intern Med* 151(10):716-726, 2009.

U.S. Preventive Services Task Force: *Screening for Cervical Cancer*. http://www.uspreventiveservicestaskforce.org/uspstf/uspscerv.htm. 2012.

U.S. Preventive Services Task Force: Screening for high blood pressure: U.S. Preventive Services Task Force reaffirmation recommendation statement, *Ann Intern Med* 147(11):783-786, 2007.

U.S. Preventive Services Task Force: Screening for osteoporosis in postmenopausal women: recommendations and rationale, *Am J Nurs* 103(1):73-80, 2003.

U.S. Preventive Services Task Force, Screening for Intimate Partner Violence and Abuse of Elderly and Vulnerable Adults: *U.S. Preventive Services Task Force Recommendation Statement, DRAFT*, 2012. http://www.uspreventiveservicestaskforce.org/uspstf12/ ipvelder/draftrecipvelder.htm.

U.S. Preventive Services Task Force: *The Guide to Clinical Preventive Services 2012 Recommendations of the U.S. Preventive Services Task Force*, 2011, AHRQ.

U.S. Preventive Services Task Force: http://www .uspreventiveservicestaskforce.org/uspstf/uspsaneu.htm.

USPSTF: Screening for testicular cancer, *Ann Intern Med* 154:483-486, 2011. http://www.uspreventiveservicestaskforce.org/uspstf10/testicular/testicuprs.htm. Epidemiology and Natural History of Penile Cancer.

Valle D: Genetics, individuality, and medicine in the 21st century, *Am J Hum Genet* 74(3):374-381, 2004.

Van Berckelaer AC, Mitra N, Pati S: Predictors of well child care adherence over time in a cohort of urban Medicaid-eligible infants, *BMC Pediatr* 11(1):36, 2011.

Van de Beek D, et al: Clinical features and prognostic factors in adults with bacterial meningitis, *N Engl J Med* 351(18):1849-1859, 2004.

Varcarolis EM: *Psychiatric nursing clinical guide: assessment tools and diagnosis*, Philadelphia, 1999, WB Saunders.

Veille JC, et al: Effects of pregnancy on the electrocardiogram in healthy subjects during exercise, *Am J Obstet Gynecol* 175:1360, 1996.

Videlefsky A: Routine vaginal cuff smear testing in post-hysterectomy patients with benign uterine conditions: when is it indicated? *J Am Board Fam Pract* 13(4):233-238, 2000.

Viera AJ, Neutze DM: Diagnosis of secondary hypertension: An age-based approach, *Am Fam Physician* 82(12):1471-1478, 2010.

Vieira AR: Unravelling human cleft lip and palate research, *J Dent Res* 87(2):119-125, 2008.

Vijayasankar D, Boyle AA, Atkinson P: Can the Ottawa Knee Rule be applied to children? A systematic review and meta-analysis of observational studies, *Emerg Med J* 26(4):250-253, 2009. Doi: 10.1136/emj.2008.063131.

Vinik AI, et al: Diabetic neuropathy in older adults, *Clin Geriatr Med* 24:4017-4435, 2008.

Visscher PM, Brown MA, McCarthy MI, et al: Five years of GWAS discovery, *Am J Hum Genet* 90(1):7-24, 2012.

Voepel-Lewis T, et al: Validity of parent ratings as proxy measures of pain in children with cognitive impairment, *Pain Manage Nurs* 6(4):168-174, 2005.

Vogel V, et al, for the National Surgical Adjuvant Breast and Bowel Project (NSABP): Effects of tamoxifen vs raloxifene on the risk of developing invasive breast cancer and other disease outcomes, *JAMA* 295:2727-2741, 2006.

Waghdhare S, Kalantri A, Joshi R, et al: Accuracy of physical signs for detecting meningitis: A hospital-based diagnostic accuracy study, *Clin Neurol Neurosurg* 112:752-757, 2010.

Wagner JM, et al: Does this patient have appendicitis? *JAMA* 276(19):1589-1594, 1996.

Wagner J: Update: Appendicitis, Adult. In Simel DL, Rennie D, editors: *The Rational Clinical Examination Evidence-Based Clinical Diagnosis*, New York, 2009, McGraw Hill.

Wall M: Idiopathic intracranial hypertension, *Neurol Clin* 28:593-617, 2010.

Wallhagen MI, et al: Sensory impairment in older adults: part 1: hearing loss, *Am J Nurs* 106(10):40-48, 2006.

Walsh S: Cardiovascular disease in pregnancy: a nursing approach, *J Cardiovasc Nurs* 2(4):53-64, 1988.

Walvoort. EC: The timing of puberty: Is it changing? Does it matter? *J Adolesc Health* 47(5):433-439, 2010.

Wardlaw GM, et al: *Contemporary nutrition*, ed 2, St Louis, 1994, Mosby.

Ware LJ, et al: Evaluation of the Revised Faces Pain Scale, Verbal Descriptor Scale, Numeric Rating Scale and Iowa Pain Thermometer in older minority adults, *Pain Manage Nurs* 7(3):117-125, 2006.

Waring WW, Jeansonne LO: *Practical manual of pediatrics*, ed 2, St Louis, 1982, Mosby.

Warner PH, et al: Shedding light on the sexual history, *Am J Nurs* 99:34-40, 1999.

Warner E, Messersmith H, Causer P, et al: Systematic review: using magnetic resonance imaging to screen women at high risk for breast cancer, *Ann Intern Med* 148(9):671-679, 2008.

Waszynski CM: Detecting delirium, *Am J Nurs* 107(12):50-59, 2007.

Watson J, Zhao M, Ring D: Predictors of Normal Electrodiagnosic testing in the evaluation of suspected carpal tunnel syndrome, *J Hand Microsurg* 2(2):47-50, 2010. Doi:10.1007/s12593-010-0012-9. Epub 2010 Oct 19.

Watts K, et al: Do skinfolds accurately assess changes in body fat in obese children and adolescents? *Med Sci Sports Exer* 38(3):439-444, 2006.

Weiner CP, Baschat AA: Fetal growth restriction: evaluation and management. In James DK, et al, editors: *High risk pregnancy: management options*, ed 2, Philadelphia, 1999, WB Saunders.

Weiss BD, Coyne C: Communicating with patients who cannot read, *N Engl J Med* 337:272-273, 1997.

Werk LN, et al: Medicine for the millennium: demystifying EBM, *Contemp Pediatr* 16:87-107, 1999.

Wexler JA, Sharretts J: Thyroid and bone, *Endocrinol Metab Clin North Am* 36:673-705, 2007.

Whooley MA, Simon GE: Managing depression in medical outpatients, *N Engl J Med* 343:1942-1950, 2000.

Wiens L, et al: Chest pain in otherwise healthy children and adolescents is frequently caused by exercise-induced asthma, *Pediatrics* 90(3):350-353, 1992.

Wieseke A, Bantz D, May D: What you need to know about bipolar disorder, *Am Nurse Today* 6(7):8-12, 2011.

Wilbourn AJ: Plexopathies, *Neurol Clin* 25(1):139-171, 2007.

Williams JW, Simel DL: Does this patient have sinusitis? diagnosing sinusitis by history and physical examination, *JAMA* 270(10):1242-1246, 1993.

Wilne S, et al: Presentation of childhood CNS tumours: a systematic review and meta-analysis, *Lancet Oncol* 8:685-695, 2007.

Wilson MEH: Keeping quiet, *Arch Pediatr Adolesc Med* 152:1054-1055, 1999.

Wilson RS, et al: The relationship between cerebral Alzheimer's disease pathology and odor identification in old age, *J Neurol Neurosurg Psychiatry* 78:30-35, 2007.

Wilson SF, Giddens JF: *Health assessment for nursing practice*, ed 3, St Louis, 2005, Mosby.

Winkleby MA, et al: Effects of an advocacy intervention to reduce smoking among teenagers, *Arch Pediatr Adolesc Med* 158:269-275, 2004.

Witting MD, Scharf SM: Diagnostic room-air pulse oximetry: effects of smoking, race, and sex, *Am J Emerg Med* 2:131-136, 2008.

Womack J: Give your sports physicals a performance boost, *J Fam Pract* 59(8):437-444, 2010.

Won AC, Ethell A: Spontaneous splenic rupture resulted from infectious mononucleosis, *Int J Surg Case Rep* 3(3):97-99, 2012.

Wong CL, et al: Does this patient have pleural effusion? *JAMA* 301(3):309-317, 2009.

Wong TY, Mitchell P: Current concepts hypertensive retinopathy, *N Engl J Med* 351:2310-2317, 2004.

Woo CK, Bahna SL: Evaluation of the Child with Immunodeficiency Disorder, *Pediatr Ann* 40(4):205-211, 2011.

Woodring JH: Distribution of pleural effusion in congestive heart failure: what is atypical? *South Med J* 98(5):518-523, 2005.

World Health Organization: *Energy and protein requirements: report of a joint FAO/WHO/UNU expert consultation*, Technical Report Series 724, Geneva, 1985, WHO.

World Health Organization: *Foodborne and waterborne health risks.* Available at www.who.int/ith/chapter03_02.html.

Wright JT: Normal formation and development defects of the human dentition, *Pediatr Clin North Am* 47(5):975-1000, 2000.

Yang AD, et al: Advance directive use among patients undergoing high-risk operations, *Am J Surg* 188:98-101, 2004.

Yang Q, Liu T, Valdez R, et al: Improvements in Ability to Detect Undiagnosed Diabetes by Using Information on Family History Among Adults in the United States, *Am J Epidemiol* 171(10):1079-1089, 2010. *doi: 10.1093/aje/kwq026* First published online: April 25, 2010.

Yernault JC, Bohadana AB: Chest percussion, *Eur Respir J* 8(10):1756-1760, 1995.

Yoshiura K, et al: A SNP in the ABCC11 gene is the determinant of human earwax type, *Nature Genet* 38(3):324-330, 2006.

Zardawi IM, et al: Effects of lubricant gel on conventional and liquid-based cervical smears [letter], *Acta Cytol* 47(4):704-705, 2003.

Zhang Y, Minassian BA: Will my Rett syndrome patient walk, talk, and use her hands? *Neurology* 70:1302-1303, 2008.

Zhang J, Savitz DA: Preterm birth subtypes among blacks and whites, *Epidemiology* 3:428, 1992.

Zink T, et al: Mothers' comfort with screening questions about sensitive issues, including domestic violence, *J Am Board Fam Med* 19(6):358-367, 2006.

Zitelli BJ, Davis HW: *Atlas of pediatric physical diagnosis*, ed 4, St Louis, 2002, Mosby.

Zitelli BJ, McIntire SC, Nowalk AJ: *Zitelli and Davis' atlas of pediatric physical diagnosis*, ed 6, St Louis, 2012, Elsevier.

Zlatnik F, et al: Vaginal ultrasound as an adjunct to cervical digital examination in women at risk for early delivery, *Gynecol Obstet Invest* 51(1):12-16, 2001.

REFERENCES AND READINGS

Glossary

abduction: Movement of the limbs toward the lateral plane or away from the axial line of a limb.

abruptio placentae: Premature separation of the placenta during pregnancy or labor before delivery of the fetus.

accommodation: Adjustment of the eye for various distances through modification of the lens curvature; negative accommodation is adjustment for far vision by relaxation of the ciliary muscle; positive accommodation is adjustment for near vision by contraction of the ciliary muscle.

acini cells: Milk-producing alveoli located in the glandular tissue of the breast.

adduction: Movement of the limbs toward the medial plane of the body or the axial line of a limb.

adenitis: Inflammation of a lymph node or a group of lymph nodes.

adnexa: Appendages (e.g., adnexa uteri are the structures adjacent to the uterus, including the ovaries, fallopian tubes, and uterine ligaments).

adventitious: Accidental or acquired; not natural or hereditary.

agoraphobia: Fear of being in an open, crowded, or public place.

alveolar ridge: Bony prominence of the maxilla and mandible that supports the teeth or dentures.

amblyopia: Reduced vision in an eye that appears structurally normal and without detectable cause when examined, including inspection with an ophthalmoscope.

amenorrhea: Absence of menses.

anacrotic: The upstroke of the pulse, which also implies a "notch" or "shoulder" on the upstroke.

anesthesia: Partial or complete loss of sensation.

aneurysm: A balloon-like swelling of the wall of an artery, vein, or heart; generally the result of a congenital defect in the wall or degenerative disease or infection (e.g., atherosclerosis or syphilis); a dissecting aneurysm is longitudinal splitting of the arterial wall with hemorrhage.

angle of Louis: The angle between the manubrium and the body of the sternum (also called the sternal angle).

anhedonia: The state in which a person appears to be involved in pleasurable activities but feels no pleasure associated with those activities.

annulus: A ring or circular structure (e.g., a tympanic annulus is a fibrous ring around the tympanic membrane that looks whiter and denser than the membrane itself).

anosmia: Absence of the sense of smell.

antalgic: Painful limp in which the patient shortens the time on the affected extremity.

anthropometry: Measurement of the size, weight, and proportions of the human body.

apex beat: The visible or palpable pulsation made by the apex of the left ventricle as it strikes the chest wall in systole; usually located in the fifth left intercostal space, several centimeters to the left of the median line (midsternal line).

aphakia: A condition in which part or all of the crystalline lens of the eye is absent, usually because of surgical removal for the treatment of cataracts.

aphasia: Impairment of language function in which speech or writing is not understood (receptive or sensory), words cannot be formed (expressive), or a combination of both.

apical: Pertaining to the apex or the area of the apex (top or tip) of a body, organ, or part.

apnea: A temporary halt to breathing.

appropriate for gestational age: A weight classification of newborns associated with better health outcomes, with the weight falling between the 10th and 90th percentiles on the intrauterine growth curve for the newborn's calculated gestational age.

apraxia: Inability to execute a skilled or learned motor act, not related to paralysis or lack of comprehension; caused by a lesion in the cerebral cortex.

arrhythmia (see dysrhythmia): A deviation from the expected rhythm of the heart.

arteriovenous fistula: A pathologic direct communication between an artery and a vein without an intervening capillary bed.

arteriovenous shunt: The passage of blood directly from an artery to a vein without an intervening capillary network.

articulation: The ability to pronounce speech sounds, words, and thoughts clearly and fluently; the junction of two or more bones; contact of the occlusal surfaces of the teeth.

ascites: Abnormal intraperitoneal accumulation of serous fluid.

asterixis: Postural tremor characterized by nonrhythmic, flapping movements of wide amplitude; extended wrist or fingers suddenly and briefly flex and then return to their original position.

astigmatism: An abnormal condition in which the light rays cannot be focused clearly in a point on the retina because of an irregular curvature of the cornea or lens.

ataxia: Impaired ability to coordinate muscular movement; usually associated with staggering gait and postural imbalance.

atelectasis: Incomplete expansion of the lung, either congenital or acquired.

atheroma: The deposit or degenerative accumulation of lipid-containing plaques on the innermost layer of the wall of an artery.

athetosis: Slow, twisting, writhing movements, with larger amplitude than chorea, that commonly involve the hands.

atrioventricular valve: Refers to the tricuspid or mitral valves.

Austin Flint murmur: A presystolic murmur, not unlike that of mitral stenosis, best heard at the apex of the heart; caused by aortic insufficiency.

autonomic nervous system: The portion of the nervous system that regulates involuntary functions supporting life; divided into the sympathetic and parasympathetic nervous systems.

baroreceptor: Sensory nerves within the walls of the atria, vena cava, aortic arch, and carotid sinus that monitor blood pressure change.

barrel chest: Increased anteroposterior diameter of the chest, often with some degree of kyphosis; commonly seen with chronic obstructive pulmonary disease.

Bartholin glands: Mucus-secreting glands located posterolaterally to the vaginal opening (also called the vestibular glands).

bifurcated: Having two branches, tines, or prongs.

bigeminal pulse: A pulse in which two beats occur in rapid succession so that they seem coupled and distinct from the succeeding set of two; each set is separated by a longer interval.

bisferiens pulse: The double-peaked systolic pulse; an arterial pulse with two palpable peaks, the second stronger than the first, but not markedly so; detected in instances of decreased arterial tension.

borborygmi: Rumbling, gurgling, tinkling noises heard on auscultation of the abdomen as a result of hyperactive intestinal peristalsis.

bossing: Bulging of the frontal areas of the skull; associated with prematurity and rickets.

boutonnière deformity: Fixed flexion of the proximal interphalangeal joint associated with hyperextension of the distal interphalangeal joint.

bradycardia: A heart rate less than 60 beats per minute.

bradykinesia: Slowing of voluntary and involuntary movements.

bradypnea: Slower than expected respiratory rate.

bronchial breathing: Harsh breathing characterized by prolonged high-pitched expiration with a tubular quality; often heard when lung tissue is consolidated.

bronchial fremitus: Adventitious pulmonary or voice sounds palpable over the chest or audible to the ear.

bronchiectasis: Persistent dilation of bronchi or bronchioles as a consequence of inflammatory disease, obstruction, or congenital abnormality.

bronchiolitis: Inflammation of the bronchioles, caused by bacteria or viruses (bronchopneumonia).

bronchogenic: Originating from the bronchi.

bronchophony: An exaggeration of vocal resonance emanating from a bronchus surrounded by consolidated lung tissue.

bronchopulmonary dysplasia: A form of chronic lung disease of uncertain cause sometimes seen in children who have had intensive respiratory support during the neonatal period.

bronchovesicular: Pertaining to the bronchial tubes and alveoli.

bruit: An unexpected audible swishing sound or murmur over an artery or vascular organ.

bruxism: Compulsive unconscious grinding of the teeth.

bubo: Inflammation and swelling of one or a group of lymph nodes, particularly in the groin or axilla, often accompanied by suppuration.

buccal mucosa: Mucous membranes inside the mouth.

bundle of His: A small band of modified heart muscle fibers that originates at the atrioventricular node and passes through the right atrioventricular junction to the interventricular septum, where the fibers divide into right and left branches and enter the respective ventricles; this bundle carries the atrial contractual rhythm to the ventricles; an interruption results in some degree of heart block.

bunion: Unexpected prominence of the medial aspect of the first metatarsal head, with bursa formation, resulting in lateral or valgus deviation of the great toe.

bursa: Disk-shaped, fluid-filled synovial sacs that develop at points of friction around joints, between tendons, cartilage, and bone; they decrease friction and promote ease of motion.

canthus: The angle at the medial or lateral margin of the eyelid; the medial canthus opens into a small space containing openings to the lacrimal duct.

caput succedaneum: An edematous swelling of the scalp of the newborn resulting from labor.

cardiac cycle: The complete sequence of cardiac action occurring from one heartbeat to the next, including both systole and diastole.

cardiac impulse: The thrust of the ventricles against the chest wall as a result of cardiac contraction.

cardiac output: The amount of blood ejected by the heart, usually stated in liters per minute, calculated by stroke volume multiplied by the number of heartbeats per unit of time.

cardiac reserve: The heart's ability to respond to demands that exceed ordinary circumstances.

carrying angle: The angle at which the humerus and radius articulate.

cellulitis: Inflammation of soft or connective tissue that causes a watery exudate to spread through the tissue spaces.

cephalohematoma: A subperiosteal hemorrhage, usually benign, along one of the cranial bones; it generally results from birth trauma.

cheilitis: Inflammation and cracking of the lips.

chemoreceptor: Any cell that is activated by a change in its chemical milieu and thereby produces a flow of nervous impulses; nerve cells sensitive to changes in the composition of the blood or cerebrospinal fluid.

choanae: A pair of posterior openings between the nasal cavity and the nasopharynx.

chordee: Ventral curvature of the penis caused by a fibrous band of tissue, often associated with hypospadias or gonorrhea.

chorea: Purposeless, involuntary rapid movements associated with muscle weakness and behavioral change; these are not tics, athetosis, or hyperkinesis. Chorea is often a delayed manifestation of rheumatic fever and may be confused with manifestations of Huntington chorea, systemic lupus erythematosus, Wilson disease, and drug reactions.

choreiform movements: Brief, rapid, jerky, irregular, and involuntary movements that occur at rest or interrupt normal coordinated movements; most often involve the face, head, lower arms, and hands.

choroid: The thin, highly vascular membrane covering the posterior five sixths of the eye between the retina and sclera.

cicatricial: Composed of scar tissue that is avascular, pale, and contracted.

ciliary body: The thickened part of the vascular tunic of the eye that joins the iris with the anterior portion of the choroid.

circumcorneal: Around the cornea.

circumduction: Circular movement of a limb (e.g., the shoulder) or the eye.

circumlocution: The use of pantomime, nonverbal expressions, or word substitutions to avoid revealing that a word has been forgotten.

clang association: Word choice based on sound so that words rhyme in a nonsensical way.

claudication: The condition resulting from muscle ischemia due to decreased arterial blood flow to an area and characterized by intermittent pain and limping.

clonus: Rapidly alternating involuntary contraction and relaxation of skeletal muscles.

coarctation: Constriction, stricture, stenosis, or narrowing, as of the aorta.

cochlea: A coiled bony structure within the inner ear; it contains the organ of Corti and perforations for the passage of the cochlear division of the auditory nerve.

cognition: The mental process of knowing, thinking, learning, and judging.

colic: Gradual onset of pain that increases in crescendo fashion until it reaches a peak of severity and then slowly subsides.

colostrum: Yellow, milky secretion from the breast that precedes the onset of true lactation; composed primarily of serum and white blood cells.

concha: A structure that is shell-shaped; the deep cavity in the auricle of the external ear containing the auditory canal meatus.

conductive hearing loss: Reduction in hearing acuity relating to interference of sound being transmitted through the outer and middle ears.

confabulation: Fabrication of detailed, plausible experiences and events to cover gaps in memory.

conjunctivitis: Inflammation of the conjunctiva caused by infectious agents or by allergies.

consolidation: Solidification of part of the lung into a firm, dense mass, particularly when the alveoli fill with fluid as a result of inflammation.

contracture: Permanent fixed flexion of a joint resulting from atrophy and shortening of muscles or from loss of skin elasticity.

coryza: Rhinitis; inflammation of the nasal mucous membranes, accompanied by swelling of the mucosa and nasal discharge.

crackle: A general term for an unexpected sound heard on auscultation of the chest; sometimes used to describe crepitus heard on auscultation.

craniotabes: An unusual softness of the skull in infants with hydrocephalus and rickets; the skull feels brittle and has a pingpong ball–snapping sensation when firmly pressed.

crepitus: A crinkly, crackling, grating feeling or sound in the joints, skin, or lungs; the quality of sound is simulated by Rice Krispies in milk; the quality of touch is somewhat simulated by rubbing hair between the fingers.

croup: An inflammation of the larynx, causing swelling of the vocal chords and sometimes severe obstruction; characterized by harsh, difficult breathing, stridor, and a hoarse cough; usually occurs in young children.

cryptorchidism: Failure of one or both testicles to descend into the scrotum.

cyanosis: A bluish or purplish color (may range from slight to intense) of the skin and mucous membranes because of insufficient oxygen levels in the blood.

deafness: Partial or complete loss of hearing.

decerebrate posturing: Rigid extension of all four extremities with hyperpronation of the forearms and plantar flexion of the feet.

dermatome: The area of skin (sensory and motor fibers) innervated by a single posterior spinal nerve.

development: The process of growth and differentiation; the acquisition of function associated with cell differentiation and maturation of individual organ systems.

dextrocardia: Location of the heart in the right hemithorax, either by displacement from disease or congenital mirror image reversal.

diastole: That time between two contractions of the heart when the muscles relax, allowing the chambers to fill with blood; diastole of the atria precedes that of the ventricles; diastole alternates, usually in a regular rhythm, with systole.

dicrotic notch: The notch in a pulse tracing between two elevations for each pulse beat.

dicrotic pulse: The double-peaked pulse; the second peak is usually weaker than the first and diastolic in timing.

diplopia: Double vision caused by defective function of the extraocular muscles or a disorder of the nerves that innervate the muscles.

dizziness: Sensation of an inability to maintain normal balance in a standing or sitting position (vertigo).

dorsiflexion: Backward bending or flexion of a joint.

dysarthria: Defective articulation secondary to a motor deficit involving the lips, tongue, palate, or pharynx.

dysfunctional uterine bleeding: Abnormal uterine bleeding not associated with tumor, inflammation, pregnancy, trauma, or hormonal imbalance; a diagnosis is given only after these causes are ruled out.

dyspareunia: Difficult or painful sexual intercourse.

dysphagia: Difficulty in swallowing.

dysphonia: A disorder in voice volume, such as hoarseness.

dyspnea: Difficult and labored breathing; shortness of breath.

dysrhythmia: Unexpected variation in the regular rhythm of the heart.

ecchymosis: A bruise, discoloration of the skin or mucous membranes as the result of hemorrhage into subcutaneous tissue.

echolalia: Automatic and meaningless repetition of another's words or phrases.

edema: Excessive accumulation of fluid in the cells, tissues, or serous cavities of the body.

edentulous: Without teeth.

effacement: The shortening of the vaginal portion of the cervix and thinning of its walls as it is stretched and dilated during labor.

effusion: Loss of fluid from the blood vessels or lymphatics into the tissues or a body cavity.

ejection murmur: A diamond-shaped systolic murmur occupying most but not necessarily all of systole; produced by the ejection of blood into the aorta or pulmonary artery.

electrocardiogram (ECG): A graphic record of the heart's electrical currents obtained with an electrocardiograph.

embolism: Obstruction of an artery by a blood clot or foreign matter.

emphysema: Pathologic accumulation of air in tissue or organs, especially the lungs.

encephalocele: A congenital gap in the skull, usually with herniation of the brain or meninges.

endocardium: The innermost membrane lining the heart cavities that is continuous with the lining of the blood vessels; its slippery surface eases the flow of blood.

epicardium: The inner visceral layer of the serous pericardium lying directly on the heart, forming the outermost layer of the heart wall.

epigastrium: The upper central region of the abdomen between the costal margins and a line drawn horizontally across the lowest costal margin.

epispadias: A congenital defect resulting in the urethral opening on the dorsum of the penis.

epulis: A tumor on the gingiva.

erythema marginatum: A distinctive evanescent pink rash, a rare manifestation of rheumatic fever; the erythematous areas have pale centers and round or serpiginous margins; they vary in size and appear mainly on the trunk and extremities, never on the face; the erythema is transient and migratory and may be induced by application of heat.

esotropia: The inward or nasal deviation of an eye (cross-eye).

eustachian tube: The cartilaginous and bony passage between the nasopharynx and the middle ear that allows equalization of air pressure between the inner ear and external pressure.

exotropia: The outward or temporal deviation of an eye (walleye).

extension: Movement that increases the angle between two adjoining bones to 180 degrees, bringing a limb toward a straight line.

external rotation: Lateral turning of a limb.

exudate: Fluid that has escaped from tissue or capillaries, usually after injury or inflammation, typically containing protein and white blood cells.

facies: Expression or appearance of the face; often used to describe characteristic expressions of disease states or congenital anomalies.

fasciculation: A localized, uncoordinated twitching of a single muscle group innervated by a single motor nerve filament; it is visible or palpable.

fibrosis: The formation of excessive connective tissue as an attempt to repair damage or as a reaction to foreign material, resulting in scarring and thickening.

flaccid: Muscles that are weak, soft, and flabby; lacking expected muscle tone.

flail chest: A flapping, unfixed chest wall caused by loss of stability of the thoracic cage after fracture of the sternum and/or ribs.

flank: The posterior part of the body below the ribs and above the ilium.

flatulence: The presence of excessive air or gases in the stomach or intestines, causing abdominal distention and resulting in rectal passage.

flexion: Movement that decreases the angle between two articulating bones, bending the limb.

floater: One or more spots that appear to drift in front of the eye; caused by a shadow cast on the retina by vitreous debris or separation of the vitreous humor from the retina.

fluctuant: A wavelike motion that is felt when a structure containing liquid is palpated.

fluency: Articulate speech that flows easily.

flutter: A rapid vibration or pulsation that impedes appropriate function.

fontanels: Membranous spaces at the juncture of an infant's cranial bones that later ossify.

foramen ovale: The communication between the two atria of the fetal heart; if it remains patent, blood shunts between the atria after birth, usually from left to right.

Fordyce spots: Ectopic sebaceous glands of the buccal mucosa appearing as small, yellow-white, raised lesions.

fornix: Arched structure (e.g., the vaginal fornix is the recess between the cervix and the vaginal wall); although one continuous structure, the vaginal fornix is anatomically divided into the anterior, posterior, and lateral fornices.

fourchette: Ridges of tissue formed by the fusion of the labia minora at the posterior aspect of the vulva.

fovea centralis: A tiny pit in the center of the macula lutea that is the area of clearest vision, permitting light to fall on the cones; it appears as an oval yellow spot on the retina and is free of blood vessels.

fremitus: A tremor vibration in any part of the body, detectable on palpation.

frenulum, lingual: Band of tissue that attaches the ventral surface of the tongue to the floor of the mouth.

friction rub: A sound audible through the stethoscope, resulting from the rubbing of opposed, inflamed serous surfaces.

functional assessment: Measurement of the abilities and activities used to perform the activities of daily living necessary for survival, vocational and social pursuits, and leisure activities.

galea aponeurotica: The fibrous sheet or tendinous material connecting the frontalis and occipitalis muscles over the skull.

gaussian distribution: A frequency distribution of observations and/or events that results in a plotted curve having the shape of a bell, reasonable symmetry, and the potential for infinite extent in either direction.

gestational age: Fetal age of a newborn, calculated from the number of completed weeks since the first day of the mother's last menstrual period to the date of birth.

gingivae: Gums of the mouth.

glaucoma: An abnormal condition of elevated pressure in the eye resulting from obstruction of the outflow of aqueous humor.

glottis: Pertaining to the vocal apparatus of the larynx, the true vocal cords, and the opening between them.

goiter: Cystic or fibrous enlargement of the thyroid gland, often related to thyroid dysfunction.

Graham Steell murmur: An early diastolic murmur of pulmonic insufficiency secondary to pulmonary hypertension.

graphesthesia: The ability to recognize symbols, shapes, numbers, and letters traced on the skin.

hallucination: A sensation (hearing, sight, smell, taste, or touch) perceived by a person while awake that is not caused by external stimuli.

helix: The prominent outer rim of the auricle of the ear.

hemangioma: A benign tumor of newly formed blood vessels that may occur anywhere in the body, most readily noticed in the skin and subcutaneous tissues.

hemianesthesia: Loss of sensation on one side of the body.

hemiplegia: Loss of motor function and sensation (paralysis) on one side of the body.

hemodynamic: Pertaining to the movement of blood and other aspects of the circulation.

hemoptysis: Coughing up blood or bloodstained sputum from the respiratory tree.

hernia: Protrusion of an organ or tissue through an opening in the muscle wall.

hilus of the lung: A hollow depression on the mediastinal surface of each lung, which is the point of entry of the bronchus, blood vessels, nerves, and lymphatics.

hirsutism: Excessive hair growth, especially an adult male pattern of hair distribution in women; usually related to heredity, hormonal dysfunction, porphyria, or medications.

holodiastolic: Occupying all of diastole.

holosystolic: Occupying all of systole.

Homan sign: Pain or discomfort behind the knee or in the calf when the ankle is gently dorsiflexed while the knee is flexed; it suggests thrombosis of the leg veins.

homonymous hemianopia: Defective vision in half of the visual field, occurring on the same side in each eye.

hydramnios: A condition of pregnancy characterized by an excess of amniotic fluid.

hydrocephaly: Enlargement of the head by an excessive accumulation of fluid dilating the cerebral ventricles, thinning the cerebral cortex, and causing separation of the cranial bones.

hyperesthesia: Unusual increased sensitivity to sensory stimuli, such as touch or pain.

hyperextension: A position of maximum extension.

hyperkeratosis: Overgrowth of the cornified layer of the skin or the cornea.

hyperkinesia: Excessive muscular activity; hyperactivity.

hypermenorrhea: Excessive bleeding during a menstrual period of usual duration.

hyperopia: A refractive error in which light rays entering the eye are focused behind the retina (farsightedness).

hyperpnea: Respiration that is deeper and more rapid than expected.

hyperresonance: Greater than expected resonance that is lower pitched in response to percussion of the chest wall or abdomen.

hyperthyroidism: Excessive activity of the thyroid gland with an increase in thyroid secretion.

hyperventilation: A state in which an increased amount of air enters the lungs, usually a result of deep and rapid breathing; if severe, it leads to alkalosis with the excessive loss of carbon dioxide.

hypesthesia: Decreased sensitivity to sensory stimuli such as touch and pain.

hypokinesia: Unusually diminished muscular activity.

hypomenorrhea: Decreased amount of menstrual flow.

hypospadias: A congenital defect in which the urethra opens on the ventral surface of the penis rather than on the glans.

hypotension: A condition in which arterial blood pressure is lower than expected.

hypothyroidism: Diminished activity of the thyroid gland with consequent reduction of thyroid hormone.

incus: One of the three ossicles of the middle ear, lying between the malleus and stapes.

induration: Excessive hardening or firmness of any body site.

infarction: An acute interruption to the blood supply of a part of the body by thrombi, emboli, extrinsic pressure, or twisting of blood vessels resulting in tissue death at the involved site.

infrapatellar fat pad: The soft tissue palpable in front of the joint space on either side of the patellar tendon.

intermittent claudication: Cramping pain and limping commonly in the calf brought on by walking; caused by ischemia of the muscles, usually from atheroma, the deposit or degenerative accumulation of lipid-containing plaques on the innermost layer of the wall of an artery that narrows the leg's arteries.

internal rotation: Medial turning of a limb.

intertriginous: An area where opposing skin surfaces touch and may rub, such as skinfolds in the axillae, fingers, toes, groin, inner thighs and beneath large breasts.

introitus: The vaginal opening.

isthmus: A narrow band of tissue connecting the two lateral lobes of the thyroid.

Janeway lesions (spots): Tiny hemorrhagic spots, a bit raised or nodular, occurring principally on the palms and soles, suggesting subacute bacterial endocarditis.

joint instability: An unusual increase in joint mobility.

jugular pulse: A pulsation in the jugular vein resulting from waves transmitted from the right side of the heart via circulating blood.

keratin: A scleroprotein that is the primary constituent of epidermis, hair, and nails.

Kiesselbach plexus: A convergence of small, fragile arteries and veins located superficially on the anterosuperior portion of the nasal septum.

Koplik spots: Small red spots with bluish white centers on the buccal mucosa opposite the molar teeth, appearing in the prodromal stage of measles.

kyphosis: An increased convex curvature of the thoracic spine.

lactation: The production and secretion of milk from the breasts.

large for gestational age (LGA): A weight classification of newborns associated with poorer health outcomes, with the weight falling above the 90th percentile on the intrauterine growth curve for the infant's calculated gestational age.

leukoplakia: Circumscribed, firmly attached, thick white patches on the tongue and other mucous membranes, often occurring as a precancerous growth.

lobule: A small lobe; the soft, lower, pendulous portion of the auricle of the ear.

locking: Inability to fully extend the joint or stiffness after being in one position for an extended time.

log-rolling: Keeping the body of the patient (i.e., similar to a log) while being turned.

lordosis: Accentuation of the lumbar curvature of the spine.

lymphangioma: A tumor composed of lymphatic vessels that vary in size and are often dilated.

lymphangitis: Inflammation of lymph vessels from bacterial infection of an extremity, characterized by fine red streaks running from the area of infection toward the groin or axilla.

lymphedema: Swelling, particularly of subcutaneous tissues, caused by obstruction of the lymphatic system and accumulation of interstitial fluid.

macroglossia: Excessively large tongue.

malleus: One of the three ossicles of the middle ear, connected to the tympanic membrane.

malocclusion: Inappropriate contact between the teeth of the upper and lower jaws.

McBurney point: In acute appendicitis, extreme sensitivity over the appendix, approximately 2 inches above the right anterosuperior iliac spine, on a line between that spine and the umbilicus.

meconium: First stools of the newborn; viscous, sticky, dark green, usually sterile and odorless.

mediastinum: The space in the thoracic cavity behind the sternum and between the two pleural sacs; contains the thoracic organs and structures.

medulla oblongata: The lowest subdivision of the brainstem, immediately adjacent to the spinal cord.

menarche: The first menstruation and initiation of cyclic menstrual function.

meninges: One of three membrane layers (dura mater, pia mater, and arachnoid) that enclose the brain and spinal cord.

meningomyelocele: A protrusion of the meninges and spinal cord through a defect in the vertebral column; also called myelodysplasia.

menorrhagia: Excessive bleeding during a menstrual period that is longer in duration than usual.

metrorrhagia: Menstrual bleeding at irregular intervals, sometimes prolonged but of expected amount.

microcephaly: An unusually small head of a newborn.

midaxillary line: A vertical line drawn midway between the anterior and posterior axillary folds.

midclavicular line: A vertical line drawn through the midpoint of the clavicle.

midsternal line: A vertical line drawn through the middle of the sternum.

miosis: Contraction of the pupil to less than 2 mm in diameter.

mitral valve: The heart valve between the left atrium and left ventricle consisting of two cusps; it allows blood to flow into the ventricle and prevents backflow.

Montgomery tubercles: Enlarged sebaceous glands located on the areola of the breast.

mucopurulent: An exudate that contains both pus and mucus.

murmur: A heart sound audible with the stethoscope, generated by disruptions in the passage of blood within the heart or blood vessels.

Murphy sign: Pain on inspiration during palpation of the liver and gallbladder that causes the patient to stop inspiration; usually a sign of gallbladder disease.

muscle tone: Level of tension or consistency of muscle mass.

myalgia: Tenderness or pain in a muscle.

myocardium: The middle and thickest of the three layers of the wall of the heart, consisting of cardiac muscle.

myopia: A condition resulting from a refractive error in which light rays entering the eye are brought into focus in front of the retina (nearsightedness).

myxedema: A condition caused by hypothyroidism characterized by dry, waxy skin, coarse hair, intolerance to cold, cognitive impairment, and slowing of the relaxation phase of deep tendon reflexes.

nasal polyp: Boggy, dependent mucosa that is rounded and elongated and projects into the nasal cavity.

nasopharynx: The portion of the pharynx extending from the posterior nares to the level of the soft palate.

neologism: A word used by a person with a mental disorder that is understood only by that person.

neurogenic: Arising from or caused by the nervous system.

nevus: A circumscribed skin lesion that is presumed to be genetic; the excess or deficient tissue may involve epidermal or connective tissue, nerve elements, or vascular elements; the nevus may be pigmented or nonpigmented.

nociception: The transmission of pain impulses from the site of injury or tissue damage to the dorsal horn of the spinal cord and brain.

nocturia: Urination at night; the individual is awakened from sleep by the need to void.

nuchal rigidity: Resistance to flexion of the neck, seen in individuals with meningitis.

nystagmus: Involuntary rhythmic movements of the eyes; the oscillations may be horizontal, vertical, rotary, or mixed.

oligomenorrhea: Infrequent menstruation.

oncotic pressure: The pressure difference between the osmotic pressure of blood and that of tissue fluid or lymph; an important force in maintaining balance between blood and surrounding tissues.

onycholysis: The loosening of the nails, starting at the border.

oropharynx: Division of the pharynx extending from behind the soft palate dorsally to the upper edge of the epiglottis.

orthostatic: Referring to an upright body position; orthostatic edema develops after standing; orthostatic hypotension occurs when the patient stands erect.

Osler nodes: Small, tender, swollen areas, varying in color from pink or red to bluish, generally in the fleshy pads of fingers or toes or in the thenar or hypothenar prominences; findings indicating subacute bacterial endocarditis.

ossification: The formation of bone.

otorrhea: Discharge, especially a purulent one, from the ear.

pack-years of smoking: An index risk for cardiac and pulmonary problems; calculated by multiplying the number of years of smoking by the number of packs smoked each day.

palpebral fissures: The elliptical opening between the upper and lower eyelids.

palpitation: Beating of the heart so vigorous that the patient is aware of it; causes include exertion, emotional stress, hyperthyroidism, and various heart diseases.

papillae: Small nipple-shaped projections; papillae on the dorsal portion of the tongue contain the taste buds.

papilledema: Edema of the optic disc resulting in loss of definition of the disc margin; the cause often is increased intracranial pressure.

paradoxic pulse: Variation in systolic pressure with respiration, diminishing with inspiration and increasing with expiration; also known as pulsus paradoxus.

paraphrasia: Speech that is incoherent or incomprehensible but that could be meaningful when carefully interpreted by a psychotherapist.

parasternal: Situated close to or beside the sternum.

parasympathetic nervous system: The division of the autonomic nervous system responsible for the protection, conservation, and restoration of body resources.

parenchyma: The functional cells of an organ, as distinguished from the supporting connective tissue framework.

paresthesia: Unusual sensation such as numbness, tingling, or burning.

parietal: Referring to the inner walls of any body cavity.

paroxysm: A sudden sharp spasm, convulsion, or attack; a sudden relapse of disease.

peak height velocity: The time during pubescence at which the tempo of growth is greatest.

peau d'orange: Dimpling of the skin that gives it the appearance of the skin of an orange.

pectoriloquy: A striking transmission of voice sounds through the pulmonary structures so that they are clearly audible through the stethoscope; commonly occurs from lung consolidation.

pectus carinatum: Forward protrusion of the sternum (pigeon chest).

pectus excavatum: Depression of the sternum (funnel chest).

pedunculated: Having a stalk or stem that acts as a means of connection.

pericardium: The fibroserous membrane covering the heart and roots of the great vessels.

perineum: The region between the thighs; in the female, between the vulva and the anus, and in the male, between the scrotum and the anus.

peristalsis: The wavelike motion by which the alimentary tract propels its contents.

petechiae: Purple or red pinpoint spots on the skin, the result of minute hemorrhages into the dermal or submucosal layers.

Peyer patches: Collections of closely packed lymphoid follicles, forming elevations on the mucous membranes of the small intestine.

philtrum: The vertical groove in the midline above the upper lip.

photophobia: Increased sensitivity to light; the condition is prevalent in albinism and disorders of the conjunctiva and cornea.

pica: A craving to eat nonfood substances such as dirt, clay, or starch; may occur with some nutritional deficiency states, pregnancy, or mental disorders.

pilonidal: Pertaining to the sacrococcygeal area.

pitch: A quality of sound that typifies its highness or lowness of tone as determined by the frequency of vibrations.

plantar flexion: Extension of the foot so that the forepart is lower than the ankle.

pleura: The serous membranes covering the lungs (visceral pleura) and lining the inner aspect of the pleural cavity (parietal pleura).

pleural cavity: The potential space between the usually closely opposed parietal and visceral layers of the pleura.

pleurisy: Inflammation of the pleura, often associated with pneumonia.

plumbism: Lead poisoning.

pneumothorax: Accumulation of air or gas in the pleural space.

polydactyly: Extra digits on the hands or feet.

polymenorrhea: Increased frequency of menstruation not consistently associated with ovulation.

postauricular: Behind the auricle of the ear.

posterior axillary line: A vertical line drawn inferiorly from the posterior axillary fold.

postmenopausal bleeding: Menstrual bleeding occurring 1 year or more after menopause.

postterm infant: An infant born after 41 completed weeks of gestation.

postural hypotension: The presence of low blood pressure when the patient stands erect (orthostatic hypotension).

preauricular: In front of the auricle of the ear.

precordium: The area of the thorax situated over the heart.

prepuce: The foreskin of the penis.

presbyopia: Hyperopia and impaired near vision from loss of lens elasticity, generally developing during middle age.

preterm infant: An infant born before 37 weeks' gestation.

primary assessment: A rapid examination of the patient's vital functions and physiologic status performed in the sequence of airway, breathing, and circulation to identify emergency physiologic dysfunction.

prodromal event: An early sign or warning of a developing disorder.

prognathism: Protrusion of the jaws, causing malocclusion of the teeth.

pronate: The act of assuming a prone position; applied to the hand, the act of turning the palm backward or downward by medially rotating the forearm; applied to the foot, turning the medial edge of the foot lower and outward by eversion and abduction of the tarsal and metatarsal joints.

proprioception: The sensation of position and muscular activity originating from within the body, which provides awareness of posture, movement, and changes in equilibrium.

proptosis, proptotic: Bulging or protrusion of an organ, such as the eyes.

pruritus: An itching sensation producing the urge to scratch.

ptosis: Prolapse of an organ or part; drooping of the upper eyelid.

pubarche: Beginning growth of pubic hair, breasts, and genitals.

pulmonary pressure: The blood pressure in the pulmonary artery.

pulmonary valve: The valve at the junction of the pulmonary artery and right ventricle consisting of three half-moon–shaped cusps; it prevents blood from regurgitating into the ventricle.

pulse: The palpable, rhythmic expansion and contraction of an artery, the result of an increased thrust of blood into the circulation each time the heart contracts; it is readily felt in the arterial component of the systemic circulation and also occurs in veins (e.g., jugular vein) and highly vascular organs (e.g., liver).

punctum: The tiny aperture in the margin of each eyelid that opens into a lacrimal duct.

purpura: Brownish red or purple discolorations on the skin as the result of hemorrhage into the tissue; also a group of disorders characterized by purpura.

pyrosis: Epigastric burning sensation; heartburn.

QRS complex: The central deflections of the electrocardiogram representing the activity of the ventricles.

radiculopathy: Nerve root pain.

rale: A general term for an unexpected sound heard on auscultation of the chest; sometimes used to denote crepitus heard on auscultation (see crackle).

regurgitation: A backward flowing (e.g., the blood between the chambers of the heart or between the great vessels and the heart); vomiting.

retrognathia: Position of the jaws behind the frontal plane of the forehead.

rhonchus: A dry, coarse sound in the bronchial tubes heard on auscultation of the chest, the result of partial obstruction; a sonorous rhonchus is low-pitched, a sibilant rhonchus is high-pitched and squeaky.

rigidity: A condition of hardness and inflexibility.

saccular: Pouched; shaped like a sac.

scapular line: A vertical line drawn through the inferior angle of the scapula.

sclerosis: Hardening or induration of body tissues, which can be the result of inflammation, particularly when it is prolonged.

scoliosis: Lateral curvature of the spine.

scotoma: A loss of vision in a defined area in one or both eyes; shimmering film appearing as an island in the visual field, often occurring as a prodromal symptom.

scrotal raphe: The line of union of the two halves of the scrotum; often more highly pigmented than the surrounding tissue.

sebum: A thick substance secreted by the sebaceous glands that consists of fat and epithelial debris.

secondary assessment: A focused assessment; an in-depth, head-to-toe examination of a patient with an emergency condition to identify anatomic problems, potentially life-threatening conditions, and the patient's previously diagnosed conditions.

semilunar valve: Refers to the pulmonic or aortic valves.

sensorineural hearing loss: Reduction in hearing acuity related to a defect in the inner ear or damage to the eighth cranial nerve.

sessile: Attached by a base rather than a stalk; a sessile lesion adheres closely to the surface of the skin or mucosa (see pedunculated).

shunt, left to right: Referring to a diversion of blood from the left side of the heart to the right (e.g., from a septal defect) or from the systemic circulation to the pulmonary circulation (e.g., from a patent ductus arteriosus).

sibilant: Having the character of a hiss or whistle.

sign: An objective finding perceived by the examiner.

simian crease: A single transverse palmar crease associated with Down syndrome.

sinus dysrhythmia: An increase in heart rate with inspiration; a physiologic response to decreased left ventricular volume during inspiration, producing a cyclic irregularity with each inspiration.

sinus rhythm: The expected regular cardiac rhythm stimulated by the sinoatrial node.

situs inversus: The inversion or transposition of the body viscera so that the heart is on the right and the liver on the left; the chest and abdominal contents become mirror images of the usual.

Skene glands: Mucus-secreting glands that open onto the vestibule on each side of the urethra (paraurethral glands).

small for gestational age (SGA): A weight classification of newborns associated with poorer health outcomes, with the weight falling below the 10th percentile on the intrauterine growth curve for the infant's calculated gestational age.

smegma: Sebaceous material secreted by the glans penis and epithelial cells desquamated from the prepuce; it appears as a cheesy white material.

spasm: Involuntary contraction of a muscle or group of muscles, interfering with usual function of that particular muscle group.

spastic: Increased muscle tone, spasms, or uncontrolled contractions of skeletal muscles causing stiff, awkward movements.

spotting: Small amounts of intermenstrual bloody vaginal discharge ranging in color from pink to dark brown.

sprain: Traumatic injury to the tendons, muscles, or ligaments around a joint.

stapes: One of the three ossicles of the middle ear, connected to the inner ear.

steatorrhea: Frothy, foul-smelling fecal matter that floats because of its high fat content; associated with malabsorption syndromes.

stellate: Shaped like a star; arranged in a rosette.

stereognosis: The ability to recognize objects by the sense of touch.

striae: Streaks or lines; skin striae result from weakening of the elastic tissue associated with pregnancy, weight gain, rapid growth periods, and high levels of corticosteroids.

stridor: A harsh, high-pitched sound during respiration caused by laryngeal or tracheal obstruction.

stroke: Common term indicating a sudden neurologic impairment of varying degree, usually related to a more or less sudden interruption of blood flow in the brain, such as from hemorrhage, thrombosis, or embolism.

stroke volume: The amount of blood pumped out of one ventricle of the heart as the result of a single contraction.

stroma: The supportive connective tissue framework of an organ as distinguished from the functional tissue (parenchyma).

sty: A purulent infection of a meibomian gland of the eyelid; often caused by a staphylococcal organism.

subaortic stenosis: Congenital narrowing of the outflow tract of the left ventricle caused by a ring of fibrous tissue or hypertrophy of the muscular septum just below the aortic valve.

subcutaneous emphysema: The presence of air or gas beneath the skin.

subcutaneous nodules: Firm and painless nodules discovered in the presence of acute rheumatic fever; these nodules occur only rarely and, when they do, usually in the presence of carditis; nodules appear over the extensor surfaces of certain joints, particularly the elbows, knees, and wrists; nodules appear over the spinous processes of the thoracic and lumbar vertebrae and in the suboccipital area; the skin over these nodules moves freely and is not inflamed.

subgaleal: The area underlying the galea aponeurotica.

subjective data: Information collected during the interview with the patient or a significant other.

subluxation: Partial or incomplete dislocation.

sulcus: A shallow groove or depression on the surface of an organ (e.g., the median sulcus of the prostate gland separating the two lateral lobes).

supernumerary nipples: Extra nipples usually not associated with underlying glandular tissue located along the embryonic mammary ridge.

supinate: To assume a supine position; applied to the arm, the act of turning the palm forward or upward by laterally rotating the forearm; applied to the foot, the act of raising the medial margin of the foot.

sutures: A fibrous joint in which the bones are closely approximated, such as between the infant's cranial bones, permitting expansion of the skull for brain growth.

swan neck deformity: Hyperextension of the proximal interphalangeal joint with fixed flexion of the distal interphalangeal joint.

sympathetic nervous system: The division of the autonomic nervous system that activates responses to physiologic or psychologic stress.

symptom: The subjective indication of disease perceived by the patient.

syndactyly: Webbing between the digits of the hands or feet.

systole: The part of the cardiac cycle during which the heart contracts, particularly the ventricles, resulting in a forceful flow of blood into both the systemic and pulmonary circulations.

tachycardia: Rapid heart rate, greater than 100 beats per minute.

tachypnea: Rapid, usually shallow, breathing.

tactile fremitus: A tremor or vibration in any part of the body detected on palpation.

tail of Spence: Upper outer tail of the breast that extends into the axilla.

term infant: An infant born between 37 and 41 weeks of gestation.

terminal hair: The pigmented coarse hair that grows on the scalp, axilla, pubis, and on the face in males.

thelarche: The beginning of female pubertal breast development.

thrill: A palpable vibration or tremor resulting from a cardiac murmur or a disruption in vascular blood flow.

thrombophlebitis: Inflammation of the wall of a vein associated with thrombus formation.

thrombosis: The formation or presence of a blood clot within a blood vessel or within one of the cavities of the heart.

thyrotoxicosis: A disease caused by excessive quantities of thyroid hormones.

tic: An involuntary movement or spasm of a small group of muscles that may be aggravated by stress or anxiety; sometimes momentarily controllable.

tinnitus: An auditory sensation in the absence of sound heard in one or both ears, such as ringing, buzzing, hissing, or clicking.

tocolysis: Suppression of premature labor with drugs.

tonus: Expected state of muscle tone, maintained by partial contraction or alternate contraction and relaxation of neighboring muscle fibers in a group of muscles.

tophus: A chalky deposit of uric acid crystals around joints or on the external ear; associated with gout.

tragus: The cartilaginous projection of the ear anterior to the auditory canal meatus.

transient ischemic attack (TIA): A transient episode of cerebral dysfunction, rapid (within minutes) in onset; usually due to vasospasm, hypotension, or a variety of events producing an ischemia that resolves usually in less than 24 hours; most often referable to the areas served by carotid and/or vertebrobasilar arteries.

transient tachypnea of the newborn: A self-limited neonatal respiratory problem characterized by a rapid respiratory rate and associated with maternal treatment with narcotics or analgesics during labor, premature labor and, at times, cesarean delivery.

tremor: Rhythmic, purposeless, quivering movements resulting from involuntary alternate contraction and relaxation of opposing muscle groups.

tricuspid valve: A heart valve between the right atrium and right ventricle, consisting of three cusps, that allows blood to flow to the ventricle and prevents backflow.

turbinates: Extensions of the ethmoid bone located along the lateral wall of the nose, covered by erectile mucous membrane.

tympanic membrane: A membranous structure separating the external ear from the middle ear (eardrum).

umbo: Landmark on the tympanic membrane created by the attachment of the tympanic membrane to the malleus.

valgus: A position in which part of a limb is twisted outward away from the midline.

Valsalva maneuver: Forced expiratory effort against a closed airway (i.e., closed mouth and nose or glottis).

varicosity: An unnaturally swollen, often tortuous, blood or lymph vessel.

varus: A position in which part of a limb is twisted inward toward the midline.

vascular: Referring to blood vessels.

vasoconstriction: A narrowing in the caliber of a blood vessel.

vasomotor: Referring to control over the dilation and constriction of blood vessels.

vasopressor: Stimulating contraction of the muscular tissues of the capillaries and arteries, causing a rise in blood pressure.

vellus hair: The soft, nonpigmented hair that covers the body.

velocity of growth: The rate of growth or change in growth measurements over a period of time.

venous hum: A continuous musical murmur heard on auscultation over the major veins at the base of the neck, particularly when a patient is anemic, upright, and looking to the contralateral side; also heard in the healthy individual, particularly the young.

venous thrombosis: Formation or presence of a blood clot within a vein.

ventilation: The movement of air into and out of the lungs, resulting in the exchange of gases between the lungs and the air.

vertigo: Sensation of dizziness, either of spinning oneself or of external objects whirling around oneself.

vesicular breath sounds: Expected breathing sounds when the patient is healthy and free of respiratory embarrassment.

vestibular function: Balance.

vestibule: The almond-shaped area enclosed by the labia minora laterally, extending from the clitoris to the fourchette anteroposteriorly.

Virchow node: A supraclavicular lymph node, particularly on the left, so enlarged that it is palpable (signal or sentinel node).

virilization: The process by which a female acquires male secondary sexual characteristics, usually as a result of adrenal dysfunction.

vulva: The visible external female genitalia consisting of the mons pubis, labia, clitoris, vaginal orifice, vestibule, and vestibular glands (pudendum).

water-hammer pulse: Full, forcible impulse and immediate collapse, providing a jerking sensation; characteristic of aortic regurgitation.

webbing: Skinfolds in the neck from the acromion to the mastoid; associated with chromosomal anomalies.

whispered pectoriloquy: The transmission of a whisper in the same way as that of more readily audible speech, commonly detected through the stethoscope when the lung is consolidated by pneumonia (see pectoriloquy).

whoop: The noisy spasm of inspiration that terminates the paroxysms of coughing characteristic of pertussis (whooping cough); caused by a sudden, sharp increase in tension of the vocal chords.

winged scapula: An outward prominence of the scapula caused by disruption of its nerves or muscles.

word salad: Meaningless, disconnected word choices often used by a person with schizophrenia or some other problem of disorientation.

xanthelasma: Xanthoma located on the eyelids.

xanthoma: Small, flat, yellowish skin plaques; the result of lipid deposition in histiocytes (cells of the reticuloendothelial system).

xiphodynia: Pain in the cartilage of the xiphoid process.

Height/Weight Growth Charts

FIGURE A-1 Physical growth curves for children ages birth to 24 months: Boys. *From: http://www.cdc.gov/ growthcharts/who_charts.htm#TheWHOCharts.*

FIGURE A-2 Physical growth curves for children ages birth to 24 months: Girls.

FIGURE A-3 Physical growth curves for ages 2 to 20 years: Boys.

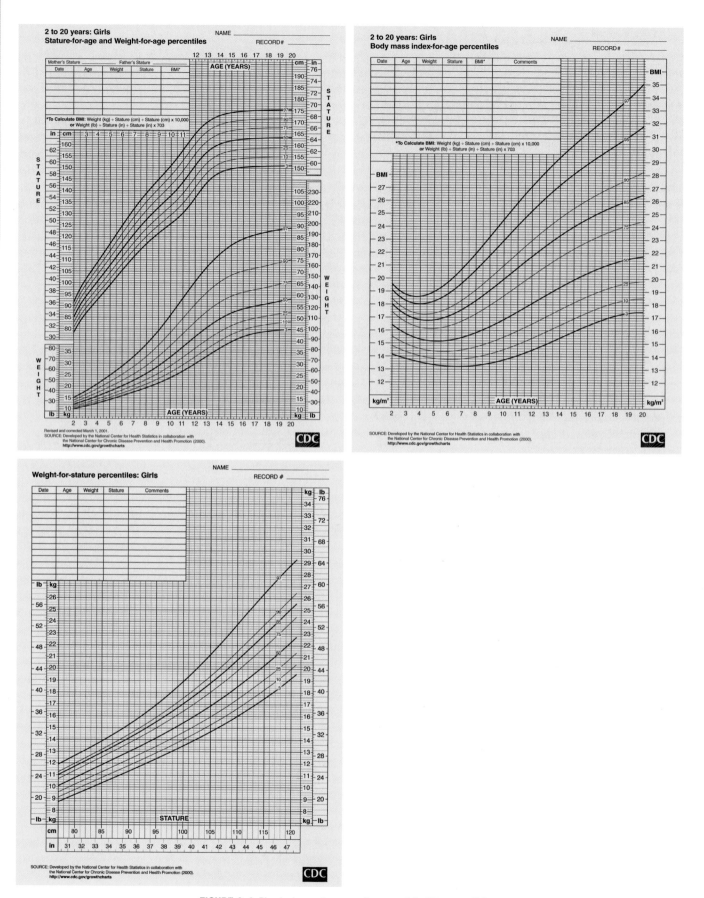

FIGURE A-4 Physical growth curves for ages 2 to 20 years: Girls.

Pediatric Blood Pressure Tables

Blood Pressure Levels for Boys by Age and Height Percentile

Age (Year)	BP Percentile ↓	Systolic BP (mmHg) ← Percentile of Height →							Diastolic BP (mmHg) ← Percentile of Height →						
		5th	10th	25th	50th	75th	90th	95th	5th	10th	25th	50th	75th	90th	95th
1	50th	80	81	83	85	87	88	89	34	35	36	37	38	39	39
	90th	94	95	97	99	100	102	103	49	50	51	52	53	53	54
	95th	98	99	101	103	104	106	106	54	54	55	56	57	58	58
	99th	105	106	108	110	112	113	114	61	62	63	64	65	66	66
2	50th	84	85	87	88	90	92	92	39	40	41	42	43	44	44
	90th	97	99	100	102	104	105	106	54	55	56	57	58	58	59
	95th	101	102	104	106	108	109	110	59	59	60	61	62	63	63
	99th	109	110	111	113	115	117	117	66	67	68	69	70	71	71
3	50th	86	87	89	91	93	94	95	44	44	45	46	47	48	48
	90th	100	101	103	105	107	108	109	59	59	60	61	62	63	63
	95th	104	105	107	109	110	112	113	63	63	64	65	66	67	67
	99th	111	112	114	116	118	119	120	71	71	72	73	74	75	75
4	50th	88	89	91	93	95	96	97	47	48	49	50	51	51	52
	90th	102	103	105	107	109	110	111	62	63	64	65	66	66	67
	95th	106	107	109	111	112	114	115	66	67	68	69	70	71	71
	99th	113	114	116	118	120	121	122	74	75	76	77	78	78	79
5	50th	90	91	93	95	96	98	98	50	51	52	53	54	55	55
	90th	104	105	106	108	110	111	112	65	66	67	68	69	69	70
	95th	108	109	110	112	114	115	116	69	70	71	72	73	74	74
	99th	115	116	118	120	121	123	123	77	78	79	80	81	81	82
6	50th	91	92	94	96	98	99	100	53	53	54	55	56	57	57
	90th	105	106	108	110	111	113	113	68	68	69	70	71	72	72
	95th	109	110	112	114	115	117	117	72	72	73	74	75	76	76
	99th	116	117	119	121	123	124	125	80	80	81	82	83	84	84
7	50th	92	94	95	97	99	100	101	55	55	56	57	58	59	59
	90th	106	107	109	111	113	114	115	70	70	71	72	73	74	74
	95th	110	111	113	115	117	118	119	74	74	75	76	77	78	78
	99th	117	118	120	122	124	125	126	82	82	83	84	85	86	86
8	50th	94	95	97	99	100	102	102	56	57	58	59	60	60	61
	90th	107	109	110	112	114	115	116	71	72	72	73	74	75	76
	95th	111	112	114	116	118	119	120	75	76	77	78	79	79	80
	99th	119	120	122	123	125	127	127	83	84	85	86	87	87	88
9	50th	95	96	98	100	102	103	104	57	58	59	60	61	61	62
	90th	109	110	112	114	115	117	118	72	73	74	75	76	76	77
	95th	113	114	116	118	119	121	121	76	77	78	79	80	81	81
	99th	120	121	123	125	127	128	129	84	85	86	87	88	88	89
10	50th	97	98	100	102	103	105	106	58	59	60	61	61	62	63
	90th	111	112	114	115	117	119	119	73	73	74	75	76	77	78
	95th	115	116	117	119	121	122	123	77	78	79	80	81	81	82
	99th	122	123	125	127	128	130	130	85	86	86	88	88	89	90

Blood Pressure Levels for Boys by Age and Height Percentile (Continued)

Age (Year)	BP Percentile	Systolic BP (mmHg) Percentile of Height							Diastolic BP (mmHg) Percentile of Height						
		5th	10th	25th	50th	75th	90th	95th	5th	10th	25th	50th	75th	90th	95th
11	50th	99	100	102	104	105	107	107	59	59	60	61	62	63	63
	90th	113	114	115	117	119	120	121	74	74	75	76	77	78	78
	95th	117	118	119	121	123	124	125	78	78	79	80	81	82	82
	99th	124	125	127	129	130	132	132	86	86	87	88	89	90	90
12	50th	101	102	104	106	108	109	110	59	60	61	62	63	63	64
	90th	115	116	118	120	121	123	123	74	75	75	76	77	78	79
	95th	119	120	122	123	125	127	127	78	79	80	81	82	82	83
	99th	126	127	129	131	133	134	135	86	87	88	89	90	90	91
13	50th	104	105	106	108	110	111	112	60	60	61	62	63	64	64
	90th	117	118	120	122	124	125	126	75	75	76	77	78	79	79
	95th	121	122	124	126	128	129	130	79	79	80	81	82	83	83
	99th	128	130	131	133	135	136	137	87	87	88	89	90	91	91
14	50th	106	107	109	111	113	114	115	60	61	62	63	64	65	65
	90th	120	121	123	125	126	128	128	75	76	77	78	79	79	80
	95th	124	125	127	128	130	132	132	80	80	81	82	83	84	84
	99th	131	132	134	136	138	139	140	87	88	89	90	91	92	92
15	50th	109	110	112	113	115	117	117	61	62	63	64	65	66	66
	90th	122	124	125	127	129	130	131	76	77	78	79	80	80	81
	95th	126	127	129	131	133	134	135	81	81	82	83	84	85	85
	99th	134	135	136	138	140	142	142	88	89	90	91	92	93	93
16	50th	111	112	114	116	118	119	120	63	63	64	65	66	67	67
	90th	125	126	128	130	131	133	134	78	78	79	80	81	82	82
	95th	129	130	132	134	135	137	137	82	83	83	84	85	86	87
	99th	136	137	139	141	143	144	145	90	90	91	92	93	94	94
17	50th	114	115	116	118	120	121	122	65	66	66	67	68	69	70
	90th	127	128	130	132	134	135	136	80	80	81	82	83	84	84
	95th	131	132	134	136	138	139	140	84	85	86	87	87	88	89
	99th	139	140	141	143	145	146	147	92	93	93	94	95	96	97

BP, Blood pressure.

*The 90th percentile is 1.28 SD, 95th percentile is 1.645 SD, and the 99th percentile is 2.326 SD over the mean.

Use the child's height percentile for the age and gender from the standard growth charts found in Appendix A. A blood pressure value at the 50th percentile for the child's age, gender, and height percentile is considered the midpoint of the normal range. A reading above the 95th percentile indicates hypertension.

National Heart, Lung, and Blood Institute, 2004.

Blood Pressure Levels for Girls by Age and Height Percentile

Age (Year)	BP Percentile ↓	Systolic BP (mmHg) ← Percentile of Height →							Diastolic BP (mmHg) ← Percentile of Height →						
		5th	10th	25th	50th	75th	90th	95th	5th	10th	25th	50th	75th	90th	95th
1	50th	83	84	85	86	88	89	90	38	39	39	40	41	41	42
	90th	97	97	98	100	101	102	103	52	53	53	54	55	55	56
	95th	100	101	102	104	105	106	107	56	57	57	58	59	59	60
	99th	108	108	109	111	112	113	114	64	64	65	65	66	67	67
2	50th	85	85	87	88	89	91	91	43	44	44	45	46	46	47
	90th	98	99	100	101	103	104	105	57	58	58	59	60	61	61
	95th	102	103	104	105	107	108	109	61	62	62	63	64	65	65
	99th	109	110	111	112	114	115	116	69	69	70	70	71	72	72
3	50th	86	87	88	89	91	92	93	47	48	48	49	50	50	51
	90th	100	100	102	103	104	106	106	61	62	62	63	64	64	65
	95th	104	104	105	107	108	109	110	65	66	66	67	68	68	69
	99th	111	111	113	114	115	116	117	73	73	74	74	75	76	76
4	50th	88	88	90	91	92	94	94	50	50	51	52	52	53	54
	90th	101	102	103	104	106	107	108	64	64	65	66	67	67	68
	95th	105	106	107	108	110	111	112	68	68	69	70	71	71	72
	99th	112	113	114	115	117	118	119	76	76	76	77	78	79	79
5	50th	89	90	91	93	94	95	96	52	53	53	54	55	55	56
	90th	103	103	105	106	107	109	109	66	67	67	68	69	69	70
	95th	107	107	108	110	111	112	113	70	71	71	72	73	73	74
	99th	114	114	116	117	118	120	120	78	78	79	79	80	81	81
6	50th	91	92	93	94	96	97	98	54	54	55	56	56	57	58
	90th	104	105	106	108	109	110	111	68	68	69	70	70	71	72
	95th	108	109	110	111	113	114	115	72	72	73	74	74	75	76
	99th	115	116	117	119	120	121	122	80	80	80	81	82	83	83
7	50th	93	93	95	96	97	99	99	55	56	56	57	58	58	59
	90th	106	107	108	109	111	112	113	69	70	70	71	72	72	73
	95th	110	111	112	113	115	116	116	73	74	74	75	76	76	77
	99th	117	118	119	120	122	123	124	81	81	82	82	83	84	84
8	50th	95	95	96	98	99	100	101	57	57	57	58	59	60	60
	90th	108	109	110	111	113	114	114	71	71	71	72	73	74	74
	95th	112	112	114	115	116	118	118	75	75	75	76	77	78	78
	99th	119	120	121	122	123	125	125	82	82	83	83	84	85	86
9	50th	96	97	98	100	101	102	103	58	58	58	59	60	61	61
	90th	110	110	112	113	114	116	116	72	72	72	73	74	75	75
	95th	114	114	115	117	118	119	120	76	76	76	77	78	79	79
	99th	121	121	123	124	125	127	127	83	83	84	84	85	86	87
10	50th	98	99	100	102	103	104	105	59	59	59	60	61	62	62
	90th	112	112	114	115	116	118	118	73	73	73	74	75	76	76
	95th	116	116	117	119	120	121	122	77	77	77	78	79	80	80
	99th	123	123	125	126	127	129	129	84	84	85	86	86	87	88

Blood Pressure Levels for Girls by Age and Height Percentile (Continued)

Age (Year)	BP Percentile ↓	Systolic BP (mmHg) ← Percentile of Height →							Diastolic BP (mmHg) ← Percentile of Height →						
		5th	10th	25th	50th	75th	90th	95th	5th	10th	25th	50th	75th	90th	95th
11	50th	100	101	102	103	105	106	107	60	60	60	61	62	63	63
	90th	114	114	116	117	118	119	120	74	74	74	75	76	77	77
	95th	118	118	119	121	122	123	124	78	78	78	79	80	81	81
	99th	125	125	126	128	129	130	131	85	85	86	87	87	88	89
12	50th	102	103	104	105	107	108	109	61	61	61	62	63	64	64
	90th	116	116	117	119	120	121	122	75	75	75	76	77	78	78
	95th	119	120	121	123	124	125	126	79	79	79	80	81	82	82
	99th	127	127	128	130	131	132	133	86	86	87	88	88	89	90
13	50th	104	105	106	107	109	110	110	62	62	62	63	64	65	65
	90th	117	118	119	121	122	123	124	76	76	76	77	78	79	79
	95th	121	122	123	124	126	127	128	80	80	80	81	82	83	83
	99th	128	129	130	132	133	134	135	87	87	88	89	89	90	91
14	50th	106	106	107	109	110	111	112	63	63	63	64	65	66	66
	90th	119	120	121	122	124	125	125	77	77	77	78	79	80	80
	95th	123	123	125	126	127	129	129	81	81	81	82	83	84	84
	99th	130	131	132	133	135	136	136	88	88	89	90	90	91	92
15	50th	107	108	109	110	111	113	113	64	64	64	65	66	67	67
	90th	120	121	122	123	125	126	127	78	78	78	79	80	81	81
	95th	124	125	126	127	129	130	131	82	82	82	83	84	85	85
	99th	131	132	133	134	136	137	138	89	89	90	91	91	92	93
16	50th	108	108	110	111	112	114	114	64	64	65	66	66	67	68
	90th	121	122	123	124	126	127	128	78	78	79	80	81	81	82
	95th	125	126	127	128	130	131	132	82	82	83	84	85	85	86
	99th	132	133	134	135	137	138	139	90	90	90	91	92	93	93
17	50th	108	109	110	111	113	114	115	64	65	65	66	67	67	68
	90th	122	122	123	125	126	127	128	78	79	79	80	81	81	82
	95th	125	126	127	129	130	131	132	82	83	83	84	85	85	86
	99th	133	133	134	136	137	138	139	90	90	91	91	92	93	93

BP, Blood pressure.

*The 90th percentile is 1.28 SD, 95th percentile is 1.645 SD, and the 99th percentile is 2.326 SD over the mean.

Use the child's height percentile for the age and gender from the standard growth charts found in Appendix A. A blood pressure value at the 50th percentile for the child's age, gender, and height percentile is considered the midpoint of the normal range. A reading above the 95th percentile indicates hypertension.

National Heart, Lung, and Blood Institute, 2004.

Conversion Tables and Anthropometric Measurements

Conversion Tables

Table C-1	Length		
IN	CM	CM	IN
1	2.54	1	0.4
2	5.08	2	0.8
4	10.16	3	1.2
6	15.24	4	1.6
8	20.32	5	2.0
10	25.40	6	2.4
20	50.80	8	3.1
30	76.20	10	3.9
40	101.60	20	7.9
50	127.00	30	11.8
60	152.40	40	15.7
70	177.80	50	19.7
80	203.20	60	23.6
90	228.60	70	27.6
100	254.00	80	31.5
150	381.00	90	35.4
200	508.00	100	39.4

1 in = 2.54 cm.
1 cm = 0.3937 in.

Table C-2	Weight		
LB	KG	KG	LB
1	0.5	1	2.2
2	0.9	2	4.4
4	1.8	3	6.6
6	2.7	4	8.8
8	3.6	5	11.0
10	4.5	6	13.2
20	9.1	8	17.6
30	13.6	10	22
40	18.2	20	44
50	22.7	30	66
60	27.3	40	88
70	31.8	50	110
80	36.4	60	132
90	40.9	70	154
100	45.4	80	176
150	66.2	90	198
200	90.8	100	220

1 lb = 0.454 kg.
1 kg = 2.204 lb.

Anthropometric Measurements

Table C-3   Body Weight in Pounds According to Height and Body Mass Index

| Height (inches) | BODY MASS INDEX (kg per m²) | | | | | | | | | | | | | |
	19.0	20.0	21.0	22.0	23.0	24.0	25.0	26.0	27.0	28.0	29.0	30.0	35.0	40.0
	Body Weight (pounds)													
58.0	90.7	95.5	100.3	105.0	109.8	114.6	119.4	124.1	128.9	133.7	138.5	143.2	167.1	191.0
59.0	93.9	98.8	103.8	108.7	113.6	118.6	123.5	128.5	133.4	138.3	143.3	148.2	172.9	197.6
60.0	97.1	102.2	107.3	112.4	117.5	122.6	127.7	132.9	138.0	143.1	148.2	153.3	178.8	204.4
61.0	100.3	105.6	110.9	116.2	121.5	126.8	132.0	137.3	142.6	147.9	153.2	158.4	184.8	211.3
62.0	103.7	109.1	114.6	120.0	125.5	130.9	136.4	141.9	147.3	152.8	158.2	163.7	191.0	218.2
63.0	107.0	112.7	118.3	123.9	129.6	135.2	140.8	146.5	152.1	157.7	163.4	169.0	197.2	225.3
64.0	110.5	116.3	122.1	127.9	133.7	139.5	145.3	151.2	157.0	162.8	168.6	174.4	203.5	232.5
65.0	113.9	119.9	125.9	131.9	137.9	143.9	149.9	155.9	161.9	167.9	173.9	179.9	209.9	239.9
66.0	117.5	123.7	129.8	136.0	142.2	148.4	154.6	160.8	166.9	173.1	179.3	185.5	216.4	247.3
67.0	121.1	127.4	133.8	140.2	146.5	152.9	159.3	165.7	172.0	178.4	184.8	191.1	223.0	254.9
68.0	124.7	131.3	137.8	144.4	151.0	157.5	164.1	170.6	177.2	183.8	190.3	196.9	229.7	262.5
69.0	128.4	135.2	141.9	148.7	155.4	162.2	168.9	175.7	182.5	189.2	196.0	202.7	236.5	270.3
70.0	132.1	139.1	146.1	153.0	160.0	166.9	173.9	180.8	187.8	194.7	201.7	208.6	243.4	278.2
71.0	135.9	143.1	150.3	157.4	164.6	171.7	178.9	186.0	193.2	200.3	207.5	214.6	250.4	286.2
72.0	139.8	147.2	154.5	161.9	169.2	176.6	183.9	191.3	198.7	206.0	213.4	220.7	257.5	294.3
73.0	143.7	151.3	158.8	166.4	174.0	181.5	189.1	196.7	204.2	211.8	219.3	226.9	264.7	302.5
74.0	147.7	155.4	163.2	171.0	178.8	186.5	194.3	202.1	209.9	217.6	225.4	233.2	272.0	310.9
75.0	151.7	159.7	167.7	175.6	183.6	191.6	199.6	207.6	215.6	223.5	231.5	239.5	279.4	319.4
76.0	155.8	164.0	172.2	180.4	188.6	196.8	205.0	213.2	221.4	229.5	237.7	245.9	286.9	327.9

From U.S. Department of Health and Human Services, 1992.

NOTE: A body mass index (BMI) of 25 is classified as overweight and 30 is classified as obesity in the National Health and Nutrition Examination Survey (NHANES II).

CONVERSION TABLES

Index

Page numbers followed by "f" indicate figures, "t" indicate tables, and "b" indicate boxes.

A
Aaron sign, 390t-391t
Abbreviations, 616, 617b
  prohibited, 616, 617t
ABCD changes in moles, 153f
ABCs (Airway, Breathing, Circulation), 637-641
Abdomen
  abnormalities, 399-415
    alimentary tract, 399-415
    children, 413-414
    hepatobiliary system, 404-406
    infants, 410-413
    kidneys, 407-415
    older adults, 415
    pancreas, 406-407
    spleen, 407
  on admission note, 630
  anatomy and physiology, 370-375, 370b, 371f-372f
  of children, 377, 394, 395f, 396t-397t, 398f
  colon cancer, 380b
  distention, 380b
  examination and findings, 377-398, 378f
    landmarks for, 378f, 379b
    recording, 625, 627-628
    sequence, 600-601, 603-604, 604f
  exposed, patient supine, 600, 600f
  of infants, 374, 377, 394, 395f, 396b, 396t-397t
  pain, 388-389, 389b, 392b, 397t
    acute, 390t-391t
    chronic, 391t
    quality and onset of, 391t
  physical examination findings, POMR, 625
  reflex, 563, 563f

Abdomen (Continued)
  review of related history, 375-377
  in secondary assessment of injured patient, 635
  signs of common conditions, 392t
  venous patterns, 378-379, 380f
Abdominal aorta, 300f
Abdominal aortic aneurysms, 388b, 390t-391t
Abdominal cavity structures, 370-375, 371f-372f
Abdominal distention, 380b
Abducens nerve (CN VI), 547t
  in children, 570t
  examination of, 553-554, 553t
  in infants, 567t
Abductor pollicis brevis, 503f-504f
Abductor pollicis longus, 503f-504f
Abscess
  lung, 286, 287f
  pelvic, suspected, 393, 394f
  perianal and perirectal, 495, 495f
  peritonsillar, 258, 258f
  renal, 408
  retropharyngeal, 258, 258f
Abstract reasoning, 69
Abuse. See also Intimate partner violence (IPV)
  of children and adolescents, 9
    patterns of injury, 164, 164f
  drug, 243b, 266, 266b
  of older adults, 9-10, 165
Acanthosis nigricans (AN), 150, 150f
Access to care, 13
Accuracy in examination, 595-596
Acetabulum, 507, 507f
Achilles reflex, 564
Achilles tendon, 504f, 522
Acne, 128f

Acne vulgaris, 161, 161f
Acoustic nerve (CN VIII)
  in children, 570t
  examination of, 553t, 556
  in infants, 567t
Acoustic stethoscope, 39, 39f
Acquired immune deficiency syndrome (AIDS), 182
Acrocyanosis, 138-139, 139f
Acromegaly, 91, 92f, 190f
Acromioclavicular joint, 505, 506f
Acromion process, 529
Acronyms, 616, 617b
Actinic keratosis, 165, 165f
Activities of daily living (ADLs)
  functional assessment, 74b, 608
  instrumental, 19
Activity, physical, 97, 98t. See also Preparation physical evaluation (PPE)
  intensity, 303b
  sports injury and, 538-543, 539b
Activity orientation, 26
Acute bronchitis, 284, 285f
Acute diarrhea, 399
Acute glomerulonephritis, 407
Acute lymphangitis, 178
Acute otitis media, 252b, 254-255, 254t
Acute pain, 50
Acute pancreatitis, 406
Acute pharyngitis, 257
Acute renal failure, 409
Acute rheumatic fever, 330, 331b
Acute suppurative lymphadenitis, 178
Addressing the patient, 2-3, 6
A-delta fibers, 51
Adenocarcinoma
  of lung, 290f
  rectal, 497

Adenoids, 170
Adie pupil, 214f
Admission note, inpatient, 628
Adnexa
　examination, 437, 439f
　　rectovaginal, 439
　ovarian cysts, 460, 461f
　tenderness, 437b
Adolescents. *See also* Children
　abdomen, 397-398, 397t
　acute abdominal pain, 397-398
　brain, 64-65
　breasts and axillae, 352-353, 352b,
　　363-364
　chest and lung abnormalities,
　　290
　concerns, 17b
　examination sequence, 596-597
　female genitalia, 422, 427
　　examination, 442
　growth, 81-82, 81f
　head and neck, 186
　identification of concerns by, 16b
　interview, 16-17
　male genitalia, 468-469
　　examination, 475, 475b
　mental status examination and, 66
　musculoskeletal system, 508
　　examination, 532-533
　nutrition, 99
　obesity in, 59b
　POMR structure for, 627
　screening tools for, 17b
　sexual maturation, 87-89, 87b,
　　422
　skin and hair, 116, 119, 140
　　abnormalities, 161, 161f
　suicide, 5b
　violence against, 9
Adoption and foster care, 16b
Adults. *See also* Older adults
　examination sequence, 596-603
　　female patient, lithotomy position,
　　　601
　　male patient, bending forward,
　　　601-602, 602f
　functional assessment, 19b
　general inspection, 597, 597f
　interviewing, 6f
　reclining 45 degrees, 599-600,
　　599f
　seated position
　　back exposed, 599, 599f
　　chest exposed, 599, 599f
　　lap draped, 600-601, 601f
　　wearing gown, 597-598, 598f
　standing position, 601, 601f

Adults (*Continued*)
　supine position
　　abdomen exposed, 600, 600f
　　chest exposed, 600
　　legs exposed, 600, 600f
Advance directive, 19, 608, 612, 628,
　642
Adventitious breath sounds, 278b
Afferent neurons, 487, 549
Aganglionic megacolon, 377, 414
Age
　gestational, 85-86, 85f, 442, 442t
　influence on patients seeking medical
　　care, 23b
Age spots, 143
Agility in older adults, 508, 534, 534b
Aging, musculoskeletal system changes
　with, 519f, 534
AIDS (acquired immune deficiency
　syndrome), 182
Air trapping, 268
Airway. *See also* Respiration
　advanced cardiac life support survey,
　　637-641
　emergency assessment, 632, 633b,
　　633f
　obstruction, upper, 642
　retractions, 270-271, 272b
Ala nasi, 233, 233f
Alcohol
　breast cancer risk and, 354b
　CAGE questionnaire for, 8, 8b
　cardiac disease and, 303
　CRAFFT questionnaire, 8, 8b
　fetal alcohol syndrome and, 191f
　TACE questionnaire for, 8, 8b
Alimentary tract. *See also* Abdomen
　abnormalities, 399-415
　anatomy and physiology, 370-372
Allen test, 340b
Allergic vaginitis, 457t
Allergy
　on admission note, 629
　eyes and chemical, 204, 212f
　latex, 30, 32b, 183
Alliance with patients, 16b, 609
Allis sign, 530, 531f
Alopecia
　areata, 154, 154f
　scarring, 155
　traction, 155
Altered mental status
　disorders of, 75
　possible abdominal pathology, 399
Alternating pulse, 341f
Alternative care, 29
Alvarado score, 389

Alveolus, 351f
Alzheimer's disease, 78
Ambiguous genitalia, 463-464, 463b,
　463f, 484, 484f
Amenorrhea, 593b
Amino acids, 96, 96b
Amphoric breath sounds, 276
AMPLE mnemonic, 635b
Amsler grid, 44-45
Amyloidosis, senile cardiac, 331
Anal cancer, 488b, 497
Anal fistula, 496
Analogies used in mental status
　examination, 67
Anal ring, 489, 490f
Anal sphincter, 438-439
Anal warts, 494, 494f
Androgens, 79
Anemia, 111t, 112
Anesthetics, local, 58b
Aneurysm
　abdominal aortic, 388b, 390t-391t
　arterial, 346, 346f
Anger, 5
Angina, 320-331
Angina pectoris, 301, 331
Angiomas
　cherry, 142-143, 142f
　spider, 124f
Anisocoria, 214f
Ankle, 507-508, 508f
　clonus, 565
　injury, acute, 524b
　inspection, 522-524, 523f
　swelling, 337
Ankylosing spondylitis, 535-538, 535f
Annular formation of lesions, 326f
Annular ligament, 505f
Anonychia, 135
Anorectal fissure, 495-496, 495f
Anorectal malformations, 486
Anorexia nervosa, 111
Antalgic limp, 560t
Anterior cerebral artery, 545f, 575f,
　575t-576t
Anterior chamber, 42f, 205f, 216b, 624
Anterior communicating artery, 545f
Anterior cruciate ligament, 507f
Anterior inferior cerebellar artery, 545f
Anterior naris, 233, 233f
Anterior rectal wall, 485-486, 490-491
Anterior spinal artery, 545f
Anterolateral spinothalamic tract, 51f
Anthrax, 151t
Anthropometrics, 100, 100b
　waist circumference, 100, 101f
　waist-height ratio, 100

Anthropometrics *(Continued)*
  waist-to-hip circumference ratio, 100-101, 101f
Antigen-antibody reaction, 183
Antihelix, 232f
Antitragus, 232f
Anus, 430
  abnormalities, 494-500
    anus, rectum, and surrounding skin, 494-498
    anatomy and physiology, 466b, 485-487, 486f
  cancer, 488b
  examination and findings, 489-493, 489b, 490f
    recording, 625, 627
  imperforate, 499, 500f
  review of related history, 487-489
Anxiety, 4, 65
  breathing and, 270b
  disorder, 77
  before female genital examination, 428b
Aorta
  abdominal, 300f
  coarctation of, 348, 348f
  palpation, 388, 388f
Aortic arch, 300f, 346, 348
Aortic dissection, 391t
Aortic regurgitation, 54-55, 303, 306b, 316
Aortic valve, 295f-296f, 297
  stenosis, 314f
Apert syndrome, 192f
Apertures, opthalmoscope, 42t
Apgar scoring system, 279, 279t
Aphasias, 71t
Apical impulse, 599, 603, 618
Apnea, 268, 272b
Apneustic breathing, 272b
Apocrine glands, 115-116
Appendages, skin, 115-117
Appendicitis
  diagnosing, 389, 390b, 390t-391t
  iliopsoas muscle test for, 393, 393f
  pain, 390t-391t
Appendix, 371f-372f
APSO notes, 620b, 621
Arachnoid, 545f
Arcus senilis, 212, 212f-213f
Areolae, 356-357
  abnormalities, 367-369, 367f-368f
  color variations, 358f
Argyll Robertson pupil, 213f
Arithmetic calculation, 69
Arms. *See* Upper extremities
Arrector pili muscle, 115f

Arrhythmia, sinus, 319, 324
Arterial aneurysm, 346
Arterial embolic disease, 347, 347f
Arterial pulse and pressure, 336, 336f, 341f
Arteries, 334f-336f
  brain, 545f, 575f
  cerebral
    anterior, 575f, 575t-576t
    middle, 575f, 575t-576t
    posterior, 575f, 575t-576t
  chest cavity, 261f
  eye, 205f
  heart, 295f
  peripheral, 338-342, 339f
  retinal, 205f
  stroke and, 575t-576t
  upper extremity, 53, 583b
Arterioles, 123b
  spasm of digital, 347
Arteriovenous fistula, 346
Arthritis
  differential diagnosis, 538t
  gout, 536, 537f
  rheumatoid, 538, 538t
Articular capsule, 506f
Articular disk, 505f-506f
Articular tubercle, 506f
Articulation, 70
Ascending spinal tracts, 547
Ascites, 388, 388b, 405f
Ascorbic acid, 103t-104t
Assessment. *See also* Examination techniques
  on admission note, 630
  critical thinking in, 610-614
  cultural, 25b
  for each problem on problem list, 625
  emergency, 632-636
    acute medical, 637-641
    advanced cardiac life support survey, 637-641
    airway and cervical spine, 632
    circulation, 633-634
    disability, 634, 634b, 634t
    head and neck, 635
    of infants and children, 638, 638b, 640b, 641t
    legal considerations, 641-642
    primary survey, 632-635, 633b
    reevaluation in, 636
    secondary, 635-636
    symptoms and risks of serious and life-threatening conditions, 639t
  fetal well-being, 443-444

Assessment *(Continued)*
  functional, 19b
    activities of daily living, 74b, 608
    for all patients, 19b
    ears, nose, and throat, 253b
    musculoskeletal system, 74b, 534b
    for older adults, 74b, 608
    Tinetti balance and gait assessment tool, 571b-572b
  musculoskeletal system, 524, 524t
    hand and wrist, 524, 524b, 525f-526f
    hips, 526-527, 527f
    knee, 527-534, 527f-528f
    lower spine, 526, 527f
    shoulder, 524-526, 526f
  neurovascular, 539b
  pain, 50, 56
    abdominal, 388-389, 389b
    behaviors, 56-60
    in children, 59-60, 59f, 61f
    in older adults, 60
    in pregnant women, 60
  past medial history, 11-12
  review of systems in, 13-14
  screening *versus*, 8b
Asthma, 283t-284t, 284
  severe episode, 644
Asymmetric tonic neck reflex, 568t-569t
Ataxia, 560t
  cerebellar, 559
Atelectasis, 283t-284t, 284, 284f
Atherosclerosis, 314t-317t, 331, 347
Athletes
  female athlete triad, 593b
  hypertension in child, 582b
Atlantoaxial instability, 582b
Atresia
  biliary, 412, 412f
  intestinal, 411
  rectal, 500f
Atrial fibrillation, 325t-327t, 347, 570b
Atrial flutter, 325t-327t
Atrial septal defect, 330, 330f
Atria tachycardia, 327f
Atrioventricular node, 326f
Atrioventricular valves, 297, 297f
Atrophic vaginitis, 457t, 465
Atrophy
  muscle, 541, 553t, 554-555, 564t
  optic, 219t, 227f
  skin, 131f
Attention-deficit/hyperactivity disorder (ADHD), 77
Attention span, 70

Attitudes
 effect on critical thinking, 611b, 612
 ethnic, toward autonomy, 26
 health belief and practices, 25b
Auditory association area, 65f
Auditory nerve, 232f
Auditory ossicles, 232f
Auricle, 232, 232f
 alignment of, 232f
 inspection of, 238-239, 239f
Auricularis anterior, 506f
Auricularis superior, 506f
Auricular sinus, 238, 239f
Auscultation, 35, 35b
 abdomen, 381, 382f, 386f, 395
 blood vessels, 340, 342b, 342f
 chest and lungs, 276-281, 276f
 head, 192, 193f
 heart, 306-319, 307b-308b, 307f,
  308t
 stethoscope for, 39-40, 39f-40f
Autism, 78
Autoimmune disorders
 Graves disease, 201
 Hashimoto disease, 201
 multiple sclerosis (MS), 573
Autonomic hyperreflexia, 37
Autonomic nervous system, 372,
  544-549
Autonomy, ethnic attitudes toward, 26
Autosomal recessive condition pedigree,
  623f
Avoidance of full story, 5
AVPU mnemonic, 634b
Axillae, 353-355
Axillary lymph nodes, 352, 352f
 breasts, 168f, 352, 352f
 palpation of, 168f, 175

B
Babinski sign, 563, 563f
Bacillus anthracis, 151f
Back
 emergency assessment, 636
 examination sequence, 599, 605, 605f
 landmarks of, 518, 518f
 pain, 509
  lower, 519b
Background diabetic retinopathy, 225,
  226f
Bacterial endocarditis, 320, 320f
Bacterial vaginosis, 457t
Balance, 559, 559f
 equilibrium, 559
 Tinetti Balance and Gait Assessment
  Tool, 571b-572b
Balance of life, 27b

Ballance sign, 390t-391t
Ballard Gestational Age Assessment
  Tool, 85
Ballottement, 393-394, 394f
 knee, 527, 527f
Band keratopathy, 223, 224f
Barlow-Ortolani maneuver, 530,
  531f
Barrel chest, 263, 268f
Barriers
 to communication, 4-5
 to critical thinking, 611-613
 language and culture, 595
Bartholin glands, 418f, 429-430, 430f
 inflammation of, 454, 455f
Basal cell cancer, 152, 152f
 risk factors, 117b
Basal ganglia system, 546
Basal metabolic rate (BMR), 97, 97t
Basic life support survey, 633b
Basilar artery, 545f, 575t-576t
Battle sign, 635, 636f
Bayes theorem, 613-614
Beard folliculitis, 145f
Beau lines, 158, 158f
Behavior
 in children, 52
 during examination, infant and
  newborn, 605
 Glasgow Coma Scale assessment of,
  634, 634t
 pain, 50b
  assessment, 56-60
Bell's palsy, 190f, 577, 577f
Benign prostatic hypertrophy (BPH),
  498, 499f
Biceps brachii
 long head, 503f-504f, 506f
 short head, 503f-504f
 tendon, 506f
Biceps femoris tendon, 507f
Biceps reflex, 564
Bicipital aponeurosis, 503f-504f
Bidigital palpation of rectal walls, 490
Bifid defect of vertebrae, 529, 530f
Bigeminal pulse, 341f
Bilateral symmetry, 510b
Biliary atresia, 412, 412f
Biliary stones, 390t-391t
Bimanual examination of female
  genitalia, 435-437, 435f-436f, 439f
Bimanual palpation
 of abdomen, deep, 385f
 adnexa, 439
 digital palpation of breasts, 360, 360f
Biochemical measurement, 108, 109t
Biologic warfare, 151, 151t

Biotin, 104
Biot respiration, 268
Birth weight, low, 86b
Bitemporal hemianopia, 228, 228f
Bladder, 373
 concerns for patients with disabilities,
  37
 palpation of, 388
 during pregnancy, 374
Bleeding
 rectal, 487, 492b
 uterine, 459, 459t
 vaginal, 423-424, 442t
  in children, 441, 441b
  during pregnancy, 465
Blepharitis, 210, 211f
Blindness, 228-230, 228f
Blisters, 128f
 genital, 426b
 sunburn, 117b
Blood
 anemia and, 111t, 112
 circulation, 332-337, 333f-335f
  advanced cardiac life support
   survey, 637-641
  emergency assessment, 633-634
  shock state, 643
 in stool, 492b, 492t
 vomiting of, 639t
Blood pressure, 50
 in children, 58-59, 59b
 hypertension and, 55-56, 62-63
 in infants, 58, 58b
 measurement, 53-56, 54b-55b,
  54f-55f, 55t
 pain and, 53-56, 54b
Blood vessels. See also Cardiovascular
  system; Heart
 abnormalities, 346-349
 anatomy and physiology, 332-337,
  332b, 333f-335f
 examination and findings, 338-345
  recording, 625, 627-628
 physical examination findings,
  POMR, 625
 review of related history, 337-338
 review of system, 13
Blumberg sign, 390t-391t
Blunt trauma, 637
Blurred vision, 209b
 during pregnancy, 206
BMI. See Body mass index (BMI)
Body language, 3-4
Body mass index (BMI), 82, 83b, 87b
 in children, 83-87
Body proportions, 81f
Boil, 145, 145f

Bones. *See also* Musculoskeletal system; Spine
   female pelvic, 419-423, 422f
   fracture of, 539, 636
   head, 184-186, 185f, 187f
   lower extremities, 507-508, 507f
   upper extremities, 505, 505f
Boutonnière deformity, 513f
Bowel
   concerns for patients with disabilities, 37
   fecal incontinence, 376
   function changes, 487-488
   movements in infants and children, 486
   sounds, 381
Bowleg, 531-532, 532f
Brachial artery, 53, 583b
Brachialis pronator teres, 503f-504f
Brachial plexus, 225, 548f
Brachioradialis, 503f-504f
Brachioradial reflex, 564
Bradycardia, sinus, 325f
Bradypnea, 53, 268
Brain
   anatomy and physiology, 64-65, 65f, 544-549, 545f
      arteries, 545f
      brainstem, 546, 546t
      cerebellum, 546
      cerebrum, 545-546, 546f
      cranial nerves, 214-216, 215f, 547, 547t
   attack (*See* Stroke)
   concussions, 588b, 589f-592f
   functional subdivisions, 65f
   growth, 80-81
   intracranial pressure, 643
   traumatic brain injury, 187-188, 588b, 589f-592f
Brainstem, 546, 546t
Branchial cleft cyst, 199, 200f
Braun von Fernwald sign, 443b
Breast feeding. *See* Lactating women
Breasts
   abnormalities, 365-369
   anatomy and physiology, 350-353, 351f
   cancer, 354b, 358b, 362f, 366, 366f
      mastectomy for, 364b
      prevention, 362b
   development, 87, 88f, 363-364
   enlargement in men, 353
   examination and findings, 355-365, 356f
      recording, 625, 627
      sequence, 599-600

Breasts (*Continued*)
   lumps, 365-369
   lymph nodes, 168f, 352, 352f
   masses, 365t
      documentation, 361b
   physical examination findings, POMR, 625
   review of related history, 353-355
   review of system, 13
   self-examination and self-awareness, 355b
Breathing
   apneustic, 272b
   emergency assessment, 632-633
      advanced cardiac life support survey, 637-641
Breath odor, 274b
Breath sounds, 276-279, 277f-278f, 277t
   adventitious, 278b
   amphoric, 276
Bridge of nose, 233, 233f
Broadening of nail, 135, 136f
Broca aphasia, 71t
Broca's area, 65f
Broken Wheel cards, 44
Bronchiectasis, 283t-284t, 293, 293f
Bronchiolitis, 292
Bronchitis, 284, 285f
   chronic, 293
   laryngotracheal, 291, 291f
Bronchovesicular breath sounds, 281
Brown-Séquard syndrome, 562
Brudzinski sign, 566, 566f
Bruises, 164, 164f
Bruits
   abdominal, 340, 381, 382f
   carotid artery, 340, 342f
   intracranial, 192, 197
   renal, 395
   temporal, 192, 193f
Buccal mucosa, 244-246, 245b, 245f-246f, 245t
Buccinator muscle, 234f
Bulbocavernosus muscle, 418f
Bulge sign, 524t, 527, 528f
Bulimia nervosa, 112
Bulla, skin, 127f
Bundle of His, 298, 299f
Bunion, 522, 523f
Burns, 164, 164f, 637, 637f
Bursitis, 537, 537f
Butterfly rash, 190f

C
Café au lait macules, 139, 139f
CAGE questionnaire, 8, 8b

Calcaneus, 508f
Calcium, 105
Calculations
   arithmetic, 69
   body mass index (BMI), 82, 83b, 87b
   midarm muscle circumference/ midarm muscle area, 108
Calculi, renal, 390t-391t, 409
Calf pain, 344b
Calipers
   skinfold thickness, 49, 49f, 107-108, 107f
   triceps skinfold thickness (TSF), 49, 49f, 107-108, 107f
Callus, 120-121, 121f
Calories, daily energy needs, 102b
Canal for central retinal vessels, 42f
Canal of Schlemm, 42f
Cancer. *See also* Tumors
   anal, 488b, 497
   breast, 354b, 358b, 362f, 366, 366f
      mastectomy for, 364b
      prevention, 362b
   cervical, 425b, 436b-437b, 457, 458f
   colon, 380b, 403, 404b, 498
   endometrial, 413, 426b
   liver, 405
   lung, 289, 290f
   male genitalia, 470b
      penile, 479, 480f
      testicular, 483
   oral cavity and oropharyngeal, 237b, 247b, 259, 259f
   ovarian, 425b, 461
   prostate, 488b, 491b, 499, 499f
      screening, 491b
   skin, 117b, 122b, 127f, 152-154, 152f, 165, 165f
   stomach, 403
   vaginal, 455
   vulvar, 456, 456f
Candida vulvovaginitis, 457t
Capillary hemangioma, 124f
Capillary refill time, 342b, 345
Capture techniques for palpating kidney, 387f
Caput succedaneum, 195, 195f
Carbohydrate, 95-96, 102, 112b
Carcinomas. *See* Cancer
Cardarelli sign, 194b
Cardiac conduction, 298-301, 299f
Cardiac cycle, 297-298, 297f-298f
Cardiac depression, 262f
Cardiac disease risk factors, 303b
Cardiac life support survey, 637-641
Cardiac tamponade, 322, 322f
Cardinal fields of gaze, 214-215, 215f

Cardiovascular system. *See also* Blood vessels; Heart
  on admission note, 630
  cardiac disease risk factors, 303b
  emergency assessment, 632
  nutrient deficiencies and, 106t-107t
Care, access to, 13
Caries, 252, 252f
Carotid artery
  bruits, 342b
  internal, 575t-576t
  palpation, 339b
  pulse, 343t
    emergency assessment, 634f
  stroke and, 575t-576t
Carpais, 505f
Carpals, 503f-504f
Carpal tunnel syndrome, 524, 525f, 536, 537t
  in pregnant women, 533
Carpometacarpal joint of thumb, 505f
Cartilage
  articular, 538
  ear, 232
  neck, 185
  nose, 233
  thyroid, 185, 186f
Cartoenemia, 119b
Caruncle, urethral, 429, 429f
Cataracts, 225, 225f
Cat scratch disease, 182
Cauda equina, 548f
Cauliflower ear, 238, 239f
Celiac trunk, 371f-372f
Cellulitis, 145, 145f
Central nervous system
  anatomy and physiology, 544-549, 545f
  disorders, 573-574
Central retinal artery and vein, 205f
Central sulcus, 65f, 546f
Cephalhematoma, 195, 195f
Cerebellar artery, 575t-576t
Cerebellar ataxia, 559
Cerebellar gait, 560t
Cerebellum, 545f, 546, 548f, 575f
  proprioception and, 556-559
Cerebral artery
  anterior, 545f, 575f, 575t-576t
  middle, 545f, 575f, 575t-576t
  posterior, 545f, 575f, 575t-576t
Cerebral cortex, functional subdivisions of, 65f
Cerebral palsy (CP), 578
Cerebrospinal fluid (CSF), 643
Cerebrovascular accident. *See* Stroke
Cerebrum, 545-546, 546f

Cerumen, 240b
Cervical adenitis, 177t
Cervical cancer, 425b
  screening after hysterectomy, 436b
  screening recommendations, 437b
Cervical enlargement of spinal nerve, 548f
Cervical nodes, 177b
Cervical plexus, 548f
Cervical spine, 516-518
  emergency assessment, 632, 633f, 636
  range of motion, 518f
Cervix, 423f
  cancer, 457, 458f
  effacement and dilation in pregnancy, 443
  examination, 431, 436, 491
  normal, 432f-433f
  polyp, 432f
C fibers, 51, 51f
Chadwick sign, 443b
Chambers of the heart, 295, 295f
Change, stages of, 613, 615t
Checklist of Nonverbal Pain Indicators, 60, 62f
Cheilitis, 244, 245f
Chemical allergy and eyes, 204, 212f
Cherry angiomas, 142-143, 142f
Chest
  on admission note, 630
  anatomy and physiology, 260-264, 260b, 261f
    anatomic landmarks, 262-264, 263f
  barrel, 263, 268f
  cavity arteries, 261f
  circumference, 85, 85f
  examination and findings, 267-281, 267f-268f, 279b, 599
    children, 607
    infants, 603, 603f
    recording, 624, 627-628
    sequence of steps, 267b
  pain, 265, 266b, 301-302, 301b-302b, 302t
  physical examination findings, POMR, 624
  review of related history, 264-267
  review of system, 13
  in secondary assessment of injured patient, 635
  wall sweep, 360, 360f
Cheyne-Stokes respiration, 268, 271f
Chickenpox, 162, 162f
Chief complaint, 11b

Chief concern, 6, 10-11, 621
  of adolescents, 16b-17b
  infants and children, 14, 14b
Child abuse, 9, 16b
  patterns of injury, 164, 164f
  sexual, 441, 441b
Children. *See also* Adolescents; Infants
  abdomen, 377, 394, 395f, 396t-397t, 398f
    abnormalities, 413-414
  adoption and foster care of, 16b
  anus and rectum, 486, 488
    abnormalities, 499-500
    examination, 491-493, 492t, 493f
  attention-deficit/hyperactivity disorder in, 77
  autism in, 78
  blood pressure in, 58-59, 59b
  blood vessels, 336-338, 345, 345f
    abnormalities, 348-349
  brain, 64
  breasts and axillae, 352-353, 352b, 363-364
    abnormalities, 369
  chest and lungs, 262-263, 266
    abnormalities, 290
    examination and findings, 280-281
  chief concern, 14, 14b
  ears, nose, and throat, 235, 238
    examination and findings, 251-252, 251f
  emergency assessment, 638, 638b, 640b, 641t
  evaluation of masturbation in, 427b
  examination sequence, 605-606
    child on parent's lap, 606-607, 606f
    child playing, 606, 606f
    child relatively supine, still on lap, diaper loosened, 607
    child returns to parent's lap, 607-608, 607f
    child standing, 607, 607f
    general inspection, 606, 606b
  eyes, 206, 207t, 208, 221-222, 222t
    abnormalities, 229-230
  family history, 15
  female genitalia, 422, 426-427, 440
  growth, 81-82, 81f
    hormone deficiency, 94, 94f
    precocious puberty, 94, 94f
  head and neck, 186, 197
    examination sequence, 607, 607f
  heart, 304, 319
    abnormalities, 328-330
    murmurs, 318b
  history of present illness, 14
  hypertension in athletic, 582b

INDEX

Children (Continued)
intellectual disability in, 77
interviews, 14-16, 14f
lower extremities examination
sequence, 606
lymphatic system, 170-172,
176-177
male genitalia, 468-469
examination, 475, 475f
measurement
arm span, 87
stature and weight, 86, 86f
upper-to-lower segment ratio, 87
memory in, 73, 73f
mental status examination, 66
musculoskeletal system, 508-509
abnormalities, 540-542
examination, 530-532, 532f
nails, 137-140
neurologic system, 549, 551-552
abnormalities, 578-579
examination, 546
nutrition, 98-99
obesity in, 59b
pain in, 52, 58-59
assessment of, 59-60, 59f, 61f
past medical history, 14-15
perceptual distortions and
hallucinations, 72-73
personal and social history, 15
premature thelarche in, 369
Problem-Oriented Medical Record
format and, 627
review of systems, 16
skin and hair, 116, 119
abnormalities, 160-164
speech milestones in, 72, 73t
upper extremities examination
sequence, 606
Chlamydia, 457t
Chloasma, 121-122, 141f
Choana, 233, 250
Cholecystitis, 390t-391t, 406
Cholelithiasis, 405
Cholesteatoma, 255, 256f
Cholesterol, 111t, 112b, 304b
lipemia retinalis and, 226, 226f
ChooseMyPlate.gov, 101-102, 101f
Chorioretinitis, 227, 228f
Choroid, 42f, 205f
Chronic bronchitis, 293
Chronic obstructive pulmonary disease,
264b, 283t-284t, 292-293, 292f
Chronic pain, 50
Chronic pancreatitis, 407
Ciliary body, 42f
Ciliary muscle, 205f

Circulation, blood, 332-337, 333f-335f
advanced cardiac life support survey,
637-641
emergency assessment, 633-634
shock state, 643
Circumcision, 471, 471f, 474b
Circus senilis, 212, 212f
Cirrhosis, 404
Clarification, 4
Classification
hypertension, 55t, 582b
malocclusion, 245f
sports according to contact, 587t
Claudication, 340
Clavicle, 506f
Claw toes, 522
Cleft lip and palate, 250-251, 250b, 259,
259f
Clinical breast examination, 358b
Clinical examination
critical thinking in, 610, 611b
validity, 613
Clitoris, 416-418, 417f, 422, 429
Clonus, 565
Closing discussion, 608-609
Clubfoot, 540, 540f
Coarctation of the aorta, 348, 348f
Cocaine abuse, 243b, 266, 266b
Coccyx, 418f, 506f, 548f
Cochlea, 232f
Cognitive abilities, 67-70, 68b,
68f-69f
abstract reasoning, 69
analogies, 67
arithmetic calculation, 69
attention span, 70
execution of motor skills, 69
intellectual disability in infants and
children and, 77
judgment, 70
writing ability, 69
Coherence, 70
Colitis, ulcerative, 402, 402f
Colon cancer, 380b, 403, 404b, 498
Color vision, 209
Columella, 233f
Columns of Morgagni, 486
Coma, 634, 634t
Common cold, 27, 28b
Communication. See also Interviews
of bad news, 609b
cultural response and, 25-28, 26b,
26f, 28b-29b
effective, 2-5, 3b, 595b, 609b
modes, 26-27, 26f
nonverbal, 67
potential barriers to, 4-5

Communication (Continued)
speech milestones and, 72, 73t
use of jargon and, 7b
Compassionate moments, 5
Competency to make medical decisions,
18b
Complementary and alternative
medicine (CAM), 23
Complete transverse lesion of the spinal
cord, 562
Complex regional pain syndrome, 63
Comprehension, 70
Compression, nipple, 363b
Concussions, sports-related, 588b,
589f-592f
Conduction, cardiac, 298-301, 299f
disturbances, 324
Conductive hearing loss, 256
Condyle of mandible, 506f
Condyloma acuminatum, 494, 494f
in men, 478, 478f
in women, 451, 452f
Condyloma latum, 453, 453f
Confidentiality, 3
for adolescents, 17
consent by proxy and, 14b
Confrontation, 4
Congenital aganglionic megacolon, 377,
414
Congenital disorders
aganglionic megacolon, 377, 414
cleft lip and palate, 250-251, 250b,
259, 259f
hypospadias, 484, 484f
klinefelter syndrome, 483-484, 483f
lymphangioma, 179
lymphedema, 178-179, 178f, 179t
spina bifida, 578, 579f
Congestive heart failure (CHF), 276b,
321
Conjunctiva, 205, 205f, 211-212,
211f-212f
Connection, seeking, 2-4
Connective tissues, abdomen, 373
Consent by proxy, 14b
Consent for treatment, 641
Constipation, 376, 391t, 398b
Contact dermatitis, 144f
Contractions, uterine, 446-447
Contracture, Dupuytren, 543, 543f
Convulsions, 550-551
Coordination, 556-559, 558f. See also
Gait
Copper, 106
Copy and paste or carry forward
(CPCF) text, 617, 617b-618b
Coracoid process, 504f

Cornea, 42f, 205f, 206, 212, 212f
Corneal ulcer, 224, 224f
Corns, 120, 120f
Coronary sinus, 296f
Coronoid process, 505f
Cor pulmonale, 323, 323f
Corpus callosum, 545f
Corrigan pulse, 341f
Cortical sensory functions, 561-562,
    562f
Costal angle, 262, 263f
Costodiaphragmatic recess, 261f
Costs of care, 1-2, 5
Cough, 264-265
    in newborns, 280
Cowper glands, 487f
Crackles, 278
Cradle transfer, 35-36
CRAFFT questionnaire, 8, 8b
Cranial nerves, 214-216, 215f, 547, 547t
    abnormalities, 577
    examination, 553-556, 553t
        in newborns and infants, 567t
        in young children, 570t
    names mnemonic, 553b
    upper and lower neuron disease,
        555b
Craniosynostosis, 203, 203f
Cremasteric reflex, 474, 564
Crepitus, 271
CRIES scale, 58
Critical thinking
    assessment, judgment, and evidence,
        610-614
    clinical examination, 610, 611b
    in decision making, 610, 611b
    evaluation and management plan and
        setting priorities, 614-615
    in evidence-based practice, 614, 614f
    possible barriers to, 611-613
    problem identification, 610-611
    valid hypotheses, 611, 612b
Crohn disease, 401, 402f
Croup, 291, 291f
Crouzon syndrome, 192f
Crust, skin, 130f
Crying, 5, 280b
Cullen sign, 636f
Cultural barriers, 595
Cultural competence, 21
    blurring of cultural distinctions and,
        23
    components of cultural response and,
        25-28, 26b, 26f
    cultural assessment guide and, 25b
    cultural humility and, 23
    dimensions of, 22b

Cultural competence (Continued)
    distinguishing physical characteristics
        and, 21-22
    overlapping concepts of patient-
        centered care and, 22f
    primacy of individual in health care
        and, 24
    questions and, 28b-29b
Cultural humility, 23
Cultural response components, 25-28,
    26b, 26f
Culture
    common cold cures and, 27, 28b
    defined, 21
    diet and nutritional practices and, 28
    family relationships and, 27-28
    health beliefs and practices and, 27,
        27b
    within health professions, 24
    impact of, 23
    impact on illness, 24
    language and, 23b
    questions that explore patient's, 24b
    value orientations and, 26b
Curiosity about the practitioner, 4
Cushing syndrome, 92, 189f
Cutaneous color changes, 121-123,
    123t
Cutaneous horns, 143, 144f
Cutaneous tags, 143, 143f
Cutis marmorata, 138-139, 139f
Cyanosis, 271
Cystic fibrosis, 290, 291f
Cystic hygroma, 179
Cysts
    branchial cleft, 199, 200f
    digital mucous, 159, 159f
    ovarian, 460, 461f
    pilonidal, 494, 494f
    skin, 128f, 239f
    thyroglossal duct, 199, 199f

D
Daily energy needs, 102b
Dance sign, 410
Darwin tubercle, 238, 239f
Deafness. See Hearing
Death and grief, 76, 629
Decision making, 610, 611b, 614, 614f
Deep pressure, 561
Deep tendon reflexes, 564-565, 564t,
    565f
Deep transverse perineal muscle, 418f
Dehydration, 140t, 141b
Delirium, 75
    differential diagnosis, 76t
Deltoid muscle, 503f-504f, 506f

Dementia, 78
    differential diagnosis, 76t
Depression, 5, 65, 76
    differential diagnosis, 76t
    Geriatric Depression Scale, 74, 75f
Depressor angulioris, 506f
Depressor labil inferioris, 506f
Dermatophytosis, 146
Dermatoscope, 48, 48f
Dermis, 115, 115f
Descending spinal tracts, 547
Diabetic retinopathy, 225-226, 225f
    background, 225, 226f
    proliferative, 226, 226f
Diagnosis. See Assessment
Diamond-shaped position for female
        genital examination, 448, 448f
Diaphragmatic excursion, 274, 274b,
    276f
Diaphragmatic hernia, 280, 280f, 290
Diarrhea, 375, 398b
    acute, 399
Diastole, 310
Diet. See also Nutrition
    adequacy determination, 101, 101f
    components of healthy, 338b
    culture and, 28
    ethnic food guide pyramids and, 102
    food diary and, 101
    review of system, 13
    twenty-four hour recall, 101
    vegetarian, 102
Dietary Guidelines for Americans, 113b
Differential diagnosis
    abdominal masses in infants and
        children, 396t
    acute abdominal pain in infants,
        children, and adolescents, 397t
    acute testicular swelling, 482t
    breast masses, 365t
    cardiac life support survey, 637, 638b
    chest pain, 302t
    comparison of osteoarthritis with
        rheumatoid arthritis, 538t
    comparison of systolic murmurs, 318t
    conditions simulating lymph node
        enlargement, 174t
    cutaneous manifestations of
        pathogens used in biologic
        warfare, 151t
    delirium, dementia, and depression,
        76t
    distinguishing characteristics of
        hernias, 477t
    headaches, 197t-198t
    immune deficiency disease in a child,
        177t

Differential diagnosis (*Continued*)
  lymphedema or edema, 179t
  mumps *versus* cervical adenitis, 177t
  neurologic signs associated with stroke by artery affected, 575t-576t
  otitis externa, otitis media with effusion, and acute otitis media, 254t
  sputum causes, 265t
  swelling, 180t
  tremors, 557t
  upper and lower motor neuron disorders, 564t
  urinary incontinence, 415t
  vaginal discharges and infections, 457t
Difficult patients, 594, 595b
Digital arterioles, spasm of, 347
Digital epiluminescence microscopy (DELM), 48
Digital mucous cysts, 159, 159f
Dilation, cervical, 443
Direct questions, 4
Disabled patients, 20, 20f
  emergency assessment, 634, 634b, 634t
  examination technique modifications for, 35-37, 36b, 597b
  female genitalia examination in, 447, 448f-449f
  sports participation by, 581, 582b
Dislocation, bone, 539
  radial head subluxation, 542
Disorders, mental status
  altered, 75
  of mood, 76-78
Disorientation and confusion, 65
Dissection, aortic, 391t
Distal interphalangeal joint, 505f
Distal phalanx, 508f
Distention, abdominal, 380b
Distorted thinking, 72b
Diverticular disease, 391t, 403, 403f
Diverticulitis, 390t-391t
Domestic violence, 8-10, 9b
Doppler, 41, 41f
Dorsal horn, 51f
Dorsal recumbent position, 32
Double vision, 209b
Down syndrome, 191f, 582b
Draping, patient, 32
  for female genital examination, 43f, 428
Drawer test, 527-528, 528f

Drugs
  abuse, 243b, 266, 266b
  cutaneous reactions to, 150, 150f
  interactions with food and nutrients, 100b
  lymph nodes and, 174b
  medications on admission, 629
Drusen bodies, 218, 219f
Duct, 351f
Duct ectasia, 367
Ductule, 351f
Duodenal ulcer, 401
Dupuytren contracture, 543, 543f
Dyspnea, 265, 265b
Dysreflexia, 37
Dystoria, 560t
Dysuria, 376
Dystrophic gait, 560t
Dysuria, 376

E
Ear drum, 232f
Ears. *See also* Hearing
  abnormalities, 254-257
  acoustic nerve, 553t, 556
  on admission note, 629
  anatomy and physiology, 231b, 232-236, 232f
  cleaning obstructed, 240b
  examination and findings, 238-242, 239f
    recording, 624, 626
    sequence, 598
  functional assessment, 253b
  lymph nodes, 168f
  otoscope for examination of, 45, 45f, 239-241, 239f
  physical examination findings, POMR, 624
  review of related history, 236-238
  review of system, 13
  tuning fork for examination of, 45-46, 46f
  tympanometer for examination of, 45, 45f
Eating disorders, 99b, 111-112
  female athletes and, 593b
Ecchymoses, 124f
Eccrine sweat glands, 115
Eclampsia, 349
Ectopic pregnancy, 390t-391t, 393b, 461, 461f
Ectropion, 210, 210f
Edema, 179t, 344-345, 344b
  peau d'orange appearance in breasts from, 356f
  pitting, 344f
Effacement, cervical, 443

Ejaculation, 469
Elbow, 505, 505f
  inspection, 515f-516f
Electrical activity of the heart, 298-301, 299f
Electrocardiogram, 298-301, 299f
Electronic environment, 613, 613b
Electronic medical record (EMR)
  copy and paste or carry forward (CPCF) text in, 617, 617b
  general guidelines, 616-619
  objective data, 618-619
  organization of note, 617-618
  replicating functions, 617
  SOAP notes, 618
  subjective data, 618
Elephantiasis, 179-180
Embolism, pulmonary, 290, 644
Emergency assessment, 632-636
  acute medical, 637-641
  advanced cardiac life support survey, 637-641
  airway and cervical spine, 632
  circulation, 633-634
  disability, 634, 634b, 634t
  head and neck, 635
  of infants and children, 638, 638b, 640b, 641t
  legal considerations, 641-642
  primary survey, 632-635, 633b
  reevaluation in, 636
  secondary, 635-636
  symptoms and risks of serious and life-threatening conditions, 639t
Emotional intimacy, 5
Emotional stability, 71-74, 71b, 595
Emphathy, 4
Emphysema, 283t-284t, 292, 292f
Empyema, 286, 286f
Encephalitis, 573
Encephalocele, 202, 202f
Endocrine system, review of system, 13
Endometrial cancer, 413, 426b
Endometriosis, 451, 451f
Endorphins, 51
Energy requirements, 97, 97t, 102, 102b
Enterobiasis, 500
Entropion, 210, 210f
Environment, 13
Epicardium, 295, 295f
Epidermis, 115, 115f
Epididymitis, 482, 482f
Epigenetic research, 81b
Epiglottis, 291, 291f
Epilepsy, 573
Epiluminescence microscopy (ELM), 48, 48f

Episcleritis, 223, 223f
Epitrochlear lymph nodes, 175-176
Epstein-Barr virus mononucleosis, 181
Equipment, examination. *See*
    Examination techniques
Erection, 468-469, 475b
Erosion, skin, 130f
Error, potential for, 596, 596b
Erythema migrans, 149f
Esophagitis, 391t, 401
Esophagus, 372
Estrogen, 79
Ethics, 612
Ethnic food guide pyramids, 102
Ethnicity of patients, 12b, 24b. *See also*
    Cultural competence
Eustachian tube, 232f
Evaluation and management plan,
    614-615
Evidence-based practice (EBP)
    acute ankle injury in adults, 524b
    acute knee injury, 528b
    cardiac murmurs in children, 318b
    cervical cancer screening after
        hysterectomy, 436b
    decision making, 614, 614f
    detection of abdominal aortic
        aneurysms, 388b
    detection of hearing loss, 238b
    diagnosis of appendicitis, 390b
    diagnosis of left-sided heart failure in
        adults, 321b
    history taking, 12b
    Mini-Mental State Examination
        (MMSE) in, 68b
    ovarian torsion, 398b
    predictors of streptococcal
        pharyngitis, 248b
    preparticipation physical evaluation,
        582b
    screening for prostate cancer, 491b
    signs of meningitis, 566b
    smoking cessation, 13b
    splenomegaly, 383b
    thyroid examination, 194b
Examination sequence, 596-597
    adults and adolescents, 596-597,
        596b
    children, 605-606
        child on parent's lap, 606-607, 606f
        child playing, 606, 606f
        child relatively supine, still on lap,
            diaper loosened, 607
        child returns to parent's lap,
            607-608, 607f
        child standing, 607, 607f
        general inspection, 606, 606b

Examination sequence (*Continued*)
    closing discussion, 608-609
    general inspection, 597, 597f
    infants, 602-608, 603f
        abdomen, 603-604, 604f
        back, 605, 605f
        behavior, 605
        chest, lungs, and heart, 603, 603f
        general inspection, 603-606, 603f
        genitals and rectum, 605
        head and neck, 604, 604f
        lower extremities, 604, 604f
        neurologic, 605
        upper extremities, 604
    measurements, 597-603
        female patient, lithotomy position,
            601
        male patient, bending forward,
            601-602, 602f
        patient reclining 45 degrees,
            599-600, 599f
        patient seated, back exposed, 599,
            599f
        patient seated, chest exposed, 599,
            599f
        patient seated, wearing gown,
            597-598, 598f
        patient sitting, lap draped,
            600-601, 601f
        patient standing, 601, 601f
        patient supine, abdomen exposed,
            600, 600f
        patient supine, chest exposed, 600
        patient supine, legs exposed, 600,
            600f
    newborns, 602
    older adults, 608
    pregnant women, 607-608
    preparation, 597
    supplies for, 596b
Examination techniques. *See also*
    Assessment
    Amsler grid, 44-45
    auscultation, 35, 35b
    calipers for skinfold thickness, 49, 49f
    dermatoscope, 48, 48f
    Doppler, 41, 41f
    equipment for, 37-49, 37f-38f
    fetal monitoring, 41-42, 42f
    goniometer, 48, 48f
    height and weight, 37-38, 37f-38f
    inspection, 32-33
    latex allergy and, 30, 32b
    modifications for disabled patients,
        35-37, 36b, 597b
    monofilament, 49, 49f
    nasal speculum, 45, 46f

Examination techniques (*Continued*)
    necessary, 31b
    neurologic hammer, 46
    nose as aid to, 33b
    ophthalmoscope, 42-43, 42f-43f, 42t
    otoscope, 45, 45f
    palpation, 33, 33b, 33t
    patient positioning and draping, 32
    for patients with spinal cord injury or
        lesion, 37
    percussion, 34-35, 34f, 34t, 35b
        hammer, 46, 47f
    photoscreening, 43
    portable ultrasound, 41
    precautions to prevent infection, 30
    pulse oximetry, 40-41, 41f
    recommendations for application of
        standard precautions for care of
        all patients in all health care
        settings, 31t
    scoliometer, 49, 49f
    sphygmomanometer, 40
    stethoscope, 39-40, 39f-40f
    tape measure, 46-47
    temperature, 39, 39f
    transilluminator, 47
    tuning fork, 45-46, 46f
    tympanometer, 45, 45f
    vaginal speculum, 47, 48f
    visual acuity charts, 43-44, 44f
    Wood's lamp, 48, 48f
Excoriation, 129f
Execution of motor skills, 69
Exercise, 97, 98t. *See also* Preparation
    physical evaluation (PPE)
    intensity, 303b
    sports injuries and, 538-543, 539b
Exophthalmos, 223, 223f
Extensor carpi radialis brevis, 503f-504f
Extensor carpi radialis longus,
    503f-504f
Extensor carpi ulnaris, 503f-504f
Extensor digiti minimi, 503f-504f
Extensor digitorum communis,
    503f-504f
External anal sphincter, 418f
External auditory canal, 232f
External ear, 232, 232f
    examination and findings, 238-239,
        239f
External eye, 205, 205f, 209-214, 210f
    abnormalities, 223-224
External nose, 242, 243f
External urethral sphincter, 418f
Extinction phenomenon, 562
Extremities. *See* Lower extremities;
    Upper extremities

Eyelids, 205, 205f, 210-211, 210f
Eyes. *See also* Vision
  abnormalities, 223-230
    external, 223-224
    extraocular muscles, 224
    internal, 225-227
    visual fields, 228-230
  on admission note, 629
  anatomy and physiology, 204-207,
    205f
    external, 205, 205f
    internal, 205-207, 206f, 207t
  examination and findings, 208-222
    external, 209-214, 210f
    extraocular muscles, 214-216
    ophthalmoscopic, 216-222, 216b
    recording, 624, 626
    sequence, 598
  impairment, 36, 70b
  muscles, 205f, 214-216, 215b, 215f
    abnormalities, 224
  nutrient deficiencies and, 106t-107t
  ophthalmoscope for examination of,
    42-43, 42f-43f, 42t
  physical examination findings,
    POMR, 624
  raccoon, 636f
  review of related history, 206
  review of system, 13
Eczematous dematitis, 144

F
Face
  examination sequence, 598, 604, 604f
  inspection, 189-192
  landmarks, 185, 185f
  muscles, 185, 185f, 506f
FACES Rating Scale, 59, 59f
Facial nerve, 232f, 553t, 555-556
Facilitation, 4
Failure to respond, pupil, 213f
Failure to thrive, 93, 93f
Fallopian tubes, 419, 419f
  pelvic inflammatory disease (PID),
    390t-391t, 462, 462f
  salpingitis, 390t-391t, 462, 462f
Falls, risk of, 552b
Family history, 6, 12. *See also* History
  abdomen, 377
  on admission note, 629
  anus and rectum, 488
  blood vessels, 338
  breasts and axillae, 355
  chest and lungs, 266
  ears, nose, and throat, 237
  eyes, 208
  female genitalia, 425

Family history (*Continued*)
  growth and measurement, 82
  head and neck, 188
  heart, 303
  infants and children, 15
  lymphatic system, 172
  male genitalia, 469
  mental status examination, 66
  musculoskeletal system, 509
  neurologic system, 551
  nutrition, 98
  pregnant women, 18
  Problem-Oriented Medical Record
    format, 622, 623f
  skin, hair, and nails, 118
Family relationships and culture, 27-28
Fascia over temporalis, 506f
Fat, dietary, 96, 102, 112b
Fat necrosis, 366, 367f
Fat-soluble vitamins, 103t
Fecal incontinence, 376, 415
Feelings and mood, 71
Feet
  abnormalities, 540-542, 540f
  bones and joints, 507-508, 508f
  club, 540, 540f
  examination sequence, 600
  inspection, 522-524, 523f
  monofilament for examination of, 49,
    49f
  plantar reflex, 563, 563f
  pronation, 522, 522f
  protective sensation, 565, 565f
Female athlete triad, 593b
Female genitalia
  abnormalities, 450-465
    lesions from sexually transmitted
      infections, 451-454
    vulva and vagina, 454-456
  anatomy and physiology
    bony pelvis, 419-423, 422f
    external genitalia, 416-423,
      416b-417b, 417f-418f
    internal genitalia, 418-419,
      418f-419f
  cancers, 425b-426b, 436b-437b
  examination and findings, 427-449
    bimanual, 435-437, 435f-436f,
      439f
    in disabled women, 447,
      448f-449f
    external, 428-430, 429f
    infants and children, 439-440,
      440f
    insertion of speculum, 430-431,
      431b, 432f
    internal, 430-435, 431b, 432f

Female genitalia (*Continued*)
  obtaining vaginal smears and
    specimens during, 431,
    433b-435b, 434f
  positioning, 428
  preparation, 427-428, 430, 438,
    447
  recording, 625, 627
  rectovaginal, 438-449
  sequence, 601, 605
  review of related history, 423-427
  self-examination, 426b
Females. *See also* Pregnant women
  athletes, 593b
  hirsutism in, 155, 155f
  review of system, 14
  sexual maturation in, 87-89, 87b,
    88f-89f, 352-353, 352b,
    363-364
Femoral anteversion, 530, 532f
Femoral hernia, 477t
Femoral nerve, 548f
Femur, 503f-504f, 507f
Fetal alcohol syndrome, 191f
Fetus. *See also* Pregnant women
  anorectal malformations in, 486
  head position, 447, 447f
  heart, 299, 299f-300f
    rate (FHR), 443-444
  monitoring equipment, 41-42, 42f
  position, 444-445, 444f
  station, 445-446, 446f
  well-being, 443-444
Fever, 52
Fibroadenoma, 366
Fibrocystic changes in breasts, 366
Fibroids, uterine, 391t, 459, 460f
Fibula, 503f-504f, 507f
Fibular collateral ligament, 507f
Fifth vital sign, 56b
Filum terminale, 548f
Financial considerations, 5
Fine motor skills, 556-559, 558f
Fingers
  clubbing, 137f
  swelling, 514f
First metatarsal, 508f
Fissure
  anorectal, 495-496, 495f
  skin, 130f
Fistula, anal, 496
Fixed splitting, 310
FLACC Behavioral Pain Assessment
  Scale, 59, 61f
Flexor carpi radialis, 503f-504f
Flexor digitorum superficialis, 503f-504f
Flexor retinaculum, 503f-504f

Fluid wave, 388, 389f
Fluoride, 106
Folate, 104
Follicle-stimulating hormone (FSH), 79
Folliculitis, 144, 145f
Foodborne infection, 400b
Food diary, 101
Food-nutrient-medication interactions, 100b
Foreign body
    in lungs, 271, 281b
    in vagina, 457t
Foreskin, retraction of, 474b
Foster care and adoption, 16b
14-step screening orthopedic examination, 581-587, 585f-586f
Fovea, 42f
Fracture, bone, 539, 636
Frenulum of lower lip, 234f
Frenulum of upper lip, 234f
Frontalis, 506f
Frontal lobe, 545f, 546
Functional assessment
    activities of daily living, 74b, 608
    for all patients, 19b
    ears, nose, and throat, 253b
    musculoskeletal system, 534b
    for older adults, 74b, 608
    Tinetti balance and gait assessment tool, 571b-572b
Fundus, 217f
    height in pregnancy, 442, 442f-443f
    pigmentation, 217b
Fungal infection
    onychomycosis, 156, 156f
    Wood's lamp for, 48, 48f
Furuncle, 145, 145f
Fusiform swelling, 514f

G
Gait, 550, 559, 559f, 570, 571f. See also Coordination
    assessment tool, 571b-572b
    cerebellar, 560t
    Parkinsonian, 560t
    unexpected patterns, 560f, 560t
Galactorrhea, 367, 368f
Gallbladder, 373, 386
Gastric bubble, 383
Gastritis, 391t
Gastrocnemius, 507f
Gastroesophageal reflux disease, 391t, 400
Gastrointestinal system
    nutrient deficiencies and, 106t-107t
    review of system, 13

Gender
    adaptations for interviews, 14-20
    patient-centeredness and physician, 27b
General inspection
    adults, 597, 597f
    children, 606, 606b
    infants, 603-606, 603f
Genital herpes
    in men, 478, 478f
    in women, 454, 454f
Genitalia. See Female genitalia; Male genitalia
Genital warts, 451, 452f
Genitourinary system
    on admission note, 629
    review of system, 13
Genome-wide association studies (GWAS), 21-22
Genu varum, 531-532, 532f
Geriatric Depression Scale, 74, 75f
German measles, 163, 163f
Gestational age, 85-86, 85f, 442, 442t
Giant cell arteritis, 346
Gibbus, 518, 519f
Gingiva, 234f, 245, 246f
Glasgow Coma Scale, 634, 634t
Glaucoma, 227
Glenohumeral joint, 505, 506f
Glenoid fossa, 506f
Glenoid labrum, 506f
Global aphasia, 71t
Glomerulonephritis, 407
Glossopharyngeal nerve, 553t, 556
Gloving, 35b, 428
Gluteus maximus muscle, 418f
Gonadotropins, 79
Goniometer, 48, 48f
Gonorrhea, 457t
Goodell sign, 443b
Goodenough-Harris Drawing Test, 72, 73f
Gout, 536, 537f
Gower sign, 532, 533f
Gracilis, 507f
Graphesthesia, 562
Graves disease, 201
Greater trochanter, 503f-504f, 507f
Greater tubercle of humerus, 506f
Grey-Turner sign, 636f
Growth and measurement
    abnormalities, 91-94
        acromegaly, 91, 92f
        Cushing syndrome, 92
        failure to thrive, 93, 93f
        growth hormone deficiency, 94, 94f

Growth and measurement (Continued)
        hydrocephalus, 93, 93f
        precocious puberty, 94, 94f
        Turner syndrome, 92, 92f
    anatomy and physiology, 79-82, 80f
    anthropometrics, 100, 100b
    charts, 84b, 86b
    differences by organ systems, 80-82, 80f
    examination and findings, 83-89
    infant and child, 81-82, 81f
    nutrition and, 107-108
        biochemical measurement, 108, 109t
        midarm muscle circumference/ midarm muscle area, 108
        mid-upper arm circumference, 108, 108f
        triceps skinfold thickness and, 49, 49f, 107-108, 107f
    pregnant women, 81-82, 88-89, 90f
    review of related history, 82-83
    sexual maturation, 87-89, 87b
    waist circumference and waist-height ratio, 100, 101f
    waist-to-hip circumference ratio, 100-101, 101f
Growth hormone deficiency, 94, 94f
Growth hormone-releasing hormone (GHRH), 79
Guidelines for Standard Precautions, 30, 31t
Guillain-Barré syndrome, 577
Gums, 244-246, 245b, 245f, 245t
Gynecomastia, 353, 369, 369f
Gyrus, 546f

H
Habits, 12
Hair
    anatomy and physiology, 116
    disorders, 154-155
        hair-pulling, 163, 163f
    examination and findings, 133-134
    family history, 118
    gray, 117
    history of present illness, 118
    nutrient deficiencies and, 106t-107t
    past medical history, 118
    review of related history, 117-119
    review of system, 13
Hallucinations and perceptual distortions, 71-74
Hamman sign, 636f

Hand
    assessment, 524, 524b, 525f-526f
    carpal tunnel syndrome, 524, 525f,
        536, 537t
        in pregnant women, 533
    dupuytren contracture, 543, 543f
    inspection, 512-524, 512f-515f
    newborn, 529, 530f
    palpation by, 33t
    veins evaluation, 343, 344f
Handshakes, 33b
Hard palate, 234f
Hashimoto disease, 201
Hawkins test, 524-526, 526f
Head
    abnormalities, 198
    on admission note, 629
    anatomy and physiology, 184-186,
        185f, 187f, 505-507, 506f
    circumference, 84-85, 85f
    examination and findings, 188-197,
        598
        children, 607, 607f
        infants, 604, 604f
        recording, 624, 626
    growth, 80-81
    inspection, 189-192
    lymph nodes, 169f, 174-175, 174f
    muscles, 506f
    physical examination findings,
        POMR, 624
    review of related history, 186-188
    review of system, 13
    in secondary assessment of injured
        patient, 635
    temporomandibular joint, 505-507,
        506f, 517f
        inspection, 516
        syndrome, 537
Headache, 187-188, 197t-198t, 198
    jolt accentuation of, 566
Health beliefs and practices, impact of
    culture on, 27, 27b
Health professionals. See Practitioners
Hearing. See also Ears
    anatomy and physiology, 232-236
    equipment for examination of, 45-46,
        45f-46f
    evaluation, 241-242, 241f-242f,
        242t
    impaired, 36-37
        female genital examination for
            women who are, 449, 449f
    loss, 236b, 238b, 256-257
Heart. See also Blood vessels;
    Cardiovascular system
    abnormalities, 320-331

Heart (Continued)
        rate and rhythm, 324-331,
            325t-327t
        risk factors, 303b
    on admission note, 630
    anatomy and physiology, 294-301,
        294b, 295f
    block, 325f
    cardiac cycle, 297-298, 297f-298f
    cardiac life support survey, 637-641
    chambers, 295, 296f, 297
    disease risk factors, 303b
    electrical activity, 298-301, 299f
    examination and findings, 304-319,
        305f, 599-600
        children, 607
        infants, 603, 603f
        recording, 625, 627-628
    failure, congestive, 276b
    fetal, 299, 299f-300f
        rate (FHR), 443-444
    murmurs, 299f, 311-312, 313t, 317b
    physical examination findings,
        POMR, 625
    review of related history, 301-304
    review of system, 13
    sounds, 307-310, 307b, 308t, 309f
        after surgical procedures, 311b
        extra, 310-311, 311f-312f, 313t
        splitting, 308-309, 310b
    structure, 295-297, 295f-296f
    thrill, 306, 306b
    valves, 297, 297b, 310
Hegar sign, 443b
Height measurement, 83
    children, 86, 86f
    devices, 37-38, 38f
    infants, 83-84, 84b
    waist-height ratio, 100
Hemangiomas, 139, 139f
Hematologic system, review of system,
    13
Hematoma, subungual, 157, 157f
Hematuria, 376
Hemolytic uremic syndrome, 414
Hemorrhage
    abdomen, 635, 636f
    eye, 204, 212f, 218, 220f, 230, 230f
    shock and, 643
    vomiting blood and, 639t
Hemorrhoids, 496, 497f
Hemothorax, 289, 289f
Hepatic artery, 373
Hepatitis, 404
    risk factors for viral, 376b
Hepatobiliary system abnormalities,
    404-406

Hepatojugular reflex, 343
Hepatomegaly, 396
Hernia, 381, 391t, 405f
    diaphragmatic, 280, 280f, 290
    femoral, 477t
    hiatal, 401
    inguinal, 472-473, 473f, 476f, 477t
Herniated lumbar disk, 535, 536f
Herpes, genital. See Genital herpes
Herpes gestationis, 160
Herpes simplex (HSV), 149, 149f, 181,
    182f
Herpes zoster, 148, 148f
Hiatal hernia, 401
Hippocratic facies, 189f
Hips, 507, 507f
    assessment, 526-527, 527f
    dislocation in infants, 530, 531f
    examination sequence, 600
    inspection, 519-520, 521f
Hirschsprung disease, 377, 414
Hirsutism, 155, 155f
History, 6. See also Family history;
    History of present illness; Review
    of systems (ROS)
    adaptations for age, gender, and
        possible disabilities, 14-20
    building the, 6-20
    chest and lungs, 264-265
    cost-containment and, 1-2
    disabled patients, 20, 20f
    evidence-based practice in physical
        examination and, 12b
    family (See Family history)
    first meeting with patients and, 594
    infants and children, 14-16
    older adults, 18-20
    outline of, 10-14
    pain and related, 52
    past medical (See Past medical
        history)
    pregnant women, 17-18
    Problem-Oriented Medical Record
        format and, 626-628
    review of systems, 13-14
    sexual, 12, 12b
    structure of, 6
    types of, 20b
History of present illness, 6, 11, 11b
    abdomen, 375-376
    on admission note, 628
    anus and rectum, 487-488
    blood vessels, 337
    breasts and axillae, 353
    eyes, 207-208
    female genitalia, 423-424
    growth and measurement, 82

History of present illness (*Continued*)
  head and neck, 187-188
  heart, 301-302, 301b-302b
  infants and children, 14
  lymphatic system, 171
  male genitalia, 468-469
  mental status examination, 65
  musculoskeletal system, 508-509
  neurologic system, 550-551
  nutrition, 97
  pregnant women, 17
  Problem-Oriented Medical Record
      format, 621-622, 627
  skin, 117-118, 117b
Hoarseness, 237
Hodgkin lymphoma, 180, 180f
Homan sign, 344
Home conditions, 13
Hordeolum, 210, 211f
Hormones, growth, 79, 80f
Horner syndrome, 225, 225f
Hot and cold conditions, 27b
HOTV chart, 44
Human immunodeficiency virus (HIV)
      infection, 172b, 182, 488b
  oral manifestations, 248f, 248t
  risk factors, 172b
Human nature orientation, 26
Human papillomavirus (HPV)
  cervical cancer and, 425b
  vaccine, 469b
Humerus, 503f-506f
Humility, cultural, 23
Hurler syndrome, 191f
Hyaloid canal, 42f
Hydrocele, 480, 480f
Hydrocephalus, 93, 93f, 191f, 202
  normal pressure, 580
Hydrocolpos, 464
Hydronephrosis, 408
Hyoid bone, 185
Hyperbilirubinemia, 137b
Hyperpigmentation, 139, 139f
Hypersensitivity, 37
Hypertension, 55-56, 62-63. *See also*
      Blood pressure
  categories, 55t, 582b
  in pediatric athletes, 582b
  pseudotumor cerebri, 574
Hypertensive retinopathy, 218, 220b
Hyperthyroid, 190f, 201, 201t
Hypodermis, 115
Hypoglossal nerve, 553t, 556, 557f
Hypospadias, 484, 484f
Hypotheses, valid, 611, 612b
Hypothyroidism, 200, 201t
Hypoxemia, 642

Hysterectomy
  cervical cancer screening after, 436b
  examining woman who has had, 436b

I
Identifying information, 621
Iliopsoas muscle test, 393, 393f
Iliotibial tract, 507f
Illustrations, 619
Immune system, 166, 177t
  serum sickness, 182
Imperforate anus, 499, 500f
Impetigo, 128f, 161, 161f
Incontinence
  fecal, 376, 415
  urinary, 376, 415t
Incremental grading, 618
Incus, 232f
Indigestion, 375
Infants. *See also* Children; Newborns
  abdomen, 374, 377, 394, 395f, 396b,
      396t-397t
    abnormalities, 410-413
  anus and rectum, 486, 488
    abnormalities, 499-500
    examination, 491-493, 492t, 493f
  blood pressure in, 58, 58b
  blood vessels, 336-338, 345
  brain, 64
  breasts, 363
  chest and lungs, 262-263, 263b, 264f,
      266
    abnormalities, 290
    examination and findings, 279-280,
        279t, 280f
  chief concern, 14, 14b
  ears, nose, and throat, 235, 250f
    examination and findings, 249-251,
        249t, 250f
  emergency assessment, 638, 638b,
      640b, 641t
  examination sequence, 602-608, 603f
    abdomen, 603-604, 604f
    back, 605, 605f
    behavior, 605
    chest, lungs, and heart, 603, 603f
    general inspection, 603-606, 603f
    genitals and rectum, 605
    head and neck, 604, 604f
    lower extremities, 604, 604f
    neurologic, 605
    upper extremities, 604
  eyes, 206, 207t, 208, 218-221, 220b,
      220f-221f
    abnormalities, 229-230, 229f-230f
  failure to thrive, 93, 93f
  family history, 15

Infants (*Continued*)
  female genitalia, 422, 426-427,
      439-440, 440f
    abnormalities, 463-464, 463b, 463f
    ambiguous genitalia, 463-464,
        463b, 463f
  gestational age, 85-86, 85f
  growth, 81-82, 81f
  head and neck, 186, 188, 195, 195f,
      200, 200f, 202-203
  heart, 299, 299f-300f, 303-304,
      318-319, 319b
    abnormalities, 328-330
  history of present illness, 14
  hyperbilirubinemia in, 137b
  intellectual disability in, 77
  interviews, 14-16
  liver, 319b
  lymphatic system, 170-172, 176-177
  male genitalia, 468-469
    ambiguous genitalia, 484, 484f
    examination, 474, 474f
  measurement, 38, 38f, 90b
    chest circumference, 85, 85f
    head circumference, 84-85, 85f
    length, 83, 84b, 84f
    weight, 84, 84b
  musculoskeletal system, 508-509
    abnormalities, 540-542
    examination, 529-530, 529f-530f
  nails, 137-140
  neurologic system, 549, 551
    examination, 566-569, 567b, 567t,
        568f
  nutrition, 98-99
  pain in, 51, 57-59
  past medical history, 14-15
  perceptual distortions and
      hallucinations, 72-73, 72f
  personal and social history, 15
  primitive reflexes routinely evaluated
      in, 568, 568t-569t
  Problem-Oriented Medical Record
      format and, 626-627
  review of systems, 16
  rolling over, 567b
  skin and hair, 116, 119, 119b
    abnormalities, 160-164
Infection
  bone, 537
  ear, 252b, 254-255, 254t, 255f
  enterobiasis, 500
  eye, 204, 210, 211f-212f
  foodborne, 400b
  fungal
    onychomycosis, 156, 156f
    Wood's lamp for, 48, 48f

Infection (*Continued*)
  Guillain-Barré syndrome, 577
  heart, 320, 320f, 322, 322f
  hepatitis, 404
  HIV, 172b
    oral manifestations, 248f, 248t
  lung, 283-293
  lymphatic system, 181-182
  prevention, 30
  skin, 161-162
  vaginal, 456, 456f, 457t
Inferior frontal gyrus, 546f
Infertility, 424, 450, 469, 476
Inflammation
  of Bartholin glands, 454, 455f
  bursitis, 537, 537f
  pelvic inflammatory disease (PID),
    390t-391t, 462, 462f
  salpingitis, 390t-391t, 462, 462f
  vulvovaginitis, 464, 464f
Influenza, 287, 288f
Information recording
  abbreviations and acronyms in, 616,
    617b
  copy and paste or carry forward
    (CPCF) text in, 617, 617b
  emergency assessment, 641
  general guidelines, 616-619, 616b,
    617t
  illustrations and, 619
  objective data, 618-619
  Problem-Oriented Medical Record
    (POMR), 618-619
  sample records, 628
  SOAP notes, 618
  subjective data, 618
Infraspinatus muscle, 503f-504f, 506f
Ingrown nails, 156, 157f
Inguinal area examination sequence,
  600-601
Inguinal hernia, 472-473, 473f, 476f,
  477t
Inguinal lymph nodes, 176, 176f
Injuries
  acute ankle, 524b
  acute knee, 528b
  child abuse patterns of, 164, 164f
  mechanisms, 636-637
  nails, 156-157
  primary assessment, 632-635
  secondary assessment, 635-636
  spinal cord, 37
    autonomic hyperreflexia, 37
    examination modifications for
      patients with, 37
    hypersensitivity and, 37
    spasticity and, 37

Injuries (*Continued*)
  sports, 538-543, 539b
  traumatic brain, 187-188
    sports-related, 588b
Inner ear, 232f, 233
Inpatient admission note, 628
Insertion of gracilis, 507f
Insertion of sartorius, 507f
Inspection, 32-33
  abdomen, 378-381, 394-395
  breasts and axillae, 355-358,
    356f-357f, 359f, 361-363,
    362f
  chest and lungs, 267-271, 267f-268f
  general
    adults, 597, 597f
    children, 606, 606b
    infants, 603-606, 603f
  head and neck, 189-197, 195f
  heart, 304-305
  lymphatic system, 169b, 172-174,
    172b, 173f, 174b
  male genitalia, 471-475, 471f-472f
  musculoskeletal system, 511f
    elbow, 513-514, 515f
    hand and wrist, 510, 512-524,
      512f-515f
    shoulders, 514-516, 516f
Instincts, respecting your, 595b
Insulin-like growth factor I (IGF-I), 79
Intellectual disability, 77
Interleukin 6 and 8 (IL-6 and IL-8), 79
Internal carotid artery, 575t-576t
Internal eye, 0, 205-207, 206f, 207t
  abnormalities, 225-227
Interphalangeal joint, 508f
Interpretation, 4
Interpreters, 4f
Intervertebral disc, 506f
Interviews. *See also* Communication,
    effective
  adaptations for age, gender, and
    possible disabilities, 14-20
  of adolescents, 16-17
  basis of understanding in, 11b
  of children, 14-16
  of disabled patients, 20, 20f
  enhancing patient responses to, 4
  interpreters used during, 4f
  of older adults, 18-20
  of pregnant women, 17-18
  questions, 2, 7
  sensitive issues in, 7-10
  setting, 6
  of young adults, 6f
Intestinal obstruction, 390t-391t
Intimacy, physical and emotional, 5

Intimate partner violence (IPV), 8-10,
  9b
Intracranial pressure, 643
  Biot respiration and, 268
Intracranial tumor, 574
Intraductal papillomas, 367
Intrapartum maternal lumbosacral
  plexopathy, 579
Intussusception, 410, 410f
Iodine, 106
Iris, 212-214
  muscle, 42f, 205f
Iritis constrictive response, 214f
Iron, 105
Irritable bowel syndrome, 391t, 400
Ischial tuberosity, 418f
Ischiocavernosus muscle, 418f
Itching, anal, 496

J
Jargon, 7b
Jaundice, 376
Jaw. *See* Temporomandibular joint
Joints. *See also* Musculoskeletal system
  capsule, 506f-507f
  cavity, 507f
  goniometer for examination of, 48,
    48f
  symptoms, 508-509
Jolt accentuation of headache, 566
Judgment, 70
Jugular venous pressure disorder,
  348-349, 348f
Jugular venous pulse and pressure,
  336-337, 337f, 342-343, 343f, 343t

K
Kaposi sarcoma (KS), 154, 154f
Kawasaki disease, 303, 349, 349f
Kehr sign, 636f
Keloids, 129f
Keratin, 115
Kernig sign, 566, 566f
Kidneys, 373, 383, 387b
  abnormalities, 407-415
  palpation, 387-388, 387f
  during pregnancy, 374
Klinefelter syndrome, 483-484, 483f
Knee, 507, 507f
  acute injury, 528b
  assessment, 527-534, 527f-528f
  examination, 520-522
Knee-chest position for female genital
  examination, 448, 448f
Knock-knee, 532, 532f
Kollonychia, 158, 158f
Koplik spots, 252

Kyphosis, 518, 519f
  in infants, 529, 529f

L
Labia majora, 416-418, 417f, 428
Labia minora, 416-418, 417f, 429, 429f
Lachman test, 528
Lacrimal gland, 205, 205f, 214
Lactating women, 353, 355, 365
Lacteriferous sinus, 351f
Lactiferous duct, 351f
Lactose intolerance, 391t
Lamina, 506f
Landmarks
  abdominal examination, 378f, 379b
  back, 518, 518f
  chest, 262-264, 263f
  eye, 205f
  facial, 185, 185f
  location of findings and, 618
  neck, 185, 186f
  thoracic, 269b, 269f
  tongue, 234f
  tympanic membrane, 232f
Language and culture, 23b
  barriers, 595
Large, bounding pulse, 341f
Large cell carcinoma of lung, 290f
Large intestine, 372
Laryngotracheal bronchitis, 291, 291f
Lateral epicondyle, 505f
Lateral patellar ligament, 507f
Lateral patellar retinaculum, 507f
Lateral rectus muscle, 205f
Lateral recumbent position, 32
Lateral sulcus, 546f
Latex allergy, 30, 32b, 183
Leading questions, 4
Leaking abdominal aneurysm,
  390t-391t
Leff scope, 41
Legal considerations in emergency
  assessment, 641-642
Legg-Calvé-Perthes disease, 541
Legs. See Lower extremities
Leiomyomas, 459
Lens, 42f, 205f, 206, 214
Leopold maneuvers, 444-445, 444f
Leptin, 79
Lesions, mouth, 237
Lesions, skin, 124f, 125-133
  annular formation of, 133f
  as clues to internal problems, 138b
  clustering, 133f
  linear formation of, 133f
  morphologic characteristics,
    131t-132t

Lesions, skin (Continued)
  primary, 126t-128t
  regional distribution of, 132b
  secondary, 129t-131t
Lesser trochanter, 503f-504f, 507f
Levator ani muscle, 418f
Levator labil superioris, 506f
LH Symbols (LEA Symbols) chart, 44
Lichenification, 129f
Life-sustaining treatment, medical
  orders for, 642
Life-threatening conditions
  hypoxemia, 642
  increased intracranial pressure, 643
  pulmonary embolism, 290, 644
  severe asthma episode, 644
  shock state, 643
  status epilepticus, 644
  symptoms and risks of, 639t
  upper airway obstruction, 642
  ventilatory failure, 643
Ligamentum teres, 507f
Limb measurement, 529-534, 529f
Limp, antalgic, 560t
Linea nigra, 374, 374f
Lipedmia retinalis, 226, 226f
Lips, 234f, 244, 245f, 271
Lithotomy position, 32
Liver, 372-373
  abnormalities, 404-406
  auscultation, 386f
  cancer, 405
  infant, 319b
  palpation, 385-388, 386f, 396
  span, 381-382, 382f
Local anesthetics, 58b
Location of findings, 618
Loeys-Dietz syndrome, 247, 248f
Lordosis, 518, 519f
Low birth weight, 86b
Lower back pain, 519b
Lower extremities
  abnormalities
    femoral anteversion, 530, 532f
    femoral hernia, 477t
    Legg-Calvé-Perthes disease, 541
    Osgood-Schlatter disease, 541
    slipped capital femoral epiphysis,
      541
  on admission note, 630
  anatomy and physiology, 507-508,
    507f
  examination, 520-522, 600
    children, 606
    infants, 604, 604f
  limb measurement, 529-534, 529f
  lymph nodes, 168f, 176, 176f

Lower extremities (Continued)
  nutrient deficiencies and, 106t-107t
  pain, 337, 344b
  range of motion, 520, 521f-522f
  reflexes, 564
  in secondary assessment of injured
    patient, 636
Lumbar curve, 281, 282f
Lumbar disk, herniated, 535, 536f
Lumbar englargement of spinal nerve,
  548f
Lumbar plexus, 548f
Lumbar spine, 518-519, 518f-519f
Lumbar stenosis, 536
Lumbosacral radiculopathy, 535, 536f
Lungs
  abnormalities, 283-293
  anatomy and physiology, 260-264,
    260b, 261f-263f, 262b
  cancer, 289, 290f
  cardiac depression, 262f
  examination and findings, 267-281
    recording, 624-625, 627-628
    sequence, 599, 603, 603f
    sequence of steps, 267b
  foreign body in, 271, 281b
  physical examination findings,
    POMR, 624-625
  review of related history, 264-267
  review of system, 13
Lyme disease, 149
Lymph, 167, 167f, 174t
Lymphadenopathy, 177b
Lymphangioma, 179
Lymphatic filariasis, 179-180
Lymphatic system
  abnormalities, 178-183
  anatomy and physiology, 166-171,
    167f
  examination and findings, 172-177,
    172b
  recording, 625-626
  growth, 80, 170-171, 171f
  review of related history, 171-172
Lymphedema, 178-179, 178f, 179t
Lymph nodes, 80, 167-169, 168f-169f,
  169b
  on admission note, 630
  breast, 168f, 352, 352f
  conditions simulating enlargement of,
    174t
  examination sequence, 600
  inspection and palpation, 172-174,
    172b-174b, 173f
  palpation, 193, 360, 360f
Lymphocytes, 169-170
Lymphogranuloma venereum, 478, 479f

Lymphoma, 180, 180f
Lymphoytes, 169-170

M
Macronutrients, 95-96
Macula, 42f, 205f
Macular degeneration, 44-45, 230
Macules, 126f, 139, 139f
Magnesium, 105
Male genitalia. *See also* Prostate gland
    abnormalities, 476-484
    on admission note, 630
    anatomy and physiology, 466-468,
        466b, 467f
    cancer, 470b
    circumcision, 471, 471f, 474b
    examination and findings, 471-475,
        471b
        recording, 625, 627
        sequence, 600-602, 605
    inspection and palpation, 471-474
        cremasteric reflex, 474
        hernia, 472-473, 473f
        penile shaft, 472, 472f
        penis, 471, 472f
        scrotum, 472, 473f
        urethral meatus, 472, 472f
    review of related history, 468-471
    self-examination, 477t
Males
    breast enlargement in, 353, 369,
        369f
    breast examination sequence, 599
    review of system, 14
    sexual maturation in, 87-89, 87b,
        90f-91f
Malignant breast tumors, 366
Malignant melanoma, 153, 153f
Malleus, 232f
Malocclusion, 244, 245t
Mania, 76
MANTRELS, 389
Markle sign, 390t-391t
Masses
    abdominal, 384-385, 385f, 396t
    breast, 361b, 365t
    objective data, 618-619
Mastectomy, 364b
Mastitis, 368, 369f
Masturbation, 427b
McBurney sign, 390t-391t
McDonald sign, 443b
McMurray test, 527, 528f
Measles, 162, 162f
Mechanistic thinking, 612-613, 613b
Meckel diverticulum, 412, 413f
Meconium ileus, 411

Medial epicondyle, 505f
Medial patellar ligament, 507f
Medial patellar retinaculum, 507f
Medial rectus muscle, 205f
Mediastinal mass, 273b
Medications. *See* Drugs
Medulla oblongata, 546f
Meibomian glands, 205, 205f
Melanoma, 117b, 122b
    malignant, 153, 153f
    risk factors, 117b
Memory
    in children, 73, 73f
    mental status and, 70, 70b
    promotion of cognitive functioning
        and, 74b
    transience of, 47b
Ménière disease, 242b, 256
Meningeal signs, 565-566
Meningitis, 574
    evidence-based practice and signs of,
        566b
    testing for, 565-566, 566f
    vaccine, 566b
Menopause, 353, 423-424
Menstruation, 419, 420f, 421t
    female athletes and, 593b
    history, 424-425
    onset of, 87
Mental retardation, 77
Mental status
    abnormalities, 75-78 (*See also*
        Depression)
        autism, 78
        delirium, 75
        dementia, 76t, 78
        disorders of altered mental status,
            75
        disorders of mood, 76-78
        intellectual disability, 77
    activities of daily living (ADLs) and,
        74b
Mental status examination
    anatomy and physiology, 64-65, 65f
    common causes of unresponsiveness
        in, 67t
    family history and, 66
    findings, 66-74, 66b, 66f
        cognitive abilities, 67-70, 68b,
            68f-69f
        emotional stability, 71-74
        importance of validation in, 67b
        memory, 70, 70b
        perceptual distortions and
            hallucinations, 71-74, 72f
        physical appearance and behavior,
            66-67

Mental status examination (*Continued*)
        speech and language skills, 70
        state of consciousness, 67
    history of present illness and, 65
    past medical history and, 66
    personal and social history, 66
    physical examination findings,
        POMR, 624
    recording, 624, 626-627
    review of related history, 65-66
Metacarpals, 503f-504f
Metacarpophalangeal joint, 505f
Metarsophalangeal joint, 508f
Metatarsals, 503f-504f
Metatarsus abductus, 540, 540f
Microcephaly, 202, 203f
Micronutrients, 96
Microtrauma and tearing of rotator cuff
    muscles, 540
Midarm muscle circumference/midarm
    muscle area, 108
Midbrain artery, 545f
Middle cerebral artery, 545f, 575f,
    575t-576t
Middle ear, 232, 232f, 251f
Middle frontal gyrus, 546f
Mid-upper arm circumference (MAC),
    108, 108f
Milia, 140, 140f
Military record, 13
Milliaria rubra, 161, 161f
Minerals, 105t-106t
Mini-Cog, 67, 69f
Mini-Mental State Examination
    (MMSE), 67, 68b, 68f
Miosis, 213f
Mitral insufficiency/regurgitation, 331
Mittelschmerz, 437b
Mnemonics
    AMPLE, 635b
    AVPU, 634b
    OLDCARTS, 622
    SOAP notes, 618, 620, 620b
Mobility impairments, 35-36, 36b
Modes of communication, 26-27, 26f
Moles, 121, 122b, 122t
    ABCD changes in, 153f
Molloscum contaglosum
    in men, 479, 479f
    in women, 452, 452f
Monofilament, 49, 49f
Mons pubis, 416-418, 417f
Montgomery tubercles, 351-352
Mood
    assessing feelings and, 71
    disorders, 76-78 (*See also* Depression)
    anxiety, 77

Mood (*Continued*)
  mania, 76
  schizophrenia, 77
Moro reflex, 568t-569t
Mouth. *See also* Throat
  abnormalities, 257-259
  anatomy and physiology, 234-236, 234f-235f
  cancer, 237b, 247b, 259, 259f
  examination and findings, 244-253, 245f, 247b, 247f
    recording, 624, 626
    sequence, 598
  lesions, 237
  physical examination findings, POMR, 624
  review of related history, 236-238
  review of system, 13
  tonsils and adenoids, 170
  vagus nerve, 553t, 556
  vestibule of, 234f
M-shaped position for female genital examination, 448-449, 449f
Multiple sclerosis (MS), 573
Mumps, 177t
Murmurs, heart, 299f, 311-312, 313t, 317b
  in children, 318b
  differential diagnosis, 318t
Muscles
  abdomen, 373
  eyes, 214-216, 215b, 215f
    abnormalities, 224
  face, 185, 185f, 506f
  head, 506f
  lower extremities, 507-508, 507f
  perineum, 430, 430f
  shoulder, 506f
  strain, 539
  strength, 511-512, 512t
    in newborns, 530, 531f
  tone, 511, 511f
  upper extremities
    anatomy and physiology, 505, 505f
    midarm muscle circumference/ midarm muscle area, 108
    trapezius, 518, 518f
Muscular dystrophy, 541
Musculoskeletal system
  abdomen, 373, 535-543
  abnormalities
    musculoskeletal, 535-538
    sports injuries, 538-543, 539b
  on admission note, 630
  anatomy and physiology, 501-508, 501b-502b, 503f-504f

Musculoskeletal system (*Continued*)
  lower extremities, 507-508
  upper extremities, 505, 505f
  bilateral symmetry, 510b
  emergency assessment, 636
  examination and findings, 510-534
    in adolescents, 532-533
    cervical spine, 516-518
    in children, 530-532, 532f
    elbow, 513-514, 515f-516f
    feet and ankles, 522-524, 523f
    hand and wrist, 505, 505f, 512-524, 512f-515f, 524b, 525f-526f
    hips, 519-520, 521f
    in infants, 529-530, 529f-530f
    knee, 520-522, 527-534, 527f-528f
    legs, 520-522
    in older adults, 519f, 534
    in pregnant women, 533, 533f
    recording, 625, 627-628
    sequence, 600
    shoulders, 514-516, 516f-517f
    temporomandibular joint, 516, 517f
  eyes, 205, 205f, 214-216, 215b, 215f, 224
  functional assessment, 74b
  growth, 80
  muscle strength, 511-512, 512t
  muscle tone, 511, 511f
  pelvis, female, 419-423, 422f
  range of motion, 511, 511f
  review of related history, 508-510
  review of system, 13
Myasthenia gravis, 576
Mydriasis, 213f
Mydriatics, 216b
Myelomeningocele (spina bifida), 578, 579f
Myocardial infarction, 323
Myocarditis, 324
Myomas, 459, 460f
Myxedema, 201
Myxedema facies, 190f

N
Nails, 117
  abnormalities
    changes associated with systemic disease, 158-159
    infections, 155-156
    injury, 156-157
    periungual growths, 159-165
  anatomy and physiology, 116, 116f
  base angle, 135
  bed adherence, 137f

Nails (*Continued*)
  color, 134
  cyanosis and, 271
  examination and findings, 134-135, 134b, 134f-136f
  family history, 118
  history of present illness, 118
  past medical history, 118
  plate, 135
  review of related history, 117-119
  review of system, 13
Nasalis, 506f
Nasal speculum, 45, 46f, 242-243, 243f
Nasopharynx, 233
Nausea, 375
Near vision charts, 44
Neck
  abnormalities, 199-203
  on admission note, 630
  anatomy and physiology, 184-186, 186f-187f
  examination and findings, 188-197, 598
    children, 607, 607f
    recording, 624, 626
  inspection, 192-197
  lymph nodes, 169f, 174-175, 174f
  physical examination findings, POMR, 624
  review of related history, 186-188
  review of system, 13
  in secondary assessment of injured patient, 635, 636f
  stiff, 188, 565-566, 566f
Necrotizing enterocolitis, 413
Neonatal Infant Pain Scale, 58
Nephroblastoma, 414
Neuroblastoma, 413
Neurologic hammer, 46
Neurologic system
  abnormalities, 573-580
    disorders of the central nervous system, 573-574
    disorders of the peripheral nervous system, 576-580
  on admission note, 630
  anatomy and physiology, 544-549, 544b
  examination and findings, 552-571, 552b
    cranial nerves, 553-556
    proprioception and cerebellar function, 556-559
    recording, 625, 627-628
    reflexes, 562-571
    sensory function, 559-562
    sequence, 600-601, 605

Neurologic system (*Continued*)
    nutrient deficiencies and,
        106t-107t
    review of related history, 550-552
    review of system, 14
    in secondary assessment of injured
        patient, 636
    upper and lower neuron disease,
        555b, 563t
Neurons, afferent, 487, 549
Neuropathic pain, 50-52, 62
Neuropathy, peripheral, 49
Neurovascular assessment, 539b
Nevi, 121, 121b, 121t, 122f
Newborns. *See also* Infants
    abdomen, 374
    brain weight, 80-81
    breasts, 363
    chest and lungs, 262-263, 263b
        examination and findings, 279-280,
            279t, 280f
    ears, nose, and throat examination,
        249-251
    examination sequence, 602
    female genitalia, 439-440, 440f
    general muscle strength, 530, 531f
    gestational age, 85-86, 85f
    hands, 529, 530f
    head and neck, 186, 188, 196f
    heart, 299, 299f-300f
    indirect cranial nerve evaluation in,
        567t
    length measurement, 83-84, 84b
    low birth weight, 86b
    nails, 137-140, 137b
    pain in, 57-59
    periodic apnea of, 272b
    skin and hair, 116, 137b, 138f
    umbilical cord, 170b
Niacin, 104
Nicotinic acid, 104
Nipple, 351-352, 351f
    abnormalities, 367-369, 367f-368f
    compression, 363b
    discharge, 353, 363f
    inspection, 356-357, 357f, 361-363,
        362f
    pore, 351f
    supernumerary, 359f
Nociceptors, 51, 51f
Nodules, skin, 127f
Nonalcoholic fatty liver disease
    (NAFLD), 406
Non-Hodgkin lymphoma, 180
Non-proliferative diabetic retinopathy,
    225, 226f
Nonverbal communication, 67

Norepinephrine, 51
Normal pressure hydrocephalus,
    580
Norms, screening based on, 24b
Nose
    as aid to physical examination, 33b
        of skin, 125b
    anatomy and physiology, 231b, 233,
        233f-234f
    bleeds, 237
    discharge, 237
    examination and findings, 242-244,
        243f-244f
        recording, 624, 626
        sequence, 598
    functional assessment, 253b
    nasal speculum for examination of,
        45, 46f, 243f
    physical examination findings,
        POMR, 624
    review of related history, 236-238
    review of system, 13
Nucleus pulposus, 506f
Nursemaid's elbow, 542
Nutrition. *See also* Diet
    abnormalities, 110-112 (*See also*
        Obesity)
        anemia, 111t, 112
        anorexia nervosa, 111
        bulimia nervosa, 112
    anatomy and physiology, 95-97
    cholesterol and, 111t, 112b
    daily energy needs, 102b
    deficiencies signs and symptoms,
        106t-107t
    determination of diet adequacy, 101,
        101f
    eating disorders and, 99b, 111-112
        female athletes and, 593b
    energy requirements, 97, 97t
    epigenetic research and, 81b
    examination and findings, 99-108
    food-nutrient-medication interactions,
        100b
    guidelines, 113b
    macronutrients, 95-96
    measures of nutrient adequacy,
        102-107, 102b, 103t-107t
    measures of nutrient analysis,
        101-102
    micronutrients, 96
    review of related history, 97-99
    special procedures, 107-108
        biochemical measurement, 108,
            109t
        midarm muscle circumference/
            midarm muscle area, 108

Nutrition (*Continued*)
        mid-upper arm circumference, 108,
            108f
        triceps skinfold thickness and, 49,
            49f, 107-108, 107f

O
Obesity, 83b, 110
    assessment and possible causes, 110t
    in children and adolescents, 59b,
        110f
    risk factors for cardiac disease, 303b
    risk factors for endometrial cancer,
        426b
    risk factors for osteoarthritis, 509b
    statistics, 99b
Objective data in EMRs, 618-619
Observation
    of patients, 597, 597f
    of respiration, 267-271
Obstetric stirrups position for female
        genital examination, 448, 448f
Obturator muscle test, 393, 394f
Occipitalis, 506f
Occipital lobe, 546, 546f
Occupation, 13
Oculomotor nerve (CN III), 553t, 554
    damage, 214f
Odor, skin, 123, 125b
Ohmann score, 389
OLDCARTS mnemonic, 622
Older adults. *See also* Adults
    abdomen, 375, 377, 398
        abnormalities, 415
    abuse of, 9-10, 165
    activities of daily living (ADLs) and,
        74b
    agility in, 508, 534, 534b
    anus and rectum, 487, 489
        examination, 493
    blood vessels, 337-338, 345
        abnormalities, 349
    brain, 65
    breasts and axillae, 353, 355, 365
    chest and lungs, 263-264, 266-267
        abnormalities, 292
        examination and findings, 281,
            282f
    competency to make medical
        decisions, 18b
    dementia in, 78
    depression in, 74, 75f
    ears, nose, and throat, 235-236, 238
        examination and findings, 252-253,
            253f
    emergency assessment, 638-641
    examination sequence, 608

Older adults (*Continued*)
  eyes, 206-208, 207b, 222
    abnormalities, 44-45, 225, 225f, 230
  female genitalia, 423, 427
    abnormalities, 465
    examination, 447
  functional assessment, 19b
  gait in, 570, 571b-572b, 571f
  growth and measurement, 83, 89
  head and neck, 186, 188, 197
  heart, 301, 304, 319
    abnormalities, 331
  history, 18-20
  lymphatic system, 171-172
  male genitalia, 468-471
    examination, 475
  mental status examination of, 66
  musculoskeletal system, 508, 508b, 510
    abnormalities, 542-543
    examination, 519f, 534
  neurologic system, 549, 552
    abnormalities, 579-580
    examination, 570-571
  nutrition, 99, 100b
  pain in, 52
    assessment of, 60
  perceptual distortions and hallucinations in, 73-74
  physical stature, 82
  Problem-Oriented Medical Record format and, 628
  skin and hair, 116-117, 119, 141-143, 141b, 141f-142f
    abnormalities, 165
  vital signs in, 60
Olecranon, 503f-505f
  bursa, 505f
Olecranon Process, 514, 516f
  bursitis, 537, 537f
Olfactory nerve, 553-556, 554f
Onycholysis, 157, 157f
Onychomycosis, 156, 156f
Open-ended questions, 2, 4
Ophthalmoscope, 42-43, 42f-43f, 42t, 216-222, 216b
Optic atrophy, 219t, 227f
Optic disc, 205f, 206, 217, 218f
Optic nerve, 42f, 205f, 553t, 554
Oral cavity. *See* Mouth
Orbicularis oculi, 506f
Orbicularis oris, 506f
Orchitis, 481, 481f
Order of cardiac valves, 297b
Orders for life-sustaining treatment, 642
Organ growth, 80-82, 80f

Oropharynx, 234-236, 234f, 248-253, 249f
  abnormalities, 257-259
Osgood-Schlatter disease, 541
Osteitis deformans, 537
Osteoarthritis, 509b, 538
  comparison with rheumatoid arthritis, 538t
Osteomyelitis, 537
Osteoporosis, 510b, 542, 542f
  female athletes and, 593b
Otitis externa, 254t, 255, 255f
Otitis media with effusion, 254-255, 254t, 255f
Otoscope, 45, 45f, 239-241, 239f
Oval window, 232f
Ovarian cancer, 425b, 461
Ovarian torsion, 398b
Ovaries, 419, 419f-420f
  cysts, 460, 461f
  examination of, 437
Oximetry, pulse, 40-41, 41f

P
Paget disease
  of bone, 537
  of breast, 368, 368f
Pain, 50-52
  abdominal, 375-376, 388-389, 389b, 392b, 397t
    acute, 390t-391t
    chronic, 391t
    quality and onset of, 391t
  anal, 487
  assessment, 50, 56-60
    in children, 59-60, 59f, 61f
    in infants, 58-59
    in newborns and infants, 58-59
    in older adults, 60
    in pregnant women, 60
  back, 509
    lower, 519b
  behaviors, 50b, 56-60
  breast, 353
  calf, 344b
  chest, 265, 266b, 301-302, 301b-302b, 302t
  children and, 52, 58-59
  complex regional pain syndrome, 63
  examination and findings, 52-60
  female genitalia and, 424, 427
  as the fifth vital sign, 56b
  head (*See* Headache)
  infants and, 51, 57-58
  leg, 337
  neurologic system, 550
  neuropathic, 50-52, 62

Pain (*Continued*)
  nociceptors and, 51, 51f
  older adults and, 52
  personal and social history and, 52
  pregnant women and, 51-52
  receptors, 51f
  rectal, 489b
  related history, 52
  scale selection, 56b
  self-report rating scales, 56
  sinus, 237
  sugar water for, 58b
  superficial, 561, 561f
  testicular, 468
  visual analogue scale, 56, 57f
Painometer, 56, 57f
Palatine tonsil, 234f
Palmar grasp reflex, 568t-569t
Palmaris longus, 503f-504f
Palpation, 33, 33b, 33t
  abdomen, 383-398, 384f-385f
    kidneys, 387f, 388
    liver, 385-388, 386f, 396
    twin pregnancy, 445, 445f
  aorta, 388, 388f
  blood vessels, 338-340, 339b, 339f
  breasts and axillae, 358-360, 360f-362f
  chest and lungs, 271-273, 272f
  eyes, 211
  head, 192, 196
  heart, 305-306, 305f-306f
  lymphatic system, 169b, 172-174, 175f, 193, 360, 360f
  male genitalia, 471-474, 472f
  musculoskeletal system, 510
  nails, 135-143
  neck, 193
  rectal walls, 490, 491f
  skin, 124-125, 125f
  thyroid, 193-195, 194b, 194f-195f
Pancreas, 373
  abnormalities, 406-407
Pancreatitis, 390t-391t, 406-407
PanOptic ophthalmoscope, 43, 43f
Pantothenic acid, 104
Pap smears, 425b, 431, 433b-435b, 434f
Papules, 126f
Paradoxic pulse, 341f
Paradoxic splitting, 310
Paraphimosis, 477, 477f
Paresthesia or weakness, 551
Parietal lobe, 546
Parkinson disease, 579, 580f
Parkinsonian gait, 560t
Paronychia, 155, 156f
Parotid gland, 199f

Paroxsmal atrial tachycardia, 327f
Partial spinal sensory syndrome, 562
Partner Violence Screen (PVS), 8-9
Past medical history, 6, 11-12
  abdomen, 377
  on admission note, 628
  anus and rectum, 488
  blood vessels, 337-338
  breasts and axillae, 353-354
  chest and lungs, 265-266
  ears, nose, and throat, 237
  eyes, 208
  female genitalia, 424-425
  growth and measurement, 82
  head and neck, 188
  heart, 302-303
  infants and children, 14-15
  lymphatic system, 171-172
  male genitalia, 469, 469b
  mental status examination, 66
  musculoskeletal system, 509
  neurologic system, 551
  nutrition, 97-98
  pregnant women, 18
  Problem-Oriented Medical Record
    format, 622, 627
  skin, 118, 118b
Patches, skin, 126f
Patella, 503f-504f
Patellar ligament, 507f
Patellar reflex, 564
Patent ductus arteriosus, 263b, 329,
  329f
Patients
  addressing, 2-3, 6
  advance directives and, 19, 608, 612,
    628, 642
  alliance with, 16b, 609
  body language, 3-4
  -centered questions, 2b
  closing discussion with, 608-609
  confidentiality, 3
  difficult, 594, 595b
  disabled, 20, 20f, 35-37, 36b
    emergency assessment, 634, 634b,
      634t
    examination technique
      modifications for, 35-37, 36b
    female genitalia examination in,
      447, 448f-449f
    sports participation by, 581, 582b
  ethnicity, 12b, 24b
  evaluation and management plan,
    614-615
  first meetings with, 594
  general information, 621
  history (See History)

Patients (Continued)
  individual primacy in health care, 24
  observing, 597, 597f
  positions and draping, 32
  relationship with
    developing, 1-5
    effective communication in, 2-5, 3b
    seeking connection in, 2-4
  unconscious, 633b-634b, 634, 634t
Pectoralis major, 503f-504f
Pectus carinatum, 267, 270f
Pediatric Appendicitis Score, 389
Pelvic bone, 507f
Pelvic floor (female), 417-418, 418f
Pelvic inflammatory disease (PID),
  390t-391t, 462, 462f
Pemphigoid gestationis, 160
Penetrating trauma, 637
Penile shaft, 472, 472f
Penis, 466-468, 467f
  abnormalities, 477-479
  cancer, 479, 480f
  curvature, 468
  inspection and palpation, 471, 472f
People-to-nature orientation, 26
Peptic ulcer, 391t
Perceptual distortions and
  hallucinations, 71-74, 72f-73f, 73t
Percussion, 34-35, 34f, 34t, 35b
  abdomen, 381-383, 382f, 382t, 384f,
    395
  chest and lungs, 273-274, 274f-275f,
    274t
  hammer, 46, 47f
  head, 192
  heart, 306
  spleen, 383f
Perforated gastric or duodenal ulcer,
  390t-391t
Perianal and perirectal abscesses, 495,
  495f
Pericarditis, 322, 322f
Pericardium, 261f, 295, 295f
Perineal body, 418f
Perineum, 430, 430f
  in secondary assessment of injured
    patient, 636
Periodic apnea of the newborn, 272b
Periodontal disease, 259
Peripheral arterial disease, 340-342, 347
Peripheral arteries, 338-342, 339f
Peripheral nervous system disorders,
  576-580
Peripheral neuropathy, 49, 578
Peripheral vasculature
  examination and findings, 342-345
  review of system, 13

Peripheral vision, 209
Peritoneal irritation, 392b
Peritonitis, 390t-391t
Peritonsillar abscess, 258, 258f
Peroneus longus, 507f
Persistent pain, 50
Personal and social history, 6, 12-13
  abdomen, 377
  on admission note, 629
  anus and rectum, 488-489
  blood vessels, 338
  breasts and axillae, 355
  chest and lungs, 266-267, 266b
  ears, nose, and throat, 238
  eyes, 208
  female genitalia, 425-427
  growth and measurement, 82
  head and neck, 188
  heart, 303-304
  infants and children, 15
  lymphatic system, 172
  male genitalia, 469-471
  mental status examination and, 66
  musculoskeletal system, 509-510
  neurologic system, 551-552
  nutrition, 98
  pain and, 52
  pregnant women, 18
  Problem-Oriented Medical Record
    format, 622, 627
  skin, hair, and nails, 118-119, 118b
Petechiae, 123, 123b, 123f-124f
Peyer patches, 170-171
Peyronic disease, 479, 479f
Phalanges, 503f-504f
Phalen test, 524, 526f
Pharyngitis, 257f
Pharynx examination sequence, 598
Phosphorus, 105
Photoscreening, 43
Physical activity, 97, 98t. See also
  Preparation physical evaluation
  (PPE)
  intensity, 303b
  sports injury and, 538-543, 539b
Physical appearance and behavior in
  mental status examination, 66-67
Physical characteristics, distinguishing,
  21-22
Physical intimacy, 5
Physicians. See Practitioners
Physiologic vaginitis, 457t
Pierre-Robin sequence, 190f
Pilonidal cyst, 494, 494f
Pinworm, 500
Piskacek sign, 443b
Pitting, nail, 159, 159f

Pitting edema, 344f
Pityriasis rosea, 147, 147f
Pivot transfer, 35
Placing reflex, 568t-569t
Plan, on admission note, 630
Plantar grasp reflex, 568t-569t
Plantar reflex, 563, 563f
Plaque, skin, 126f
Pleural effusion and/or thickening, 283t-284t, 285, 286f
Pleurisy, 285, 285f
Pneumonia, 287, 287f
    consolidation, 283t-284t
Pneumothorax, 283t-284t, 288, 289f
Point location, 562
Polyps
    anal, 497, 497f
    cervical, 432f
Pons, 545f
Popliteal lymph nodes, 176, 176f
Portable ultrasound, 41
Positions, patient, 32
    female patient, lithotomy position, 428, 601
        in disabled patients, 448-449, 448f
    male patient, bending forward, 601-602, 602f
    patient reclining 45 degrees, 599-600, 599f
    patient sitting, lap draped, 600-601, 601f
    patient standing, 601, 601f
    patient supine, abdomen exposed, 600, 600f
    patient supine, chest exposed, 600
    patient supine, legs exposed, 600, 600f
    for rectal examination, 489
    seated, back exposed, 599, 599f
    seated, chest exposed, 599, 599f
    seated, with gown, 597-598, 598f
Postcentral gyrus, 65f, 546f
Posterior auricular muscle, 506f
Posterior cerebral artery, 545f, 575f, 575t-576t
Posterior chamber, 42f
Posterior communicating artery, 545f
Posterior cutaneous nerve of thigh, 548f
Posterior inferior cerebellar artery, 545f
Posterior root ganglion, 51f
Posterior spinal artery, 545f
Postpartum period, 18, 375
Postpolio syndrome, 580
Posturing, 566-571, 567f
Potassium, 105
Potential for error, 596, 596b

Practitioners
    accuracy, 595-596
    basis of understanding, 11b
    closing discussion with patient, 608-609
    communication of bad news by, 609b
    effective communication by, 2-5, 3b, 609b
    enhancing patient responses, 4
    knowing yourself, 2
    patients' curiosity about, 4
    professional cultures within health professions and, 24
    professional dress and grooming, 3b
    respecting your instincts, 595b
    seeking connection with patients, 2-4
    vulnerability of, 30b
Preauricular skin tag, 238, 239f
Precentral gyrus, 546f
Precocious puberty, 94, 94f
Preeclampsia, 338b, 349
Prefrontal area, 65f
Pregnant women. See also Females; Fetus
    abdomen, 374-375, 374f, 377, 398
    anus and rectum, 487, 489
        examination, 493
    blood vessels, 337-338, 338b, 345
        abnormalities, 349
    breasts and axillae, 353, 355, 364, 364f
    chest and lungs, 263, 266
        examination and findings, 281
    early signs of pregnancy and, 443b
    ears, nose, and throat, 235-236, 238
        examination and findings, 252
    ectopic pregnancy and, 390t-391t, 393b, 461, 461f
    examination sequence, 607-608
    eyes, 206, 208, 222
    family history, 18
    fetal monitoring equipment, 41-42, 42f
    genitalia, 422-423, 423f, 427
        abnormalities, 465
        examination, 442
    gestational age and, 85-86, 85f, 442, 442t
    growth and measurement, 81-82, 88-89, 90f
    head and neck, 186, 188, 197
    heart, 299-301, 300t, 304, 319
    history of present illness, 17
    interview, 17-18
    lymphatic system, 171-172
    musculoskeletal system, 508, 510
        examination, 533, 533f

Pregnant women (Continued)
    neurologic system, 549, 552
        abnormalities, 579
        examination, 570
    nutrition, 99
    pain in, 51-52
        assessment of, 60
    past medical history, 18
    perceptual distortions and hallucinations in, 73
    personal and social history, 18
    postpartum period and, 18
    Problem-Oriented Medical Record format and, 627-628
    review of systems, 18
    risk assessment, 18
    skin and hair, 116, 119, 140-141, 141f
        abnormalities, 160
    vital signs, 60
Premature Infant Pain Profile (PIPP), 58
Premature rupture of membranes (PROM), 465
Premature thelarche, 369
Premenstrual symptoms, 424
Premenstrual syndrome (PMS), 450
Premotor area, 65f
Preparticipation physical evaluation (PPE)
    classification of sports according to contact and, 587t
    examination form, 583f-584f
    female athlete triad and, 593b
    14-step screening orthopedic examination, 581-587, 585f-586f
    goal of, 581
    recommended components of, 583b
    settings for, 581
    special Olympics and, 582b
    sports-related concussions and, 588b, 589f-592f
    value of, 582b
Pressure ulcers, 142t
Prevention, 15b
    cancer, 362b
    infection, 30
    stroke, 570b
Priaprism, 472, 472f
Primary apnea, 272b
Primary auditory area, 65f
Primary hepatocellular carcinoma, 405
Primary sensory functions, 561, 561f
Primary skin lesions, 126t-128t
Primary survey in emergency assessment, 632-635, 633b

Primary taste area, 65f
PR interval, 298-301, 299f
Priority setting, 614-615
Prior surgery admission note, 629
Privacy. *See* Confidentiality
Probabilistic thinking, 612-613, 613b
Problem identification, 610-611
Problem-Oriented Medical Record
    (POMR), 618-619
    APSO notes, 620b, 621
    assessment, 620
    comprehensive health history and
        physical examination, 619
    notes from subsequent evaluations,
        621
    plan, 620
    problem list, 619-620
    SOAP notes, 620, 620b
Problem-Oriented Medical Record
    (POMR) format, 621-628
    assessment, 625
    children and adolescents and, 627
    history, 621-622, 626-628
    infants and, 626-627
    older adults and, 628
    physical examination findings,
        624-625
    plan, 625-628
    pregnant women and, 627-628
    review of systems, 622-624
Problems, allergies, medications, and
    immunizations (PAMI) List,
    621
Procerus, 506f
Professional dress and grooming, 3b.
    See also Practitioners
Progressive postpoliomyelitis muscular
    atrophy, 580
Prohibited abbreviations, 616, 617t
Proliferative diabetic retinopathy, 226,
    226f
Pronation of feet, 522, 522f
Prone position, 32
Proprioception and cerebellar function,
    556-559
Prostate gland. *See also* Male genitalia
    abnormalities, 498-500
    anatomy and physiology, 486, 487f
    cancer, 488b, 491b, 499, 499f
        screening, 491b
    enlargement, 491b
    examination, 491, 491b
Prostatitis, 498, 498f
Protective sensation, 565, 565f
Protein, 96, 96b, 102-107, 112b
Proximal interphalangeal joint, 505f
Proximal phalanx, 508f

Pruritic urticarial papules and plaques
    of pregnancy (PUPPP), 160
Pruritus ani, 496
Pseudotumor cerebri, 574
Psoriasis, 147, 147f
    of nails, 159, 159f
Psychiatric assessment, review of system,
    14. *See also* Mental status
    examination
Pterygium, 212, 212f-213f
Ptosis, 210, 210f
Puberty
    in boys, 87-89, 87b, 90f-91f, 468
    in girls, 87-89, 87b, 88f-89f, 352-353,
        352b, 363-364, 422, 427, 442
    hormones and, 79
    precocious, 94, 94f
Pudendal nerve, 548f
Pulmonary embolism, 290, 644
Pulse
    abnormalities, 341f
        alternating, 341f
        bigeminal, 341f
        large, bounding, 341f
        paradoxic, 341f
        pulsus bisferiens, 341f
    arterial pulse and pressure, 336, 336f,
        341f
    carotid artery, 343t
        emergency assessment, 634f
    jugular venous pulse and pressure,
        336-337, 337f, 342-343, 343f,
        343t
    rate, 50
        pain and, 53, 53f
Pulse, water-hammer, 341f
Pulse oximeter, 40-41, 41f
Pulsus bisferiens, 341f
Pupil, 205f, 212-214
    abnormalities, 213t-214t
Pustules, 128f
P wave, 298-301, 299f
Pyelonephritis, 408
Pyloric stenosis, 410, 411f
Pyridoxine, 104

Q
QRS complex, 298-301, 299f
QT interval, 298-301, 299f
Questions
    about sexuality, 4-5
    about spirituality, 10
    alcohol use, 8, 8b
    building history through, 7
    CAGE questionnaire, 8, 8b
    CRAFFT questionnaire, 8, 8b
    culturally competent, 28b-29b

Questions (*Continued*)
    direct, 4
    enhancing patient responses to, 4
    intimate partner violence, 8-10, 9b
    leading, 4
    open-ended, 2, 4
    patient-centered, 2b
    TACE questionnaire, 8, 8b
    that explore patient's culture, 24b

R
Raccoon eyes, 636f
Race
    acute otitis media and, 252b
    cerumen and, 240b
    cleft lip and palate and, 250-251,
        250b
    eye protrusion and, 215b
    fundus and, 217b, 217f
    strabismus and, 221
Radial head subluxation, 542
Radiocarpal joint, 505, 505f
Radioulnar joint, 505f
Radius, 503f-505f
Ramus of mandible, 506f
Range of motion, 511, 511f
    cervical spine, 518f, 519
    elbow, 516f
    feet and ankle, 522, 523f
    lower extremities, 520, 521f-522f
    shoulder, 517f
    temporomandibular joint, 517f
    thoracic spine, 519, 520f
Rating scales, pain, 56
Raynaud phenomenon, 347, 347f
Rebound tenderness, abdomen,
    391-393, 393f
Reclining position, 599-600, 599f
Recording information. *See* Information
    recording
Rectal atresia, 500f
Rectal examination in children,
    441-442
Rectal walls
    anterior, 485-486, 490-491
    bidigital palpation, 490
    examination, 490, 490f-491f
    rectovaginal septum and, 439
Rectovaginal examination, 438-449
Rectum
    abnormalities, 494-500
    anatomy and physiology, 466b,
        485-487, 486f
    examination and findings, 489-493,
        489b, 490f
    recording, 625, 627
    review of related history, 487-489

Rectum (*Continued*)
  in secondary assessment of injured
      patient, 636
Rectus femoris tendon, 507f
Red eye, 207-208
Red herrings, 611b
Reflection, 4
Reflex apnea, 272b
Reflexes, 562-571
  abdominal, 563, 563f
  cremasteric, 474, 564
  deep tendon, 563t-564t, 564-565,
      565f
  plantar, 563, 563f
  primitive, 568, 568t-569t
  superficial, 562-564, 563t
Reflex hammer, 46, 47f
Regurgitation, aortic, 54-55, 303, 306b,
    316
Relational orientation, 26
Relationship with patients
  closing discussion and, 608-609
  developing, 1-5
  effective communication in, 2-5, 3b,
      595b
  first meeting with patients and, 594
  seeking connection in, 2-4
Religious and cultural preferences, 10,
    13
Renal abscess, 408
Renal calculi, 390t-391t, 409
Respiration
  abnormalities, 283-293
  airway
    emergency assessment, 632, 633b,
        633f
    retractions, 270-271, 272b
  biot, 268
  breath sounds, 276-279, 277f-278f,
      277t, 278b
  difficulties, 265, 265b, 268b
    air trapping and, 268
    emergency assessment, 632-633
    in newborns, 281b
  observation of, 267-271
  patterns, 268, 271f
  risk factors for disability, 268b
  ventilatory failure, 643
Respiratory rate, 50, 268, 270b
  pain and, 53
Resting energy expenditure (REE), 97,
    97t
Retardation, mental, 77
Retina, 42f, 205f-206f, 206-207, 217,
    217f
  unexpected findings, 219t
Retinal artery, 205f

Retinal hemorrhages in infancy, 230
Retinal vein, 205f
Retinitis pigmentosa, 227, 227f
Retinoblastoma, 229, 229f
Retinol, 103t
Retinopathy of prematurity (ROP),
    229, 229f
Retraction, airway, 270-271, 272b
Retropharyngeal abscess, 258, 258f
Review of systems (ROS), 6, 13-14
  on admission note, 629
  infants and children, 16
  pregnant women, 18
  Problem-Oriented Medical Record
      format, 622-624
Rheumatic fever, 303, 330, 331b
Rheumatoid arthritis, 538
  comparison with osteoarthritis, 538t
Rhinophyma, 148f
Rhonchi, 278
Rhythm disturbance, 318-319
Riboflavin, 104
Rinne test, 241-242, 242f, 242t
Risk assessment
  ovarian cancer, 425b
  pregnancy, 18
Risk factors
  anal cancer, 488b
  basal and squamous cell cancer, 117b
  breast cancer, 354b
  cardiac disease, 303b
  cataract formation, 207b
  cervical cancer, 425b
  colon cancer, 380b
  eating disorders, 99b
  endometrial cancer, 426b
  falls in older adults, 552b
  hearing loss, 238b
  HIV infection, 172b
  melanoma, 117b
  oral cavity and oropharyngeal cancer,
      237b
  osteoarthritis, 509b
  osteoporosis, 510b
  possible medication effects on
      nutritional intake and status,
      100b
  preeclampsia, 338b
  prostate cancer, 488b
  respiratory disability, 268b
  severe hyperbilirubinemia in infants,
      137b
  sports injury, 539b
  stroke, 551b
  suicide, 71b
  varicose veins, 338b
  viral hepatitis, 376b

Rolling over in infant development,
    567b
Romberg test, 559, 559f
Rooting reflex, 568t-569t
Rosacea, 148, 148f
Rosenbaum Pocket Vision Screener,
    209
Roseola infantum (HHV-6), 181
Rotator cuff, 524, 526f
  muscles microtrauma and tearing,
      540
  tear, 540
Round window, 232f
Roundworm, 500
Rovsing sign, 390t-391t
Rubella, 163, 163f
Rubeola, 162, 162f
Ruptured ovarian cyst, 390t-391t

S
Sacral plexus, 548f
Sacrotuberous ligament, 418f
Sacrum, 506f
Salivary gland tumor, 198
Salpingitis, 390t-391t, 462, 462f
Sample records, 628
Sartorius, 507f
Scales, skin, 128f
Scales, weight, 37-38, 37f-38f
Scarring alopecia, 155
Scars, 129f, 379b
Schamroth technique, 135f
Schizophrenia, 77
Sciatic nerve, 548f
Scissoring gait, 560t
Sclera, 42f, 205f, 206, 214, 214f
Scoliometer, 49, 49f
Scoliosis, 541, 542f
Screening, 8b. *See also* Assessment;
    Examination techniques
  for adolescent issues, 17b
  breast cancer, 354b, 358b
  colorectal cancer, 404b
  considering the "norm" with care and,
      24b
  mental status, 66-74, 66b, 66f
  neurologic, 552b
  prostate cancer, 491b
  sexually transmitted infections, 488b
Scrotum, 467f
  abnormalities, 480-484
  inspection and palpation, 466, 472,
      473f-474f
Seated position, 32
  back exposed, 599, 599f
  chest exposed, 599, 599f
  for examination of breasts, 359f, 360

Seated position (*Continued*)
  with gown, 597-598, 598f
  lap draped, 600-601, 601f
Sebaceous cysts, 239f
Sebaceous glands, 115f, 116
  on scrotum, 472, 473f
Sebaceous hyperplasia, 142,
    143f
Seborrheic dermatitis, 160, 160f
Seborrheic keratoses, 142, 143f
Secondary apnea, 272b
Secondary assessment of injured
    patients, 635-636
Secondary skin lesions, 129t-131t
Seduction, 5
Seizures, 550-551
  disorder, 573
Selenium, 106
Self-awareness, breast, 355b
Self-care, 12
Self-examination
  breast, 355b
  genital
    female, 426b
    male, 477t
Self-report pain rating scales, 56
Semicircular canals, 232f
Senile cardiac amyloidosis, 331
Senile hyaline plaque, 214, 214f
Senile purpura, 123, 123b, 123f-124f
Sensitive issues, 7-10
Sensitivity and specificity, 613, 613f
Sensorineural hearing loss, 256
Sensory ataxia, 560t
Sensory function, 559-562, 561f
  cortical, 561-562, 562f
  impairment, 36-37, 595
    female genital examination in
        women with, 449, 449f
  patterns of loss, 562b
Serotonin, 51
Serum sickness, 182
Sesamoid bone, 508f
Setting, interview, 6
Severe asthma episode, 644
Sexual abuse, 441, 441b
Sexuality
  questions about, 4-5
  sexual history, 12, 12b
Sexually transmitted infections, 493b
  condyloma acuminatum
    in men, 478, 478f
    in women, 451-454, 452f
  condyloma latum, 453, 453f
  genital herpes
    in men, 478, 478f
    in women, 454, 454f

Sexually transmitted infections
    (*Continued*)
  lymphogranuloma venereum, 478,
      479f
  molluscum contagiosum
    in men, 479, 479f
    in women, 452, 452f
  screening in men who have sex with
      men (MSM), 488b
  syphilitic chancre
    in men, 477, 477f
    in women, 453, 453f
Sexual maturation, 87-89, 87b
  in boys, 87-89, 87b, 90f-91f
  in girls, 87-89, 87b, 88f-89f, 352-353,
      352b, 363-364, 422
Sexual maturity rating (SMR), 87
Shaken baby syndrome, 579
Shifting dullness, 388, 389f
Shingles, 148, 148f
Shock state, 643
Shortness of breath, 265, 265b
Shotty nodes, 172-173
Shoulder
  assessment, 524-526, 526f
  inspection, 505, 505f-506f, 516f
  joint, 514-516, 517f
  muscles, 506f
Sickle Cell Disease, 276b
Sick sinus syndrome, 324
Silence, 4-5
Sims position, 32
Sinus bradycardia, 325f
Sinuses, 233, 243-244, 249-250, 252
  abnormalities, 257
  pain, 237
  transillumination, 244, 244b, 244f
Sinusitis, 257
Sinus rhythm with first-degree AV
    block, 295f
Skene, 429-430, 430f
Skin
  abnormalities
    caused by biologic warfare, 151
    cutaneous reactions, 150
    inflammatory and infectious
        conditions, 144-149
    malignant/neoplastic, 152-154
  on admission note, 630
  anatomy and physiology, 114-117,
      115f
  calipers for measuring thickness of,
      49, 49f, 107-108, 107f
  cancers, 117b, 122b, 127f, 152-154,
      152f
  dermatoscope for examination of, 48,
      48f

Skin (*Continued*)
  examination and findings, 119-133,
      120b-121b, 120f-121f, 121t
    recording, 624, 626, 628
  family history, 118
  history of present illness, 117-118,
      117b
  lesions, 124f, 125-133
    annular formation of, 133f
    as clues to internal problems, 138b
    clustering, 133f
    linear formation of, 133f
    morphologic characteristics,
        131t-132t
    primary, 126t-128t
    regional distribution of, 132b
    secondary, 129t-131t
  monofilament for examination of, 49,
      49f
  nutrient deficiencies and, 106t-107t
  odor, 123, 125b
  palpation, 124-125, 125f
  past medical history, 118, 118b
  personal and social history, 118-119
  physical examination findings,
      POMR, 624
  review of related history, 117-119
  review of system, 13
  self-examination, 118b
  sunscreen for, 119b, 133b
  tag, preauricular, 239f
  turgor, 125, 125f, 140, 140f, 142f
  type, 118b
  Wood's lamp for examination of, 48,
      48f, 133
Sleep
  apnea, 272b
  position and SIDS, 196b
Slipped capital femoral epiphysis, 541
Small cell carcinoma of lung, 290f
Small intestine, 372
Smallpox, 151t
Smoking, 264b, 303
  cessation, 13b
Snellen alphabet, 43, 44f, 208-209
Snoring, 237
SOAP notes, 618, 620, 620b
Sodium, 105
Soft palate, 234f
Solar keratosis, 165, 165f
Solar lentigines, 143, 144f
Soleus, 507f
Somatic sensory association area, 65f
Somatostatin, 79
Spastic diplegia, 560t
Spastic hemiparesis, 560t
Spasticity, 37

Special Olympics, 582b
Specificity and sensitivity, 613, 613f
Speculum
    nasal, 45, 46f
    vaginal, 47, 48f, 430-431, 432f, 435
Speech
    impaired, 36-37
    and language skills, 70, 71t
    milestones in children, 72, 73t
    vocal resonance and, 279-281, 279b
Spermatocele, 480, 480f
Sphincter, 489
Sphygmomanometer, 40
Spider angioma, 124f
Spina bifida, 578, 579f
Spinal accessory nerve, 553t, 556
Spinal artery, 575t-576t
Spinal cord
    anatomy and physiology, 547, 548f
        spinal nerves, 547-549, 548f-549f
        spinal tracts, 547
    complete transverse lesion of, 562
    injury
        autonomic hyperreflexia, 37
        examination modifications for patients with, 37
        hypersensitivity and, 37
        spasticity and, 37
    reflex arc, 549, 550f
Spinal nerves, 547-549, 548f-549f
Spine
    anatomy and physiology, 505-507, 506f
    cervical, 516-518, 518f
        emergency assessment, 632, 633f, 636
        range of motion, 518f
    curvature, 518, 519f
    examination sequence, 601
    kyphosis, 518, 519f
        in infants, 529, 529f
    lumbar, 518-519, 518f-519f
    scoliometer for examination of, 49, 49f
    scoliosis, 541, 542f
    thoracic, 518-519, 518f-520f
Spinothalamic tracts, 547
Spinous process, 506f
Spirituality, 10, 13
Spleen, 170, 176-177, 373, 383, 383b, 383f
    abnormalities, 407
    palpation, 386-387, 387f
    rupture, 390t-391t, 407
Splenomegaly, 383b
Splitting, heart sounds, 308-309, 310b

Sport Concussion Assessment Tool, 589f-592f
Sports injury, 538-543, 539b. See also Preparation physical evaluation (PPE)
    concussions, 588b, 589f-592f
Sputum, 265, 265t
Squamous cell cancer, 117b, 152, 152f, 165, 165f
    anal, 497
    of lung, 290f
    on tongue, 259, 259f
Stages of change, 613, 615t
Stapes, 232f
Staphylococcal infection of eye, 210, 211f
Stasis dermatitis, 165, 165f
State of consciousness, 67
Status asthmaticus, 644
Status epilepticus, 644
Steppage, 560t
Stepping reflex, 568t-569t
Stereognosis, 562
Sternocleidomastoid muscles, 506f, 518, 518f
Sternum, xiphoid of, 378f
Stethoscope, 39-40, 40f, 276-281, 276f
    acoustic, 39, 39f
Stiff neck, 188, 565-566, 566f
Stomach, 372
    cancer, 403
Stool
    blood in, 492b, 492t
    changes in pregnancy, 493b
    examination, 491-493, 492b, 492t
    fecal incontinence, 376
    infant and child, 486
    rectovaginal examination, 439
StrabismoScope, 43, 43f, 215-216, 215f
Strabismus, 215-216, 216f, 221, 224
Strain, muscle, 539
Stratum corneum, 115, 115f
Stratum germinativum, 115, 115f
Stratum lucidum, 115, 115f
Strength, muscle, 511-512, 512t
    in newborns, 530, 531f
Streptococcal pharyngitis, 248b
Stridor, 280
Stroke, 574, 575f
    differential diagnosis by artery affected, 575t-576t
    prevention, 570b
    risk factors, 551b
ST segment and T wave, 298-301, 299f
Stye, 210, 211f
Styloid process, 506f
Stylomandibular ligament, 506f

Subacromial bursa, 506f
Subarachnoid space, 545f
Subdeltoid tendon, 506f
Subjective data in EMRs, 618
Subscapularis muscle, 506f
Substantia gelatinosa, 51f
Subtalar joint, 508f
Subungual hematoma, 157, 157f
Sucrose solutions for pain, 58b
Sudden infant death syndrome (SIDS), 196b
Suicide, 71b
    adolescent, 5b
Sunscreen, 119b, 133b
Superficial pain, 561, 561f
Superficial reflexes, 562-564, 563f
Superficial transverse perineal muscle, 418f
Superior cerebellar artery, 545f
Superior frontal gyrus, 546f
Superior temporal gyrus, 546f
Supernumerary nipples, 359f
Supine position, 32
    abdomen exposed, 600, 600f
    chest exposed, 600
    for examination of breasts, 360-365, 361f
    legs exposed, 600, 600f
Supraspinatus muscle, 506f
Supraventricular tachycardia, 327f
Surgery, prior, 629
Suspensory ligaments of Cooper, 351f
Swallowing, 237
Sweat glands, 115-117, 115f
Swelling, 180t
    acute testicular, 482t
    ankle, 337
    finger, 514f
    hemorrhoids, 496, 497f
    inguinal area, 468
Symphysis pubis, 416-418, 417f-418f
Syncope, 13-14
    abdominal disorders and, 401, 407
    heart abnormalities and, 320, 322-324
    in older adults, 304
    during pregnancy, 304
Synovial sheath, 506f
Syphilitic chancre
    in men, 477, 477f
    in women, 453, 453f
Systemic lupus erythematosus, 190f
Systole, 308, 309b

T
TACE questionnaire, 8, 8b
Tachypnea, 268

Tactile fremitus, 272-273, 273f
Talipes equinovarus, 540, 540f
Talonavicular joint, 508f
Tanner stages, 352, 508
Tape measure, 46-47
Tarsals, 503f-504f
Tarsometatarsal joint, 508f
Taste sensation, 556b, 556f
Teeth, 235f, 237, 244-246, 245b, 245f, 245t. *See also* Mouth; Throat
   caries, 252, 252f
Telangiectasias, 123, 123b, 123f-124f, 128f
Temperature, 39, 39f, 50
   pain and, 52
   sensory function and, 561
Temporal arteritis, 346
Temporal gyrus, 546f
Temporal lobe, 545f, 546
Temporomandibular joint, 505-507, 506f, 517f
   inspection, 516
   syndrome, 537
Tendonitis, 539
Tenosynovitis, 539
Tension, moments of, 4-5
Teres minor muscle, 506f
Terry nails, 158, 158f
Testes, 466-468
   cancer, 483
   inspection and palpation, 473-474, 473f
   swelling, 482t
   torsion, 482-483
   tumor, 483f
Testosterone, 79
Tetralogy of Fallot, 328, 328f
Thalamus, 548f
Thermogenesis, 97
Thermometers, 39, 39f
Thiamin, 103t-104t
Thoracic spine, 518-519, 518f-519f
   range of motion, 519, 520f
Thorax. *See also* Chest
   inspection, 267-271, 267f-268f
   landmarks, 269b, 269f
Thought process and content, 71
Thrill, 306, 306b
Throat. *See also* Mouth
   anatomy and physiology, 234-236, 234f-235f
   examination and findings, 238-253
      recording, 624
   functional assessment, 253b
   physical examination findings, POMR, 624
   review of system, 13

Throat (*Continued*)
   sore, 237
   streptococcal pharyngitis, 248b
Thrombosis, 343
Thymus, 170, 170f
Thyroglossal duct cyst, 199, 199f
Thyroid, 185, 188, 194b
   abnormalities, 200-203, 201t
   hormone, 79
   hyper-, 190f, 201, 201t
   hypo-, 200, 201t
   palpation, 193-195, 194b, 194f-195f
Tibia, 503f-504f, 507f-508f
Tibial collateral ligament, 507f
Tibialis anterior, 507f
Tibial torsion, 531, 532f
Tibiotalar joint, 507-508, 508f
Tic douloureux, 577
Ticklishness, 384b
Tinea, 146, 146f
Tinetti Balance and Gait Assessment Tool, 571b-572b
Tip of nose, 233f
Tobacco use, 264b, 303
   risk factors for cardiac disease, 303b
   risk factors for cervical cancer, 425b
   risk factors for oral cavity and oropharyngeal cancer, 237b
   risk factors for stroke, 551b
Tocopherols, 103t
Tone, muscle, 511, 511f
Tongue, 234f, 246-248, 247f, 248b
   glossopharyngeal nerve, 553t, 556
   hypoglossal nerve, 553t, 556, 557f
   lymph nodes, 169f
   squamous cell cancer on, 259, 259f
   taste sensation, 556b, 556f
Tonic pupil, 214f
Tonsilitis, 253f, 257f
Tonsils, 170, 252, 253f
Tophi, 239f
Torsion, testicular, 482-483
Torticollis, 200, 200f
Toxoplasmosis, 181
Trachea, 193f, 262f, 273, 273b, 273f
Tracheomalacia, 292
Traction alopecia, 155
Tract of Lissauer, 51f
Transillumination, 47
   male genitalia, 475
   sinuses, 244, 244b, 244f
   skull, 196-197, 196f
Transverse acetabular ligament, 507f
Transverse gyrus, 65f
Trapezius muscles, 506f, 518, 518f

Trauma
   blunt, 637
   in childhood, 16b
   due to violence, legal considerations, 641-642
   penetrating, 637
   primary emergency assessment, 635
   signs that indicate serious injury associated with, 636f
Traumatic brain injury, 187-188, 588b, 589f-592f
Treacher-Collins syndrome, 191f
Tremor, 551, 557t
Trendelenburg sign, 527, 527f
Triceps
   lateral head, 503f-504f
   long head, 503f-504f
   medial head, 503f-504f
Triceps reflex, 564
Triceps skinfold thickness (TSF), 49, 49f, 107-108, 107f
Trichomoniasis, 457t
Trichotillomania, 163, 163f
Trigeminal nerve (CN V), 553t, 554-555, 554f
Trigeminal neuralgia, 577
Triplets, 14b
Trochlear nerve (CN IV), 553t, 554
Tubal pregnancy, 390t-391t, 393b, 461, 461f
Tuberculosis, 288, 288f
Tumbling E chart, 44, 44f
Tumors. *See also* Cancer
   abdominal, 414, 414f
   intracranial, 574
   parotid gland, 199f
   salivary gland, 198
   skin, 127f
   testicular, 483f
   uterine, 391t, 459, 460f
Tuning fork, 45-46, 46f
Turgor, skin, 125, 125f, 140, 140f, 142f
Turner syndrome, 92, 92f
Twenty-four hour recall diet, 101
Twins, 14b, 445, 445f
Two-person transfer, 36
Two-point discrimination, 562
Tympanic membrane, 232, 232f, 240f, 241t, 251f
   on admission note, 629
Tympanometer, 45, 45f

U
Ulcerative colitis, 402, 402f
Ulcers
   corneal, 224, 224f
   gastric or duodenal, 390t-391t, 401

Ulcers (*Continued*)
    peptic, 391t
    skin, 224, 224f
    venous, 349, 349f
Ulcers, skin, 130f, 142t
Ulna, 505f
Ultrasound, portable, 41
Umbilical cord, 170b, 395b
Umbilical hernia, 405f
Umbilical ring, 385
Uncertainty, 596
Unconscious patients, 633b-634b, 634,
        634t
Understanding, basis of, 11b
Upper airway obstruction, 642
Upper and lower neuron disease, 555b,
        563t-564t
Upper extremities
    on admission note, 630
    anatomy and physiology, 505, 505f
    examination sequence, 598
        children, 606
        infants, 604
    lymph nodes, 168f, 175-176, 176f
    midarm muscle circumference/
            midarm muscle area, 108
    mid-upper arm circumference, 108,
            108f
    nutrient deficiencies and, 106t-107t
    reflexes, 564
    in secondary assessment of injured
            patient, 636
    span measurement, 87
    triceps skinfold thickness (TSF), 49,
            49f, 107-108, 107f
Upper motor neurons, 547
Upper-to-lower segment ratio, 87
Ureters, 373
Urethral caruncle, 429, 429f
Urethral meatus, 472, 472f
Urethral opening
    female, 416-418, 417f, 429, 429f
    male, 466, 467f
Urinary frequency, 376, 424
Urinary incontinence, 376, 415t
Uterine fibroids, 391t, 459, 460f
Uterus
    bleeding, 459, 459t
    contractions, 446-447
    endometriosis, 451, 451f
    examination of, 418-419, 418f-419f,
            491
        bimanual, 437, 438f
    myomas, 459, 460f
    pelvic inflammatory disease (PID),
            390t-391t, 462, 462f
    in pregnancy, 422-423

Uterus (*Continued*)
    prolapse, 458, 458f
    rectovaginal examination, 439
    size in pregnancy, 442-443, 442t
Uvea, 205f, 206
Uvula, 234f
U wave, 298-301, 299f

V
Vaccines, 566b
Vagina, 418-419, 418f, 422
    abnormalities, 454-456
    bleeding
        in children, 441, 441b
        during pregnancy, 465
    cancer, 455
    discharge, 424, 427
        in children, 441
        differential diagnosis, 457t
    infections, 456, 456f
    in pregnancy, 422-423
    smears and specimens, 431, 433b-
            435b, 434f
    vaginal speculum for examination of,
            47, 48f, 430-431, 432f, 435
Vaginal introitus, 429
Vaginal orifice, 416-418, 417f
Vaginal speculum, 47, 48f, 430-431,
        432f, 435
Vaginal vestibule, 416-418, 417f
Vaginitis, 457t
    atrophic, 465
Vagus nerve (CN X), 553t, 556
Validation, 67b
Valid hypotheses, 611, 612b
Validity of clinical examination, 613
Values
    critical thinking and, 612
    orientations among cultural groups,
            26b
Valves, heart, 297, 310
    order of, 297b
Varicella, 162, 162f
Varicocele, 481, 481f
Varicose veins, 338b, 345
Varus and valgus stress test, 528, 528f
Vascular dementia, 78
Vasculature, abdominal, 373-375
Vastus medialis, 507f
Vegetarian diets, 102
Veins, 334f-336f
    hand, 343, 344f
    obstruction and insufficiency
            assessment, 343-345
    peripheral, 342-345
    retinal, 205f
    varicose, 338b, 345

Venous hum, 342b
Venous star, 124f
Venous thrombosis, 348
Venous ulcers, 349, 349f
Ventilatory failure, 643
Ventricular fibrillation, 327f
Ventricular septal defect, 328, 329f
Vernix caseosa, 116
Vertebrae, 505-507, 506f
    bifid defect of, 529, 530f
    location of spinal nerves in relation
            to, 548f
Vertebral artery, 545f
Vertigo, 236-237, 257
Vesicles
    seminal, 487f
    skin, 127f
Vestibular bulb, 418f
Vestibular glands, 416-418, 417f
Vestibule, nose, 233f
Vibration, 561, 561f
Violence
    in childhood, 9, 16b
    intimate partner, 8-10, 9b
    legal considerations and trauma due
            to, 641-642
    against older adults, 9-10
Viral hepatitis, 376b
Vision. *See also* Eyes
    abnormalities, 228-230
    blurred *versus* double, 209b
    color, 209
    development in infants and children,
            206, 207t
    examination and findings, 208-209,
            209b, 209f
        assessment of near vision, 44, 209
    impaired, 36, 70b
        female genital examination for
                patients who are, 449, 449f
        history of present illness and, 207
    in older adults, 206-207, 207b
    peripheral, 209
    during pregnancy, 206
Visual acuity charts, 43-44, 44f,
        208-209
Visual analogue scale, 56, 57f
Visual association area, 65f
Visual cortex, 65f
Vital signs, 50
    abnormalities, 62-63
    on admission note, 629
    anatomy and physiology related to,
            50-52
    in children, 58-59
    examination and findings, 52-60
    in newborns and infants, 57-58

Vital signs (Continued)
  in older adults, 60
  in pregnant women, 60
  review of related history, 52
Vitamin A, 103
Vitamin B$_1$, 103
Vitamin B$_2$, 104
Vitamin B$_6$, 104
Vitamin B$_{12}$, 104
Vitamin C, 103
Vitamin D, 103
Vitamin E, 103
Vitamin K, 103
Vitamins
  fat-soluble, 103t
  water-soluble, 103t-104t
Vitiligo, 121-122, 122f
Vitreous, 42f
  body, 205f
Vocal resonance, 279-281, 279b
Voice quality, 70
Volvulus, 390t-391t
Vomiting, 375
  of blood, 639t
V-shaped position for female genital
    examination, 449, 449f
Vulva, 416-418, 417f, 423f
  abnormalities, 454-456
  cancer, 456, 456f
Vulvovaginitis, 464, 464f

W
Waddling, 560t
Waist circumference, 100, 101f

Waist-height ratio, 100
Waist-to-hip circumference ratio,
    100-101, 101f
Warts, 159, 159f, 452f
  anal/genital, 451, 494, 494f
Water, 96
  -soluble vitamins, 103t-104t
Water-hammer pulse, 341f
Weakness or paresthesia, 551
  generalized muscle, 533f
  neurologic-specific, 574
  sudden, 551
Weber test, 241-242, 241f, 242t
Wedge method of breast palpation,
    361
Weight
  body mass index (BMI) and, 82-87,
      83b, 87b
  control, 83b
  daily energy needs and, 102b
  gain, 97
    during pregnancy, 81-82
  loss, 97
    history of present illness and,
        375
  low birth, 86b
  measurement, 83, 100, 100b
    children, 86
    infants, 84, 84b
  obesity, 83b
    in children and adolesents, 59b
    statistics, 99b
  scales, 37-38, 37f-38f
Wernicke aphasia, 71t

Wernicke's area, 65f
Wet mount procedure, 433b-435b
Wheals, 126f
Wheezes, 278
Whispered voice test, hearing, 241
White banding (Terry nails), 158,
    158f
White blood cell count, 457t
Wide splitting, 310
Wilms tumor, 414, 414f
Wong/Baker Faces Rating Scale, 59,
    59f
Wood's lamp, 48, 48f, 133
Wrist, 512-524
  assessment, 524, 524b
  carpal tunnel syndrome, 524, 525f,
      536, 537t
    in pregnant women, 533
  inspection, 505, 505f, 512f-513f
Writing ability, 69
Wry neck, 200f

X
Xanthelasma, 210, 210f
Xiphoid process, 260, 261f, 263f
  of sternum, 378f

Y
Young adults, interviewing of, 6f

Z
Zinc, 106
Zygomaticus major, 506f
Zygomaticus minor, 506f

Special Features

Clinical Pearls

"Unique," Originally Derived from Latin "Unus," Meaning "One," 1
The Patient Relationship, 1
Professional Dress and Grooming, 3
Adolescent Suicide, 5
Watch the Use of Jargon, 7
Screening, 8
Chief Complaint or Chief Concern?, 11
Who Are You?, 12
The Five Ps of a Sexual History, 12
Twins or More, 14
Putting Prevention into Practice, 15
Identification of Concerns by Adolescents, 16
Language Is Not All, 23
The Impact of Gender, 27
Complementary and Alternative Treatments for the Common Cold, 28
The Headache, 33
Right-Sided Examination?, 33
Unexpected Findings, 35
The Transience of Memory, 47
Transillumination, 47
The Fifth Vital Sign, 56
Selection of Pain Scale, 56
Blood Pressure in Infants, 58
Obesity in Children and Adolescents, 59
The Importance of Validation, 67
Testing Memory in the Visually Impaired, 70
Distorted Thinking, 72
Using the Correct Growth Chart, 84
Reliability of Length Measurements, 84
Uses of Growth Charts, 84
Special Growth Charts, 86
Eating Disorders, 99
"Rule of Thumb" Estimates for Calculating Daily Energy Needs, 102
Sunscreen, 119
Carotenemia, 119
Telangiectasias: Capillary Spider/Spider Angioma, 123
Bald Spots in Children and Infants, 140
Hydration Status in Older Adults, 141
Umbilical Cord, 170
Reminders About Nodes, 173
Not Always Pathology, 174
Drugs and Nodes, 174

Vaccinations and Nodes, 176
Cervical Nodes, 177
Cardarelli Sign and Oliver Sign, 194
Is It the Thyroid Gland?, 194
Examining the Head, 195
Is It Blurry or Is It Double?, 209
Factors That Affect Visual Acuity Testing, 209
Fundus Pigmentation, 217
Examining an Infant's Eyes, 220
Cleaning an Obstructed Auditory Canal, 240
Ménière Disease, 242
Cocaine Abuse, 243
Use of a Tongue Blade, 248
Patent Ductus Arteriosus (PDA), 263
Chest Pain, 266
Pain from Cocaine, 266
The Sequence of Steps, 267
Clue to a Mediastinal Mass, 273
Congestive Heart Failure, 276
Sickle Cell Disease, 276
Vocal Resonance, 279
The Sobbing Baby, 280
Foreign Body, 281
Order of Valves, 297
Heart Sounds, 307
Heart Sounds after Surgical Procedures, 311
The Infant Heart and Liver, 319
Carotid Palpation, 339
Calf Pain, 344
Edema, 344
Nipple Compression, 363
Scars, 379
Abdominal Distention, 380
Assessing Liver Size, 383
Ectopic Pregnancy, 393
Umbilical Cord, 395
Palpating an Infant's Abdomen, 396
Enlarged Liver, 396
Constipation with Diarrhea, 398
Anxiety, 428
Gloving, 428
Mittelschmerz and Adnexal Tenderness, 437

Continued

Clinical Pearls—cont'd

Looks Can Be Deceiving, 463
Retraction of the Foreskin, 474
Concerns of Adolescence, 475
In Pain?, 489
Stool Changes in Pregnant Women, 493
Unexplained Fever, 498
Bilateral Symmetry, 510
Mnemonic for Cranial Nerve Names, 553
Upper and Lower Neuron Disease, 555

Evaluating Taste Sensation, 556
Infant Development—Rolling Over, 567
Atlantoaxial Instability, 582
Hypertension in the Pediatric Athlete, 582
Respecting Your Instincts, 595
Mnemonic AVPU, 634
Delay Secondary Assessment to Resuscitate, 635
Mnemonic AMPLE, 635

DIFFERENTIAL DIAGNOSES

Distinguishing Characteristics of Aphasias, 71
Distinguishing Characteristics of Delirium and Dementia and
    Depression, 76
Cutaneous Manifestations of Two Pathogens That May Be Used in
    Biologic Warfare, 151
Conditions Simulating Lymph Node Enlargement, 174
Mumps Versus Cervical Adenitis, 177
How to Discover an Immune Deficiency Disease in a Child, 177
Lymphedema or Edema?, 179
When the Body Swells, 180
Comparison of Various Types of Headaches, 197-198
Otitis Externa, Otitis Media with Effusion, and Acute Otitis Media,
    254
Some Causes of Sputum, 265
Comparison of Some Types of Chest Pain, 302
Comparison of Systolic Murmurs, 318
Signs and Symptoms of Breast Masses, 365
Abdominal Masses in Infants and Children, 396
Causes of Acute Abdominal Pain in Infants, Children, and
    Adolescents, 397
Urinary Incontinence, 415
Vaginal Discharges and Infections, 457
Distinguishing Characteristics of Hernias, 477
Acute Testicular Swelling, 482
Comparison of Osteoarthritis with Rheumatoid Arthritis, 538
Tremors, 557
Characteristics of Upper and Lower Motor Neuron Disorders, 564
Neurologic Signs Associated with Stroke by Artery Affected,
    575-576

Evidence-Based Practice in Physical Examination

Screening for Abuse and Intimate Partner Violence, 9
History Taking, 12
Smoking Cessation, 13
Mini-Mental State Examination, 68
Thyroid Examination, 194
Detection of Hearing Loss, 238
Predictors of Sinusitis, 244
Predictors of Streptococcal Pharyngitis, 248
Is There a Plural Effusion?, 272
Cardiac Murmurs in Children, 318
Can the Clinical Examination Diagnose Left-Sided Heart Failure in
    Adults?, 321
Breast Cancer Screening, 358
Detecting Splenomegaly, 383
Detecting Abdominal Aortic Aneurysms, 388
Detecting Ascites, 388
Diagnosing Appendicitis, 390
Abdomen, 398
Screening for Colorectal Cancer, 404
Lubricating the Speculum, 431
Cervical Cancer Screening After Hysterectomy?, 436
Screening for Prostate Cancer: The Controversy, 491
Acute Ankle Injury in Adults, 524
Carpal Tunnel Syndrome, 524
Acute Knee Injury, 528
Signs of Meningitis, 566
The Particular Value of a Careful History, 582

Sample Documentation

Mental Status, 74
Growth and Measurement, 90
Nutrition, 108
Skin, Hair, and Nails, 143
Lymphatic System, 177
Head and Neck, 197
Eyes, 222
Ears, Nose, and Throat, 254
Chest and Lungs, 281

Heart, 320
Blood Vessels, 345
Breasts and Axillae, 365
Abdomen, 399
Female Genitalia, 450
Male Genitalia, 476
Anus, Rectum, and Prostate, 493
Musculoskeletal System, 534
Neurologic System, 571